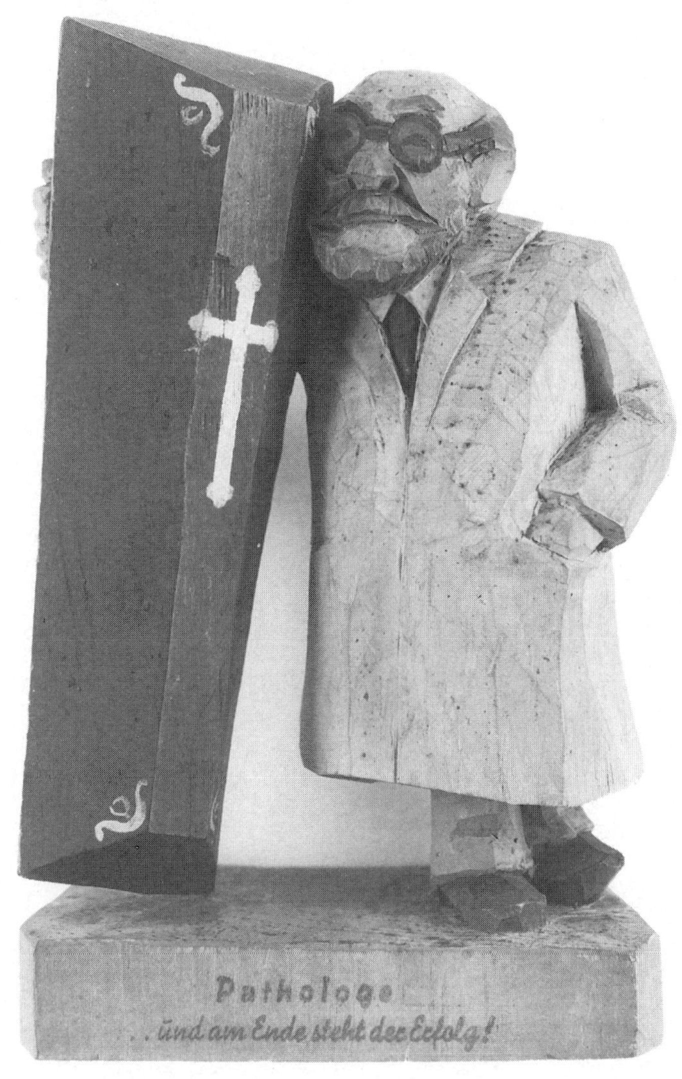

PATHOLOGIST

... and in the end, you see what happened.

This wooden figurine of Rudolf Virchow stood in a pawn shop in the Bronx, New York City. Literally translated, the inscription says: "Pathologist—and in the end stands success," which seems to mean here, success in discovering the cause of diseases.

Handbook
of
Autopsy Practice

3rd Edition

Jurgen Ludwig, MD

Emeritus Consultant,
Department of Laboratory Medicine and Pathology,
Mayo Clinic;
Emeritus Professor of Pathology,
Mayo Medical School,
Rochester, MN

Humana Press 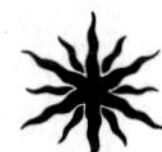 **Totowa, New Jersey**

For additional copies, pricing for bulk purchases, and/or information about other Humana titles, contact Humana at 999 Riverview Drive, Suite 208, Totowa, NJ 07512 or at any of the following numbers: Tel.: 973-256-1699; Fax: 973-256-8341; E-mail: humana@humanapr.com; Website: http://humanapress.com

As new scientific information becomes available through basic and clinical research, recommended treatments and drug therapies undergo changes. The authors and publisher have made all reasonable attempts to make this book accurate, up to date, and in accord with accepted standards at the time of publication. The authors, editors, and publisher are not responsible for errors or omissions or for consequences from application of the book, and make no warranty, expressed or implied, in regard to the contents of the book. Any practice described in this book should be applied by the reader in consultation with a physician and taking regard of the unique circumstances that may apply in each situation. The reader is advised always to check product information (package inserts) for changes and new information regarding dose and contraindications before administering any drug. Caution is especially urged when using new or infrequently ordered drugs. Nothing in this publication implies that Mayo Clinic endorses the products or equipment mentioned in this book.

All articles, comments, opinions, conclusions, or recommendations are those of the author(s) and do not necessarily reflect the views of the publisher or of Mayo Clinic.

This publication is printed on acid-free paper. ∞
ANSI Z39.48-1984 (American Standards Institute) Permanence of Paper for Printed Library Materials.

Acquisitions Editor: Thomas H. Moore.

Cover design by Patricia F. Cleary.

Production Editor: Mark J. Breaugh.

Printed in the United States of America. 10 9 8 7 6 5 4 3 2 1

Library of Congress Cataloging in Publication Data
Handbook of autopsy practice / edited by Jurgen Ludwig.--3rd ed.
p. ; cm
Rev. ed. of: Current methods of autopsy practice / Jurgen Ludwig. 2nd ed. 1979.
Includes bibliographical references and index.
ISBN 1-58829-169-3 (alk. paper)
1. Autopsy. I. Ludwig, Jurgen, 1931- II. Ludwig, Jurgen, 1931-. Current methods of autopsy practice.
[DNLM: 1. Autopsy--methods. QZ 35 H236 2002]
RB57 .L8 2002
616.07'59--dc21

2001051893

Preface

The second edition of *Handbook of Autopsy Practice* appeared in 1979 under the title *Current Methods of Autopsy Practice* (W. B. Saunders Company); that edition was out of print in the early 1980s. Now, over 20 years later, it appeared timely to thoroughly update the material in a third edition by adding what we have learned in the meantime and eliminating text that has become obsolete. There is an acute need for a complete and readily accessible resource for autopsy work because few pathologists still specialize in autopsy practice and, as a consequence, expertise in autopsy technology and autopsy pathology has declined. Our colleagues in the forensic field have remained the only large group of autopsy practitioners. For most other pathologists, the economic situation, time constraints, and the steadily decreasing autopsy rates have made a career in autopsy pathology unattractive. This state of affairs is perpetuated by a lack of interest among many of our young colleagues, partly because the teaching of autopsy pathology and autopsy techniques during most residencies is insufficient. Numerous articles have bemoaned this situation, but the trend, I fear, is irreversible. Still, autopsies will be requested, particularly in complex and difficult situations where the questions remaining after the death of the patient might challenge even experienced autopsy pathologists. Under these circumstances, this *Handbook of Autopsy Practice* should meet a particular need by providing the prosector with a source of information when it is most required—in the autopsy room. Thus, the text is written primarily for practicing pathologists with at least some autopsy experience; this is not an introductory teaching manual.

The principal organization of the original book has been maintained. Part I is a general text on autopsy methods and all their corollary activities. This part has been updated but also shortened considerably because many methods that were described in detail in the second edition have become obsolete—partly because of the decline of the classical pathology museums, partly because of our increased awareness of the toxic hazards of many chemicals that were used in pathology museums of only a few decades ago. Files of 35-mm slides or disks with digitalized images have largely replaced the museum because funds are lacking—museum space and personnel are costly—and also because interest in museum-type specimen display has waned. We have lost something here, no doubt, but a realistic evaluation of the situation caused me to condense Part I. Nevertheless, many old references were reprinted so that access to the classical techniques would not become too difficult. At the same time, some new developments needed to be addressed, such as the principles of quality assurance and the increased safety precautions that were prompted by the resurgence of potentially fatal infectious diseases.

Part II represents the most important resource during work in the autopsy room by providing tabulations of technical procedures recommended in specific diseases or conditions and by listing expected findings in these situations. Thus, the authors assumed that one or several clinical diagnoses had been rendered, and on this basis, we tabulated the "what to look for" and the "how to dissect and preserve it."

Part III concludes with updated tabulations of weights, measurements, and related data. Major changes include the combination of several tables from the second edition with data from fetuses, infants, and children. Most cardiac weights and measurements were culled from current sources.

I acknowledge with pleasure the contributions of Mr. Darrell Ottman and his fellow technologists, and of all colleagues, past and present, in the Mayo Clinic Autopsy Service. Many colleagues in other Mayo Clinic Departments, and in institutions outside the Mayo Clinic, provided much helpful advice. Drs. Lawrence J. Burgart and Jeffrey L. Myers, both from the Mayo Clinic Division of Anatomic Pathology, critically reviewed the text in Part II on many hematological and respiratory disorders, respectively. I am particularly indebted to Dr. Hagen Blaszyk who, in addition to compiling the weight tables, provided much needed support during the preparation of the manuscript. Drs. Thomas V. Colby from Mayo Clinic Scottsdale and Theresa S. Emory at the Armed Forces Institute of

Pathology helped with the compilation of addresses of tumor and disease registries. Dr. Wayne Duer and Dr. Julia Martin, both from the Hillsborough County Medical Examiner Department, contributed to the discussion of toxicological autopsies and rape cases, respectively. We hope that the book will serve its purpose. I also would like to thank Mr. Thomas H. Moore and his colleagues at Humana Press for their expert support.

Jurgen Ludwig, MD

Contents

Preface ..... *v*

Contributors ..... *ix*

Part I: Autopsy Techniques, Laboratory Procedures, and Data Processing *1*

1 Principles of Autopsy Techniques, Immediate and Restricted Autopsies, and Other Special Procedures
Jurgen Ludwig *3*

2 Medicolegal Autopsies and Autopsy Toxicology
Vernard I. Adams *7*

3 Cardiovascular System
William D. Edwards *21*

4 Tracheobronchial Tree and Lungs
Jurgen Ludwig *45*

5 Esophagus and Abdominal Viscera
Jurgen Ludwig *53*

6 Nervous System
Caterina Giannini and Haruo Okazaki *65*

7 The Eye and Adnexa
R. Jean Campbell *85*

8 Skeletal System
Jurgen Ludwig *95*

9 Autopsy Microbiology
Brenda L. Waters *101*

10 Chromosome Study of Autopsy Tissues
Gordon W. Dewald *107*

11 Autopsy Chemistry
Vernard I. Adams *113*

12 Autopsy Roentgenology and Other Imaging Techniques
Jurgen Ludwig ... *117*

13 Autopsy of Bodies Containing Radioactive Materials
Kelly L. Classic ... *123*

14 Fixation, Color Preservation, Gross Staining, and Shipping of Autopsy Material
Jurgen Ludwig and Brenda L. Waters ... *129*

15 Museum Techniques and Autopsy Photography
Jurgen Ludwig and William D. Edwards ... *137*

16 Organization, Maintenance, and Safety Concerns of the Autopsy Service; Tissue Registries; Interviews With the Next of Kin
Jurgen Ludwig ... *143*

17 Autopsy Documents, Data Processing, and Quality Assurance
Jurgen Ludwig ... *151*

18 Autopsy Law
Vernard I. Adams and Jurgen Ludwig ... *159*

19 The State of Autopsy Practice: *An Annotated Bibliography*
Jurgen Ludwig ... *167*

PART II: ALPHABETIC LISTING OF DISEASES AND CONDITIONS ... *169*
Jurgen Ludwig with Vernard I. Adams (Medicolegal and Toxicologic cases),
William D. Edwards (Cardiovascular cases),
Caterina Giannini (Neuropathologic cases),
and Brenda L. Waters (Pediatric and Infectious Disease cases)
Organization of Part II ... *171*
Special Histological Stains ... *172*
Listing ... *175*

PART III: NORMAL WEIGHTS AND MEASUREMENTS
Weights and Measurements
Hagen Blaszyk, Jurgen Ludwig, and William D. Edwards ... *551*
Weights and Measurements in Fetuses, Infants, Children, and Adolescents ... *553*
Weights and Measurements in Adults ... *567*

Index ... *573*

Contributors

VERNARD I. ADAMS, MD • *Medical Examiner Department, Hillsborough County; Department of Pathology and Laboratory Medicine, University of South Florida, Tampa, FL*

HAGEN BLASZYK, MD • *Department of Pathology and Laboratory Medicine, MCHV Campus, University of Vermont, Burlington, VT*

R. JEAN CAMPBELL, MD • *Division of Anatomic Pathology, Mayo Clinic, Rochester, MN*

KELLY L. CLASSIC, MS • *Section of Safety, Mayo Clinic, Rochester, MN*

GORDON W. DEWALD, PhD • *Division of Laboratory Genetics, Mayo Clinic, Rochester, MN*

WILLIAM D. EDWARDS, MD • *Division of Anatomic Pathology, Mayo Clinic, Rochester, MN*

CATERINA GIANNINI, MD • *Division of Anatomic Pathology, Mayo Clinic, Rochester, MN*

JURGEN LUDWIG, MD • *Division of Anatomic Pathology, Mayo Clinic, Rochester, MN*

HARUO OKAZAKI, MD • *Division of Anatomic Pathology, Mayo Clinic, Rochester, MN*

BRENDA L. WATERS, MD • *Department of Pathology and Laboratory Medicine, MCHV Campus, University of Vermont, Burlington, VT*

Autopsy Techniques, Laboratory Procedures, and Data Processing

I

1 Principles of Autopsy Techniques, Immediate and Restricted Autopsies, and Other Special Procedures

JURGEN LUDWIG

CLASSIC AUTOPSY TECHNIQUES

The review by Rössle *(1)* remains the most comprehensive text on classic autopsy techniques and their variations and combinations. The techniques of Albrecht, Fischer, Ghon, Heller, Letulle, Nauwerck, Rokitansky, Virchow, and Zenker, among others, are described. The review is written in German and is not readily available. For a comprehensive English text with abundant references on autopsy techniques and related matters, readers should consult the manual *Autopsy—Performance and Practice,* compiled by the College of American Pathologists *(2)*. Four principal autopsy techniques can be distinguished:

TECHNIQUE OF R. VIRCHOW Organs are removed one by one. This method has been used most widely, often with some modifications. Originally, the first step was to expose the cranial cavity and, from the back, the spinal cord, followed by the thoracic, cervical, and abdominal organs, in that order.

TECHNIQUE OF C. ROKITANSKY This technique is characterized by *in situ* dissection, in part combined with the removal of organ blocks. Only second-hand descriptions are available. The term "Rokitansky's technique" is used erroneously by many pathologists to designate the removal techniques by Ghon and Letulle, as described in the next paragraphs.

TECHNIQUE OF A. GHON Thoracic and cervical organs, abdominal organs, and the urogenital system are removed as organs blocks ("en bloc" removal). Modifications of this technique are now widely used.

TECHNIQUE OF M. LETULLE Thoracic, cervical, abdominal, and pelvic organs are removed as one organ block ("en masse" removal) and subsequently dissected into organ blocks *(3)*. This technique requires more experience than the other methods but has the great advantage that the body can be made available to the undertaker in less that 30 min without having to rush the dissection. Unfortunately, the organ mass is awkward to handle.

From: *Handbook of Autopsy Practice,* 3rd Ed. Edited by: J. Ludwig © Humana Press Inc., Totowa, NJ

CURRENT ROUTINE AUTOPSY TECHNIQUES

GENERAL POLICIES Autopsy techniques are learned from a preceptor in the autopsy room. This time-honored method still is integrated in the training of all anatomic pathologists and therefore, printed or audiovisual teaching aids, referenced in the earlier editions of this book, have played no appreciable role. Thus, a detailed description of autopsy techniques is beyond the scope of this book. Nevertheless, some recent guidelines may be helpful *(2,4,5)*. Pathologists generally achieve the best results if they use the methods with which they are most familiar, even if the situation at hand would cause the expert to choose a different approach. Special considerations in *medicolegal autopsies* are discussed in Chapter 2.

ADULT AUTOPSIES After the external descriptions, the body is weighed and body length is determined; roentgenographic studies may be needed at this time. This is followed by the Y-shaped primary incision and, if indicated, removal of material from the abdomen for microbiologic study. Subsequent steps include collection of abdominal effusions and exudates; search for hernias; incision of anterior abdominal musculature and breasts; search for pneumothorax (see under that heading in Part II); cutting the lower ribs so that chest plate can be lifted and fluid in pleural cavities can be collected; removal of chest plate; removal of thymic fat pad; incision of pericardial sac and collection of pericardial contents; and, if indicated, removal of blood for microbiologic, serologic, biochemical, or toxicological studies (the descending thoracic aorta often is a good puncture site, particularly in cases of extensive postmortem clotting). In some institutions, ligatures are placed to identify the carotid, subclavian, and femoral arteries for the convenience of the embalmer.

At this point, the techniques may be varied according to personal preference or the type of lesion. En masse removal (Letulle technique) yields the best results if pathologic lesions are expected to involve or pass through the diaphragmatic plane, as in the presence of acute aortic dissection. The preparation is then carried out from the posterior aspect of the organ mass. Organ blocks (Ghon technique) are removed routinely or only when pathologic processes make the preservation of vascular supplies desirable. In all other cases, Virchow's organ-by-organ removal technique can be followed.

Special attention must be paid to the removal of the *neck organs and the floor of the mouth*. Whether these structures are removed together with the chest organs or as a separate tissue block, lacerations of the skin in the neck area or even of the lips may occur if the prosector is inexperienced or works hastily. Furthermore, the prosector can easily cut or stab the assisting hand during the removal of the soft palate and the floor of the mouth. These procedures should not be attempted without the guidance of an experienced preceptor; work should be slow and deliberate in these areas. (*See* also below under, "Lesions of Face, Arms, or Hands.") In medicolegal autopsies, particularly in cases of suspected strangulation, extensive skin incisions of the neck area are indicated and permitted *(6)*. In these instances, the brain should be removed first so that blood is drained from the neck and the chance of an artifactual hemorrhage is minimized *(6)*. For further details, see references by V.I. Adams in Chapter 2. The central nervous system, peripheral nerves, muscles, bones, and joints usually are exposed at the end of the autopsy, before or after embalming.

The routine selection of organs and tissues for histologic study depends on the macroscopic findings, clinical diagnoses, teaching obligations, research protocols, personal attitudes, institutional policies, and, linked to all of them, economic considerations. If an institution has a very restrictive policy for the histologic study of autopsy material, it is particularly important that samples of all major organs and tissues are saved in formalin or, preferably, in paraffin blocks. This also should be done if histologic study is done primarily with frozen sections *(7)*.

PEDIATRIC AUTOPSIES Perinatal and pediatric autopsy techniques and related reporting procedures differ in some important aspects from adult autopsies *(8–10)*. It is often preferable if such autopsies are performed by pathologists experienced in perinatal pathology. Excellent texts are available *(11–15)*. A perinatal autopsy protocol, published in 1995 by the Armed Forces Institute of Pathology, and the manual on pediatric autopsies from the same institution, reprinted in 1997, can be ordered from the American Registry of Pathology Sales Office, AFIP, Room 1077, Washington, DC 20306-6000.

The external examination, particularly of fetuses and newborns, has to concentrate on the search for malformations such as cleft palate, choanal atresia, or stenosis and atresia of the anus and vagina. Face, ears, and hands may show characteristic changes—for instance, in Down's syndrome, renal agenesis, or gargoylism. The placenta, fetal membranes and umbilical cord must be studied in all autopsies of fetuses and newborns *(8)*. For further details, *see* "Stillbirth" in Part II of this book.

The removal of the brain in fetuses and newborns is described in Chapter 6. Dr.Waters, the coauthor of the pediatric disease procedures in Part II, recommends a horizontal cut over the occiput from behind one ear to the other, combined with a midline cut, running caudally from the first cut. This leaves the face unmarred and allows support for the brain as the attachments are being cut. This procedure appears most suitable for preterm infants and demonstration of the Arnold-Chiari malformation.

In infants, the whole chest cavity can be opened under water in order to demonstrate a pneumothorax. However, only a chest roentgenogram can provide a reliable permanent record (*see* also under "Pneumothorax" in Part II). For organ removal, any of the described techniques may be suitable but for the demonstration of rare malformations such as anomalous pulmonary venous connections in fetuses and infants, the en masse removal (after Letulle) is recommended.

As a minimum requirement for pediatric autopsies, histologic sections should be taken from lungs, liver, kidney, thymus, costochondral junction of a rib, and brain. In fetuses and newborns, placenta, fetal membranes and umbilical cord should be added.

SPECIAL AUTOPSY TECHNIQUES

POSTOPERATIVE AUTOPSIES Few autopsies present more difficulties because the pathologist is rarely familiar with all operative techniques that may have been used, the complications that were encountered, including anesthesia-related and drug-induced mishaps, and the postoperative events that may completely obscure the immediate surgical results. Possible medicolegal implications must be considered also *(16)*. The following general guidelines should be observed.

1. In any team, the most experienced autopsy pathologist should do postoperative cases. At least one assistant should be available.
2. The surgeon or one surgical assistant who participated in the operation should attend the autopsy. If this cannot be arranged, a telephone conversation, prior to the autopsy, between pathologist and surgeon is essential. Frequently, the main questions of the surgeon are not at all obvious from the written notes.
3. More important than in most other situations, the case history, the surgical report, and the results of roentgenographic and laboratory studies should be studied prior to the autopsy.
4. The autopsy technique should be changed as required by the specific situation. *Incisions* should not be carried through operative wounds. Instead, wounds should be viewed from their outer and inner aspects and then opened to find possible suture abscesses. To determine whether a *dehiscence* developed before or after death, the sutured region should be widely excised and fixed for preparation of properly oriented histologic sections for evaluation of vital tissue reactions. For the exclusion of *air embolism*, see Part II. Chest roentgenograms or other appropriate tests for *pneumothorax* should be performed also. *Fistulas* should be filled with a stained contrast medium so that their course can be demonstrated by roentgenograms and dissection. *Drains* should not be removed before their precise location has been established, always from an incision distant to the drain. At repeated and appropriate intervals, smears should be prepared and material removed for microbiologic examination (*see* Chapter 9). This may be of considerable help in determining the source of an infection. Some authors

prefer en block removal for dissection after abdominal surgery *(17)*. We would recommend this only under exceptional circumstances and only if great care is taken to avoid trauma to the operative sites during the excision of the organ block.

5. Instructive views of all decisive phases of the autopsy should be documented by photographs.
6. Protocols of postoperative autopsies should be dictated during the actual inspection and dissection of organs and tissues. At a later time, surgically significant findings often cannot be recalled and described accurately. For the measurements of volumes, lengths and weights, the metric system should be used (mL, cm, g).
7. During the autopsy, the pathologist should describe the findings but not interpret or comment on them. Hasty conclusions are often proved wrong by subsequent histologic studies or additional clinical information.

IMMEDIATE AUTOPSIES FOR SPECIAL LABORATORY PROCEDURES SUCH AS ELECTRON MICROSCOPY, CYTOCHEMISTRY, AND TISSUE CULTURE For the preservation of cytological detail or growth in tissue culture, autopsies often prove unsuited unless the postmortem interval is very short. For microbiologic studies and many other laboratory techniques, immediate autopsies also are indicated. Whenever possible, the prosector should be assisted by technicians who process the freshly removed samples and do the necessary paper work.

The first phase of the autopsy begins immediately after death has been pronounced and appropriate permissions have been obtained. Through a modified "Y" incision, organs and tissues are sampled for rapid processing. If there is no time to bring the body to the morgue, samples often can be removed with surgical instruments through mini-incisions. Depending on the purpose of the study, the specimens are immediately snap-frozen (e.g., for subsequent biochemical analysis), prepared and fixed for electron and light microscopic study, and transferred to tissue culture media (*see* Chapter 10) or other solutions as indicated by the intended procedures. Blood samples also can be collected during this phase of the autopsy. If a patient died from a hematologic disorder, procurement of good bone marrow preparations may be the most important autopsy technique. This can be achieved by injecting, shortly after death, 10 mL B-5 fixative into the sternum. The method is described further in Chapter 8.

For the examination of the central nervous system by electron microscopy, the intracranial vasculature is rinsed through an internal carotid artery with a solution of isotonic sodium chloride, followed by in situ fixation with a buffered solution of glutaraldehyde. The perfusion work in the neck can be done while another prosector procures tissue from other sites. In neonates, Zamboni's solution can be injected percutaneously into the lateral ventricles and drained through an intrathecal spinal needle *(18)*.

Once samples for electron microscopy have been collected, and in some instances revived in a tissue-culture medium (*see* Chapter 10), methods of fixation and specimen preparation for transmission or scanning electron microscopy do not differ from those used with biopsy material. Energy-dispersive X-ray microanalysis can then be used to identify metals and other elements (*see* Chapter 14). For immunohistochemisty and other special studies described in Chapter 14, samples should be collected with the same speed that often is needed for tissue culture and electron microscopy.

The second phase of the "immediate autopsy" is the routine dissection procedure, which can be delayed as necessary. An alternative to the "immediate autopsy" is described in the next paragraphs.

NEEDLE AUTOPSIES Needle biopsies in the immediate postmortem interval may be used to obtain tissue samples when more invasive procedures, as described under "immediate autopsies," are not possible. This may be the case in tropical countries *(19)*, if proper infection precautions cannot be taken *(20)*, or if all efforts to obtain permission for a regular autopsy fail *(21)* but the next of kin agree to multiple sampling by needle. Obviously, needle autopsies are inferior to conventional autopsies but they may be an acceptable alternative in selected cases *(22,23)*. Wide-core needles give the best results, either biopsy needles from the hospital supply or special autopsy needles (with a projecting trocar), which should be 10–15 cm in length with a bore of 2–3 mm. A large syringe should be used to provide appropriate suction. Liver, heart, lung, and kidneys usually can be biopsied successfully with this technique *(22)*. Specimens from large tumors also may be easy to obtain.

A variant of these methods can be used to prefix tissues prior to a routine autopsy. For example, if electron microscopic study of pulmonary tissue is intended, stained glutaraldehyde can be injected through the chest wall into the lungs during the immediate postmortem period. The staining permits identification of the fixed tissue at the time of autopsy.

ENDOSCOPIC AUTOPSIES The indications may be the same as those for needle autopsies, described in the previous paragraphs. Neoplasms and traumatic lesions with or without intraperitoneal or thoracic hemorrhages can be readily identified with these techniques *(23–25)*.

RESTRICTION OF SKIN INCISIONS Autopsy permission may be restricted to the re-opening of a surgical incision or it may specify that only an abdominal incision may be made. Many and often remote organs and tissues can be removed or at least sampled through these incisions, provided next of kin consent to such extended procedures.

LESIONS OF FACE, ARMS, OR HANDS The face is essentially "off limits" for the autopsy pathologist. Small specimens of facial skin tumors occasionally can be taken, particularly if the tumor is large enough to cover the defect. Lesions of facial soft tissues or bones may be removed only with special permission; removal of minute samples may be hardly noticeable but after excision of large specimens, reconstruction usually is difficult *(26)*.

Accidental damage such as cuts into facial tissues during an autopsy may be very traumatic to the next of kin. If such a mishap does occur, delicate suturing, cream and powder may render the damage nearly invisible. A plastic surgeon and a sympathetic mortician may provide much needed help in such a situation.

Tissues of the arms and hands should be removed only with special permission. If bones, joints or soft tissues of the hands are to be removed, the incision should be placed at the volar surfaces. A prosthesis may be needed to restore the contours (*see* Chapter 8).

DEATH MASKS In very rare instances, a pathologist may be asked to prepare or aid in the preparation of a death mask *(27)*. First, oil or petroleum jelly is applied to the face, and hair is protected with gauze. The nostrils are closed with gauze or other material. Next, a cardboard with an oval opening for the face is placed over the head to provide a frame that determines how far back the death mask should reach—for example, whether the ears will be included. Plaster of Paris or plastic molding material (also used in dentistry for moldings needed for the preparation of dentures) is placed over the face and allowed to harden. The facial mold is then greased and used to create the actual mask.

REFERENCES

1. Rössle R. Technik der Obduktion mit Einschluß der Meßmethoden an Leichenorganen. In: Abderhalden E, ed. Handbuch der biologischen Arbeitsmethoden, vol. VIII, part I (2). Urban & Schwarzenberg, Berlin, 1935, pp. 1093–1246.
2. Hutchins GM, ed. Autopsy. Performance and Technique. College of American Pathologists, Northfield, IL, 1990.
3. Saphir O. Autopsy Diagnosis and Technic, 4th ed. Paul B. Hoeber, New York, 1958.
4. Cotton DWK, Cross SS. The Hospital Autopsy. Butterworth Heinemann, Oxford, 1993.
5. Hutchins GM. Practice guidelines for autopsy pathology, autopsy performance. Autopsy Committee of the College of American Pathologists. Arch Pathol Lab Med 1994;118:19–25.
6. Vanezis P. ACP Broadsheet No. 139. Post mortem techniques in the evaluation of neck injury. J Clin Pathol 1993;46:500–506.
7. McCarthy EF, Gebhardt F, Bhagavan BS. The frozen-section autopsy. Arch Pathol Lab Med 1981;105:494–496.
8. Chamber HM. The perinatal autopsy: a contemporary approach. Pathology 1992;24: 45–55.
9. Bove KE. Practice guidelines for autopsy pathology: the perinatal and pediatric autopsy. Autopsy Committee of the College of American Pathologists. Arch Pathol Lab Med 1997;121:368–376.
10. ACOG committee opinion. Genetic evaluation of stillbirth and neonatal deaths. Int J Gynaecol Obstet 1997;56:287–289.
11. Valdéz-Dapena MA, Huff DS. Perinatal Autopsy Manual. Armed Forces Institute of Pathology, Washington, DC, 1983.
12. Dimmick JE, Kalousek DK. Developmental Pathology of the Embryo and Fetus. JB Lippincott, New York, 1992.
13. Gilbert-Barnes E, ed. Potter's Pathology of the Fetus and Infant. Mosby, St. Louis, MO, 1997.
14. Stocker JT, Dehner LP. Pediatric Pathology. J.B. Lippincott, Philadelphia, PA, 1992.
15. Wigglesworth JS, Singer DB. Textbook of Fetal and Perinatal Pathology. Blackwell Scientific Publications, Boston, MA, 1991.
16. Start RD, Cross SS. Pathological investigation of deaths following surgery, anaesthesia, and medical procedures. J Clin Pathol 1999; 52:640–652.
17. Culora GA, Roche WR. Simple method for necropsy dissection of the abdominal organs after abdominal surgery. J Clin Pathol 1996; 49:776–779.
18. Bass T, Bergevin MA, Werner AL, Liuzzi FJ, Scott DE. In situ fixation of the neonatal brain and spinal cord. Pediatr Pathol 1993;13: 699–705.
19. Marsden PD. Needle autopsy. Revista da Sociedade Brasileira de Medicina Tropical 1997;30:161–162.
20. Baumgart KW, Cook M, Quin J, Painter D, Gatenby PA, Garsia RJ. The limited (needle biopsy) autopsy and the acquired immunodeficiency syndrome. Pathology 1994;26:141–143.
21. Huston BM, Malouf NN, Azar HA. Percutaneous needle autopsy sampling. Mod Pathol 1996;9:1101–1107.
22. Forudi F, Cheung K, Duflou J. A comparison of the needle biopsy post mortem with the conventional autopsy. Pathology 1995;27:79–82.
23. Damore LJ II, Barth RF, Morrison CD, Frankel WL, Melvin WS. Laparoscopic postmortem examination: a minimally invasive approach to the autopsy. Ann Diagn Pathol 2000;4:95–98.
24. Avrahami R, Watemberg S, Daniels-Philips E, Kahana T, Hiss J. Endoscopic autopsy. Am J Forens Med Pathol 1995;16:147–150.
25. Avrahami R, Watemberg S, Hiss Y, Deutsch AA. Laparoscopic vs. conventional autopsy. A promising perspective. Arch Surg 1995;130: 407–409.
26. De Jonge HK, van Merkesteyn JP, Bras J. Reconstruction of the lower half of the facial skeleton after removal of the mandible at autopsy. Int J Oral Maxillofac Surg 1990;19:155–157.
27. Jansen HH, Leist P. The technique of death masks making. Beitr Pathol 1977;161:385–390.

2 Medicolegal Autopsies and Autopsy Toxicology

VERNARD I. ADAMS

MEDICOLEGAL AUTOPSIES

DEFINITION OF MEDICOLEGAL AUTOPSIES In the broadest sense, a medicolegal autopsy generates an evidentiary document that forms a basis for opinions rendered in a criminal trial, deposition, wrongful death civil suit, medical malpractice civil suit, administrative hearing, or workmen's compensation hearing. Because any autopsy report can become such a document, all autopsies could be considered medicolegal. However, for the purposes of this chapter, a medicolegal autopsy is more narrowly defined as an autopsy that is performed pursuant to the provisions of a medical examiners or coroners act of a state.

FORENSIC PATHOLOGISTS, MEDICAL EXAMINERS, AND CORONERS Ideally, medicolegal autopsies should be carried out by trained forensic pathologists—that is, experts in the physical effects of mechanical, chemical, baro-, and electrical trauma. Although the shortage in this country of board-certified members of this specialty has eased in recent years *(1,2)*, many general pathologists still perform medicolegal autopsies.

In the States and Territories of the United States, medical examiners (22 states) or coroners (11 states) are in charge of death investigation systems, and in 11 states, both systems operate *(3)*. In general, medical examiners are appointed by state or county governments, and are required to be physicians, pathologists, or forensic pathologists, depending on locale. Coroners are elected, and, in general, the only requirement is to be a registered voter. Forensic pathologists are employed as medical examiners and, in the more populous coroner jurisdictions, as coroners' pathologists.

ACTIVITIES RELATED TO MEDICOLEGAL AUTOPSIES Particularly challenging are death investigations involving blunt impact to the head or neck, infant deaths, postoperative deaths, and drug-related deaths. Investigation of this last group has become easier with the advent of sophisticated methods of analysis, as mentioned later in this chapter. Medical examiner autopsies sometimes are requested by next-of-kin who are dissatisfied with the medical care that was rendered to a decedent. Life insurance companies also rely on medicolegal autopsies. Finally, both plaintiff and defense attorneys in the medical malpractice field and hospital risk managers prefer to have autopsies in as many deaths as possible.

ERRORS IN MEDICOLEGAL INVESTIGATION In many instances, a seemingly trivial error can have unforeseen disastrous consequences. Every pathologist who works in this field should benefit enormously by reading and rereading the examples given in Moritz' classic paper *(4)*.

Although nonforensic pathologists generally understand the purpose of the descriptive (objective) part of the autopsy report, they have little or no training in opinion formation. The essentials are set forth in the following paragraphs.

DEFINITIONS OF DEATH First, one must understand the terms "cause of death," "manner of death," and "mechanism of death." The *cause of death* is the disease or injury that sets in motion the physiologic train of events culminating in cerebral and cardiac electrical silence. "Carcinoma of the Pancreas," and "Gunshot Wound of the Head with Perforation of the Skull and Brain" are underlying causes of death. "Bronchopneumonia" and "Pulmonary Embolism" are *immediate* causes of death, being in almost all cases the consequence of underlying injuries or diseases such as Alzheimer's disease or femoral neck fracture.

The *manner of death* is a pseudo-judicial classification of deaths dating back to Norman England, when the property of suicide victims was seized by the Crown. The four manners of death are natural, accident, suicide, and homicide. *Natural* deaths are caused exclusively by disease. *Accidents* are deaths in which trauma causes or contributes to the cause of death, and the harm inflicted is not intentional. A *homicide* is death at the hands of another person, with intent to cause harm. *Suicide* is the intentional unnatural death of one's self, by one's self.

The *mechanism of death* is the physiological derangement set in motion by the causes of death that leads to the cessation of cellular electrical activity. Common mechanisms of death are ventricular fibrillation, adult respiratory distress syndrome, and cerebral edema. When clinicians use the term "cause of death," they usually mean the mechanism of death.

From: *Handbook of Autopsy Practice,* 3rd Ed. Edited by: J. Ludwig © Humana Press Inc., Totowa, NJ

The cause and the mechanism of death are interrelated and one may explain the other. For example, an autopsy reveals atherosclerotic heart disease, and the toxicological studies reveal concentrations of benzodiazepines and opioid narcotics somewhat above the therapeutic ranges. If the history is that of a man who was alert, oriented, and who suddenly collapsed in view of witnesses, one may infer a ventricular arrhythmia as the mechanism and atherosclerotic heart disease as the cause of death. If, for the same set of findings, the history is that of a man who became somnolent, gradually comatose, and then had a diminishing tidal volume followed by respiratory arrest, and then a brief period of persistent cardiac activity, then one may infer that the mechanism is respiratory depression and the cause of death is intoxication by the effects of the drugs.

In a criminal proceeding, opinions must be to a *reasonable degree of certainty*. This means that there can be no other reasonable possibilities—that is, the opinion is beyond a reasonable doubt. Speculation is not allowed. For example, it is *conceivable* that the defense attorney and the pathologist in a case might be on the next space shuttle, but such a possibility is obviously speculative.

In a civil proceeding, the opinion by an expert is to the standard of *probable*—that is, *more likely than not*. Under this standard, one need not eliminate competing reasonable possibilities. It is necessary only that the competing possibilities be less likely than the favored one. Speculation is not allowed in civil proceedings either.

For death certificates, the required degree of certainty is not well-defined, but is generally understood to require a more-likely-than-not probability. In a homicide, the death certificate should meet the standard of reasonable medical certainty. Otherwise, the death certificate might be used to impeach one's trial testimony.

In the formation of opinions, three principal errors are often made.

First, a pathologist seizes onto one particularly interesting finding but ignores equally compelling evidence that points to a contrary explanation. Unwarranted criminal or civil suits may result. Moritz described this approach as the substitution of intuition for a scientifically defensible interpretation *(4)*.

Second, errors are caused by the failure to appreciate the distinctions between various degrees of opinion and probability. Thus, a mere reasonable possibility is introduced as if it were a probability, or a speculative idea is presented as a reasonable possibility.

Third is the failure to appreciate the unspoken underlying assumptions. In the absence of facts, they point to one opinion or another and guide pathologists in the right direction most of the time. For instance, a pathologist conducting a second autopsy must start with the rebuttable presumption that the findings of the first autopsy are correct. Likewise, in the absence of facts, or in the presence of conflicting facts, a decedent is entitled to the rebuttable presumption of a natural death for the purpose of the formation of the final cause-of-death opinion. This is perfectly compatible with an initial investigative presumption of homicide because this ensures a careful investigation. A violent death creates the rebuttable presumption of an accidental manner, as opposed to suicide or homicide.

Numerous sources describe the technical aspects of medicolegal autopsies *(5–8)*.

PRONOUNCEMENT OF DEATH Failure to ascertain that death has in fact occurred has on occasion led to serious embarrassments and repercussions. The findings supporting a pronouncement of death are briefly recapitulated here. With few exceptions—for example, mitochondrial poisoning by cyanide —the vast majority of deaths are met by either a rapid cardiac mechanism or a slow central nervous system mechanism *(9)*. Many findings are self-evident. Ordinary citizens recognize a putrefied body as being dead. Most police patrolmen recognize dependent lividity and rigor mortis. Emergency medical technicians and paramedics will usually recognize early dependent lividity in bodies that have not yet developed rigor mortis, and will opine death without resorting to a cardiac monitor. However, a still, cool body with no livor requires the demonstration of the absence of cardiac electrical activity before death is confirmed.

In practice, by the time the medical examiner arrives at the scene, enough time has elapsed that livor will be present. Medical professionals such as nurses who actually observe deaths uninterrupted by resuscitation efforts will observe the following:

1. Cessation of respiration. As a slow death approaches, the person frequently breathes in gasps. Intervening apneic periods rarely last for more than 30 s; their presence can be ruled out by extending the examination over a 10-min period.
2. Cessation of circulation. In slow deaths, the lack of a peripheral pulse does not necessarily denote cardiac arrest, and the heartbeat does not necessarily cease as soon as breathing stops *(10)*. In contrast, in persons with a rapid cardiac death, ventricular fibrillation or asystole leads to immediate cessation of blood flow to the brain and immediate cessation of the pulse. Cessation of respiratory efforts, voluntary muscle activity, and consciousness all follow within 13 s.

DEATHS FROM NATURAL CAUSES Not all medicolegal autopsies deal with violent or unnatural deaths. For example, in two major medical examiner districts in Florida, 45 and 44% of deaths investigated, respectively, were found to be from natural causes wherein death occurred suddenly, unexpectedly, or in an unusual manner *(11)*. Atherosclerotic and hypertensive vascular diseases in their cardiac and cerebral manifestations were the most common diseases causing natural deaths *(12)*. One cannot necessarily conclude that the manner of death was natural merely because a natural disease was demonstrated, because the natural disease may be an immediate cause of death that resulted from an underlying traumatic cause of death. Table 2-1 provides a checklist of natural diseases that can be the sequelae of mechanical or chemical trauma.

EVALUATION OF THE SCENE AND CIRCUMSTANCES OF DEATH Investigation of the scene where the body was found may provide critical environmental evidence, allow the preservation of medicaments, and allow the medical examiner to take witness accounts that are crucial to interpreting the autopsy findings. A body thought by police to have bled from a homi-

Table 2-1
Some Common Natural Diseases and Their Possible Violent Antecedents

Disease	*Possible underlying injury, acute or chronic*
Central nervous system	
Meningitis; cerebral abscess	Fracture of skull, jaw, facial bones; injuries to middle ear, nasopharynx, air sinuses; infection introduced by surgical, anesthetic, roentgenologic, chemotherapeutic, diagnostic procedures
Intracerebral hemorrhage	Cerebral contusion enlarged by alcoholic coagulopathy, masquerading as hypertensive bleed
Subarachnoid hemorrhage	Blunt impact to head or neck; laceration of vertebral artery
Subdural hematoma	Blunt impact to head from fall
Cardiovascular system	
Coronary artery insufficiency	Emotional or strenuous physical effort related to occupation, or threat of assault
Ruptured heart valve; aortic aneurysm	Strenuous physical effort or blunt impact
Congenital anomalies	Teratogenic drugs
Seizure disorder, "Vasovagal attacks"	Shock; fright
Respiratory system	
Pneumothorax; subcutaneous and mediastinal emphysema; hemopneumothorax	Traumatic intubation, artificial ventilation with bag-mask, aspiration of foreign body, SCUBA diving, premature putrefaction in the setting of sepsis
Pneumonia; pulmonary embolism	Trauma, immobilization
Pulmonary fibrosis; mesothelioma; pneumoconiosis	Exposure to radiation; drugs; asbestos; industrial exposure
Alimentary system	
Ruptured viscus; perforated ulcer; peritonitis; intestinal obstruction	Impact to abdominal wall; burns; strenuous physical effort; foreign bodies by mouth or rectum, or left at laparotomy; diagnostic or therapeutic endoscopy; paracenteses; peritoneal dialysis
Fulminant toxic hepatitis; massive hepatic necrosis	Exposure to drugs; poison, anesthetic agents; pesticides; shock
Genitourinary system	
Renal tubular necrosis; papillary necrosis	Poisons; drugs; heavy metals; burns; shock; dehydration
Cystitis; pyelonephritis; ruptured bladder; ruptured uterus; ruptured ectopic pregnancy	Impact to abdomen; abortion; injudicious instrumentation
Hematopoietic and reticuloendothelial system	
Hemolytic anemia	Incompatible blood transfusion
Aplastic anemia; agranulocytosis; thrombocytopenia; leukemia	Drugs; poisons; pesticides; industrial and laboratory chemicals; antibiotics
Miscellaneous	
Malnutrition; failure to thrive	Negligence; parental cruelty; eccentric or unusual religious beliefs
"Crib death"	Accidental or homicidal suffocation

cidal wound may be putrefied with pulmonary purging, dead from apparent natural causes. In this situation, an opinion by a medical examiner at the scene prevents an unnecessary full-scale criminal investigation.

Physicians responsible for investigating scenes of violent death should foster police policies directed toward the end of ensuring that nothing in the vicinity of the body is disturbed before their arrival. The uninstructed patrolman will instinctively remove a firearm from the body of a suicide. On the other hand, such a policy need not be transmitted to the fire department. A well-trained fireman will pull a freshly dead, viewable body off a pile of smoldering tires, making identification easy, whereas a well-trained detective will not disturb the scene. If the medical examiner arrives at a death scene before the police technicians and detectives, masterly inactivity is required until they are ready for the body to be disturbed. In busy jurisdictions, the medical examiner is summoned after detectives have arrived, preliminary statements have been taken, and crime scene technicians have completed measurements and photographs in the vicinity of the body. In jurisdictions with few homicides, the medical examiner will often be summoned immediately by the first uniformed police officer to arrive at the scene.

The position of the body, the distribution of blood lost by the victim or the assailant, or objects in the neighborhood of the body may offer important clues for the reconstruction of the fatal events, especially in cases of blunt impact or bludgeoning, and in cases of industrial accidents. Scene investigation is much more apt to yield clues as to the approximate time of death than is the autopsy (see below) and may help in the estimation of the interval that may have elapsed between injury and death.

Pathologists without training or appreciable forensic experience should not hesitate to secure help from statewide law-enforcement agencies. Homicide detectives and crime-scene technicians from large police departments are familiar with death-scene investigations; patrolmen and detectives from small police jurisdictions usually have very limited experience in this area.

Pathologists who do not examine the site where the body was found must rely on the written or oral reports of the circumstances of death, and photographs or illustrating sketches, if they are available.

A forensic autopsy should not begin before the known circumstances surrounding the death have been reviewed. However, the quantity of information available in homicides is generally much less than that available in accidental and suicidal deaths, because the person with the best and most complete information is usually the killer, who in most cases has not made a statement at the time the medical examiner is conducting the scene investigation.

ESTIMATION OF THE TIME OF DEATH The postmortem interval is determined by asking the police investigator when the decedent was last known to be alive and when the decedent was found dead. An opinion can be given with assurance that the subject died in that time frame. Because the onset of the signs of death varies widely, the physician can only in some cases opine that death occurred more toward one end of that time spectrum than the other. The physical signs that may help in this regard are described in the following paragraphs.

Livor Mortis (Postmortem Lividity) After cessation of circulation, the blood drains to the most dependent vessels, and becomes deoxygenated. The external manifestation of this process is the appearance of a faint pink erythema of the dependent skin surfaces, visible after 30–60 min in bright light in Caucasians, and later with poor lighting or when the skin is pigmented.

As the blood continues to pool under the influence of gravity, a distinct purple appearance develops on the dependent surfaces. Up until roughly 12–24 h after death, the livor can be blanched by pressing a finger or instrument against the skin surface. Livor is usually absent at pressure points, such as the skin over the scapulae and buttocks in a supine body.

Then, as blood pigment migrates extravascularly, the lividity becomes fixed. In a body whose position is changed before the onset of fixation of livor, the blood will shift to the newly dependent areas. If the livor has become entirely fixed, it will not shift, and the pattern of the livor will be inconsistent with the position of the body.

Livor mortis is of most use in determining that death has in fact occurred. It is occasionally helpful in determining whether the body has been moved after death. Less commonly, it is of use in determining the postmortem interval. The full fixation of livor, in the experience of the author, usually coincides with the passing of rigor and the onset of the earliest signs of putrefaction. Livor mortis is pink in the presence of substantial concentrations of carboxyhemoglobin. Refrigeration of bodies frequently induces a change in the color of lividity from purple to pink.

Rigor Mortis (Postmortem Rigidity) The maintenance of a loose, supple quality in muscle fibers requires energy in the form of adenosine triphosphate and glycogen. The low-energy state of muscle fibers is manifested by stiffness. In dead bodies, the stiffness is customarily termed rigor mortis. The strength of the rigor is entirely dependent on the mass of muscle; grading rigor as weak, moderate, and strong is a useless exercise. Thus, muscular young men who are dead have impressively strong rigor mortis that is difficult to break, whereas a frail elderly woman with little muscle mass seems to have weak rigor mortis. More important to note is whether the rigor is present or absent, and if present, whether it is oncoming, fully developed, or passing.

Rigor mortis ordinarily makes its first appearance 2–4 h after death. Its detectable appearance is hastened by antemortem depletion of muscular energy stores. Thus, vigorous physical activity or convulsions immediately before death can result in the almost instantaneous onset of muscle stiffening. Rigor may begin at identical times in two bodies, but will be apparent earlier in the body with the greatest muscle mass. It becomes fully developed in roughly 4–10 h. The onset and passing of rigor are hastened by high ambient temperatures, and delayed by cold ambient temperatures. This is most often manifested by the maintenance of rigor in bodies maintained under refrigeration. Rigor begins to fade simultaneously with the onset of putrefaction. Rigor is easily and reliably ascertained by attempting to open the mouth by pressing on the mandible. In the extremities, especially the upper limbs, rigor often has been broken prior to transportation of the body because elbows, hips, and knees had to be straightened.

Algor Mortis (Postmortem Cooling) The rate of cooling of a dead body is dependent on the temperature gradient between the body and the environment; the body mass in relation to its surface area; the rate at which air or water moves across the body surfaces; and the extent to which insulation is afforded by shelter, clothing, and adipose deposits. This multiplicity of variables results in wide variation in the rate of cooling. Published tables and formulas for estimating the postmortem interval generally take into account only the temperature gradient. Such formulae seem to enjoy popularity in cool climates where most people die indoors in structures with indoor heating and fairly uniform temperatures. In Florida, where outdoor deaths occur throughout the year, the formulas are largely ignored. The author's practice is to palpate the torso with the back of the gloved hand, and to estimate whether the body is warm, cool, cold, or at ambient temperature. In most cases, warm bodies are recently dead; or hyperthermic from sepsis, cocaine intoxication, or neuroleptic medication, or from obesity. Cool bodies of adults usually are dead for some time and often have livor or rigor mortis.

Stomach Contents and State of Digestion Under normal conditions, the stomach empties a medium weight meal in approx 3 h. Emptying time is delayed by a heavy meal. Significant craniocerebral trauma can delay gastric emptying for days. Carbohydrate foods such as potatoes and bread are readily dissolved by swallowed salivary amylase. Vegetable matter and meat are recognizable for a few hours. Mushrooms seem to stand up to gastric juices the longest.

In a homicide for which the time of injury is not known, the gastric contents not needed for toxicologic analysis can be strained and rinsed to facilitate naked-eye identification of food matter. The information gained can be correlated with investigative information to help establish whether or not the decedent was alive at certain times or present at certain meals.

Autolysis Within 3 or 4 h after death, the corneas begin to cloud. This effect is most useful in determining whether or not death was very recent. The degree of cloudiness is of no real use. Corneal clouding is extreme in burned bodies, in which the corneas have been baked. Such high temperatures tend to render all irises a cloudy blue, regardless of the initial color.

Skin slippage, or postmortem blistering, is a sign of autolysis that develops simultaneously with putrefaction. But under subtropical sun, or if the skin is near a heat source, slippage can be evident within a half hour after death.

Putrefaction Putrefaction is caused by the migration of bacteria from the gut into the blood, where they multiply, consume the blood, and produce a variety of gases as metabolic products. The volume of gases produced can be enough to float bodies that have been tied down with iron weights. In most cases hydrogen sulfide is produced. This gas combines with the iron in hemoglobin and myoglobin to produce black-green discoloration of the blood, viscera, and cutaneous livor.

The earliest visible effect of putrefaction is often blue-staining of the skin of the right lower quadrant of the abdomen, over the cecum, and black staining of the inferior aspect of the right lobe of the liver, adjacent to the hepatic flexure of the colon. Because putrefaction follows the blood, it is most pronounced in areas of dependent lividity, where it first manifests as ruddy and then green-black marbling, also termed venous suggillations. With fully developed putrefaction, the face and genitalia become grotesquely swollen with gas, the eyes bulge, the skin acquires extensive green-black discoloration, and a foul putrid odor becomes evident. The body cavities are filled with putrid gases under tension, which escape with a rush when the cavities are opened. The soft tissues and viscera are softened, darkened, mottled, and riddled with gas bubbles.

Exsanguination removes the principal nutrient source for bacteria and greatly retards putrefaction. In temperate climates, putrefactive changes begin to be evident roughly 3 d after death. In subtropical climates, they can be evident within 24 h. Putrefaction is hastened by obesity, because the viscera are insulated from cooling; and delayed in infants, whose bodies cool rapidly.

Mummification When the body cools rapidly, the warmth needed to sustain putrefactive bacterial growth is denied. The ears, nose, lips, toes, and fingers, and in extreme cases, the calves and forearms shrivel and darken as the water content evaporates from the tissue. This change is of little use in determining the postmortem interval. Mummification is more common in children and small-framed adults, and in a cold or dry environment.

Adipocere This substance is a rancid semisolid product of fat decomposition. Adipocere is found most often on bodies which have decomposed without having been exposed to air. Its presence is not useful in determining postmortem interval.

Entomologic Evidence Dead bodies attract flies, which lay eggs, particularly near the eyes, nostrils, mouth, genitalia, and wounds. The eggs hatch into larvae, which are popularly termed "maggots." Maggots consume soft tissue, leaving behind bone, cartilage, gristle, and some but not all of the dermis. The maggots molt one or more times, going through stages of development termed "instars," and finally crawl off the body to pupate in nearby soil. The maggots are eaten by other insects. When the soft tissues have been largely removed and the partly skeletonized remains have dried somewhat, beetles move in to consume the cartilage, gristle, and dried dermis. The order of their appearance depends on the local fauna present at that particular time of year. Maggots mature more rapidly in warm weather. A forensic entomologist can make these interpretations, but generally requires baseline data for the local area, including the time of appearance of local species, and data on temperature ranges. An entomologist can narrow the date-of-death window down to a few days in some cases, whereas the forensic pathologist working with the signs of decomposition can only give broad estimates of numbers of weeks or months in cases of advanced decomposition.

Chemical Evidence Mathematical formulas have been devised to estimate the postmortem interval from the concentration of nitrogenous compounds in cerebrospinal fluid, and from potassium in vitreous. In practice, the formulas produce wider time frames than are provided by acquiring from the police the times last known alive and found dead, and are of academic interest only *(13,14)*.

IDENTIFICATION OF THE BODY A Polaroid photograph of the face is useful for the purpose of identification of a viewable body by friends or relatives. Burned bodies often have one or two printable fingers, and may be identifiable by dental comparison or comparison of antemortem and postmortem somatic roentgenographs. Dismembered bodies that are recovered piecemeal require the separate identification of the major elements. The head can be identified by dental comparison or plain roentgenographs, which portray the unique outlines of the frontal sinuses. The upper extremities can be identified by fingerprinting. The torso can be identified by chest, abdominal, and pelvic roentgenographs, if antemortem films exist. Virtually any part of the body can be used for a DNA match. Serologic studies, performed by the crime laboratory, can differentiate human from animal blood or tissue.

Fingerprinting may become difficult if the skin is shriveled, macerated from immersion, or charred. If there is no ridge elevation, but the pattern is visible, the whorl pattern can be photographed with a macro lens. If there are ridges, but the fingerpads do not roll well because of maceration or desiccation, the fingerpads can be built up with injectable compounds, including formalin, found on the shelves of all funeral directors with embalming facilities.

Blood typing will be done by the crime laboratory in cases of serologic interest, such as bludgeonings. In criminal cases with no immediately perceived serologic interest, such as homicidal gunshot wound deaths, it has been the practice of the author's office to have the crime laboratory do preliminary typing, and prepare a blood stain on filter paper. The paper is then stored long-term at room temperature, and the tube of blood is discarded according to local policy.

Sex determination can be made from most skeletal remains from the contours of the pelvis and skull. Age determination can be based on evaluation of epiphyses, laryngeal and sternocostal cartilages, sacral, hyoid, and cranial bone sutures, and the condition of joints and teeth. Stature is reconstructed by anthropologic measurements and formulas *(15,16)*.

THE FORENSIC AUTOPSY PROTOCOL To ensure that all details, no matter how irrelevant, are captured, the protocol can be dictated concurrently with the progress of the autopsy. However, many experienced pathologists make notes on a body diagram and dictate the external and internal examinations only after the completion of the internal examination. This style tends to produce a concise, well-organized prose narrative.

If the protocol is dictated directly at the time of examination, and there are no handwritten notes, it should be promptly typed and proofread. If notes have been made, the need for a prompt proofing is still apparent for lengthy protocols with multiple gunshot wounds, or combinations of injurious modalities, such as impact, strangulation, and stabbing. The most common error made by experienced pathologists is the transposition of the words "left" and "right."

Because it is the testimony that is offered into evidence at trial, and not the autopsy report, mistakes in the protocol can be corrected at any time. However, the concerned attorneys must be notified immediately of any change that affects an opinion. If a change is cosmetic, it is sufficient to notify the attorney who has called the pathologist, just before the pathologist takes the witness stand. The attorney can choose whether to elicit testimony concerning the change on direct examination, or to ignore it. The subjective and objective sections of the protocol should be clearly separated from each other. The subjective portion comprises the cause of death opinion, the diagnoses, and the prose summary and opinion if there is one. The objective portion comprises the macro- and microscopic descriptions.

The gross protocol should contain objective descriptions with which no reasonable, trained pathologist would disagree. No revision of the gross description should be necessary after the microscopic slides are reviewed and further medical history and investigative information becomes available. Diagnostic terms may be used if the diagnosis will never be in question. For instance, if the lungs have obvious bronchopneumonia, and it is clear that the diagnosis will not be changed by subsequent microscopic studies, the end of communication is best served by including the term "bronchopneumonia" in the description of the lesion.

The opinion section, which includes the cause-of-death opinion, the line diagnoses, and any prose opinions, should be clearly labeled as opinion. The opinions contained in this section are based on all the available information, including medical history and circumstantial information. Unlike the data in the gross protocol, which should never change, the opinions *can* change if there are changes in circumstantial and historical information on which the opinions are based.

Identifying features must be recorded in detail for bodies that are unidentified "John Does." In contrast, a brief mention of iris color, hair color and distribution, facial hair, and significant scars is adequate for bodies for which identification is not in question. For instance, this author is satisfied to describe the lengths of scars as small, medium, and large in relation to the involved body regions for identified bodies.

Descriptions of endotracheal tubes, central venous catheters, and other devices of therapy are best clustered in a single paragraph that has both the external and internal aspects of the descriptions of the locations of the devices. For instance, "An endotracheal tube runs from the mouth to the trachea." The observations in this paragraph need not be repeated in the external and internal sections of the report.

Finally, the protocol should contain another separately titled section for all the external and internal data on any penetrating wounds, such as gunshot wounds and stab wounds *(17)*. I use the same device for blunt impact wounds, with separate sections for head and neck, torso, and extremities. The wound descriptions are *not* repeated in the customary sections for external examination and internal examination.

Measurements are made metrically or in the English system, depending on the purpose to which the measurements will be put. Lesions caused by *disease* and anatomical measurements of interest only to physicians should be measured metrically. *Wounds* can be measured metrically or by the English system, at the discretion of the pathologist. The author measures wounds metrically, unless the wound is patterned, and is being matched to an impacting object that was manufactured to English system specifications. However, the old axiom that wounds must be measured in inches no longer holds; jury pools now contain citizens educated in the metric system.

In the United States, distances between wounds and anatomic landmarks such as the top of the head, the median sagittal plane, and the soles of the feet should be recorded in inches because police investigators will be using feet and inches to measure the distances between bullet holes in walls and floors.

In the USA, body length and weight should be in the English system, because the parties who use this information are most often attorneys. Readers of the autopsy report who must perform physiologically oriented calculations based on body weight or length will be capable of converting the English measurements to metric measurements.

Measurements should be preceded by a qualifying adjective to indicate whether the number is actually measured, or is estimated (e.g., "A measured 1200 mL of dark red clot is in the left pleural cavity," "A measured 85 grams of clot is in the subdural space on the left side," "An estimated 100 mL of liquid blood is in the retroperitoneal soft tissues," "An estimated 50 grams of the heart weight is attributable to increased epicardial fat"). Blood accumulations in the retroperitoneal or mediastinal soft tissues must be estimated because they cannot be measured by any reasonable means.

For organ descriptions, terms such as "Normal," "Unremarkable," and "Within normal limits" may be used, but a reviewing pathologist will have more confidence in the report if the normal organs are briefly described, e.g., "The myocardial cut surfaces are the usual red-brown." The written description of external wounds should be supplemented by sketches on pre-printed diagrams and by photographs. Suitable diagrams of the external surface anatomy, the skeleton, dentition, and organs are available from the Armed Forces Institute of Pathology. Diagrams are particularly useful in jogging the memory while reviewing old cases, because they depict the wounds not as the camera saw them, but as the pathologist perceived them.

The availability of roentgenographs varies with the equipment and personnel of the facilities in which autopsies are conducted (*see* Chapter 12). In addition to roentgenographs for the detection of foreign objects in penetrating wounds, the author routinely takes chest roentgenographs to detect venous air embolism in all victims of traffic crashes who are dead at the scene or around the time when they arrived at the hospital, and all victims of penetrating neck trauma. The common portals of air entry are dural sinuses lacerated by skull fractures, and penetrating wounds of the jugular and subclavian veins *(18)*.

It is useful to have an internal scale near a lesion being photographed to get a sense of scale, but the internal scale cannot be used to measure the lesion in the picture, owing to the distorting effect of photographing a curved surface. Attorneys have at times raised the question of what lesions might be obscured by the scale, so it is good practice to have a companion photograph without a scale or other objects.

THE CHAIN OF CUSTODY In all criminal or noncriminal cases, medicolegal or hospital-derived, the chain of custody of the body should be documented by a record that includes the names of the transport driver, the log-in technician, the log-out technician, and the driver for the funeral home to which to body is released; and the dates and times of each transfer. Care must be taken that no one tampers with the body without authorization. If possible, a lock should be put on the cooler in which the body is kept.

Likewise, a record of the chain of custody must be kept of physical evidence such as bullets, hair and fingernail exemplars, trace evidence, and toxicologic specimens. (For the chain of custody of toxicologic evidence, *see* also below under "Autopsy Toxicology.") Such material should be saved in containers labeled with the case number, the name of the deceased if known, the date the specimen was impounded, the name of the specimen and the site from which it was removed, and the name of the medical examiner.

Bullets can be inscribed on the base or nose, but not on the sides. Any mark or symbol serves to take a bullet out of the legal category of fungible items. Pathologists in court frequently recognize their bullets not by the faded, tarnished marks made months before, but by the writing on the evidence envelope or by comparing the bullet to photographs taken of the bullet before it was sealed in the evidence envelope. The author routinely photographs all removed bullets with a macro lens.

THE EXTERNAL EXAMINATION When available, clothing from victims of gunshot wounds and pedestrians struck by vehicles that fled the scene should be examined for soot and gunpowder, and transfer of paint and trace evidence, respectively. Victims of bludgeoning, brawls, and strangulation should be examined for transferred hairs and fibers before the body is stripped and cleaned. Clothing can be examined at the scene and placed into police custody, or transported on the body to the autopsy facility and re-examined in good light, at the discretion of the pathologist. For apparent natural deaths, the clothing can be stripped by the autopsy room technicians, and retained for later examination by the pathologist in the unlikely event that it becomes necessary.

The inspection of the external body surfaces and orifices should be sufficient to detect old suicidal wrist scars, partial finger amputations, needle tracks, conjunctival petechiae, cutaneous contusions, and open wounds of the hair-bearing aspects of the scalp. However, when the hair is thick and tightly coiled, perforations of the scalp are easily obscured. Cutaneous contusions are made less evident by skin pigmentation.

Roentgenographs Head, neck, chest, abdominal, and pelvic roentgenographs should be taken before the internal examination in unviewable bodies, because they may be needed for identification purposes. If an unviewable body has decomposed severely and thus, trauma cannot be precluded with confidence, then roentgenographs of the extremities should be prepared also.

Chest roentgenographs should be obtained in cases of motor vehicle accidents with head trauma, and in victims of stabbing of the neck, to detect venous air embolism from torn dural sinuses, unless the victim has lived long enough to have had spontaneous circulation of blood. For the detection of pneumothoraces, *see* under that heading in Part II and below under "Internal Examination." Pelvic roentgenographs are helpful in traffic fatalities, because they are more sensitive than the autopsy in detecting pelvic fractures. Chest roentgenographs are not needed to detect rib fractures because the autopsy is more sensitive in this regard. Likewise, roentgenographs are less sensitive for the detection of skull fractures than is direct observation after reflection of the galea and stripping of the dura. Cervical roentgenographs will show cervical dislocations that are obvious at autopsy, but are inferior to posterior neck dissection in detecting lethal craniocervical derangements in which there is no residual static dislocation.

Photographs Photographs of external wounds should be taken with a 35 millimeter camera. Pathologists customarily use Ektachrome or Kodachrome transparency film for three reasons: the slides are small and store easily, there is no need to develop prints, and they are suitable for projection at lectures. Police customarily use print film, and develop the prints only if a court appearance is anticipated. Some pathologists and police photographers now use digital cameras.

THE INTERNAL EXAMINATION A postmortem examination should include examination and removal of the thoracic, abdominal, pelvic and neck organs, and the intracranial contents. So-called limited autopsies, which omit the opening of the skull, examination of the neck organs, or examination of the chest or abdominal organs, permit only limited opinions to be made, and are merely specimen retrievals. An autopsy conducted pursuant to statute should never be limited. It is often preferable to have no postmortem examination at all than to be responsible for an examination that cannot answer the anticipated questions.

The standard Y-shaped incision will permit a thorough examination of the anterior neck organs, and removal of the tongue *(6)*. After retracting skin and muscles of the anterior chest, a pleural window should be created to detect pneumothoraces by scraping the intercostal muscle off the external aspect of the parietal pleura. This should be done on both sides of the anterior aspect of the chest, usually near the third ribs.

In cases of third and fourth degree burns, it is usually necessary to make a European-style midline incision to the chin, because the tissue is contracted and indurated. For the same reason, the testes must often be removed through scrotal incisions in these bodies. This is not a problem for the undertaker because these bodies are not viewable.

Layerwise examination of the anterior neck structures is desirable in all cases, and is accompanied by sequential *in situ* photography in cases of suspected strangulation. Layerwise examination of the posterior neck structures is required for traffic fatalities in which there is insufficient trauma elsewhere to account for death, or in which there is an unexplained laceration of the brainstem, or hemorrhage in the prevertebral fascia. Posterior neck dissection is necessary to rule out craniocervical derangement in cases of suspected suffocation in traffic accidents, and is recommended in all infant deaths that occur outside the hospital. The pathologist opening an infant spinal canal for the first time may be surprised to find that the delicate and loosely supported epidural venous plexus has become so hypostatically congested that the blood has extravasated into the loose fibrofatty tissue of the epidural compartment. The absence of sprain hemorrhages in the supporting ligaments and muscles of the vertebral column permits the exclusion of the diagnosis of true epidural hemorrhage.

For special procedures for the diagnosis of arterial and venous air embolism or pneumothorax, see under these headings in Part II.

The method of evisceration should be the one with which the pathologist is most comfortable. Some experienced forensic pathologists remove thoracic and abdominal organ blocks prior to dissection (*see* Chapter 1) but others remove organs in sequence (Virchow's technique), with equally good results. Many crucial observations can be made only during the evisceration. Therefore, it is important for the pathologist not to delegate the evisceration procedure. If this is neglected, an attorney might convince the judge, the jury, and the press that the autopsy was actually performed by the technician, and that the doctor merely looked at removed specimens. The helper in these cases may be called to testify, because the observations that were passed on to the pathologist are hearsay.

The order of examination of the organs is not critically important. The pathologist who does only occasional autopsies should use the same order consistently so that no change of dissection techniques is necessary. Some pathologists prefer to dissect the heart first, arguing that the most important findings in an apparent cardiac death should be brought to light first. The author's preference in such cases is to dissect the heart last, to decrease the time interval between the observations and the recording of these observations.

EMBALMING For the autopsy pathologist, embalming is much to be desired in an exhumed body, but much to be avoided in a fresh body. Embalming involves two phases.

Arterial embalming involves the introduction of a catheter into a common carotid artery, usually the right, following which the blood vessels are flushed with embalming fluid. If the embalmer observes that the embalming fluid is not perfusing an extremity, he will expose the brachial and femoral arteries as necessary. Poor perfusion generally results from luminal obstruction by postmortem clots. In the United States, arterial embalming fluid is generally a mixture of methanol, formaldehyde, and red dye.

Obviously, embalming creates challenges for the toxicologist. After the arteries have been thoroughly flushed, there is no usable blood available. Ocular fluid, bile, and urine are available as liquid specimens, but will have artifactual concentrations of methanol appearing in the gas chromatograph. Technical problems abound in these situations.

Arterial embalming produces soft formalin fixation and artifactual pink coloration of the tissues. It produces artifactual effusions in the body cavities, and hardens intravascular clots. At the same time, it induces contraction of the tunica media in the walls of blood vessels, which then contract around any postmortem clots, producing an appearance similar to or indistinguishable from that of a distending thrombus.

Trocar embalming involves the introduction of a sharp-tipped hollow metal pipe through the abdominal wall. The trocar is used to aspirate any liquids and to inject cavity embalming fluid; this fluid has no dyes, and usually has more methanol than does the arterial fluid. After trocar embalming, the liver, stomach, mesenteries, and loops of bowel have numerous perforations. The lungs and heart generally have fewer perforations, depending on the diligence of the embalmer. The tissue along the perforations is firm and gray, unlike the tissue fixed only by the arterial embalming fluid. The perforations of the diaphragm and pericardial sac produce communication paths among body cavities. The body cavities can contain substantial formalin collections mimicking effusions. More troublesome are real effusions and blood collections that are diluted by the embalming fluid. Fixed feces is often found floating in the peritoneal fluid.

The practice of permitting arterial embalming before an autopsy is mentioned only to discourage it. At the Mayo Clinic, where the autopsy suite includes an embalming room, the neck organs are removed after arterial embalming has been accomplished, which facilitates the work of the embalmer. Embalming before examination of the neck organs should not be permitted for medicolegal autopsies.

EXHUMATION AND OTHER SPECIAL PROCEDURES Recently exhumed bodies differ from the embalmed bodies described above only by the presence of colorful growths of mold on the skin surfaces. The internal findings are similar to those of yet-to-be-buried embalmed bodies. Long-buried bodies have variable degrees of decomposition, and can be virtually skeletonized.

Many special procedures, from "Abortion" to "Strangulation" are listed in Part II in alphabetical order of the condition.

AUTOPSY TOXICOLOGY

Most autopsies in which toxicologic analysis is performed are conducted pursuant to statute, toward the end of determining the cause of death. For additional details, *see* Chapter 11.

INVESTIGATION OF CIRCUMSTANCES OF POISONING Frequently, medical examiner investigators or police detectives can use directed interview questions to elicit information

Table 2-2
Investigative Information Useful for Suspected Poisoning Cases[a]

Date deceased was last known to be in good health
Date and time last known to be alive
Date admitted to hospital
Date and time pronounced dead in hospital, or
Date and time found dead
Date, time, and content of last meal
Prescribed drugs (append medication record if indicated)
Known drugs of abuse
Suspected drug of ingestion
Symptoms: nausea, vomiting, diarrhea, constipation, thirst, loss of weight, jaundice, blindness, cyanosis, shivering, hallucinations, convulsions, pupillary dilatation or contraction, delirium, drunkenness, sweating, unconsciousness

[a]Adapted with permission from ref. *(19)*.

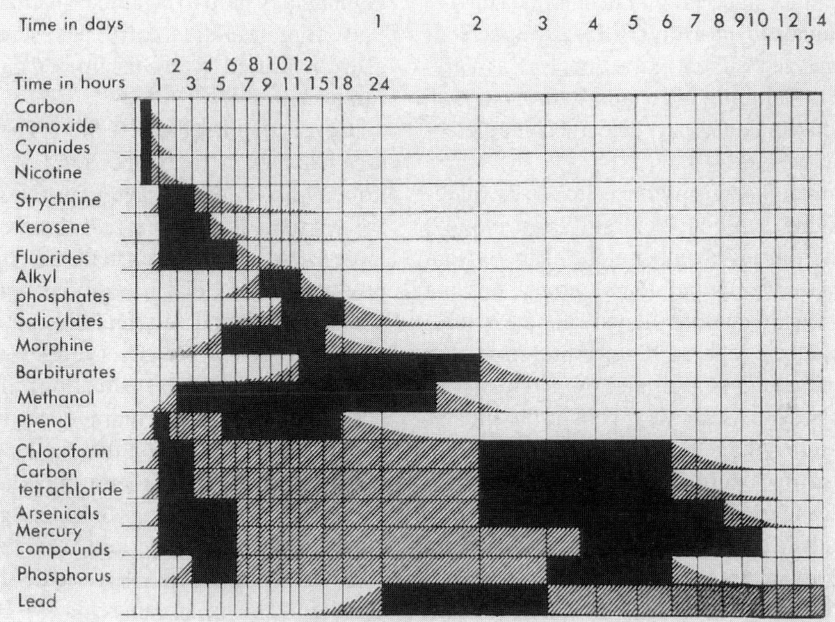

Fig. 2-1. Average time of death after ingestion or inhalation of fatal dose of poison. Solid regions indicate interval in which most deaths occur. Shaded regions indicate intervals in which death occurs occasionally but less commonly. Adapted with permission from ref. *(21)*.

that is helpful to further a toxicologic investigation, once poisoning is suspected (*see* Table 2-2). Of particular interest is the time interval between the alleged intake of the poison and the death of the decedent *(20)*. Figure 2-1 shows that this time interval may be too long or too short to make death from a specific poison likely.

CONTAINERS To prevent contamination of specimens by cleaning or embalming agents, previously unused polyethylene or glass containers are preferable in most situations. With time, highly volatile compounds such as the accelerants used by arsonists will diffuse through polyethylene and escape the container. Glass containers are susceptible to breakage during transport. If glass containers are to be used, they must be washed with dichromate. Dichromate can activate the glass surface and cause adsorptive loss or low concentrations of drugs and metabolites. In the laboratory, this type of adsorptive loss is reduced by silyzation, silanization, or siliconization of the glassware prior to use. The pathologist should always be present if a funeral director obtains tissues for toxicologic study.

The label for each specimen container should state the date the material was secured, the name of the decedent, the case number, and the name of the organ or liquid sample. Samples added to containers with preservatives should be inverted several times to disperse the preservative through the sample. Samples should be kept refrigerated before and during transport to the toxicology laboratory. After analysis, deep-freeze storage is preferable to refrigeration. In the future, weighing and freeze-drying may permit storage of specimens at room temperature.

ROUTINE SAMPLING OF TOXICOLOGIC MATERIAL In the author's office, it is usual practice in all autopsies to save 50 mL each of central blood, bile, urine, liver, and brain, plus available femoral vein blood up to 50 mL, and all retrievable vitreous. Approximately half the blood is placed in containers with sodium fluoride as a preservative. Sodium fluoride inhibits both bacterial growth and serum esterases which hydrolyze cocaine postmortem. If commercially available gray-top Vacutainer® tubes are not used, 250 mg of NaF can be added to 30 mL containers.

Urine Urine is aspirated with a syringe through the dome of the bladder after the peritoneal cavity has been opened. If the bladder is nearly empty, it can be secured by hemostats before incising the dome to facilitate aspiration of the bladder lumen under direct vision. Toxicologists often prefer urine as a specimen for enzyme-multiplied immunotechnique (EMIT) and enzyme-linked immunosorbent assay (ELISA) drug screening, because it can be analyzed without extraction. NaF as a preservative is optional; as an inhibitor of cocaine hydrolysis NaF is unnecessary, because the immunoassays detect cocaine metabolites rather than parent cocaine.

Blood Central luminal blood is preferred to cavity (pleural, pericardial, or peritoneal) blood. Central ("heart blood") specimens are aspirated from any chamber of the heart, or from the intrapericardial thoracic aorta, pulmonary artery, or vena cava. However, for a growing number of analytes, most notably tricyclic antidepressants, peripheral blood is preferred over central blood. Peripheral blood is aspirated by percutaneous puncture before autopsy, from the femoral vein or the subclavian vein. The author prefers the femoral approach in order to avoid any question of artifact in the diagnosis of venous air embolism. Peripheral blood can be obtained by a technician as soon as the body is received. If cocaine intoxication is likely, it is highly desirable to obtain this specimen in a tube with NaF as soon as possible, in order to inhibit postmortem hydrolysis of cocaine. The term, "cavity blood" is used for blood ladled or aspirated from a hemothorax, hemopericardium, hemoperitoneum, or from the pooled blood left in the common cavity after removal of the heart and lungs. Cavity blood analyses should be supplemented by peripheral blood, vitreous, or solid tissue analyses, because of the real possibility of contamination from gastric contents.

Vitreous Vitreous is an excellent specimen for alcohol and drug analysis. The protected location in the orbit renders the fluid less susceptible to putrefaction than blood, and the problem of site-dependent variation in concentrations in blood specimens is avoided. Two to three mL of vitreous from one or both eyes is gently aspirated from the lateral angle of the eye with a 5 mL clean syringe. The tip of the needle should lie near the center of the eyeball. The procedure is illustrated in Chapter 7 (Fig. 7-1). Forceful aspiration must be avoided because it may detach retinal cells, which cloud the specimen and give spuriously high potassium values. Before dilution, the chemist must invert the specimen 10 or 12 times to ensure thorough mixing.

Gastrointestinal Tract After removal of the stomach, duodenum, pancreas, and esophagus, the gastric contents are squeezed out through the esophagus, or through an incision in the stomach, into a 1-L container. A representative 50-mL specimen is satisfactory for the toxicologist, unless the stomach contents have a nonuniform slurry of solid and liquid elements, in which case a higher volume is desirable. If the solid elements seem to be fragments of medicaments, then nearly all the contents should be saved for the toxicologist, except for what is needed to strain and inspect the material to identify food matter. In suspected suicides, in which death may have followed ingestion by several hours, it can be useful to ligate a length of jejunum before removing it and draining it into a specimen container. The jejunum in such circumstances may have a higher concentration of analyte than the stomach.

The establishment of toxicity in adults cannot be done from analysis of gastric content; investigative information and analysis of tissue or body fluids are needed. Analysis of gastric content may help to establish suicidal intent and to investigate poisoning in infants. In infants, screening of gastric contents also can be used to save the limited quantities of blood for quantitative analysis.

Cerebrospinal Fluid (CSF) The practice of removing CSF (*see* Chapter 6) by suboccipital or lumbar puncture is mentioned only to discourage it. Although pathologists certainly vary in their skill levels, and some can make a clean puncture more often than not, even in the best hands blind punctures often produce blood-lined tracks that render the interpretation of posterior neck and vertebral dissections problematic. Vitreous, like CSF, is a low-protein erythrocyte-free substitute for blood, and is preferred in most situations. If CSF must be drawn, it is best taken from the cerebral cisterns after the skull has been opened is such a fashion that the leptomeninges are relatively intact and the CSF has not run out. The situation most often calling for a CSF specimen is the meningitis autopsy with no urine available for a latex agglutination test for bacterial antigens.

Bile Bile is aspirated by needle after the abdomen is opened and before the organs are removed. Because the mucosa of the gallbladder is lush and easily becomes ensnared in the needle tip, it is helpful to aspirate with gentle vacuum, and to use the free hand to milk the gallbladder. Bile is a useful substitute for blood when the analyte of interest is an opiate or an alcohol. In rapidly fatal opiate intoxications, the offending opiate may be detectable only in bile.

Other Liquid Specimens In hospitalized decedents, the highest concentrations of toxic substances may be found in dialysis and lavage fluids, if they have not been discarded after death.

Solid Organs Liver is the solid organ of choice when no liquid specimens are available. Reference values are available for the lethal concentrations of numerous types of drugs in liver tissue. Liver specimens from the right lobe of the liver are preferred to specimens from the left lobe, to avoid spuriously high concentrations from diffusion from the stomach *(22)*. Brain tissue is useful for alcohol determinations in the absence of a useful liquid specimen.

In putrefied bodies, blood and bile are usually absent, and the only specimens available may be solid organs, such liver, brain, and skeletal muscle. Skeletal muscle from the least decomposed extremity is preferred.

In fire deaths, arson investigators occasionally request specimens for accelerant analysis. For this purpose, lung tissue is sealed in an unused lidded metal can of the style used by paint manufacturers.

Hair Hair is a useful specimen in suspected chronic arsenic poisoning, and may be useful in the determination of chronic drug abuse. Hair should be pulled from the scalp, to include the roots. A large sample, about 10 grams, should be tied in a lock to identify the root end of the specimen.

Skin If it is suspected that a poisonous substance has been injected, the skin around the needle-puncture site can be excised at a radius of 2–4 cm from the injection site. If a poisonous substance might have been taken up by absorption, the skin is excised in the area where the absorption is thought to have occurred, and from a distant, preferably contralateral area as a control. Skin samples are saved with the expectation that the toxicologist will prefer to obtain the information necessary to opine the cause of death by first analyzing the customary liquid specimens.

CHAIN OF CUSTODY The continuity of the custody of the specimens should be documented. A blank space on the specimen transmittal form (see next paragraph) can be used for tracking custody from the pathologist to an in-house toxicology laboratory.

Transmittal Sheet Specimens submitted to a toxicology laboratory should be accompanied by a transmittal sheet and a summary of the investigative information as it is known at that time. The transmittal sheet contains case identifying information, a list of specimens, supplementary information necessary to select analytical methods, and signatures to indicate the chain of custody. It should state whether the body is embalmed or decomposed and indicate the duration of hospitalization (during which an alcohol or drug is metabolized). An example is in Table 2-3.

If a courier is used to transport a sealed container with multiple specimens from multiple cases to an outside laboratory, an additional, separate, single transmittal form can be devised that lists all the case numbers; omits specimen details; and has signature/date lines for the in-house technician, the courier, and the receiving clerk at the laboratory.

METHODOLOGY Although the techniques of toxicologic analysis are beyond the scope of this book, a brief summary of current methods is in order.

Volatiles by Gas Chromatography The analyte most frequently tested is ethyl alcohol. Toxicologists in medical examiner offices generally detect and quantify ethyl alcohol by gas chromatography, as part of a general panel designed to capture numerous volatile compounds, including ethyl, methyl, and isopropyl alcohols, and ketones. Tertiary butyl alcohol is often used as an internal standard, because it does not occur naturally. Hospital and clinical laboratories most often use the alcohol dehydrogenase method, which measures any substance capable of being dehydrogenated by the enzyme. It does not distinguish methyl, ethyl, and isopropyl alcohols and it has a larger experimental error than does gas chromatography. The dichromate method, which measures oxidizing activity, is nonspecific and mainly of historical interest.

Specific Drug Screening by Enzyme-Multiplied Immunoassay (EMIT) Drugs of abuse are commonly detected but not quantified by EMIT (Enzyme Multiplied ImmunoTechnique), in which the activities of selected families of drugs are measured by antibody interaction. The panels are selected depending on local drug-abuse patterns. Panels are available for cocaine metabolites, tricyclic antidepressants, barbiturates, cannabinoids, amphetamines, opiates, and propoxyphene. Not detectable are drugs present in parts per billion, such as fentanyl.

Specific Drug Screening by Enzyme-Linked Immunosorbent Assay (ELISA) Gradually supplanting the EMIT technique is the ELISA technology, which also uses antibodies, but is capable of detecting drugs whose concentrations are in parts per billion.

Drug Screening by Thin-Layer Chromatography (TLC) Although EMIT and ELISA panels detect the most commonly occurring abused drugs, they are not general drug screens. The technically simplest general drug screen utilizes the TLC so familiar to high school chemistry students. Specimens are prepared for TLC by extracting into solvents under acidic, neutral, or basic conditions, in order to bring different classes of drugs into the extraction solvents.

General Drug Screening, Identification and Quantitation by High-Performance Liquid Chromatography (HPLC) Supplanting TLC is high-performance liquid chromatography, in which the chromatograph is a thin column with packing material and a liquid solvent. HPLC can be linked to a computer database of hundreds of drugs to provide spectral identification and quantification. Historically, HPLC has been used by most laboratories for assaying specific classes of drugs such as tricyclic antidepressants. A few laboratories have developed extraction methods and columns that permit HPLC to be used as a general screen. HPLC, with its cool injection ports, is often a preferred quantitative method when compared to gas chromatography/mass spectrometry (GC/MS) (see below), which uses hot injection ports in the gas chromatograph to volatilize drugs. The heat decomposes drugs such as methocarbamol and propoxyphene.

Specific Drug Identification and Quantitation by Gas Chromatography (GC) Linked to Mass Spectrometry (MS) The gold standard for identifying drugs is gas chromatography linked to mass spectroscopy (GC/MS). GC utilizes a gaseous medium to separate the analyte drugs in a column. The output of the column is fed into a mass spectrometer, which breaks compounds into ionic subunits, whose weights form a bar-graph spectrum that can be specific for each compound.

Carbon Monoxide Tests Carboxyhemoglobin is detected in most medical examiner toxicology laboratories by visible spectrophotometry. In hospitals, carboxyhemoglobin is frequently detected and reported in the course of routine arterial blood gas analysis. Some medical examiner laboratories use GC for the determination of carboxyhemoglobin.

Metals Heavy metals can be detected by qualitative tests. For example, the Reinsch test primarily detects arsenic, and is an insensitive test for mercury, antimony, and bismuth. Quantifica-

Table 2-3
Toxicology Specimen Transmittal Sheet

Toxicology Specimen Transmittal Sheet
(Name of Medical Examiner Agency)
(Address and Telephone Number of Medical Examiner Agency)

Medical Examiner Case Number: *97-012345*
Name of Decedent: *Joe Doe*
Date Specimens Obtained: *5/3/97*

Duration of Hospitalization: *36 hours* Embalmed? *No*
Decomposition (circle): None 1+ 2+ 3+ 4+
Check here to retain specimens and issue a report that states "Toxicology Testing Not Indicated" *X*

X	Blood, heart[a]
X	Blood, peripheral
	Blood, cavity
	Liquid from heart or vessels (embalmed)
X	Bile
X	Urine
X	Gastric content
	Bowel content
X	Vitreous
X	Liver
	Lung
X	Brain
	Kidney
	Skeletal muscle
	Other:____________________

Other information or instructions:

Pathologist name and date:
Laboratory receipt of specimen; name and date:

[a]An "X" indicates specimen collected.

tion and specific metal identification is done by atomic absorption spectroscopy, usually by a reference laboratory.

Cyanide A good screen for cyanide is the nose of a person who is capable of smelling the ion. Because only a minority of persons can smell cyanide, it is helpful to know in advance if any person in an office or laboratory can smell cyanide. Textbooks state that hydrogen cyanide gas smells like bitter almonds; forensic pathologists who can smell the compound state that it has its own specific odor, which is not comparable to any other (Davis JH, personal communication, 1984).

SAMPLING FOR SPECIFIC TOXICOLOGIC SUBSTANCES Pertinent procedures have been listed in Part II, under the name of the substances involved, from "Alcohol Intoxication and Alcoholism" to "Poisoning, Thallium."

ACKNOWLEDGMENT

Wayne Duer, PhD, Chief Forensic Toxicologist for Hillsborough County, Florida, reviewed the manuscript, suggested improvements, and corrected errors in the toxicology section. Any remaining errors are those of the author.

REFERENCES

1. Curran WJ. The status of forensic pathology in the United States. N Engl J Med 1970;283:1033–1034.
2. Hartmann W. for the American Board of Pathology. Personal communication, March 13, 1997.
3. Combs DL, Parrish RG, Ing R. Death Investigation in the United States and Canada, 1995. U.S. Department of Health and Human Services, Centers for Disease Control and Prevention, Atlanta, GA, 1995, p. 11.
4. Moritz AR. Classical mistakes in forensic pathology. Am J Clin Pathol 1956;26:1383–1397. (Reprinted in Am J Forensic Med Pathol 1981;2:299–308.)
5. Wetli CV, Mittleman RE, Rao VJ. Practical Forensic Pathology. Igaku-Shoin, New York, 1988.
6. Adams VI. Autopsy techniques for neck examination: I. Anterior and lateral compartments and tongue. Pathol Annu 1990;25(2):331–349.
7. Adams VI. Autopsy technique for neck examination: II. Vertebral column and posterior compartment. Pathol Annu 1991;26(1):211–226.
8. U.S. Department of Defense. Army Department: Autopsy Manual. U.S. Government Printing Office, Washington, DC, 1981.
9. Davis JH, Wright RK. The very sudden cardiac death syndrome: a conceptual model for pathologists. Hum Pathol 1980;11:117–121.

10. Atlee WL and the Medical Faculty of Lancaster. Report of a series of experiments made by the medical faculty of Lancaster, upon the body of Henry Cobler Moselmann, executed in the jail yard of Lancaster County, PA, on the 20th of December, 1839. Am J Med Sci 1840(May):51:13–34.
11. Medical Examiners Commission. 1995 Annual Report. Florida Department of Law Enforcement, FL, p. 18.
12. Medical Examiner Department Computer Database for 1995 and 1996, Public Records of Hillsborough County, Florida.
13. Ihm P, Schleyer F. Fehlerkritische Betrachtungen über die Todeszeitberechnung anhand biochemischer Komponenten im Zisternenliquor and Serum. Arch Klin Med 1967;214:20–33.
14. Lie JT. Changes of potassium concentration in the vitreous humor after death. Am J Med Sci 1967;254:136–143.
15. Bass WM. Human Osteology: A Laboratory and Field Manual, 3rd ed. Missouri Archaeological Society, Special Publication, 1987.
16. Ubelaker DH. Human Skeletal Remains: Excavation, Analysis, Interpretation, 2nd ed. Teraxacum, Washington, DC, 1989.
17. Hirsch CS. The format of the medicolegal autopsy protocol. Am J Clin Pathol 1971;55:407–409.
18. Adams VI, Hirsch CS. Venous air embolism from head and neck wounds. Arch Pathol Lab Med 1989;13:498–502.
19. Churg A. Poison Detection in Human Organs, 2nd ed. Charles C. Thomas, Tallahassee, FL, 1969.
20. Moritz AR, Morris CR. Handbook of Legal Medicine, 3rd ed. C.V. Mosby, St. Louis, MO, 1970.
21. Moritz AR, Morris CR. Handbook of Legal Medicine, 3rd ed. C.V. Mosby, St. Louis, MO, 1970.
22. Pounder DJ, Fuke C, Cox DE, Smith D, Kuroda N. Postmortem diffusion of drugs from gastric residue. Am J Forensic Med Pathol 1996;17:1–7.

AN ANNOTATED REFERENCE LIST FOR THE OCCASIONAL FORENSIC PATHOLOGIST

Bass WM. Human Osteology: A Laboratory and Field Manual, 3rd ed. Special Publication No. 2 of the Missouri Archaeological Society, Columbia, MO, 1987.
A useful handbook when examining skeletal remains, especially when the skeleton is fragmentary.

Baselt RC, Cravey RH. Disposition of Toxic Drugs and Chemicals in Man, 4th ed. Chemical Toxicology Institute, Forest City, CA, 1995.
Has well-organized descriptions of metabolism, procedures, therapeutic concentrations, and concentrations found in fatalities.

Spitz WU, ed. Spitz and Fisher's Medicolegal Investigation of Death: Guidelines for the Application of Pathology to Crime Investigation, 3rd ed. CC Thomas, Springfield, IL, 1993.
A standard textbook of forensic pathology.

Froede RC, ed. Handbook of Forensic Pathology. College of American Pathologists, Northfield, IL, 1990.
A general reference on applied forensic pathology.

Wetli CV, Mittleman, RE, Rao VJ. Practical Forensic Pathology. Igaku-Shoin, New York, 1988.
Descriptions of practical procedures and the rationales behind them.

3 Cardiovascular System

William D. Edwards

REMOVAL OF THE HEART FROM THE CHEST

INITIAL STEPS Before the autopsy is begun, a radiogram of the chest may be performed (*see* Chapter 12). The removal of the chest plate has been described in Chapter 1. In patients who have had previous open-heart surgery via a median sternotomy, diffuse pericardial adhesions are common, which requires careful dissection of the heart away from the sternum so as not to disrupt any surgical sites. Pericardial exudate should be cultured (*see* Chapter 9). Pericardial blood clots should be weighed. If it is necessary to distinguish between blood and serosanguinous fluid, a hematocrit can be obtained.

CHOOSING THE METHOD OF REMOVAL Normal hearts and most hearts with acquired disease can be excised separately. In the presence of extracardiac disorders such as pulmonary or esophageal carcinoma or ascending aortic dissection, the heart should be removed with the *thoracic organs en bloc* (*see* Chapter 1). For congenital heart disease, the thoracic contents should be removed en bloc, regardless of the age of the patient.

DESCRIPTION OF THE HEART Cardiac *size* may be normal or enlarged (cardiomegaly) due to hypertrophy or dilatation (or both) and can involve one or more chambers. Overall cardiac *shape* may be conical (normal), globoid, or irregular (as with a ventricular aneurysm), and one or more chambers may be abnormal in shape. The *color* of the subepicardial myocardium may be gray with an old infarct, pale with chronic anemia, and mottled or hemorrhagic with an acute infarct or rupture. Left ventricular *consistency* can be firm (due to hypertrophy, fibrosis, amyloidosis, calcification, or rigor mortis) or soft (due to acute myocardial infarction, myocarditis, dilated cardiomyopathy, or decomposition).

EVALUATION OF THE CORONARY ARTERIES

Before any of the many forms of cardiac dissection is applied *(1–14)*, coronary arteries should be inspected for calcification and tortuosity. If angiography is indicated, the procedure must be performed before dissection of the coronary vessels and preferably before fixation of the heart.

From: *Handbook of Autopsy Practice,* 3rd Ed. Edited by: J. Ludwig © Humana Press Inc., Totowa, NJ

POSTMORTEM CORONARY ANGIOGRAPHY This important method is described in detail in Chapter 12.

DISSECTION OF CORONARY ARTERIES In subjects younger than 30 yr, in whom the cause of death is noncardiac, the coronary arteries may be opened longitudinally. Otherwise, the vessels should be cut in cross-section at 3–5 mm intervals. Calcified vessels that cannot be readily cut with a scalpel should be stripped off the heart and decalcified for at least 24 h before cutting.

GRADING OF CORONARY OBSTRUCTION A four-point system is applied, by 25% increments of narrowing in cross-sectional area *(15)*. A grade-4 lesion indicates stenosis of at least 75% and is considered severe, whereas a grade-4 lesion of 90% represents critical stenosis. As a rule, grade-4 lesions should be documented microscopically. Depending on the number of major epicardial vessels with grade-4 lesions, a heart may have severe 1-vessel, 2-vessel, or 3-vessel disease. Severe left main disease is equivalent to 2-vessel disease, and its coexistence with grade-4 disease in the other three coronary arteries represents severe 4-vessel disease.

DISSECTION METHODS OF THE HEART

Many older methods *(7)* are impractical for routine diagnostic pathology. Only the inflow-outflow and short axis (bread slice) methods have withstood the test of time; the latter technique is applicable to virtually any form of heart disease. In addition, some recently described methods are useful for teaching purposes and correlations with current cardiac imaging *(8–14)*.

INFLOW-OUTFLOW METHOD OF CARDIAC DISSECTION This technique is suitable primarily for normal hearts. For each side of the heart, the atrium is opened first, and then the ventricle is opened along its inflow and outflow tracts, following the direction of blood flow (Fig. 3-1). Valves are cut between their commissures.

Using scissors, the initial cut is made from the inferior vena cava to the right atrial appendage, sparing the superior vena cava with the region of the sinus node. The right ventricular inflow tract is opened with a knife or scissors from the right atrium, through the posterior tricuspid leaflet, running parallel to and about 1 cm from the posterior ventricular septum. The outflow tract is opened in a similar fashion, approx 1 cm from

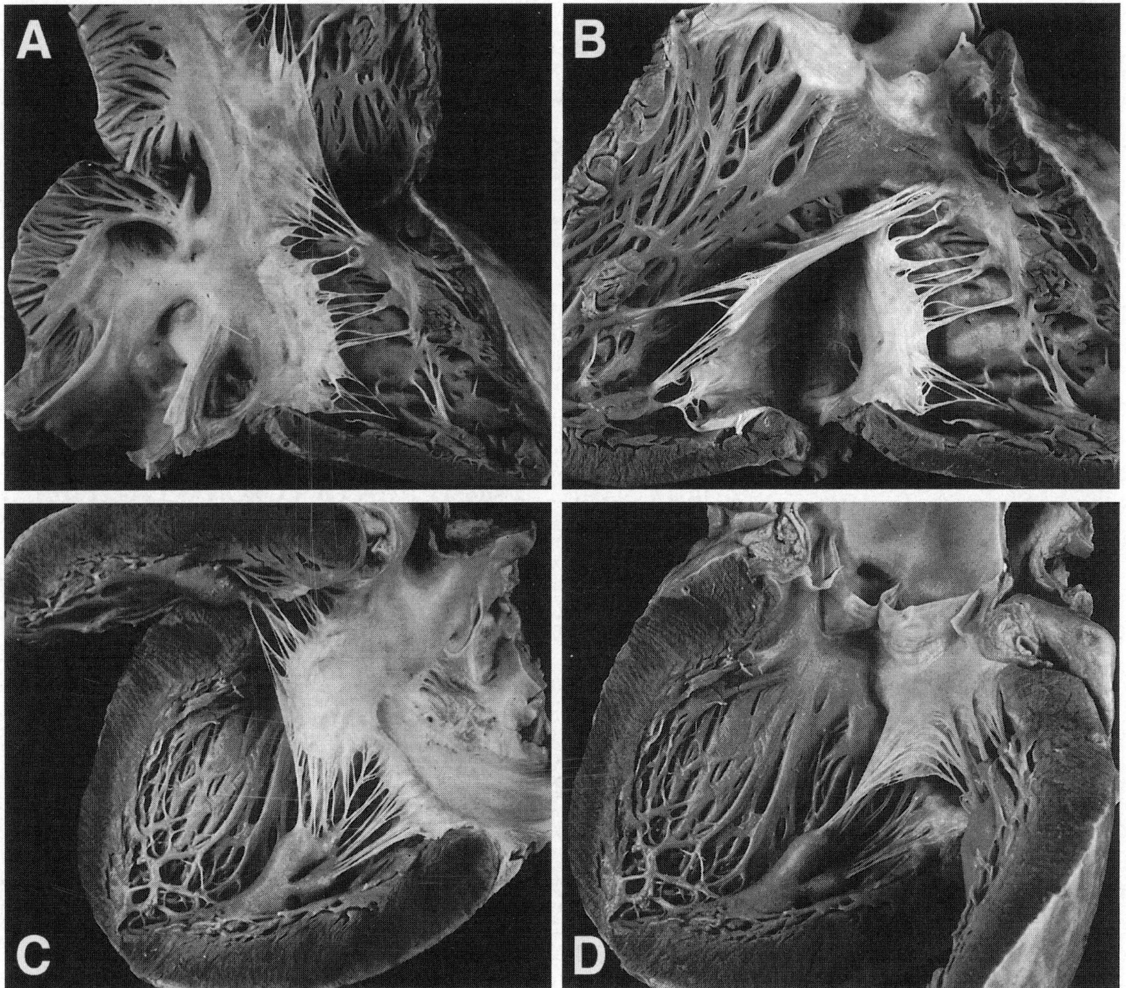

Fig. 3-1. Inflow-outflow method of cardiac dissection. The method is shown in a normal heart. (**A**) Opened right atrium and right ventricular inflow tract. (**B**) Opened right ventricular outflow tract and pulmonary artery. (**C**) Opened left atrium and left ventricular inflow tract. (**D**) Opened left ventricular outflow tract and aorta.

the anterior ventricular septum, extending through the anterior pulmonary cusp and into the main pulmonary artery.

The left atrium is opened with scissors between the right and left upper pulmonary veins and then between the upper and lower veins on each side. The incision can be extended into the left atrial appendage to assess for mural thrombus. The left ventricular inflow tract is opened with a long knife along the inferolateral aspect through the left atrial wall near its appendage, through the midportion of the posterior mitral leaflet, between the two mitral papillary muscles, and through the apex. The outflow cut travels parallel to the anterior ventricular septum and about 1 cm from it. This curved cut is best accomplished with a scalpel; care should be taken not to cut into either the anterior mitral leaflet or the ventricular septum. Scissors can be used to extend the cut across the left aortic cusp and into the ascending aorta, to one side or the other of the left coronary ostium. Further slicing into the myocardium is not recommended.

SHORT-AXIS METHOD OF CARDIAC DISSECTION This is the method of choice not only for the evaluation of ischemic heart disease *(2,5,15)* but for virtually any other cardiac condition, because the slices expose the largest surface area of myocardium. They correspond to the short-axis plane produced clinically by two-dimensional echocardiography *(8–14)*.

For this method, the flat diaphragmatic aspect of the heart is placed on a paper towel to prevent slippage, and cuts 1.0–1.5 cm thick are made with a sharp knife, parallel to the atrioventricular groove. One firm slice should be used, or two slices in the same direction, avoiding sawing motions that leave hesitation marks. Each slice is viewed from the apex toward the base (Fig. 3-2), analogous to echocardiographic imaging. The basal third of the ventricles is left attached to the atria. The basal portion is then opened according to the inflow-outflow method, as described earlier.

OTHER TOMOGRAPHIC METHODS OF DISSECTION AND REPAIRING MISTAKES For teaching purposes, the

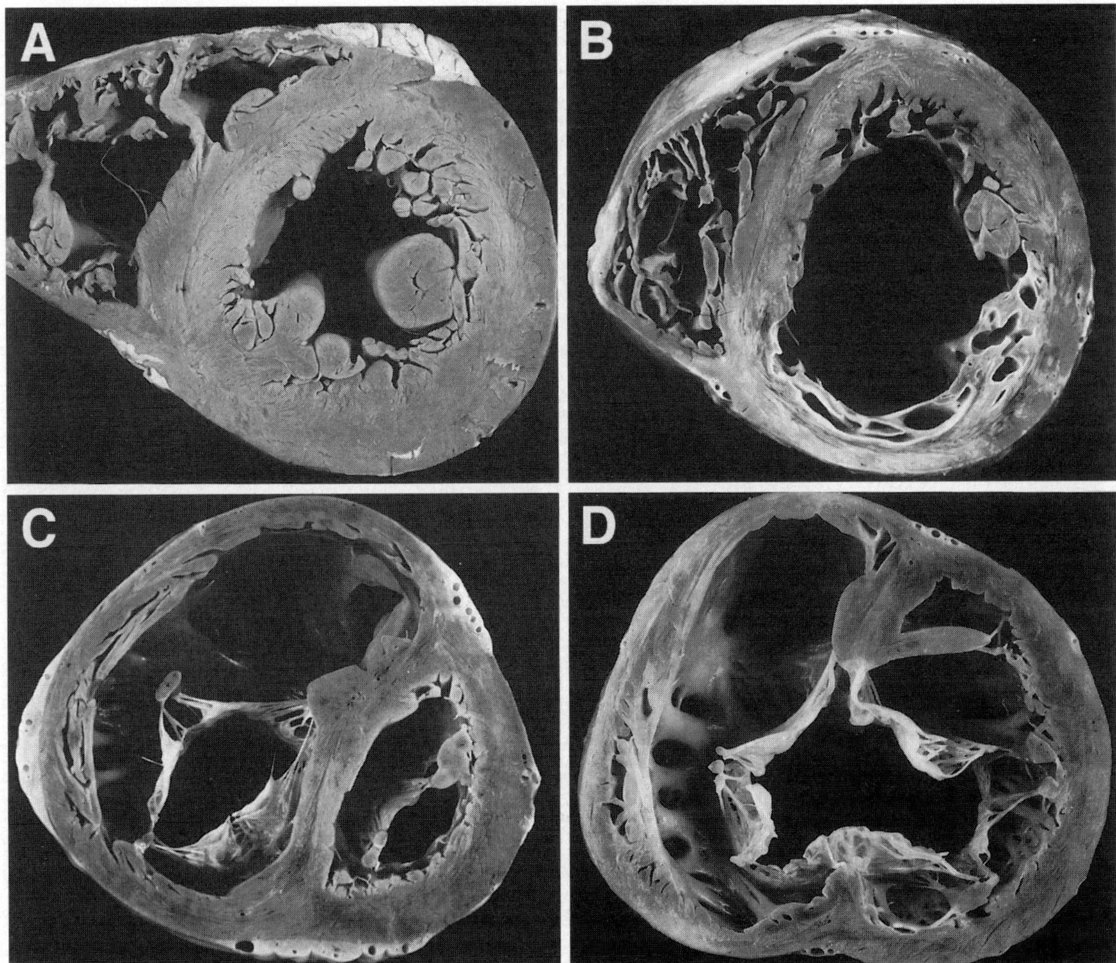

Fig. 3-2. Short-axis method of cardiac dissection. (**A**) Normal heart, with ventricular cross-section oriented for evaluation. (**B**) Old transmural myocardial infarct, involving inferior wall of left ventricle, with secondary left ventricular dilation. (**C**) Right ventricular hypertrophy and dilation due to chronic pulmonary hypertension. (**D**) Complete atrioventricular septal defect, showing the common atrioventricular valve.

short-axis, long-axis, and four-chamber planes are ideally suited for demonstrating cardiac pathology *(10,11)*. Additional planes that have proven useful clinically and at autopsy include right ventricular long axis, left-sided two-chamber, right-sided two-chamber, transverse (horizontal, or foreshortened four-chamber), frontal (or coronal), lateral (or parasagittal), and others. Hearts should first be fixed in a distended state, either by perfusion fixation (*see* Chapters 4 and 5) or by chamber distention with cotton or paper towels.

Repairing Mistakes If *mistakes* are made in attempting tomographic dissection, pieces can be glued back together and then recut in a more desirable plane of sectioning. For most purposes, any of the commercially available cyanoacrylate glues (such as Superglue® or Krazy Glue®) will suffice *(12,13)*.

Four-Chamber Method Using a long knife and beginning at the cardiac apex, a cut is extended through the acute margin of the right ventricle, the obtuse margin of the left ventricle, and the ventricular septum (Fig. 3-3). Cutting is then extended through the mitral and tricuspid valves and through the atria. This will divide the heart into two pieces, both of which show all four chambers. The upper half can then be opened along both ventricular outflow tracts, according to the inflow-outflow method previously described.

Long-Axis Method For this cut, the plane is best demarcated with three straight pins before making the cut. The first pin is placed in the cardiac apex, the second in the right aortic sinus (adjacent to the right coronary ostium), and the third near the mitral valve annulus, between the right and left pulmonary veins. The heart can then be cut along this plane, from the apex toward the base (or in the opposite direction), passing through both the mitral and aortic valves (Fig. 3-4).

Base of Heart Method This method displays all four valves intact at the cardiac base and thus is ideal for demonstrating anatomic relationships between the valves themselves and between the valves and the adjacent coronary arteries and the atrioventricular conduction system. The technique is best

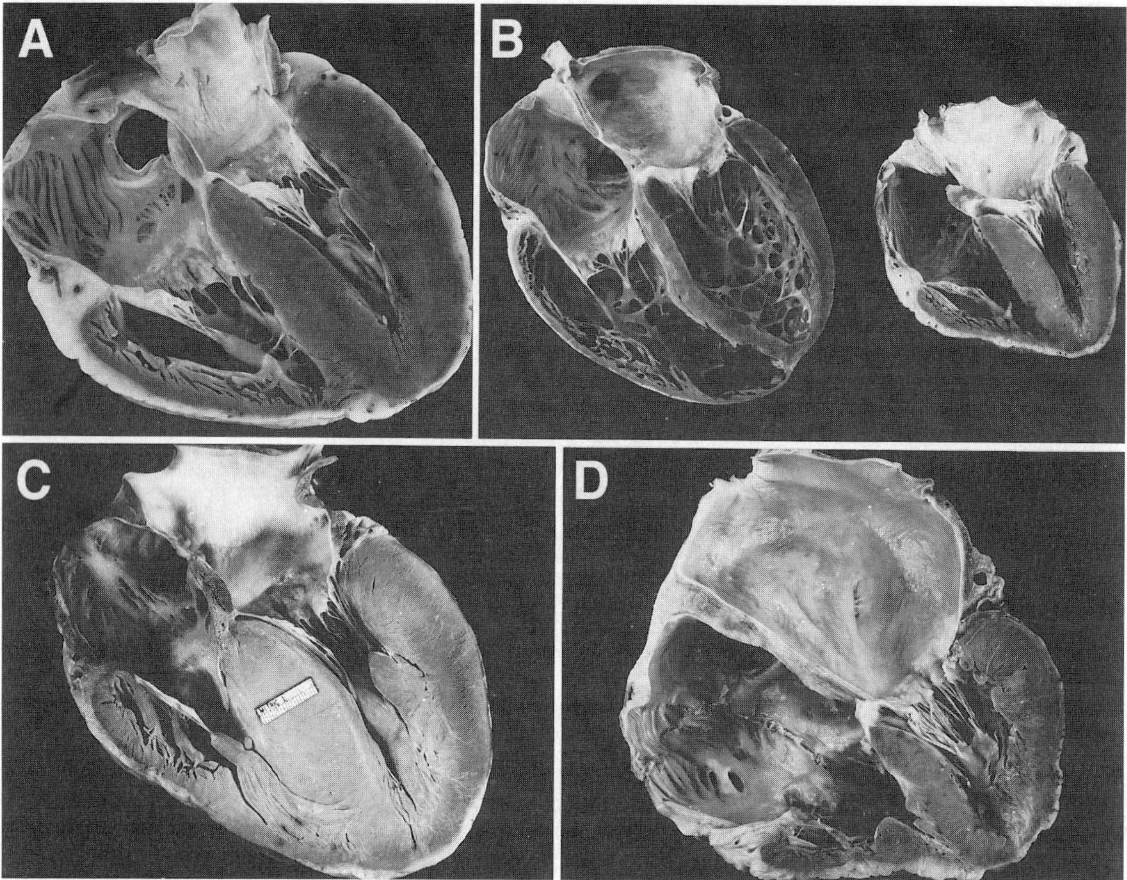

Fig. 3-3. Four-chamber method of cardiac dissection. (**A**) Normal heart, showing both atrioventricular valves and all four cardiac chambers. (**B**) Idiopathic dilated cardiomyopathy, with dilatation of all four chambers, compared with a normal heart (to the right). (**C**) Hypertrophic cardiomyopathy, with disproportionate ventricular septal hypertrophy. (**D**) Restrictive cardiomyopathy, with biatrial dilatation.

applied to hearts with prominent valvular disease, including prosthetic valves (Fig. 3-5) *(10,11)*.

The left anterior descending coronary artery can be evaluated before dissecting the base of the heart, but the right and circumflex arteries are best left uncut until afterward. The ventricles are sliced in the short-axis plane before the cardiac base is dissected, and slices can extend above the level of the tips of the mitral papillary muscles. With the cut surface of the ventricles placed on a paper towel, the atria are removed. Begin at the inferior vena cava with scissors and cut into the right atrium, staying about 0.5–1.0 cm above the tricuspid valve annulus. Cut only through the atrial free wall, taking care not to injure the adjacent right coronary artery. End the cut at the upper aspect of the atrial septum, adjacent to the ascending aorta.

For the left atrium, first locate the ostium of the coronary sinus, near the inferior vena cava, and cut in a retrograde fashion along the outer wall of the coronary sinus in the left atrioventricular groove. Then, use scissors or a scalpel to cut through both the inner wall of the coronary sinus and the adjacent left atrial free wall. This cut should extend from the lower aspect of the atrial septum to the level of the left atrial appendage. Continue the cut between the mitral valve annulus below and the appendage above, dissecting the left atrial wall away from the ascending aorta. At the upper border of the atrial septum, the left atrial cut should meet that from the right atrium. Cut through the atria septum, from its upper to lower aspects, and remove the two atria from the cardiac base.

Transsect the two great arteries along their sinotubular junctions, at the level of the valve commissures. After removing the ascending aorta and pulmonary artery, the arterial sinuses can be trimmed away with scissors to better demonstrate the two semilunar valves. The aortic valve is located centrally and abuts against the other three valves. After photographs have been taken, the right and circumflex coronary arteries can be evaluated for obstructions.

Window Method This method is useful for the preparation of dry cardiac museum specimens, using paraffin and other materials *(5,16,17)* or plastination, which is the currently favored method (*see* Chapter 15) *(18)*. Hearts should be perfusion-fixed, as described in Chapters 4 and 5. Windows of various sizes can be removed from the chambers or great vessels with a scalpel (Fig. 3-6). The blocks of tissue that are removed in this manner can be used for histologic study. Windows should initially be made small. Then, by looking inside the heart, one can determine how much to enlarge the opening to best demonstrate the lesion of interest.

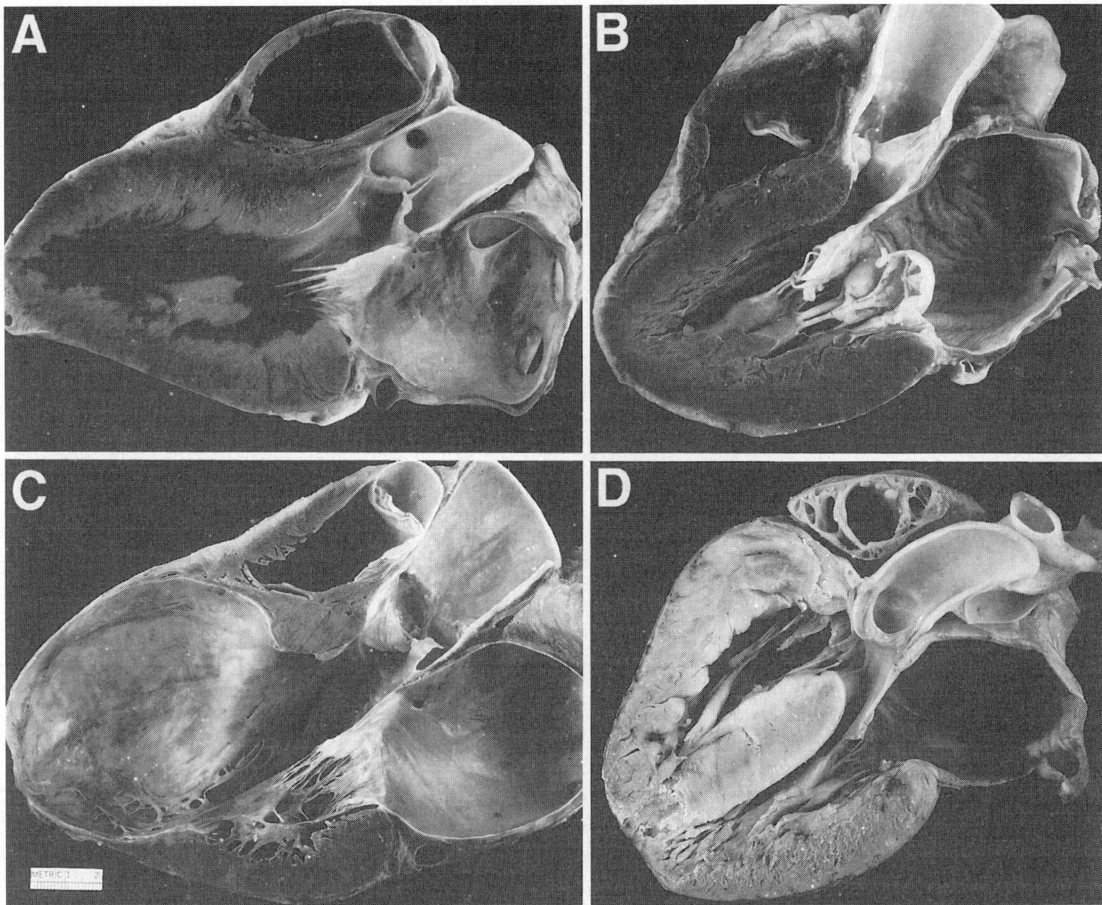

Fig. 3-4. Left ventricular long-axis method of cardiac dissection. (**A**) Normal heart, showing left ventricular inflow and outflow tracts, left atrium, ascending aorta, and right ventricular outflow tract. (**B**) Myxomatous mitral regurgitation, with prolapse of the posterior leaflet. (**C**) Old transmural myocardial infarct, with a large apical anteroseptal aneurysm. (**D**) Membranous ventricular septal defect.

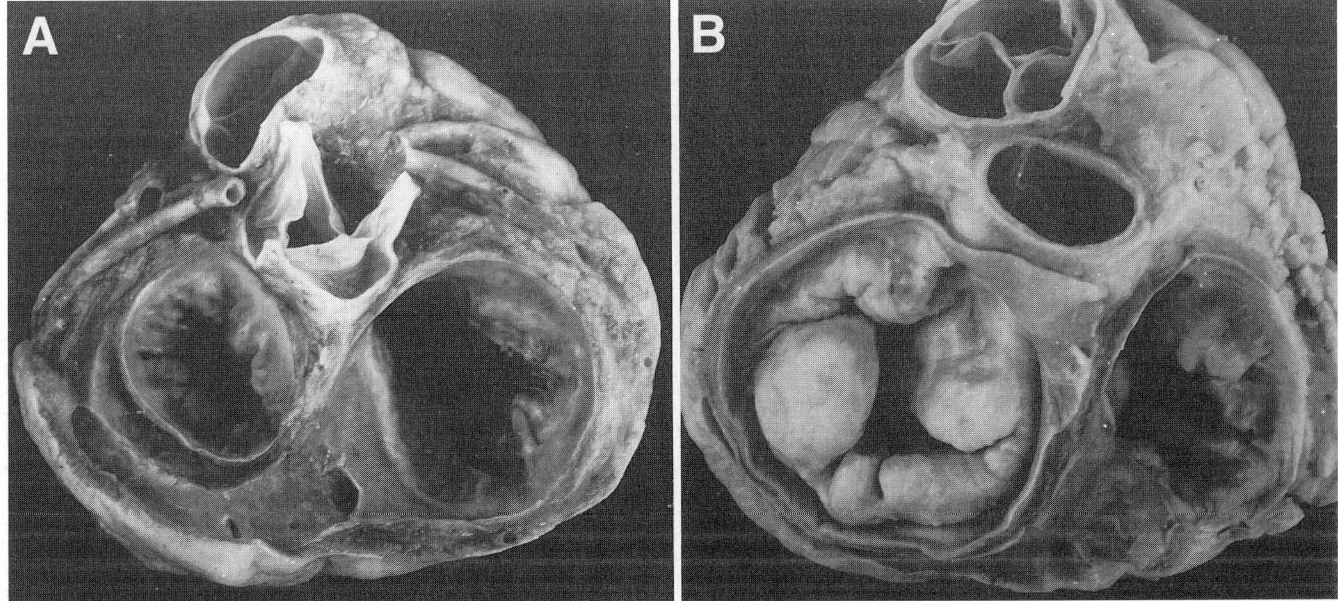

Fig. 3-5. Base-of-heart method of cardiac dissection. (**A**) Normal heart. (**B**) Myxomatous mitral valve disease.

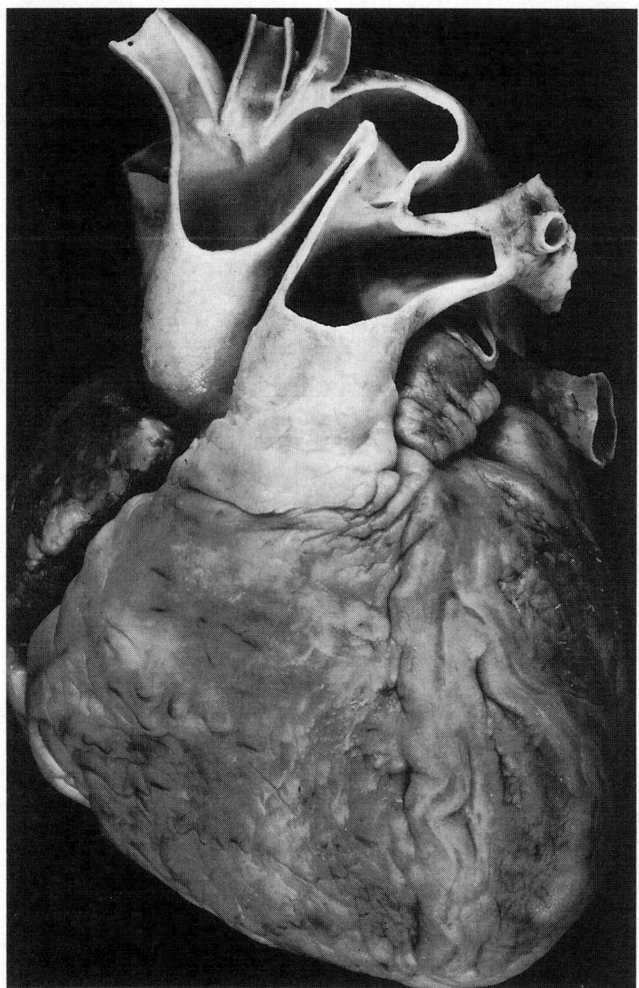

Fig. 3-6. Window method of cardiac dissection. Window in the great arteries, showing a widely patent ductal artery.

Unrolling Method This technique can be used to demonstrate opacified epicardial arteries in a single plane. Following postmortem coronary angiography, the ventricular septum and free walls are unrolled by one of three techniques *(7)*. The method of Rodriguez and Rainer *(19)* is the simplest and is best accomplished on fresh hearts. All unrolling techniques cause considerable mutilation of the heart and should be reserved for research studies.

Partition Method Partitioning techniques are used to weigh each ventricle separately for detailed assessment of ventricular hypertrophy *(6,7,20)*. Because these techniques also mutilate the specimen, it is recommended to first evaluate the heart diagnostically by the short-axis method, as described earlier. Partitioning begins with the stripping of epicardial fat and coronary vasculature from the specimen. Next the atria and great arteries are removed. Excision of the valves is optional. Finally, the ventricular free walls are separated from the ventricular septum. The weight of each cardiac segment can now be compared to tables of normal values *(6,7)*.

Injection-Corrosion Method Plastic or latex is injected into the coronary vasculature or into the cardiac chambers and great vessels *(5,7,21–24)*. Casts made from silicon rubber are resilient and nonadhesive and can therefore be extracted from the coronary arteries or cardiac chambers without resorting to corrosion of the specimen *(23)*. For further details on injection-corrosion methods, *see* Chapter 15.

Dissection of the Cardiac Conduction System *In situ* demonstration of the glycogen-rich left bundle branch with Lugol's iodine solution is possible but only within 90 min after death *(5)*. The atrioventricular (AV) bundle and proximal portion of the right bundle lie too deep to be shown by this technique. However, the AV node, AV (His) bundle, and right bundle branch can be observed by gross dissection *(5,25,26)* although the procedure is of no practical diagnostic value. The sinus node cannot be identified in this manner.

Many descriptions exist of the microscopic evaluation of the conduction system in normal and abnormal hearts *(2,5,6, 25,26)*. In practice, such an examination is rarely necessary, except for cases of nontraumatic death in which toxicologic studies are negative and no anatomic cause of death can be found. Another example is complete heart block. In such cases, the sinus node and the atrioventricular conduction tissues should be evaluated microscopically.

To remove a block of tissue that consistently contains the sinus node, the first cut should be made with scissors just anterior to the terminal crest, cutting through the numerous pectinate muscles (Fig. 3-7). This cut should extend to the upper border of the right atrial appendage. The second cut, perpendicular to the first, courses along this upper border and into the superior vena cava. The third cut, roughly perpendicular to the second and parallel to the first, travels along the right atrial wall, where it joins the atrial septum, and is directed from the superior vena cava toward the inferior vena cava. This cut should be about 2 cm long. The fourth cut completes the rectangular shape of the tissue block.

From this block, 6–8 sections are made with a scalpel, parallel to the second and fourth cuts. This cuts the sinus node artery, which usually can be seen grossly, in cross section. All sections can usually be submitted in 2 or 3 (consecutively labeled) cassettes. Because the node contains substantially more collagen than the adjacent myocardium, a trichrome or Verhoff-van Gieson stain will aid in its identification. Between the ages of 10 and 90 yr, the percentage of collagen normally expected in the sinus node is approx the same as one's age *(25)*.

To remove a tissue block that consistently contains the AV conduction system, the dissection should commence from the right side of the heart. The AV node is located just above the tricuspid valve annulus, between the coronary sinus ostium and the membranous septum, within the triangle of Koch. First, orient the heart with the right-sided chambers opened such that the right atrium is positioned above and the right ventricle below (Fig. 3-8). Using a scalpel, remove a rectangular block of tissue, approx 2.0 cm in height, that extends laterally from the coronary sinus ostium to the far right side of the membranous septum. Within the tissue block, the tricuspid annulus should

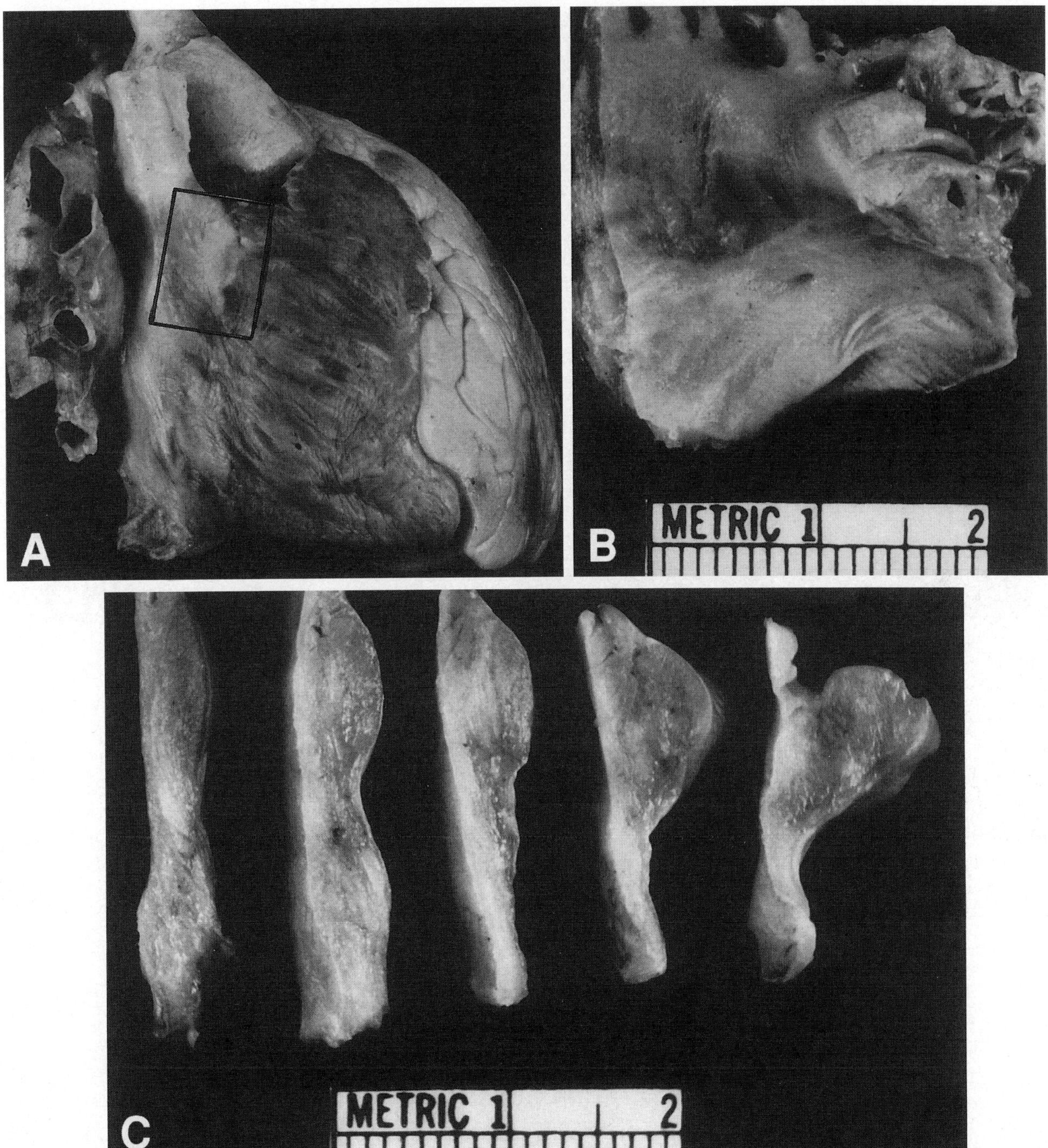

Fig. 3-7. Dissection of the sinus node for microscopy. (**A**) Right lateral view of the right atrium, showing the rectangular region (black lines) to be removed. (**B**) Excised tissue block, showing the endocardial aspect. (**C**) Sections cut for microscopy.

be skewed upward, such that about 1.5 cm of *atrial* septum is included at the side near the coronary ostium and 1.5 cm of *ventricular* septum is present at the side of the membranous septum.

The excised tissue block will contain much of the septal tricuspid leaflet and portions of the mitral and aortic valves; only the pulmonary valve should remain uncut. Valves can be trimmed back to within 0.5 cm of their annuli. For right-handed cutting, rotate the specimen 180°, with the right atrium closer to the prosector than the right ventricle and the left-sided chambers against the cutting board. Using a scalpel, cut 6–10 sections about 3 mm thick, beginning at the side nearest to the coronary sinus ostium and progressing toward the side with the membranous septum. Place tissues, in that order, into cassettes labeled AV-1, AV-2, and so on. Depending on the thickness of the ventricular septum, each cassette may hold 1–3 specimens.

Generally, each paraffin block from the conduction system needs to be cut only at one level. Trichrome or Verhoff-van Gieson stains are most suitable to identify the conduction sys-

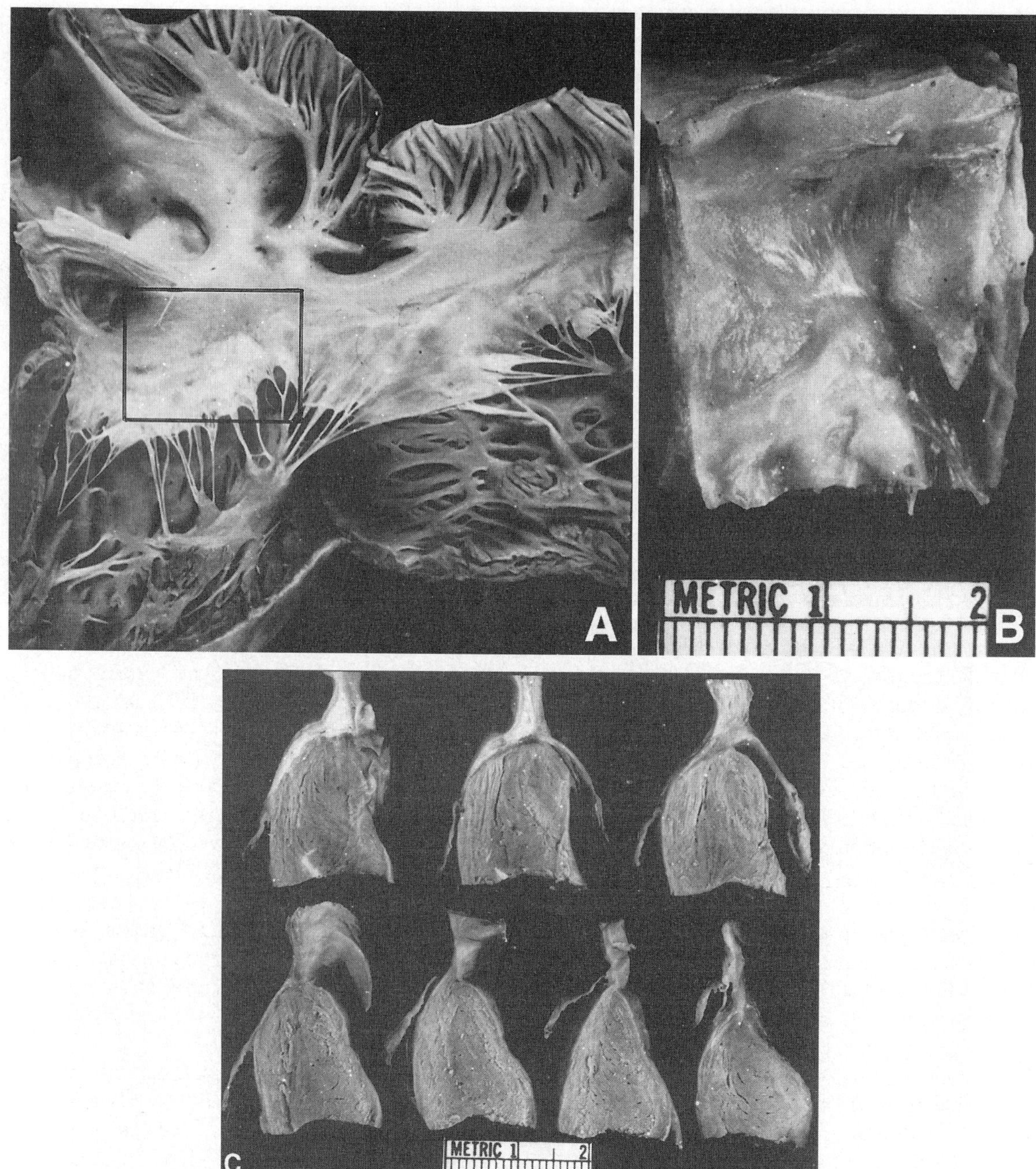

Fig. 3-8. Dissection of the atrioventricular (AV) conduction tissues for microscopy. (**A**) Opened right atrium (above) and right ventricle (below), showing the rectangular specimen (black lines) to be removed. (**B**) Excised tissue block, showing its right-sided aspect. (**C**) Sections cut for microscopy.

tem because it is insulated with collagen. In rare instances, such as iatrogenic injury to the conduction system, one or two blocks may be cut at several levels to better delineate the damage, but exhausting the block to make slides from every 10th to 40th section is indicated only for detailed research investigations.

Perfusion Fixation of the Heart The method is recommended for dissections that are to be used for teaching purposes, including both museum specimens and photographs *(10,11)*. In general, perfusion-fixation is indicated for the tomographic and window types of dissection, and several methods have been described *(27–29)*. Even without perfusion apparatus, hearts can be fixed in an apparent distended state by filling the chambers and vessels with cotton *(30)*. For more detailed descriptions of perfusion fixation techniques, *see* Chapters 4 and 5.

QUANTITATIVE MEASUREMENTS OF THE HEART

HEART WEIGHT *Total heart weight is the most reliable single measurement at autopsy for correlation with cardiac disease states (7)*. The assessment must take into account the size of the patient. Other described measurements such as linear external dimensions, surface areas, and volume of the entire heart or myocardium *(7)* are less useful than the total heart weight.

Hearts are weighed after the parietal pericardium has been removed, the great vessels have been trimmed to about 2 cm in length, and postmortem clots have been removed from the cardiac chambers. Weights are recorded to the nearest gram *(3,6)* (or at least to the nearest 5 g in adults). For subjects younger than 1 yr, scales should be used that weigh accurately to the nearest 0.1 g. Fixation may alter heart weight by 5–10% *(31, 32)*. Among the numerous available tables of normal values *(5–7,32–34)* the variation has generally been less than 10%.

Normal expected heart weights are related to age, gender, and body size *(32–34)* (*see* also Part III of this book). Normal heart weight usually correlates better with body weight than with age or height *(33,34)*. In some settings, for instance if patients received massive fluid therapy for shock or had a recent amputation, expected heart weight should be based on height or on the body weight before fluid therapy or amputation.

CARDIAC WALL THICKNESS Left ventricular thickness has usually been measured 1–2 cm below the mitral annulus *(5)*, but because wall thickness is greatest at the base and least at the apex, the most reliable average measurement is found at the level of the papillary muscles. The ventricular septum and the right ventricle should be measured at the same level. All three values can readily be attained from hearts dissected by the short-axis method. Trabeculations and papillary muscles should not be included in the measurements. Fixation may increase left ventricular wall thickness by 10% *(31)*. Right ventricular thickness is usually greater inferiorly than anteriorly. Normal values should only be compared to nondilated hearts (*see* Part III of this book) *(31,33,34)*.

With the rare exception of stone heart (intractable systolic contracture), the heart at death stops in asystole, not systole or diastole. Initially, the heart is flaccid *(7)* but within an hour, it begins to develop rigor mortis. Therefore, the left ventricular wall thickness and chamber dimensions generally resemble those in end-systole *(35)*. About 24 h after death, rigor mortis remits, left ventricular wall thickness decreases again, and the chambers dilate, a condition not to be confused with dilated cardiomyopathy.

CARDIAC CHAMBER SIZES After death, chamber sizes may change considerably because of rigor mortis (*see* above) or fixation (which *decreases* ventricular volumes by about 50%) or because of perfusion fixation (which may *increase* them appreciably) *(36)*. This makes the interpretation of chamber volumes difficult. From the internal long-axis length (L) and short-axis diameter (D), a formula ($\pi LD^2/6$) may be used to calculate left ventricular volume.

CARDIAC HYPERTROPHY AND DILATATION For nondilated hearts from adults who show rigor mortis, hypertrophy is generally present if left ventricular wall thickness exceeds 1.5 cm or if right ventricular wall thickness exceeds 0.5 cm *(7)*. For dilated hearts, however, these measurements are not reliable. Thus, total heart weight is the best gross indicator of cardiac hypertrophy, when compared to expected normal weight (*see* p. 568 in Part III of this book) *(37)*. For research studies, the partition method is recommended, with comparison to tables of normal values for each chamber *(6,7,20)*.

There is no gross or microscopic difference between physiologic hypertrophy of athletes and pathologic hypertrophy that results from disease states *(6)*. However, in athletes, the heart weight is rarely increased more than 25% above the expected value. Ischemic heart disease alone, without coexistent hypertension, generally produces only mild hypertrophy, affecting all four chambers, and a heart weight of <550 g *(38)*.

In chronic disorders such as systemic hypertension, aortic stenosis, dilated or hypertrophic cardiomyopathy, and congenital heart disease, the heart often weighs 2.0–2.5 times the expected value, or about 600–900 g in adults. Weights exceeding 1000 g may be found in hypertrophic cardiomyopathy, chronic aortic regurgitation, and acromegaly with hypertension. Isolated right ventricular hypertrophy due to pulmonary hypertension rarely produces a heart weight above 500 g.

Volume hypertrophy (avoid the potentially misleading term, eccentric hypertrophy *[37]*) of the left ventricle is always accompanied by chamber dilatation and secondary wall thinning. In hearts from adults of average size with rigor mortis, the short-axis internal dimension of the left ventricle is normally ≤2.5 cm. This measurement can be used to estimate the severity of left ventricular dilatation (*see* p. 570 in Part III of this book). The wall thickness of a *dilated* left ventricle cannot be used as an accurate indicator of hypertrophy *(37,39)*; instead, the overall heart weight is used for this purpose. The other three cardiac chambers are normally thin-walled; thus, hypertrophy and dilatation are not as readily quantitated as for the left ventricle, and pressure hypertrophy is often attended by substantial dilatation. All dilated chambers should be evaluated for mural thrombi, particularly within atrial appendages, ventricular apices, and ventricular aneurysms.

CARDIAC VALVE SIZE Valve function is difficult to evaluate at autopsy *(6)*. Regurgitation can be assessed to some extent by filling the chambers with water to check for retrograde flow through the intact valve. Stenosis is best evaluated by measuring the effective orifice size.

For intact hearts, valve *diameters* can be measured with a ruler or a calibrated cone (Fig. 3-9A) *(32)*. A cone will distort the elliptical orifices of the mitral and tricuspid valves, producing minor inaccuracies. In stenotic valves, cones measure orifice size rather than annular size.

Most pathologists measure valve *circumferences* (rather than diameters) along the annulus of the atrioventricular valves and at the arterial sinotubular junction of the semilunar valves. Measurements should be to the nearest 0.1 cm. Standard fixation may decrease valvular circumferences by 10–25% *(31)*, whereas perfusion fixation generally increases the measurements, particularly for the right-sided valves. For a given body size, women have slightly larger valves than men *(34)*. Valve circumferences, particularly those of the semilunar valves, progressively dilate during adult life *(34,40)*. The thickness and area of leaflets and cusps also increase with age. For normal values and their interpretation, and for further references, *see* Part III of this book *(32–34,40)*.

PATENCY OF THE FORAMEN OVALE Postnatally, the foramen ovale closes either anatomically or only functionally,

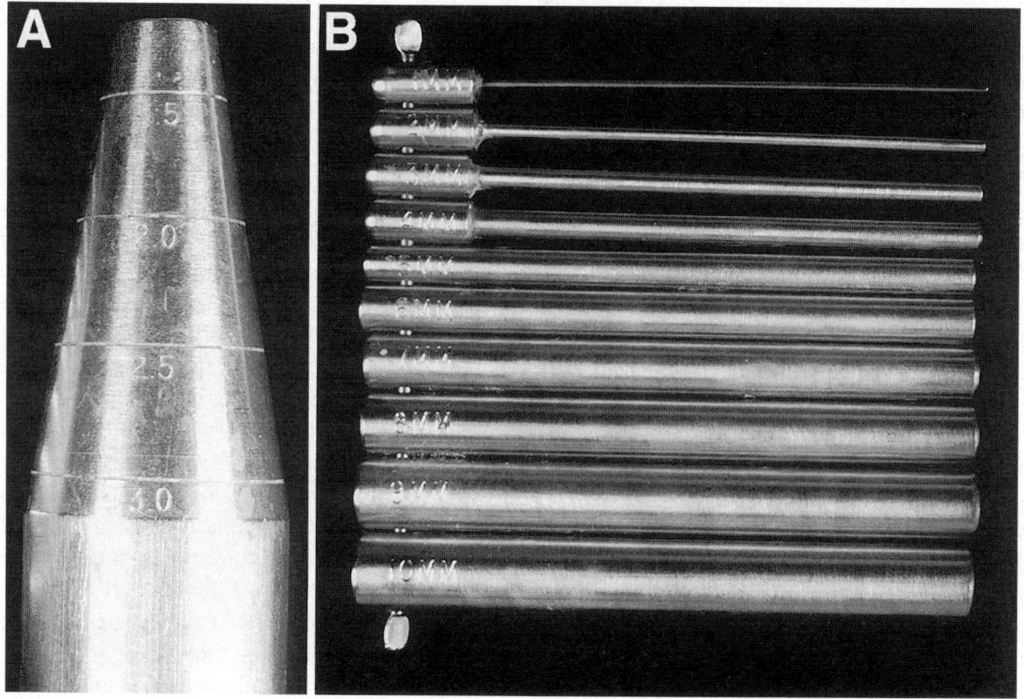

Fig. 3-9. Calibrated measuring devices. (**A**) Metal cone, with markings for diameters ranging from 1.0–3.0 cm. (**B**) Metal probes, ranging from 1–10 mm in diameter.

as a flap-valve. A patent foramen ovale may later serve as an avenue of paradoxical embolization and, therefore, its presence should be recorded. If an interatrial passageway is present, a probe can be passed from the right atrium between the valve and limb of the fossa ovalis, or from the left atrium from the ostium secundum. The maximum potential diameter of the foramen ovale is best established using graduated probes (Fig. 3-9B). For normal values *(41)*, *see* Part III of this book.

STANDARD GROSS AND MICROSCOPIC EXAMINATION

Many suggestions have been made for sections to be taken for microscopic examination *(3,42)*; most current policies are determined by the clinical history, the gross findings, special interests of the prosector *(7)*, and cost restraints.

GENERAL RECOMMENDATIONS For operated hearts and cases with a cardiac cause of death, a photograph of the heart should be taken before its dissection is begun. Preferably, the heart should be fixed in formalin for at least 5 min (to dull the surface) and then oriented as it is normally positioned in the chest. If it is dissected by the short-axis method, at least one photograph of the largest slice should be obtained, with the specimen viewed from the apex toward the base and with a short ruler (*see* Fig. 3-2).

For autopsy cases with a noncardiac cause of death and a grossly normal heart, no histologic slides may be needed or only a single section from the left ventricle, preferably including one of the papillary muscles. All microscopic samples should be transmural, about 1.5 cm wide and 0.3 cm thick. Rectangular sections are preferred because they contain more subendocardial tissue, where ischemic injury most commonly occurs. Specimens should be labeled in detail according to their location (Fig. 3-10).

Coronary arteries and valves should be stained with Verhoff-van Gieson. For conduction tissues, a trichrome stain is optional. Routine stains suffice for most other cardiac sections. In the first week after open heart surgery, low-output failure without an obvious morphologic cause, either grossly or microscopically, is common *(43)*.

ISCHEMIC HEART DISEASE Coronary artery disease, ischemic myocardial changes, and, in some cases, the effects of surgical and nonsurgical interventions must be evaluated *(2,15, 44,45)*. Postmortem coronary angiography is optional; perfusion fixation is only necessary in research studies. The arteries are cut in cross sections at 3–5 mm intervals. Heavily calcified vessels should be removed and decalcified prior to sectioning. Microscopy may be performed to document chronic grade-4 obstructions and acute lesions such as plaque rupture and thrombosis (Table 3-1).

Segments with nonsurgical interventions such as percutaneous transluminal coronary angioplasty (PTCA), stent placement, or atherectomy may also be evaluated microscopically. For bypass grafts, sections should include the most obstructed areas of the graft body, coronary anastomosis, and distal coronary artery (Fig. 3-11). In most cases, all sections from one graft can be placed into one cassette (*see* Appendix 3-1). At the anastomosis, the coronary artery should be cut in cross-section, regardless of the angle of the graft.

Hearts should be dissected by the short-axis method (*see* Fig. 3-2B) *(7,11,42,46,47)*. Only for teaching purposes are

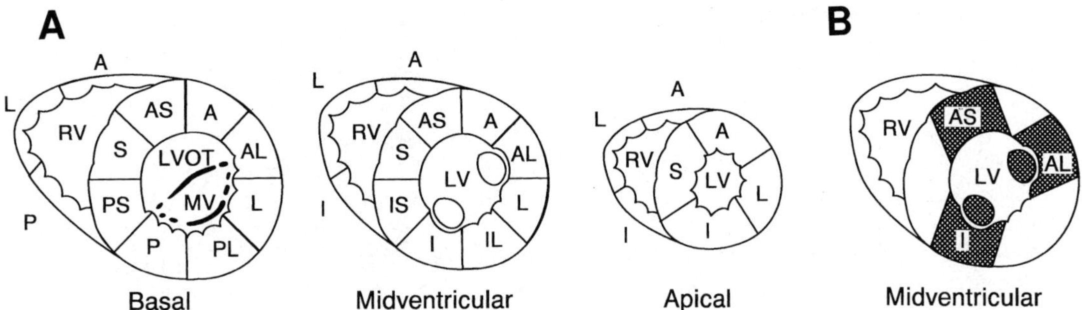

Fig. 3-10. Schematic diagram of the left (LV) and right (RV) ventricular regions. (**A**) Abbreviations for ventricular regions. (**B**) Three standard sections for microscopic evaluation. (A, anterior; AL, anterolateral; AS, anteroseptal; I, inferior; IL, inferolateral; IS, inferoseptal; L, lateral; P, posterior; PL, posterolateral; PS, posteroseptal; S, septal.)

Table 3-1
Correlation Between Clinical Manifestation of Coronary Artery Disease and Pathologic Features of Atherosclerotic Plaques[a]

Clinical state	*Microscopic features of coronary atherosclerosis*
Asymptomatic	Stable plaques, grades 1–3; occasionally, grade 4 stable plaques (generally one-vessel disease).
Angina pectoris	
Chronic stable (exertional)	Stable grade 4 plaques (usually two-vessel or three-vessel disease).
Variant (Prinzmetal's)	Stable plaques, of any grade; evidence of plaque progression; occasionally an unstable atheroma.
Microvascular (syndrome X)	No significant disease of epicardial coronary arteries; medial and intimal thickening of intramural arteries; swollen capillary endothelial cells.
Unstable (preinfarction)	Unstable plaque, of any grade, with rupture and acute nonocclusive platelet-rich thrombus; also stable grade 4 plaques (usually three-vessel disease).
Myocardial infarction (MI)	
Acute myocardial ischemia[b]	Unstable plaque, of any grade, with rupture and acute thrombus, either nonocclusive or occlusive; often associated with other stable grade 4 plaques.
Acute subendocardial MI	Same as for unstable angina.
Acute transmural MI	Unstable plaque, of any grade, with rupture and acute occlusive fibrin-rich thrombus; also stable grade 4 plaques (usually two-vessel or three-vessel disease).
Chronic myocardial ischemia[c]	Stable grade 4 plaques (usually two-vessel or three-vessel disease).
Old healed MI (scars > 1 cm)	Stable grade 4 plaques (usually two-vessel or three-vessel disease); old organized thrombus, especially with transmural infarcts.
Chronic heart failure	Stable grade 4 plaques (usually two-vessel or three-vessel disease); old organized thrombus; evidence of plaque progression.
Sudden death	Unstable plaques, of any grade, with rupture and acute thrombus, either nonocclusive or occlusive; associated with other stable grade 4 plaques (two-vessel or three-vessel disease in 80%, one-vessel disease in 15%, and four-vessel disease in 5%).

[a]Represents autopsied cases only (a source of bias). *See* the section on "Evaluation of Coronary Arteries" for a description of the grades of obstruction. Unstable plaques are characterized by a thin fibrous cap, a large lipid-rich core, subendothelial clusters of monocytes or foam cells, atherophagocytosis, or adventitial or intimal lymphocytes.

[b]Characterized microscopically by contraction band necrosis or by nuclear pyknosis and intense sarcoplasmic staining with eosin, occurring in the absence of an infiltrate of neutrophils or, with reperfusion, macrophages. These features generally represent preinfarction changes in which the patient died before leukocytic infiltration occurred.

[c]Characterized microscopically by patchy subendocardial collections of vacuolated myocytes or by small (<1 cm) subendocardial patches of fibrosis or granulation tissue.

Adapted from Edwards *(15)*.

other methods recommended (*see* Fig. 3-4C). Grossly, both old and acute infarcts should be described in terms of extent (transmural or subendocardial), location (anteroseptal, inferior, or lateral), and level (apical, midventricular, or basal).

For the macroscopic demonstration of acute myocardial ischemia, various dyes have been used, the most popular of which have been nitro-blue tetrazolium (NBT) and triphenyl tetrazolium chloride (TTC) *(46–49)*. Nevertheless, the best and least expensive method, within 4 h after injury, is a slide well-stained with hematoxylin-eosin. The microscopic features of acute and chronic myocardial ischemia *(50–53)* and of acute myocardial infarction of various ages (Table 3-2) *(54–56)*, have

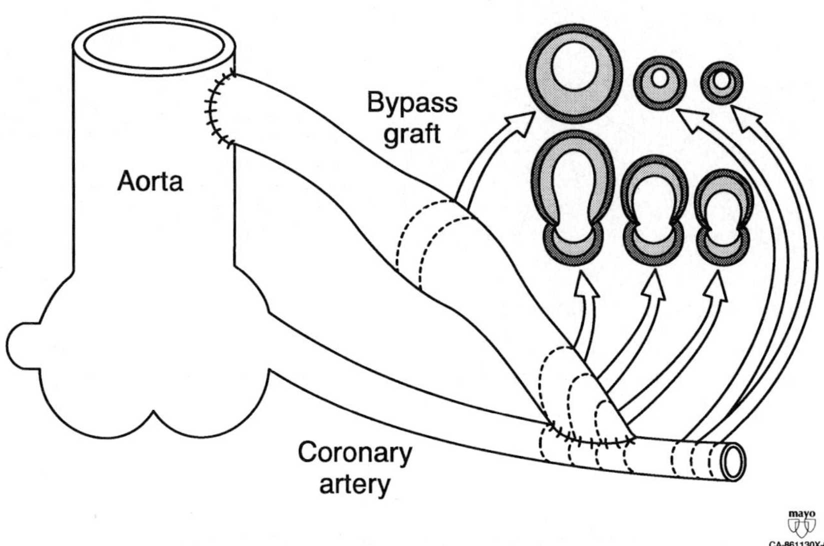

Fig. 3-11. Schematic diagram of a coronary artery bypass graft and the recommended sites for microscopic evaluation.

Table 3-2
Age-Related Features of Myocardial Infarction

Age	*Gross features*	*Light microscopy*
<4 h	No change.	No change.
4–12 h	Slight mottling, with areas of dark discoloration.	Intense sacroplasmic eosinophilia and nuclear pyknosis; contraction bands (with reperfusion).
12–24 h	Mottled and mildly edematous, with bulging cut surface.	As above, with early interstitial edema and neutrophilic infiltrates.
2–4 d	Soft yellow-tan core with mottled border.	Maximum neutrophilic infiltrate; nuclear loss and sarcoplasmic coagulation.
5–7 d	Yellow-tan core and irregular hyperemic red-brown border.	Basophilic interstitial debris; early macrophage infiltration; dilated capillaries at border.
8–10 d	Yellow-gray core and red-brown border; depressed cut surface.	Numerous macrophages, with active phagocytosis; pigmented macrophages filled with lipofuscin.
11–14 d	Yellow-gray core and red-gray border; depressed cut surface.	Granulation tissue along border; ongoing phagocytosis at core.
2–4 wk	Core becoming smaller; border becoming larger, grayer, firmer, and less gelatinous; less depressed cut surface.	Ongoing scar formation, dense at outer border; chronic inflammation; dilated peripheral small vessels; central core of necrotic tissue.
>1 mo	Firm gray-white or red-gray scar, with scar retraction and variable wall thinning.	Mature scar (dense collagen, focal elastin, and hypercellularity); focal lymphocyte.

Adapted from Edwards *(15)*.

been described, although reperfusion alters the pattern *(15,57, 58)*. All current methods of detecting early myocardial infarctions have recently been reviewed *(52)*.

If ischemic heart disease is suspected as the cause of death, at least three histologic sections should be taken at the midventricular level and include the anteroseptal, anterolateral, and inferior walls, with both mitral papillary muscles. If mottled or obviously infarcted areas are identified grossly, these should also be evaluated. Sections from inferoseptal infarcts should also include the inferior wall of the *right* ventricle.

VALVULAR HEART DISEASE For cases of suspected endocarditis, vegetations can be cultured as described in Chapter 9. Other disorders of native or prosthetic valves are best demonstrated using a combination of the short-axis and base-of-heart methods of dissection (*see* Fig. 3-5B). For aortic and mitral valve disease, the left ventricular long-axis approach can also be used (*see* Fig. 3-4B). For the distinguishing features of various prosthetic valves, *see* Table 3-3 *(59–62)*.

For microscopic examination of infected valves, large or multiple sections should be taken to increase the likelihood of detecting organisms. After treatment with antibiotics, a Grocott methenamine silver stain may better demonstrate dead bacteria in the vegetations than a Gram stain.

Left-sided valve disease may be associated with myocardial ischemia, due to inadequate coronary perfusion, coronary obstruction from embolic valvular vegetations, or injury to a coronary

Table 3-3
Types of Prosthetic Heart Valves Likely to Be Encountered at Autopsy

Mechanical	*Bioprosthetic*
Bileaflet	Porcine Aortic Valve
CarboMedics	Carpentier-Edwards
St. Jude	Hancock
Tilting Disk	Bovine Pericardial Valve
Bjork-Shiley	Carpentier-Edwards
Lillehei-Kaster	Ionecu-Shiley
Medtronic-Hall	Cadaveric Homograft Valve
Omniscience	CryoLife
Sorin	Red Cross
Caged Ball	Autograft
Starr-Edwards	Ross Procedure[a]

[a]Involves using the patient's own pulmonary valve in the aortic position.

Table 3-4
Modified Heath-Edwards Classification of Plexogenic Pulmonary Hypertension in Congenital Cardiac Left-to-Right Shunts

Grade	*Lesion*	*Reversible*
1A	Muscularization of arterioles	Yes
1B	Medial hypertrophy of arteries	Yes
1C	Loss of intra-acinar arteries	Yes
2	Concentric intimal proliferation	Borderline
3	Concentric laminal intimal fibrosis	Borderline
4[a]	Plexiform lesions	No
5	Dilatation (angiomatoid) lesions	No
6	Fibrinoid degeneration of arteries	No
6	Necrotizing arteritis	No

[a]Grade 4 plexiform lesions are now thought to represent the aftermath of necrotizing arteritis and microaneurysm formation and, hence, follow rather than precede grade 5 and 6 lesions.

Adapted with permission from Edwards *(63)*.

artery during valve surgery. Accordingly, the myocardial sections recommended for cases of valvular heart disease are the same as those for ischemic heart disease, particularly if there is a valvular vegetation, valvular prosthesis, or history of sudden death.

Additional recommendations for specific valvular lesions are listed in Part II of this book.

CARDIOMYOPATHIES For most cases of dilated cardiomyopathy, arrhythmogenic right ventricular cardiomyopathy, and hypertrophic cardiomyopathy, the heart should be dissected by the short-axis method. In contrast, the four chamber method is ideal for demonstrating biatrial dilatation in the eosinophilic and noneosinophilic forms of restrictive cardiomyopathy. Occasionally, it can also be used for dilated or hypertrophic cardiomyopathy (*see* Fig. 3-3B,C). The long-axis method of dissection is useful for demonstrating the anatomic substrate for left ventricular outflow tract obstruction in some patients with hypertrophic cardiomyopathy.

The heart from any adult with suspected cardiomyopathy should be evaluated for coexistent coronary atherosclerosis. For dilated cardiomyopathy in adults, an iron stain is recommended for the evaluation of possible hemochromatosis, and an amyloid stain is suggested for cases with suspected hypertrophic cardiomyopathy. (For macroscopic staining methods, *see* Chapter 14.) Diffusely vacuolated myocytes may be indicative of an underlying storage disease, such as Fabry's disease; transmission electron microscopy is indicated in such cases.

Additional recommendations for specific types of cardiomyopathy are listed in Part II of this book.

CONGENITAL HEART DISEASE The evaluation should include study of the underlying malformation, its secondary effects on the heart and lungs, and review of diagnostic or therapeutic procedures and their effects or complications *(63)*. Chronic lesions such as aortic root dilatation (with conotruncal anomalies) or myxomatous valves (with single functional ventricles), in operated patients who have survived into adulthood, may also be encountered at autopsy.

Detailed descriptions of the specific forms of congenital heart disease can be found in Part II of this book. Synonyms abound for cardiovascular anomalies, and these are listed in Appendix 3-2, as well as with each individual malformation in Part II. For cardiac anatomy and for congenital cardiac anomalies, Anglicized terms rather than Latin names are currently preferred, and these are listed in Appendix 3-3. Common eponyms for various surgical procedures applied to malformed hearts, and their explanations are supplied in Appendix 3-4. In Appendix 3-5, a two-page form is provided that can be used during the autopsy evaluation of complex cases of congenital heart disease *(63–65)*.

In general, the thoracic organs should be removed en bloc but if the vascular connections are normal, the tracheobronchial tree, lungs, and esophagus can be removed from the heart. Section from the upper and lower lobes of both lungs should be evaluated for pneumonia and hypertensive pulmonary vascular disease. Note that the modified Heath-Edwards classification of plexogenic pulmonary hypertension is applicable only for subjects with congenital left-to-right shunts (*see* Table 3-4). In operated patients, the lesions of pulmonary venous hypertension are more common than plexogenic disease.

The major epicardial coronary arteries should be examined for anomalies in origin and distribution and for obstruction, especially if operative procedures have been performed nearby. Cardiomegaly is a common feature; even years after surgical repair of congenital heart disease, residual ventricular hypertrophy and dilatation may be striking. Asymmetric septal hypertrophy in conotruncal anomalies should not be misinterpreted as coexistent hypertrophic cardiomyopathy.

Congenitally malformed hearts may be opened by the inflow-outflow method but in postoperative cases, the short-axis method is best (*see* Fig. 3-2D). In selected circumstances (*see* Fig. 3-4D and 3-6), the four-chamber, long-axis, base-of-heart, and window methods are also useful *(10)*. In general, microscopic sections should be taken from both ventricles for the evaluation of fibrosis and recent ischemic injury, particularly in the subendocardial region of hypertrophied hearts.

UNEXPLAINED SUDDEN DEATH The coronary arteries should be examined carefully throughout their length, to document any anomalies or obstructions, including ostial flaps. Hearts with appreciable ischemic, valvular, cardiomyopathic, or congenital lesions should be dissected as described earlier.

If the heart appears grossly normal, at least four slides should be taken for microscopy from the left ventricle, and two from the right ventricle. If no myocarditis or acute myocardial ischemia is detected microscopically, the cardiac condution system should be evaluated as described earlier in this chapter. Though rare, mesothelioma of the AV node or sarcoidosis of the AV node or AV (His) bundle may cause sudden death. In some fatal arrhythmic disorders, such as the long QT syndrome, the heart may be normal grossly and microscopically *(66)*. This syndrome has been implicated in some incidents of drowning and near drowning *(67)*. *See* also under "Death, sudden unexpected, ..." in Part II of this book.

EVALUATION OF THE VASCULATURE

Examination of coronary arteries was described earlier in this chapter. For the study of vessels in other organs, see the appropriate chapter. Microscopic evaluation of vascular diseases should include a Verhoff-van Gieson stain.

AORTA AND OTHER MAJOR ARTERIES In general, the thoracic and abdominal portions of the aorta are opened posteriorly, between the origins of the right and left intercostal and lumbar arteries. In cases of congenital heart disease, the thoracic aorta is left attached to the heart. If an acute aortic dissection is suspected, the heart and the entire aorta should be removed intact; transsection of the ascending aorta may distort or destroy the intimal tear. For the evaluation of renovascular disease, the kidneys and renal arteries are best kept together with the abdominal aorta.

Measure all aneurysms in length and diameter. They may be dissected either longitudinally or by cross-section, noting the amount of mural thrombus and the size of the residual lumen. Rupture sites should be studied microscopically for any underlying disease processes. Most forms of obstructive arterial disease are best evaluated by cross-section, but in fibromuscular dysplasia, longitudinal sections are recommended both grossly and microscopically.

Although the mesenteric arterial system can be more rapidly examined by opening the vessels longitudinally, cross-sections are better for the documentation of obstructions. If vasculitis is suspected, multiple cross-sections from the distal portion of the mesentery will reveal many small arteries for microscopic evaluation. The celiac arterial system is best demonstrated by arteriography (*see* Chapter 5), followed by dissection of the major branches.

Atherosclerosis of the longitudinally opened aorta is graded according to the percentage of intimal surface area that contains plaques. Four grades of disease exist, based on 25% increments of involvement. Grade 4 implies that more than 75% of the surface area is involved by plaques. Grade 0 indicates an absence of lesions. Mural thrombus, ulceration, calcification, and aneurysm do not affect the grade but are described individually. Usually, the grade is stated separately for the thoracic and abdominal regions (or for the suprarenal and infrarenal regions), because infrarenal disease is often more severe.

Atherosclerosis of aortic branches (such as coronary, renal, and mesenteric arteries) is graded according to the percentage of obstruction in *cross-sectional area*. Thus, a four-point grading system is applied to cross sections of these vessels, based on 25% increments of involvement. Grade-4 disease indicates a region of stenosis in which more than 75% of the expected cross-sectional area has been obstructed; this often leads to ischemic injury. Total occlusion (100% obstruction) should be specified; it is generally the result of old or acute plaque rupture and thrombosis.

Older methods of evaluating atherosclerosis require longitudinally opened vessels. The intima is stained with Sudan IV solution *(68)* to facilitate grading, or the vessels are compared with a panel of photographs prepared by the American Heart Association *(69)*. These methods still may be used for research studies.

The patency of grafts and anastomoses should be recorded. Arterial and venous anastomoses in transplanted organs should be inspected for obstruction, including internal thrombosis and external compression or stricture. Synthetic vascular grafts may also compress or erode into adjacent structures. Infected grafts or aneurysm can be cultured, as described in Chapter 9.

POSTMORTEM ANGIOGRAPHY Arteriographic methods are described in Chapter 12.

OBTAINING VESSELS AFTER EMBALMING In general, the vessels of the neck, face, arms, and legs are inaccessible to the prosector until after embalming. For removal of the neck vessels, *see* Chapter 6. Temporal arteries may be resected from the subcutaneous aspect of the skin flap made during removal of the brain. The femoral and popliteal vessels can be removed without having to make skin incisions along the legs *(70)*. For this method, an aluminum tube is used, which measures approx 1.5 cm in internal diameter and 75 cm in length and which has been sharpened distally to form a cutting edge (Fig. 3-12). A string is tied around the femoral artery and vein, just proximal to the inguinal ligament, and passed through the metal tube. By pulling on the string, a constant pressure is placed on the vessel, while the tubing is pushed down the thigh, with a twisting motion, toward the popliteal fossa. Then the tension on the string is released, and the vessels are cut distally by twisting the sharpened edge of the tube. Femoral and popliteal vessels are removed intact with the tube. Veins can be opened longitudinally and inspected for thrombus, particularly in the pockets of the venous valves, but arteries should be cut in cross section.

EVALUATION OF AIR AND FAT EMBOLISM Diagnostic autopsy methods are described in Part II of this book (*see* "Embolism, air" and "Embolism, fat").

EVALUATION OF LYMPHATIC VESSELS Under normal circumstances, only the thoracic duct and its main tributaries can be evaluated. Distended small lymphatic vessels can be identified in conditions such as lymphatic carcinomatosis, congestive heart failure, and cirrhosis of the liver.

The thoracic duct lies in the adipose tissue behind the descending aorta and is best dissected from the left side. It usually travels

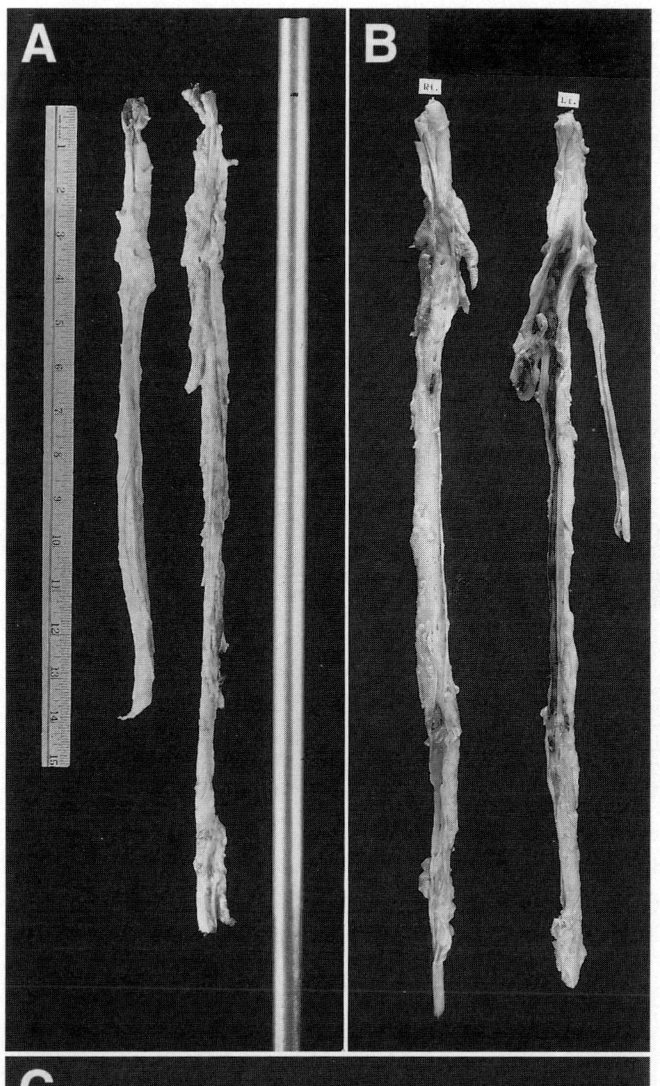

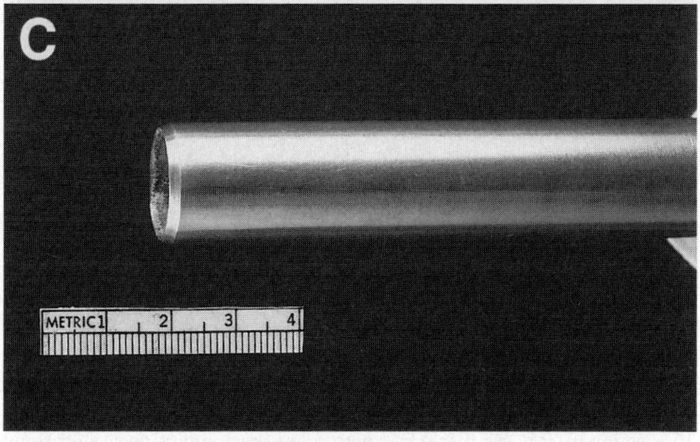

Fig. 3-12. Aluminum tube for the removal of the femoral and popliteal vessels. (**A**) Extracted femoral-popliteal vessels, with metal tube (to the right). (**B**) Bilateral venous thrombosis, in opened femoral and popliteal veins. (**C**) Cutting edge of the metal tube.

medial to the azygos vein and crosses over to the left side of the vertebral column at the level of the aortic arch. For exposure, the left lung is either lifted upward (and held there by an assistant) or removed from the chest cavity. The intercostal arteries are transsected close to the aorta, and the descending thoracic aorta is pulled rightward so that the thoracic duct can be dissected from the surrounding fat tissue (Fig. 3-13). Care must be taken not to lacerate it, particularly near the aortic arch, to which it is closely related. Dissection is facilitated by injecting saline or gelatin solution, with or without dye. Contrast medium may be injected for lymphangiography (*see* Chapter 12).

Some pathologists prefer to dissect the thoracic duct after the chest organs have been removed from the body. To avoid laceration of the duct, the mediastinal tissues must be separated from the spine immediately above the vertebral periosteum. If injection of the duct and its tributaries is planned, this must be done before the thoracic organs are removed.

Peripheral lymphatics can be demonstrated at autopsy by lymphangiography. Because retrograde injection is rarely successful, a peripheral lymphatic channel must be identified. It is then cannulated with a 27-gauge needle. For contrast medium, one can use Ethiodol, stained with a few drops of oil paint, or a dilute barium sulfate mixture *(71)*. Owing to the thick medium and small needle caliber, the required injection pressure may be quite high (500–600 mm Hg).

Lymphatic channels can also be demonstrated by applying a 3% solution of hydrogen peroxide onto the surface of an organ or tissue, which will cause after a short time the spontaneous inflation of lymphatics with oxygen. The results may be unimpressive but can be improved if the tissues are first aged for 12–24 h and then soaked for 4–8 h in a 1:10 dilution of a stock solution of 10 gallons of water, 20 lb of crystalline phenol, 5 lb of potassium nitrate, 1.5 lb of sodium arsenite, 1.5 gallons of glycerin, 1.5 gallons of ethanol, and 0.5 gallon of formalin. After this, the samples are immersed for several minutes in 1% hydrogen peroxide *(72)*.

REFERENCES

1. Edwards WD. Cardiac anatomy and examination of cardiac specimens. In: Allen HD, Gutgesell HP, Clark EB, Driscoll DJ, eds. Moss and Adams' Heart Disease in Infants, Children, and Adolescents, 6th ed. Lippincott Williams & Wilkins, Philadelphia, PA, 2001, pp. 80–117.
2. Virmani R, Ursell PC, Fenoglio JJ. Examination of the heart. Major Probl Pathol (Cardiovasc Pathol) 1991;23:1–20.
3. Silver MM, Silver MD. Examination of the heart and of cardiovascular specimens in surgical pathology. In: Silver MD, Gotlieb AI, Schoen FJ, eds. Cardiovascular Pathology, 3rd ed. Churchill Livingstone, New York, NY, 2001, pp. 1–29.
4. Hutchinson GM, ed. Autopsy: Performance and Technique. College of American Pathologists, Northfield, IL, 1990.
5. Ludwig J, Lie JT. Heart and vascular system. In: Ludwig J, ed. Current Methods of Autopsy Practice, 2nd ed. W.B. Saunders, Philadelphia, PA, 1979, pp. 21–50.
6. Davies MJ, Pomerance A, Lamb D. Techniques in examination and anatomy of the heart. In: Pomerance A, Davies MJ, eds. The Pathology of the Heart. Blackwell Scientific Publications, Oxford, 1975, pp. 1–48.
7. Reiner L. Gross examination of the heart. In: Gould SE, ed. Pathology of the Heart and Great Vessels, 3rd ed. Charles C. Thomas, Springfield, IL, 1968, pp. 1111–1149.
8. Seward JB, Khandheria BK, Freeman WK, Oh JK, Enriquez-Sarano M, Miller FA, et al. Multiplane transesophageal echocardiography: image orientation, examination technique, anatomic correlations, and clinical applications. Mayo Clin Proc 1993;68:523–551.

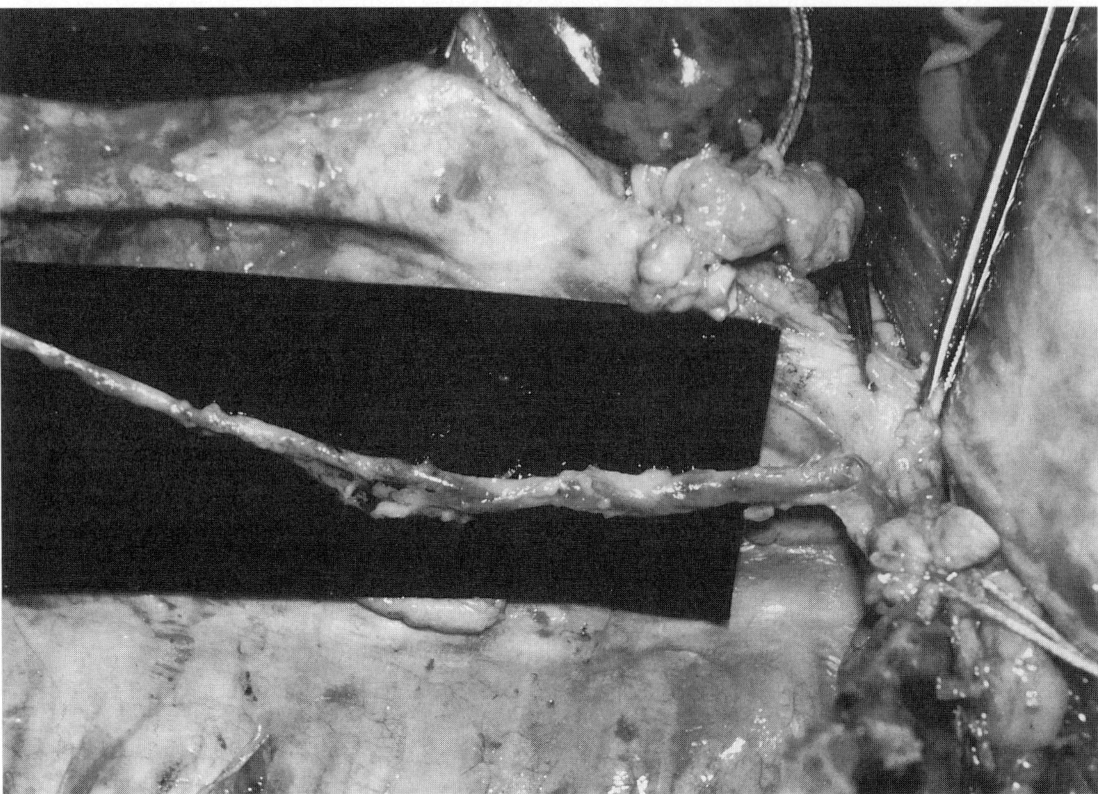

Fig. 3-13. Removal of the thoracic duct. The approach is from the left side. The left lung has been lifted out of the thoracic cavity, and the descending thoracic aorta has been dissected free and retracted rightward. The thoracic duct, displayed on black cardboard, has been dissected away from the retroaortic adipose tissue.

9. Seward JB, Khandheria BK, Edwards WD, Oh JK, Freeman WK, Tajik AJ. Biplanar transesophageal echocardiography: anatomic correlations, image orientation, and clinical applications. Mayo Clin Proc 1990;65:1193–1213.
10. Ackermann DM, Edwards WD. Anatomic basis for tomographic analysis of the pediatriac heart at autopsy. Perspect Pediatr Pathol 1988;12:44–68.
11. Edwards WD. Anatomic basis for tomographic analysis of the heart at autopsy. Cardiol Clin 1984;2:485–506.
12. Silverman NH, Hunter S, Anderson RH, Ho SY, Sutherland GR, Davies MJ. Anatomical basis of cross sectional echocardiography. Br Heart J 1983;50:421–431.
13. Edwards WD, Tajik AJ, Seward JB. Standardized nomenclature and anatomic basis for regional tomographic analysis of the heart. Mayo Clin Proc 1981;56:479–497.
14. Tajik AJ, Seward JB, Hagler DG, Mair DD, Lie JT. Two-dimensional real-time ultrasonic imaging of the heart and great vessels: technique, image orientation, structure identification, and validation. Mayo Clin Proc 1978;53:271–303.
15. Edwards WD. Pathology of myocardial infarction and reperfusion. In: Gersh BJ, Rahimtoola SH, eds. Acute Myocardial Infarction, 2nd ed. Chapman & Hall, New York, NY, 1997, pp. 16–50.
16. Kramer FM. Dry preservation of museum specimens: a review, with introduction of simplified technique. J Tech Methods 1938;18: 42–51.
17. Gross L, Leslie E. Paraffin infiltration of hearts: a permanent method for preservation. Am Heart J 1931;6:665–671.
18. Tiedemann K, von Hagens G. The technique of heart plastination. Anat Rec 1982;204:295–299.
19. Rodriguez FL, Reiner L. A new method of dissection of the heart. Arch Pathol 1957;63:160–163.
20. Bove KE, Rowlands DT, Scott RC. Observations on the assessment of cardiac hypertrophy utilizing a chamber partition technique. Circulation 1966;33:558–568.
21. Baroldi G, Scomazzoni G. Coronary Circulation in the Normal and the Pathologic Heart. US Government Printing Office, Washington DC, 1967, pp. 1–96.
22. James TN. Anatomy of the Coronary Arteries. Paul B. Hoeber, Inc./ Harper & Brothers, New York, 1961, pp. 3–161.
23. Kilner PJ, Ho SY, Anderson RH. Cardiovascular cavities cast in silicone rubber as an adjunct to post-mortem examination of the heart. Int J Cardiol 1988;22:99–107.
24. Dübel H-P, Romaniuk PA. A simple technique for producing cast specimens of the cardiac ventricles. Cardiovasc Intervent Radiol 1980; 3:131–133.
25. Davies MJ, Anderson RH, Becker AE. The Conduction System of the Heart. Butterworths, London, 1983, pp. 9–94.
26. Anderson RH, Becker AE. Anatomy of the conduction tissues revisited. Br Heart J 1978;40(Suppl):2–16.
27. Thomas AC, Davies MJ. The demonstration of cardiac pathology using perfusion-fixation. Histopathology 1985;9:5–19.
28. McAlpine WA. Heart and Coronary Arteries: An Anatomical Atlas for Clinical Diagnosis, Radiological Investigation, and Surgical Treatment. Springer-Verlag, Berlin, 1975, pp. 1–8, 133–209.
29. Glagov S, Eckner FAO, Lev M. Controlled pressure fixation apparatus for hearts. Arch Pathol 1963;76:640–646.
30. Rosenberg HS, Marcontell J. Whole-mount paraffin embedding as a method for preservation of congenitally malformed hearts. Am Heart J 1964;67:379–382.
31. Eckner FAO, Brown BW, Overll E, Glagov S. Alteration of the gross dimensions of the heart and its structures by formalin fixation: a quantitative study. Virchows Arch [Pathol Anat] 1969;346:318–329.

32. Hutchins GM, Anaya OA. Measurements of cardiac size, chamber volumes and valve orifices at autopsy. Johns Hopkins Med J 1973; 133:96–106.
33. Scholz DG, Kitzman DW, Hagen PT, Ilstrup DM, Edwards WD. Age-related changes in normal human hearts during the first 10 decades of life. Part I (growth): a quantitative anatomic study of 200 specimens from subjects from birth to 19 years old. Mayo Clin Proc 1988;63:126–136.
34. Kitzman DW, Scholz DG, Hagen PT, Ilstrup DM, Edwards WD. Age-related changes in normal human hearts during the first 10 decades of life. Part II (maturity): a quantitative anatomic study of 765 specimens from subjects 20 to 99 years old. Mayo Clin Proc 1988;63:137–146.
35. Maron BJ, Henry WL, Roberts WC, Epstein SE. Comparison of echocardiographic and necropsy measurements of ventricular wall thicknesses in patients with and without disproportionate septal thickening. Circulation 1977;55:341–346.
36. Sairanen H. Post mortem measurement of ventricular volumes of the heart: an analysis of errors and presentation of a new method. Acta Pathol Microbiol Immunol Scand [Sect A] 1985;93:109–113.
37. Edwards WD. Applied anatomy of the heart. In: Giuliani ER, et al. eds. Mayo Clinic Practice of Cardiology, 3rd ed. Mosby, St. Louis, MO, 1996, pp. 422–489.
38. Dean JH, Gallagher PJ. Cardiac ischemia and cardiac hypertrophy: an autopsy study. Arch Pathol Lab Med 1980;104:175–178.
39. Murphy ML, White HJ, Meade J, Straub KD. The relationship between hypertrophy and dilatation in the postmortem heart. Clin Cardiol 1988;11:287–302.
40. Schenk KE, Heinze G. Age-dependent changes of heart valves and heart size. Recent Adv Studies Cardiac Structure Metabol 1975;10: 617–624.
41. Hagen PT, Scholz DG, Edwards WD. Incidence and size of patent foramen ovale during the first 10 decades of life: an autopsy study of 965 normal hearts. Mayo Clin Proc 1984;59:17–20.
42. Lie JT, Titus JL. Pathology of the myocardium and the conduction system in sudden coronary death. Circulation 1975;52(Suppl III): 41–52.
43. Lee AHS, Gallagher PJ. Post-mortem examination after cardiac surgery. Histopathology 1998;33:399–405.
44. Waller B. Morphology of percutaneous transluminal coronary angioplasty used in the treatment of coronary heart disease. Major Probl Pathol (Cardiovasc Pathol) 1991;23:100–133.
45. Virmani R, Atkinson JB, Forman MB. Aortocoronary bypass grafts and extracardiac conduits. In: Silver MD, ed. Cardiovascular Pathology, 2nd ed. Churchill-Livingstone, New York, 1991, pp. 1607–1648.
46. Lichtig C, Glagov S, Feldman S, Wissler RW. Myocardial ischemia and coronary artery atherosclerosis: a comprehensive approach to postmortem studies. Med Clin North Am 1973;57:79–91.
47. Baroldi G, Hatt PY, Málek P, Milam J, Paulin SJ, Pearse AGE, et al. The pathological diagnosis of acute ischaemic heart disease: report of a WHO scientific group. WHO Techn Rep Ser 1970;441:1–27.
48. Klein HH, Puschmann S, Schaper J, Schaper W. The mechanism of the tetrazolium reaction in identifying experimental myocardial infarction. Virchows Arch [Pathol Anat] 1981;393:287–297.
49. Feldman S, Glagov S, Wissler RW, Hughes RH. Postmortem delineation of infarcted myocardium: coronary perfusion with nitro blue tetrazolium. Arch Pathol Lab Med 1976;100:55–58.
50. Teraoka K, Kaneko N, Takeishi M. Clinical and pathologic studies on contraction band lesion: relation to acute myocardial infarction and unexplained sudden death. Mod Pathol 1991;4:6–12.
51. Bouchardy B, Majno G. Histopathology of early myocardial infarcts. Am J Pathol 1974;74:301–330.
52. Vargas SO, Samson BA, Schoen FJ. Pathologic detection of early myocardial infarction: a critical review of the evolution and usefulness of modern techniques. Mod Pathol 1999;12:635–645.
53. Geer JC, Crago CA, Little WC, Gardner LL, Bishop SP. Subendocardial ischemic myocardial lesions associated with severe coronary atherosclerosis. Am J Pathol 1980;98:663–680.
54. Fishbein MC, Maclean D, Maroko PR. The histopathologic evolution of myocardial infarction. Chest 1978;73:843–849.
55. Lodge-Patch I. The ageing of cardiac infarcts, and its influence on cardiac rupture. Br Heart J 1951;13:37–42.
56. Mallory GK, White PD, Salcedo-Salgar J. The speed of healing of myocardial infarction: a study of the pathologic anatomy in seventy-two cases. Am Heart J 1939;18:647–671.
57. Cowan MJ, Reichenbach D, Turner P, Thostenson C. Cellular response of the evolving myocardial infarction after therapeutic coronary artery reperfusion. Hum Pathol 1991;22:154–163.
58. Roberts CS, Schoen FJ, Kloner RA. Effect of coronary reperfusion on myocardial hemorrhage and infarct healing. Am J Cardiol 1983; 52:610–614.
59. Mehlman DJ. A pictorial and radiographic guide for identification of prosthetic heart valve devices. Prog Cardiovasc Dis 1988;30:441–464.
60. Morse D, Steiner RM. Cardiac valve identification atlas and guide. In: Morse D, Fernadnez J, eds. Guide to Prosthetic Cardiac Valves. Springer-Verlag, New York, 1985, pp. 257–346.
61. Silver MD, Datta BN, Bowles VF. A key to identify heart valve prostheses. Arch Pathol 1975;99:132–138.
62. Schoen FJ. Pathologic considerations in replacement heart valves and other cardiovascular prosthetic devices. In: Schoen FJ, Gimbrone MA, eds. Cardiovascular Pathology: Clinicopathologic Correlations and Pathogenetic Mechanisms. USCAP Monograph in Pathology, No. 37. Williams & Wilkins, Baltimore, MD, 1995, pp. 194–222.
63. Edwards WD. Congenital heart disease. In: Damjanov I, Linder J, eds. Anderson's Pathology, 10th ed. Mosby Year Book, St. Louis, MO, 1996, pp. 1339–1396.
64. Edwards WD. Classification and terminology of cardiovascular anomalies. In: Allen HD, Gutgesell HP, Clark EB, Driscoll DW, eds. Moss & Adams' Heart Disease in Infants, Children, and Adolescents, Including the Fetus and Young Adult, 6th ed. Williams & Wilkins, Philadelphia, PA, 2001, pp. 118–142.
65. Anderson RH, Becker AE, Freedom RM, et al. Sequential segmental analysis of congenital heart disease. Pediatr Cardiol 1984;5:281–288.
66. Davies MJ. The investigation of sudden cardiac death. Histopathol 1999;34:93–98.
67. Ackerman MJ, Porter CJ. Identification of a family with inherited long QT syndrome after a pediatric near-drowning. Pediatrics 1998; 101:306–308.
68. Guzman GA, McMahan CA, McHill HC Jr, Strong JP, Tejada C, Restrepo C, et al. Selected methodologic aspects of the International Atherosclerosis Project. Lab Invest 1968;18:479–497.
69. McGill HC, Brown BW, Gore I, McMillan GC, Paterson JC, Pollak OJ, et al. Grading human atherosclerotic lesions using a panel of photographs. Circulation 1968;37:455–459.
70. Becking RE Jr, Titus JL. Laboratory suggestion: a method for the autopsy study of the femoral-popliteal vessels. Am J Clin Pathol 1967; 47:652–653.
71. Ludwig J, Linhart P, Baggenstoss AH. Hepatic lymph drainage in cirrhosis and congestive heart failure: a postmortem lymphangiographic study. Arch Pathol 1968;86:551–562.
72. Parke WW, Michels NA. A method for demonstrating subserous lymphatics with hydrogen peroxide. Anat Rec 1963;146:165–171.

Appendix 3-1
Examples for Abbreviations Used for Labeling Microscopic Slides[a]

Abbreviation	Meaning
Aorta and Selected Arteries (Excluding Coronaries)	
Br-Ceph Art	Brachiocephalic (innominate) artery (or BCA or Innom Art)
Ductal Art	Patent ductal artery (patent ductus arteriosus) (or PDA)
Ductal A Lig	Ductal artery ligament (ligamentum arteriosum)
Asc Aorta	Ascending aorta
Desc Thor Ao	Descending thoracic aorta
Abd Aorta	Abdominal aorta
Truncal Art	Persistent truncal artery (truncus arteriosus)
Cardiac valves	
Ao Valve-L	Left cusp of aortic valve (or AV-L)
Ao Valve-P	Posterior cusp of aortic valve (or AV-P)
Ao Valve-R	Right cusp of aortic valve (or AV-R)
Aortic Valve	Aortic valve
Com AV Valve	Common atrioventricular valve (or CAVV)
Mitral Valve	Mitral valve
Pulm Valve	Pulmonary valve
Pulm Valve-A	Anterior cusp of pulmonary valve (or PV-A)
Pulm Valve-L	Left cusp of pulmonnary valve (or PV-L)
Pulm Valve-R	Right cusp of pulmonary valve (or PV-R)
Tric Valve	Tricuspid valve (or TV)
Tric Valve-A	Anterior leaflet of tricuspid valve (or TV-A)
Tric Valve-P	Posterior leaflet of tricuspid valve (or TV-P)
Tric Valve-S	Septal leaflet of tricuspid valve (or TV-S)
Trunc Valve	Truncal valve (or Truncal Valv)
Coronary arteries	
AVNA	AV nodal artery
LAD	Left anterior descending
LAD-D	Unspecified diagonal branch of LAD
LAD-D1	First diagonal branch of LAD
LAD-FSP	First septal perforating branch of LAD
LCX	Left circumflex
LCX-OM	Unspecified obtuse marginal branch of LCX
LCX-OM1	First obtuse marginal branch of LCX
LCX-OM2	Second obtuse marginal branch of LCX
LCX-PD	Posterior descending branch of LCX (with left dominance)
LMA	Left main coronary artery
IA	Intermediate artery (with trifurcating LMA)
RCA	Right coronary artery
RCA-PD	Posterior descending branch of RCA
Coronary arteries *(continued)*	
RCA-PL	Posterolateral branch of RCA
SNA	Sinus nodal artery
Coronary artery bypass grafts	
LAD-GEA	Gastroepiploic artery to LAD
LAD-LIMA	Left internal mammary (thoracic) artery to LAD
LAD-LIMA-RA	LIMA to radial artery segment to LAD
LAD-SVG	Saphenous vein graft to LAD
LAD-D1-SVG	Saphenous vein graft to LAD-D1
LCX-SVG	Saphenous vein graft to LCX
LCX-OM1-SVG	Saphenous vein graft to LCX-OM1
RCA-RIMA	Right internal mammary (thoracic) artery to RCA
RCA-SVG	Saphenous vein graft to RCA
RCA-PD-SVG	Saphenous vein graft to RCA-PD
RCA-PL-SVG	Saphenous vein graft to RCA-PL
Myocardium	
Atrial Sept	Atrial septum
AV-1	Atrioventricular conduction tissue (first cassette); AV-2 (second cassette), etc.
LA	Left atrial free wall
LAA	Left atrial appendage
LA-MV-LV	Left atrium, mitral valve, and left ventricle (one specimen)
LV-AV-Ao	Left ventricle, aortic valve, and ascending aorta (one specimen)
LV-I apex	Inferior wall of left ventricle at apical level
LV-PS base	Posteroseptal wall of left ventricle at basal level
LV-S mid	Ventricular septum at midventricular level
RA	Right atrial free wall
RAA	Right atrial appendage
RA-TV-RV	Right atrium, tricuspid valve, right ventricle (one specimen)
RV-A base	Anterior wall of RV at basal level (or RVOT, for RV outflow tract)
RV-A,L mid	Anterior and lateral walls of RV at midventricular level
RV-I mid	Inferior wall of right ventricle at midventricular level
RV-PV-PA	Right ventricle, pulmonary valve, pulmonary artery (one specimen)
SN-1	Sinus node (first cassette); SN-2 (second cassette), etc.

[a]All abbreviations listed above have 12 or fewer characters, in accordance with automated slide labeling systems that generally allow only 12 characters per line.

For abbreviations for veins, find their arterial counterpart and replace "Artery, Art, or A" with "Vein or V."

Appendix 3-2
Synonyms for Commonly Used Diagnostic Terms in Congenital Heart Disease

Preferred term	*Synonyms*
Anomalous pulmonary venous connection	Anomalous pulmonary venous drainage or return (not always anatomically accurate).
Aortopulmonary septal defect	Aortopulmonary window or fenestration; aorticopulmonary window or septal defect.
Asplenia syndrome	Right isomerism; visceral heterotaxy; Ivemark's syndrome (eponyms should be avoided).
Atrioventricular discordance	Ventricular inversion; L-loop ventricles.
Atrioventricular septal defect	AV canal defect; endocardial cushion defect; AV commune; common AV orifice.
Common inlet right ventricle	Cor biloculare (no longer an acceptable term).
Complete transposition of the great arteries	D-transposition; d-loop transposition; simple regular transposition; transposition of the great vessels.
Congenitally corrected transposition of the great arteries	L-transposition; corrected transposition of the great arteries; physiologically corrected transposition.
Double outlet right ventricle with subpulmonary VSD	Taussig-Bing heart (eponyms should be avoided).
Double chamber left atrium	Subdivided left atrium; triatrial heart; cor triatriatum (a term to avoid).
Double inlet left ventricle	Single left ventricle; univentricular heart; common ventricle (exceedingly rare); cor triloculare biatriatum (no longer an acceptable term).
Double inlet left ventricle with normally related great arteries	Holmes heart (eponyms should be avoided).
Extrathoracic heart	Ectopic heart; ectopia cordis.
Inlet VSD	Subtricuspid, AV canal, or AV commune VSD.
Membranous VSD	Paramembranous, perimembranous, or infracristal VSD.
Muscular VSD	Persistent bulboventricular foramen.
Outlet or infundibular VSD	Subarterial, subaortic, subpulmonary, supracristal, conal, or doubly-committed juxta-arterial VSD.
Patent ductal artery	Patent arterial duct; patent ductus arteriosus; persistent ductus arteriosus.
Persistent truncal artery	Persistent arterial trunk; truncus arteriosus; truncus arteriosus communis.
Polysplenia syndrome	Left isomerism; visceral heterotaxy.
Primum ASD	Ostium primum ASD; partial AV septal defect.
Pulmonary atresia with VSD	Tetralogy with pulmonary atresia (pseudotruncus and type IV truncus are no longer acceptable terms).
RPA or LPA from ascending aorta	Hemitruncus (no longer an acceptable term).
Secundum ASD	Ostium secundum ASD, or fossa ovalis ASD.
Sinus venosus defect	Sinus venosus ASD, Juxtacaval ASD; sinoseptal defect.
Superoinferior ventricles	Over-and-under heart; upstairs-downstairs heart.
Tricuspid atresia	Single inlet left ventricle; absent right atrioventricular connection.
Twisted atrioventricular connection	Criss-cross heart.

ASD, atrial septal defect; AV, atrioventricular; d, dextro; l, levo; LPA, left pulmonary artery; RPA, right pulmonary artery; VSD, ventricular septal defect.

Adapted from Edwards *(63)*.

Appendix 3-3
Latin Terms and Their Anglicized Equivalents for Cardiovascular Structures

Latin term (Plural)	*Anglicized equivalent (Plural)*
Annulus (annuli); anulus (anuli)	Annulus (annuluses), or anulus, or ring
Aorta (aortae)	Aorta (aortas)
Atrium (atria)	Atrium (atriums)
Chorda tendinea (chordae tendineae)	Tendinous cord (cords)
Conus arteriosus	Right ventricular outflow tract, or infundibulum
Cor triatriatum	Triatrial heart, or double chamber left atrium
Cor triatriatum dexter	Double chamber right atrium
Crista supraventricularis	Supraventricular crest or ridge
Crista terminalis	Terminal crest or ridge
Ductus arteriosus (ductus arteriosi)	Ductal artery, or arterial duct
Ductus venosus	Ductal vein, or venous duct
Ectopia cordis	Ectopic heart, or extrathoracic heart
Foramen ovale	Oval foramen
Fossa ovalis	Oval fossa
Inferior vena cava	Inferior caval vein
Infundibulum (infundibula)	Infundibulum (infundibulums)
Ligamentum arteriosum	Arterial ligament, or ductal artery ligament
Ligamentum venosum	Venous ligament, or ductal vein ligament
Limbus fossae ovalis, or annulus ovalis	Limb or rim of the oval fossa
Ostium (ostia)	Ostium (ostiums), or orifice
Ostium primum	First ostium or orifice
Ostium secundum	Second ostium or orifice
Patent ductus arteriosus	Patent ductal artery
Patent foramen ovale	Patent oval foramen
Septum (septa, not septae or septi)	Septum (septums)
Septum primum	First septum
Septum secundum	Second septum
Sinus venosus	Venous sinus, or sinus vein
Situs ambiguous	Isomerism, or indeterminate sidedness
Situs inversus	Mirror-image sidedness
Situs solitus	Normal sidedness
Superior vena cava	Superior caval vein
Trabecula septomarginalis	Septal band, or moderator band
Trabecula carnea (trabeculae carneae)	Trabeculation(s)
Truncus arteriosus	Truncal artery, or arterial trunk

Adapted from Edwards *(63)*.

Appendix 3-4
Eponyms for Surgical Procedures for Congenitally Malformed Hearts

Eponym	*Description of procedure*	*Cardiovascular anomalies*
Blalock-Hanlon shunt	Partial atrial septectomy (posterosuperior region).	Complete TGA with intact ventricular septum.
Blalock-Taussig shunt	Subclavian-to-pulmonary artery (classic: end-to-side anastomosis; modified: interposed synthetic graft).	Conditions with decreased pulmonary blood flow (tetralogy, PA-VSD, and DORV or DILV with PS).
Damus-Kaye-Stansel procedure	Proximal PT to ascending aorta (end-to-side anastomosis); conduit from RV to distal PT; VSD closure.	Complete TGA without PS and with or without VSD.
Glenn anastomosis	SVC to RPA (end-to-side); ligation of SVC at RA; ligation of proximal RPA (bidirectional Glenn: no ligation of RPA).	Tricuspid atresia, or DILV with PS.
Fontan procedure (modified)	Anastomosis of SVC, RA, or RV to RPA or LPA; may include intra-atrial conduit from IVC to SVC.	Hearts with single functional ventricle (e.g., tricuspid atresia or DILV).
Jatene procedure	Transection and switching of great arteries and coronary arteries.	Complete TGA, and DORV with subpulmonary VSD.
Konno procedure	Outlet (infundibular) septostomy, with patch enlargement of LV and RV outflow tracts, and aortic valve replacement.	Tunnel subaortic stenosis, and severe hypertrophic cardiomyopathy.
Mustard procedure	Resection of atrial septum; intra-atrial baffle directing caval blood flow to LV, and pulmonary venous blood to RV.	Complete TGA.
Norwood procedure	*Stage 1* (atrial septectomy; PDA ligation; PT transection; aortic incision; reconstruction of aorta with allograft; aorta-PT shunt). *Stage 2* (modified Fontan operation).	Aortic atresia (hypoplastic left heart syndrome).
Potts shunt	Descending thoracic aorta to LPA (side-to-side anastomosis).	Same as for Blalock-Taussig shunt.
Rastelli procedure	VSD closure directing LV blood to aorta; conduit from RV to distal PT; ligation of proximal PT.	PA-VSD, PTA, complete TGA with VSD and PS, and DORV with PS.
Senning procedure	Use of atrial septum to fashion intra-atrial baffle, similar to Mustard procedure.	Complete TGA.
Waterston shunt	Ascending aorta to RPA (side-to-side anastomosis).	Same as for Blalock-Taussig shunt.

DILV, double inlet left ventricle; DORV, double outlet right ventricle; IVC, inferior vena cava; LPA, left pulmonary artery; LV, left ventricle, PA-VSD, pulmonary atresia with a ventricular septal defect; PDA, patent ductal artery; PS, pulmonary stenosis; PT, pulmonary trunk; PTA, persistent truncal artery; RA, right atrium; RPA, right pulmonary artery; RV, right venricle; SVC, superior vena cava; TGA, transposition of the great arteries; VSD, ventricular septal defect.

Adapted with permission from Edwards *(63)*.

Appendix 3-5
Standardized Form for the Autopsy Evaluation of Congenital Heart Disease

GENERAL INFORMATION CASE NO.: ____________
Patient Name: ______________________ Age, Gender: ____________
Patient I.D. No.: ______________________ Date of Death: ____________

CARDIAC ARRANGEMENT
Thoracic Position ☐ Left-Sided ☐ Right-Sided ☐ Midline ☐ Unknown ☐ Ectopic ________
Apical Direction: ☐ Left-Sided ☐ Right-Sided ☐ Midline ☐ Other: ________
Displacement: ☐ None ☐ Leftward ☐ Rightward ☐ Midline ☐ Unknown
Morphologic RA: ☐ Right-Sided ☐ Left-Sided ☐ Bilateral ☐ Absent ☐ Indeterminate
PULMONARY ARRANGEMENT
Morphology of Right-Sided Lung: ☐ Right ☐ Left ☐ Indeterminate No. of Lobes: ________
Morphology of Left-Sided Lung: ☐ Left ☐ Right ☐ Indeterminate No. of Lobes: ________
ABDOMINAL ARRANGEMENT
Spleen: ☐ Single ☐ Accessory ☐ Polysplenia ☐ Asplenia ☐ Unknown
Liver: ☐ Right-Sided ☐ Left-Sided ☐ Midline ☐ Unknown ☐ Other: ________
Bowel: ☐ Normal ☐ Malrotation: ________
VISCERAL SIDEDNESS
Cardiac: ☐ Normal ☐ Mirror-Image ☐ R. Isomerism ☐ L. Isomerism ☐ Indeterminate ________
Pulmonary: ☐ Normal ☐ Mirror-Image ☐ R. Isomerism ☐ L. Isomerism ☐ Indeterminate ________
Abdominal: ☐ Normal ☐ Mirror-Image ☐ R. Isomerism ☐ L. Isomerism ☐ Indeterminate ________
ATRIUMS
Right-Sided: ☐ RA ☐ LA ________
Left-Sided: ☐ LA ☐ RA ________
Septum: ☐ Intact ☐ POF ☐ ASD: ________
Cor. Sinus: ☐ Present ☐ Absent ☐ Other: ________
ATRIOVENTRICULAR VALVES
Right-Sided: ________ % to RV ________ % to LV Morphology: ________
Left-Sided: ________ % to RV ________ % to LV Morphology: ________
Common: ________ % to RV ________ % to LV Morphology: ________
VENTRICLES
Morphologic RV: Orientation: ☐ Normal ☐ Mirror-Image Position: ________
Morphologic LV: Orientation: ☐ Normal ☐ Mirror-Image Position: ________
Hypoplastic: ☐ RV ☐ LV ________
Septal Position: ☐ Vertical ☐ Angled ☐ Horizontal ☐ Twisted ☐ Other: ________
Septum: ☐ Intact ☐ VSD: ________
SEMILUNAR VALVES
Pulmonary: ________ % to RV ________ % to LV Morphology: ________
Aortic: ________ % to RV ________ % to LV Morphology: ________
Truncal: ________ % to RV ________ % to LV Morphology: ________
AORTIC VALVE POSITION RELATIVE TO PULMONARY VALVE
☐ R. Post. ☐ Dextroposed ☐ R. Lat. ☐ R. Ant. ☐ Ant. ☐ L. Ant. ☐ L. Lat. ☐ L. Post. ☐ Post.
GREAT ARTERIES
Pulm. Artery: ☐ Present ☐ Atretic ☐ Hypoplastic ☐ Absent ☐ Other: ________
Systemic Collaterals: ☐ Absent ☐ Present: ________
Thoracic Aorta: ☐ L. Arch ☐ R. Arch ☐ Coarctation ☐ Other: ________
Ductal Artery: ☐ Patent ☐ Absent ☐ Ligament ☐ Other: ________
CORONARY ARTERIES
Ostiums: ☐ Normal ☐ Other: ________
Distribution: ☐ Normal ☐ Mirror-Image ☐ Other: ________

CONNECTIONS

Venoatrial	(Systemic Veins):	☐ Normal Veins	☐ Other: ______		
	(Pulmonary Veins):	☐ Normal Veins	☐ Other: ______		
Atrioventricular	(Biventricular):	☐ Concordance	☐ Discordance	☐Ambiguous:	______
	(Univentricular):	☐ Double Inlet	☐ Single Inlet	☐ Common Inlet	______
Ventriculoarterial	(Two Arteries):	☐ Concordance	☐ Discordance	☐ Double Outlet	______
	(One Artery):	☐ Single Outlet (Atretic PT)		☐ Common Outlet (Truncal Artery)	

CARDIAC MEASUREMENTS

Body Size:	Height (cm) ______	Weight (kg) ______	BSA (m2) ______
Weights (g):	Heart & Lungs ______	R. Lung ______	L. Lung ______
	Heart ______	(Normal Mean ______	and Range ______)
Wall Thickness (cm):	LV ______	RV ______	VS ______
Valves (cm):	Aortic ______	Pulmonary ______	Truncal ______
	Mitral ______	Tricuspid ______	Common ______

Shunts (cm): POF ______ ASD ______ AVSD ______ VSD ______ PDA ______

SECONDARY CARDIAC EFFECTS

	Hypertrophy	Dilation	Atrophy	Fibrosis	Mural Thrombus
LV:	______	______	______	______	______
RV:	______	______	______	______	______
LA:	______	______	______	______	______
RA:	______	______	______	______	______

SECONDARY PULMONARY EFFECTS

Plexogenic Pulmonary Hypertension: ______

Pulmonary Venous Hypertension: ______

Other Pulmonary Hypertension: ______

Pulmonary Infection: ______

Other Microscopic Features: ______

INTERVENTIONAL PROCEDURES

Procedure (Date): ______

Appearance at Autopsy: ______

Procedure (Date): ______

Appearance at Autopsy: ______

Procedure (Date): ______

Appearance at Autopsy: ______

DIAGRAMS

Adapted from Edwards *(63)*.

4 Tracheobronchial Tree and Lungs

JURGEN LUDWIG

DISSECTION AND FIXATION TECHNIQUES

UPPER RESPIRATORY TRACT AND DISSECTION OF LARYNX The removal of the neck organs has been briefly described in Chapter 1. The organ block should contain not only trachea, larynx, and cervical esophagus but also the floor of the mouth, tongue, soft palate, and tonsils. For special studies of the upper respiratory tract, the posterior portions of the nasal cavities and adjacent sinuses can be removed together with the neck organs. In these instances, the brain must be removed first and the nasal and perinasal bony structures must be separated from the rest of the base of the skull with an oscillating saw (*see* Chapter 6) *(1)*. If properly done, the contours of the face are not affected by this procedure.

Routinely, the *larynx* is opened along the posterior midline, and the lateral portions are pulled apart to expose the mucosa. In adults, this maneuver may require breakage of the ossified laryngeal cartilage. If the cartilage is not or only minimally ossified, the larynx can be cut into serial cross-sections, which yields good histologic specimens for the demonstration of mucosal changes and also of the cricoarytenoid joint. This joint is found just beneath the level of the vocal cords, at both sides of the posterior midline of the larynx. These joints are readily available at autopsy and can be studied, together with the sternoclavicular joints, in suspected systemic arthritis. After suspected strangulation, the hyoid bone must be identified for evidence of fracture and the larynx examined for hemorrhages (*see* "Strangulation" in Part II). Some authors try to facilitate inspection by cutting the larynx in two halves along the sagittal midline *(2)*.

DISSECTION OF TRACHEA AND MAIN BRONCHI The trachea and main bronchi usually are opened along their posterior membranous walls. Anterior incisions *in situ* may be indicated in cases of aspiration and drowning. Tracheoesophageal fistulas also are best demonstrated by anterior midline incision or complete removal of the anterior half of the trachea (Fig. 4-1).

DISSECTION OF FRESH LUNGS

Dissection from Hilus The pulmonary arteries and bronchi are opened from the hilus toward the periphery of the mediastinal surface of the lung. Subsequently, the lungs are cut into several sagittal slices, that is, parallel with the mediastinal surface. This method permits study of many cross-sections of bronchovascular units and gives a good overall view of the parenchyma. Unfortunately, the continuity of the organs is lost so that it may be difficult to identify the original site of individual slices. More important, vessels and bronchi running in a more frontal plane cannot be opened without at least partly destroying the slices.

Dissection from Incisions Along Lateral Surface of Lung After separation from the mediastinum, a bronchopulmonary cuff should remain on the lungs. The hilus of the lungs with this cuff is held in the hand of the prosector. An incision is made from the apex to the base of the pulmonary lobes along their longest lateral axis. For the right middle lobe, this axis lies almost in the horizontal plane. The incisions into the upper and lower lobes reach toward but not into the hilus and are connected by a third incision that lies at a right angle to the first and second. This third incision divides part of the wall of a main pulmonary artery, which usually shines through the pleura in the interlobar fissure close to the hilus. One blade of a pair of scissors is introduced into this opening and the pulmonary arteries are opened radially in all directions. The cuts made by the scissors should include the periphery of the pulmonary parenchyma and the parietal pleura so that the lungs can be laid out well (Fig. 4-2). Subsequently the bronchial tree is dissected in the same fashion (Fig. 4-3). During this last maneuver, the prosector must cut through many pulmonary artery branches.

This method requires more practice than the dissection from the hilus, but it leaves the dissected lung in continuity and permits easy reconstruction of the original position of pulmonary lesions. If the lungs had been separated from the main bronchi too close to the hilus, it may be difficult to leave the hilar structures intact. In order to preserve the continuity of most arteries and bronchi, this method can be combined with dissection from the hilus *(3)*.

Histologic Sampling For routine histologic sampling, a container can be used with three compartments for the right pulmonary lobes and two compartments for the left lobes. Whatever method is used, the origin of every lung section should be identified. For electron microscopic studies, rapid collection and fixation of samples is recommended. For fixation prior to routine autopsy, *see* Chapter 1 "Immediate Autopsies for

From: *Handbook of Autopsy Practice,* 3rd Ed. Edited by: J. Ludwig © Humana Press Inc., Totowa, NJ

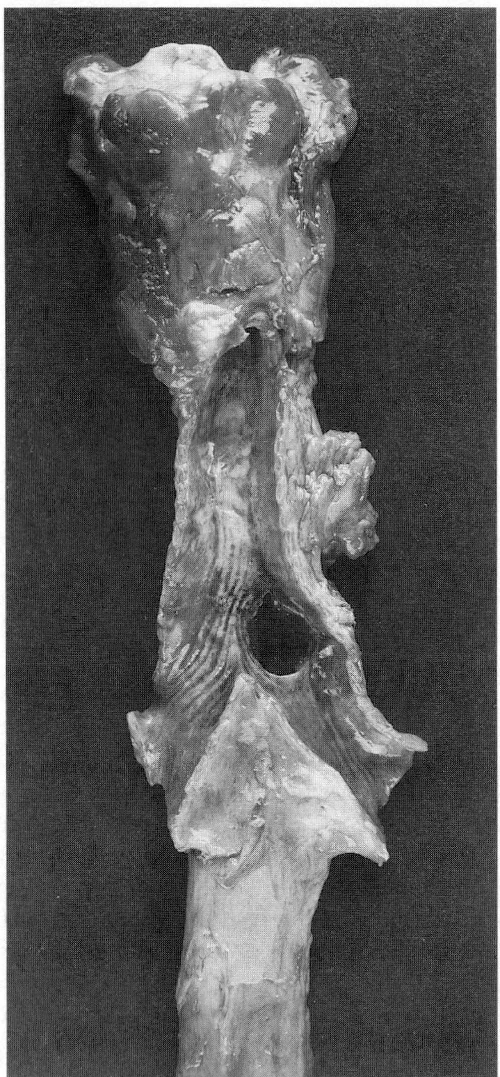

Fig. 4-1. Larynx, trachea with carina, and esophagus with anterior half of trachea and adjacent main bronchi removed. Note perforation of carcinoma of esophagus into left main bronchus at carina.

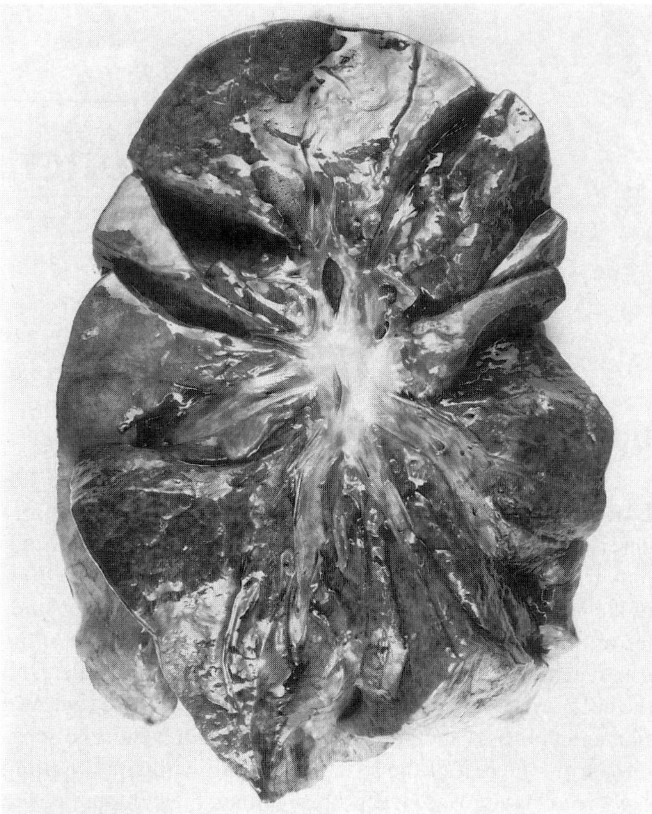

Fig. 4-2. Cut surface of lung dissected from incisions along lateral surfaces of lobes. Hilus is left intact. Pulmonary artery tree has been opened lengthwise in radial fashion.

Special Laboratory Procedures such as Electron Microscopy, Cytochemistry, and Tissue Culture" and "Needle Autopsies."

WET FIXATION OF LUNGS Formalin fixation of lungs with a perfusion apparatus (*see* below) provides excellent specimens, both by reconstituting the size of the lung at full inspiration and by providing good fixation for histologic study. A prudent approach is to perfuse one lung and dissect the other in the fresh state to obtain material for microbiologic study and for smears, for instance when *Pneumocystis carinii* infection is suspected. Also, pulmonary edema and embolism are best assessed in the fresh lung.

If no perfusion apparatus is available, lungs can be reinflated with 10% formalin solution through the main bronchus. About 2 L of formalin solution is needed for an adult lung. The inflation can be done with a large syringe or, better still, from a bottle 30–50 cm above the specimen. Subsequently, the main bronchus is clamped and the lung is floated in a formalin bath. It should be noted that the organ shrinks again during this period.

Removal and Preparation of Lungs Prior to Wet Fixation For most special studies of isolated lungs, it is essential not to lacerate the organ during removal. We usually first produce a pneumothorax through a small parasternal incision. In many instances, the chest plate can then be removed safely. If one wants to protect the lungs even better, the anterior attachments of the diaphragm to the rib cage should be incised so that the hand of an assistant can be introduced to hold back the lung during removal of the chest plate. The remaining rib ends should be covered with a thick towel or plastic sheet because the severed bone may lacerate the pleura (and also the skin of the persons working on the cadaver!). Before the lungs are removed, adhesions must be carefully dissected as close to the parietal pleura as possible. This is particularly difficult at the posterior base of the lower lobes, where adhesions are frequently encountered. If adhesions are extensive, one may attempt to remove the lungs with the parietal pleura that must be dissected from the bony and muscular parts of the chest wall. Small rents in the pleura should be tied off or sealed with wound spray ("artificial skin").

Connection of the lung with the perfusion apparatus is greatly facilitated if an extrapulmonary bronchoarterial cuff is left attached to the lung. It is also possible to leave the lungs

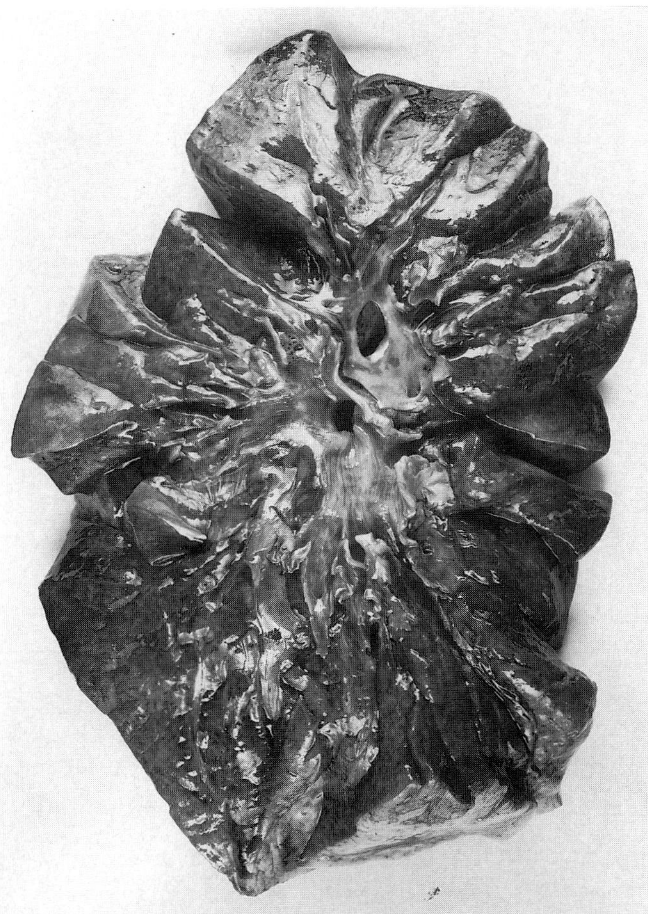

Fig. 4-3. Same lung as in Fig. 4-2. Bronchial tree has been opened lengthwise in radial fashion, sacrificing continuity of some overriding arteries.

attached to the trachea and thus perfuse them simultaneously. Similarly, pulmonary angiograms can be prepared by leaving the lungs attached to the main pulmonary artery. Both procedures can be carried out *in situ*.

Before perfusion, mucus and purulent material should be suctioned from the bronchi. If this cannot be done successfully, the lungs should be perfused through the pulmonary vessels.

Fixation Time Complete perfusion fixation requires about 3 d. Consolidated and fibrosed lungs may need longer. Plugging of bronchi may completely prevent proper expansion and fixation. In such an event, the affected portions of the lung will not inflate.

Formalin Perfusion Techniques (Pressure Fixation) In the previous edition of this book, several apparatuses were described and illustrated. More recently *(4)*, a fixation apparatus for surgically obtained lungs has be described that undoubtedly would also be suitable for autopsy lung. With this apparatus, the perfusion pressure can be set in a range from 15–95 cm H_2O. However, for routine purposes, our cascade perfusion system which has been in use for more than 25 years, has been most satisfactory. Therefore, only this system and its operation shall be described here *(5,6)*. The apparatus can also be used to perfuse livers *(5)* and other organs such as heart and kidneys, either from the autopsy service or from the surgical pathology laboratory.

In the perfusion apparatus shown in Fig. 4-4, the fixative cascades through stacked plastic containers and flows through nozzles tied into the main bronchus or the trachea. An electric pump causes the fixative to circulate. As fixative, we often use modified Kaiserling's solution (*see* Chapter 14) but neutral buffered formalin is suitable also. Angiograms can be prepared before or after fixation. Prior to the perfusion fixation, we flush the lungs with 10% buffered formalin. This helps to keep the actual perfusion solution reasonably clean. After 3 or more days of continuous cascade perfusion, the lungs are sliced with an extra-long knife (*see* below), which is needed to avoid cutting marks. It should be noted that the perfusion apparatus shown in Fig. 4-4 was assembled in the Mayo Clinic engineering shop; the complete system is not commercially available but modifications undoubtedly can be built without too much difficulty.

OTHER WET, GASEOUS, AND DRY PRESERVATION METHODS Pressure-free perfusion fixation at predetermined states of expansion *(7)*, fixation with formaldehyde gas, or formalin steam fixation have been used in the past, mostly for research purposes. These and other methods have been illustrated in the second edition of *Current Methods of Autopsy Practice (8)*. They include air-drying of lungs, which is obsolete but still would be justified if no other preservation method is available. After air-drying, the macroscopic features of the lungs are remarkably well-preserved but histologic samples are unsatisfactory. Museum specimens have been prepared by this method, using infiltration of lungs with paraffin or diglycol stearate; this probably has no place in current autopsy practice.

SLICING OF FIXED LUNGS We use a special knife and slicing board (Fig. 4-5) The cork slicing board is mounted in a metal tray where the draining formalin solution collects. The knife has a 78-cm long blade that in many instances permits the whole lung to be cut with one uninterrupted pulling motion. This ensures a smooth and even cut surface without knife marks. This knife also works well to prepare even slices of livers or large spleens. The lung usually is cut in the frontal or sagittal plane in slices about 1.5 cm thick. For frontal sectioning, the lung is placed so that the hilus is uppermost. We usually make the first cut immediately adjacent to the hilus. If the cut section is to be along the axis of a bronchus, the knife is guided along metal probes or glass rods previously inserted into the major airways. For the preparation of large and very thin slices, gelatin infiltration is required (*see* below under "Paper-Mounted Sections").

IMPREGNATION AND STORAGE OF LUNG SLICES

BARIUM SULFATE IMPREGNATION This method renders pulmonary tissue opaque and thus makes it considerably easier to quantitate lung changes such as in pulmonary emphysema. After impregnation with barium sulfate, the lung slices sink in water and can easily be photographed and studied with the naked eye or with a dissecting microscope.

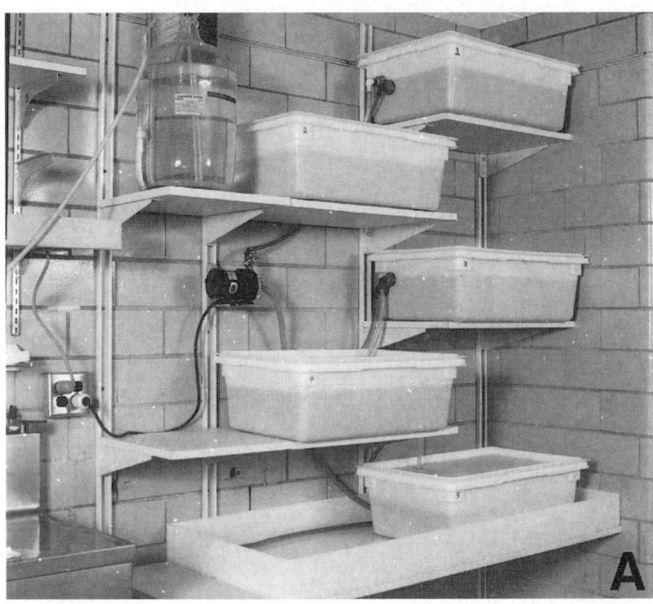

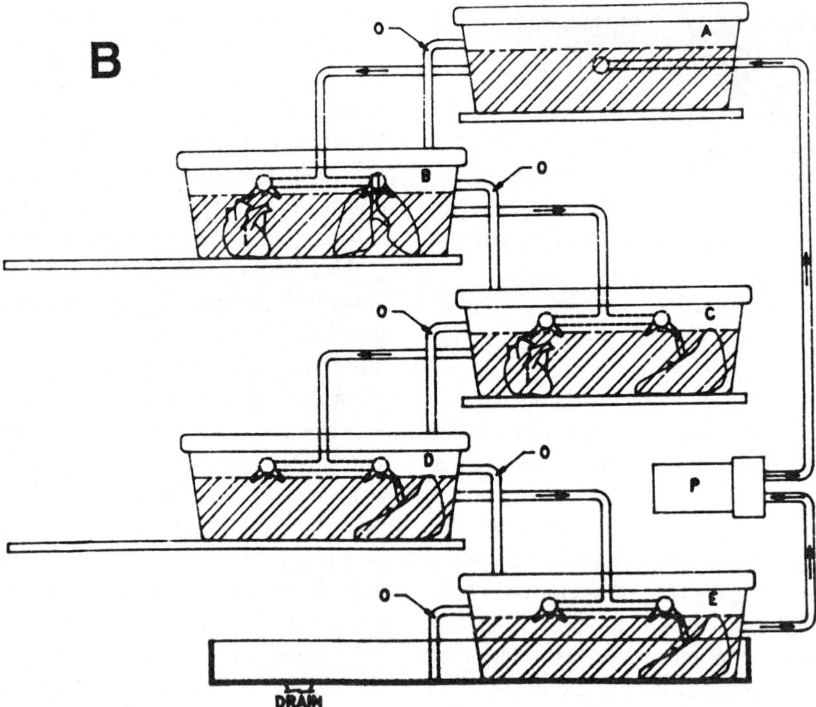

Fig. 4-4. Perfusion system for lungs and other organs. (**A**) Four plastic containers are stacked on adjustable shelves. An electric pump is mounted to one of the center rails. Some of the tubing between the containers is visible. The large flask in the upper left corner of the picture contains neutral buffered 10% formalin solution that is used to gravitate-perfuse the specimens before they are placed in the containers with the circulating fixative (*see* text). The floor space occupied by the system is 160 × 60 cm. (**B**) Schematic drawing of perfusion system. *P,* electric pump (TEEL magnetic drive pump with 5/8' outer diameter inlet and outlet, Dayton Electric Manufacturing Co., Chicago, IL). The direction of the fixative flow is indicated by arrows. The solution cascades from containers *A* to *E*, flowing through any organ that is attached to one of the nozzles. The distance between one container and the next lower one is 30–33 cm, and thus the perfusion pressure is 30–33 cm H_2O. If an outflow opening in one of the containers becomes plugged, the fluid level rises until it reaches the opening to the overflow tube, *O*, which leads into the next-lower container. Tube *O* of container *E* drains into a large base pan that is normally empty. However, that pan has a drain that can be opened manually. Note the nozzles inside containers *B* to *E*. In the example drawn, one pair of lungs, three livers, and two hearts are attached to the system. Adapted with permission from ref. *(5)*.

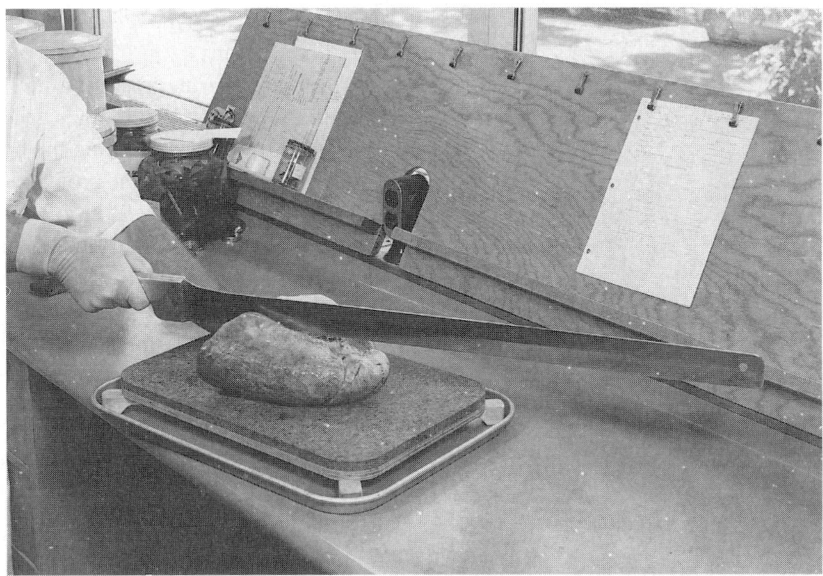

Fig. 4-5. Slicing of lung with special long-bladed knife. The lung is cut with an uninterrupted pulling motion, which avoids knife marks on cut surface. Cork cutting board rests on metal tray that collects draining formalin solution.

Method of Heard *(9)* A slice of fixed lung is placed in a solution of 75 g of barium nitrate dissolved in 1 L of warm water. The lung tissue is slightly squeezed so that the solution penetrates the tissue. After about 1 min, the slice is taken out of this solution and excess fluid is squeezed out.

Next, the tissue is submerged in a solution of 100 g sodium sulfate dissolved in 1 L of warm water. The lung tissue is again slightly squeezed and then taken out of the solution, drained, and returned to the barium nitrate bath. This procedure is repeated several times until all air bubbles have been squeezed out and the barium sulfate precipitate has rendered the lung tissue opaque and grayish white (Fig. 4-6).

STORAGE Fresh lungs can be stored in a refrigerator for a few days at temperatures just above the freezing point. Fresh lungs also can be kept deep frozen for months but it is recommended to obtain samples for histologic study prior to snap-freezing. Fixed lungs are best sliced and stored flat in heat-sealed plastic bags filled with 5–20% formalin solution. Several slices can be stored in a stack without distorting the lung tissue.

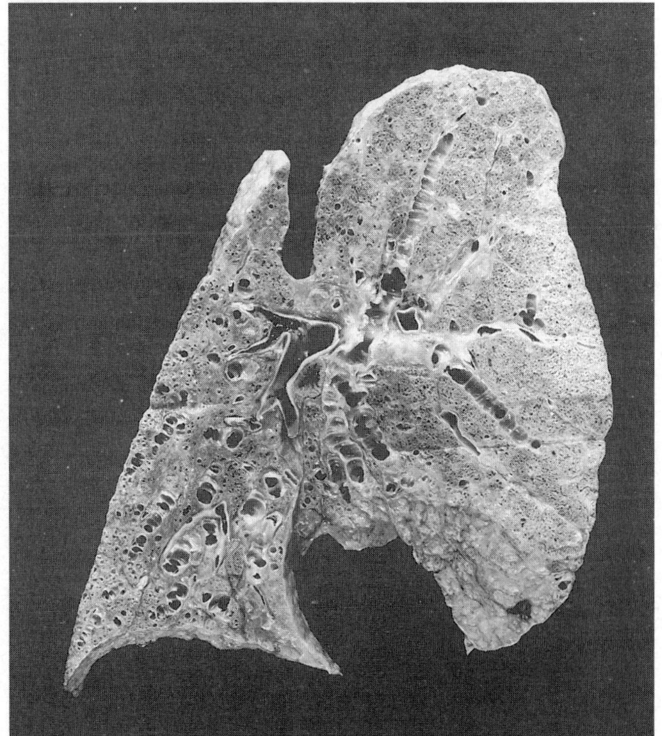

Fig. 4-6. Slice of perfusion-fixed lung. The left lung was cut in a sagittal plane. The slice shown was impregnated under water with barium sulfate as described by Heard (*see* text). Note multiple tubular bronchiectases.

PAPER-MOUNTED SECTIONS

This method was pioneered by Gough and has undergone several modifications *(10)*. The technique yields very instructive, detailed, esthetically appealing, and extremely durable views of pulmonary abnormalities. After perfusion fixation with formalin and sodium acetate, 2-cm thick slices of the lungs are washed and embedded in a gelatin mixture that contains a disinfectant. After the gelatin mixture has penetrated the tissue, the block is frozen and large, 400-μm sections are cut, refixed, and transferred to another gelatin mixture, and eventually mounted on paper. Routine stains can be applied without difficulty. The technique also can be applied to other organs such as liver. For further details, the second edition of this book *(8)* or the original publications should be consulted. Readers will find that paper-mounting requires some skill; it also is work-intensive (the original method of Gough required 11 d, although other authors have achieved comparable results in

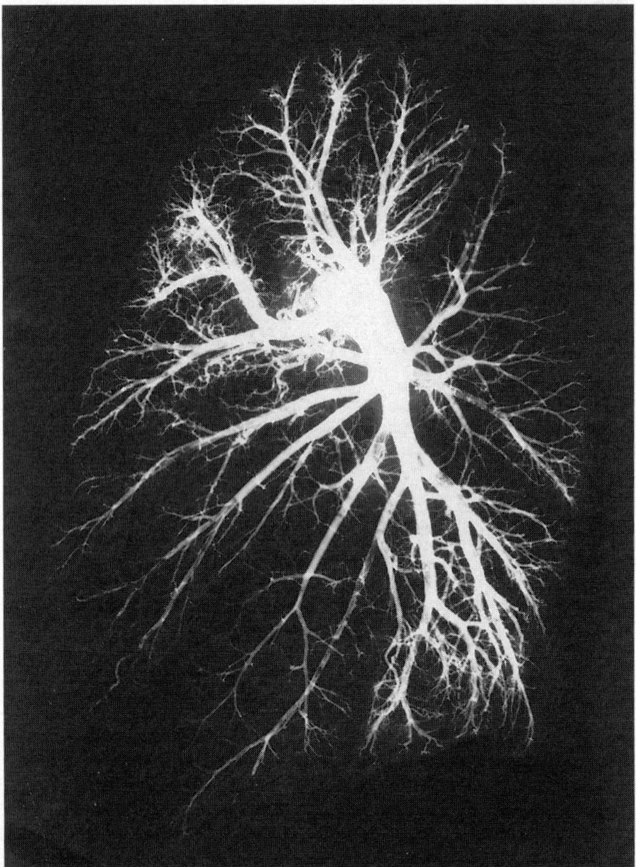

Fig. 4-7. Arteriogram of left lung. Lung inflated with carbon dioxide and pulmonary artery injected with barium sulfate-gelatin mixture. Note marked rarefication of vascular tree of this emphysematous lung.

2 d *[11]*), and thus costly. Despite its didactic and esthetic appeal, the method has been largely replaced by photography of perfusion-fixed specimens.

POSTMORTEM PULMONARY ANGIOGRAPHY AND BRONCHOGRAPHY

Satisfactory injection can be achieved only with inflated lungs. Therefore, careful removal of the lungs and sealing of accidental lacerations of the pleura is essential.

PULMONARY ARTERIOGRAPHY Barium-gelatin mixtures are the preferred media. Because the viscosity of the gelatin preparations depends on many factors, the optimal concentration of gelatin will vary and has to be tested. For further details, *see* Chapter 12. The pulmonary arteries can be injected *in situ* by introducing a 13-gauge needle just above the pulmonary valve. This technique is particularly useful when tumors, adhesions, or other pathologic conditions prevent the removal of intact lungs. It may be necessary, however, to place the cadaver for some time in a refrigerator to allow the gelatin to set; the lungs can then be removed without causing much leakage from minor lacerations.

The preferred method is pulmonary arteriography on isolated lungs (Fig. 4-7). Tubing is tied with glass or plastic cones into the pulmonary artery and the bronchus, respectively. The lung is inflated through the bronchus with air or carbon dioxide at a pressure of approx 20 mm Hg (the lung should attain its normal volume). The barium-gelatin medium is warmed to about 60°C and injected into the pulmonary artery of the inflated lung at a pressure of about 70–80 mm Hg. Again, some experimentation may be necessary because required injection pressures vary depending on the viscosity of the medium, temperature, types of syringes, and other factors. With the methods described here, we have consistently filled the peripheral pulmonary artery branches (Fig. 4-8), down to vessels with an internal diameter of about 60 μm. The study of even smaller vessels requires very low-viscosity gelatin mixtures or nonconsolidating contrast media. For an average-sized lung, about 150 mL of medium is needed. The injection takes 5–10 min. When the vascular tree is filled, the pressure increases suddenly; hence this endpoint cannot easily be missed. The lung should be kept warm during the injection so that the gelatin does not set too quickly. The techniques described here are for adult lungs but they also can be applied to infant lungs *(12)*.

PULMONARY VENOGRAPHY AND LYMPHANGIOGRAPHY The injection technique for the venography is basically similar to that for pulmonary arteriography. *In situ* filling can be achieved by tying glass cones into these veins at their connection to the left atrium. The same technique may be used on heart-lung blocks or on isolated lungs. In the last instance, the procedure is facilitated if a part of the left atrium has been left attached to the lung so that glass or plastic tubes or cones are easier to tie into the veins. Injection pressures may vary between 20 and 70 mm Hg.

For lymphangiographic studies, stained sodium tritrizoate (*see* Chapter 15) is injected into pleural lymphatics with a no. 30 lymphangiography needle while the lung is kept at an inflation pressure of about 18 cm H_2O *(13)*.

BRONCHIAL ARTERIOGRAPHY Similar to the pulmonary vessels, the bronchial arteries can be injected *in situ* but this method is not recommended because multiple aortic branches must be tied first and because the origin of the bronchial arteries is not constant. In isolated lungs, the bronchial arteries usually can be cannulated at the posterosuperior aspect of the main bronchus. A 30-gauge polyethylene catheter is tied into the isolated bronchial artery or arteries. The lung is then inflated with carbon dioxide or air, and the contrast medium (*see* "Pulmonary Arteriography") is injected through the catheter. The injection pressure is 150 mm Hg. The end point of the injection has been discussed in the previous section. Bronchial arteriograms clearly show these vessels (Fig. 4-9). After bronchopulmonary anastomoses have opened, bronchial arteriograms may also show segments of pulmonary arteries.

BRONCHOGRAPHY High-viscosity barium-gelatin mixtures can be used but clinical contrast media give better results. Ideally the contrast medium should be instilled while the lung is expanded in a vacuum chamber.

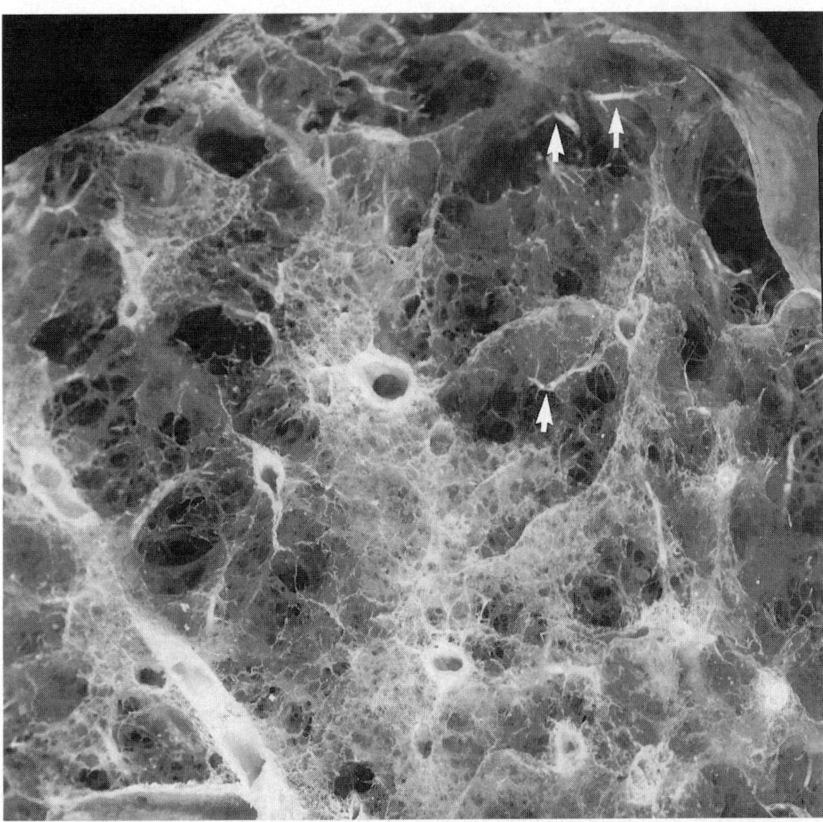

Fig. 4-8. Slice of perfusion-fixed lung with advanced destructive centrilobular emphysema. Note pulmonary artery branches containing white contrast medium (arrows). A barium sulfate-gelatine mixture was used as contrast medium. Photographed specimen is under water.

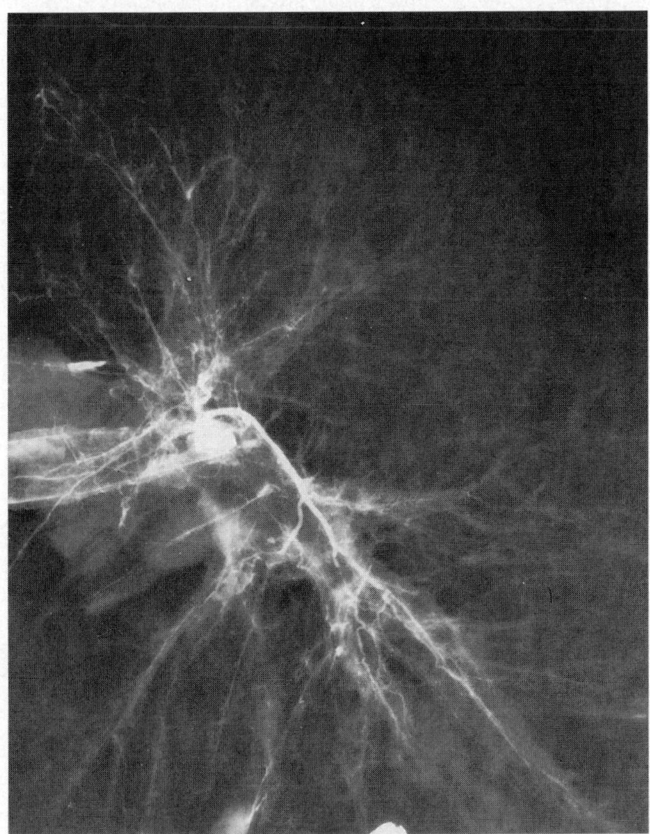

Fig. 4-9. Bronchial arteriogram.

PREPARATION OF PULMONARY VASCULAR AND BRONCHIAL CASTS

Polyvinyl Chloride Corrosion may yield excellent instructive casts. *Wood's metal,* a low-melting alloy of lead, tin, bismuth, and cadmium, also has been used for this purpose. Tissues for histologic study must be secured after plastic injection and before the lung tissue is destroyed by the corrosion. Details of the methods are supplied by the factories that sell the plastic. Principally, the injection methods resemble those used for angiography or bronchography. Again, the lungs should be injected in an inflated state. After the plastic has set, the casts are prepared by chemically dissolving the lungs (generally by immersing them for 1 or 2 d in concentrated hydrochloric acid or a 40% solution of potassium hydroxide).

Latex Injection does not require corrosion. The cast can be studied in relation to the surrounding tissues. Details of the methods again must be obtained from the factories that sell the latex mixtures.

MEASUREMENTS OF PULMONARY BLOOD AND AIR VOLUMES AND OTHER SPECIAL STUDIES

These methods were described in detail in the last edition of this book *(8)*; they played an important role in research conducted at that time. However, there is little current need for investigations of this type, either because the data already have been obtained or because more sophisticated in vivo methods are now available. In the studies described in the last edition, pulmonary air content, total pulmonary blood content, pulmonary arterial and venous blood volume, bronchial vascular blood volume, capillary blood volume, and physical properties such as tissue elasticity and surface tension were determined.

PARTICLE IDENTIFICATION

HISTOLOGIC ANALYSIS Many types of particles can be identified histologically if they are within the resolution limits of the light microscope. The "Particle Atlas" may be most helpful in such a situation *(14)* (unfortunately, no new edition is available). Inorganic particles can be isolated and concentrated for morphologic study by holding an unstained, uncovered paraffin section over a flame until the organic tissue has been incinerated.

QUANTITATIVE STUDIES In most cases, light microscopic observation with polarizing lenses provides sufficient semiquantitative information. However, for research purposes and other special circumstances, mineral particles in lung tissue can be analyzed quantitatively by a multitude of methods, either in bulk (macroanalytic) by X-ray diffraction, X-ray fluorescence, neutron activation analysis, atomic absorption spectroscopy, or proton-induced X-ray emission spectroscopy, or with microanalytic techniques such as energy-dispersive X-ray spectroscopy and wavelength dispersive X-ray spectroscopy. Many of the advanced methods of microprobe analysis such as ion microprobe mass spectrometry are not readily available. Experts such as Dr. Andrew Churg (The University of British Columbia, Vancouver Hospital, Vancouver, British Columbia) or Dr. Victor L. Roggli (Duke University School of Medicine, Durham, North Carolina) may provide helpful consultation. For an excellent review of these methods, *see* ref. *(15)*. It should be noted that the results of any quantitative method must be interpreted with some caution because particles tend to be distributed unevenly, which adversely affects the results of quantitative studies, particularly if the samples are small.

For the quantitative evaluation of asbestosis, ferruginous bodies are harvested from the fixed or unfixed lungs by digesting the tissue in 5.25% sodium hypochlorite. The solid residues are collected on membrane filters. The characteristic features of asbestos bodies allow reasonably accurate counts. For a detailed description of current digestion techniques and other methods of counting asbestos bodies, ref. *(16)* should be consulted. For the semiquantitative demonstration of asbestos bodies, dried scrapings from lung sections are often studied. Ferruginous bodies also can be viewed electron microscopically *(17)*.

REFERENCES

1. Lamprecht J, Hegemann S, Hauptmann S. Vorteile einer HNO-gebietsspezifischen Sektionstechnik. HNO 1994;42:233–235.
2. Maxeiner H, Dietz W. Anleitung für eine vollständige Kehlkopfpräparation. Zeitschrift für Rechtsmedizin. J Legal Med 1986;96: 11–16.
3. McCulloch TA, Rutty GN. Postmortem examination of the lungs: a preservation technique for opening the bronchi and pulmonary arteries individually without transsection problems. J Clin Pathol 1998; 51:163–164.
4. Barberà JA, Ramírez J, López FA, Roca J, Rodriguez-Roisin R. New design for fixation of surgically obtained lungs specimens. Path Res Pract 1989;184:630–634.
5. Ludwig J. Laboratory suggestion: cascade system for space-saving perfusion fixation of lungs. Am J Clin Pathol 1973;59:117–118.
6. Ludwig J, Ottman DM, Eichmann TJ. Methods in pathology: the preparation of native livers for morphologic studies. Modern Pathol 1994;7:790–793.
7. Hartung W. Gefrier-Groβschnitte von ganzen Organen, speziell der Lunge. Zentralbl Allg Pathol 1969;100:408–413.
8. Ludwig J. Current Methods of Autopsy Practice, 2nd ed. W.B. Saunders, Philadelphia, PA, 1979.
9. Heard BE. Pathology of pulmonary emphysema: methods of study. Am Rev Resp. Diseases 1960;82:792–799.
10. Gough J. Twenty years' experience of the technique of paper mounted sections. In: Liebow AA, Smith DE, eds. The Lung. Williams & Wilkins, Baltimore, MD, 1968, pp. 311–316.
11. Whimster EF. Rapid giant paper sections of lungs. Thorax 1989;24: 268–273.
12. Davies G, Reid L. Growth of the alveoli and pulmonary arteries in childhood. 1970;25:669–681.
13. Hendin AS, Greenspan RH. Ventilatory pumping of human pulmonary lymphatic vessels. Radiology 1973;108:553–557.
14. McCrone WC, Draftz RG, Delly JG. The Particle Atlas: A Photomicrographic Reference for the Microscopical Identification of Particulate Substances. Ann Arbor Science Publishers, Ann Arbor, MI, 1967.
15. Churg A, Green FHY. Analytic methods for identifying and quantifying mineral particles in lung tissues. In: Churg A, Green FHY, eds. Pathology of Occupational Lung Disease, 2nd ed. Williams and Wilkins, Baltimore, MD, 1998.
16. Roggli VL, Greenberg SD, Pratt PC. Pathology of Asbestos-Associated Diseases. Little, Brown and Company, Boston, MA, 1992.
17. Churg A, Sakoda N, Warnock ML. A simple method for preparing ferruginous bodies for electron microscopy. Am J Clin Pathol 1977; 68:513–517.

5 Esophagus and Abdominal Viscera

JURGEN LUDWIG

ESOPHAGUS

For the demonstration of tracheoesophageal fistulas or infiltrating tumors, the esophagus should be left attached to the mediastinal organs. Tracheoesophageal fistulas are demonstrated by opening the esophagus along its posterior wall and opening the trachea anteriorly (Chapter 4, Fig. 4-1). Infiltrating tumors are best demonstrated by cutting properly oriented sections through the previously fixed mediastinal organs. Intraluminal tumors or strictures are well-displayed on fixed specimens.

DEMONSTRATION OF ESOPHAGEAL VARICES

Mucosal Inversion and Injection The esophagus should be left attached to the stomach, which should be opened along the greater curvature. A string is tied to the upper end of the unopened esophagus and then pulled through the lumen to evert the esophagus. Varices will shine through the mucosa and are accentuated by subsequent formalin fixation.

The features can be further enhanced by injecting the varices with barium sulfate-gelatin, either directly or after inflating the veins with air. Unless autolytic changes are severe, points of hemorrhage are easily demonstrated by this method. It should be noted that in general, esophageal varices still can be successfully injected and roentgenographs prepared (Fig. 5-1) if the esophagus has not been inverted but opened conventionally, that is, lengthwise. Of course, some leakage must be expected at the free edges of the specimen.

Other Methods Air-drying and clearing techniques *(1–3)* have been used in the past, primarily to prepare museum specimens (Fig. 5-2). They are probably no longer practiced and shall not be described here further.

DEMONSTRATION OF LOWER ESOPHAGEAL RINGS

Lower esophageal rings (Schatzki rings) can be palpated or objectively demonstrated by roentgenography *(4)*. The lower half of the esophagus is removed with the upper half of the stomach and an attached ring of diaphragm. The stomach is clamped across the corpus. The preparation is then filled and slightly distended with a mixture of barium sulfate and 10% formalin solution. Roentgenograms should be prepared as soon as possible after death. Subsequently, the specimen should be fixed in the distended state. We suspend it in a formalin tank until it is to be cut.

This method also can be used for other types of strictures and stenoses of the esophagus.

STOMACH

The stomach routinely is opened along the greater curvature. Penetrating ulcers or infiltrating tumors are best displayed by fixing and sectioning the stomach together with the pancreas, a portion of the liver, or whatever the infiltrated tissue might be. Tumors with predominantly intraluminal growth and the associated obstruction can be displayed after formalin fixation of the unopened specimen and subsequent dissection. The stomach is inflated with formalin while it is suspended in a formalin bath. Microscopic studies of the mucosa or macroscopic staining methods for intestinal metaplasia *(5)* often are unsatisfactory because of autolytic changes.

ARTERIOGRAPHY For gastric arteriography, the organs supplied by the celiac artery should be removed en masse. The splenic and hepatic arteries are tied as far distally as possible. A barium preparation is injected through the celiac artery. After injection, the stomach is isolated, opened *along the middle of the anterior surface* parallel with the longitudinal axis of the organ, spread out on an X-ray plate, and roentgenographed.

INTESTINAL TRACT

In the presence of tumors or other pathologic lesions involving the duodenum, papilla of Vater, head of pancreas, or hepatoduodenal ligament, the duodenum should be opened *in situ*. Precise orientation may become impossible after removal of these organs. This is particularly important in postoperative autopsies.

Routinely, the intestinal tract is opened with an enterotome, that is, large scissors with one blunted branch that lies in the lumen of the intestine. The procedure is greatly facilitated when the mesentery has been cut close to the wall of the small intestine. The specimen usually is opened in a sink under running water. If possible, specimens for histologic study should be obtained before they are exposed to tap water. We no longer use or recommend the use of the stationary enterotome, illustrated in the last edition, mainly because of the risk of injury during cleaning of this instrument.

From: *Handbook of Autopsy Practice,* 3rd Ed. Edited by: J. Ludwig © Humana Press Inc., Totowa, NJ

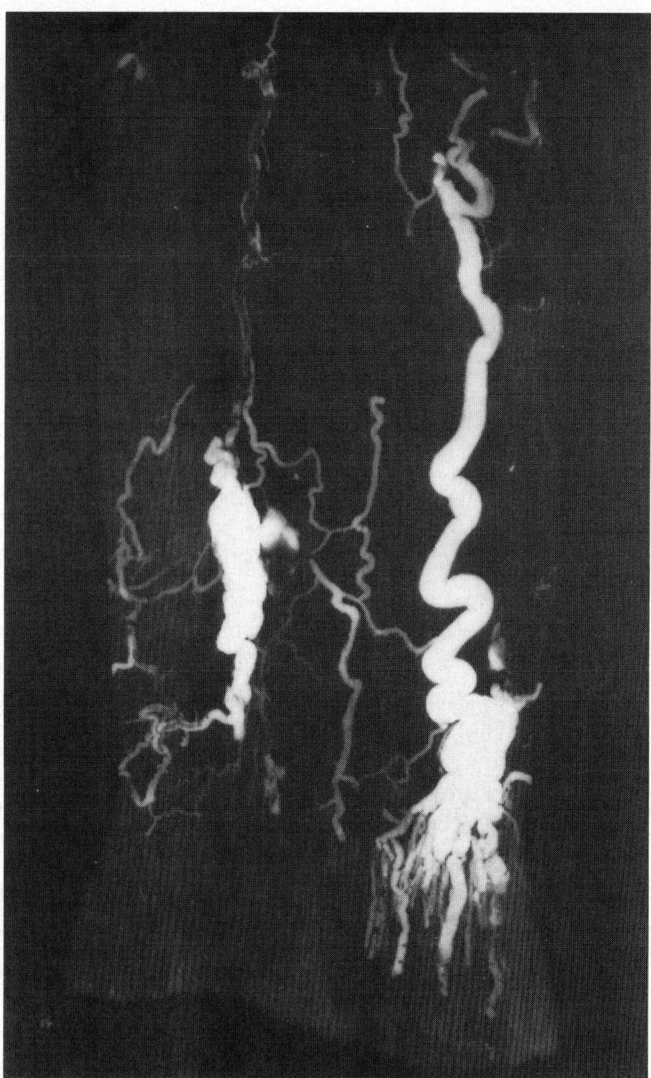

Fig. 5-1. Esophageal varices, injected with barium sulfate-gelatine mixture. Varices stand out and are white; the features are enhanced in a roentgenogram.

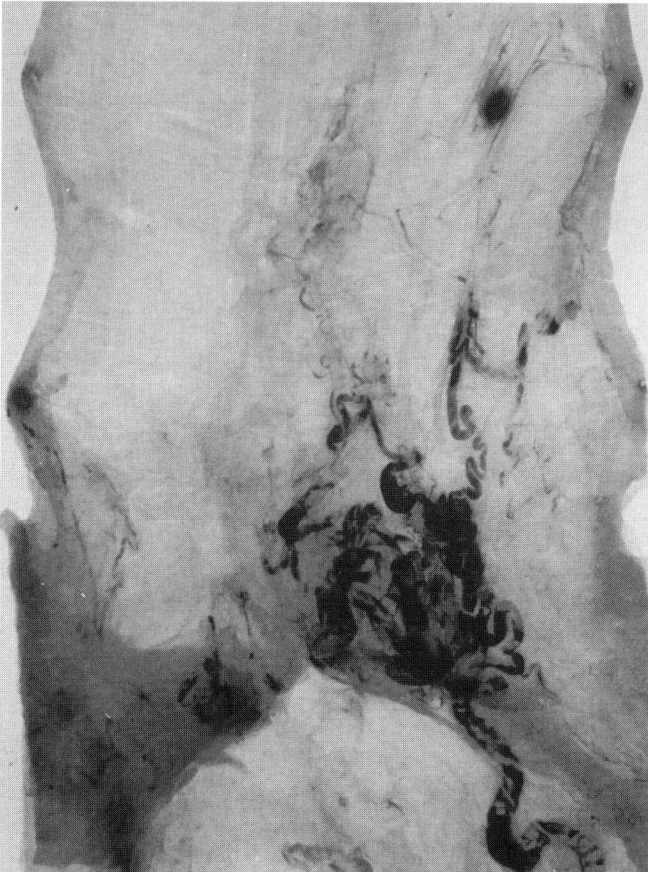

Fig. 5-2. Esophageal varices in cleared specimen. The mucosal layer has been stripped from the muscularis and cleared in benzene, as described in ref. *(2)*.

A tumor with predominantly intraluminal growth and its associated obstruction can be displayed after formalin fixation of the unopened specimen and subsequent dissection. A glass tube at the hose from an elevated formalin container is simply tied into the hollow viscus; the other end is clamped or tied off. The whole preparation is suspended in a formalin bath.

For proper histologic orientation, long strips of gastric or intestinal mucosa can be cut parallel with the long axis of the organ, fixed, and embedded in a spiral fashion, for example, with the proximal end at the center. Isolated histologic specimens of gastrointestinal tract should always be fixed on corkboard or cardboard to keep the samples flat. This will allow embedding and cutting the specimens properly on edge.

PRESERVATION OF SMALL INTESTINAL MUCOSA The small bowel is tied at the duodenojejunal junction and at the terminal ileum close to the cecum. A cannula is inserted into the most superficial presenting loop of the small intestine. Concentrated formalin (40% formaldehyde) solution is instilled through the cannula until the small bowel is distended. During this procedure, the small intestine should be handled as little as possible. The formalin-filled bowel should be left untouched as long as possible. The bowel is then removed and soaked for another 24 h in 10% formalin solution. Satisfactory results can be expected if the fixation is begun within 6 h after death *(6)*.

PREPARATION OF SPECIMENS FOR STUDY UNDER DISSECTING MICROSCOPE Postmortem autolysis causes the loss of intestinal epithelium. Thus, the dissecting microscope often shows villi that appear thinner than the ones seen on biopsy specimens. The openings of the crypts become more prominent. In spite of these differences, the extent and character of abnormal mucosal patterns can easily be evaluated with a dissecting microscope.

Specimens can be viewed after they have been rinsed in saline or they can be processed further *(7)* by pinning square pieces of corkboard, and fixing them in buffered 10% formalin solution. After at least 24 h of fixation, the specimens are put into one change of 70% alcohol and two changes of 95% alcohol for 2 h each. The specimens are stained with 5% alcoholic eosin for 4 min and subsequently treated with two changes of absolute alcohol for 2 h each. The fixed stained and dehydrated intestinal wall is placed in xylol. The preparation is now ready

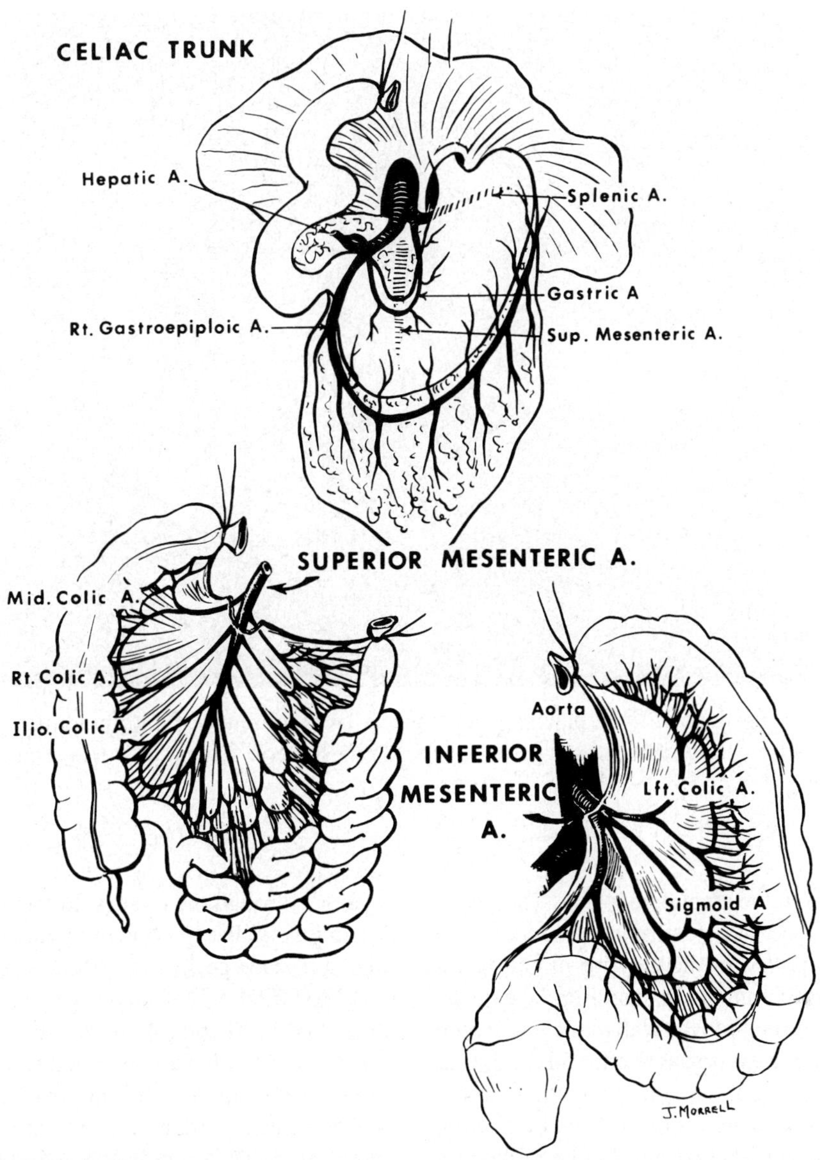

Fig. 5-3. Partitioned abdominal viscera for celiac and mesenteric arteriography. *Celiac trunk specimen*: Note rotation and upward sweep of duodenum. Root of superior mesenteric artery remains with celiac artery but is hidden behind pancreas. *Superior mesenteric artery specimen*: This includes intestine from middle of first jejunal loop to middle of transverse colon. *Inferior mesenteric artery specimen*: This extends from middle transverse colon to anus; pelvic viscera (uterus and bladder) are attached. Adapted from ref. *(9)*.

for examination. Unstained specimens or specimens stained with a hematoxylin-alum solution *(8)* also can be studied.

DRY PRESERVATION Air-drying or paraffin infiltration yields interesting permanent museum specimens. After rinsing the unopened bowel with saline, glass tubes are tied into both ends. One tube is connected to a tank with compressed air, the other tube is connected to a rubber hose that can be slowly clamped while the air inflated the organ. After 1–3 d, air-drying is completed. No fixation is necessary. Lesions such as diverticula are well-displayed by this method but again, histologic specimens become unsatisfactory and interest in this technique has waned.

MESENTERIC ANGIOGRAPHY The celiac, superior mesenteric, or inferior mesenteric artery can be injected with a barium sulfate-gelatin mixture, either *in situ* or after en block removal of the abdominal viscera. If all three vessels are injected (Fig. 5-3), the abdominal organ block must be partitioned so that the three vascular compartments can be displayed properly *(9)*.

Clearing methods and India ink or latex injection techniques are largely obsolete.

LIVER AND HEPATODUODENAL LIGAMENT

Before removal of the liver, the hepatoduodenal ligament should be dissected. First, the common bile duct is incised and

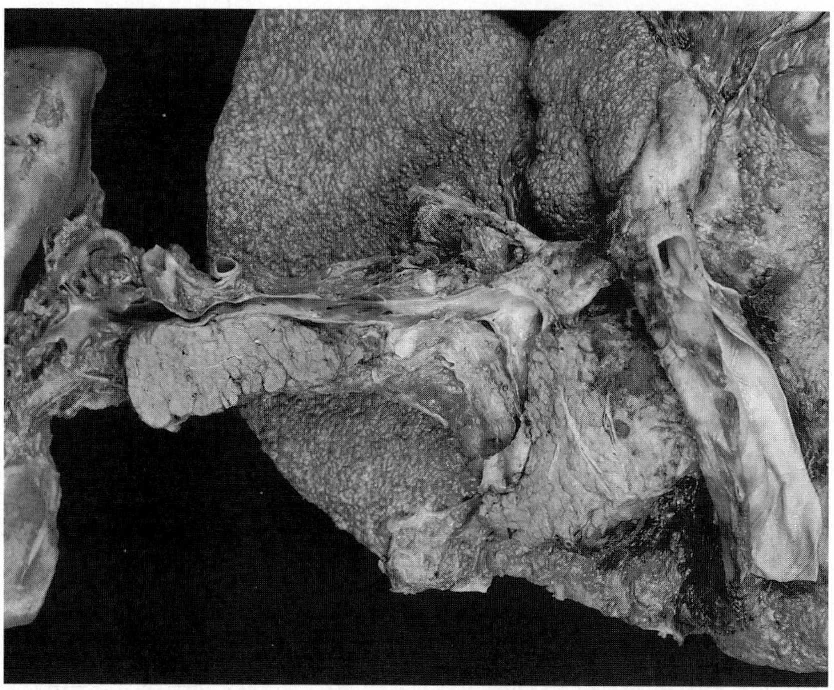

Fig. 5-4. Posterior view of portions of liver, pancreas, and spleen. Note presence of micronodular cirrhosis. The splenic vein has been opened and the confluence with the portal vein the superior mesenteric vein is shown, together with the partially opened inferior vena cava.

opened toward the hilus and the ampulla of Vater. The lowermost portion of the common bile duct runs retroduodenally. The duodenum must be pulled in the anterior direction and somewhat to the left if the common bile duct is to be exposed in its full length without cutting into the wall of the duodenum. Again, the best specimens can be prepared after formalin fixation. In fetuses and newborns, dissection of the common bile duct is difficult, and its patency is easier to check by opening the duodenum and observing whether bile can be milked out through the papilla. This is a useful test, particularly when biliary atresia is suspected.

The hepatic artery lies to the left of the common bile duct and can easily be dissected from the anterior aspect of the hepatoduodenal ligament. For the demonstration of the portal vein and its tributaries or of the inferior vena cava, dissection from the posterior aspect gives the most instructive results (Fig. 5-4). In these instances, en bloc or en masse removal (page 3) is recommended.

SLICING It is almost impossible to slice livers with normal-sized knives without leaving knife marks on the cut surface. Smooth cut sections of cirrhotic livers are even more difficult to prepare. We use a knife with a 78-cm blade (its use for lungs is illustrated Chapter 4, Fig. 4-5), which in most instances permits slicing of the whole organ with an uninterrupted pulling motion.

Usually, the liver is sliced in the frontal plane, each slice being about 2 cm thick. The hilar structures may remain attached to one of the central slices. However, it is sometimes necessary to expose, on one cut section, a large parenchymatous surface or leave the hilar structures intact. In these instances, horizontal sections through the liver is the methods of choice (Fig. 5-5). We routinely slice livers in this manner if they had been prefixed in our cascade perfusion system (*see* below).

FIXATION The cascade perfusion system for lungs that is described in Chapter 4, works also very well with surgically removed livers that are obtained from the liver transplant program. The failure rate with autopsy livers is greater than the rate with surgically obtained livers, undoubtedly because of postmortem clotting. Nevertheless, if the recently described methods are applied properly, many autopsy livers can be fixed successfully with this machine. For the preparation of large histologic sections, perfusion fixation of the whole liver yields the best results. If large slices of fresh livers are placed in a formalin bath, the fixative often does not penetrate deep enough. If the slices are only 3–4 mm thick, they fix readily but usually with considerable distortion.

GROSS STAINING FOR IRON This method *(11)* is used particularly in cases of genetic hemochromatosis. Excessive hemosiderin storage in other organs (pancreas, myocardium) also can be demonstrated by this technique. The actual staining procedure is described in Chapter 14, page 133.

HEPATIC ARTERIOGRAPHY, PORTAL VENOGRAPHY, AND CHOLANGIOGRAPHY Barium sulfate gelatin mixtures give excellent results. For angiography, it is safe to remove the liver together with the diaphragm, the hepatoduodenal ligament, and a long segment of inferior vena cava. Vessels or bile ducts can be injected with contrast medium either before or after perfusion fixation. Fig. 5-6 (A) shows nozzles that are needed for the infusion of the contrast medium. The figure (Fig. 5-6, B) shows such a nozzle in place. After the vessels

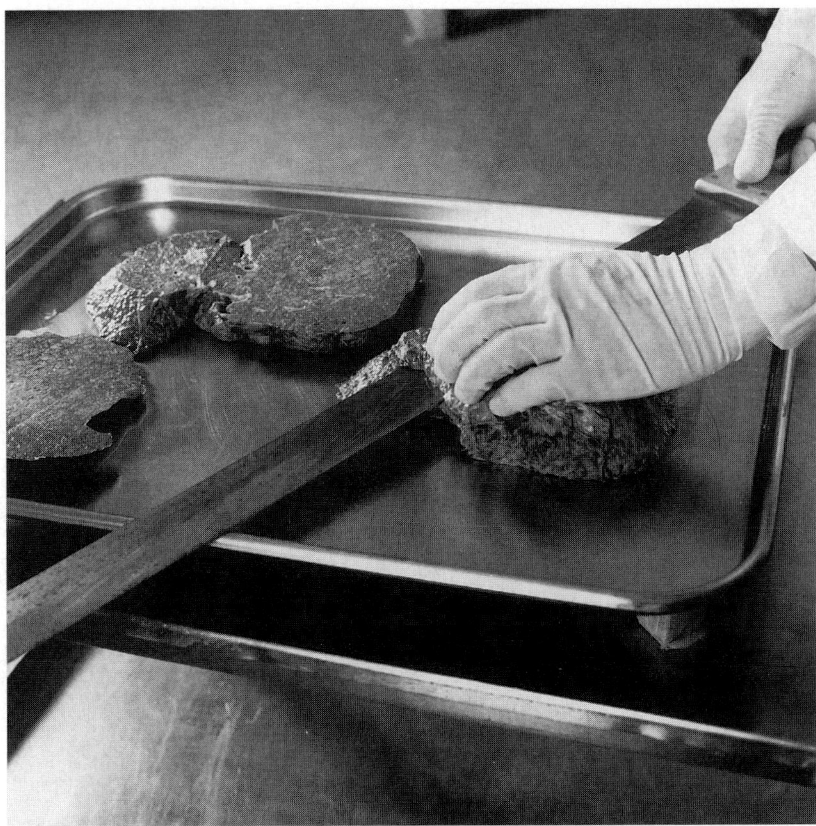

Fig. 5-5. Cutting a perfusion-fixed liver in a horizontal plane. Note that the rims of the metal tray are used to guide the long-bladed knife. Adapted with permission from ref. *(10)*.

have been cannulated, blood and blood clots are flushed out with saline. Cholangiography is facilitated if a sufficiently long sleeve of the common hepatic duct remains attached so that a cannula can easily be tied into the lumen. Removal of the gallbladder prior to cholangiography may lead to leakage of contrast medium from the gallbladder bed and therefore it may be better to fill the gallbladder together with the bile ducts (Fig. 5-7); it can be removed after the gelatin has solidified. If the contrast mixture has a low gelatin content and thus low viscosity, small vessels and ducts (below 100 µm diameter) can be filled. In autopsy livers, cholangiography sometimes leads to simultaneous filling of portal vein branches, probably because of autolytic changes. This is not observed in surgically removed livers.

For the preparation of hepatic venograms, see below under "Renal Venography."

Preparation of Corrosion Casts Vinylite corrosion and Latex injection are the most commonly used methods. Differently colored media often were used to identify the various vascular compartments and the bile ducts. Details of the methods are supplied by the factories that sell the plastic.

GALLBLADDER

To avoid spilling of bile and the discoloration of organs, the gallbladder usually is removed from its bed intact and opened in a fine-meshed strainer over a collecting vessel. If liver and gallbladder are to be fixed in a block, it is advisable to first remove the bile from the unopened gallbladder with a syringe. Before the tissue block is submerged in the formalin bath, the gallbladder and the extrahepatic bile ducts are partially opened and stuffed with formalin-soaked cotton in order to preserve the normal shape of the structures. The cystic duct is very difficult to dissect because of its numerous folds.

Gallstones sometimes can be cut fresh but often need a 24-h fixation period in concentrated formalin to harden them sufficiently. If the stones are too hard to cut, a fine scroll saw may be needed to prepare an instructive cut surface.

PANCREAS

The parenchyma usually is best exposed by cutting the organ in the frontal plane. Parallel sagittal sections are preferred when the pancreatic duct is dilated. When only one routine section of pancreatic tissue is to be studied, the tail of the pancreas is usually selected because of the abundance of islets in this region. For the demonstration of lipomatosis, a slice can be stained with Sudan III (*see* page 133). For the accentuation of fat tissue necroses, a slice of formalin-fixed tissue is placed in a copper acetate solution. After 1 d in the incubator or several days at room temperature, the fat tissue necroses turn blue green *(12)*.

Arteriograms require injection of the celiac and superior mesenteric artery system, as described earlier. The retrograde

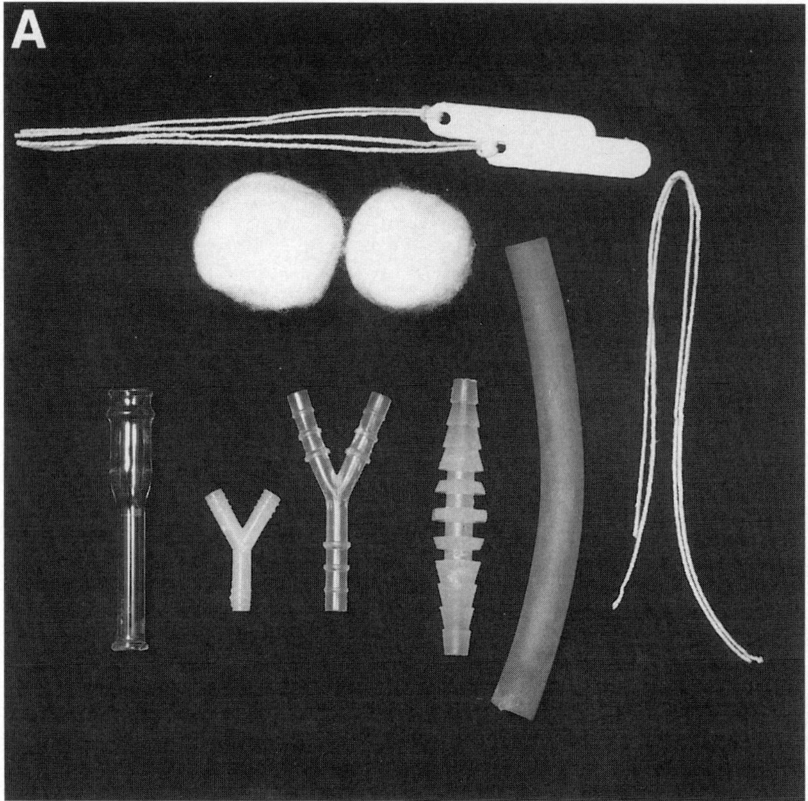

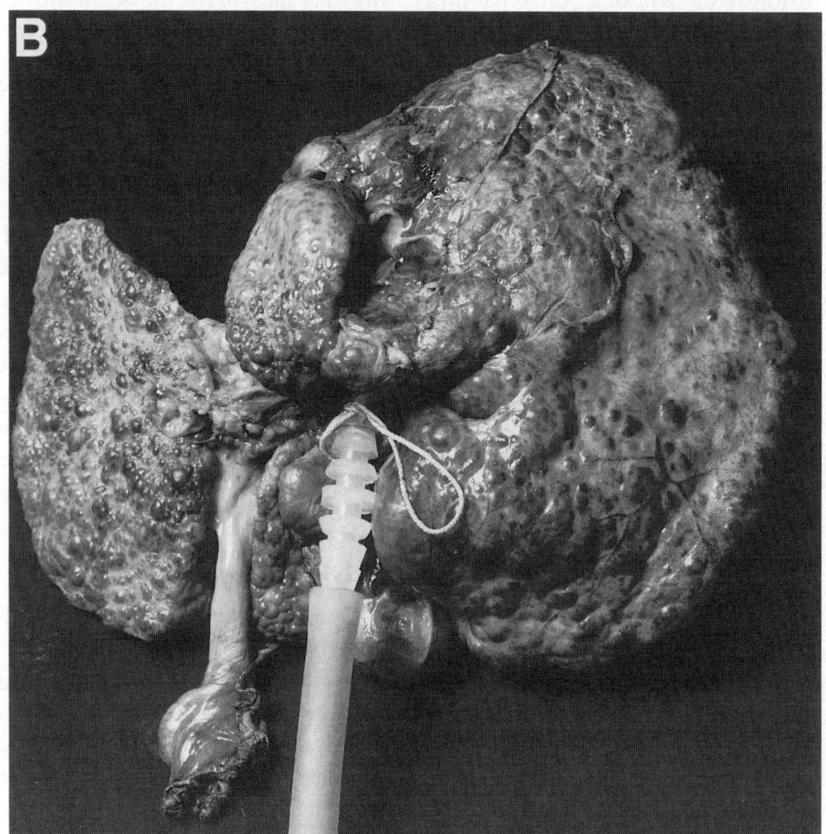

Fig. 5-6. Preparation for angiography and cholangiography. (**A**) Straight and bifurcated nozzles for hilar vessels and bile ducts; rubber hose for attaching specimens to perfusion apparatus, cotton wads for plugging hepatic veins, and ligature with needle to secure nozzles. Two identification tags are also shown. (**B**) Cirrhotic liver with nozzle tied into portal vein. Adapted with permission from ref. *(10)*.

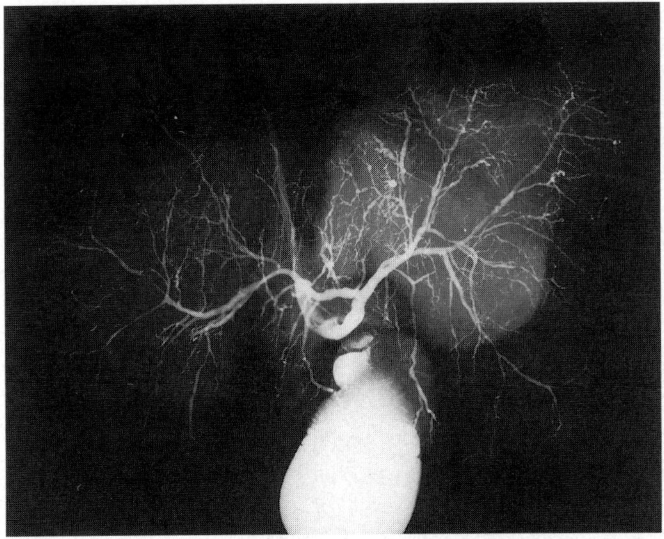

Fig. 5-7. Postmortem specimen cholangiogram. Note that in this case, the gallbladder has been left in place and is filled with contrast medium.

injection of radiopaque medium from the papilla of Vater provides excellent roentgenograms of the pancreatic duct system. The pancreatograms show concrements and other duct abnormalities quite clearly *(13)*.

SPLEEN

Frontal or horizontal sections are prepared, by the same principles used for sectioning the liver. Formalin perfusion of the intact organ through the splenic vessels has proved unsatisfactory unless the blood has been previously removed (*see* below). Some areas tend to remain unfixed. If formalin fixation is intended, care must be taken that the slices are very thin. Fixative does not penetrate well into the splenic pulp. The splenic reticulum is best studied by washing the blood out of the pulp. This also facilitates fixation of the whole organ. The spleen is first perfused through the splenic artery or vein with 0.9% saline. If the injection pressure is about 100 mm Hg, the splenic pulp will turn white after about 1 h. The perfusion is now continued with 10% formalin solution. In some instances it may be useful to fix the organ at more than its normal volume by tying the efferent vessels.

Injection into the celiac artery or directly into the splenic artery is used for splenic arteriography.

URINARY AND GENITAL SYSTEM

KIDNEYS AND URETERS Renal vessels usually are opened lengthwise from the aorta or inferior vena cava to the hilus. We routinely incise the kidneys *in situ*. The fibrous and adipose capsule is tripped, using the unsevered renal vessels as anchor. This prevents the organs from slipping out of one's hand after they have been removed from the retroperitoneal fat tissue. The kidneys are then excised from their convexity toward the hilus, exposing the renal pelvis. During this procedure the organ can be held in a firm grip by applying some tension to the renal vessels.

The ureters are opened lengthwise, starting from the renal pelvis and, if necessary, cutting through some undissected parenchyma at the lower pole of the kidneys. The renal vessels and ureters can now be severed, or the kidneys can be removed together with the aorta, inferior vena cava, and pelvic organs. Blocks for histologic examination should include renal cortex, medulla with a papilla, and a portion of the renal pelvis.

If retroperitoneal disease processes involve more than one organ, for example, after rupture of abdominal aortic aneurysms or after renal cell carcinomas have spread into veins (Fig. 5-8) it may be necessary to remove an organ block for proper dissection.

Perfusion Fixation A cannula is tied into the renal artery and the kidneys are perfused with 10% formalin solution. Because the renal veins often contain blood clots, perfusion with 0.9% saline, followed after 20 min by perfusion with 7% formalin-saline has been recommended *(14)*.

Renal Arteriography Arteriograms can be prepared in situ (Fig. 5-9), after en block removal of the abdominal aorta and kidneys, or on isolated organs. Clinical contrast media or barium sulfate-gelatin mixtures give excellent results. A catheter is tied into the celiac artery *in situ* or after removal of the organ block and all nonrenal arteries are tied and both ends of the aorta are clamped.

Renal Venography The techniques are essentially similar to the ones used for arteriography. We have prepared *in situ* venograms by injection of contrast medium into a segment of the inferior vena cava that was sealed off by inflatable cuffs (Fig. 5-10). The tube with the cuffs can be introduced from the iliac or femoral veins without handling of the inferior vena cava system. By moving the cuffs higher, excellent *hepatic venograms* can be prepared.

Urography Retrograde urograms are easy to prepare with any of the conventional contrast media. The ureter is cannulated either from the urinary bladder or through the wall of the distal ureter. This can be particularly helpful for the detection of congenital urethral valves (Figs. 5-11 and 5-12).

Preparation of Plastic Casts Plastic casts can be used for the demonstration of the renal vasculature, the pelvic system, and cysts or other abnormal cavities. The methods are similar to those described for other organs. Again, the instructions supplied by the manufacturer should be followed carefully.

PELVIC ORGANS Intravascular formalin injection or freezing methods have been used to harden pelvic organs in their natural position *(16)*. The vascular system of the pelvic can be injected from the internal iliac artery. Corrosion specimens are prepared by the usual techniques.

Urinary Bladder Fixation in the distended position is achieved by injecting formalin solution through a catheter. Urine in the bladder must be removed first. The urinary bladder is left intact until fixation is completed. The upper half of the bladder is then removed and the base of the bladder is exposed. This technique is particularly recommended in cases of benign prostatic hyperplasia with urethral obstruction or urinary bladder tumors in the area of the trigone. Some tumors or abscesses are better exposed by frontal sections through the base of the urinary bladder and prostate.

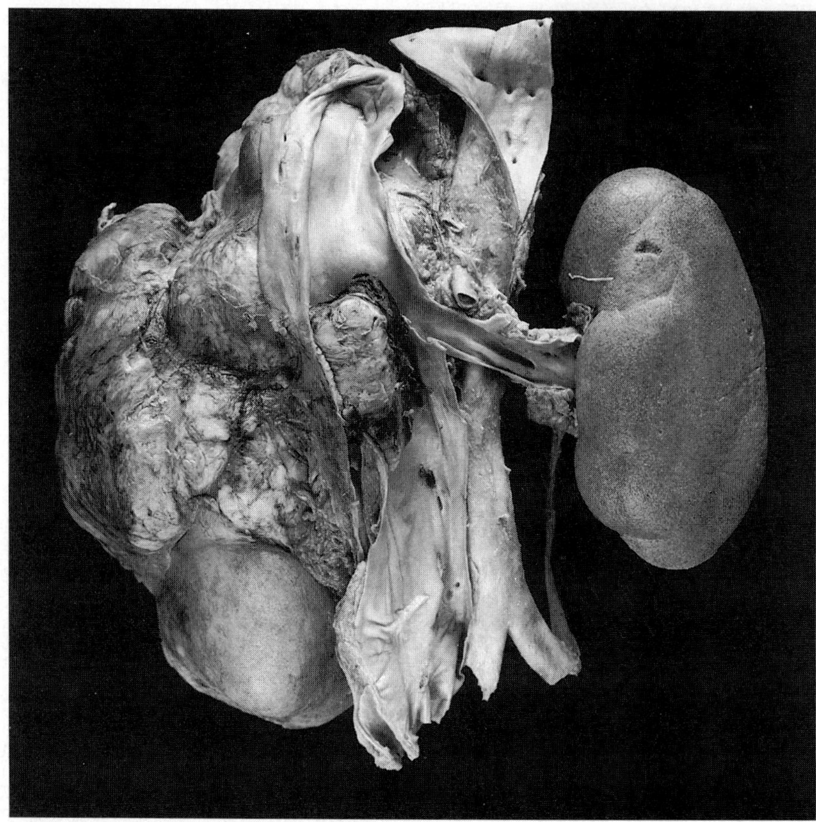

Fig. 5-8. Anterior view of kidneys, inferior vena cava, and abdominal aorta. Note renal cell carcinoma in upper pole of right kidney and large tumor nodule in the lumen of the inferior vena cava, just below the entrance of the left renal vein.

Penis and Male Urethra Most pathologists do not routinely dissect these organs. Congenital urethral valves (Figs. 5-11 and 5-12), strictures, and tumors are the main indications for study. The penis, usually without surrounding skin, should be left attached to the urinary bladder. This can be achieved by either sawing out a portion of the pubic bone or by pulling the penis through the pubic arch. These maneuvers require preparatory dissection of soft tissue and appropriate incisions of the skin of the penis. The urethra should be opened lengthwise in the anterior midline. Histologic sections through urethra and corpora cavernosa are usually taken in a frontal plane, that is, perpendicular to the axis of the urethra.

Urethra valves can best be located by injecting radiopaque material into the urinary bladder (Fig. 5-11). The urethra should then be opened along the anterior midline against the direction of the flow of urine (Fig. 5-12). This will help prevent laceration of the delicate valves.

Fixation of the corpora cavernosa can be achieved by injecting formalin solution or gelatin-formalin through the vena dorsalis penis.

Uterus The pregnant uterus can be fixed by first puncturing the uterus through the anterior abdominal wall and replacing the amniotic fluid with formalin solution. After the prefixed uterus has been opened, the fetus is perfused with formalin solution through the umbilical cord. If one intends to preserve uterus and fetus as one specimen, a formalin-gelatin mixture is injected into the cavity of the uterus.

Placenta In some institutions the placenta is routinely discarded. Autopsy pathologists should discourage such practices, especially with autopsies on stillbirths (*see* Part II, "Stillbirth") and neonates. In these cases, pathologists always need to study the placenta also. The following procedures for gross examination are suggested *(17,18)*.

First, the placenta should be weighed because both low placental weight and overweight placentas generally are associated with other fetal or neonatal abnormalities *(19)*. For expected placental weights, see Part III, Appendix (page 556). If the placenta cannot be studied further after delivery, it should be stored in a closed container in the refrigerator. If one wants to ascertain the original position of the placenta by demonstrating the site of the uterine cornua and the point of rupture of the membranes, one can begin the examination with the reconstruction, in a tank of saline, of the fetal membranous bag. The narrowest width of membranes is measured. If there are no velamentous vessels, the bag is trimmed from the placenta. A sausage-shaped roll of membrane is fixed for histologic study, with the site of the rupture innermost. The cord is then measured and its surface and cross-sections inspected; the vessels are counted on cross-sections. A segment of the umbilical cord is fixed for histologic study. After the cord is cut near its insertion and the

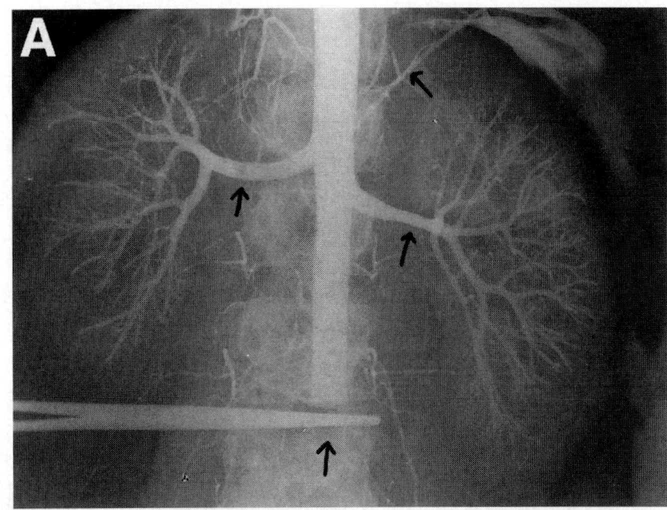

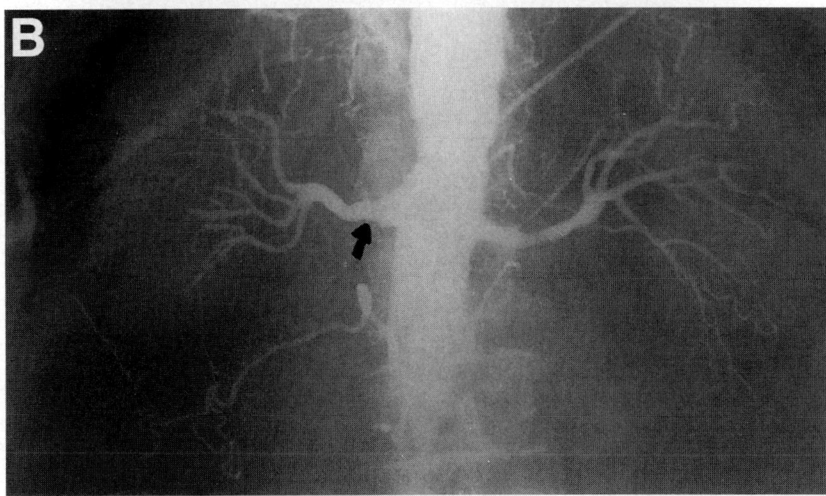

Fig. 5-9. *In situ* renal arteriograms. (**A**) Polyethylene catheter in superior mesenteric artery. Main renal arteries had minimal histologic evidence of atherosclerosis (arrows). Cross-clamping of aorta is evident at base of film (arrow). (**B**) Evidence of narrowing in both renal arteries but more pronounced in right renal artery (arrow). Histologically, stenosis was graded as severe. Adapted with permission from ref. *(15)*.

membranes removed, the placenta is weighed and measured. The placenta should be kept moist. The fetal and maternal surfaces are inspected. The yolk sac is searched for. If cotyledons are missing, milk injection (*see* below) or other injection procedures help to distinguish true tissue defects from artifacts of handling. The placenta is then cut into thin slices with a long-bladed knife. Blood is wiped off and the cut surfaces are inspected. Grossly abnormal areas are placed in Bouin's solution for histologic study; after a few hours, the tissue is trimmed and refixed. Routinely, three section are taken from central areas of the placenta where chorionic vessels can be included.

The examination of *placentas in multiple pregnancies* requires special precautions. A longitudinal strip is cut from the portion of fusion or approximation of the membranous sacs, leaving the placenta intact, and a roll is prepared for histologic study. (One also can prepare a "T-section"—that is, an area of fused twin placenta with dividing membranes extending above that may show two amnions or two amnions and two chorions. Unfortunately, T-sections interfere with subsequent vascular injection.) The dividing membranes are then peeled apart with the aid of forceps. If two chorions are present, separation attempts will disrupt villous placental tissue. The placenta is now weighed and measured.

Vascular injection is necessary to separate the vascular beds of the fused dichorionic placenta. Injections also are used to decide whether vascular communications exist and to determine their nature and number. Because of artifactual villous disruptions, usually only selected areas can be injected, using milk or other injection media. Shunts are absent in all dichorial twins but will be seen in almost all monochorial twin placentas. The "vascular equator" can be identified after the amniotic membranes have been stripped. At various sites in this area, milk is injected into arteries near presumed common vascular channels. About 30–50 mL of milk usually is necessary at each site to determine whether fluid returns to the same infant or its partner through anastomoses. During the injection, blood must be allowed to escape from where the umbilical cords have been cut near their insertions.

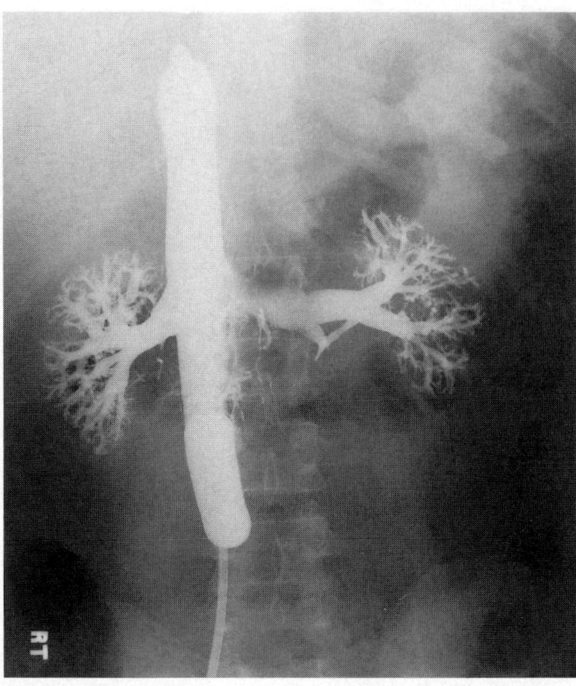

Fig. 5-10. Normal renal venogram. Rubber tube with two inflatable cuffs was introduced to seal off inferior vena cava above and below renal veins. Barium sulfate-gelatin mixture was injected through midportion of tube. There is also filling of lumbar, prevertebral, adrenal, and left testicular veins.

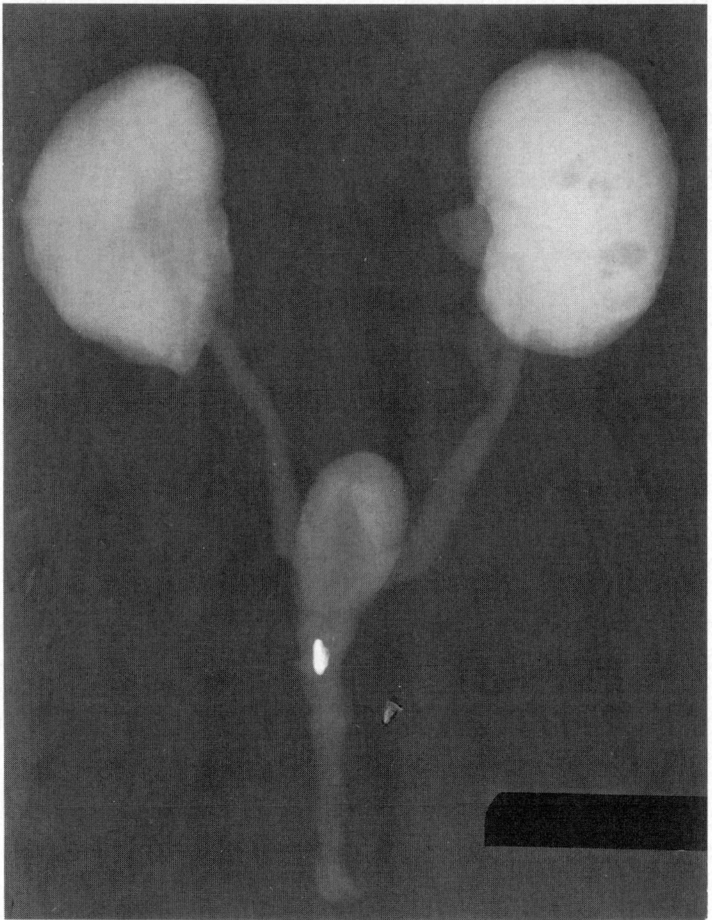

Fig. 5-11. Urogram in patient with congenital urethral valves. Some radiopaque material was injected into the urinary bladder and attempts were made to squeeze it onto the urethra. The radiograph shows that this was not possible.

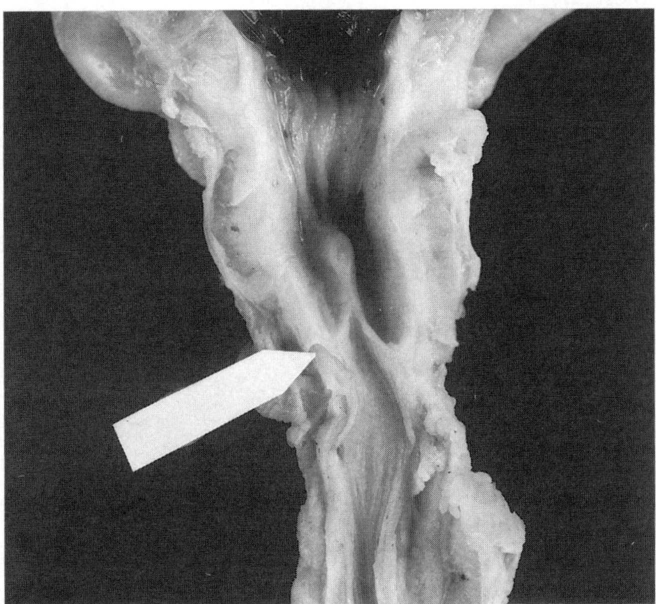

Fig. 5-12. Urethra with congenital valves. The penis and urinary bladder have been removed in continuity as described in the text, and opened in the anterior midline. The arrow shows the delicate urethral valves.

REFERENCES

1. Abramowsky CR, Gonzalvo AA. Postmortem demonstration of esophageal varices by a simple method. Am J Clin Pathol 1975;64: 672–677.
2. Chomet B, Gach BM. Demonstration of esophageal varices in museum specimens. Am J Clin Pathol 1969;51:793–794.
3. Chomet B, Hart LM, Reindl FJ. Demonstration of esophageal varices by simple technique. Arch Pathol 1960;69:185–187.
4. Goyal RK, Glancy JJ, Spiro HM. Lower esophageal ring (first of two parts). N Engl J Med 1970;282:1298–1305.
5. Stemmermann GN, Hayashi T. Intestinal metaplasia of the gastric mucosa: a gross and microscopic study of its distribution in various disease states. J Natl Cancer Inst 1968;41:627–634.
6. Wilson JP. Post-mortem preservation of the small intestine. J Pathol 1966;92:229–230.
7. Loehry CA, Creamer B. Post-mortem study of small-intestinal mucosa. BMJ 1966;1:827–829.
8. Dymock JW, Gray B. Staining method for the examination of the small intestinal villous pattern in necropsy material. 1968;21:748–749.
9. Reiner L. Mesenteric vascular occlusion studied by postmortem injection of the mesenteric arterial circulation. In: Sommers S, ed. Pathologic Annual 1966, vol. I. Appleton-Century-Crofts, New York, 1966, pp. 193–220.
10. Ludwig J, Ottman DM, Eichmann TJ. The preparation of native livers for morphological studies. Mod Pathol 1994;7:790-793.
11. Pulvertaft RJV. Museum techniques: a review. J Clin Pathol 1950; 3:1–23.
12. Benda C. Eine makro- und mikrochemische Reaction der Fettgewebs-Nekrose. Virchows Arch [Pathol Anat] 1900;161:194–198.
13. Schmitz-Moormann P, Himmelmann GW, Brandes J-W, Fölsch UR, Lorenz-Meyer H, Malchow H, et al. Comparative radiological and morphological study of human pancreas. Pancreatitis like changes in postmortem ductograms and their morphologic pattern. Possible implications for ERCP. Gut 1985;26:406–414.
14. Tracy RE, Overll EO. Arterioles of perfusion-fixed hypertensive and aged kidneys. Arch Pathol 1966;82:526–534.
15. Holley KE, Hunt JC, Brown AL Jr, Kincaid OW, Sheps SG. Renal artery stenosis: a clinical-pathologic study in normotensive and hypertensive patients. Am J Med 1964;37:14-22.
16. Loeschke H, Weinnoldt H. Methoden zur morphologischen Untersuchung des Genitalapparates, Nebennieren. In: Abderhalden E. Handbuch der biologischen Arbeitsmethoden, vol. VIII, part I (I). Urban & Schwarzenberg, Berlin, 1924, pp. 651–660.
17. Benirschke K. Examination of the placenta. In: Race GJ, ed. Laboratory Medicine, vol. 3. Harper & Row, Hagerstown, MD, 1974.
18. Benirschke K, Kaufmann P. The Pathology of the Human Placenta. Springer-Verlag, New York, 1995.
19. Naeye RL. Do placental weights have clinical significance? Hum Pathol 1987;387–391.

6 Nervous System

CATERINA GIANNINI AND HARUO OKAZAKI

REMOVAL OF BRAIN IN ADULTS

INCISION OF SCALP The head is elevated slightly with a wooden block or a metal headrest attached to the autopsy table. The hair is parted with a comb along an imaginary coronal plane connecting one mastoid with the other over the convexity (Fig. 6-1). A sharp scalpel blade can then be used to cut through the whole thickness of the scalp from the outside. The incision should start on the right side of the head (the "viewing-side" in most American funeral parlors) just behind the earlobe, as low as possible without extending below the earlobe, and extend to the comparable level on the other side. This will make reflection of the scalp considerably easier. Sufficient tissue should be left behind the ear to permit easy sewing of the incision by the mortician.

The anterior and posterior halves of the scalp are then reflected forward and backward, respectively, after short undercutting of the scalp with a sharp knife, which permits grasping of the edges with the hands. The use of a dry towel draped over the scalp edges facilitates further reflection, usually without the aid of cutting instruments. If the reflection is difficult, a scalpel blade can be used to cut the loose connective tissue that lags behind the reflecting edge as the other hand continues to peel the scalp. The knife edge should be directed toward the skull and not toward the scalp. The anterior flap is reflected to a level 1 or 2 cm above the supraorbital ridge. The posterior flap is reflected down to a level just above the occipital protuberance.

SAWING OF CRANIUM The cranium is best opened with an oscillating saw. Because aerolization of bone dust poses a risk of infection (*see* Chapter 16), the procedure should be done within a protective device such as inside a plastic bag *(1,2)*. (Fig. 6-2) Alternatively, a handsaw can be used, especially for cases of suspected Creutzfeldt-Jakob disease *(3,4)*. Various saw cuts are in use but we recommend the method illustrated in Fig. 6-3; the configuration of the saw cut minimizes slippage of the skull cap during restoration of the head by the embalmer. Naturally, the saw cut may have to be modified after some neurosurgical procedure(s) or in the presence of skull fracture(s). The temporalis muscle should be cut with a sharp knife and cleared from the intended path of the saw blade.

From: *Handbook of Autopsy Practice,* 3rd Ed. Edited by: J. Ludwig © Humana Press Inc., Totowa, NJ

Ideally, sawing should be stopped just short of cutting through the inner table of the cranium, which will easily give way with the use of a chisel and a light blow with a mallet. Leaving the dura and underlying leptomeninges intact allows to view the brain with the overlying cerebrospinal fluid (CSF) still in the subarachnoid space. To obtain this view, after removal of the skull cap, the dura must be cut with a pair of scissors along the line of sawing and reflected.

To protect the brain, the extended index finger of the hand that holds the neck of the oscillating saw should gauge the distance of the blade penetration. The oscillating blade should be moved from side to side during cutting to avoid deep penetration in a given area. Our saw (Lipshaw Co.) is equipped with a guard (*see* Chapter 8) and can be used with little training, without fear of deep penetration.

The frontal point of sawing should start approx two fingerbreadths above the supraorbital ridge. While the lateral aspects of the skull are being cut, turning the head to the opposite side permits the brain to sink away from the cranial vault and thereby diminishes the chance of injury to the brain.

When the dura is left intact, as in the method described earlier, the skull cap can be peeled away easily. A twist of a chisel placed in the frontal saw line will admit the fingers inside the skull cap. A blunt hook may be used to pull the skull cap away from the underlying dura. A hand inserted between the skull and the dura (periosteum) helps the blunt separation of these while the other hand is pulling the skull cap. If the dura adheres too firmly to the skull, it can be incised along the line of sawing and the anterior attachment of the falx to the skull can be cut between the frontal lobes. The posterior portion of the falx can be cut from inside after the skull cap is fully reflected. The dura is then peeled off the skull cap. The superior sagittal sinus may be opened with a pair of scissors at this time. Routinely, the dorsal dural flaps on both sides can be removed easily from the brain by severing the bridging veins. In the presence of epi- or subdural hemorrhage and neoplasia, it is best to leave the dural flaps attached to the dorsal brain and section them together.

DETACHMENT OF BRAIN The frontal lobes are gently raised and the olfactory bulbs and tracts are peeled away from the cribriform plates. The optic nerves are cut as they enter the optic foramina. Under its own weight, the brain is allowed to

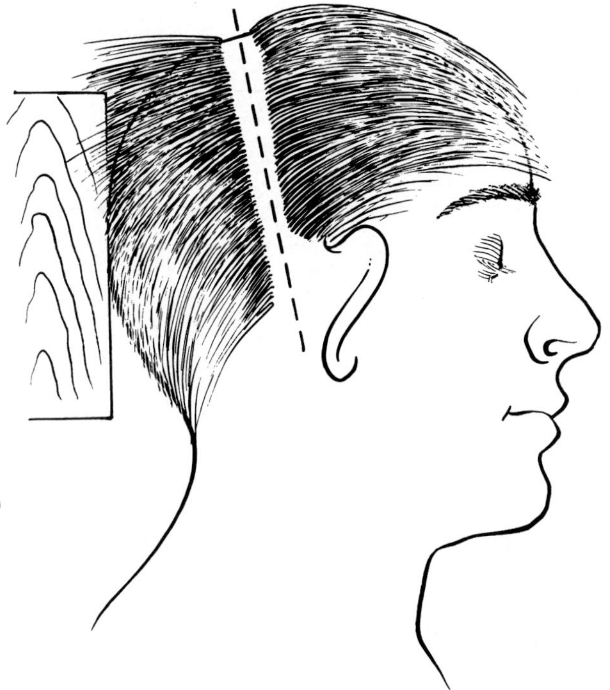

Fig. 6-1. Scalp incision. Dotted line indicates coronal plane of the primary incision. It starts on right side over the mastoid just behind earlobe and passes over palpable posterolateral ridges of parietal bones to reach opposite mastoid. This line is slightly tilted backward from plane parallel with face.

fall away from the floor of the anterior fossa, while it is being supported with the palm of one hand. The pituitary stalk is cut, followed by the internal carotid arteries as they enter the cranial cavity. Cranial nerves III, IV, V, and VI are severed as close to the base of the skull as possible. Subdural communicating veins are also severed. Next, the attachment of the tentorium along the petrous ridge is cut on either side with curved scissors. At this time, the brain must not drop backward excessively because this will cause stretch tears in the cerebral peduncles. This also can be prevented by raising the head very high from the beginning, with pronounced flexion of the neck, using a wooden pillow or a metal support attached to the table.

Cranial nerves VII, VIII, IX, X, XI, and XII are then cut identifying each one in sequence. The vertebral arteries are severed with scissors as they emerge into the cranial cavity. Then, the cervical part of the spinal cord is cut across as caudally as possible, but too oblique a plane of sectioning should be avoided. Curved scissors will be best for this purpose. If a critical lesion exists in the region, a cross-section perpendicular to the neuroaxis at the pontomedullary junction or higher may be elected in order to preserve the integrity of the abnormality.

The brain can then be reflected further back by using the support hand to deliver the brain stem and cerebellum from the posterior fossa without causing excessive stretching at the rostral brain stem level. The brain is pulled away from the base of the skull after cutting the lateral attachment of the tentorium to the petrous bones. The pineal body must not be left behind during this maneuver.

REMOVAL OF BRAIN IN FETUSES AND INFANTS

When the sutures are not closed and the cranial bones are still soft, Beneke's technique is used to open the cranium. The scalp is reflected as in adults. Starting at the lateral edge of the frontal fontanelle, the cranium and dura on both sides are cut with a pair of blunt scissors along the line indicated in Fig. 6-4A. (In this age group, the skull is often difficult to separate from the underlying dura in the manner described for adults.) This cut leaves a midline strip approx 1 cm wide, containing the superior sagittal sinus and the falx, and an intact area in the temporal squama on either side, which serves as a hinge when the bone flap is reflected. The older the infant, the narrower the sagittal strip will be because ossification advances toward the midline.

An alternate method of cutting, which follows the cranial suture lines, is illustrated in Fig. 6-4B and B'. With this method, fracture lines will be created along these bone flaps on their reflection; an optional cut along the posterior base of the frontal bone on either side will facilitate the procedure. The falx is then sectioned in a manner similar to that described for adults.

To minimize brain distortion during removal, several methods have been proposed *(4–9)*. In an early stage of the autopsy, fixatives such as 10% formalin in 70% alcohol can be infused through the neck arteries; this increases the consistency of the brain and facilitates its removal *(7)*. The fixative also can be injected percutaneously into the lateral ventricles, through the lateral margin of the anterior fontanelle, while the CSF fluid is allowed to exit via an intrathecal spinal needle *(5,7)*. Zamboni's fixative, which is yellow, shows whether the injection is sufficient. All these methods interfere with microbiologic examination.

In a modification of Beneke's method the skull is incised lightly along the cranial sutures and at the fontanelles *(7)*. By reversing the scalpel and passing it under the bones, the bones are separated from the underlying dura. The bone flaps are reflected after a small nick is made at the base in each of the bones. This procedure is similar to the method illustrated in Fig. 6-4 and B'. The dura is then cut as close to the base of the skull as possible. This method has the advantage of protecting the usually friable surface of the infant brain from damage during its removal. Damage to the brain can be minimized further if the scalp and calvarium are opened and the falx sectioned with the body in a sitting position and the infant's head being supported by an assistant. The tentorium and vein of Galen are transected in this position by gently separating the parieto-occipital lobes. After the tentorium is sectioned, the body is suspended upside down by the assistant, the brain being supported during the movement by the hand of the prosector.

The brain is cut away from the base of the skull in this upside-down position, which minimizes movement of the brain and damage to the brain substance and its surfaces. The bone flaps can be repositioned in their normal position on one side; supporting the head with the hand on this side, the brain can be freed on the other side. This is repeated on the opposite side. The brain is not touched directly during these procedures and,

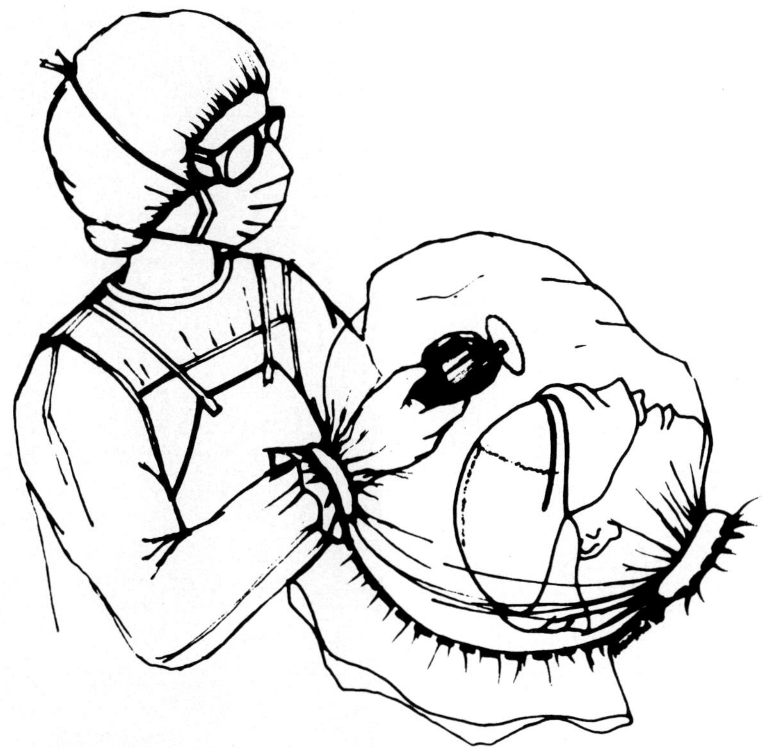

Fig. 6-2. Protective device. Prosector's hand holds saw inside bag. Dashed line indicates tape-seal of bag to, from left, prosector's gown, opposite side of the bag and neck of deceased. Adapted from ref. *(1)*.

when all attachments are severed, it is allowed to fall free, preferably into a body of water and not on to a hard surface.

Beneke's method of leaving the tentorium and removing the cerebral hemispheres from the brain stem and cerebellum is controversial *(9)*. We keep the brain as intact as possible at this stage but inspect the tentorium and neighboring structures during the removal procedure.

REMOVAL OF SPINAL CORD IN ADULTS

Removal of the spinal cord has been traditionally neglected by general pathologists but can be accomplished very easily within 10–15 min by the use of an oscillating saw, as described below. This should be part of every autopsy.

POSTERIOR APPROACH The body should be placed in the prone position with blocks under the shoulders. The head is rotated forward in a flexed position. Towels are placed under the face to avoid damage. A midline incision is placed over the spinous processes, muscles are resected, and bilateral laminectomies are made with the use of a saw (Fig. 6-5).

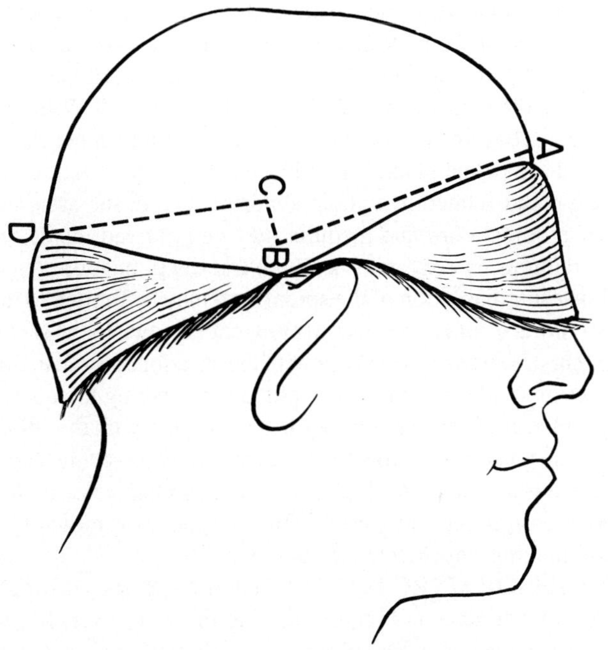

Fig. 6-3. Lines of saw cuts for skull cap removal. Frontal point (**A**) is approx two fingerbreadths above supraorbital ridges. Temporal point (**B**) is at the top of ear in its natural position before scalp reflection. Point (**C**) is approx 2 cm above (B). Occipital point (**D**) is approx two fingerbreadths above external occipital protuberance (inion). If (A) is too low, there is danger of cutting into the roof of the orbit; if (B) is too low, saw will enter petrous portion of temporal bone. Either of these will make removal of skull vault difficult. When (D) is too low, saw line will be below attachment of the tentorium.

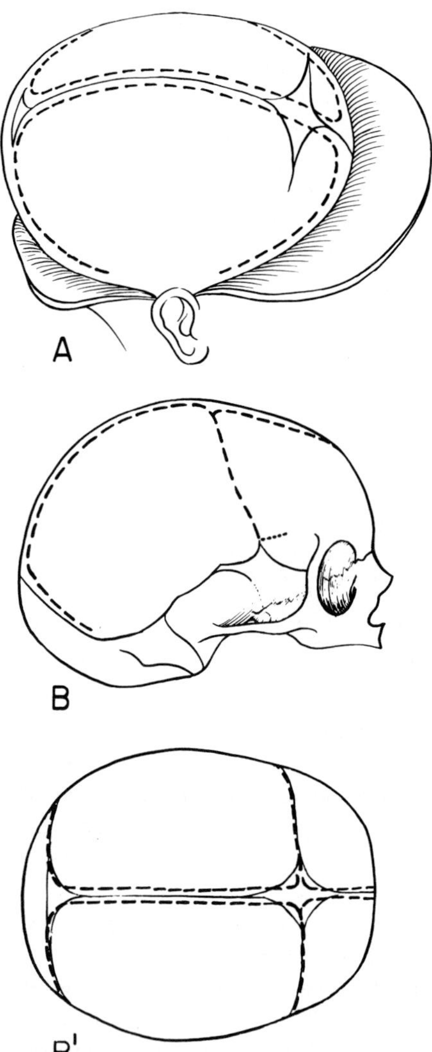

Fig. 6-4. Two methods of opening the calvarium in fetus and neonate. (**A**) illustrates Beneke's technique as described in text. In method shown in (**B**) and (**B'**), reflection of frontal bone flaps will result in fracture lines along their base. Optional cut may be made into posterior portion of these flaps as indicated by dots in (**B**).

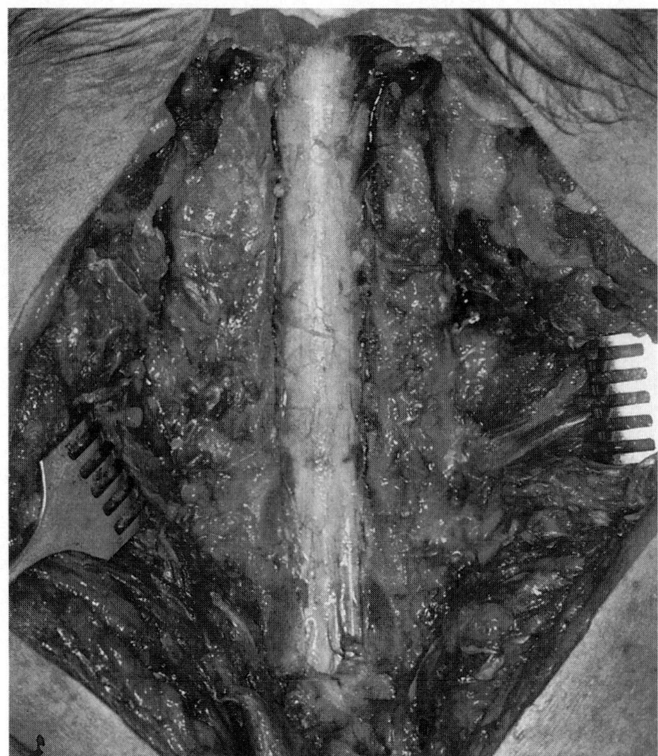

Fig. 6-5. Posterior approach to spinal cord. The spinal cord inside the dura after the removal of vertebral arches C1–C7 is shown.

This methods allows easy exposure of the uppermost cervical spine and allows direct visualization of the craniocervical junction; it is therefore recommended in cases in which neck injuries are suspected (flexion and extension neck injuries), in cases of craniocervical instability and in special situations, for example, when an occipital encephalocele needs to be excised or *in situ* exposure of an Arnold-Chiari malformation is required. A myelomeningocele also can be removed more easily by the posterior approach (*see* below). Many morticians object to the routine use of this method, because embalming fluids tend to leak from the incision on the back. Therefore, if embalming is planned, this approach should be chosen only when strictly indicated. Posterior dissection reveals the posterior muscles of the neck, ligaments, vertebrae (spinous and transverse processes as well as the vertebral bodies), and vertebral arteries. Deep contusions with blood extravasation, injuries to ligaments, and fractures of posterior parts of vertebral bodies also are demonstrated by this method *(10)*. After the spinal cord has been removed, the spinal canal can be readily examined. With this approach, continuity between lower brainstem and upper cervical cord can be maintained, if indicated. To study sites of compression and related histologic abnormalities in the area, the cervical spinal cord and medulla may be removed inside the bony column, in continuity with the fora-men magnum *(11)*.

Posterior dissection of the spinal cord may be limited to the upper thoracic and cervical cord or extended down to the sacral segments. However, compared with the anterior approach, this dissection method is much less suited for pursuing the course of peripheral nerves for any length in contiguity with the spinal cord. The posterior approach is used by us only on special occasions such as excision of an occipital encephalocele, *in situ* exposure of an Arnold-Chiari malformation, or removal of a spinal meningomyelocele (*see* below).

ANTERIOR APPROACH The anterior approach is simple and quick and does not require turning the body over. It also permits removal of the spinal cord and peripheral nerves in continuity when indicated. Immediate examination of the vertebral bodies is an added advantage. Kernohan's hemivertebral section method, devised as a quick anterior approach with the advantage of providing rigidity to the spinal column, fails to expose one side of the spinal cord *(7)*. Consequently, it restricts removal of the spinal cord, nerve roots, and dural covering. For

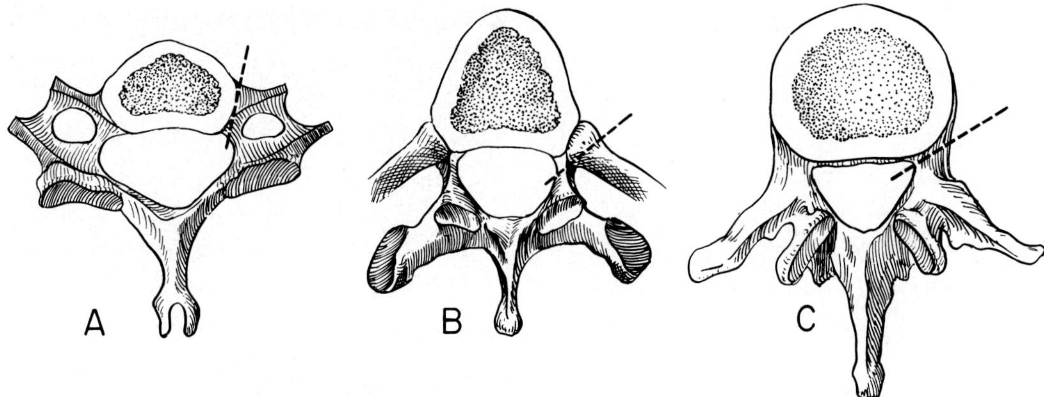

Fig. 6-6. Anterior approach to spinal cord. Dotted lines between vertebral body and arch indicate planes of saw cut adjusted to shapes of different levels of vertebral column. (**A**) Cervical. (**B**) Thoracic. (**C**) Lumbar.

the preferred method, that is, complete removal of these structures, *see* below.

After evisceration is completed, the first cut is made across the uppermost part of the thoracic region (T-1 or T-2). The head is dropped back by removing the head support or placing a wooden block behind the back under the midthoracic region, which straightens the spinal column and facilitates the procedure. The next cut is placed on either side of the upper thoracic spine, caudal to the first, for approx 10–15 cm along the line indicated in Fig. 6-6A. The sawing should be stopped as soon as one feels a "give," to prevent cutting into the spinal cord. Sectioning over the proximal ends of the ribs *(7)* has the advantage of creating a wider opening for the spinal cord and of giving easier access to the spinal ganglia and the peripheral nerves. The freed portion of the thoracic spine readily snaps up toward the prosector, especially when the spine has been straightened as described earlier.

It is better to saw both sides of the spine for short distances, instead of one side all the way down to the lumbar area, followed by the other side. With the latter technique, one cannot be certain whether the line of cut is being placed properly. If the upper thoracic spine fails to snap up because of faulty sectioning, a remedied cut can be placed at this early stage. Grasping the freed spine with the left hand and pulling it toward the prosector makes the further caudal extension of the cuts easier.

As one proceeds toward the lumbar area, the angle of the blade should be changed by adjusting to the shape of the vertebrae as illustrated in Fig. 6-6B and C. The muscles in this area should be cut away from the spine, down to the level of emerging nerves but without dividing them before sawing. Since removal of the L-5 body with the rest of the spine is often difficult because of the angulation of the spine at this level, L5 can be removed separately from the sacral bone with relative ease but first, the lumbar spine at the L4-5 interspace must be transected with a slightly curved short knife. Twisting a broad chisel in the saw tracts helps to separate the vertebral bodies away from the rest of the spine. In most instances, the cauda equina roots can be transected at either L-4 or L-5.

Freeing the rest of the cauda equina from the sacral bone is time-consuming, because it is difficult to manipulate the saw within the pelvic cavity. In rare instances, one has to cut a wedge of bone near the midline with an oscillating saw blade and remove the remaining lateral portion of the sacral bone with a rongeur to avoid damage to the nerve roots in the foramina.

The exposed portion of the spinal cord and the cauda equina encased by the dura mater is lifted off the spinal canal with as many spinal ganglia as possible. When indicated, the spinal cord can be removed with all spinal ganglia and the nerves of the lumbar plexuses and beyond by extending the process of freeing these structures from the bony and soft-tissue encasement more peripherally (Fig. 6-7). A string and a label tied to one of the lumbar roots allows future identification.

The cervical spinal cord can be removed by Kernohan's extraction technique (*see* below), without removing the cervical spine. However, cervical spinal roots or posterior spinal ganglia cannot be obtained by this technique and therefore, when these structures must be examined, the dissection of the spine must be extended upward. The carotid arteries are pushed to the side and the cervical plexuses are exposed in the same manner as used in lumbar area. The spine is then cut along the plane shown in Fig. 6-8 on either side up to the level of C2-3 interspace, where it is transected with a scalpel blade (Fig. 6-8 upper). Alternatively, the cervical spine is simply reflected cephalad and fractured (Fig. 6-8 lower). This method should only be applied in the absence of important antemortem bony lesions in this area.

A slight lateral tilting of the blade facilitates the removal of the spinal ganglia in this region. With excessive tilting, accidental cutting of the spinal cord may occur. Another common mistake is to deviate the line of cutting toward the midline cephalad, ending up with the pointed tip. This easily results in damage to the underlying cervical cord. To facilitate the insertion of the oscillating saw blade underneath the skin flap, we have cut off the top portion of the circular blade. Adequate exposure of the neck region requires a primary chest incision from shoulder to shoulder and freeing the skin flap from the underlying muscles and connective tissue.

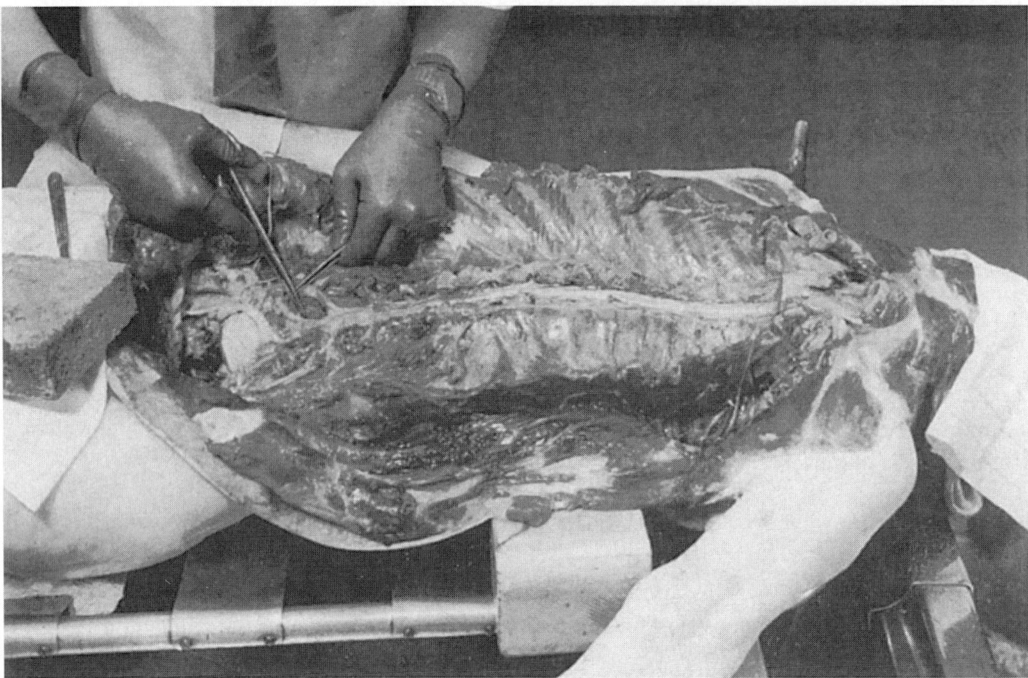

Fig. 6-7. Freeing of lumbar roots and plexus. It is convenient at this time to place a string and label around L4 or L5 root for future identification of spinal cord segments.

In order to remove the upper cervical cord and its roots from the intact bony canal one needs to approach it from the cranial cavity to free the dural attachment from the foramen magnum as high as possible. First, one makes a circular cut here. The dura is then peeled away from the bones caudad. Holding the freed dura taut with a hemostat or forceps facilitates this procedure. Usually, no special tools are required other than a pair of long scissors. On occasion, we have made use of semicircular chisels.

If the remaining portion of the spine needs to be removed, one can use a wire-saw passed through the spinal canal or a jigsaw with a long blade to complete the section. The latter instrument may injure the spinal cord, whereas the wire-saw can be used safely while the cervical cord is still in place. This will permit removal of the cervical spine in one piece. Although the upper cervical cord can be safely removed by the anterior approach, we would advocate the safer posterior approach if examination of higher cervical segments is critical.

After the cervical spine has been removed and the cervical cord exposed, the spinal cord and brain can be removed in continuity. This may be desirable in rare situations, as in the case of a tumor of the medulla and spinal cord. Of course, the usual transection at the lower medulla may not be made earlier. In this situation, it is better to expose and loosen the spinal cord completely before working on the removal of the brain *(7)*.

Routinely or when difficulties are encountered in reaching the high cervical level, it is advisable to cut across the cervical spine at a lower level and to extract the spinal cord by *Kernohan's method* after cutting the dura circumferentially at the exposed edge and opening it longitudinally along the midline below this level. The spinal cord and dura are wrapped in a moist towel. The right hand grasps the lower portion of the spinal cord and provides a gentle, steady, caudad pull while the fingers of the left hand are placed close to the top of the exposed spinal cord to minimize angulation at this point. It is possible to remove most of the spinal roots from the cervical enlargement by this method. Although some plucking of the nerve roots (especially the posterior ones) from the cord occurs, the often-expressed fear that the cord itself may be seriously damaged by this method is unfounded, based on our experience. The most frequent damage is caused by an inexperienced prosector who places the right thumb over the upper thoracic cord and proceeds to bend the cord at this level instead of pulling it caudally along the long axis. This extraction method is a compromise to encourage the routine removal of the entire length of the cord. Finally, the posterior base of the skull also can be removed together with the cervical spine and spinal cord *(11)*. For removal of the central nervous system in toto, undisturbed within the bony cage, *see* ref. *(12)*.

REMOVAL OF SPINAL CORD IN INFANTS

ANTERIOR APPROACH The basic principle is the same as in adults. The incomplete calcification of the spinal column permits the use of a scalpel blade instead of an oscillating saw blade.

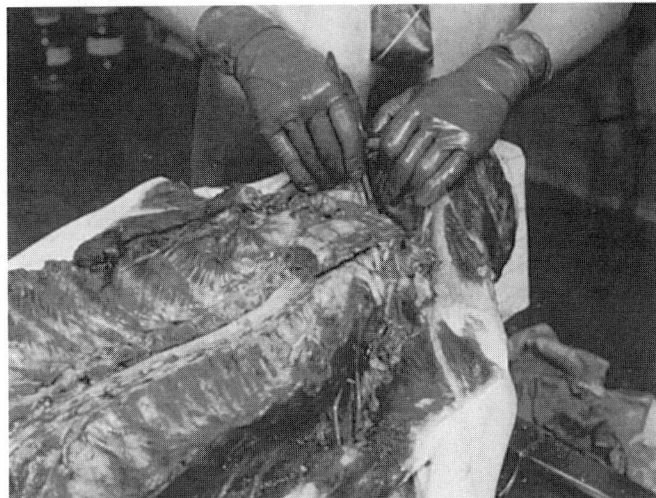

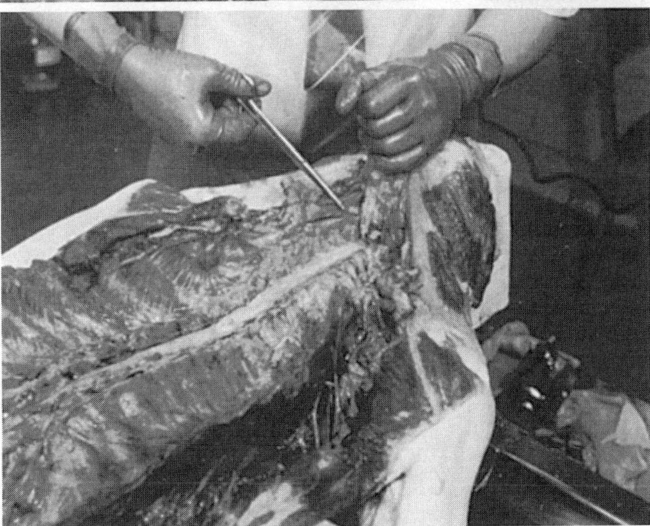

Fig. 6-8. Removal of cervical spine. Upper, scalpel blade is used to separate bone block at an intervertebral disk. Lower, bone block to be removed is reflected upward forcefully to break off at high cervical level. This method is faster, but not suitable when examination of the cervical spine (e.g., for fractures or disk protrusion) is necessary. Notice continuity of cervical roots with spinal cord.

COMBINED APPROACH For complete removal of a meningocele, meningomyelocele, or other lesion related to a midline fusion defect, it is best to combine the anterior and posterior approaches. After evisceration, the body is turned over and an incision is made around the meningomyelocele or other defect to allow en bloc removal of the lesion with the entire spinal column and cord. That task can be approached either posteriorly by extending a midline incision over the spinous processes, or anteriorly. In either case, the ribs are separated from the spine and the sacral bone is cut away from the rest of the pelvic bones. A transection is made across the upper thoracic spine and the entire block is freed from soft-tissue attachments. For retaining the continuity of the cervical spine, the posterior approach obviously is the method of choice. The method can be used regardless of the position of the midline defect. A similar approach is suitable for the removal of an occipital meningocele or encephalocele. An Arnold-Chiari malformation should be exposed with its posterior aspect within the bony cavity and for this, the posterior portion of the occipital bone is cut off, followed by laminectomy of the upper cervical spine. The skull is opened in a routine fashion.

EXAMINATION AND REMOVAL OF STRUCTURES AT BASE OF SKULL

VENOUS SINUSES, GANGLIA, AND DURA The venous sinuses including the cavernous sinuses are opened with curved scissors after removal of the brain. The Gasserian ganglia can be removed at this time. The dura at the base of the skull should be thoroughly stripped. This procedure is essential for exposing fracture lines. Before the dura is stripped, chisel and hammer should be used with caution because they may create artifactual fractures. Removal of the cavernous sinuses with their contents may be indicated, as in a case of aneurysm of the internal carotid artery, and in such a case, the method described next for the *in situ* removal of the pituitary gland can be used.

PITUITARY GLAND The margins of the diaphragma sellae should be incised before the posterior clinoid is knocked off with a small chisel. The tip of the chisel is placed at the crest of the dorsum sellae. The chisel can be directed either posteriorly (downward) over and nearly parallel to the midline anterior fossa or nearly perpendicular to it. If the chisel is placed perpendicularly, the pituitary remains visible during the procedure but a tap is needed over the broad side of the chisel near the tip, instead of a tap on the end of it. The diaphragma must be freed first or the tension on it may result in squeezing of the tissue in the pituitary fossa. A pair of forceps is applied to the edge of the diaphragma and the pituitary is dissected out, with a sharp blade, away from the base of the fossa. The pituitary gland may be removed with its bony encasement, for example, in a case of pituitary adenoma. For this, saw cuts are made along the lines indicated in Fig. 6-9 and the entire block is lifted off the base of the skull. With normal pituitary glands, removal from the fossa becomes more difficult after fixation, because the gland enlarges and the dura adheres firmer to the sella. For histologic examination, it is best to cut the pituitary gland after fixation.

A method to remove the hypothalamus and the pituitary gland and its bony encasement in continuity is available also *(13)*. Should this be indicated, most the brain is resected and only the hypothalamus and pituitary gland are left *in situ*. The block is lifted with the cavernous sinuses and posterior lining of the sella attached. For better preservation of the cerebral tissue, one can remove the frontal lobes, along the coronal plane at the level of the lamina terminalis, and free the pituitary from the pituitary fossa by sharp dissection and, if necessary, with use of a small rongeur to chip some of the bones. The remainder of the brain is removed as usual.

PARANASAL SINUSES AND NASOPHARYNX Various paranasal sinuses can be entered in tracranially for inspection or removal of specimens for histologic observation. The ethmoid sinuses can be approached by breaking the cribriform

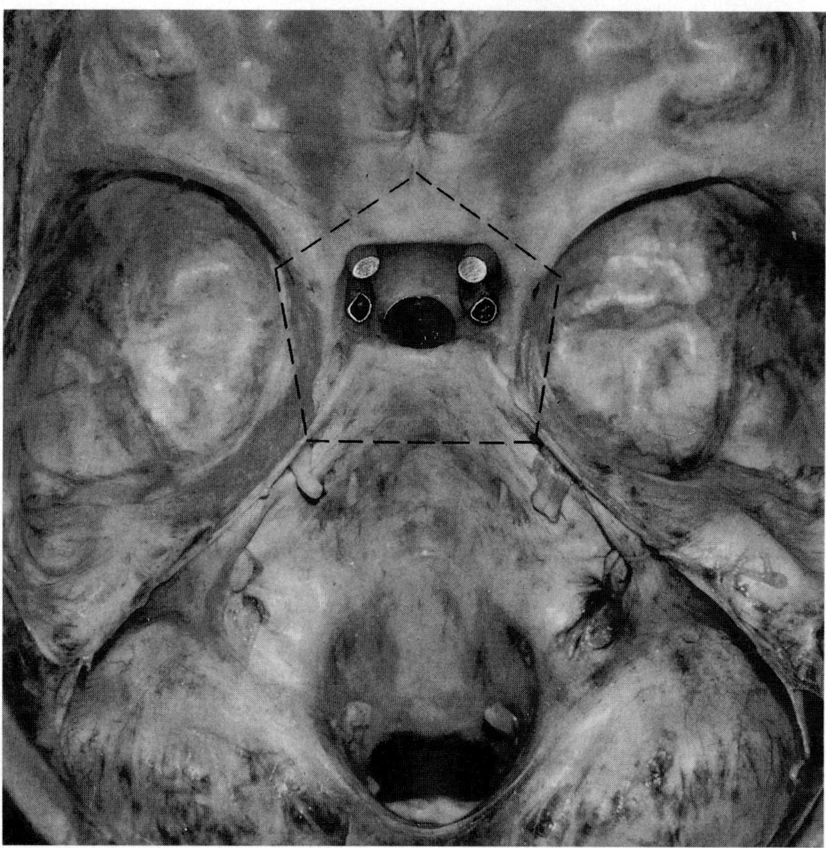

Fig. 6-9. Removal of pituitary gland with its bony encasement. Pentagonal block is cut out along the lines indicated, with saw blade directed roughly perpendicular to bone surfaces.

plate with a chisel and mallet. Continued chiseling leads into the maxillary sinuses. The frontal sinuses are entered by chiseling away their posterior walls close to the midline. The sphenoidal sinuses can be inspected after the anterior wall and the floor of the pituitary fossa have been exposed. If the block of bone containing the pituitary fossa is removed (Fig. 6-9) with an oscillating saw, the sphenoidal sinuses are exposed even better. The nasopharynx and the throat can be entered by extending this dissection. For an excellent review of nasopharyngeal dissection methods, *see* ref. *(14)*. More recently, en bloc resection of all ENT-relevant organs without disfiguring the body has been described *(15)*.

EAR Even when there is no indication for removing the auditory and vestibular apparatus in one piece, it is still a good practice to look into the middle and inner ear, particularly in the presence of an inflammatory process within the cranial cavity. This can be done simply by the use of a large rongeur over the posterolateral portion of the petrous ridge. A primary focus of infection may be found within the ear structures. When total removal of the ears is indicated, we apply the method described in the pamphlet from the Temporal Bone Bank *(16)*. The use of an oscillating saw facilitates the procedure.

The cut is made along the lines indicated in Fig. 6-10A. The block of bone thus sectioned is lifted with a bone-holding forceps, and the connective tissue bands anchoring the block are cut with curved scissors. When the temporal bone is freed, chisel and hammer should be used with caution. The internal carotid artery stump should be ligated or, simpler still, plugged with clay to help the embalmer. Alternatively, a bone-plug cutter attached to the vibrating saw (Fig. 6-10B) can be used. The Temporal Bone Bank recommends the use of 20% formalin solution, approx 400 mL, for fixation in a refrigerator for 1 d and fresh 10% formalin solution daily for 2 additional days. Refrigerated specimens can be saved indefinitely. Following a short decalcification, the specimen can be sliced and processed for light microscopy *(17)*.

FIXATION

The best routine fixative that allows the widest choice of stains for the nervous tissue is formalin, usually as a 10% solution (*see* Chapter 14). In fetuses and infants, the addition of acetic acid to the fixative solution appears to be helpful. Acetic acid increases the specific gravity of the fixative and allows the brain to float in the solution; it also makes the tissue firmer without altering its histologic characteristics *(18)*.

IMMERSION METHODS For detailed anatomic studies of the nervous system it is best to fix the specimen, with a minimum of prior handling, in a large amount of freshly pre-

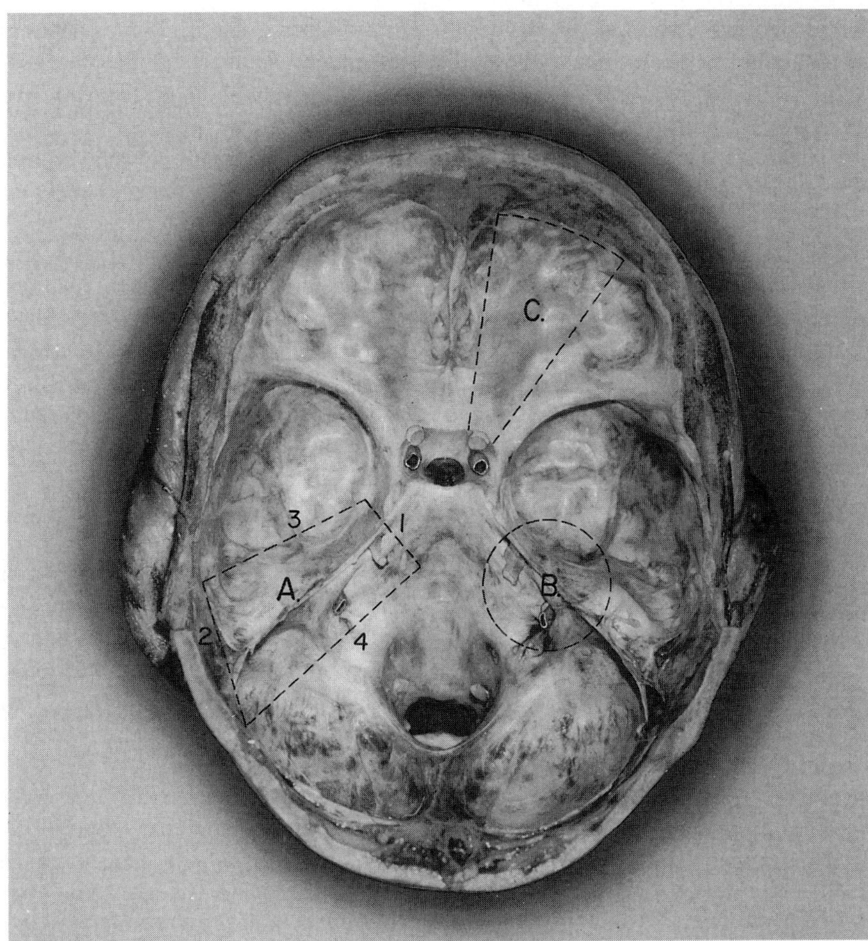

Fig. 6-10. Removal of inner and middle ear and eye. (**A**) line 1 is placed near the apex of petrous bone as possible, roughly at right angle to superior edge of petrous bone. Line 2 is over mastoid region, as close to lateral wall as possible. Line 3 is placed, with blade held vertical to floor. (**B**) Circle indicates block to be removed with bone-plug cutter. (**C**) Dotted line indicates area of bone removal to approach orbital content intracranially.

pared 10% formalin solution. We use plastic buckets that hold 8 L. (These are readily available at local stores at a considerably lower price than traditional glass or earthenware jars, which also are heavier and break more easily). We suspend the brain to prevent distortion during fixation by passing a thread underneath the basilar artery in front of the pons. Inevitably, the vessel is slightly pulled away from the brain substance. If this is undesirable, as in the case of pontine infarcts or other lesions in this region, a thread can be passed under the internal carotid or middle cerebral arteries on both sides, provided that no pathologic lesions are suspected in these regions.

Alternatively, the dorsal dura can be used as an anchoring point. A thread is passed through the short dural flaps on either side of the falx, and the brain is suspended right-side-up. However, a minor pull may deform the parasagittal brain tissue and cause an abnormally pointed dorsal midline surface of the brain. Generally, suspension from blood vessels deforms the parenchyma less than dural suspension. In rare instances, we suspend the brain upside down with a pair of threads tied to the edge of the entire dorsal dural flap on either side. With all these methods, the ends of the thread(s) are tied to the attachments of the bucket handle, care being taken not to allow the specimen to touch the bottom or sides of the bucket. Another safe method makes use of the plastic brain support described below for perfusion. Placing several holes in the dome-shaped receptacle will ensure proper fixation of the contact surface of the brain.

We do not recommend any method based on tying a thread around any portion of the brain substance, such as the stump of the medulla or the midbrain, nor do we recommend sectioning of the corpus callosum for alleged improved entry of fixative into the ventricles.

Formalin solution should be replaced within the first 24 h, but this not mandatory if a large amount of fixative is used. If the fixative becomes very bloody, prompt replacement with fresh solution is indicated; this also prevents undue discoloration of the specimen.

Approximately 10–14 d are required for satisfactory fixation. If the brain is dissected earlier, the central portion may still be pink, even though the consistency may be satisfactory.

PERFUSION METHODS The brain can be perfused with fixative through the arterial stumps before further fixation by immersion, as described earlier. This shortens the fixation time and ensures adequate fixation of deeper portions of the brain. When it is necessary to dissect the brain at the time of autopsy, this preliminary perfusion fixation makes the tissue firmer and thus facilitates the dissection and decreases the surface wrinkling and tissue warping that are inevitable under these circumstances.

Large volumes of formalin (for example, 1,000 mL) improve fixation but with too much fixative, large lakes of fluid may accumulate, particularly in the areas weakened by a pathologic process (e.g., infart, hemorrhage, metastasis), and the specimen may become asymmetric because of uneven perfusion. Even without these gross distortions, excessive volumes of fixative may produce annoying perivascular zones of tissue rarefaction microscopically, in addition to unnatural dilatation of small blood vessels. Obstructing emboli or thrombosis also might be obscured. The weight changes induced by perfusion fixation are described in Part III (Appendix) of this book. Injection of 150 mL of isotonic saline followed by 150 mL of 10% formalin solution causes the least problems *(19)*. This can be done manually with a syringe connected to a simple tubing system *(7)*. For easy handling and better preservation of the contour of the specimen, we use a plastic holder during the procedure. Satisfactory fixation for dissection can be obtained in 7–10 d. However, earlier dissection may be possible if one can tolerate some degree of incomplete fixation, which is manifested mainly by central areas of softness and pink coloration. For perfusion of a large amount of fixative, an embalmer's pump may be used. For a simple gravity-feed method, one may use an infusion bottle raised 150–180 cm above the specimen.

DISSECTION OF BRAIN AND SPINAL CORD

Brain weight in the fresh and fixed state should be recorded. It is not necessary to use a very large knife to dissect the brain. We prefer a single-blade autopsy knife about 25 cm long and 2 cm wide.

DISSECTION OF FRESH BRAIN IN ADULTS The most exacting examination of brain in terms of recognition of lesions and correlation of their topography with clinical symptoms and images generated by computerized trans-axial tomography (CT) or magnetic resonance imaging (MRI) techniques can be achieved only when the brain is sectioned after adequate fixation *(20–22)*. At times, however, the fresh brain must be dissected, particularly when microbiologic and chemical investigations are of prime importance or when an immediate diagnosis is needed (this speed unfailingly leads to distortion of the cut surface during subsequent fixation). As a compromise, we limit fresh dissection to three or four coronal cuts through the cerebral hemispheres, leaving more complicated anatomic structures such as the basal ganglia and upper brain stem (thalamus and midbrain) as undisturbed as the circumstances permit. This preliminary dissection usually reveals the presence of large lesions, directly or indirectly, by showing distortion of the ventricular system or other anatomic landmarks.

Further judiciously selected sections may be made into the primary slices of the brain tissue to expose the suspected hidden lesions. The central portion of the cerebral hemispheres is left connected with the brain stem, and this block is suspended by a string, as described earlier. It may be necessary to sever the brain stem and cut into the infratentorial structures; one horizontal cut through these structures usually suffices for preliminary examination. Even with several cuts, one should not be satisfied solely with fresh dissection of the brain because many small lesions are easily missed and subtle lesions such as an early infarct, small or large, can be overlooked. Every brain should be reexamined with new dissection after adequate fixation.

Preliminary perfusion or cooling of the brain in a refrigerator for about 30 min, preferably in a contoured support as described earlier, makes the brain firmer and dissection easier. If diffuse, roughly symmetric lesions are expected, as in lipidoses, "degenerative diseases," "demyelinating" disorders, other inborn or acquired toxic-metabolic diseases, or widespread infectious conditions, the brain may be bisected along the sagittal plane, one half being further sectioned and submitted for chemical or microbiologic investigations while the other half is retained for later sectioning and histologic examination. This latter half must be fixed either by suspension or by letting it lie on its midsagittal plane to avoid undesirable distortions.

Dissection of fresh brain (according to the aforementioned procedure) may be required by brain-banking protocols or specific research protocols (e.g., Alzheimer's disease), in order to provide adequate material for histological, immunocytochemical, biochemical, and molecular biology studies. References *(23)* and *(24)* provide a general overview regarding procedures involved in "brain banking."

We find no use for the classical *Virchow method* of fresh dissection. Any brain subjected to this method would look, after adequate fixation, like a book immersed in water and subsequently dried.

DISSECTION OF FRESH BRAIN IN FETUSES AND INFANTS Without an overriding need to secure unfixed samples for chemical or microbiologic examination, fetal and infantile brains are best kept intact until after proper fixation, because of their pronounced softness and ease of bruising. Our method is essentially similar to that described for adult brains. To increase consistency to fetal or infantile brains, we use as fixative 20% formalin solution containing 1% glacial acetic acid. No additional measures such as one or two changes of alcohol are needed.

DISSECTION OF FIXED BRAIN After a careful inspection of the external surface of the brain, the arteries at the base of the brain may be exposed through tears made into the arachnoid membrane and followed for a short distance distally to check for pathologic conditions such as thrombosis, embolism, or aneurysm. This procedure should be omitted when pathologic processes in this region may be disturbed. Routine removal of the arterial tree from the brain substance has no merit in a

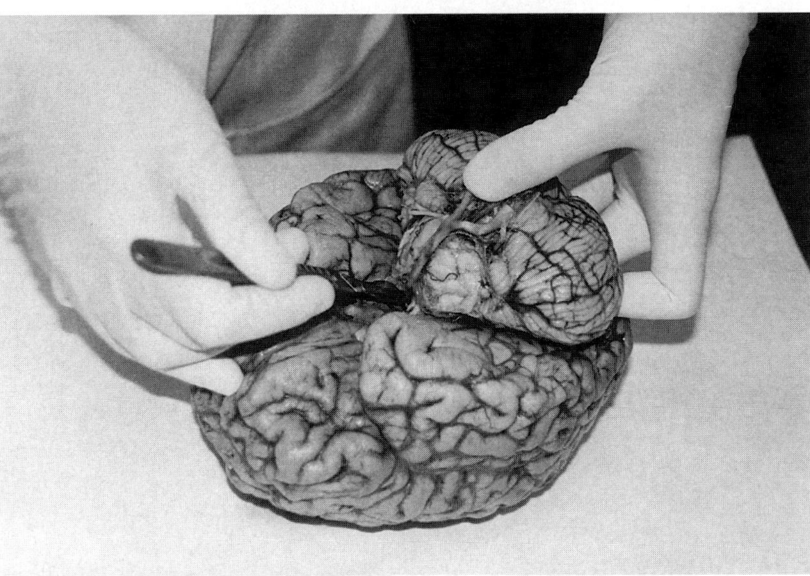

Fig. 6-11. Sectioning brain stem at midbrain level.

thorough pathologic examination because this separates vascular lesions from the resulting areas of parenchymal damage.

After adequate external examination, the brain stem and the cerebellum are separated from the cerebral hemispheres. In rare instances, it is better to retain this continuity, for example, for display of the distorting effect of a supratentorial lesion on the brain stem needs. It is essential to section through the midbrain along a flat surface perpendicular to the neuroaxis. For this purpose, with the brain placed upside down, the cerebellum should be held between the index finger of the one hand with the tip in proximity of the pineal gland and the thumb on the inferior surface of cerebellum (Fig. 6-11). With the scalpel in a pen-holding position, the cutting hand rests on the ventral aspect of the frontal lobes to provide the proper angle. The blade is held toward the prosector with its tip in front of the distant cerebral peduncle a few millimeters above the tip of the mammillary body. The blade enters the midbrain in the midline, aiming toward the pineal gland until the scalpel barely passes through the thickness of the brainstem; the blade is then brought toward the prosector (resulting in sectioning through half of the midbrain). The scalpel is now flipped over and moved forward along the same plane cutting the other half of the midbrain. A gentle pull with the holding hand on the brain stem and cerebellum during the procedure helps to complete the sectioning. Placing a knife over the temporal lobe and cutting the midbrain from the side should be avoided since this will result in a roof-shaped midbrain; this complicates the evaluation of the midbrain and makes its complete cross-sectional representation on histologic slides impossible.

Attempts to sever the midbrain too rostrally often result in an uneven or incomplete cut because the cerebral peduncles widen rapidly in the rostral portion. In order to avoid this, one may place a preliminary section close to the pontomesencephalic junction; then, under direct visualization, a parallel slice of the midbrain can be removed more rostrally.

Coronal sectioning of the cerebral hemispheres is the most common and safest method for any contingencies. We prefer free cuts, without use of a cutting apparatus. Before sectioning, the central sulci should be marked by carefully cutting, with the tip of a scalpel blade, into the leptomeninges bridging over them, without injuring the underlying brain substance. This gives a valuable point of reference on multiple coronal sections.

As an initial step we hold the brain on its convexity with the orbital lobes and occipital poles in an horizontal plane. The first section is made through the mammillary body and cut surfaces are examined for symmetry (Fig. 6-12A). Attempts to slice with a single motion of the knife often exerts undue pressure toward the cutting board, which may squash or tear various structures, while the vessels are dragged into the softer brain tissue. Multiple slicing excursions without undue downward pressure produce a clean-cut surface more effectively. The knife handle should be held lightly, as this will facilitate smooth gliding movements of the blade. A firm grip tends to cause knife marks on the surfaces of brain slices.

Alternatively, the first cut can be made just in front of the temporal poles, exposing the anterior ventricular horns. This may be important in cases of hydrocephalus, in which this view may disclose an obstruction of the foramen of Monro (e.g., by a colloid cyst or a third ventricular tumor) and still allow a change in sectioning technique to better demonstrate the obtruction *(25)*.

Brain slices should be approx 1 cm thick. We like to section the halved brain pieces by holding them down on the cut surface and by moving the knife side to side from the inferior surface of the brain toward the convexity (Fig. 6-12B,C). A

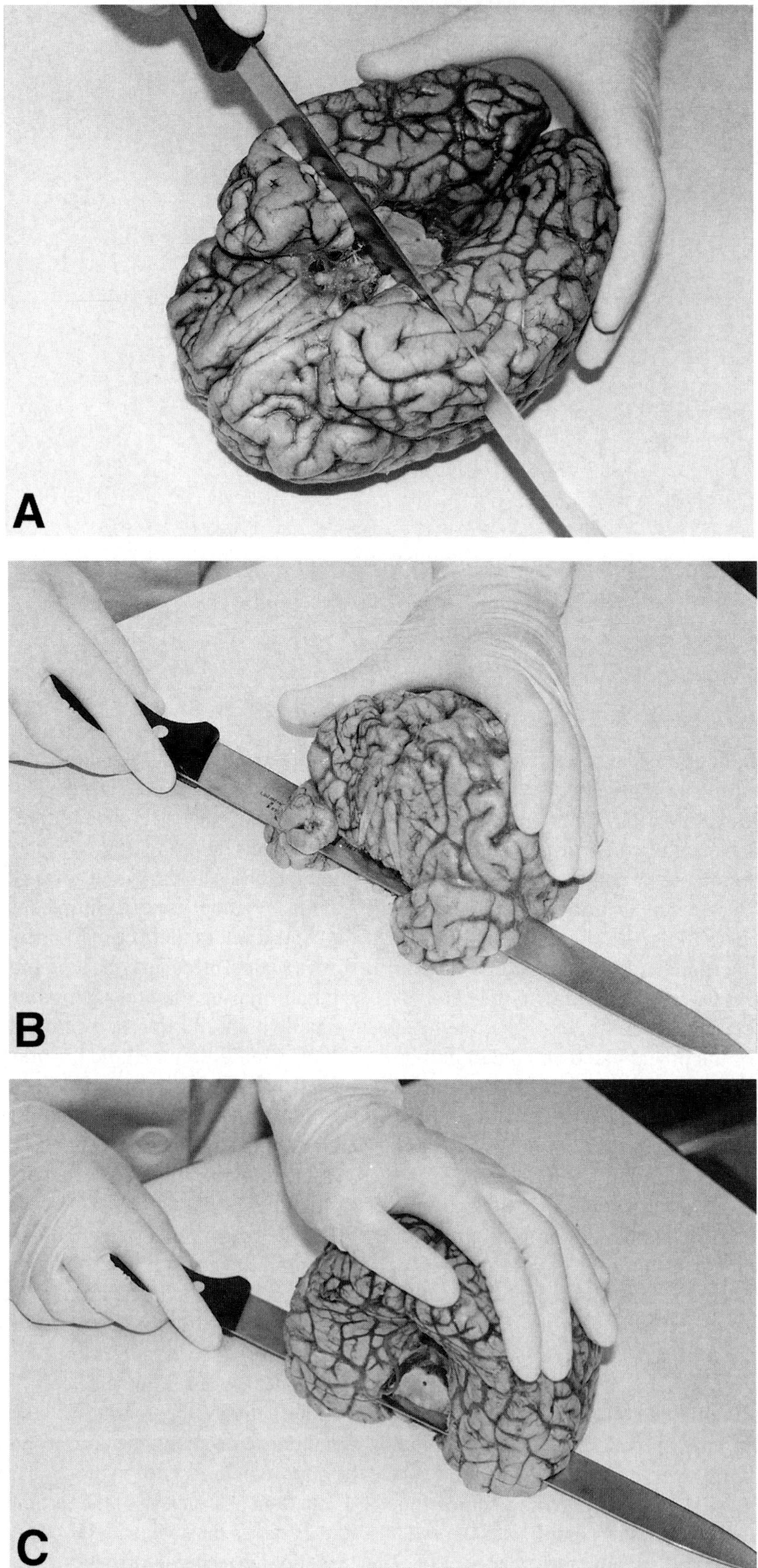

Fig. 6-12. Sectioning of cerebral hemispheres. (**A**) initial cut is placed through mammillary bodies. (**B,C**) the halved brain pieces are held down on the cutting board and sliced from the inferior surface toward the convexity. Cloth or paper towels under the brain will prevent the board surface becoming slippery from fluid dripping from the brain. When slicing cerebral hemispheres in this fashion, the "limp" optic nerves need to be propped up to avoid cutting them longitudinally.

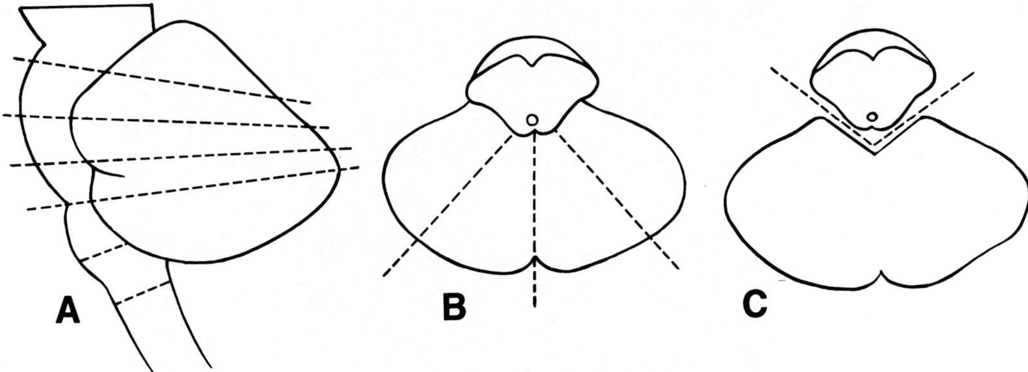

Fig. 6-13. Approach to routine dissection of brain stem and cerebellum. (**A**) Brain stem and cerebellum are dissected together by series of cuts roughly perpendicular to neuroaxis. For consistency, base line is made through pontomedullary junction and posterior ridges of cerebellar hemispheres. This will give a flat surface on which to rest the brain stem and cerebellum, which makes the subsequent sections easy. (**B**) Midline incision is made in vermis, and wedge of tissue is removed from each cerebellar hemisphere. Hemispheres are further sectioned through vertical planes perpendicular to external lines of cerebellar cortex. Brain stem and rest of cerebellum are sectioned as in (A). (**C**) Cerebellum is separated from brain stem. Latter is sectioned as in (A). Cerebellum is sectioned either horizontally or vertically as in (B).

slicing guide (*see* below) can be used for particularly delicate specimens. It is also important to examine each new cut surface before the next slice is made so that any necessary adjustment can be made in the next plane of section. The slices are displayed on a board, with the right side of the specimen on the left side of the prosector. Although the classical pathologists' approach to the brain corresponded to viewing one's own brain from behind (and therefore, right side of the specimen on the right side of the prosector), we prefer the frontal view because of current neuroimaging practice, which is similar to that of the physician who sees the living patient face to face. A large cutting board is needed because slices should not overlap. Sufficient space for display is mandatory for adequate examination of the brain.

Several different approaches can be used in routine dissection of the brain stem and cerebellum (Fig. 6-13). The brain stem is best sectioned perpendicular to its axis, which is slightly curved. Consequently, the planes of section should be adjusted. The cerebellum can be sectioned in horizontal planes or in planes perpendicular to the folial orientation, with the converging point in front of the cerebellum. The latter method gives the best histologic orientation of the cortical structures. A combination of both methods also can be used.

Display of the brain stem and cerebellum should be consistent with the principle used for the cerebral hemispheres. There are two options to achieve this end (*see* below) and either method can be suitably used under different circumstances.

Since the advent of CT and MRI, sections of the brain along the planes of tomography have become important for clinicopathologic correlation *(26)*. For this purpose, we use a simply constructed device made of plexiglass, shown in Fig. 6-14. The table (Fig. 6-14A) has a small opening to admit the cerebellum and brain stem. The guide on top of the table can be moved up and down so that the most desirable inclination on the initial cut can be selected, based on the imaging prints. After the initial cut (Fig. 6-14B), the halved brain pieces are sectioned serially on the board (Fig. 6-14C), which has 13-mm guides on its edge. Guides half as tall as these can be attached on the other side of the board. The display slices should correspond to the printed CT images.

We consider the coronal sectioning of the cerebral hemispheres and the horizontal sectioning of the brain stem and cerebellum the best routine method for the brain in that the slices obtained will display most advantageously the pattern of vascular supplies and the relationship of the internal structures. This holds true even in the absence of corresponding neuroimages.

DISSECTION OF SPINAL CORD For routine examination, after the dura has been opened along the anterior midline and the cord surface has been examined, series of cross-sections are prepared. Marking the right side of the cord with India ink may help later when segmental and long pathway pathology need to be reconstructed. The dura should be left attached to the cord to keep the sectioned spinal cord and roots together. This allows to orient roots for cross sections during embedding. When specific radicular-level involvement has been reported premortem, the involved roots should be identified and processed separately (*see* "Peripheral Nerves"). With a sharp scalpel blade, the spinal cord is sectioned approx at 1-cm intervals. Occasionally, longitudinal sections can be made to emphasize the rostral-caudal extent of the lesion, such as in traumatic contusion. However, it is often difficult to get a straight plane of section. In most instances, the cross-sectional extent of the lesion at any given segmental level is more important for understanding clinical symptoms. A combination of the two methods

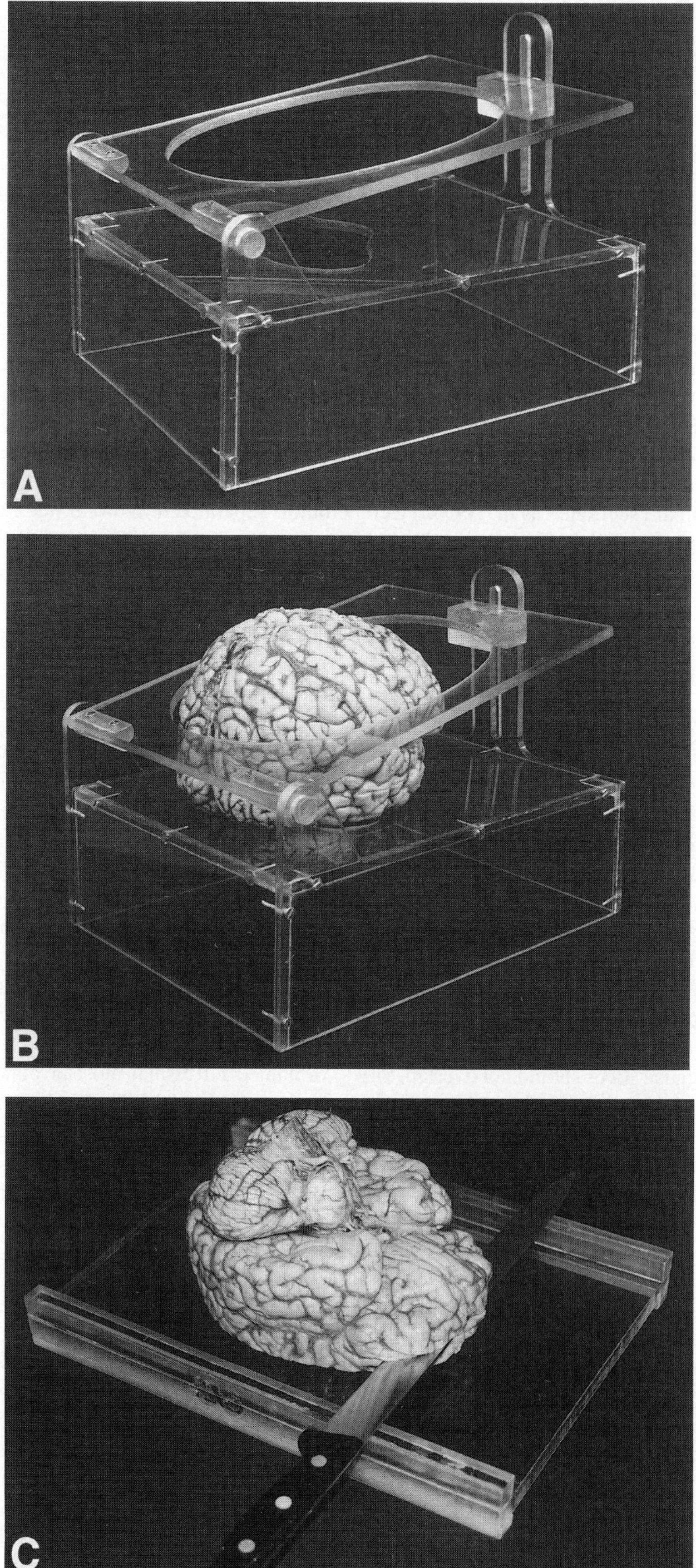

Fig. 6-14. Device for sectioning brain along planes of tomography. (**A**) Plexiglass table with opening for cerebellum and brain stem and movable guide. (**B**) Brain in position for initial cut. (**C**) Halved brain positioned on board for serial sectioning.

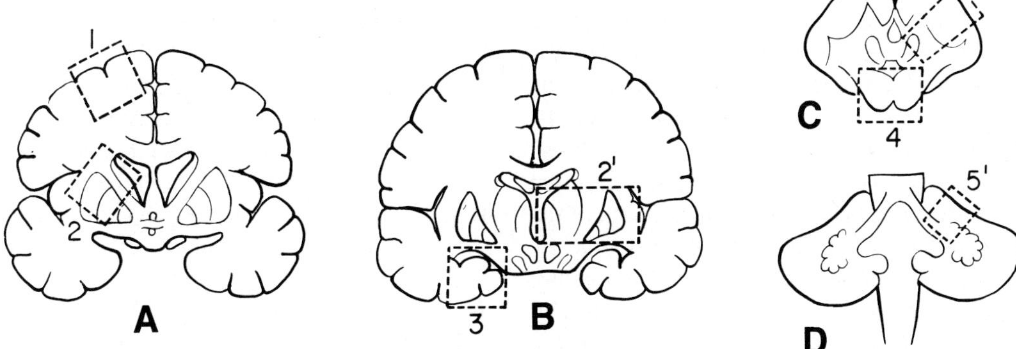

Fig. 6-15. Selection of tissue blocks. (**A**) 1 = superior and middle frontal gyri. This is an arterial border ("water-shed") zone most likely to arbor small ischemic lesions. This also may reveal atrophic or "senile" changes such as senile plaques or neurofibrillary tangles. 2 = basal ganglia. Vascular changes and their effects on parenchyma are likely to be found here, as are other "degenerative changes." (**B**) 2' = basal ganglia together with thalamus. 3 = hippocampus and adjacent neocortex. This is often a sensitive indicator of anoxic-ischemic changes. Neurofibrillary tangles, neuritic plaques, and the "aging" changes make their first appearance here. (**C,D**) 4 = pons. Vascular (particularly small arterial) changes are found more frequently here than in other portions of brain stem. 5 and 5' = cerebellum. Ischemic and toxic metabolic conditions are often reflected in cerebellar cortex.

may be used by taking a cross-sectional slice at the point of maximal damage and slicing the rest longitudinally along the frontal plane. Of course, unorthodox and creative sectioning may, in rare instances, display some lesions at their best.

SELECTION OF TISSUE BLOCKS FOR HISTOLOGIC EXAMINATION

BRAIN AND SPINAL CORD When the lesions in the *brain* are obvious, selection of the appropriate blocks is simple. For orientation and for possible evidence of pathologic involvement, some recognizable structures from the surrounding and presumably normal areas should be included. When gross lesions cannot be found despite the presence of clinical neurologic signs or symptoms, one must be familiar with the topographic distribution of the lesions expected in a given disease or syndrome to be able to select appropriate sections. Familiarity with the patient's clinical history must be accompanied by some basic knowledge of where the lesions are to be expected.

It is difficult to define what constitutes adequate selection of sections in "routine normal cases." No universally accepted standards exist, but whatever choices are made, selections should be consistent topographically. The areas shown in Fig. 6-15 are our minimal requirements; the reasons for this selection are given in the legend. It is best to store the whole brain until the microscopic examination is completed and the clinicopathologic correlation is satisfied.

In most cases, the size of the sections can be limited to be suitable for the standard 1- by 3-inch glass slides. We use tissue capsules of different sizes for automatic processing machines. We try not to "mutilate" the original brain slices and therefore, if photographs are taken of crosssectional surfaces, we select tissue blocks from the same surface of the adjoining slice so that photography can be be repeated. Alternatively, the brain slab can be sliced thinly up to the area of block removal while the knife blade protects the lower half of the slab and vertical cuts are made into the upper slab. Experienced prosectors can prepare complete thin slices and lay them on the cutting board before blocks are removed. It is not a good practice to hold a thick slab in the hand and to try to undercut a centrally located block through one of the vertical cuts, as this will invariably result in an uneven "dig" into the remaining tissue.

In the absence of known *spinal cord* abnormalities, one section each from the cervical, thoracic, and lumbosacral levels is appropriate. When spinal cord lesions are expected, pathologists should attempt to localize the "radicular-segmental" or "vertebral-body" level of the lesion. Keeping in mind that the conus medullaris generally ends at the level of the upper part of the L2 vertebral body, the Ll and L2 dural root exits can be localized. Cephalad from this point, spinal cord roots and vertebral body levels can be counted. For correct localization of the levels, the dural sac and the exit zones must be intact (*see* "Removal of spinal cord" and "Dissection of the spinal cord").

PERIPHERAL NERVES The cervical and lumbar plexuses can be removed totally and in continuity with the spinal roots and ganglia, as outlined for removal of the spinal cord. As a routine procedure, this is too time-consuming.

A quicker method is to cut the nerves as they emerge from the intervertebral foramina and to sample selected nerves as the clinical signs dictate. Routinely, lengths of the sciatic and femoral nerves or any other portions of the lumbosacral plexuses proximal to their exits from the pelvic and abdominal cavities can easily be removed without creating new incisions. Similarly, sampling of the brachial plexuses and their distal extensions can be achieved from the supraclavicular axillary regions. Care should be exercised to preserve the brachial arteries for embalming.

In cases in which detailed clinical studies were performed on the peripheral nervous system, the affected nerves should be sampled at autopsy. When incisions are made in the extremities for sampling of muscles, as described in the next section, the nerves innervating them can be removed conveniently. In a diffuse neuropathic condition, one may select the sciatic nerve and its distal ramifications for detailed studies. To this end, the body is turned over and an incision is made in the back of the thigh to free the sciatic nerve, which has been severed previously at its pelvic exit. The incision may be extended caudally to allow the removal of the peroneal and tibial nerves in the leg. More conservatively, a 15-cm longitudinal incision in the popliteal region exposes these nerves at their bifurcation. The arteries in the vicinity must not be lacerated, as this would interfere with the embalming procedure. To assist the embalmer, we have also removed the sciatic nerve by incising the anterior surface of the thigh and leg. Sawing away a portion of the pelvic bone (mainly the ischium) helps to free the nerve without pulling it up or down behind the bone. This approach is cumbersome, but a bonus is the easy removal of the femoral nerve and its branches.

One of the most accessible peripheral nerve is the sural nerve, which has been biopsied in many clinical studies. Therefore, its removal at autopsy through a small incision behind the lateral malleolus gives an excellent base for comparison. For removal and fixation techniques, *see* ref. *(27)*. A useful adjunct to diagnostic studies of the peripheral nervous system is a fiber-teasing method that has become a standard procedure in many research laboratories. After fixation, a portion of nerve is stained with 1% osmium tetroxide and macerated in 60% glycerol, and individual fibers are teased out under a dissecting microscope. This method allows to examine fibers three-dimensionally and to evaluate axonal degeneration and demyelination *(27)*. For best preservation of these nerves, autopsies should done within 6 h after death.

SKELETAL MUSCLE In the absence of specific diseases affecting the neuromuscular system, skeletal muscle is rarely sampled. One or two specimens should be stored in the "routine" autopsy. The ileopsoas muscle is easily accessible and shows the effects of general systemic disease on the skeletal muscles.

In cases of known or suspected neuromuscular diseases, more extensive sampling is required. For primary myopathies, the selection has to be based on clinical findings and the status of the muscles at the time of autopsy. Sections should be taken from muscles that are severely affected, that show early but active involvement, and that are grossly uninvolved. A list of muscles to be sampled in cases of neurogenic muscle atrophy is shown in ref. *(28)*. Table 6-1 lists muscles that are accessible without major procedures and will give an adequate diagnostic sampling.

The specimens should be cleanly excised or neatly trimmed to about 3.0 × 1.0 × 0.5 cm. Placing the samples on a piece of cardboard does not completely prevent shrinkage of the tissue during fixation. A corkboard with two narrow strips of cork fastened to it provides ridges to which multiple muscle samples can be pinned. This eliminates the problem of poor fixation of the underside of the specimens. Parts of wooden applicator stick may be used to support smaller pieces of muscle, which are tied to it with suture material at both ends. We consider 10% neutral formalin solution the most satisfactory all-purpose fixative, particularly if staining of the nervous tissue in the specimen is important. Additional pieces can be fixed in Bouin's solution to improve trichrome stains; fresh-frozen cryostat sections can be prepared for Gomori's trichrome stain and for staining with hematoxylin and eosin, after 2 min fixation in 10% formalin solution on a cover slip (Engel AG, personal communication).

Teasing the removed specimens lengthwise after fixation, rather than cutting with a knife blade, sometimes produces a better longitudinal arrangement of the muscle on histologic slides. As with peripheral nerves, both cross and longitudinal aspects of the muscle should be represented.

Table 6-1
Suggested Muscles for Sampling at Autopsy

Muscle	*Comment*
Extraocular muscles	Obtained through orbital plate intracranially or anteriorly with or without the globe.
Tongue	Removed with pharynx and larynx; small pieces can be removed through mouth.
Sternocleidomastoid; diaphragm; pectoralis major	No new incision required; pectoralis major is preferred over deltoid because previous intramuscular injection into deltoid may have caused abnormalities.
Biceps; triceps	Removed through incision in axillary aspect of upper arm or by subcutaneous extension of primary incision into arm.
Forearm muscles	Morticians generally consider skin incision on the forearm undesirable, particularly in females. Incision in ulnar side of palmar aspect of forearm is least objectionable.
Intercostal; psoas major	No new incision required.
Quadriceps	Removed through incision in ventral aspect of thigh.
Anterior tibialis; gastrocnemius	Removed through incision in lateral aspect of lower leg.

SPECIAL TECHNIQUES

ARTERIOGRAPHY Adequate examination of the extracranial portions of the cerebral arteries is important. The simplest method consists of injecting water through the proximal stumps to test patency. This test is conclusive only when vessels are completely occluded; luminal narrowing cannot be appreciated by this method.

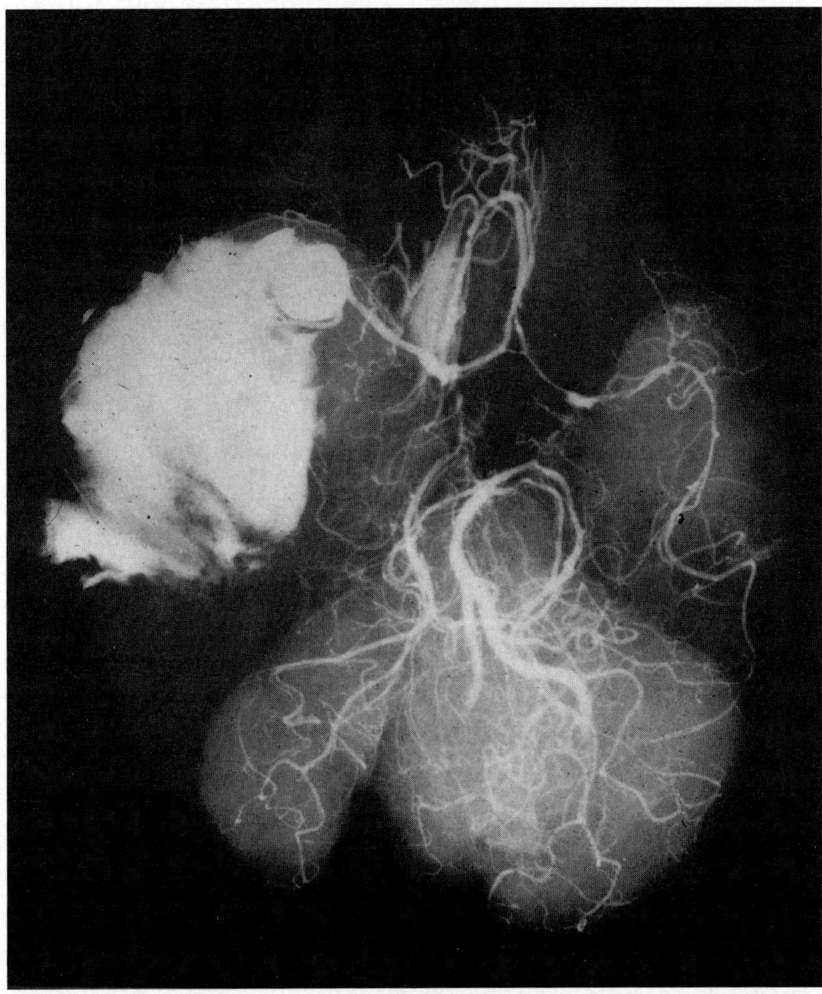

Fig. 6-16. Postmortem angiography. Usefulness of the method is demonstrated by this case in which large temporal lobe hematoma is associated with ruptured saccular aneurysm of right middle cerebral artery at "trifurcation".

Many postmortem angiographic studies of cerebral arteries have been described *(29–31)*. We remove the neck vessels in most instances and thus, angiographic studies are not performed routinely. When indications for them do arise, we clamp the external carotid arteries and inject 5–10 mL of warm barium sulfate-gelatin mixture into the common carotid arteries and roentgenograms are made in the autopsy room (Chapter 12). In a similar fashion, the vertebral arteries can be injected at their origins. Injection from the intracranial stumps of the internal carotid arteries also has been described *(29)*. We have injected a 40% solution of potassium iodide in Karo corn syrup, approximately at systolic pressure. The contrast medium temporarily distends the injected vessels and then dissipates rapidly, which does not interfere with satisfactory embalming of the face and with proper evaluation of the arteries and brains by the pathologist.

To opacify the intracranial cerebral arteries, we prefer to inject them after removal of the brain, so that the lesions can be inspected first. We routinely use a barium sulfate-gelatin mixture (Chapter 12), with or without addition of red or blue dye. When a cerebral aneurysm or vascular malformation is suspected but not immediately visualized by external inspection and careful flushing of the blood from the basal subarachnoid space, we prefer to inject the opacifying material before attempting to "dig out" the lesion. Successful roentgenographic demonstration (Fig. 6-16) obviates excessive "picking" of the brain substance. After roentgenographic demonstration of these lesions, the brain is best left intact until fixation is completed. Postmortem angiography is also useful in cases of surgically treated vascular lesions, for example, clipping of an aneurysm. Angiography shows whether the vascular system is patent, that is, whether contrast medium appears beyond the site of clipping.

VENOGRAPHY Injection of the venous system *in situ* or after removal of the brain appears to have little diagnostic use, although it provides background information for neuroradiologists who study the deep cerebral venous system in order to localize lesions. Radiopaque material is injected into the straight sinus or vein of Galen, preferably through a buff hole, before the brain is removed from the cranial cavity. The external venous system of various cranial sinuses and the superficial cerebral veins can be examined directly.

VENTRICULOGRAPHY Outlining the ventricular system of the brain by injection of various materials has been attempted

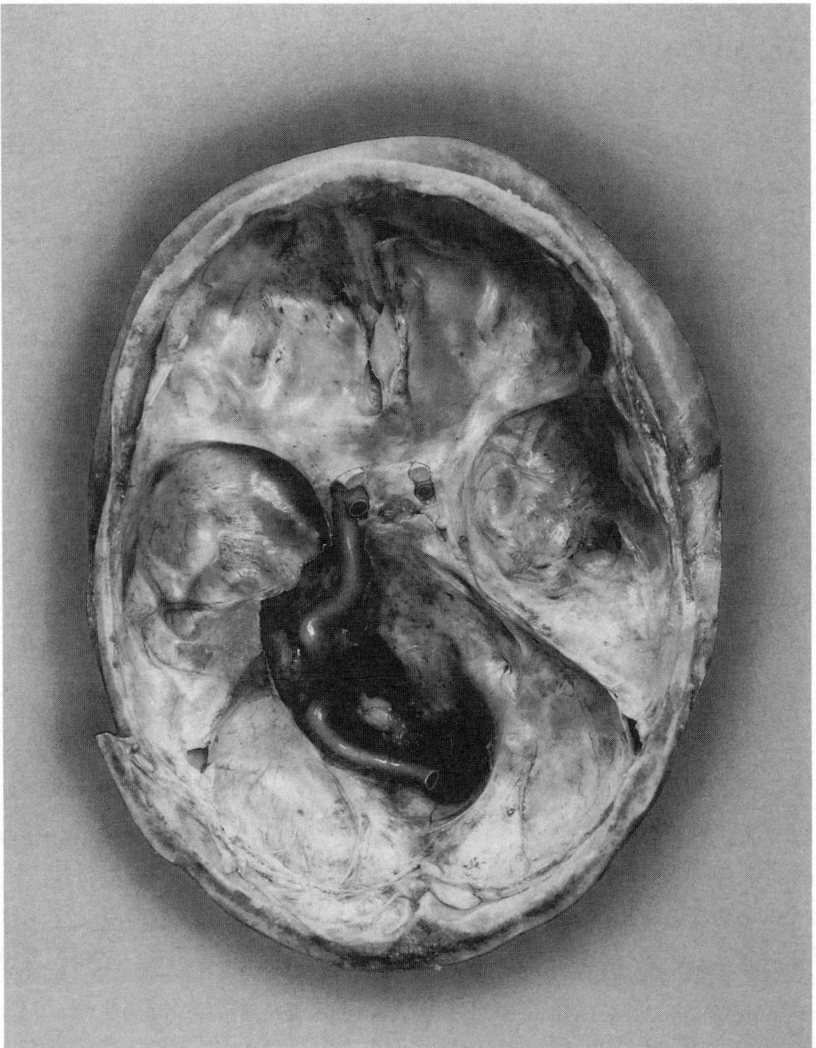

Fig. 6-17. Intracranial freeing of internal carotid and vertebral arteries. Portion of basal cranial bones to be removed is shown. Horizontal portion of carotid artery is exposed first down to carotid canal. Latter is exposed along with entrance of vertebral artery.

in the past mostly for preparation of anatomic specimens. Because pneumoencephalography and ventriculography are of historical interest only, these casting methods have ceased to be of interest for diagnostic neuropathology. For the technique of making casts, *see* ref. *(32)*.

REMOVAL OF NECK VESSELS For fear of interfering with subsequent embalming, neck vessels are rarely removed completely in the United States. We remove the neck organs and arteries after the embalming procedure, which is performed by private morticians in rooms adjoining the autopsy room. In some institutions, the common and internal carotid arteries are removed from the neck and a small rubber or plastic catheter is placed in the proximal external carotid artery for subsequent embalming at funeral homes *(30)*.

After the primary incision, the skin flap is reflected over the face while subcutaneous tissue is severed by blunt dissection with scissors. Keeping the neck straight or slightly overextended facilitates the approach to the arteries. The common carotid arteries are followed upward by blunt dissection, with occasional snips of scissors, up to the bifurcation. Then, the external and internal carotid arteries are isolated and the dissection is continued along the latter up to as close to the base of the skull as possible. The cavernous and petrous portions of the arteries are freed from the bony enclosure intracranially by chiseling or rongeuring the bone away. The carotid canal may be enlarged and the artery freed from the soft tissue in this region. This can be accomplished by removing a vertical strip of bone mesial to the canal and just above the entrance of the vertebral artery. This is preparatory for the complete removal of the latter. Use of an oscillating saw in part will facilitate the procedure. Then, the neck arteries can be pulled down from below.

Dissection of the vertebral arteries is a little more time-consuming *(33)*. First, portions of the occipital and temporal bones above the lateral and posterior parts of the atlas are removed intracranially by chiseling along the line shown in Fig. 6-17. We use the common bony defect to free intracranially the carotid and vertebral arteries. The posterior process of the superior articular surface of the atlas, which hides the artery, is chiseled

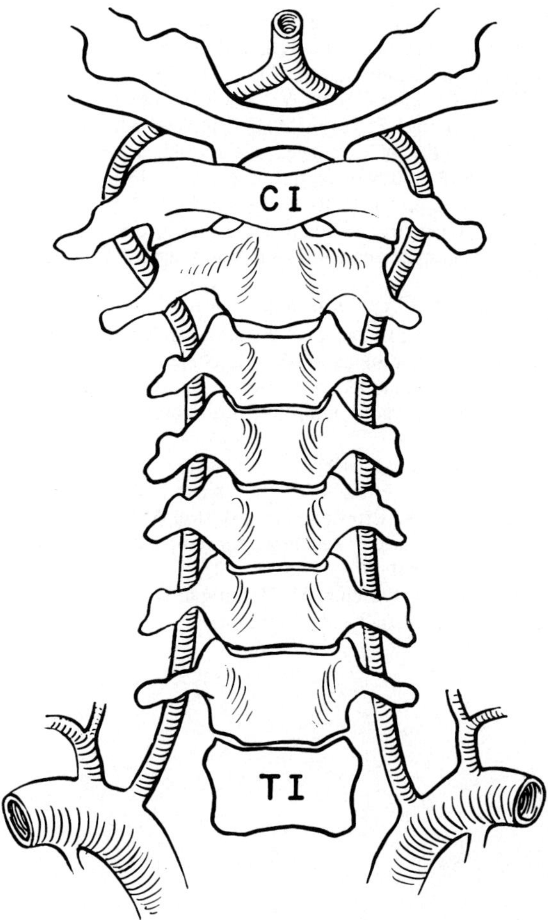

Fig. 6-18. Course of vertebral artery in neck.

away. The artery is then dissected free from the dura to the transverse process of the atlas. Second, in the neck (Fig. 6-18), the transverse foramina of the cervical spine up to the C-3 level are opened with a chisel; the transverse processes are broken, exposing the vertebral artery. The chisel should now be directed upward and laterally to follow the course of the artery in C-2. Because of the fibrous fixation of the artery to the transverse process of the atlas, the process is chiseled off medial to the artery and removed with the latter.

Alternatively, the cervical portion of the carotid and vertebral arteries can be removed together with the cervical spine (from the atlas to the seventh cervical vertebra), preceded by the injection of a barium sulfate-gelatine mixture (Chapter 12) into these arteries *(7)*. Because this interferes with the embalming procedure, the method proved impractical in our institution.

The removed arteries are examined either before or after adequate fixation. A method of perfusing the neck arteries under constant pressure (120–150 mm Hg) *(34)* supposedly preserved the vessels in the shape and degree of distention present in the systolic phase. Longitudinal sections of these vessels reveal the nature and extent of an atheromatous process, but the degree of narrowing of affected arterial segments cannot be assessed by this method. Also, this method of opening will create artifactual fractures on the surface of extensive plaques, and the condition of the luminal surface will be difficult to evaluate. Some particularly fragile atheromatous material will be lost. Of course, when occlusion is complete, this method of opening cannot be continued without destroying the pathologic process. To avoid these difficulties and to demonstrate the degree of luminal narrowing or the presence of thrombotic occclusion, cross-sectioning is preferred and generally causes less regret. Calcified neck vessels can be fixed in a formalin solution containing ethylenediamine tetraacetic acid (EDTA); this greatly reduces crush artifacts at the time of sectioning.

ACKNOWLEDGMENT

The authors would like to thank Drs. Vincenzo Caronia and Fabio Ricagna for their help with some of the illustrations.

REFERENCES

1. Mac Arthur S, Jacobson R, Marrero H, Rahman Z, Schneiderman H. Autopsy removal of the brain in AIDS. A new technique (Correspondence). Hum Pathol 1986;17:1296–1297.
2. Towfighi J, Roberts AF, Foster NE, Abt AB. A protective device for performing cranial autopsies. Hum Pathol 1989;20:288–289.
3. Brown P. Guidelines for high risk autopsy cases: special precautions for Creutzfeldt-Jakob disease. In: Autopsy Performance and Reporting. College of American Pathologists, Northfield, IL, 1990, pp. 68–74.
4. Budka H, Aguzzi A, Brown P, Brucher JM, Bugiani O, Gullota F, Haltia M. Tissue handling in suspected Creutzfeldt-Jakob disease and other human spongiform encephalopathies. Brain Pathol 1995;5: 319–322.
5. Isaacson G. Postmortem examination of infant brains (techniques for removal, fixation and sectioning). Arch Pathol Lab Med 1984; 108:80–81.
6. Bass T, Bergevin MA, Werner AL, Liuzzi FJ, Scott DE. In situ fixation of the neonatal brain and spinal cord. Ped Pathol 1993;13:699–705.
7. Okasaki H. Nervous system. In: Ludwig J, ed. Current Methods of Autopsy Practice. W.B. Saunders, Philadelphia, PA, 1979, pp. 96–129.
8. Wigglesworth JS. Performance of perinatal autopsy. In: Bennington JL, ed. Perinatal Pathology, vol. 15. Major Problems in Pathology. W.B. Saunders, Philadelphia, PA, 1984, pp. 37–39.
9. Towbin A. Neonatal neuropathologic examination. In: Tedeschi CG, ed. Neuropathology: Methods and Diagnosis. Little, Brown and Co., Boston, MA, 1970, pp. 215–224.
10. Adams VI. Autopsy technique for neck examination II. Vertebral column and posterior compartment. Pathol Annu 1991;26:211–226.
11. Geddes JF, Gonzales AG. Examination of spinal cord in diseases of the craniocervical junction and high cervical spine. J Clin Pathol 1991;44:170–172.
12. Laurence KM, Martin D. A technique for obtaining undistorted specimens of the central nervous system. J Clin Pathol 1959;12:188–190.
13. Sheehan HL. Neurohypophysis and hypothalamus. In: Bloodworth JMB Jr, ed. Endocrine Pathology. Williams & Wilkins, Baltimore, MD, 1968, pp. 12–74.
14. Szanto PB. A modified technique for the removal of the nasopharynx and accompanying organs of the throat. Arch Pathol 1944;38:313–320.
15. Lamprecht J, Hegemann S, Hauptmann S. Advantages of ENT-specialty-specific autopsy technique [German] HNO 1994;42:233–235.
16. Temporal Bone Banks Program for Ear Research. Technique for acquiring and preparing the human temporal bone for the study of middle and ear pathology. Tran Am Acad Ophthalmol Otolaryngol 1966;70:871–878.

17. Michaels L, Wells M, Frohlich A. A new technique for the study of temporal bone pathology. Clin Otolaryng 1983;8:77–85.
18. Thompson SW. Selected Histochemical and Histopathological Methods. Charles C. Thomas, Springfield, IL, 1966, pp. 13–14.
19. Tedeschi CG. Neuropathology: Methods and Diagnosis. Little, Brown and Co., Boston, MA, 1970.
20. Simpson RHW, Berson SD. The postmortem diagnosis of diffuse cerebral injuries, with special reference to the importance of brain fixation. S Afr Med J 1987;71:10–14.
21. Katelaris A, Kencian J, Duflou J, Hilton JMN. Brain at necropsy: to fix or not to fix? J Clin Pathol 1994;47:718–720.
22. Powers JM. Practice guidelines for autopsy pathology. Autopsy procedures for brain, spinal cord and neuromuscular system. Autopsy Committe of the College of American Pathologists. Arch Pathol Lab Med 1995;119:777–783.
23. Alafuzoff I, Winblad B. How to run a brain bank: potentials and pitfalls in the use of human post-mortem brain material in research. J Neural Transm 1993;39:235–243.
24. Duyckaerts C, Sazdovitch V, Seilhean D, Delaere P, Hauw JJ. A brain bank in a neuropathology laboratory (with some emphasis on diagnostic criteria). J Neural Transm 1993;39:107–118.
25. Lindenberg R. Forensic neuropathology. In: Minckler J, ed. Pathology of the Nervous System. McGraw-Hill, New York, 1972, pp. 2726–2740.
26. Nguyen JP, Gaston A, Louarn F, Marsault C, Bargiotas E, Wallman J, Poirier J. CT of brain: technique for comparative postmortem slicing. Am J Neuroradiol 1983;4:191–193
27. Dyck PJ, Giannini C, Lais A. Pathologic alterations of nerves. In: Dyck PJ, Thomas PK, Low PA, Griffin JW, Poduslo JF, eds. Peripheral Neuropathy. W.B. Saunders, Philadelphia, PA, 1993, pp. 514–595.
28. Beckwith JB. Sampling of muscle at autopsy in cases of lower motor neuron disease. Am J Clin Pathol 1964;42:92–93.
29. Choi SS, Crampton A. Atherosclerosis of arteries of neck: postmortem angiographic and pathologic study. Arch Pathol 1961;72:379–385.
30. Stein BM, Svare GT. A technique of postmortem angiography for evaluating arteriosclerosis of the aortic arch and carotid and vertebral arteries. Radiology 1963;81:252–256.
31. Karhunen PJ, Mannikko A, Penttila A, Liesto K. Diagnostic angiography in postoperative autopsies. Am J Forens Pathol 1989;10:303–309.
32. Thompsett DH, Tedeschi CG. Museum preparations of brain and spinal cord. In: Tedeschi CG, ed. Neuropathology: Methods and Diagnosis. Little, Brown and Co., Boston, MA, 1970, pp. 215–224.
33. Bromilow A, Burns J. Technique for removal of the vertebral arteries. J Clin Pathol 1985;38:1400–1402.
34. McCormick WF, Stein BM. Technique for study of extracranial arteries. Arch Pathol 1962;74:52–56.

7 The Eye and Adnexa

R. JEAN CAMPBELL

As the eye and the adnexal structures may be involved by systemic disease, as well as by direct extension from adjacent structures, it is important to consider their removal and study in the autopsy procedure *(1,2)*. Primary pathology that involves the eye will obviously require the removal of these structures. Such primary pathology embraces not only neoplasms but congenital abnormalities, primary open angle glaucoma, and a host of retinal diseases for which the pathology may not hitherto have been described. In addition to the value of correlative information, the eyes provide valuable teaching material for those in training. Fresh tissue allows research procedures of the corneal endothelium and cells of the trabecular meshwork.

Forensic investigation may require sampling of the vitreous for toxicology and biochemical studies *(3,4)*. The eye may also be injured directly or show the effects of a nonaccidental death such as child abuse *(5)*. Legal and ethical considerations will vary from country to country and, within North America, from state to state, but the same health and safety considerations are utilised as for the general autopsy procedure.

VITREOUS SAMPLING

Sampling of the vitreous for toxicological and other forensic investigation *(3,4)* or for microbiologic studies *(6)* is best performed on an eye that is intact and without known structural intraocular pathology, such as a retinal detachment. A 15-gauge needle is inserted at an oblique angle through the sclera at a point 5 mm lateral to the limbus (corneo-scleral junction) (Fig. 7-1). The needle will traverse the pars plana and enter the vitreous body. Damage to the retinal cells will result in a falsely high potassium value (the correct vitreous potassium concentration can be used for a rough estimation of the postmortem interval) and thus *gentle* aspiration of 2–3 mL of vitreous is required. The material, which is drawn into a 10 mL sterile syringe may be stored at 4°C for up to 48 h (*see also* p. 16 and 113).

In *suspected child abuse*, vitreous should *never* be aspirated because there is a risk of artifactual damage to the retina. Instead, prior to the removal of the eye (*see* below), the fundus should be photographed. It is the retina that bears the brunt of the injury in child abuse and the assessment and position of retinal hemorrhages is of prime importance.

From: *Handbook of Autopsy Practice,* 3rd Ed. Edited by: J. Ludwig © Humana Press Inc., Totowa, NJ

REMOVAL OF THE EYE AND ORBITAL CONTENTS

ANTERIOR APPROACH In the vast majority of instances, the eye is removed by the anterior approach. (For the removal of orbital contents, *see* below under "Intracranial Approach.") The eyelids are held apart with the aid of retractors (Fig. 7-2). Using curved scissors, the conjunctival attachments to the limbus are severed, care being taken not to cut the eyelids. Tenon's capsule is left intact to avoid leakage into the empty socket. The four rectus muscles are cut so that approx 5.0 mm of muscle are left attached to the globe; this allows orientation of the globe at a later time. The inferior oblique muscle is then severed. Rotation of the eye temporally by traction on the stump of the inferior oblique muscle allows access to the optic nerve and ensures that a long piece of the intraorbital portion of the optic nerve is obtained. It is not deemed necessary to ligate the optic stalk as only a portion of the leakage after enucleation arises from the severed end of the optic nerve. The socket is dried with a towel and a silastic mold is placed in position (Fig. 7-3). The disadvantage of this anterior approach is that it excludes adequate examination of the orbital contents and the lacrimal gland.

INTRACRANIAL APPROACH (EXENTERATION PROCEDURE) This method is advisable when there is pathology of the orbit *and* the eye. Such conditions include inflammation, neoplasia, vascular disease, and disease of the orbital portion of the optic nerve. The method consists of first cutting the conjunctival attachments at the limbus by the anterior approach as outlined earlier, and using the intracranial approach to expose the orbital contents.

After removal of the brain, two saw cuts are made, one vertically downward opposite the cribriform plate of the ethmoid and the second downward and medially, immediately anterior to the lateral end of the lesser wing of the sphenoid. The orbital plate is broken with a chisel and hammer and the bone is removed piecemeal with the aid of bone forceps. Care must be taken not to damage the optic nerve and other contents of the optic foramen as this area is exposed. Curved scissors are used to free the globe and its attached muscles. The superior oblique muscle is cut from the body of the sphenoid bone and the inferior oblique muscle is cut from the floor of the medial orbit. Freeing of the conjunctival attachments must proceed with caution in order to avoid damage to the eyelids and anterior chamber of the eye.

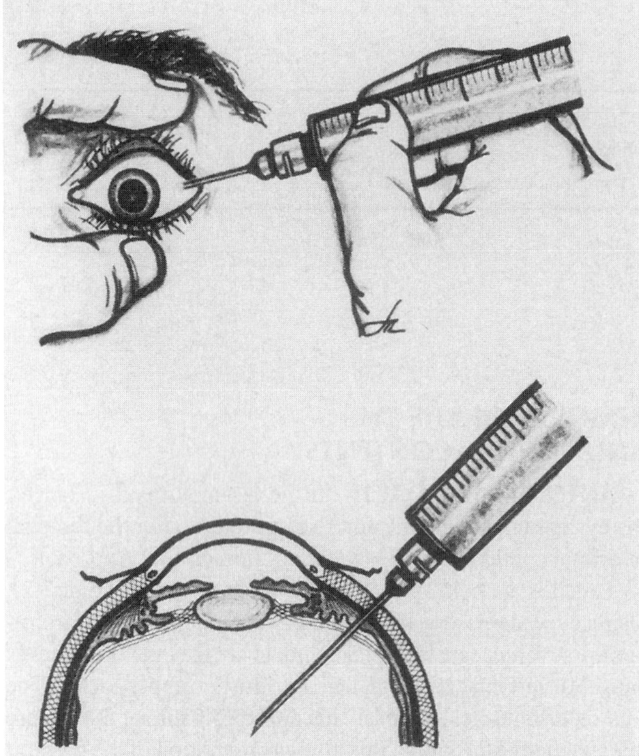

Fig. 7-1. Aspiration of vitreous. Upper, Needle inserted 5 mm lateral to the limbus (corneo-scleral junction). Lower, Needle enters vitreous through pars plana of ciliary body.

The eye with optic nerve, surrounding nerves, muscles, and fat, are freed from the walls of the orbit. Again, Tenon's capsule is left intact in order to avoid leakage into the empty socket. The orbit and lacrimal fossa should be palpated after the exenteration procedure to determine the presence or absence of any abnormality such as a neoplasm.

REMOVAL OF CORNEA FOR TRANSPLANTATION

CONTRAINDICATIONS The Eye Bank Association of America (EBAA) *(7)* and the Food and Drug Administration (FDA) have stringent standards and regulations for tissue that is to be used for transplantation. This has made it necessary for trained personnel who are aware of the ever-changing requirements to be responsible for the retrieval and processing of such tissue.

At the time of writing, the EBAA has a list of absolute contraindications that includes HIV, hepatitis B and C (social conditions that put the donor at risk for these entities are also considered contraindications), Creutzfeld-Jakob disease, ocular and intraocular inflammation, rabies, malignant tumors of the anterior segment, leukemia, lymphoma, and retinoblastoma.

The EBAA Medical Standards define the minimum standards of practice for the procurement, preservation, storage, and distribution of eye tissue for transplantation as determined by the ophthalmic medical community.

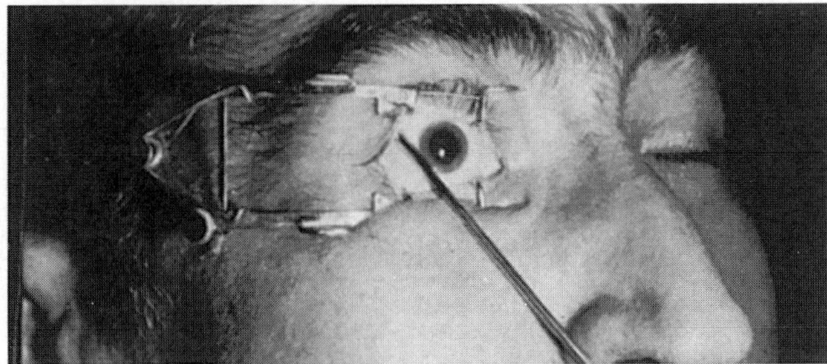

Fig. 7-2. Eyelids held apart by Weeks' speculum. This allows enucleation or biopsy of the lacrimal gland.

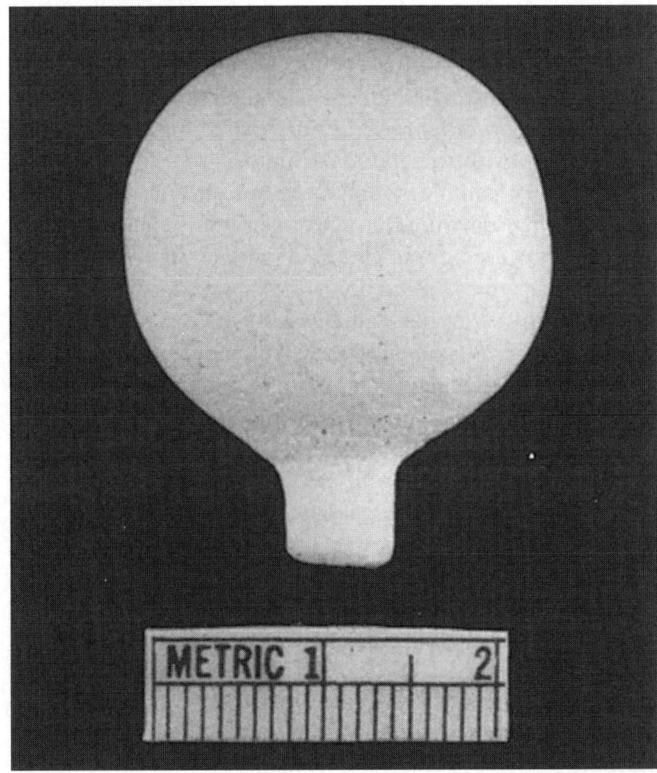

Fig. 7-3. Prosthetic mold. The material is composed of "Coecal Buff" dental stone (Coe Laboratories, Inc., Chicago, IL) that is placed in empty socket after removal of eye.

TECHNICAL ASPECTS Preferably, the enucleation is performed before the general autopsy procedure has commenced. The eye is removed by the anterior approach under aseptic conditions as soon as possible after death but within 24 h.

The eye is placed with the cornea directed upwards in a glass receptor that contains sterile saline (Fig. 7-4). The specimen is kept at 2–6°C in a refrigerator. If the eye is to be transported out of town, the moist chamber jar is placed in a Styrofoam container with plastic bags that contain chipped ice. Blood is collected from the donor (7–10 mL) for required serological testing. Contact with the local police or highway patrol will facilitate rapid transport to its destination.

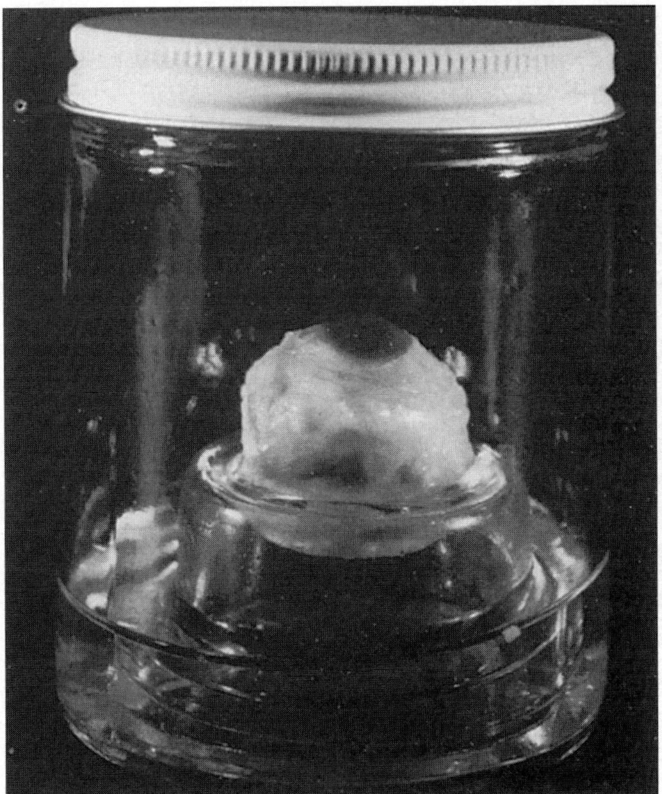

Fig. 7-4. Eye for corneal transplantation. Eye positioned in sterile glass receptor with cornea directed upward. Sterile jar contains sterile saline to maintain moisture to cornea.

REMOVAL OF SCLERA FOR TRANSPLANTATION

The same requirements must be met that are used for the retrieval of other tissues for transplantation. Before embalming, the eye is enucleated by either of the methods previously outlined. The enucleated globe is opened immediately and the anterior segment, choroid, retina, and vitreous are removed. As much as possible of the darkly pigmented choroid is removed with the aid of a cotton swab. The remaining sclera is cut into suitable portions for surgical use (halves, quarters, or thirds). Each portion is packaged separately in a plastic bag (Fig. 7-5) and is sterilized by exposure to gamma rays from a cobalt-60 unit (Neutron Products, Inc. Dickerson). After completion of sterilization by this method, one batch of sclera is cultured as a control to check that sterilization has been satisfactory.

REMOVAL OF THE LACRIMAL GLAND

The lobulated, bean-shaped lacrimal gland lies in the lateral part of the upper orbit in the hollow of the medial side of the zygomatic process of the frontal bone and is adjacent to the roof (Fig. 7-6). The gland may be obtained either before or after removal of the globe. The lacrimal nerve and artery, which lie in the fat at the junction of the roof and lateral wall of the orbit, may be traced to the lacrimal gland. The concave medial surface of the gland lies on the superior levator and lateral rectus muscles; these may also be traced to the gland. Curved scissors are used to free the gland from the adjacent muscles and the short fibrous bands that bind it to the orbital margin.

If only a limited autopsy is permitted, a specimen of lacrimal gland may be obtained by inserting a biopsy needle beneath the upper eyelid and aiming it upward and laterally toward this gland.

PROCESSING OF OCULAR SPECIMENS

FIXATION, ORIENTATION, DOCUMENTATION OF LESIONS AND SECTIONING The enucleated eye is placed in 20–25 times its volume of 10% buffered formalin for 48 h of fixation. The neck of the container should be approximately twice the diameter of the globe for ease of removal of the specimen (Fig. 7-4). Injection of fixative into the globe is *not* necessary and should be avoided as it introduces artifact into the globe.

If the eye and orbital contents have been removed in toto, the eye should be dissected from the orbital contents and placed in a separate container because otherwise, its fixation will be delayed. The orbital contents are fixed separately.

After 48 h fixation, the eye is rinsed in running water to allow easier handling by persons sensitive to formalin. It is then placed in 60% alcohol until it is sectioned, a period of 16–20 h.

Orientation with regard to side is determined by observation of the following (Fig. 7-7):

1. The horizontal plane is characterized by the posterior ciliary vessels; the more prominent vessels lie on the nasal side.
2. The temporal side is characterized by the insertion of the inferior oblique muscle, which is usually fleshy and extends inferiorly from the optic nerve.
3. The superior aspect is characterized by the tendinous insertion of the superior oblique muscle, which underlies the superior rectus muscle.

The superior pole is marked with a grease pencil to allow continued quick orientation with subsequent handling (Fig. 7-8). The anteroposterior, horizontal, and vertical planes are measured with a caliper (Fig. 7-9). If the presence of calcium, bone, or a foreign body is suspected, a roentgenogram of the globe is helpful (Fig. 7-10).

A phthisical eye contains bone and thus requires decalcification. This is performed using Formic Acid Decal which is a 20% solution of formic acid in 10% neutral buffered formalin. Orbital bone requires a stronger decalcification solution. The rapid method with Decalcifier ll (Surgipath) is effective but once the bone is placed in this solution, it must be examined every 2 h and cannot be left in the solution overnight. Adequate decalcification is determined by repeat roentgenograms.

The external appearance of the eye should be documented. Surgical and accidental penetrating or perforating wounds need to be noted. Transillumination of the globe is then performed. If a defect in transillumination is present, such as may be caused by an intraocular tumor, the area is outlined with a grease pencil, the size of the opacity determined, and the plane of section is made accordingly to give the best information.

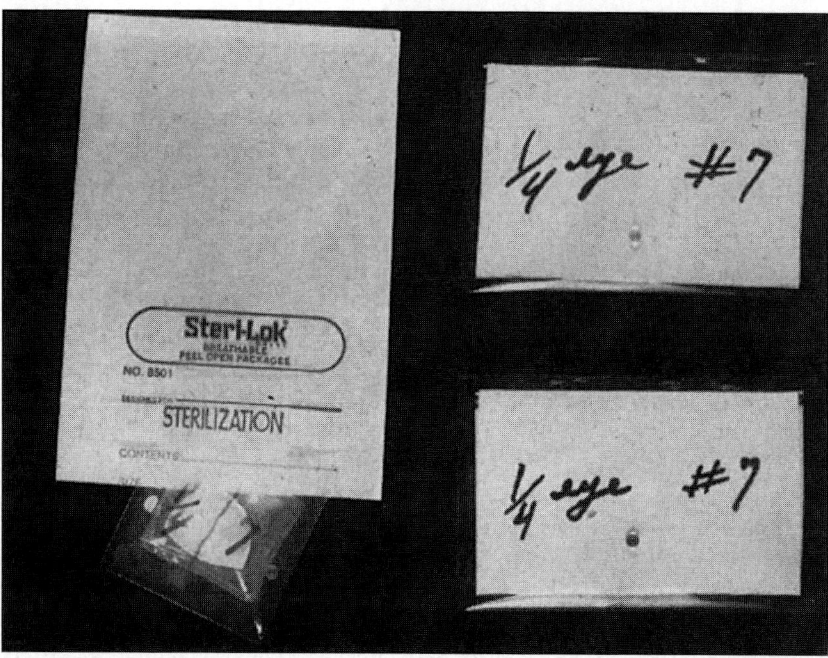

Fig. 7-5. Scleral tissue for transplantation. Left, Sclera sealed in double plastic container is placed within containing jacket (Steri-Lok package) for sterilization. Note glass bead, which is clear before radiation process. Right, Upper package contains nonsterile sclera with a clear glass bead that indicates the tissue has not yet been exposed to radiation and is therefore not sterile. Lower package contains sterile sclera with darkened bead, which indicates exposure to radiation.

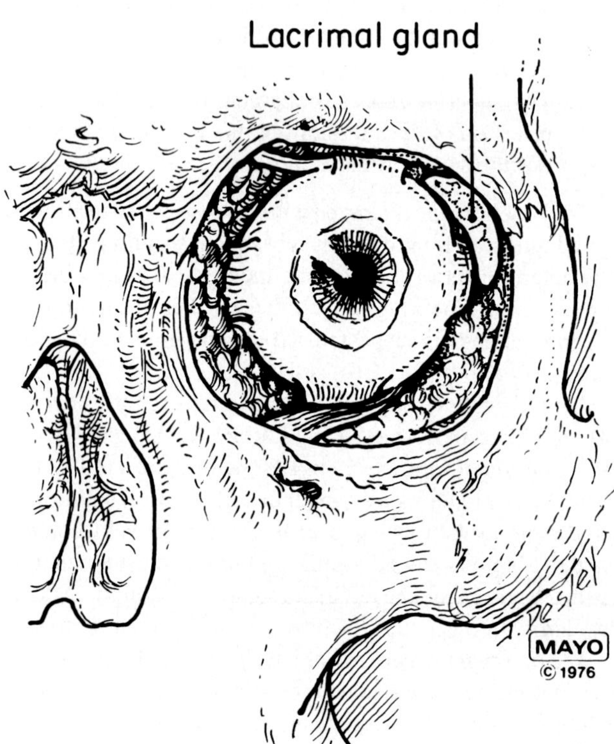

Fig. 7-6. Diagram of left orbit viewed from front. Note position of lacrimal gland in lacrimal fossa.

A transverse section of the optic nerve is made only if the length of the optic nerve is such that the back of the globe will not be opened by the cut (Fig. 7-11).

Sectioning is performed on a piece of dental wax, to which the escaping vitreous does not adhere; thus the attachment of the retina to the choroid is maintained. The eye is positioned so that the cornea is against the wax and the optic nerve projects upwards. The inferior 'cap' or calotte is removed by placing a razor blade immediately abutting the inferior aspect of the optic nerve (Fig. 7-12). With a smooth motion, the blade is directed toward the limbal edge of the cornea. The inferior calotte, together with the remaining globe, is examined in 60% alcohol under a dissecting microscope (Fig. 7-13). Pathological conditions and photography are recorded at this time.

Most eyes are sectioned in the horizontal plane (Fig. 7-14). This is known as the PO section (pupil/optic disc) and will show the macula as well as the optic disc and pupil. For eyes that have been traumatized or contain a neoplasm, such a horizontal cut may not show the pathology to advantage and an oblique or vertical cut may be required.

The larger portion of the globe with the superior pole is then placed with its flat surface on the dental wax. The razor blade is placed immediately adjacent to the optic nerve and the second cut is made parallel to the first; this mid-section of the globe, approx 3 mm thick, is submitted for processing. A diagram for sectioning the globes is shown in Fig. 7-15. The instruments used for sectioning are shown in Fig. 7-16.

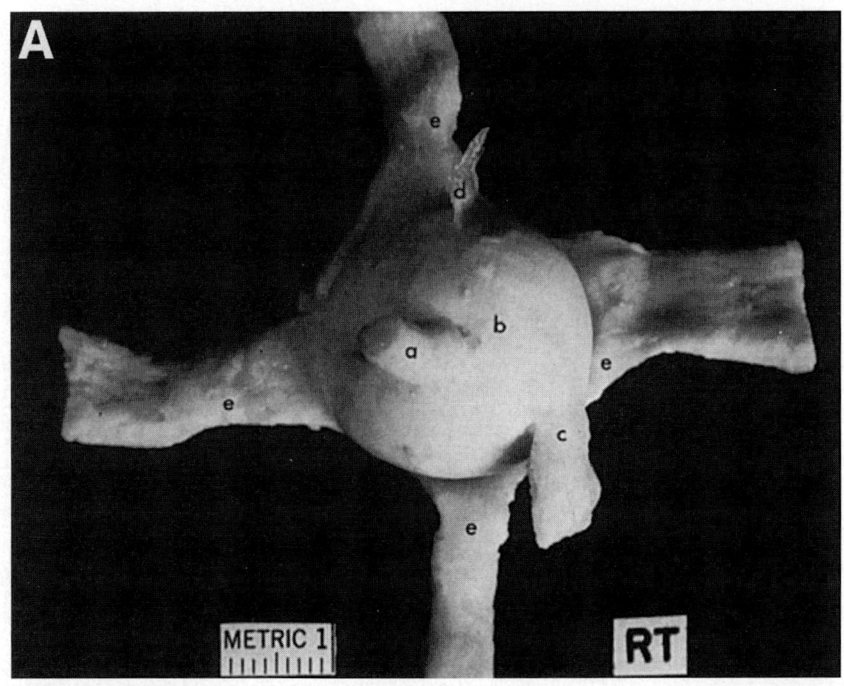

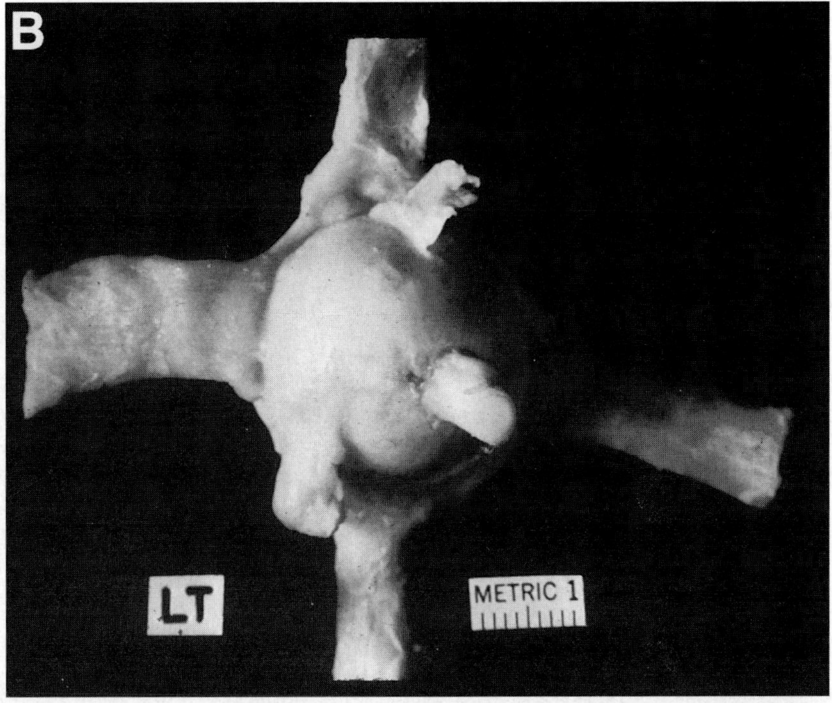

Fig. 7-7. Eyes enucleated at autopsy. (**A**) Right eye. (**B**) Left eye. Note (a) optic nerve, (b) posterior ciliary vessels running horizontally, (c) inferior oblique muscle, (d) superior oblique muscle, and (e) rectus muscles.

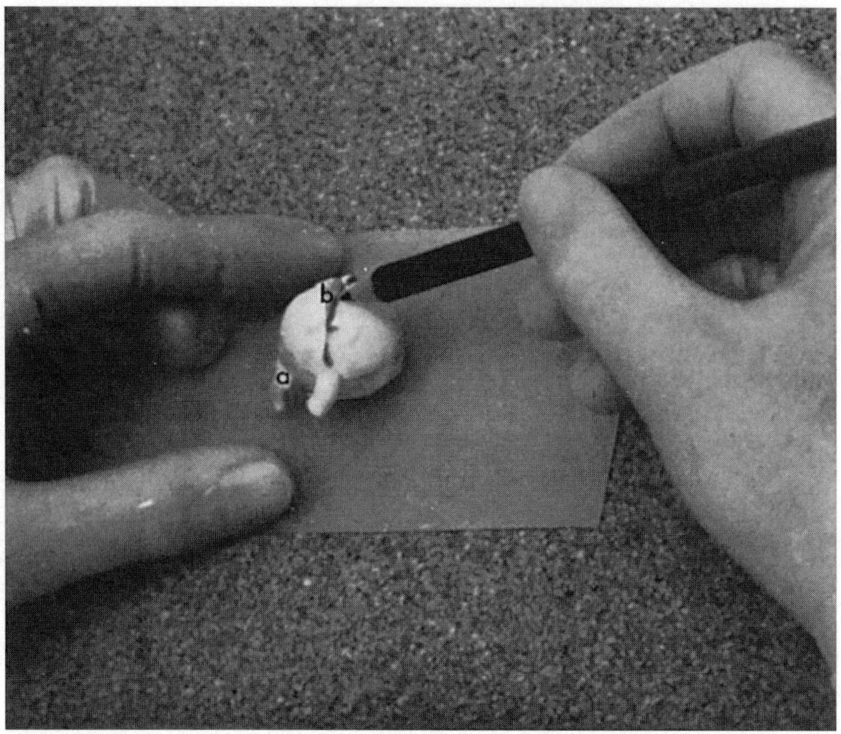

Fig. 7-8. Left eye in position on piece of dental wax. Superior pole is marked with a grease pencil. Note inferior oblique muscle (a) and superior oblique muscle (b).

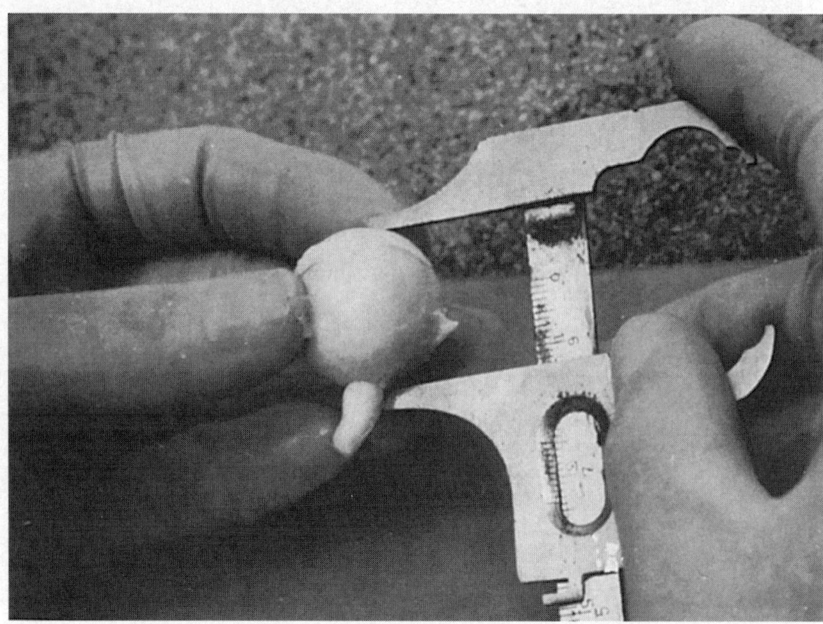

Fig. 7-9. Measurement of globe. Eye is measured in three planes: anteroposterior, horizontal, and vertical.

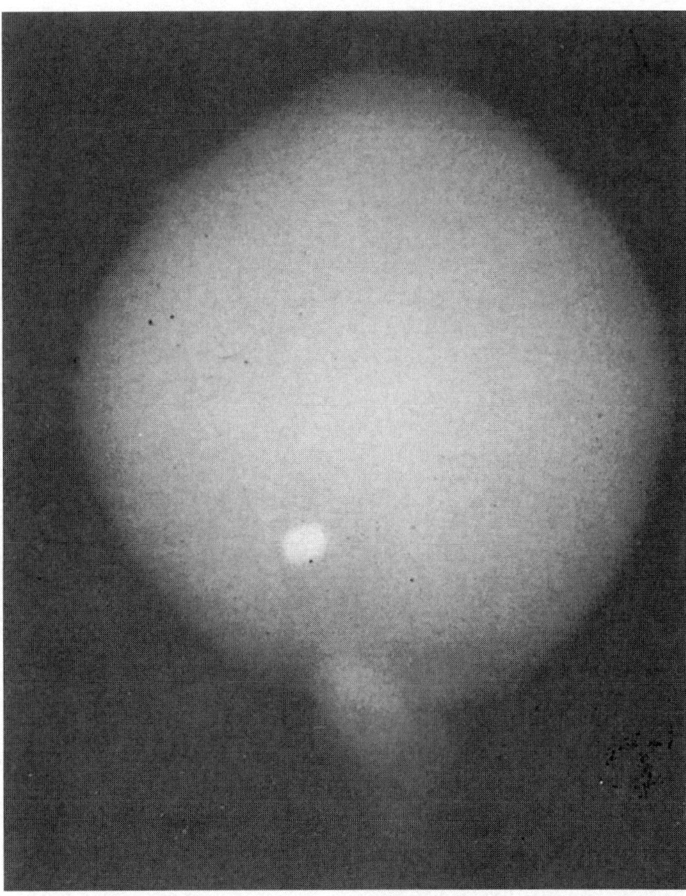

Fig. 7-10. Roentgenogram of globe showing foreign body (portion of bullet).

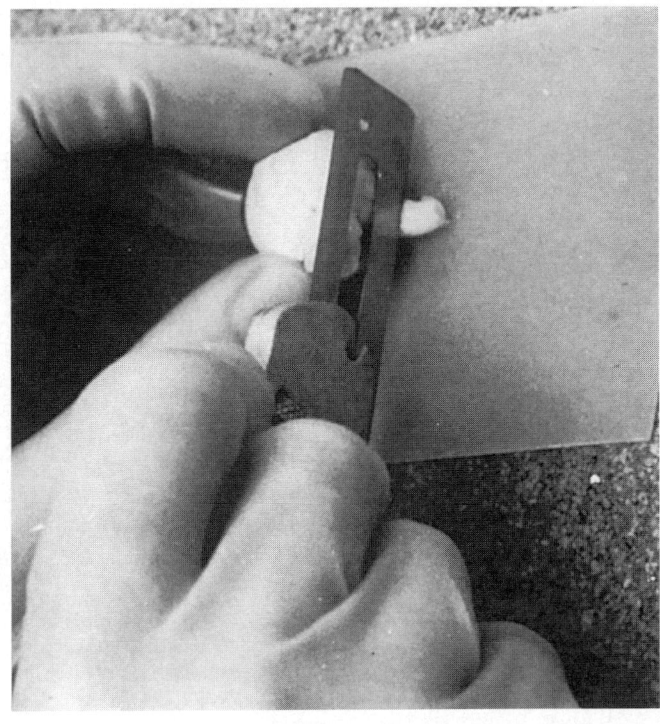

Fig. 7-11. Eye in position on dental wax. Blade in position for transverse section of optic nerve.

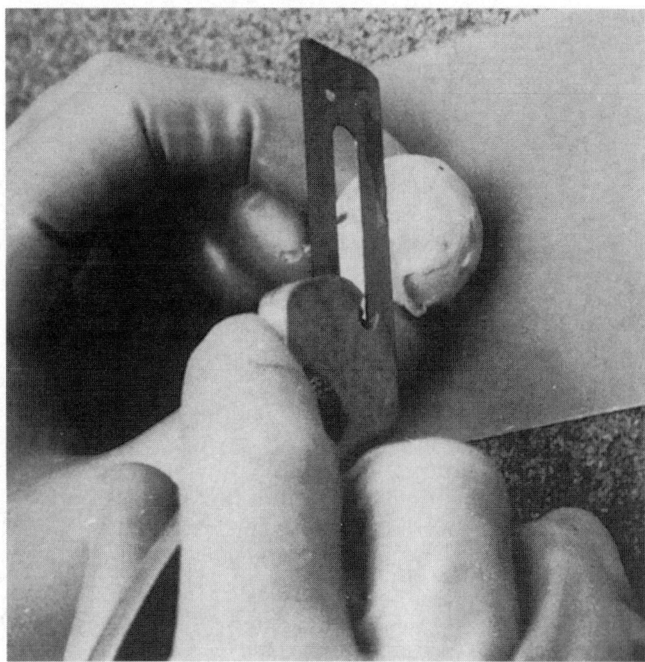

Fig. 7-12. Sectioning of globe. Eye is positioned with cornea facing down on dental wax and superior pole with grease pencil mark is to left. Razor blade is placed parallel to the horizontally running posterior ciliary vessels and immediately abutting the optic nerve. This cut removes the inferior calotte.

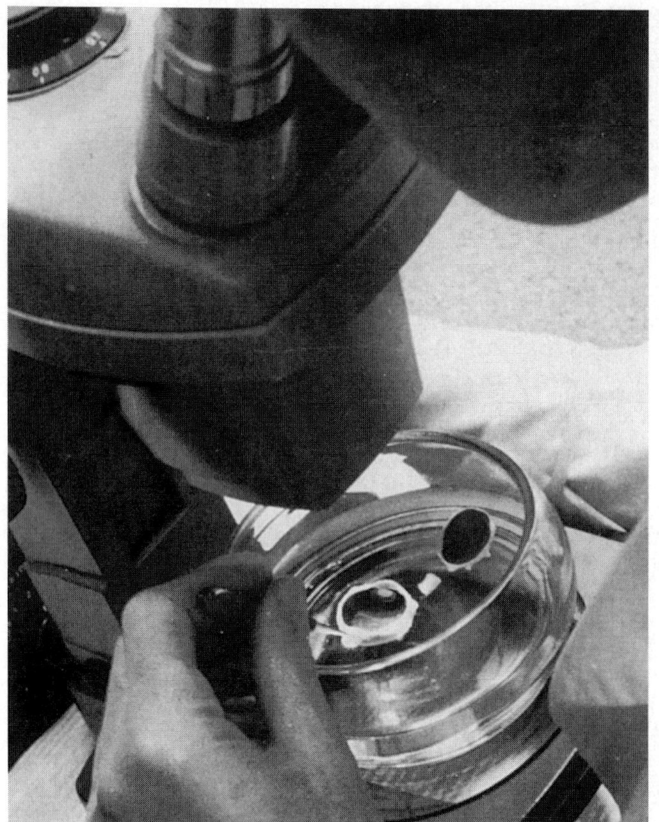

Fig. 7-13. Sectioned globe. Inferior calotte and remaining globe are placed in 60% alcohol and examined with a dissecting scope.

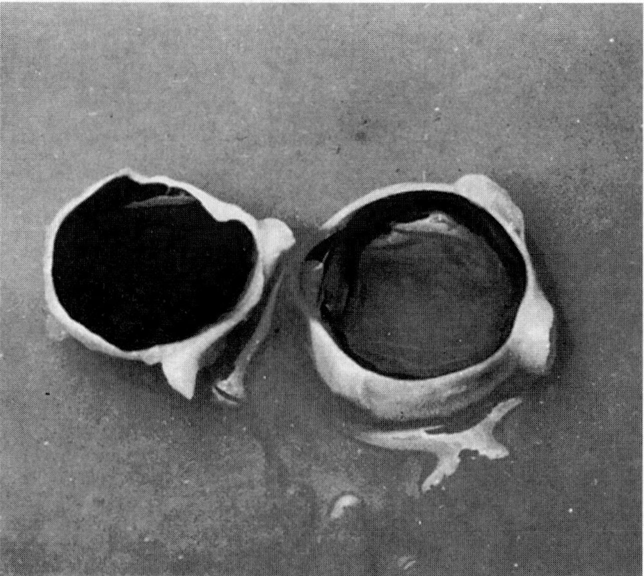

Fig. 7-14. Sectioned globe. The 3-mm thick horizontal section is on the right. The superior calotte is on the left.

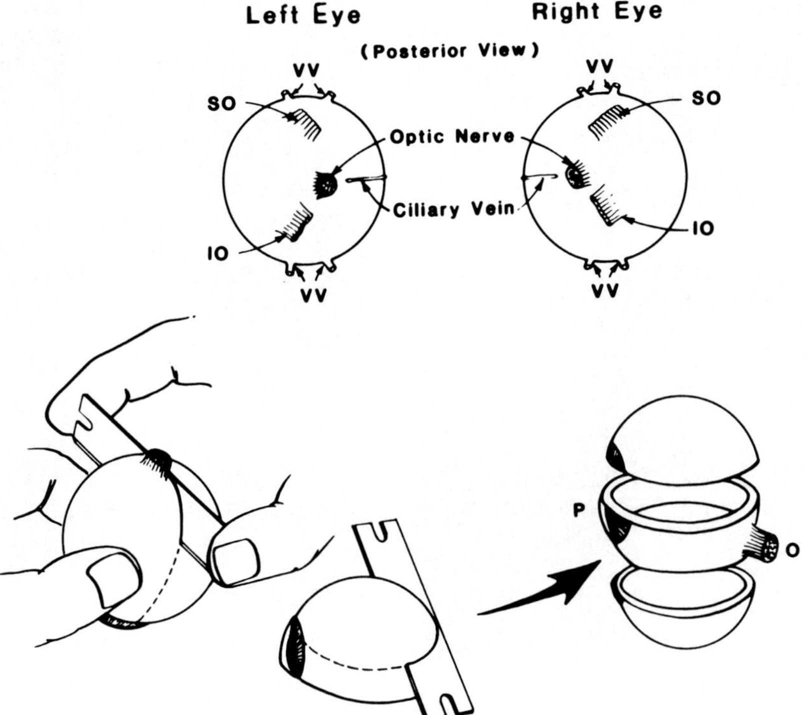

Fig. 7-15. Diagram demonstrating sectioning of the globe.

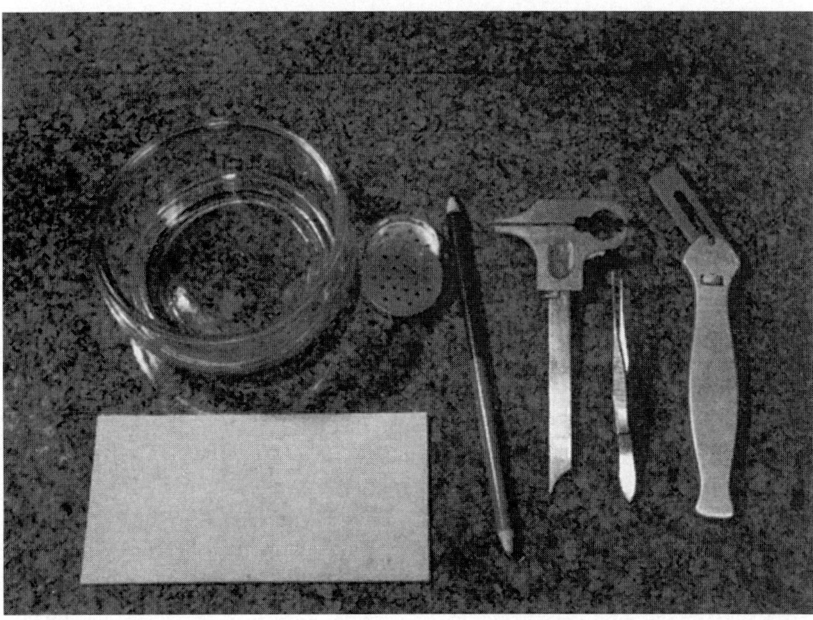

Fig. 7-16. Instruments used for sectioning globe. From left to right: glass bowl, tissue button, grease pencil, caliper, forceps, and razor blade. Piece of dental wax is in foreground.

EYES CONTAINING AN INTRAOCULAR PROSTHESIS (IOL) It is recommended that such specimens are opened in the coronal plane. The anterior segment is processed as a whole. Chloroform, as a clearing agent, will dissolve the plastic prosthesis and other plastic substances such as a scleral buckle or a Molteno shunt. The paraffin-infiltrated specimen is then trisected to display the position of the hapics that have anchored the prosthesis within the eye. All pieces sectioned are embedded. The posterior portion of the globe is sectioned in the horizontal plane.

STAINING PROCEDURES Routine stains include hematoxylin and eosin and the periodic acid Schiff reaction. The latter gives adequate examination of Descemet's membrane, the lens capsule, Bruch's membrane, and other materials with CHO groupings such as glycogen.

PREPARATION FOR ELECTRON MICROSCOPY The eye is opened immediately upon removal from the body and the specimen is placed promptly into a 3% solution of glutaraldehyde. With the aid of the dissecting microscope, sections that are 2 mm square, are cut from the area selected for examination.

REFERENCES

1. Eye Bank Association of America. Medical Standards. Eye Bank Association of America, Washington, DC, 1996.
2. Forrest AR. ACP Broadsheet no. 137: April 1993. Obtaining samples at post mortem examination for toxicological and biochemical analyses. J Clin Pathol 1993;46:292–296.
3. Green MA, Lieberman G, Milroy CM, Parsons MA. Ocular and Cerebral trauma in non-accidental injury in infancy: underlying mechanisms and implications for paediatric practice. Br J Ophthalmol 1996; 80:282–287.
4. Lee WR. Examination of the globe: technical aspects. In: Lee WR, ed. Ophthalmic Histopathology. Springer-Verlag, London, 1993, pp. 1–23.
5. McKinney PE, Phillips S, Gomez HF, Brent J, MacIntyre M, Watson WA. Vitreous humor cocaine and metabolite concentrations: do postmortem specimens reflect blood levels at the time of death? J Forensic Sci 1995;40:102–107.
6. Mietz H, Heimann K, Kuhn J, Wieland U, Eggers HJ. Detection of HIV in human vitreous. Int Ophthalmology 1993;17:101–104.
7. Parsons MA, Staut RD. ACP Best Practice no. 164. Necropsy techniques in ophthalmic pathology. J Clin Pathol 2001;54:417–427.

8 Skeletal System

JURGEN LUDWIG

DISSECTION AND REMOVAL OF BONE SPECIMENS

Routine preparation of gross and microscopic bone specimens can be carried out only on a limited scale. However, portions of rib with costochondral junction, sternum, vertebral body, or iliac crest, and sternoclavicular joint should be removed and permanently saved in every autopsy. Specimens suggested for study in cases of metabolic or other systemic bone and joint diseases are indicated below. The site of a circumscribed neoplastic or inflammatory bone lesion can be determined from clinical or roentgenological examination. Circumscribed osteolytic processes in the ribs or in the calvarium can often be identified by viewing these specimens against a bright light.

Specimens consisting of both bone and soft tissue may be difficult to prepare for satisfactory preservation. The best method is to freeze the fixed specimen and to cut the solidly frozen tissue with a band saw. The sliced specimen is placed in a tank of alcohol. The layer, on the cut surface, of frozen fat and sawdust is removed with a brush or will float off spontaneously. The alcohol treatment will also restore the color in specimens fixed in Kaiserling I solution *(1)* (*see* Chapter 14).

SAWING Handsaws and chisels have become obsolete and at present, only two types of saws are in general use.

Oscillating Saws The Stryker autopsy saw (Stryker Corporation, 420 Alcott Street, Kalamazoo, MI) still is the most popular tool in this class. The blade of this saw cuts bone by high-speed oscillation. Blades of various shapes with round cutting edges can be attached to the arbor, depending on the size and location of the bone specimen to be removed. One of the largest blades (#1105) is used for the anterior removal of the *spinal column* (*see* Chapter 6). *Temporal bones* are removed with a trephine (Schuknecht temporal trephine, Stryker Corporation). According to the specifications, this trephine cuts about 4.5 cm deep and removes a specimen about 3.7 cm in diameter.

The Lipshaw autopsy saw (saw no. 450; Lipshaw Manufacturing Company, 7446 Central Ave., Detroit, MI) differs from the Stryker saw because its motor is not in the handpiece but separated from the instrument by a cable. Lipshaw blades also can be used with the Stryker saw; these blades generally are less expensive.

A disadvantage of oscillating saws is the production of bone dust, both in the air and in the structures of the cut surface. Inhalation should be prevented by wearing a face shield or hood and by removing the calvarium inside a plastic bag *(2,3)* (*see* Chapters 16 and 6, respectively). After use of oscillating or other saws, bone dust on the cut surface can in part be brushed off, but histologic sections must be from deep within the block to avoid the dust particles. Use of cold saline during sawing will wash away some bone dust and will also prevent heating of bone.

All oscillating saws become hot after prolonged use. Occasional greasing of the moving parts is advisable.

Band Saws This type of saw is ideal if one wishes to prepare even section through large bones such as the femur or the spinal column. Band saws also are preferred for cutting small specimens into thin slices for histologic preparations. Unfortunately, they are difficult to clean and hazardous to operate. Because of the increased concerns related to infection control, we no longer use a band saw on fresh specimens.

PREPARATION OF HISTOLOGIC SPECIMENS To achieve optimal fixation with minimal exposure to decalcifying agents, bone specimens for histologic study should not be thicker than 3 mm. However, bone dust from sawing machines may have been ground into all levels of such a specimen, so that somewhat thicker sections may be required. Thin sections are easier to prepare with a band saw, which also grinds less bone dust into the section than does an oscillating saw. For the hazards of band saws, see previous paragraph. Brushing and flushing of the cut surfaces with saline and submerging the specimen in alcohol help to remove superficial bone dust. Excellent results can also be achieved by freezing the specimens in water and then sawing them in a solid block of ice until pieces of the desired shape and thickness are obtained. The plane of the saw sections will usually be perpendicular to articular, periosteal, or other surfaces. Buffered neutral formalin (Chapter 14) is a recommended fixative. Additional fixing in 20% formalin may be indicated, particularly for large specimens.

SAMPLING PROCEDURES

Ribs Usually, they are sawed in a horizontal plane. The section should include costal cartilage, costochondral junction, and bony rib.

Sternum A sagittal midline slice through the manubrium is usually saved. Fragments of bone marrow can be dug out

From: *Handbook of Autopsy Practice,* 3rd Ed. Edited by: J. Ludwig © Humana Press Inc., Totowa, NJ

with a sturdy knife. These fragments should contain only cancellous bone so that minimal decalcification time is required.

Vertebrae We prepare a sagittal saw section through the center of a vertebra after the anterior half of the spinal column has been removed for exposure of the spinal cord. Intervertebral disk tissue should be part of the slice selected for histologic study, particularly in the presence of degenerative diseases, ochronosis, or ankylosing spondylitis. In this latter condition, costovertebral and costotransverse joints should be included.

Iliac Crest This site is particularly recommended for the study of metabolic bone disease. A slice of iliac crest tissue can easily be removed with an oscillating hand saw. The plane of sawing should be perpendicular to the iliac crest surface.

Calvarium This is an important part of the skeleton to study metabolic bone diseases, neoplastic involvement (myeloma, metastatic carcinoma, or multifocal Langerhans cell histiocytosis), and certain hemolytic anemias (thalassemia). A strip of calvarium should be removed so that it includes the external and internal tables and the diploë.

Bones of Extremities Removal of the femur requires a long lateral skin incision. The knee joint is exposed by flexing the knee and cutting the quadriceps tendon, the joint capsule, and the cruciate ligaments. The muscular attachments are dissected from the shaft of the femur, starting at the distal end and continuing toward the hip. The capsule of the hip can be palpated and then incised by flexing and rotating the femur.

If only the femoral head, neck, and trochanter region are needed, essentially the same procedure is used except that the femoral shaft is sawed off about 10 cm below the trochanter major.

The upper femoral shaft and the bone marrow in this region are usually exposed from an anterolateral incision. A 5-cm portion of the anterior half of the femoral shaft is then removed with an electric saw. The continuity of the bone can thus be preserved.

The humerus can be dislocated anteriorly in the humeroscapular joint. In this way the muscle attachments of the proximal humerus can be dissected away from the whole circumference of the bone without additional skin incisions. The upper shaft of the humerus is then exposed and sawed off. For removal of the complete bone, a skin incision down to the elbow is necessary.

The bones of the distal extremities, particularly of the hands, should be exposed from the volar surfaces (*see* Chapter 1).

DISSECTION AND REMOVAL OF JOINTS

The best joint sections are prepared by shelling out the whole joint and sawing across the proximal and distal bones, staying far enough from the joint space so as not to cut into the joint capsule. The whole specimen is then sawed, usually in the frontal plane. Good saw sections should include articular cartilage, synovium, meniscus, capsule, epiphysis, metaphysis, and a small portion of diaphysis of the adjacent long bones.

Complete removal and sectioning of the intact joint might be impractical because of the size of the specimen, prosthetic problems, or limitations of the autopsy permission. In these instances the joint space can be exposed and specimens of articular cartilage with adjacent bone, joint capsule, synovium, and disks or meniscus can be excised for histologic study. The joint space can be palpated, tapped, incised, and exposed by bending the joint in the direction opposite to the site of the intended puncture or incision.

Infectious Arthritis Both exudate and synovial tissue should be cultured.

Gout and Pseudogout For the identification of crystals *(4)*, a small drop of synovial fluid or exudate is placed, with a 1-mm bacteriologic wire loop, on a clean glass slide and is immediately covered. The cover slip is rimmed with clear nail polish to prevent the specimen from drying. The crystals can be analyzed with the polarizing microscope.

For macroscopic demonstration of urate deposits in joints and soft tissues, see Chapter 14.

STERNOCLAVICULAR JOINTS These joints are easily accessible and should be saved routinely. Study of them is recommended in all cases of rheumatoid arthritis and related diseases. The area around the joint is freed from soft tissue. The sternum is split in the midline and halfway across the side where the joint is to be removed. This cross-section is made about 1 cm below the level of the joint. The clavicle is sawed apart about 1 cm lateral from the joint space. The specimen is now sawed with a band saw in a horizontal plane to expose the joint spaces and disks.

ACROMIOCLAVICULAR AND HUMEROSCAPULAR JOINTS These can be reached and excised from the conventional skin incisions.

ATLANTO-OCCIPITAL JOINTS It is possible to remove the posterior base of the skull together with the cervical spine *(5)* but the procedure is rarely indicated.

LARYNGEAL JOINTS These, and particularly the cricoarytenoid joints, are very useful in the study of *rheumatoid arthritis* and related disorders. Good sections of these small joints can be prepared from sagittal sections through the entire posterior wall of the larynx, in a paramedian plane. The cricoarytenoid joints are found at or just beneath the level of the vocal cords. Dissection of the larynx is further discussed in Chapter 4.

JOINTS OF THE MIDDLE EAR The incudostapedial and incudomalleal joints are synovial joints that may be affected by *rheumatoid arthritis* and allied diseases. For removal of the middle ear, *see* Chapter 6.

BONE MARROW PREPARATIONS

SECTIONS Sections from sternum, ribs, vertebrae, and iliac crest usually show abundant red bone marrow. In the presence of hematologic disorders, femoral bone marrow should be included. Good fixation is essential; for instance, in B-5 fixative (Chapter 14).

Excellent bone marrow preparations can be made by injecting, shortly after death, B-5 or another suitable fixative into the bone marrow that was selected for later study. The fixative is injected slowly, preferably from two or more sites so as to avoid mechanical damage of the marrow by the fixative.

Exposure to decalcifying agents should be kept to a minimum by careful end-point determination (*see* below) or can even be avoided altogether if marrow can be squeezed out from cancellous bone fragments. Such fragments can be dug out, with a sturdy knife, from the vertebral bodies or sternum. Marrow also can be squeezed from ribs with a pair of pliers.

SMEARS Smear preparations or imprints of bone marrow, spleen, or lymph nodes should be prepared within 3 h after death although cellular detail on occasion is retained up to 15 h. We use a stronger solution of Wright's stain (0.6%) than is ordinarily used. Smears are made in the usual way.

PROSTHESES

Skeletal contours and continuity of tubular bones or of the spinal column must be restored after the autopsy. An assortment of wooden prostheses should be available for insertion in place of the removed bone. A simple substitute is a wooden rod with two nails protruding from both ends. After the heads of the nails are sawed off, the nails are inserted into the wooden rod. The tips of the nails are then driven into the proximal and distal portions of the bone. Complete segments of the spinal column can be replaced by such prostheses. Wooden spokes may serve this purpose. For replacing the hip, angular metal rods are useful. Plaster of Paris provides a good prosthesis for the calvarium. Simple wood dowels and plastic tubing is recommended as replacement for bones and joints of fingers and toes. As stated in Chapter 1, procedures involving the extremities require special permission. Incisions should not be visible when the body is viewed; normal contours, particularly of the hands, must be restored. Most pathologists are now very reluctant to remove samples from such areas.

DECALCIFYING PROCEDURES

Decalcification is required for preparing histologic sections of bone, dentine, cementum, calcified vessels, and calcification in lesions, such as granulomas and tumors. Decalcification solutions are commercially available but we found formic acid decalcification optimal for most purposes. The solution is easy to prepare, inexpensive, and causes little tissue damage. The composition of the solution is as follows:

FORMIC ACID DECALCIFICATION FLUID Formic acid decalcification fluid: 80 mL Neutral buffered formalin (see page 130), 20 mL Formic acid.

For very soft bone specimens and autopsy samples that do not need to be processed urgently, ethylenediamine tetraacetic acid (EDTA) is recommended:

EDTA DECALCIFICATION FLUID EDTA Decalcification Fluid: 4 g Disodium ethylene diamine tetra acetic acid (EDTA); 40 mL Neutral buffered formalin (see page 130).

PROCESSING OF SPECIMENS The samples should not be thicker than 3 mm. For each piece, 100 mL of decalcification fluid should be used. Change and agitate solution daily or more often. Exact end-point determination is essential because staining properties will be lost if fluid is not washed out immediately after decalcification is completed. Formic acid decalcification should not last longer than 2 d; EDTA decalcification may last 2–5 d. The formic acid must be removed by washing the specimen for 30 min in running tap water; EDTA preparations should be processed without washing in tap water.

Fixation with an aqueous solution of calcium acetate, glutaraldehyde, and formalin, followed by decalcification in neutral 10% EDTA reportedly prevents the loss of antigens and the fading of ferritin iron and enzymes *(6)*.

Decalcification time depends on numerous factors such as the size and texture of the specimen, the type and temperature of the solution, and the use of agitation and electrolysis. A small specimen in an acid bath that is exposed to the heat and agitation of the Autotechnicon will be decalcified in little more than 2 h; a protective acid-resistant insert must be used. The speed of decalcification can also be increased by electrolysis. The specimen is placed in acid decalcifying fluid with platinum electrodes; the acid serves as the electrolyte. Use of *ultrasound* is another method to increase the speed of decalcification. With this method, the fixation process can be combined with the use of acid or chelating decalcifiers *(7)*.

To achieve histologic slides of the best quality, the decalcification process should not be unnecessarily prolonged. Piercing the sample with a needle or blade or bending the specimen usually permits one to judge roughly when decalcification is complete. Another indicator is the decrease or disappearance of CO_2 bubbles from the specimen. Among the many methods for end-point determination of decalcification, serial roentgenograms permit the most precise control. For small specimens, dental films can be used.

For additional decalcification methods as well as information on fixation, staining, and other procedures, the reader should consult one of the current textbooks and manuals listed in the beginning of Part II.

PREPARATION OF UNDECALCIFIED SECTIONS AND MICRORADIOGRAPHY

Bone specimens fixed in buffered formalin are dehydrated in alcohol, as in routine histologic preparations, and then embedded in methyl methacrylate *(8)*. Specimens are cut to a thickness of 75–125 μm, usually with a diamond or carborundum-embedded wheel. For quantitative microradiography, sections are ground to a thickness of 100 μm (±5 μm). Kodak high-resolution plates (Eastman Kodak Company, Rochester, NY) can be used, preferably with a vacuum cassette, which ensures that the specimen is placed flat against the emulsion *(9)*. Undecalcified bone can also be prepared for electron microscopy *(10)*.

MACERATION OF BONE

Maceration of bone yields instructive specimens that are esthetically satisfying and of unlimited durability.

The specimens shown in Figs. 8-1, 8-2, and 8-3 (Courtesy, the late Prof. Dr. E. Uehlinger) were prepared in the Department of Pathology, Zürich, Switzerland, by the antiformin maceration technique.

METHOD OF ANTIFORMIN MACERATION (Pathology Laboratory Zürich; Bürgi, personal communication).

1. Clean attached soft tissue mechanically from bone (avoid knife marks).
2. Immerse specimen in a glass jar with 3% antiformin solution. (Antiformin stock solution: 1,400 mL sodium

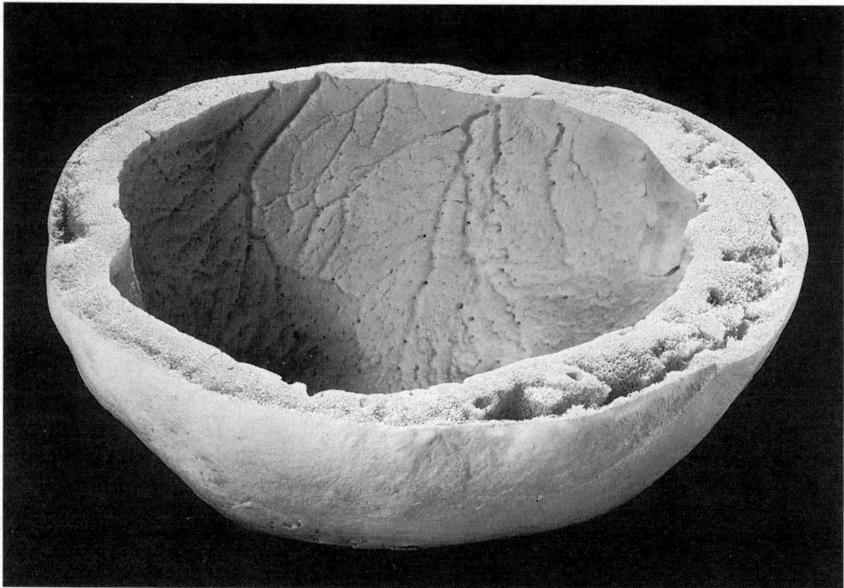

Fig. 8-1. Macerated calvarium. Paget's disease involving the cranium: 64-yr-old woman.

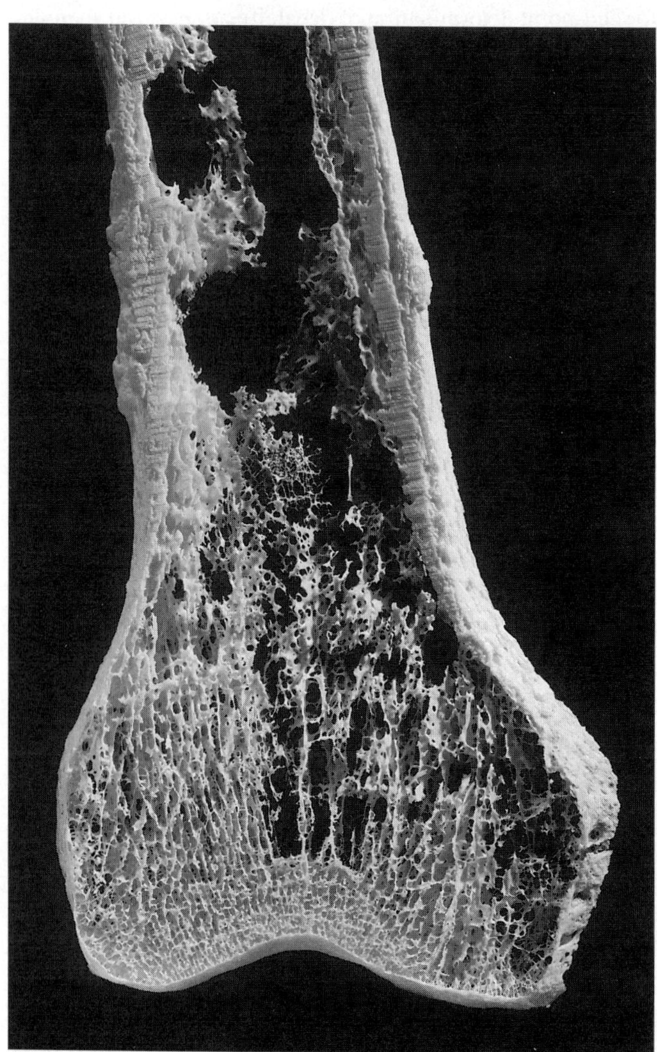

Fig. 8-2. Macerated humerus. Severe destruction of cancellous bone by multiple myeloma: 61-yr-old man.

hypochlorite, 10% solution; 1,400 mL distilled water; 4,200 mL potassium hydroxide, 45% (w/w). For maceration of bones, 1, 2, and 3% dilutions of this stock solution are prepared.) Place the jar in an incubator (embedding oven) at 70–80°C for 3–4 h. The time of incubation may be less with small or more with large specimens.

3. Decant antiformin and flush specimen with hot water. The remaining fragments of soft tissue are removed by blowing compressed air through the specimen and by scratching them from the surface of the bone with a knife. Occasionally, the specimen has to be incubated again in 1 or 2% antiformin. Check the progress every 30 min. Repeat step 3.
4. Bleach bone with 3% hydrogen peroxide solution in an incubator at 70–80°C. Bleaching time is 12–24 h. Flush in hot water.
5. Place specimen in cotton and dry at room temperature.
6. Place specimen in ether for about a week. This is to remove fat that has remained in the bone. The duration of ether treatment depends on the amount of fat in the tissue. Subsequently, the tissue is air-dried. Specimens can also be degreased with carbon tetrachloride or tetrachloroethylene. These are excellent fat solvents (*Caution*: proper ventilation is needed).

OTHER METHODS Maceration also can be achieved by prolonged putrefaction, by treatment with 0.25 *N* NaOH at 90°C, or by autoclaving with 1 *N* NaOH *(11)*. Repeated checking and mechanical removal of soft tissue are essential in all methods.

A slow but safe method is to boil the specimen until only the bone is left. If the bone is very fatty, incubation for 2 d in 50% ether-acetone will remove the fat and facilitate removal of the organic material. Some mineral is lost by this procedure. This

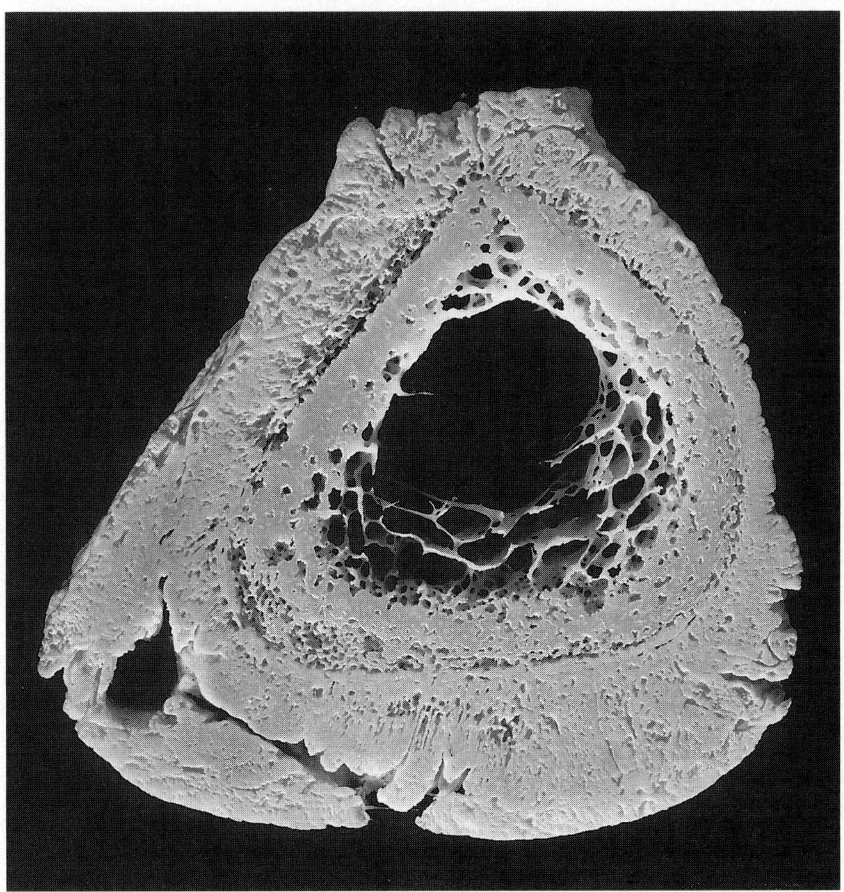

Fig. 8-3. Macerated tibia (horizontal section). Periosteal new bone formation in hypertrophic osteoarthropathy associated with carcinoma of breast and multiple metastases: 58-yr-old woman.

method is particularly recommended if one is dealing with a very valuable specimen.

Enzymatic maceration *(12)* is carried out with 0.1% papain in isotonic saline. The specimen is incubated for 24 h at 37°C. washed, and bleached in hydrogen peroxide.

FOR STUDY OF EXHUMED BONES Boiling is the method of choice. Maceration may permit otherwise unobtainable diagnoses, not only in medicolegal autopsies on bodies that had been buried for months and years but also for historic and prehistoric material.

REFERENCES

1. Baker SL. A freezing method for preparing museum specimens composed of bone and soft tissue. J Tech Methods 1940;20:42–47.
2. Mac Arthur, Jacobson R, Marrero H, Rahman Z, Schneiderman H. Autopsy removal of the brain in AIDS. A new technique (Correspondence). Hum Pathol 1986;17:1296–1297.
3. Towfighi J, Roberts AF, Foster NE, Abt AB. A protective device for performing cranial autopsies. Hum Pathol 1989;20:288–289.
4. Phelbs P, Steele AD, McCarty DJ Jr. Compensated polarized light microscopy: identification of crystals in synovial fluid from gout and pseudogout. JAMA 1968;203:508–512.
5. Becker V. Zur Sektionstechnik der Halswirbelsäule. Virchows Arch [Pathol Anat] 1959;332:384–388.
6. Schaefer HE. Die histologische Bearbeitungstechnik von Beckenkammbiopsien auf der Basis von Entkalkung und Paraffineinbettung unter Berücksichtigung osteologischer und hämatologischer Fragestellungen. Pathologe 1995;16:11–27.
7. Milan L, Trachtenberg MC. Ultrasonic decalcification of bone. Am J Surg Pathol 1981;5:573–579.
8. Islam A, Frisch B. Plastic embedding in routine histology. I: Preparation of semi-thin sections of undecalcified marrow cores. Histopathology 1985;1263–1274.
9. Jowsey J, Kelly PJ, Riggs BL, Bianco AJ Jr, Scholz DA, Gershon-Cohen J. Quantitative microscopic studies of normal and osteoporotic bone. J Bone Joint Surg [Am] 1965;47:785–806.
10. Schulz A. Embedding of undecalcified bone tissue for electron microscopic investigation. Beitr Pathol 1975;156:280–288.
11. Pulvertaft RJV. Museum techniques: a review. J Clin Pathol 1950;3: 1–23.
12. Edwards JJ, Edwards MJ. Medical Museum Technology, Oxford University Press, London, 1959.

9 Autopsy Microbiology

Brenda L. Waters

GENERAL COMMENTS

CLINICAL DISEASE AND POSTMORTEM CULTURE RESULTS The medical literature is replete with examples of discrepancies between clinical evidence of infection and postmortem culture results *(1–6)*. These discrepancies have been attributed to contamination during specimen collection *(5,6)*, transmigration of bacteria from the gut into surrounding tissues and blood *(2,4)*, and even the presence of indigenous bacteria in normal, healthy tissue *(7)*. Of these explanations, contamination is most frequently implicated and remains a major obstacle in meaningful postmortem microbiology. The theory of transmigration has never been substantiated. Articles published as early as 1921 offered evidence to disprove it *(8)*. As for the presence of indigenous bacteria in normal tissue, this theory has never gained much support.

Given the lack of specificity inherent in postmortem microbiology, it is necessary for the prosector to be very judicious in the selection of specimens for culture. This will optimize the information obtained as well as limit the cost of microbiologic assessment. Moreover, judicious use of cultures in the autopsy service will foster a good working relationship with the microbiology laboratory.

A thorough knowledge of gross pathology is the best tool for determining what specimens to submit for culture. In most patients whose immunologic status is intact, a grossly visualized host response, such as pneumonia, abscess, caseating granuloma, or collection of cloudy fluid is the best indication for culture. As a rule, one should not culture if there is no host response and no clinical information to raise suspicion of infection. Positive cultures from tissues that show no inflammation histologically generally are the result of contamination and, thus are meaningless.

CONSIDERATIONS IN IMMUNOCOMPROMISED PATIENTS These cases require a different approach at autopsy because infections may not be grossly evident. Thus, the selection of specimens for microbiological assay must be directed by a thorough understanding of the clinical history, close communication with the physicians who cared for the patient, and a carefully thought-out differential diagnosis of possible etiologic agents. At the autopsy table, the pathologist should carry a higher index of suspicion and thus may be prompted to submit cultures from organs that show no gross features of infection. Moreover, the variety of organisms to which these patients are susceptible is greater, requiring a larger scope of microbiological methods to isolate and characterize them. As a result, specimens might be collected for bacterial, mycobacterial, and fungal culture, and tissue submitted in transport media for viral culture. Immediate placement of tissue in fixative for electron microscopy, freezing of tissue at –70°C, and obtaining air-dried smears or touch preparations also may be indicated.

THE GRAM STAIN IN AUTOPSY STUDIES A powerful tool in the autopsy pathologist's armamentarium is the Gram stain. This stain is very inexpensive, easy to perform, and can be done by the pathologist with little inconvenience to the clinical laboratory staff. Moreover, Gram stains of touch preparations or smears demonstrate bacterial morphology much better than Gram stains of 5-μm paraffin sections. With just a brief examination of the smear, an experienced pathologist can characterize the inflammatory response or identify a neoplasia. Such findings may direct the focus of further investigation.

If the presence of an infection is in doubt, tissue or fluid samples may be submitted to the clinical microbiology laboratory with the instruction to "culture for bacteria if Gram stain shows inflammation." Although this instruction may sound vague, it encourages dialogue between the microbiology staff and the autopsy physicians; it also demonstrates the commitment of the autopsy service to minimize unnecessary cultures.

Touch preparations of tissue for Gram staining are best obtained from a 1-cm^3 sample from which excess blood is removed by touching the specimen once or twice with a paper towel. Then, the tissue fragment is blotted 2 or 3 times onto different areas of a slide. Following air-drying and heat fixation, the touch preparations are ready to Gram stain and examine. The "pull-prep" method is useful in preparing smears of fluid or pus for Gram staining. In this procedure, a single drop of fluid is placed onto the center of a slide. A second slide is pressed against the first, keeping the slides essentially congruent, and then the two are pulled apart, thereby spreading the fluid into a thin layer. It is best to place the drop of fluid in the center of the slide so as to maximize the area over which the fluid will be spread. In most cases, a single small drop of fluid is sufficient.

From: *Handbook of Autopsy Practice,* 3rd Ed. Edited by: J. Ludwig © Humana Press Inc., Totowa, NJ

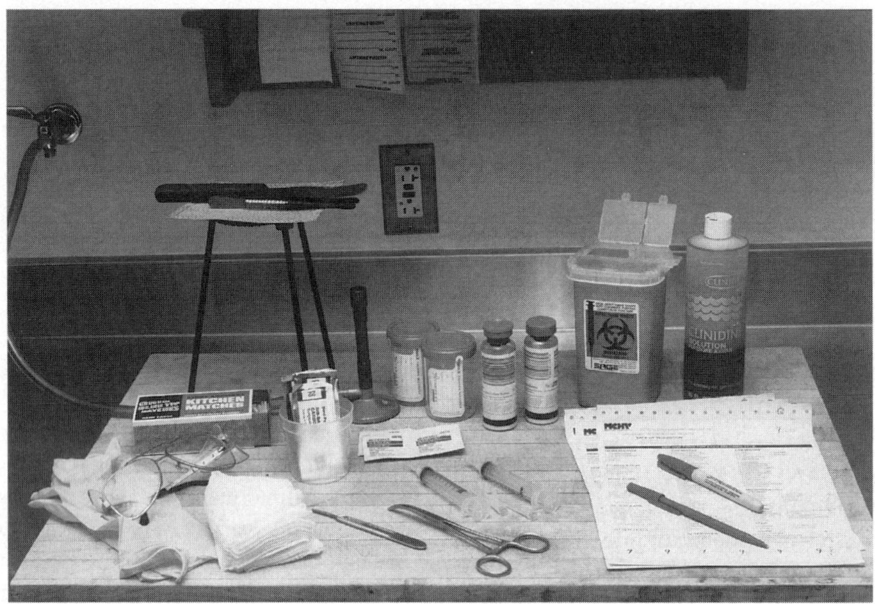

Fig. 9-1. Equipment for processing autopsy specimens for culture. These tools should be stored and readily available in the autopsy room. See text for detailed description.

PRINCIPLES OF SUBMISSION AND CULTURE OF SPECIMENS In most situations, the use of swabs for collecting specimens is inadequate. Fluids or exudates should be collected in needle-less syringes, which may be conveniently sealed with the cap that accompanied them. Two to three milliliters of fluid are sufficient. This volume allows storage of leftover specimens for future use, should new questions arise. Some laboratories may find it useful to freeze and store leftover tissue for several weeks in case histologic examination reveals an unexpected finding, such as viral inclusions or granulomatous inflammation. Tissue specimens should measure at least 1–2 cm^3. If the sample is too small, it may dry during transportation to the microbiology laboratory.

The tools needed to obtain specimens for culture at autopsy (Fig. 9-1) include a Bunsen burner, spatula, forceps that can be sterilized in the flame, scalpels, sterile syringes and needles, sterile containers and blood culture bottles, povidone iodine and alcohol swabs, an appropriate container for disposal of sharps, and the necessary writing utensils to label the containers and requisition slips. Protective eyewear (*see* Chapter 16) and gloves are also required. Glass slides should be available for smears and touch preparations. Any grinding or surface decontamination of tissues is best performed in a biosafety cabinet by microbiology technologists.

Finally, both safety and courtesy demand that all specimen containers departing the autopsy suite be clean and dry on the outside. Given the nature of the autopsy procedure, this standard may take more effort to achieve but it must be no less inviolable. It is often helpful to have an assistant with clean, gloved hands who can fill the blood culture bottles and handle the containers while the prosector procures the specimens.

SPECIMEN COLLECTION

BLOOD CULTURES Postmortem blood cultures are frequently obtained but they rarely provide useful information. A recent study *(5)* from a general hospital showed that in 54% of patients with negative antemortem blood cultures, positive blood cultures were obtained postmortem although the patients had no infectious disease that could be considered a cause of death. Of patients with confirmed antemortem bacteremia/fungemia, only 34% had a postmortem blood culture from which the same organisms were isolated. Moreover, of patients without cultures or with negative or contaminated antemortem blood cultures, all had positive postmortem cultures; 76% of the isolates were considered contaminants and 22% of the isolates were of indeterminate significance *(5)*. Thus, the decision to obtain a postmortem blood culture should rely on a strong clinical suspicion of sepsis in the absence of a pathogen-isolated antemortem. Because the results of in vivo blood cultures generally are quite reliable, a known bloodstream pathogen rarely needs to be isolated again at autopsy.

Hospitalized patients commonly receive antibiotics prior to phlebotomy for blood cultures. This is frequently prompted by new fever spikes or acute deterioration in clinical status. Despite such treatment, organisms may still be isolated at autopsy from these patients *(1)*.

Blood may be obtained from the right atrium, inferior vena cava, or from the aorta. In patients in whom thoracic dissection is not possible, as with a restricted autopsy permission, blood may be obtained from the femoral vein. Although the theory of bacterial transmigration through the bowel wall is largely dismissed, traditional autopsy protocol recommends that blood be obtained prior to manipulation or removal of the bowel. Searing the area with a hot spatula will sterilize the site of needle entry. In cases requiring a femoral stick, sterilize the skin with povidone iodine. In fetuses and neonates, a portion of liver may be submitted in place of blood, since searing of the heart or great vessels may damage the thoracic organs.

LUNG CULTURES The lungs' gross appearance should direct the pathologist to the best site for culture. The most common evidence of acute infectious pneumonia is pleural fibrinous exudate and parenchymal consolidation. Palpation of the lungs while they are still *in situ* is the best method for detecting this change. The surface of the lungs may be sterilized by searing with a heated spatula. Four stabbing motions, 90° to each other with a sterile blade, will mobilize a cube of tissue that can then be lifted up with a sterile forceps. The blade can then make the final cut to free the tissue block. The tip of the forceps should not be too hot as the tissue will stick, making it difficult to drop the specimen into the container. Providing that the lung has not been perfused with formalin, areas of consolidation may still be cultured after the lung is sliced. Again, the surface should be sterilized by searing. In patients with moderate to severe emphysema, pneumonia may be more difficult to visualize grossly. Thus, in these patients, the prosector's index of suspicion should be raised.

It is standard practice in most microbiology laboratories that with all cultures of tissues a Gram stain is performed as well. If the prosection occurs in the morning, the results of the Gram stain may be available to be included in the preliminary autopsy report. Any Gram stains performed and read by the pathologist may also provide other valuable information for the preliminary autopsy report—for example, the presence of a coexisting lymphoma.

Oral and gastric contents may enter the bronchial tree agonally or during transit of the body to the autopsy room. This contamination may change the gross appearance of the pulmonary cut surface as well as add more bacteria to the lung parenchyma. However, the lack of consolidation will help the pathologist to conclude that the discoloration is not pneumonia. Should the pathologist obtain a lung culture of such an area, the Gram stain will yield the correct interpretation.

ABSCESSES During evisceration or dissection of organs, abscesses may be found unexpectedly. In such a case, the prosector should immediately aspirate some of the pus with a needle and syringe. An attempt should be made to take material from the center of the abscess. Even though the abscess is contaminated at this time, the specimen is still acceptable since any organisms in the abscess will likely far outnumber those introduced during the course of the dissection. The Gram stain will aid in this interpretation.

There is no reason to culture acute perforations of bowel since both Gram stain and culture will point to fecal flora. Only when a host response is seen, such as an abscess, should the lesion be cultured.

CARDIAC VALVULAR VEGETATIONS The microbiologic examination of endocarditis is a special challenge for the pathologist, because it competes with the other components of a complete examination, that is, photography and histology. If a vegetation is suspected clinically, the task is easier. In the case of an aortic or pulmonic valve vegetation, the ascending aorta or main pulmonary artery may be cut carefully away so as to visualize the valve leaflets (Fig. 9-2). Following photography, a portion of the vegetation may be removed with sterile forceps and scalpel or scissors and sent for culture. Enough material should be collected to allow for an adequate Gram stain to be prepared as well. Since the amount of tissue is usually scant, it should be sent to the microbiology laboratory as soon as possible to prevent drying.

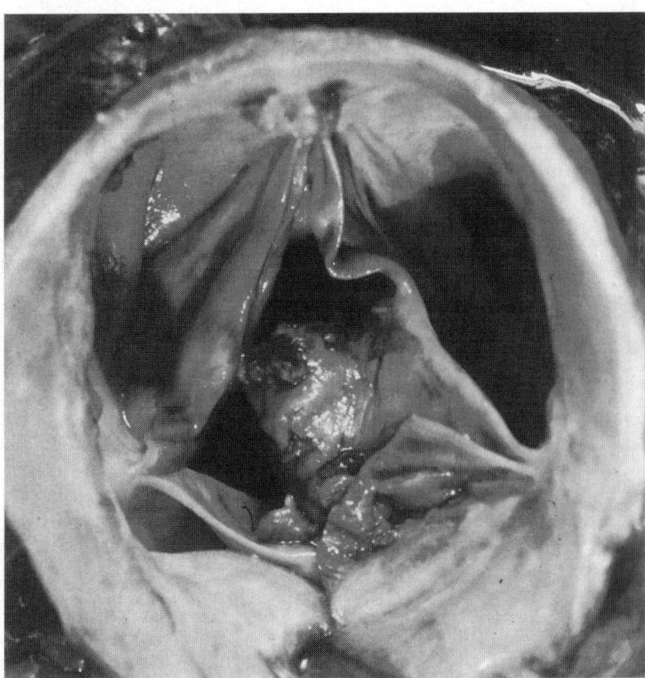

Fig. 9-2. Aseptic exposure of aortic valve vegetation. The aorta has been trimmed away to allow good visualization of the aortic valve. Photography and collection of a portion of the vegetation (center of field) for culture and Gram stain was easily accomplished. (Courtesy Dr. W.D. Edwards.)

In suspected infective endocarditis with mitral or tricuspid vegetation, the outside of the heart need not be seared as this would cause disfigurement of the heart. Rather, the ventricle is incised along the acute or obtuse margin (right and left ventricles, respectively) with a sterile scalpel until the ventricular chamber is entered (Fig. 9-3). The cut across the atrial-ventricular groove is then extended so that it will be easier to splay open the valve ring. It may be necessary to have an assistant to keep the ventricle open. After taking photographs, a portion of the vegetation is obtained for culture and Gram stain.

If the suspected endocarditis appears to be accompanied by coronary atherosclerosis and myocardial infarctions, the prosector may find it more appropriate to examine (or remove) the coronary arteries prior to addressing the valve pathology. Manipulation of the heart should be minimized. The pathologist may then begin to breadloaf the heart, keeping the slices at 1-cm thickness. When the slices have reached the tip of the papillary muscles, the valve may be viewed from below and specimens may be procured for Gram stain and culture.

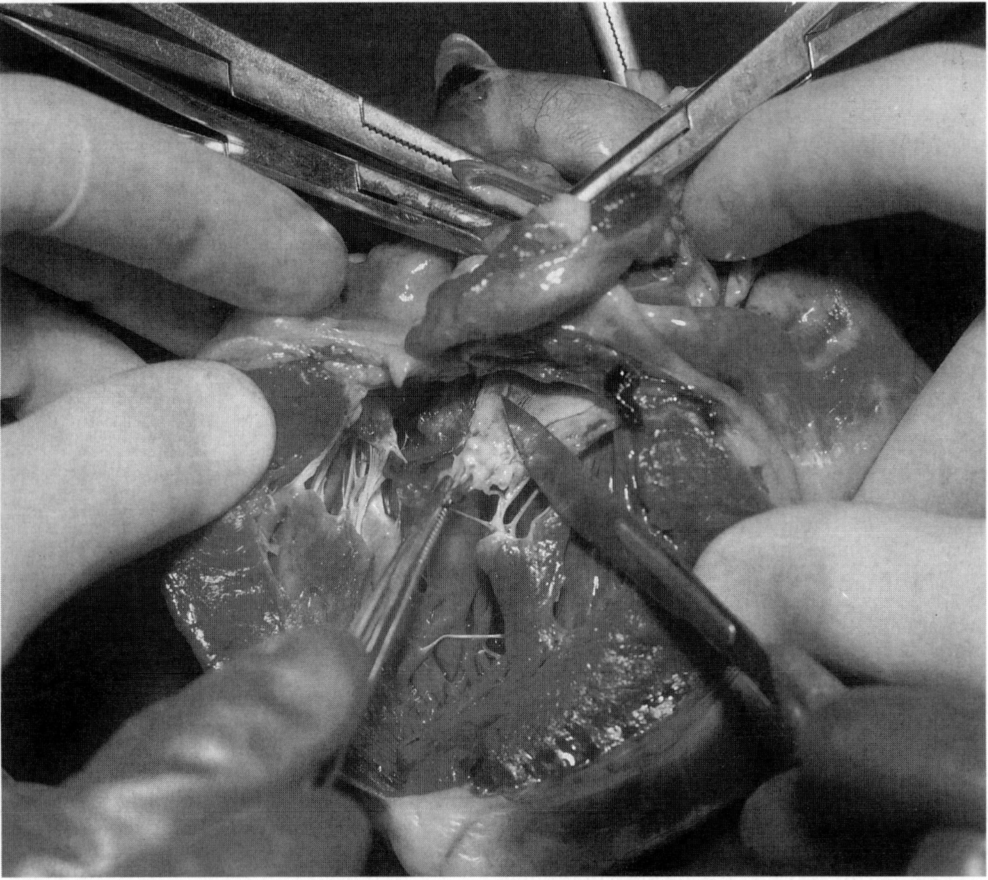

Fig. 9-3. Aseptic exposure of mitral valve from left ventricle. With an incision into the left ventricle along the obtuse margin, the mitral valve is readily available for photography and collection of a vegetation for culture and Gram stain.

When infective vegetations are encountered unexpectedly, the pathologist should submit tissue for culture and Gram stain, despite the expected contamination. Important information can still be obtained because the repertory of expected pathogens is limited and the Gram stain will be very helpful in interpreting the culture results.

DRAINING SINUSES Since draining sinuses are usually continuous with the skin surface, they may be heavily contaminated with skin flora. Thus, the material closest to the skin surface should be wiped away with sterile gauze. The purulent material that is present in the deeper sections of the sinus will be much more informative. This material may be aspirated with a large bore needle and syringe, a scalpel or, as a last resort, a swab. The Gram stain is critically important in the interpretation of the organisms isolated. The presence of acute inflammation will differentiate true infection from colonization. When the clinical history suggests *Actinomyces*, the prosector should examine a portion of the pus for "sulfur granules." If they are found, they may be pressed between two slides and then the two slides may be pulled apart, as with the "pull-prep." Since sulfur granules are more solid and require more force to spread out, it is safer to press the two slides together on a counter top, to avoid breaking the slides.

CEREBROSPINAL FLUID (CSF) When infectious meningitis is suspected but not confirmed prior to death, the prosector may find it necessary to procure CSF. This is most easily accomplished by performing a cisternal tap. The procedure entails placing the body in a prone position making sure that there is adequate padding under the face so as to avoid disfigurement. After vigorous cleansing of the skin with iodine and then alcohol (the alcohol must be allowed to evaporate), a 12-gauge needle is inserted at the midline below the base of the occipital bone and directed slightly superiorly, toward the eyes. The needle is pushed forward slowly and carefully, with frequent attempts to aspirate fluid. Unnecessary movement of the syringe should be avoided so as to prevent bleeding. (As stated in Chapter 2, aspiration of blood, together with CSF, is common, even among experienced prosectors.) If no or only blood-tinged CSF is aspirated, it is still possible to collect a satisfactory specimen after removal of the calvarium. For that purpose, a needle may be inserted in the subarachnoid space. Should this fail, a tissue specimen of meninges and a small amount of underlying brain may be taken. Pus tends to collect in the inferior aspect of the brain, thus making collection of material possible.

If a brain abscess is suspected, the prosector can try to localize the lesion by palpation. Should the site be determined, the brain surface can be sterilized by searing and aspiration can be attempted with a long, large-bore needle. In certain situations, hemisection of the brain (*see* Chapter 6) and fresh cutting of one half may be indicated.

REFERENCES

1. Koneman EW, Minckler TM, Shires DB, de Jongh DS. Postmortem bacteriology: II. Selection of cases for culture. J Clin Pathol 1971;55:17–23.
2. Nehring JR, Sheridan MF, Funk W. Postmortem bacteriology: II. The use of tracer organisms to evaluate the possibility of postmortem bacterial transmigration. Am J Clin Pathol 1971;56:133–134.
3. Koneman EW, Davis MA. Postmortem bacteriology: III. Clinical significance of microorganisms recovered at autopsy. Am J Clin Pathol 1974;61:28–40.
4. Kellerman GD, Waterman NG, Scharfenberger LF. Demonstration *in vitro* of postmortem bacterial transmigration. Am J Clin Pathol 1976; 66:911–915.
5. Wilson SJ, Wilson ML, Reller, LB. Diagnostic utility of postmortem blood cultures. Arch Pathol Lab Med 1993;117:986–988.
6. Wilson ML. Clinically relevant, cost-effective clinical microbiology. Strategies to decrease unnecessary testing. Am J Clin Pathol 1997;107: 154–167.
7. Minckler TM, Newell GR, O'Toole WF, Niwayama G, Levine PH. Microbiology experience in collection of human tissue. Am J Clin Pathol 1966;45:85–92.
8. Giordano AS, Barnes AR. Studies in postmortem bacteriology. Value and importance of cultures made postmortem. J Lab Clin Med 1921; 7:538–546.

10 Chromosome Study of Autopsy Tissues

GORDON W. DEWALD

INDICATIONS

IN ADULTS Various aneuploidies of the sex chromosomes are the most common chromosome abnormalities encountered in autopsies of adults. The Turner (usually 45,X but mosaicism is common) and Klinefelter (47,XXY) syndromes are two examples *(1)*. Deletions or unbalanced translocations and inversions are rarely seen at autopsies in adults because patients with these abnormalities seldom survive into adulthood. Approximately 1/500 adults carries a genetically balanced abnormality of chromosome structure. These balanced chromosome anomalies may affect the reproductive history of an individual, but rarely affect the phenotype *(2)*. Some adults have sporadic chromosome changes as part of a chromosome breakage syndrome such as Fanconi anemia *(3)*, ataxia-telangiectasia *(4)*, Bloom syndromes *(5)*, and others.

Chromosome analysis may be done at autopsy to eliminate a specific diagnosis; thus, establishing that the karyotype of the deceased is normal can be useful. Chromosome studies may be done at autopsy to establish the karyotype of specific tissues when chromosome mosaicism is suspected *(6)*. Cytogenetic studies may be useful in the same setting to help resolve issues of malignant disorders. Chromosome studies can help establish the presence of an abnormal clone, classify neoplastic disorders, assess disease progression, and detect the emergence of therapy related neoplasms. At least 215 different chromosome abnormalities have been strongly associated with specific malignant disorders *(7–9)*. In these cases, it is important that the tissue(s) selected for chromosome studies be derived from the neoplasm in question. Sometimes autopsy chromosome studies are done as part of research protocols.

IN NEONATES, INFANTS, AND CHILDREN Chromosome analysis should be done when the malformations correspond to well-established chromosome syndromes, especially when the diagnosis is doubtful. The syndromes associated with aneuploidy are the most common and easily recognized at autopsy. Three of the more frequently encountered conditions in autopsies of newborns are the Down (trisomy 21) *(10)*, Patau (trisomy 13), and Edwards (trisomy 18) syndrome *(11)*. Presence of ambiguous genitalia is also a common indication of a genetic problem and may be a clue to gonadal dysgenesis, true hermaphroditism, and other abnormalities or gene mutations involving the sex chromosomes *(1,12)*.

As a group, deletions, translocations, and inversions are the most common chromosome abnormalities in newborns; they also are the most difficult to recognize clinically. Anomalies of chromosome structure can involve more than one chromosome and they can involve any part of any chromosome. Structural anomalies in neonates are often private mutations, i.e., found only in the deceased or some of their blood relatives. For this reason, genetic imbalances resulting from structural anomalies are inconsistent among individuals and the clinical presentation is generally nonspecific. Because structural anomalies usually are associated with multiple congenital anomalies, postmortem chromosome analysis may be done in severely malformed neonates. Three rare syndromes that involve abnormalities of chromosome structure and may be encountered at autopsy of neonates are Cri du Chat *(13)*, Wolf- Hirschhorn *(14)*, and Langer-Giedion syndromes *(15)*, but many others are known.

It is particularly important to do chromosome studies of neonates when a family has a history of frequent spontaneous abortions, as the results can be useful in genetic counseling of living relatives *(2)*. Structural abnormalities of chromosomes can be familial when one of the parents is a balanced carrier. When this occurs, the parents of the deceased and other relatives may be at considerable risk to produce abnormal offspring and this information is important in family planning and the application of prenatal genetic testing with further pregnancies *(2)*.

IN SPONTANEOUS ABORTIONS Chromosome analyses on spontaneous abortuses can be an emotional benefit to patients, both in having the cause of death explained or in ruling out an identifiable inherited abnormality. Chromosome studies of spontaneous abortions may be done to define the cause of fetal demise, collect information on familial chromosome anomalies, and identify molar pregnancies *(16,17)*. From 1991 to 1993, we studied 1,502 spontaneous abortuses; some were associated with recognizable fetal tissue but others did not contain discernible fetal tissue. We successfully completed chromosome studies on 1,164 of these specimens: 414 (36%) had a chromosome abnormality.

Chromosome anomalies in abortuses with identifiable tissue included any kind of trisomy involving an autosome (47%), triploidy (17%), and 45,X (Turner syndrome, 16%). The remaining chromosome anomalies included unbalanced translocations,

From: *Handbook of Autopsy Practice,* 3rd Ed. Edited by: J. Ludwig © Humana Press Inc., Totowa, NJ

aneuploidy of multiple chromosomes, mosaicism, tetraploidy, and balanced translocations. These results are consistent with other investigations of spontaneous abortions *(16)*.

Of the 33 abnormal spontaneous abortuses without recognizable fetal tissue, 5 had triploid karyotypes. This karyotype is often associated with partial hydatidiform moles. In the remaining 28 spontaneous abortuses, 6 carried anomalies which could have been familial. Potentially familial chromosome anomalies would include any unbalanced or balanced structural abnormality. In these cases, family members and subsequent pregnancies should be studied because of the risk that a similar chromosome abnormality will recur. Chromosome abnormalities identified in the remaining cases included trisomies and monosomies, and were the probable cause of fetal demise.

It is possible to calculate the statistical probability that future pregnancies of a couple will involve a chromosome abnormality based on the karyotype of the spontaneous abortus and the parents. In general, if the spontaneous abortus has an abnormal karyotype and the parents have a normal karyotype, the risk for a future abortion due to chromosome abnormalities is about 1%. Prenatal studies are often recommended in subsequent pregnancies when the spontaneous abortus has a trisomy or monosomy that has been associated with a classic syndrome.

Complete and partial hydatidiform moles are genetically aberrant conceptuses that have the potential to develop into malignancies *(17)*. Usually, complete moles have a diploid karyotype with only paternal chromosomes. Most partial moles have 69 chromosomes (triploidy), including 23 of maternal origin and 46 of paternal origin. Differentiation between complete and partial moles is important, as they have different potentials for clinical persistence, malignant transformation, recurrence, and presence of a fetus. The complete mole consists of abnormal, cystic chorionic villi with no fetal tissue present. Retained fragments after an incomplete spontaneous abortion may evolve into choriocarcinoma. The risk of recurrence is about 1%. The partial mole also has cystic chorionic villi, but a fetus is always present initially. The fetal tissue may or may not survive up to the time of diagnosis. The recurrence risk for triploid partial hydatidiform moles is unknown. Subsequent pregnancies should be studied with either finding.

Any structural chromosome abnormality found in a spontaneous abortion requires chromosome studies on the parents to determine whether the abnormality is familial or a *de novo* mutation *(2)*. When the spontaneous abortus has a duplication or deletion not found in the parent, the recurrence risk is <0.5%. Thus, during subsequent pregnancies, studies are not strongly indicated. When the spontaneous abortus has an unbalanced inversion, and one parent is the carrier, recurrence risk in subsequent pregnancies ranges from 0.5% with a paracentric inversion to 5–10% with a pericentric inversion. In the latter case, prenatal studies are indicated for all future pregnancies. If the spontaneous abortion has a translocation, either balanced or unbalanced, prenatal studies would be indicated only if one of the parents carries the balanced translocation.

Approximately 80% of the spontaneous abortions without recognizable fetal tissue in our study were chromosomally normal females. We suspect many of these studies were done on maternal cells. This points out the importance of attempting to collect specimens that contain fetal tissues even though this is not always possible. When unidentifiable tissue is all that can be collected, the cytogenetic laboratory should attempt to further isolate embryonic or extra-embryonic tissue using a dissecting microscope. The rational to do chromosome analyses on unidentified tissues is not always clear. In our study, 11 of the 33 products of conception had chromosome anomalies, which may have explained the fetal demise or led to useful chromosome studies on the parents.

COSTS

Since cytogenetic studies are expensive, they should be applied to autopsies in a frugal manner, but they certainly are indicated if chromosome analysis is the only means to obtain pertinent medical information. The cost of chromosome analysis varies among cytogenetic laboratories and ranges from a few hundred dollars to over $1,000, depending on the type of tissue studied.

SPECIMEN COLLECTION, TRANSPORT, AND PROCESSING

Most chromosome studies require living tissues to obtain successful cell culture for chromosome studies *(18)*. For this reason, it is important to use sterile procedures to collect specimens. Whole blood and other tissues have been cultured successfully from mailed-in specimens for clinical purposes. Thus, it is not necessary for the autopsy pathologist to have ready access to a cytogenetic laboratory. Since living cells are involved, it is important to transport specimens to the cytogenetic laboratory in 1 or 2 d. Moreover, exposure of the specimen to temperature extremes (freezing or >30°C) can prevent a successful chromosome study. The specimens should not be frozen or packed on ice for delivery.

The cytogenetic laboratory is often used to culture cells from autopsies with evidence of a molecular or biochemical genetic disorder. In these cases, it is important that the prosector informs the cytogenetic laboratory to the need for molecular or biochemical genetic testing. This will assure that the cytogenetic laboratory processes the specimen correctly and forwards the cultured cells to another laboratory for appropriate genetic testing.

The following procedures may be used to prepare and mail specimens collected at autopsy for cytogenetic studies. When other tissues are needed, the collection procedure and mode of transportation should be discussed with personnel from the cytogenetic laboratory to enhance chances of a successful result.

BLOOD Blood is generally the preferred specimen for chromosome analysis when a congenital disorder is suspected and it is possible to collect an appropriate specimen. Obtain 5–10 mL of unclotted, uncontaminated blood in a sterile fashion. Mix the blood sample with 1 mL of sodium heparin in a small sterile vial and send it to the cytogenetic laboratory.

In the cytogenetic laboratory, the cells are incubated for 66–72 h at 37°C with a T-cell mitogen such as phytohemagglutinin. The cells are then harvested for chromosome analysis using ethidium bromide, colcemid, and hypotonic solution and then fixed with glacial acetic acid and methanol.

A few factors may interfere with processing blood for chromosome analysis. Cells may be lysed due to forcing the blood quickly through a needle. An improper anticoagulant (sodium heparin is best) or not mixing the blood with the anticoagulant can cause the blood cells to clot. Rare patients have blood T-lymphocytes that do not respond to mitogens used to cause cells to undergo mitosis.

FIBROBLASTS Specimens for fibroblast cultures should be collected at autopsy when a congenital disorder is suspected and blood is either unavailable or alternative tissues are needed to answer a medical question. Fibroblast cultures are generally more expensive than other chromosome studies because they require more time and culture maintenance. The prosector should make a longitudinal incision through the skin of the anterior thigh and dissect down to the fascia lata. A 5–15 mm^2 sample of the fascia lata is then removed, together with about 2–3 mm thickness of underlying muscle. The tissue is wrapped in sterile gauze moistened with Hank's balanced salt solution (HBSS) and placed it in a small sterile vial for transportation to the chromosome laboratory.

Upon arrival in the cytogenetic laboratory, the specimen is cut into small pieces and treated with enzymes *(19)*. The tissue is then placed into a culture flask with Chang and MEM-alpha-medium containing 20% fetal bovine serum (FBS) and antibiotics. After 5–14 d, the fibroblasts are processed for chromosome analysis with ethidium bromide, colcemid, hypotonic solution, and fixed with glacial acetic acid and methanol.

The most common problems with these specimens are lack of viable cells and bacterial contamination. These problems can interfere with attempts to establish fibroblast cultures.

BONE MARROW Bone marrow specimens may be required for chromosome studies at autopsy when a question of malignant hematological disorder is involved. Approximately 1 mL of bone marrow should be obtained in a sterile fashion and mixed with 1 mL of sodium heparin in a small sterile vial, and then sent to the cytogenetic laboratory.

In the cytogenetic laboratory, bone marrow specimens may either be processed for chromosome analysis directly or by a short-term (24–72 h) culture method *(19,20)*. In either case, the bone marrow is harvested for chromosome analysis by using ethidium bromide, colcemid, and hypotonic solution and then fixed with glacial acetic acid and methanol.

PRODUCTS OF CONCEPTION OR STILLBIRTH These specimens should be collected when a congenital disorder is suspected and blood is unavailable. A 1-cm^3 biopsy of muscle and fascia from the thigh, a 1-cm^3 biopsy of lung, and 20–30 mg of chorionic villi should be obtained. Each biopsy sample is placed in a separate 15 mL sterile centrifuge tube with 10 mL of transfer culture media. In situations where the fetus is not identifiable, the specimen is placed in a single sterile container with 10 mL of HBSS or a similar solution.

Upon arrival in the cytogenetic laboratory, these specimens are cut into small pieces and treated with enzymes *(19)*. The tissues are then placed into separate tissue flasks with Chang and MEM-alpha-medium containing 20% FBS and antibiotics to establish a fibroblast culture. After 5–14 d, the fibroblasts are processed with ethidium bromide, colcemid, hypotonic solution, and fixed with glacial acetic acid and methanol.

Chromosome analysis may be unsuccessful in some specimens because of a lack of viable cells or bacterial contamination. In our experience this occurs in up to 20% of cases and is usually due to a lack of viable cells. Sometimes maternal cells are cultured and analyzed rather than fetal cells.

SOLID TUMORS These specimens should be collected for chromosome studies only when the medical question relates to a solid tumor. The specimen should be representative of the solid tumor as the neoplastic chromosome abnormalities are rarely congenital or present in normal tissues. Using sterile procedures, a 5-mm^3 or larger tumor biopsy is submitted. The specimen is placed in a transport container with 5 mL of HBSS or a similar solution.

In the cytogenetic laboratory, the tissue is dissociated using enzymes and/or mechanical means and then transferred to culture flasks *(19)*. The cultures are incubated at 37°C with 5% CO_2, 5% O_2 and 90% N_2 for 1–2 d depending on cell growth. The cells are harvested for chromosome analysis with ethidium bromide, colcemid, hypotonic solution, and fixed with glacial acetic acid and methanol.

Normal cells are often present in and around tumor tissue. In culture, these cells may grow better than neoplastic cells and result in the study of normal somatic cells.

METHODS OF CHROMOSOME ANALYSIS AND INTERPRETATION OF RESULTS

The methods to analyze chromosomes are numerous, sophisticated, and vary among laboratories. Today, the cytogenetic laboratory must be proficient with many forms of culture techniques, more than 20 different chromosome staining methods, and have expertise with fluorescence-labeled DNA probes and *in situ* hybridization (FISH) *(18,21–24)*. Typical examples are shown in Fig. 10-1. Metaphases are usually stained with G-banding, but other staining methods are frequently employed as needed. Twenty metaphases are typically examined for structure and number of chromosomes, but structural chromosome abnormalities are subtle and can be missed. In cases where mosaicism is suspected, 30 or more metaphases are often analyzed but true mosaicism still is sometimes missed because of metaphase sampling error. Representative metaphases are photographed and karyotypes are prepared from at least two cells.

In the case of malignant neoplasms, two or more metaphases with the same structural abnormality or extra chromosome, or three or more metaphases lacking the same chromosome, are regarded as minimal evidence for the presence of an abnormal clone *(25)*. In some neoplastic disorders, abnormal clones may be missed when the malignant cells are not dividing *(9)*. In solid tumors, numerous complex chromosome anomalies sometimes make it difficult to identify specific chromosome abnormalities associated with certain neoplasms, but it is usually possible to identify the presence of an abnormal clone *(26)*.

The results of chromosome studies are usually provided according to a complicated but well-defined nomenclature *(25)*. In addition, cytogeneticists usually provide a narrative report that can be readily appreciated by a physician who is not expert in genetics. A cytogenetic report is usually issued after about 5–7 d for peripheral blood and bone marrow, 2–4 wk for fibroblast cultures, and about 10 d for solid tumors.

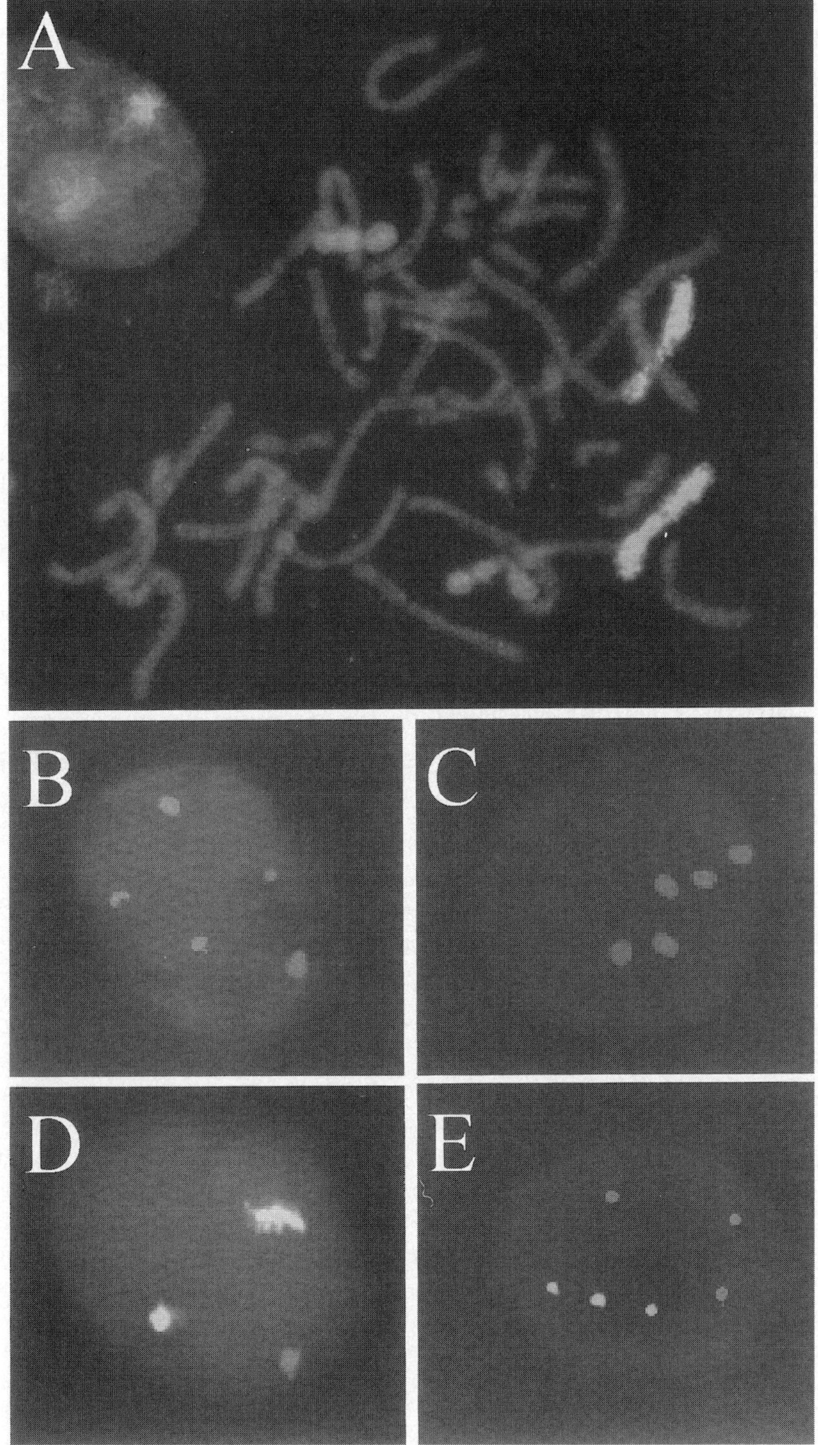

Fig. 10-1. The utility of fluorescence *in situ* hybridization (FISH). (**A**) FISH with spectrum green whole chromosome paint 16 and spectrum orange whole chromosome paint 9 demonstrating an unbalanced 9;16 translocation in a metaphase from an amniotic fluid specimen. (**B**) FISH with spectrum green locus-specific probes for chromosome 13 band q14 and spectrum orange locus specific probes for chromosome 21 band q11.2-q22.2 in an interphase cell with trisomy 13 from an amniotic fluid specimen. (**C**) FISH with spectrum green locus-specific probes for chromosome 13 band q14 and spectrum orange locus-specific probes for chromosome 21 q11.2-q22.2 in an interphase cell with trisomy 21 from an amniotic fluid specimen. (**D**). FISH with spectrum green centromere-specific probes for the X chromosome and spectrum aqua centromere-specific probes for chromosome 18 in an interphase cell with monosomy X from an amniotic fluid specimen. (**E**) FISH with spectrum green locus-specific probes for chromosome 21 band q11.2-q22.2 in an interphase cell from an amniotic fluid specimen with triploidy.

REFERENCES

1. Dewald GW, Spurbeck JL. Sex chromosome anomalies associated with premature gonadal failure. Semin Reprod Endo 1983;1:79–92.
2. Dewald GW, Michels VV. Recurrent miscarriages: cytogenetic causes and genetic counseling of affected families. Clin Obst Gyn 1986;29:865–885.
3. Kuffel D, Zinsmeister A, Lindor N, Litzow M, Dewald GW. Mitomycin C chromosome stress test to identify hypersensitivity to bifunctional alkylating agents in patients with Fanconi anemia or aplastic anemia. Mayo Clin Proc 1997;72:579–580.
4. Dewald GW, Noonan KJ, Spurbeck JL, Johnson DD. T-lymphocytes and 7;14 translocations: frequency of occurrence, breakpoints, and clinical and biological significance. Am J Hum Genet 1986;38:520–532.
5. Dicken CH, Dewald GW, Gordon H. Sister chromatid exchanges in the Bloom syndrome. Arch Dermat 1978;114:755–760.
6. Lindor NM, Devries EMG, Michels VV, Schad CR, Jalal SM, Donovan KM, et al. Rothmund-Thomson syndrome in siblings: evidence for acquired in vivo chromosome mosaicism. Clin Genet 1996;49:124–129.
7. Dewald GW, Schad CR, Lilla VC, Jalal SM. Frequency and photographs of HGM11 chromosome anomalies in bone marrow samples from 3,996 patients with malignant hematologic neoplasms. Can Genet Cytogenet 1993;68:60–69.
8. Dewald GW, Stupca P. 154 chromosome anomalies in hematologic malignancies. Leuk Res 2000;24:487–489.
9. Dewald GW, Morris MA, Lilla VC. Chromosome studies in neoplastic hematologic disorders. In: McClatchey KD, ed. Clinical Laboratory Medicine, Williams and Wilkens, Baltimore, MD, 1993, pp. 703–740.
10. Rex A, Preus M. A diagnostic index for Down syndrome. J Pediatr 1982;100:903–906.
11. Nagahana H, Haamoto Y, Takeuchi T. An autopsy case of the 18 trisomy syndrome. Bull Osaka Med Sch 1974;20:26–33.
12. Dewald G, Haymond MW, Spurbeck JL, Moore SB. Origin of chi 46,XX/46,XY chimerism in a human true hermaphrodite. Science 1980;207:321–323.
13. Niebuhr E. The cri du chat syndrome: epidemiology, cytogenetics, and clinical features. Hum Genet 1978;44:227–275.
14. Tachdjian G, Fondacci C, Tapia S, Huten Y, Blot P, Nessmann C. The Wolf-Hirschhorn syndrome in fetuses. Clin Genet 1992;42:281–287.
15. Fryns JP, Emmery L, Timmermans J, Pedersen JC, van den Berghe. Tricho-rhino-phalangeal syndrome type II: Langer-Giedion syndrome in a 2.5-year-old boy. Am J Hum Genet 1980;28:53–56.
16. Warburton D, Kline J, Stein Z, Hutzler M, Chin A, Hassold T. Does the karyotype of a spontaneous abortion predict the karyotype of a subsequent abortion? Evidence from 273 women with two karyotyped spontaneous abortions. Am J Hum Genet 1987;41:465–483.
17. Lindor NM, Ney JA, Gaffey TA, Jenkins RB, Thibodeau SN, Dewald GW. A genetic review of complete and partial hydatidiform moles and nonmolar triploidy. Mayo Clin Proc 1992;67:791–799.
18. Dewald GW. Modern methods of chromosome analysis and their application in clinical practice. In: Homberger H, Batsakis JG, eds. Clinical Laboratory Annual, vol. 2, Appleton-Century Crofts, Norwalk, CT, 1983, pp. 2:1–29.
19. Spurbeck JL, Carlson RO, Allen JE, Dewald GW. Culturing and robotic harvesting of bone marrow, lymph nodes, peripheral blood, fibroblasts, and solid tumors with *in situ* techniques. Can Genet Cytogenet 1988;32:59–66.
20. Dewald GW, Broderick DL, Tom WW, Hagstrom JE, Pierre RV. The efficacy of direct, 24-hour culture, and mitotic synchronization methods for cytogenetic analysis of bone marrow in neoplastic hematologic disorders. Can Genet Cytogenet 18:1–9, 1985.
21. Crifasi PA, Michels VV, Driscoll DJ, Jalal SM, Dewald GW. DNA fluorescent probes for diagnosis of velocardiofacial and related syndromes. Mayo Clin Proc 1995;70:1148–1153.
22. Jalal SM, Law ME. Detection of newborn aneuploidy by interphase fluorescent in situ hybridization. Mayo Clin Proc 1997;72: 705–710.
23. Jalal SM, Law ME, Carlson RO, Dewald GW. Prenatal detection of aneuploidy by directly labeled multicolored probes and interphase fluorescence in situ hybridization. Mayo Clin Proc 1998;73:132–137.
24. Jalal SM, Law ME, Dewald GW. Atlas of Whole Chromosome Paint Probes: Normal Patterns and Utility for Abnormal Cases. Mayo Foundation for Medical Education and Research, Rochester, MN, 1996, 145 pp.
25. International system for cytogenetic nomenclature. Mitelman F, ed. S. Karger, Basel, 1995.
26. Kimmel DW, O'Fallon JR, Scheithauer BW, Kelly PJ, Dewald GW, Jenkins RB. Prognostic value of cytogenetic analysis in human cerebral astrocytomas. Ann Neur 1992;31:534–542.

11 Autopsy Chemistry

VERNARD I. ADAMS

DEFINITIONS, INDICATIONS AND LIMITATIONS OF THE METHOD

Autopsy chemistry, or postmortem chemistry, is the term applied to the measurement of endogenous constituents in dead bodies. Toxicologic tests, which measure concentrations of drugs and exogenous toxins, are discussed in Chapter 2. Postmortem chemical studies provide *direct* information concerning derangement of physiology. In contrast, customary gross and histological autopsy examinations are primarily tests of structural derangement, from which physiologic derangements may sometimes be inferred. Chemical testing may not only establish the cause of death but may contribute to the evaluation of the physiologic effects of recognizable anatomic lesions. For example, the extent of uremia can be determined in a case of polycystic kidney disease.

Although any clinical laboratory test may be applied to postmortem material, only a limited number of tests yield results that can be interpreted. Useful tests fall into two groups; those that measure analytes that are stable after death, toward the end of estimating the antemortem concentrations; and those that measure a diagnostically useful postmortem rise or fall in the concentration of the analyte. For many biochemical substances, interpretation of postmortem tests is precluded by the total absence of published data.

Our understanding of postmortem chemistry has been considerably enhanced by the pioneering work of Dr. Coe *(1)*, a forensic pathologist who showed that the vitreous, which is normally unavailable for clinical testing, is the substrate of choice for what have become the most frequently used postmortem chemical tests. Because the eye is mechanically isolated and well-protected by the orbit, vitreous is usually preserved even if serious trauma to the head had occurred. Vitreous is less subject to putrefaction than is blood, and is not subject to diffusion of drugs and alcohol. Like cerebrospinal fluid, it is nearly free of erythrocytes, but it is more accessible and artifacts of procurement are easier to recognize.

In this chapter, we give only an overview of autopsy chemistry. For methodological details, the reader should consult standard textbooks and manuals of laboratory medicine as well as pertinent references in the review articles by Coe *(1)* and Kleiner et al. *(2)*. Many of the data presented here are derived from Dr. Coe's work.

From: *Handbook of Autopsy Practice,* 3rd Ed. Edited by: J. Ludwig © Humana Press Inc., Totowa, NJ

SELECTION AND COLLECTION OF SPECIMENS FOR ANALYSIS

Specimens for biochemical and toxicological analysis must be retrieved, labeled, stored, and analyzed under established, standardized conditions *(3)*. In most cases, the time of sample procurement is the documented time of autopsy. For this reason, the recorded time of autopsy should be the time that the internal examination is commenced. If a postmortem sample is drawn either before or after the internal autopsy examination, the time of procurement should be separately noted. Interpretation of postmortem chemistry is also enhanced by the routine recording of early putrefactive changes.

BLOOD This is the substrate of choice for testing for hemoglobin S, hormones, cholinesterase, and abnormal metabolites in infants with suspected inborn errors of metabolism. Blood can be used to measure the concentrations of creatinine, urea nitrogen and bilirubin if vitreous, the specimen of choice, was not procured. All postmortem serum or plasma samples have some degree of hemolysis, and laboratories differ in their tolerance for specimens of this type. As a practical matter, the autopsy pathologist ordinarily need not be concerned with the distinction between plasma and serum; the laboratory separates the red cell mass from the supernatant and labels it as it sees fit. Postmortem concentrations of many analytes vary considerably with the anatomic locations of the sampling sites. Unlike the situation with postmortem toxicology, this variation has not been well-studied for endogenous substances, with the exception for glucose, for which the sample of choice is vitreous, rather than blood. The sampling and labeling policies required for toxicologic analysis are more than adequate for postmortem chemical analysis. The choice of container is dictated by the test to be undertaken, as in clinical testing. A common screening panel for inborn errors of metabolism requires three drops of blood on a filter paper.

VITREOUS This is the most frequently used specimen for postmortem chemical analysis. Typically, a panel of six tests is run, comprising sodium, potassium, chloride, urea nitrogen, creatinine, and glucose. Bilirubin may be added to the panel if

Table 11-1
Common Changes of Postmortem Chemical Values[a]

Substances[b]	*Body fluids or tissues analyzed*	*Interpretation*
Bilirubin	Serum	Slight increase after death.
Chloride	Serum and vitreous	Serum chloride values decrease after death; vitreous sodium is stable. (*See* Table 11-2 under "Dehydration" and "Uremia.")
Cholesterol	Serum	Stable after death (but *not* cholesterol esters).
Cholinesterase (true and pseudo-cholinesterase)	Serum	Stable after death (important for diagnosis of organic phosphorus or carbofuran poisoning).
Creatinine	Serum and vitreous	Values stable after death.
Desoxyribonucleic acid (DNA)	Tissues (unspecified)	More stable than ribonucleic acid; analyzed by Southern blotting. Small fragments can be amplified with PCR.
Glucose	Serum and vitreous	High values in vena cava and right heart chambers; vitreous values more reliable. (*See* Table 11-2 under "Diabetes mellitus" and "Hypoglycemia.")
Hypoxanthine	Vitreous	Values increase steadily after death; has been used to determine postmortem interval (*see* also "Potassium.").
Lactic acid	Serum and vitreous	Values increase after death. (*See* Table 11-2 under "Asphyxia.")
Lipoproteins		(*See* "Triglycerides and lipoproteins.")
Potassium	Vitreous	Values increase steadily after death; has been used to determine postmortem interval. (*See* also "Hypoxanthine.")
Proteins	Serum	Electrophoretic patterns remain stable.
Ribonucleic acid (RNA)	Tissues (unspecified)	Less stable than DNA (*see* above) but mRNA may be stable for several hours after death.
Sodium	Serum and vitreous	Serum sodium values decrease after death; vitreous sodium is stable.
Triglycerides and lipoproteins	Serum	Erratic changes after death.
Urea nitrogen	Serum and vitreous	Values stable after death.

[a]Data from refs. *(1)* and *(2)*. Numerous other substances (e.g., ammonia, amino acids, creatine, magnesium, phosphates, sulfates, trace elements, uric acid, xanthine) have been studied in various body fluids but are not listed here because tests in the postmortem setting are unreliable or are rarely of practical importance.

[b]In alphabetical order.

the gross autopsy is equivocal for the diagnosis of jaundice. If no postmortem chemical testing is contemplated, routinely drawn vitreous specimens can be sent to the toxicologist, who will use them for volatiles analysis and drug screening. The technique of drug screening is described in Chapter 2. Depending on the analytical technique used, centrifugation of the vitreous may be required to obtain a supernatant sample, to avoid clogging the analytical instruments.

INTERPRETATION OF POSTMORTEM CHEMICAL DATA

The most important changes of body-fluid components after death are compiled in Table 11-1. A synopsis of postmortem chemical findings in diseases such as diabetes mellitus is shown in Table 11-2. The tables show that glucose is best determined in vitreous because blood glucose values may increase dramatically in the agonal period, particularly after resuscitation attempts *(1)*. Hyperglycemia and diabetic ketoacidosis can be diagnosed readily but hypoglycemia cannot be confirmed by postmortem testing. The dehydration pattern (Table 11-2) has provided a compelling basis for the diagnosis of dehydration in cases of homicidal deprivation of food and water.

ADVANCED ANALYTICAL METHODS APPLIED TO POSTMORTEM SAMPLES

Although experiences are still limited, authors have shown in a number of publications that the following methods may be applicable under selected circumstances. In the autopsy setting, most of these tests still are used mainly for research purposes *(2)*. Some pertinent references are given in the following paragraphs. For additional diagnostic techniques, *see* Chapter 2. Other special laboratory procedures such as *in situ* hybridization, X-ray microanalysis, and autoradiography are described in Chapter 14.

HIGH-PERFORMANCE LIQUID CHROMATOGRAPHY (HPLC) Postmortem adrenaline and noradrenaline concentrations were determined by this method *(4)*.

IMMUNOCHEMISTRY Recombinant immunoblot assay (RIBA) *(5)* has been used for the detection of the human immunodeficiency virus.

IMMUNOHISTOCHEMISTRY Techniques in this field are widely applied and appropriate textbooks should be consulted for specific methods. Immunohistochemistry sometimes allows analysis of gene expression in archival tissue in paraffin

Table 11-2
Postmortem Chemical Changes in Pathological Conditions[a]

Diseases or conditions	*Body fluids analyzed*	*Interpretation*
Acidosis and alkalosis	Serum	Postmortem measurements of pH values probably not reliable. For ketoacidosis, *see* "Diabetes mellitus."
Dehydration	Vitreous	High sodium (>155 meq/L) and chloride (>135 meq/L) values with moderate increase (above 40 mg/dL) of urea nitrogen concentration.
Diabetes mellitus	Vitreous	High glucose (>200 mg/dL or >11.1 mmol/L) and ketone concentrations in diabetic ketoacidosis.
Endocrine disorders	Serum and other body fluids	The concentration of many pituitary, adrenal cortical, and some other hormones reflects the antemortem values. Epinephrine and insulin are unstable.
Hepatic coma	Cerebrospinal fluid	Glutamine concentrations increased.
Hyperglycemia		*See* "Diabetes mellitus."
Hypoglycemia	Serum, cerebrospinal fluid, and vitreous	No reliable way to diagnose hypoglycemia.
Inborn errors of metabolism[c]	Blood	Abnormal metabolites are found.
Liver diseases (See also "Hepatic coma")	Serum	Aminotransferases and other enzyme activities increase erratically after death and cannot be used for diagnosis. The albumin-globulin ratio can be estimated reliably.
Low-salt pattern	Vitreous	Low sodium, chloride, and potassium concentrations common in fatty change or cirrhosis of the liver.
Postmortem change unrelated to clinical disease (decomposition pattern)	Vitreous	Low sodium and chloride concentrations but *high* potassium values (>20 mEq/L).
Uremia	Vitreous	Marked increase of urea nitrogen and creatinine concentrations with sodium and chloride values near the normal range. (*See* also "Dehydration.")

[a]Data from ref. *(1)*.
[b]In alphabetical order.
[c]Examples are maple syrup urine disease, methylmalonic acidemia, medium chain acyl-CoA dehydrogenase deficiency.

blocks *(6)*. See also under "Immunohistochemistry" in Chapter 14 and below under "Polymerase chain reaction."

POLYMERASE CHAIN REACTION (PCR) This method has become a particularly powerful tool to study gene expression *(7,8)*, viral antigen *(9–11)*, as well as deoxyribonucleic acid (DNA), ribonucleic acid (RNA), and proteins in other settings *(2)*.

ATOMIC ABSORPTION SPECTROSCOPY This method, together with inductively coupled plasma emission spectroscopy and inductively coupled plasma mass spectroscopy has been used to analyze iron, copper, and other essential elements in fresh and formalin-fixed autopsy tissues *(12)*.

REFERENCES

1. Coe JI. Postmortem chemistry update. Emphasis on forensic application. Am J Forensic Med Pathol 1993;14:91–117.
2. Kleiner DE, Emmert-Buck MR, Liotta LA. Necropsy as a research method in the age of molecular pathology. Lancet 1995;346:945–948.
3. Forrest AR. Obtaining samples at post mortem examination for toxicological and biochemical analyses. ACP Broadsheet no 137: April 1993. J Clin Pathol 1993;46:292–296.
4. Hirvonen J, Huttunen P. Postmortem changes in serum noradrenalin and adrenalin concentrations in rabbit and human cadavers. Int J Legal Med 1996;109:143–146.
5. Little D, Ferris JA. Determination of human immunodeficiency virus antibody status in forensic autopsy cases in Vancouver using a recombinant immunoblot assay. J Forensic Sci 1990;35:1029–1034.
6. Terada T, Shimizu K, Izumi R, Nakanuma Y. Methods in pathology. p53 expression in formalin-fixed, paraffin-embedded archival specimens of intrahepatic cholangiocarcinoma: retrieval of p53 antigenicity by microwave oven heating of tissue sections. Mod Pathol 1994; 7:249–252.
7. Palacios J, Ezquieta B, Gamallo C, Limeres MA, Benito N, Rodrigues JI, Molano J. Detection of delta F508 cystic fibrosis mutation by polymerase chain reaction from old paraffin-embedded tissues: a retrospective autopsy study. Mod Pathol 1994;7:392–395.
8. Manci EA, Culberson DE, Chen GJ, Mankad V, Joshi VV, Fijimura FK. Polymerase chain reaction facilitates archival autopsy studies of sickle cell disease. Pediatr Pathol 1993;13:75–81.
9. Sei S, Kleiner DF, Kopp JB, Chandra R, Klotman PE, Yarchoan R, et al. Quantitative analysis of viral burden in tissues from children with symptomatic human immundeficiency virus type I infection assessed by polymerase chain reaction. J Infect Dis 1994;170:325–333.
10. Skowronski EW, Mendoza A, Smith SC Jr, Jaski BE. Detection of cytomegalovirus in paraffin-embedded coronary artery specimens of heart transplant recipients by the polymerase chain reaction: implications of cytomegalovirus association with graft atherosclerosis. J Heart Lung Transplant 1993;12:717–723.
11. Turner PC, Bailey AS, Cooper RJ, Morris DJ. The polymerase chain reaction for detecting adenovirus DNA in formalin-fixed, paraffin embedded tissue obtained postmortem. J Infect 1993;27:43–46.
12. Bush VJ, Moyer TP, Batts KP, Parisi JE. Essential and toxic element concentrations in fresh and formalin-fixed human autopsy tissues. Clin Chem 1995;41:284–294.

12 Autopsy Roentgenology and Other Imaging Techniques

JURGEN LUDWIG

Roentgenology provides one of the most important supplements of modern autopsy technology. Many applications of postmortem roentgenography, in particular, angiographic procedures, have been described in Chapters 2–8. In addition, numerous indications for the use of autopsy roentgenology are listed throughout Part II. Therefore, in this chapter, only a brief overview shall be provided.

COMMON APPLICATIONS OF AUTOPSY ROENTGENOLOGY

MEDICOLEGAL CASES The use of roentgenographs in medicolegal autopsies is further discussed in Chapter 2; they are used *(1)* primarily for

- Identification purposes;
- The diagnosis of traumatic bone lesions;
- The identification of bullets and other foreign bodies; and
- Identification of gas in body cavities, vessels, and other sites.

Comparison of postmortem dental roentgenograms with in vivo films is the most common method of identification, particularly in the presence of advanced decomposition. Fractures and other bone lesions generally can be identified with greater accuracy in roentgenograms than by dissection. In fact, bone lesions of the extremities often cannot be studied in any other way. Most important, bullets and other radiodense objects may be impossible to find by any method other than roentgenography (Fig. 12-1). It should be noted, however, that a prosector still may have the greatest difficulties to find a small metallic object such as a bullet, even if it is clearly visible in the roentgenogram. In such an instance, the tissue with the foreign object should be removed and subdivided. Roentgenograms of the smaller samples will allow location of the area where the object can be found. If the tissue with the foreign object cannot be removed, additional roentgenographs with placement of radiodense markers is helpful. Finally, roentgenograms are most helpful to identify gas, for example, if one wants to determine whether a newborn was breathing and thus has air in the lungs and the gastrointestinal tract *(1)*. For other examples, *see* below.

From: *Handbook of Autopsy Practice,* 3rd Ed. Edited by: J. Ludwig © Humana Press Inc., Totowa, NJ

CLINICAL CONDITIONS DEMONSTRABLE BY POSTMORTEM ROENTGENOGRAMS

Principally, most roentgenologic diagnostic methods that do not require cooperation of the patient or a functioning circulation can be done in the autopsy setting. The most important indications and methods are listed here. It should be noted that many of the indications may have medicolegal implications.

- Gas embolism, pneumothorax, pneumomediastinum, and pneumoperitoneum generally are easy to identify in appropriate roentgenograms. Without this technique, these conditions may be totally missed or the diagnosis must be based on a fleeting impression because only roentgenograms can provide a permanent record. However, the important distinction between air and putrefaction gases must be made. Whereas the changes in a tension pneumothorax are diagnostic (for an illustration, *see* "Pneumothorax" in Part II), air embolism may be simulated by putrefaction gases. The presence of other putrefactive changes and the analysis of the gas (page 290) should provide the correct diagnosis;
- Angiographically demonstrable vascular abnormalities. Coronary artery disease (*see* below), congenital coronary abnormalities, pulmonary vascular disease *(2)*, mesenteric, splenic *(3)*, or hepatic artery occlusion, cerebral artery aneurysm, or arteriovenous malformations *(4)*, renal artery stenosis or renal vein thrombosis, vascular tumors, and many other arterial and venous lesions that can be demonstrated *in situ* or on isolated organs;
- Cholangiography. Typical indications are primary sclerosing cholangitis and Caroli's disease *(5)*;
- Postoperative autopsies. Roentgenographic techniques, including angiography *(6)*, may be most helpful to find and document operative mishaps or postoperative complications such as anastomotic arterial occlusion or iatrogenic tension pneumothorax as described earlier;

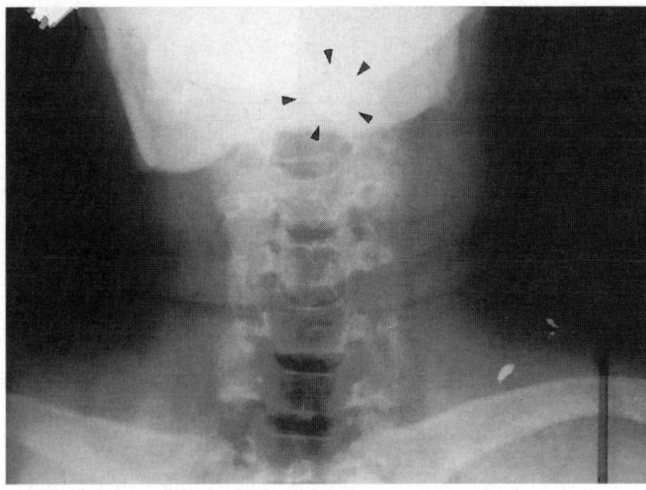

Fig. 12-1. Use of roentgenogram in medicolegal cases: deflected bullet lodged at base of skull. The entrance wound of this 38 caliber bullet was found on the back, over the left scapula, but during dissection at autopsy, the bullet could not be found. The roentgenogram shows two small bullet fragments, clearly visible in the soft tissue of the left shoulder but the remainder of the bullet had been deflected upward and was found in a deformed state at the level of the foramen magnum (arrow heads), just to the left of the midline.

- Postinfectious, dystrophic calcification as in pulmonary tuberculosis *(1)* or parasitic diseases, or metastatic calcifications (e.g., in lungs, stomach, or kidneys) in hyperparathyroidism;
- Traumatic, neoplastic, metabolic, and other skeletal diseases.

EQUIPMENT IN THE AUTOPSY ROOM

We use a modified and shielded autopsy room as shown in part in Fig. 12-2. A Machlett Super Dynamax Tube (1-mm and 2-mm focal spots) has been installed. We are using a Picker X-ray table. A 300-mA Keleket machine (140-kV generator) is in an adjacent room. Films are processed in a small darkroom with a Kodak RP X-OMAT processor, which permits one to monitor injection procedures by reviewing films while the injection is still under way.

We are using this facility for chest roentgenography before most autopsies, for roentgenographic surveys in medicolegal cases, and occasionally for *in situ* angiographic or other studies. In the last case, the autopsy or parts of the autopsy are done on the X-ray table. Most angiographic or cholangiographic studies are carried out on isolated organs such as heart, lungs, liver, kidneys, or brain.

The modifications of an autopsy room with shielding and new installations may be forbiddingly expensive. However, less elaborate setups are available. For years we worked with an old transportable Keleket machine and had satisfactory results. In order to bring the cassette into proper position, we used a special sturdy rack, on which bodies' autopsies could be done. It consisted of an aluminum frame with channels at the inside, for sliding cassettes back and forth, and a top layer of X-ray Bakelite (Fig. 12-3).

If X-ray equipment is used by the autopsy service, the facilities and procedures must be reviewed and approved by a radiation safety officer. For the decontamination of X-ray tables, racks, cassettes, and other tools for autopsy roentgenology, the principles apply that are described in Chapter 16.

ANGIOGRAPHIC TECHNIQUES

Postmortem angiography is among the most important applications of roentgenologic methods in the autopsy room. For contrast media, *see* Chapter 15. Because of its importance, postmortem coronary angiography is described here. Similar methods, applied to other organ systems, have been presented in Chapters 4–6.

POSTMORTEM CORONARY ANGIOGRAPHY Many contrast media have been used in the past *(7,8)* but barium sulfate with gelatin is now preferred *(9,10)*, although iodinated dyes can also be used *(11)*. For quantitative studies, a radioisotope dilution method has been reported *(12)*. Double-contrast techniques and in situ angiography (Fig. 12-4) have also been described *(13–15)*. Radiopaque dyes used clinically are applicable to the coronary arteries at autopsy (Chapter 15). A setup for controlled-pressure coronary angiography is shown in Fig. 12-5. For this procedure, the heart is removed with 2–4 cm of the major vessels attached. Postmortem clots are removed by irrigation with saline. Cannulas of suitable size are placed into the coronary ostia. Care is taken to identify an independent ostium. Ligatures are placed around the coronary arteries and are tied as near as possible to the origins.

The cannulated heart is suspended in isotonic saline or Kaiserling I solution at about 45°C. The coronary arteries are perfused at a low pressure with isotonic saline. This is continued for several minutes, with use of 100–200 mL, until the return through the coronary sinus is free of blood.

The previously prepared barium-gelatin mixture (Chapter 15) is drawn into two 30-mL syringes. These are attached, via three-way stopcocks, to the apparatus shown in Fig. 12-5, and the actual injection is begun. Care is taken to avoid introduction of air bubbles at any stage of the procedure. While the system is kept supplied with contrast medium by way of the syringes, the pressure is increased almost simultaneously to a maximum of 110 mm Hg. Lacerated vessels may require ligation at this stage, but these are rare in our experience. A control roentgenogram can be prepared at this time. The heart chambers may be irrigated to remove any contrast material that enters into the lumens. With the coronary cannulas still in place and maintaining a pressure of 100–120 mm Hg, the chambers are packed with formalin-soaked cotton to their approximate normal size and shape and the specimen is immersed in cold Kaiserling I or formalin solution (Chapter 14). The heart is cooled for 1–3 h to permit the gelatin to set and then roentgenograms are prepared.

Angiography may underestimate the severity of obstruction if the narrowed region is compared to an adjacent segment that is considered normal but is actually stenotic. Conversely, microscopy can overestimate the degree of narrowing if the effect

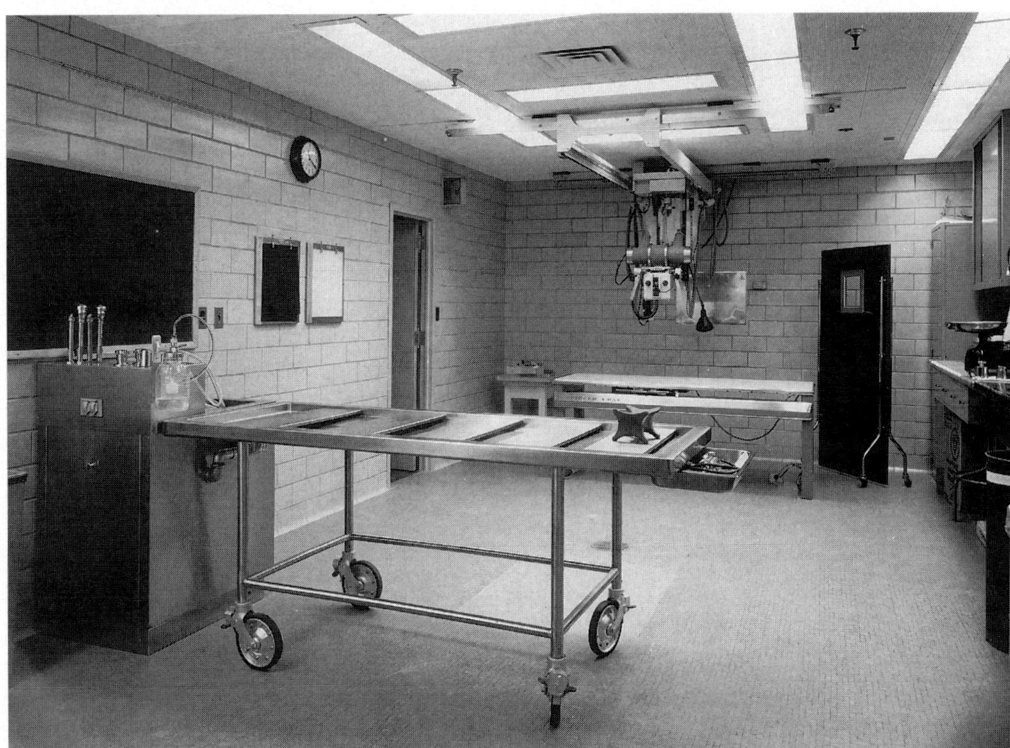

Fig. 12-2. Shielded autopsy room for roentgenologic examination. In the background is a Machlett Super Dynamax Tube and a Picker X-ray table. In adjacent room to the left, a 300-mA Keleket X-ray machine with a 125-kV generator is installed. In the foreground is a mobile autopsy table with a separate service island.

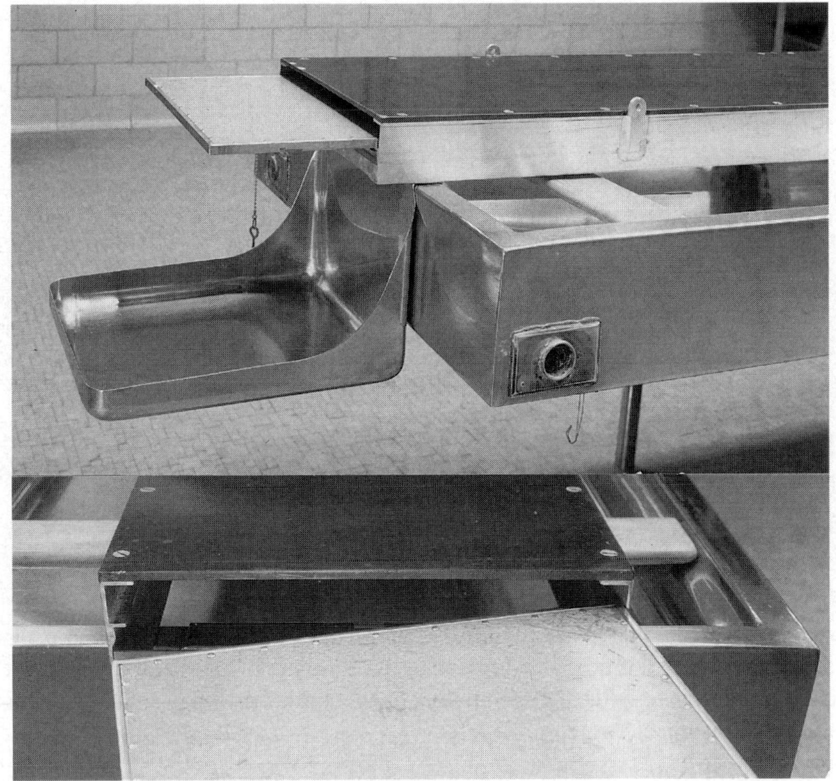

Fig. 12-3. Autopsy rack for postmortem roentgenography with transportable X-ray machines. This rack is 198 by 40 cm and consists of an aluminum frame (upper) with channels that permit the X-ray casette to slide to the desired position. The casette is inserted at the end of the rack and can be moved by hand from below (lower). The rack is covered with X-ray Bakelite, 0.64 cm thick. The Bakelite seams are watertight so that autopsies can be done on this rack and contamination of the inside can be kept to a minimum.

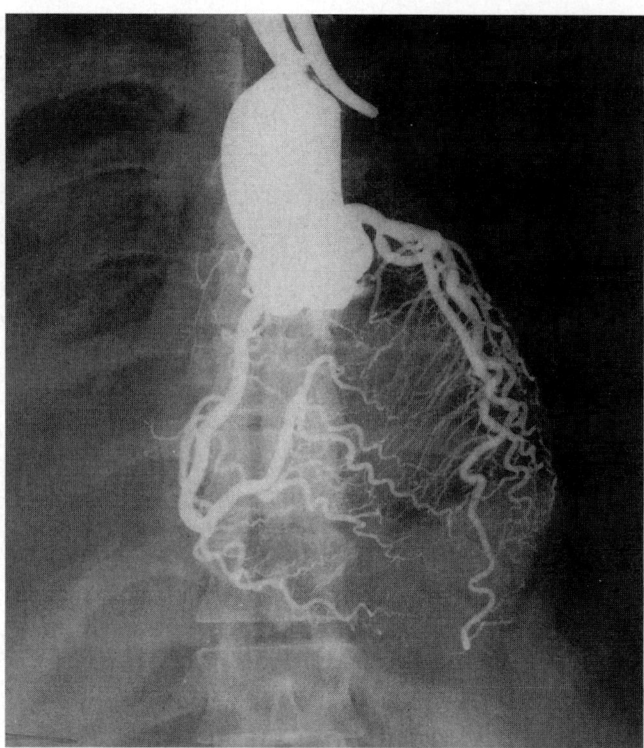

Fig. 12-4. Normal coronary angiogram *in situ*. The sternum was split in the midline and about 300 mL of barium sulfate-gelatin mixture was injected into the ascending aorta without pressure regulation, by hand with a large syringe. Superior portion of ascending aorta has been clamped off.

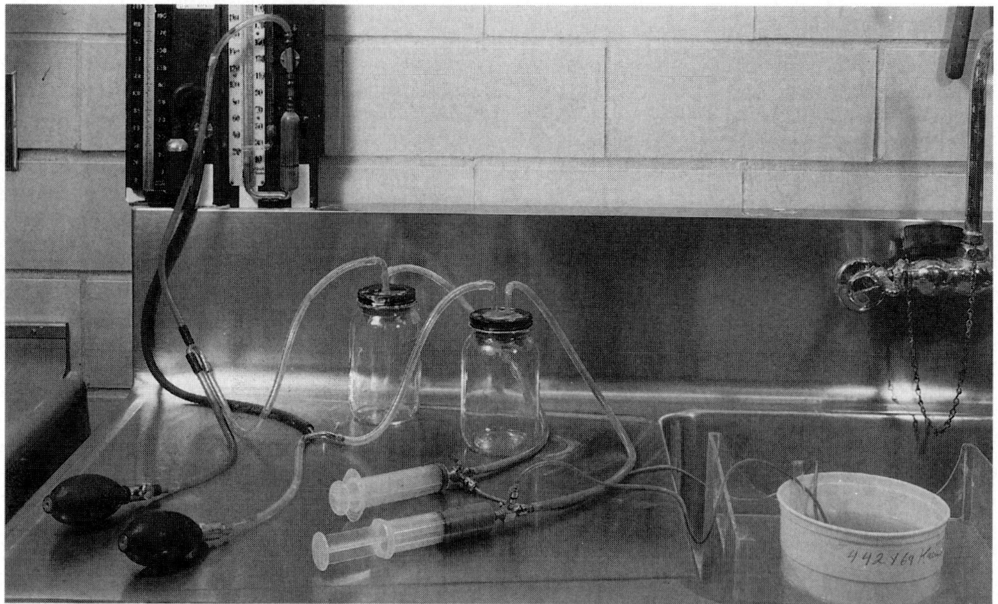

Fig. 12-5. Setup for controlled pressure injection of contrast medium into coronary arteries. In this instance, each syringe contains chromopaque of a different color and is connected to one of the coronary orifices and the pressure-regulating system. The heart is suspended in Kaiserling solution or saline in the container on the right, which is in an ice-water bath. The two independent pressure-regulating systems with manometers are on the left.

of compensatory dilatation of atherosclerotic segments is not considered *(16)*. Thus, coronary angiography does not replace microscopy. Although arteriography localizes obstructive lesions, microscopy is still necessary to determine its nature—for example, chronic atherosclerosis vs acute plaque rupture with stenosis.

The arteries of the extremities can be studied by angiography with a pressure-controlled system *(17)*, resembling the system used with coronary arteries. As mentioned in Chapter 3, phlebography and lymphangiography (Fig. 12-6) can also be performed at autopsy. Intraosseus phlebography can be used for

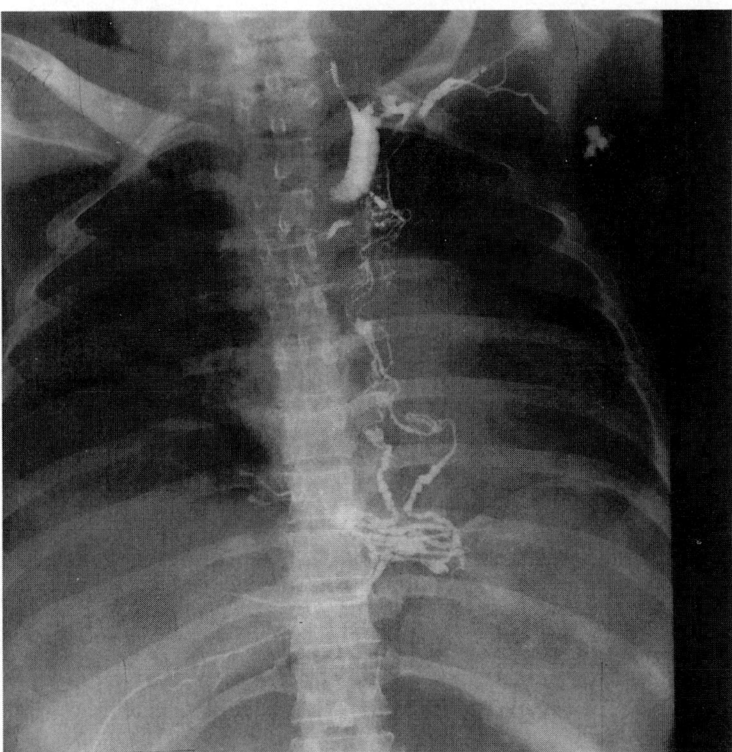

Fig. 12-6. Postmortem lymphangiography showing dilated lymphatics in the hepatoduodenal ligament and the anterior mediastinum in a patient with liver cirrhosis and congestive heart failure. The lymphatics drain in the subclavian vein as shown by the presence of contrast medium in this vessel. Adapted with permission from ref. *(18)*.

the evaluation of thrombosis of deep leg veins, but the method is a bit cumbersome *(19)*.

ANGIOGRAPHY OF OTHER ORGANS Pulmonary angiography and bronchography is described in Chapter 4; the demonstration of esophageal varices and mesenteric angiography is presented in Chapter 5; in Chapter 6, cerebral arteriography, venography, and ventriculography are discussed; and in Chapter 15, the use of angiographic methods in the study of museum specimens is shown. Roentgenologic and other imaging techniques in specific clinical or forensic diseases and conditions are also shown in Part II.

APPLICATION OF OTHER IMAGING TECHNIQUES

Except for ultrasonography which probably could be used in many autopsy settings without too much difficulty, other imaging techniques have also been widely used in recent years.

MAGNETIC RESONANCE IMAGING (MRI) This has been used particularly as a supplement to perinatal autopsies *(20)*, autopsies in stillbirth *(21)*, and pediatric autopsies in cases of suspected child abuse *(22)*. MRI was useful in directing the autopsy and, particularly, the brain cutting to focal areas of abnormality *(22)*. In a limited number of comparisons which included two adults, MRI was equal to autopsy in detecting gross cranial, pulmonary, abdominal, and vascular pathology, and superior in detecting air and fluid in potential body spaces *(21)*.

COMPUTERIZED TOMOGRAPHY (CT) CT images produced in vivo are widely used in autopsy studies, primarily in brain cutting (*see* Chapter 6). The method also has been used to compare diagnostic yields of CT and MRI (*see* above) *(23)* and other research endeavors but we are not aware of routine use in autopsy settings.

ULTRASONOGRAPHY Use of this method in fetuses often failed to detect anomalies that were identified during autopsy *(24)*.

REFERENCES

1. Schmidt G, Kallieris D. Use of radiographs in the forensic autopsy. Forensic Sci Int 1982;19:263–270.
2. Resnik JM, Engeler CE, Derauf BJ. Postmortem angiography of catheter-induced pulmonary artery perforation. J Forensic Sci 1992; 37:1346–1351.
3. Karhunen PJ, Penttila A. Diagnostic postmortem angiography of fatal splenic artery haemorrhage. Zeitschrift für Rechtsmedizin. J Legal Med 1989;103:129–136.
4. Karhunen PJ, Penttila A, Erkinjuntti T. Arteriovenous malformation of the brain: imaging by postmortem angiography. Forensic Sci Int 1990;48:9–19.
5. Terada T, Nakanuma Y. Congenital biliary dilatation in autosomal dominant adult polycystic disease of the liver and kidneys. Arch Pathol Lab Med 1988;112:1113–1116.
6. Karhunen PJ, Manniko A, Penttila A, Liesto K. Diagnostic angiography in postoperative autopsies. Am J Forensic Med Pathol 1989; 10:303–309.

7. Reiner L. Gross examination of the heart. In: Gould SE, ed. Pathology of the Heart and Great Vessels, 2nd ed. Charles C. Thomas, Springfield, IL, 1968, pp.1111–1149.
8. Saphir O. Gross examination of the heart: injection of coronary arteries; weight and measurements of heart. In: Gould SE, ed. Pathology of the Heart and Great Vessels, 2nd ed. Charles C. Thomas, Springfield, IL, 1960, pp. 1043–1066.
9. Schlesinger MJ. A new radiopaque mass for vascular injection. Lab Invest 1957;6:1–11.
10. Hales MR, Carrington CB. A pigment gelatin mass for vascular injection. Yale J Biol Med 1971;43:257–270.
11. Suberman CO, Suberman RI, Dalldorf FG, Gabrielle OF. Radiographic visualization of coronary arteries in postmortem hearts: a simple technic. Am J Clin Pathol 1970;53:254–257.
12. Davies NA. A radioisotope dilution technique for the quantitative study of coronary artery disease postmortem. Lab Invest 1963;12: 1198–1203.
13. Ludwig J, Lie JT. Heart and Vascular System. In: Ludwig J, ed. Current Methods of Autopsy Practice, 2nd ed. W.B. Saunders Co., Philadelphia, PA, 1979, pp. 21–50.
14. Rissanen VT. Double contrast technique for postmortem coronary angiography. Lab Invest 1970;23:517–520.
15. Davies MJ, Pomerance A, Lamb D. Techniques in examination and anatomy of the heart. In: Pomerance A, Davies MJ, eds. Blackwell Scientific Publications, Oxford, 1975, pp. 1–48.
16. Edwards WD. Pathology of myocardial infarction and reperfusion. In: Gersh BJ, Rahimtoola SH, ed. Acute Myocardial Infarction, 2nd ed. Chapman & Hall, New York, 1997, pp. 16–50.
17. Ross CF, Keele KD. Post mortem arteriography "normal" lower limbs. Angiology 1951;2:374–385.
18. Ludwig J, Linhart P, Baggenstoss AH. Hepatic lymph drainage in cirrhosis and congestive heart failure. A postmortem lymphangiographic study. Arch Pathol 1968;86:551–562.
19. Lund F, Diener L, Ericsson JLE. Postmortem intraosseous phlegogaphy as an aid in studies of venous thromboembolism. Angiology 1969;20:155–176.
20. Brookes JA, Hall-Craggs MA, Sams VR, Lees WR. Non-invasive perinatal necropsy by magnetic resonance imaging. Lancet 1996;348: 1139–1141.
21. Ros PR, Li KC, Baer H, Staab EV. Preautopsy magnetic resonance imaging: initial experience. Magn Reson Imaging 1990;8:303–308.
22. Hart BL, Dudley MH, Zumwalt RE. Postmortem cranial MRI and autopsy correlation in suspected child abuse. Am J Forensic Med Pathol 1996;17:217–224.
23. Westesson PL, Katzberg RW, Tallents RH, Sanchez-Woodworth RE, Svensson AS. CT and MR of the temporomandibular joint: comparison with autopsy. Am J Roentgenol 1987;148:1165–1171.
24. Weston J, Porter HJ, Andrews HS, Berry PJ. Correlation of antenatal ultrasonography and pathological examination in 153 malformed fetuses. J Clin Ultrasound 1993;21:387–392.

13 Autopsy of Bodies Containing Radioactive Materials

KELLY L. CLASSIC

Current practice in medicine uses a variety of radioactive sources; they are introduced into a human body intentionally for medical research, diagnosis and therapy, or when there is an accident involving radioactive materials. Because the latter is fortunately rare, medical procedures are the main cause of radioactivity in a dead body. Each year, nearly ten million medical procedures involve injection or ingestion of radioactive materials by patients *(1)*. Since most affected patients are in an older age group (e.g., 81% for heart studies with radioactive material are done in patients past 45 yr of age), deaths and hence embalming, autopsies, and cremation of radioactive cadavers are likely to occur with increasing frequency.

GENERAL POLICIES

Some patients who received therapeutic doses of liquid radiopharmaceuticals must remain under the control of the licensed facility *(2)*. In these cases, the person in charge of the radiation safety program (usually designated as the radiation safety officer) would be notified immediately—that is, prior to release of the deceased to a morgue or funeral home. The radiation safety officer or designee attaches a tag to the dead body indicating that it is radioactive and stating whether special precautions are necessary (Fig. 13-1). Other patients who have received therapeutic activities can—under appropriate conditions—be released immediately from a licensed facility *(2)*. Administration of liquid radiopharmaceuticals for diagnostic purposes rarely requires that patients remain under the control of a licensed facility. Diagnostic procedures are outpatient procedures and under normal circumstances, patients are not considered a hazard to other members of the public.

Patients with radioactive implants (radioactive material in a solid form) may or may not be under the control of a licensed facility. If they die while in a facility, the implant generally will be removed prior to release of the body. The deceased is no longer radioactive after removal of the implant and thus, no special precautions are required while working on or around it. If patients with permanent radioactive implants are released from a medical facility *(3)*, radiation exposure from these persons is not considered hazardous to the general public. However, family members are instructed to contact the prescribing radiation oncologist if the patient dies at home or in another hospital to assure that appropriate measures are taken with regard to the implant.

From: *Handbook of Autopsy Practice,* 3rd Ed. Edited by: J. Ludwig © Humana Press Inc., Totowa, NJ

HAZARD TYPES

Radioactive bodies present two types of hazard: external exposure and radioactive contamination. The risks depend on the type and activity of radiation, whether the body will be opened, the number of days since administration of the radioactive material, and the time that persons spend in the vicinity of the body. External exposure is the primary concern if the body will not be opened. Individuals will rarely encounter high exposures around bodies of patients who were released from a hospital. However, exposure rates from bodies directly from a medical center may be appreciable; the appropriate tag will provide this information. Table 13-1 shows unshielded dose rates at two distances for some radioisotopes that may be encountered. The radioactivity level chosen for the first entry (^{99m}Tc) is typical administered activity and the level for the last four entries is activity below which a patient can be released from the hospital *(3)*. Beta-emitting radioisotopes (^{32}P, ^{89}Sr, ^{90}Y) are not considered external exposure hazards when the body cavity will not be opened so they are not addressed in Table 13-1. The listed dose rates will decrease significantly as time after administration of radioactive materials with short half-lives (6 h and 2.7 d for ^{99m}Tc and ^{198}Au, respectively) increases. The same holds true for radioactive materials that are rapidly metabolized (^{99m}Tc and ^{131}I). Activity in implants will decrease only by half-life.

Radiation exposure limits for members of the general public have been determined by federal regulatory agencies and radiation protection consensus groups *(4,5)*. Individuals who are infrequently exposed to sources of radiation, for example, funeral home directors, are allowed to receive 100 mrem whole body annually. Individuals who are frequently exposed may receive 500 mrem whole body annually. Hands are relatively insensitive to radiation and therefore have a recommended annual limit of 5,000 mrem.

RADIOACTIVITY
PRECAUTIONS
Radionuclide ____________
Administered Activity ____________ mCi
Final Measured Dose Rate ____________ mR/h
Date ____________
Tag is not to be removed until:
1) Radioactive material is removed from patient, or
2) Authorization is received from Radiation Safety Officer.
Signature ____________
Radiation Safety Officer

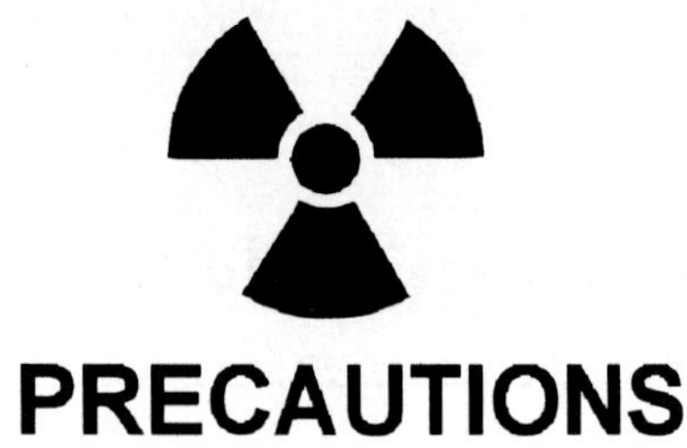

Fig. 13-1. Tag for radioactive deceased person.

Table 13-1
Unshielded Dose Rates at 30 and 100 cm for Common Radioactive Materials

		Dose rate (mrem/h)	
Radioisotope	*Activity (mCi)*	*30 cm*	*100 cm*
^{99m}Tc	20	16	2
^{103}Pd (implant)	40	33	3
^{125}I (implant)	9	7	1
^{131}I	33	78	7
^{198}Au	93	237	21

If the body will be opened for an autopsy, both external exposure and radioactive contamination are of concern. The dose rates in Table 13-1 still apply but in addition, precautions to minimize or prevent contamination must be practiced.

GENERAL PRECAUTIONS

Reducing time, increasing distance, and using shields are methods to reduce radiation exposure. Keeping the time of exposure at a minimum is the principal method of dose reduction for autopsy personnel. Extremity distance can be achieved through the use of long-handled instruments. Shielding with a radiology lead apron (0.5 mm lead equivalent thickness) would provide some protection for gamma radiation from ^{99m}Tc and ^{125}I but would do little for highly penetrating gamma rays from ^{103}Pd, ^{131}I, ^{182}Ta, and ^{198}Au.

Common barrier protection as determined by consensus standards *(6)* includes numerous items that minimize external radiation exposure from beta-emitting radioisotopes (when body cavities are opened) and assist in the prevention of personal contamination. These include double-gloves, hair covers, long-sleeved jump suits that are fluid resistant, foot covers, and facial protection (splash guards). Any wound sustained during procedures on a radioactive body should be attended immediately. The wound should be débrided, if necessary, and rinsed thoroughly to remove as much radioactivity as possible. For further details on safety measures, *see* Chapter 16.

Placing plastic-backed paper on the floor around the autopsy table will facilitate decontamination and prevent further spread of contamination. Autopsy tools can be wrapped in plastic for the same reasons.

PROCEDURE-SPECIFIC TECHNIQUES

If a deceased patient had received therapeutic amounts of radioisotopes and was hospitalized, it is likely that a knowledgeable person (radiation safety officer or designee) will accompany the body to the funeral home or morgue. The officer should provide specific directions that will prevent contamination and reduce exposure. Hospitalized patients who die with radioactive implants will have them removed; no residual radioactivity remains in their body fluids. Imbedded permanent implants require special handling (*see* below) but the body fluids of the deceased are not radioactive.

EMBALMING

Liquid Radioisotopes In the presence of liquid radioisotopes, simple embalming using standard aspiration and injection methods minimizes the likelihood of contamination and will not expose the embalmer to appreciable amounts of radiation. Fluids should be removed by means of a trocar and tubing in a manner that does not require an individual to hold either item or be close to the body while the fluid is draining. Fluids from the body can be drained directly into the sewage system unless directed otherwise by the radiation safety officer. Collection and handling of body cavity fluids should be done only under the direction of a knowledgeable person as these procedures may increase radiation exposures. Depending on the radioisotope and route of administration, the fluid may contain high radioactivity levels and must be handled accordingly—for example, stored in shielded containers (*see* below).

Embalming may or may not appreciably reduce activity levels within the body. Early after administration, ^{131}I is circulating throughout the body. Twenty-four hours after administration, only trace amounts are circulating because most of the material has been excreted or taken up by the thyroid gland. Similarly, ^{89}Sr that has not been excreted is found in the skeleton after only a few days. Therefore, 2–3 d after administration, these radioisotopes would be found only in minimal concentrations in embalming fluid. However, patients who have received radioisotopes (e.g., ^{32}P, ^{198}Au) intrapleurally or intraperitoneally

Table 13-2
Dose to Hands in Peritoneal Cavity[a]

	Dose (mrem/min)					
	^{198}Au			^{32}P or ^{90}Y		
Activity (mCi)	*No gloves*	*Surgical gloves*	*Double gloves*	*No gloves*	*Surgical gloves*	*Double gloves*
1	12	7	2	13	8	5
5	60	35	10	65	40	25
10	10	70	20	130	80	50
25	300	175	50	325	200	125
50	600	350	100	650	400	250

[a]Adapted from ref. *(7)*.

will have a large portion of the activity removed with the pleural or ascitic fluids, respectively *(7)*.

Urine may contain some radioactivity depending on the time since administration, the radioisotope that was administered, and the route of administration. Within a few days of administration, the urine may contain appreciable radioactivity and, unless directed otherwise, should be drained directly into the sewer system, similar to pleural and ascitic fluid during embalming. It should be noted, however, that activity levels may not be reduced by removal of residual urine. After the first 2 d of the administration of ^{131}I and ^{89}Sr, more than half the activity would normally be excreted through the urine *(8)* though the patient's medical condition may sometimes delay this process. Draining urine from the bladder of these patients prior to autopsy procedures may reduce radiation exposure. Radioisotopes in the pleural or peritoneal cavities will be much less affected by removal of urine.

AUTOPSY

Liquid Radioisotopes If radioisotopes had been administered intraperitoneally (^{32}P, ^{90}Y, ^{198}Au), much activity will be removed with pleural and ascitic fluids but some activity will remain on serous surfaces *(7)*. Drying the open cavity with sponges can reduce the radioactivity level. Double gloving or thick rubber gloves should be used. Table 13-2 shows dose to the hands from work performed in the peritoneal cavity. Whenever possible, the use of long-handled instruments is recommended. With beta emitters, distances of as little as 15 cm of air or 2.5 cm of tissue can appreciably reduce extremity exposure.

For handling an autopsy case with a high ^{131}I radioactivity burden, emphasis must be placed on reducing external exposure levels and contamination potential of the dead body while it is still at the hospital and before it is released to a local funeral home where regulatory exposure limits for the general public apply *(4,9)*. Risks to persons outside the hospital appear to be reduced by removal of organs with high activity burdens. During these procedures, external exposure should be monitored by issuing each individual one dosimeter to be worn on the torso and one to be worn on the dominant hand under gloves. When this was tested, the highest doses were received by the lead pathologist (who worked on the cadaver with high activity organs still in place); doses were 22 mrem to the whole body and 550 mrem to the hand, well below annual permissible dose levels. Precautions designed to reduce radiation exposure of employees included the use of personal protective equipment, limiting personnel time (20-min rotations), instructing staff to maintain increased distance from the cadaver when feasible, and general methods to reduce room contamination. When this was tested, employees other than the lead pathologist received a maximum of 13 mrem to the whole body and 59 mrem to the hand *(9)*.

Other recommended precautions in such a setting included preselection of surgical instruments that were either easy to clean or disposable, controlled access to the autopsy room, and complete stocking of the room so that personnel did not need to exit for supplies *(10)*. Action-specific procedures were similar to those used at a decontamination facility—that is, correct donning and removal of personal protective equipment, use of a "clean" (not radioactively contaminated) area, and frequent personal surveys with a portable radiation detection monitor. When this was tested, the pathologist received 20 mrem to the whole body and 70 mrem to the hand *(10)*. In that study, radioactive organs were not removed nor was the body embalmed; instead, the funeral director placed the body directly into a commercial casket liner made of steel and sealed it shut. Although radiation levels could still be detected through the casket, they diminished rapidly due to the short (8 d) half-life.

Synopsis of Precautions Based on the aforementioned experiences and consensus standard recommendations *(7)*, the following procedures should be followed for bodies containing high levels of radioactivity:

1. Supervision by an individual knowledgeable in radiation (local institution radiation safety officer);
2. External exposure monitoring of personnel (whole body and hand);
3. Use of disposable tools or tools that are easy to clean;
4. Storage of sufficient supplies in the autopsy room;
5. Secured area access;
6. Personnel time limits (rotation of personnel);
7. Bioassay of personnel at conclusion of procedure (to assure contamination was not inhaled, absorbed, or ingested);
8. Surveys of personnel with portable instrumentation upon exit from secured area;
9. Survey and decontamination of area and all equipment;
10. Observance of the procedures for proper disposal of radioactive waste items; and
11. Use of personal protective equipment, which includes
    a. double gloves,
    b. face mask,
    c. eye splash protection,
    d. surgical hats,
    e. plastic gowns,
    f. plastic shoe covers, and
    g. lead aprons (if they are expected to reduce exposure levels).

Removal of highly radioactive organs depends on anticipated disposition of the body. If a full autopsy will be performed, removal of the organs is encouraged to limit pathologist

Table 13-3
Radiation Exposure Rates From Radioactive Implants

	Exposure rates (rem/h) for 50 mCi							
	^{125}I		^{103}Pd		^{182}Ta		^{198}Au	
Distance (cm)	*No shielding*	*Tissue[a] shielding*	*No shielding*	*Tissue[a] shielding*	*No shielding*	*Tissue[a] shielding*	*No shielding*	*Tissue[a] shielding*
3	3.9	1.2	0.17	0.12	37.8	28.8	15.5	11.1
8	0.55	0.02	0.02	0.008	5.3	2.6	1.8	0.74
13	0.2	0.001	0.009	0.002	2.1	0.66	0.7	0.17
20	0.08	Negligible	0.004	Negligible	0.83	0.13	0.28	0.03
30	0.04	Negligible	0.002	Negligible	0.38	0.02	0.13	0.005

[a]Tissue shielding assumes that the distance in column 1 is all body tissue.

exposure. For embalming, removal of organs would reduce exposures but because this procedure involves only short periods of time next to the cadaver and because greater distances are kept during the procedure itself, the embalmer would receive minimal exposure with the organs in place while an individual who might remove the organs could receive higher exposure. The staff must consider exposure to all personnel during each step to keep collective exposure as low as possible. If the embalmer intends to do cosmetic restoration of the face and the thyroid is the highly radioactive organ, removal of the thyroid and adjacent contaminated tissue might be indicated.

Procedures in the Presence of Implants Radioactive implants, sometimes referred to as "seeds," generally are small pieces of radioactive wire or small capsules containing the radioactivity. If the location of the implant is known and no need exists to expose them during the autopsy, removal may involve more radiation exposure than leaving the implants undisturbed and working quickly when near them. Table 13-3 shows unshielded and shielded (with body tissue) radiation exposure rates at chosen distances from radioisotopes that are commonly used as permanent implants. The numbers represent possible extremity exposures. Permanent implants of beta emitters and low-energy gamma emitters—for example, ^{125}I or ^{103}Pd, do not normally present major radiation hazards and therefore typically do not require removal prior to an autopsy *(11)*.

If a prosector wants to remove the radioactive implants, with or without the surrounding tissue, a radiograph of the area should be prepared to show their current location because the implants may have shifted from their original site. After removal of the material, a second radiograph should confirm that all radiation sources had been removed. Source removal should be done rapidly and with long-handled instruments. If an entire organ or a large tissue sample can be removed with the radiation sources intact, individuals performing the procedure would receive much less exposure. Exposures of pathologists at an institution performing procedures on an average of 16 autopsy cases with permanent implants each year remained below maximum permissible limits for the general public *(12)*.

Explanted radiation sources should be placed together in a container and stored in an area not frequented by personnel. Active sources should be disposed of by approved methods *(4,13)*. This can be accomplished by contacting and returning the sources to the institution where they were implanted, contacting a local institution licensed to receive and dispose of the radioisotope, or contacting the radiation control section at the State Board of Health.

CREMATION Bodies containing radioisotopes will contaminate the crematorium and, in most cases, will leave contaminated ashes. These ashes must be removed and handled by personnel wearing appropriate protective equipment. In three accidents involving contamination in crematoriums, the ash collection worker wore a heat-resistant jacket, leather gloves, and a dust mask, and used long-handled (3–4 m) tools to rake and sweep the ashes toward the front of the oven *(14)*. Because this individual was still found to have internal contamination, most likely from inhalation, it is recommended that respirators be worn while collecting ash.

Whether the radioactive burden should be reduced prior to cremation, depends on the level of radioactivity remaining in the deceased. One consensus group states that no radiation hazard would exist if a crematorium were to handle a total of up to 200 mCi ^{131}I or 2,000 mCi of all other radioisotopes annually *(7)*. Another group would require no special precautions for cremation of individual bodies containing less than 30 mCi ^{131}I or ^{198}Au, or 10 mCi ^{32}P *(15)*. However, both groups state that attempts should be made to remove permanent implants prior to cremation.

RADIOACTIVE TISSUES: SECTIONING AND STORAGE

Tissue removed from a radioactive body may contain some of the radioisotope. Outside the primary organ (defined as the organ where the radioactive material localizes), tissues would contain negligible amounts of radioactive material and would not present a major hazard. However, precautions should include minimal handling time, double gloving, and wearing splash protection and protective gowns to prevent contamination of personnel. If death occurred within 2 d of administration of the radioactive material, the primary organ—for example, the thyroid in ^{131}I cases, should be manipulated with long-handled tools in order to minimize contact as much as possible. Formalin jars with tissue samples from a patient who received ^{131}I therapy read 5 mrem/h on the surface of the jars *(10)*.

The choice of containers for storage of radioactive tissue depends on the activity in the sample or organ. Most samples are rather harmless; organs and tissues with high radioactivity ("primary organs") require leaded containers available from a local radiation safety professional. Radioactivity will diminish with storage time, eventually eliminating the need for lead containers.

DECONTAMINATION

INSTRUMENTS AND CLOTHING Generally, instruments and clothing must be cleaned and decontaminated (vs becoming radioactive waste) by repeated soaking in water with detergents. Some items, as determined by the radiation safety professional, may need to be held for decay of the radioisotope; they should placed in a plastic bag and properly marked to identify the isotope, the date the item became contaminated, and the level of activity. The bag should be stored in a remote location.

WASTE PRODUCTS All contaminated items to be disposed must be bagged and properly marked to identify the isotope, the date the radioactive waste products were produced, and the level of activity. If the half-life is short, the materials can be held for decay and disposed as nonradioactive *(4)*. If the half-life is long, the radiation safety professional should determine the most appropriate way to store or dispose of the materials.

REFERENCES

1. National Council on Radiation Protection and Measurements. Exposure of the U.S. population from diagnostic medical radiation. Report No. 100. NCRP, Bethesda, MD, 1989.
2. U.S. Nuclear Regulatory Commission. Code of Federal Regulations, Title 10, Part 35. U.S. Government Printing Office, Washington, DC, 1988.
3. U.S. Nuclear Regulatory Commission. Regulatory Guide 8.39: Release of patients administered radioactive materials. U.S. Government Printing Office, Washington, DC, 1997.
4. U.S. Nuclear Regulatory Commission. Code of Federal Regulations, Title 10, Part 20. U.S. Government Printing Office, Washington, DC, 1992.
5. National Council on Radiation Protection and Measurements. Limitation of exposure to ionizing radiation. Report No. 116. NCRP, Bethesda, MD, 1993.
6. National Committee for Clinical Laboratory Standards. Protection of laboratory workers from infectious disease transmitted by blood, body fluids, and tissue. NCCLS Document M29-T2. 1991, pp. 62–70.
7. National Council on Radiation Protection and Measurements. Precautions in the management of patients who have received therapeutic amounts of radionuclides. Report No. 37. NCRP, Bethesda, MD, 1970.
8. International Council on Radiological Protection. 1990 Recommendations of the International Commission on Radiological Protection. ICRP Publication 60; Ann. ICRP 21(1–3). Pergamon Press, Oxford, 1991.
9. Parthasarathy KL, Komere KM, Quain B. Necropsy of a cadaver containing 50 mCi of sodium ^{131}iodide. J Nucl Med 1982;23:777–780.
10. Johnston AS, Minarci J, Rossi R, Pinsky S. Autopsy experience with a radioactive cadaver. Health Phys 1979;37:231–236.
11. National Council on Radiation Protection and Measurements. Protection against radiation from brachytherapy sources. Report No. 40. NCRP, Bethesda, MD, 1972.
12. Laughlin JS, Vacirca SJ, Duplissey JF. Exposure of embalmers and physicians by radioactive cadavers. Health Phys 1968;15:451–455.
13. National Council on Radiation Protection and Measurements. Radiation protection for medical and allied health personnel. Report No. 105. NCRP Bethesda, MD, 1989.
14. Kaufman KA, Hamrick B. Contamination events in crematoriums. RSO Mag 1997; January/February:23–25.
15. International Council on Radiological Protection. The handling, storage, use and disposal of unsealed radionuclides in hospitals and medical research establishments. ICRP Publication 25; Ann. ICRP 1(2). Pergamon Press, Oxford, 1977.

14 Fixation, Color Preservation, Gross Staining, and Shipping of Autopsy Material

JURGEN LUDWIG AND BRENDA L. WATERS

FIXATION FOR LIGHT MICROSCOPY

Some fixatives are superior for the demonstration of certain histologic details; others are specifically required (or specifically contraindicated) for certain special stains. Special indications are listed with the various fixative recipes. For routine purposes, excellent fixation can be achieved with almost all the mixtures listed below; the choice will depend on availability, costs, technical help, and increasingly, on environmental concerns. Every effort should be made to reduce the use of toxic substances such as mercury.

The smaller the specimen, the sooner the fixation will be completed. The acceptable thickness of tissue is listed with the various fixation mixtures. Larger specimens may remain completely unfixed in the center. The use of small volumes of fixation fluid for large specimens is the most frequent cause of poor tissue preservation. The minimal acceptable volume of fixation fluid is about 15–20 times the volume of the specimen.

No matter what type of fixative is used, the tissues should not touch each other or be pressed against the bottom or walls of the jar. Suspension of larger specimens or use of a cushion of cotton for smaller specimens will permit optimal exposure. If the fixative becomes stained, cloudy, or diluted by blood or other tissue fluids, it must be replaced.

Heating will accelerate the fixation process but, at the same time, will enhance autolytic changes in the unfixed portion of the tissue. Boiling will result in rapid fixation and has been used to prepare rapid-fixed frozen sections. We prefer to use unfixed tissues or formalin-fixed tissues (after routine penetration fixation of small samples) for frozen sections. *Decalcification procedures* are described in Chapter 8.

FIXATION MIXTURES Many fixatives have been modified by various authors and institutions. However, it seems that the improvements, if any, are minor compared with the results that will be achieved if size and exposure of the specimen and volume and freshness of the fixation fluid are appropriately controlled. Most of the recipes and specifications described here have not been changed since they were listed in the last edition. Several current sources *(1,2)* provide additional details.

From: *Handbook of Autopsy Practice,* 3rd Ed. Edited by: J. Ludwig © Humana Press Inc., Totowa, NJ

Alcohol

1. Indications. Preservation of urates, glycogen, sulfhydryl groups of protein, and water-soluble pigments; enzyme studies. If alcohol is used to preserve water-soluble substances, no aqueous staining procedures can be used.
2. Composition. Absolute ethyl alcohol.
3. Procedure. Fix slices, not thicker than 5–6 mm, in 20 volumes of absolute alcohol. The fixation time will be about 4 h. Transfer to 70% ethyl alcohol for another 72 h. For enzyme studies, 70% alcohol should not be used, but instead use two additional treatments (12 h each) with absolute ethyl alcohol.
4. Storage. Fixed tissue should be stored in 70% alcohol.

Bouin's Fixative

1. Indications. May serve as a general-purpose fixative but proper use is time-consuming. Excellent for subsequent trichrome staining. Glycogen is retained. Erythrocytes are lysed. Excellent for histologic demonstration of pulmonary edema fluid. Recommended for immunohistochemical studies (*see* below).
2. Composition. Stock solution: 750 mL saturated aqueous picric acid, 250 mL formaldehyde solution (36–40%).

   Preparation of aqueous picric acid for stock solution: 20 g picric acid (trinitrophenol, USP), 1,000 mL distilled water.

   Heat until picric acid dissolves. Cool and decant supernate. Prepare fixative just before use, by mixing: 95 mL stock solution, 5 mL glacial (99.7%) acetic acid.
3. Procedure. Fix slices not thicker than 3–5 mm. If the tissue is very soft, thin slices can be cut from larger pieces after about 2 hours of fixation. The fixation must be completed in 12–24 h. Transfer to 50% ethyl alcohol for another 6–24 h. The alcohol should be changed when it becomes yellow.
4. Storage. Fixed tissue should be stored in 70% alcohol.

B-5 Fixative

1. Indications. Preserves excellent nuclear details, particularly in lymph node pathology. Autolytic changes in autopsy specimens are not reversed.

2. Composition. Stock solution: 5 g sodium acetate, 24 g mercuric chloride, 360 mL distilled water.
   Heat until crystals dissolve, let stand for 24 h and filter into brown glass bottle. Prepare fixative just before use, by mixing: 45 mL stock solution, 5 mL concentrated formalin (*see* below).
3. Procedure. Fix slices not thicker than 3 mm. Transfer slices after 90–120 min into buffered formalin to avoid overfixation causing the tissue to shrink and become brittle. Because of its mercury content, special disposal procedures must be followed.
4. Storage. Fixed tissue should be stored in buffered formalin (*see* below).

Carnoy's Fixative

1. Indications. Preservation of nuclei and other structures rich in nucleic acids, protein sulfhydryl groups, and glycogen.
2. Composition. 640 mL absolute ethyl alcohol, 120 mL chloroform, 40 mL glacial (99.7%) acetic acid.
   Prepare fixative just before use.
3. Procedure. Slices up to 1.5 cm in thickness can be fixed. The fixation time will vary from 2–20 h. Transfer into absolute ethyl alcohol.
4. Storage. Fixed tissue should be stored in cedar oil (reagent grade or USP) or lightweight liquid petrolatum.

Formalin Solutions Formalin is a 36–40% solution of gaseous formaldehyde (HCHO) in water. One usually uses a 10% solution, which is a 4% solution of gaseous formaldehyde in water. The term "formalin" is also frequently used for the 10% solution. Thus, "formalin" and "10% formalin" have become synonymous. The 36–40% solution of formaldehyde in water is then referred to as "concentrated formalin."

In this chapter, the term "formalin" or "concentrated formalin" means a 36–40% solution of gaseous formaldehyde in water. The usual 10% formalin solution is referred to as "10% formalin solution" or "formalin solution." When tissue are referred to as "formalin-fixed" it also means that a 10% formalin solution was used.

Formalin solution is by far the most widely used fixative. For regulations designed to prevent toxic effects, *see* Chapter 16.

1. Indications. Ten percent formalin solution is the most widely used fixative, recommendable for most purposes; it is cheap, and requires little attention. Formalin-calcium solution is used for the preservation of phospholipids, and formalin ammonium bromide solution is recommended for fixation of central nervous system tissue when impregnation with gold and silver is intended. It should be noted that formalin-fixed tissues should not be frozen because during thawing, the tissue cannot absorb water normally and thus, extracellular ice crystals persist and severely interfere with subsequent microscopic study *(3)*. Frozen section, however, are quite satisfactory.
2. Composition.
   a. Unbuffered formalin (10% solution): 100 mL formalin, 900 mL tap water.
   b. Formalin-saline: 100 mL formalin, 8.5 g sodium chloride, 900 mL tap water.
   Unbuffered acid formalin solutions or unbuffered neutralized formalin solutions should *not be used for routine fixation* and storage of tissue because of the formation of formalin pigment and its interference with various stains. Buffered neutral formalin solution is preferred. For *in situ* hybridization and immunohistochemistry, buffered 10% formalin solution also works quite well.
   c. Buffered neutral formalin solution: A crude method is to add an excess of calcium and magnesium carbonate to unbuffered 10% formalin solution. Neutral formalin solution (buffered at pH 6.8–7.0): 6.5 g dibasic sodium phosphate (Na_2HPO_4), 4.0 g monobasic sodium phosphate (NaH_2PO_4), 10 mL formalin, 90 mL distilled water.
   d. Formalin-alcohol: 100 mL formalin, 900 mL ethyl alcohol, 95%, 0.5 g calcium acetate (added if neutralization is required).
   e. Formalin-calcium: 10 mL formalin, 1 g calcium chloride, anhydrous ($CaCl_2$), distilled water to make 100 mL, piece of chalk, 3–5 cm long.
   Dissolve the calcium chloride in part of the water. Add the formalin and then make to volume with water. Add the chalk to the mixture to maintain the pH, which should be approx 4.7–4.9.
   f. Formalin-formic acid: 100 mL formalin, 900 mL 4 *N* formic acid.
   g. Formalin-acetic acid-alcohol: 100 mL formalin, 50 mL glacial (99.7%) acetic acid, 850 mL ethyl alcohol, absolute.
3. Procedure. Fix slices not thicker than 6 mm in 20 volumes of formalin solution. The fixation time will be about 6–18 h. However, the tissues may remain in formalin solution for unlimited periods. Change the formalin solution until the fixative remains clear.
4. Storage. Fixed tissue should be stored in formalin solution.
   h. Modified Millonig's Formalin: 100 mL concentrated formalin, 900 mL distilled water, 18.6 g monobasic sodium phosphate ($NaH_2PO_4{\cdot}H_2O$), 4.2 g sodium hydroxide.
   Procedure and storage. The solution has a pH of 7.4 and can serve as a general fixative that allows electron microscopy of stored tissue. Sectioning of paraffin blocks may not be as easy as after fixation with other formalin solutions.

Formalin Replacements Increasing concerns about possible toxic effects of formaldehyde gases (*see* Chapter 16) have created a market for commercially available solutions that closely resemble formalin but do not share many of its toxic effects. Although some seem to work well and appear to be suitable for histochemical studies *(4)*, they generally are much more expensive and have not yet stood the test of time.

Glutaraldehyde

1. Indications. This is a fixative for electron microscopic studies and certain histochemical methods (*see* below)

but phosphate-buffered glutaraldehyde also can be used as an all-purpose fixative. Glutaraldehyde produces less irritating fumes than formalin, is well-suited for perfusion of large specimens, and yields excellent cytological details. Connective tissue stains are well differentiated. The dye uptake is increased in glutaraldehyde-fixed sections. Sectioning artifacts are less frequent. The fixative is more expensive than formalin.

2. Composition. The final preparation represents a 2% glutaraldehyde solution: 50 mL purified glutaraldehyde, 25%, 575 mL Sorenson's phosphate buffer 0.1 *M*, pH 7.4.
3. Procedure. Fix slices not thicker than 4 mm in 20 volumes of 4% glutaraldehyde solution. The fixation time at room temperature will be 6–24 h. Cold fixation with glutaraldehyde for histochemical enzyme location yields complete fixation after 6 h but only in the outer 1 mm of tissue.
4. Storage. Use 2% or 4% glutaraldehyde solution; store at 4°C.

Helly's Fixative

1. Indications. This is an excellent fixative for bone marrow and organs containing much blood. It is superior to Zenker's fixative in terms of penetration. Still, most hematopathologists now prefer the B5-fixative.
2. Composition. 2.5 g potassium dichromate ($K_2Cr_2O_7$), 5.0 g mercuric chloride ($HgCl_2$), 1.0 g sodium sulfate, anhydrous (Na_2SO_4), 100 mL distilled water, 5–6 mL formalin.
3. Procedure. Fix slices not thicker than 6 mm in 20 volumes of fixative. The fixation time will be about 12–24 h. Tissues must then be washed for 14–16 h. Transfer to 80% alcohol. Residues of mercuric chloride must be removed from the sections with 0.5% aqueous iodine (5 min) followed by 5% aqueous sodium thiosulfate (5 min).
4. Storage. Use 70% ethyl alcohol for short-term storage. For long-term preservation, dehydration and paraffin embedding are the methods of choice.

Orth's Solution

1. Indications. General purpose fixative but most suitable for the demonstration of chromaffin granules in adrenal medulla and pheochromocytomas.
2. Composition: 2.5 g potassium dichromate ($K_2Cr_2O_7$), 1.0 g sodium sulfate (Na_2SO_4), 100 mL distilled water.
   Just before use, add 10 mL concentrated formalin.
3. Procedure. Fix slices not thicker than 4 mm in 20 volumes of fixative. The fixation time will be about 24 h to 48 h. Wash in running water for 24 h. Transfer to 70% ethyl alcohol.
4. Storage. Store in 70% alcohol.

Regaud's Fixative

1. Indications. For the demonstration of rickettsiae.
2. Composition: 80 mL potassium dichromate ($K_2Cr_2O_7$), 3% aqueous solution, 20 mL formalin.
3. Procedure. Fix slices not thicker than 4 mm in 20 volumes of fixative. The fixation time will be about 24–48 h. Wash in running water for 24 h. Transfer to 70% ethyl alcohol.
4. Storage. Store in 70% ethyl alcohol.

Zamboni's Solution

1. Indications. General purpose fixative. Allows secondary fixation with osmium, which makes it suitable as a primary fixative for electron microscopy.
2. Composition. Stock solution: 20.0 g paraformaldehyde, 150 mL saturated aqueous (double filtered) picric acid.
   Heat to 60°C. After the paraformaldehyde is dissolved, add drops of 2.5% aqueous sodium hydroxide to render the solution alkaline. Filter solution and allow to cool.
   Add phosphate buffer to solution to make 1,000 mL. Composition of phosphate buffer: 3.32 g monobasic sodium phosphate ($NaH_2PO_4 \cdot H_2O$), 17.88 g dibasic anhydrous sodium phosphate (Na_2HPO_4), 1,000 mL distilled water.
   If the final pH is not 7.3, the value must be adjusted.
3. Procedure and storage. Similar to formalin.

Zenker's Fixative

1. Indications. Similar to Helly's fixative. Recommended for staining of cytoplasmic inclusions and for use with the Feulgen stain.
2. Composition. Stock solution: 50 g mercuric chloride ($HgCl_2$), 25 g potassium dichromate ($K_2C_2O_7$), 10 g sodium sulfate, anhydrous (Na_2SO_4), 1,000 mL distilled water.
   Just before use, the stock solution is mixed with either acetic acid or formic acid: 95 mL stock solution, 5 mL glacial (99.7%) acetic acid, or 95 mL stock solution, 5 mL formic acid (88%, analytical grade).
3. Procedure. Fix slices not thicker than 6 mm in 20 volumes of fixative. The fixation time will be about 24 h. Thick specimens should be postfixed for 2 h in a 2.5% aqueous solution of potassium dichromate. Tissues must then be washed for 14–16 h. Transfer to 80% alcohol. Residues of mercuric chloride must be removed from the section with 0.5% aqueous iodine (5 min) followed by 5% aqueous sodium thiosulfate (5 min).
4. Storage. Use 70% ethyl alcohol for short-term storage. For long-term preservation, dehydration and paraffin embedding is recommended.

FIXATION BY MICROWAVE HEATING This technique has been used successfully both for light and electron microscopy *(5)*. Heating of samples in saline to 58°C leads to good fixation for routine light microscopy but also for immunohistochemical reactions. For electron microscopy, samples should be placed in 2.5% glutaraldehyde and irradiated for 90 s to achieve a temperature of 58°C.

COLOR PRESERVING FIXATION MIXTURES

Most fixatives and fixation mixtures turn the natural color of organs into a uniform gray. Many color-preserving mixtures have been in use before the decline of the pathologic museum.

Color photography has largely replaced these techniques. Kaiserling's and Jores' solutions still are used in some institutions. Modifications of the Kaiserling solution have been published by Lundquist *(6)*, Meiller *(7)*, and others. Modifications of Jores' solution exist also *(8)*.

The following solutions are among Kaiserling's own final modifications.

KAISERLING'S SOLUTIONS

1. Composition.
   a. Kaiserling I: 85 g potassium acetate, 45 g potassium nitrate (KNO_3), 4,800 mL formalin solution (3–4%).
   b. Kaiserling II: ethyl alcohol, 80–95%.
   c. Kaiserling III: 200 g potassium acetate, 300 mL glycerin, 900 mL tap water.
2. Procedure. Fix specimen for 1–5 d in Kaiserling I. Fixation time will vary with the thickness of the organ. Excessive perfusion with Kaiserling I solution causes loss of natural color because too much blood is rinsed out. Transfer to Kaiserling II for a few hours. Acid hematin will turn into alkaline hematin, which approximates the color of hemoglobin.
3. Mounting. Use Kaiserling III solution.

MODIFIED KAISERLING'S SOLUTION AFTER LUNDQUIST *(6)* This method was developed to avoid the use of alcohol which tends to add to the stiffening and contraction of the specimens.

1. Composition.
   a. Kaiserling I: 200 g potassium acetate, 45 g potassium nitrate (KNO_3), 80 g chloral hydrate, 444 mL formalin 4,000 mL tap water.
2. Procedure. Suspend the specimen in 10–20 times its volume of fluid. Just after the fixation is completed (avoid overfixation), wash thoroughly in running water and retrim so that all cut surfaces are resurfaced. Transfer to mounting solution for 12 h. Change solution for permanent mounting.
3. Mounting: Kaiserling III: 10 g potassium acetate, 5 g chloral hydrate, 10 mL glycerin, 90 mL tap water.

JORES' SOLUTION

1. Composition: 10 g sodium chloride (NaCl), 20 g magnesium sulfate ($MgSO_4$), 20 g sodium sulfate (Na_2SO_4), 1,100 mL formalin solution (2–4%).
2. Procedure. Fix specimen for 1 or 2 d or longer. Rinse in 95% ethyl alcohol. Leave in 95% ethyl alcohol for 24 h or until red color has returned.
3. Mounting. Mount specimen in a solution of equal parts of glycerin and water.

REJUVENATION OF OLD FORMALIN-FIXED SPECIMENS

REJUVENATION SOLUTION

1. Composition: 100 g sodium chloride (NaCl), 5 g sodium sulfate (Na_2SO_4), 50 mL glycerin, 1,000 mL tap water.
2. Procedure. Sodium chloride and sodium sulfate are dissolved in the water and the solution is filtered. Then the glycerin is added. Just before the jar containing this solution is resealed, a few drops of alcoholic camphor are added. There will be a temporary cloudiness of the solution. For another rejuvenation fluid, *see* ref. *(8)*.

CARBON MONOXIDE REJUVENATION This method *(9)* cannot be recommended because of the risk of carbon monoxide poisoning for those who work with the gassing apparatus.

FIXATION FOR ELECTRON MICROSCOPIC STUDIES, HISTOCHEMISTRY, IMMUNOHISTOCHEMISTRY, *IN SITU* HYBRIDIZATION, AND OTHER SPECIAL LABORATORY PROCEDURES

GENERAL PRINCIPLES For processing autopsy material, the same standard laboratory methods are used that would be applied to biopsy samples. However, compared with the work up for light microscopy (*see* above), much more attention must be paid to the rapid procurement of the material to keep postmortem changes at a minimum. This is described in Chapter 1 under "Immediate Autopsies for Special Laboratory Procedures Such as Electron Microscopy." Needle biopsies in the immediate postmortem period (Chapter 1) also may provide samples without or with minimal autolytic changes.

TRANSMISSION ELECTRON MICROSCOPY Fixation with 2% glutaraldehyde buffered with Millonig's phosphate buffer at pH 7.4 (*see* also above under "Formalin Solutions" and under "Glutaraldehyde") has been recommended for *transmission electron microscopy* but paraformaldehyde or a mixture of 10% formalin solution and 1% phosphate-buffered glutaraldehyde are also suitable fixatives *(10)*. The samples should not exceed 1 mm^3 and should not remain in glutaraldehyde for more than 4 d. For long-term storage, the tissue should be embedded and kept in the plastic blocks. One can also place the glutaraldehyde-fixed specimens in buffered formalin solution (*see* above). For comprehensive discussions of fixatives in electron microscopy, *see* refs. *(11)* and *(12)*. If no tissue had been saved for electron microscopy but the need arises at a later time, tissue from the exposed surfaces of formalin-fixed tissue can be obtained and postfixed prior to processing. The same can be done with tissues from paraffin blocks; they are postfixed after the samples were deparaffinized. Obviously, the quality of the electron micrographs suffers considerably under these circumstances. However, depending on the questions at hand, answers still can be obtained in some instances.

SCANNING ELECTRON MICROSCOPY Glutaraldehyde, formalin solution or other fixatives can be used. We have obtained excellent electron micrographs of tissue samples that had been stored in formalin solution for some time. Again, it is most important to keep autolysis at a minimum.

HISTOCHEMISTRY Most histochemical stains can be applied to autopsy tissues that had been obtained after the usual postmortem intervals and that were fixed in formalin solution. If new histochemical applications are used on postmortem material, pilot experiments have to be carried out to determine the effect of postmortem changes. Other aspects of histochemistry and related analytical methods are presented in Chapter 11.

IMMUNOHISTOCHEMISTRY Tissue samples should be obtained as soon as possible after death (*see* also above under "General Principles"), snap-frozen, or placed in formalin solution. Other authors recommend Bouin's solution of B-5. The sections should be thin enough to permit rapid penetration of the fixative; if formalin is used, they should be removed after 12–18 h and if Bouin's solution is used, 4–6 h suffice. If the tissue sample is thick, a thin slice should be obtained from the exposed tissue surface after the recommended fixation time. If antigens need to be identified that are sensitive to the chemical action of fixatives or if immunofluorescent staining is intended, snap-freezing is the method of choice *(13)*. Other aspects of immunohistochemistry and related analytical methods are presented in Chapter 11.

***IN SITU* HYBRIDIZATION** Buffered formalin, pH 7.0, serves as an excellent fixative for this technology. Fixatives with picric acid (Bouin's) or heavy metals (Zenker's) may interfere with subsequent *in situ* hybridization. Paraffin-embedded tissue is quite suitable for many commercially available DNA probes.

X-RAY MICROANALYSIS (ENERGY-DISPERSIVE X-RAY MICROANALYSIS) Conventional transmission or scanning electron microscopes may also be able to identify elements such as copper, iron, sulfur, or thorium *(14)* (elements 5–99 can be identified in this fashion). It is best to use glutaraldehyde-fixed tissue but formalin-fixed tissue can also be used, including, as a last resort, tissue from paraffin blocks or tissues lifted from hematoxylin-eosin stained slides. For further applications, *see* refs. *(12)* and *(15)*.

AUTORADIOGRAPHY Postmortem material can be used for the identification and localization of radioactive material. Postmortem changes and choice of fixative have little effect on the quality of the autoradiograms. The demonstration of thorium dioxide contrast medium (Thorotrast) used to be the main application of this method. Presently, electron micrography with energy-dispersive X-ray microanalysis (*see* above) is a faster and more specific method. For the preparation of autoradiograms, the reader is referred to appropriate textbooks.

STAINING OF GROSS TISSUES AND SELECTED TUMORS

Historically, gross staining of tissues was used to enhance the quality of museum specimens (Chapter 15). Thus, most of the methods reproduced here, mention the appropriate mounting media. In current autopsy practice, stained specimens are photographed, shown at a conference, and then stored out of sight or discarded. Thus, mounting media are rarely needed.

TISSUES

Hematoxylin or Eosin Stains Tissues such as the intestinal mucosa can be stained with alcoholic eosin or hematoxylin *(16,17)*.

Fat and Lipoid Stains Fat stains are used either as differential tissue stains—for example, to outline malignant lesions infiltrating fat tissue—or to identify fat and lipids in organs or pathologic lesions.

When differential fat staining is desired, the freshly trimmed, fresh or formalin-fixed specimen is immersed in a saturated solution of Sudan III or Scharlach R in 70% alcohol *(18)*. The fat will stain bright red. Nonfatty structures are decolorized by placing the specimen in 95% alcohol. After the differentiation is complete, the tissue is washed and mounted in formalin solution. A variant of this method *(19)* uses formalin-fixed specimens, which are soaked for 1 d in 50% alcohol, followed by staining for 1 or 2 d in a saturated solution of Sudan III in 70% alcohol. After the fat has become deep orange red, the specimen is returned to 50% alcohol solution until all nonfatty tissues return to their normal color.

Staining of Myelinated and Nonmyelinated Fibers of Brain These methods *(20)* have been largely replaced by the use of histologic macrosections. Therefore, they will not be described here.

Stain for Iron (Hemosiderin) The reaction of Fe^{3+} with ferrocyanide has been used most widely for the demonstration of tissue iron in hemochromatosis and other iron overload states. Slices of liver, pancreas, heart, or other tissues are placed for several minutes in a 1–5% aqueous solution of potassium ferrocyanide and then are transferred to 2% hydrochloric acid. One can also use a solution of equal parts of 10% HCl and 5% aqueous ferrocyanide *(21)*. The specimens are then washed for 12 h in running water. In the presence of abundant hemosiderin, the tissue will rapidly turn dark blue. Mount in 5% formalin-saline. It should be noted that in hemochromatosis specimens the color tends to fade out.

Amyloid Stains

1. Iodine stain. Immerse the specimen in a solution made up of 1 g of iodine, 2 g of potassium iodide, 1 mL of sulfuric acid, and 100 mL of water. Amyloid will turn blue. The specimen is then washed in tap water. Museum specimens are mounted in liquid paraffin. This technique is said to prevent fading of the stained amyloid; without sulfuric acid, amyloid will turn brown.

   Edwards and Edwards *(22)* suggested that the specimens should not be washed but should be put in 70% alcohol until the differentiation is complete. The specimen is then removed from the jar and the alcohol is allowed to evaporate. Subsequently, the tissue, which should be almost dry, is placed in liquid paraffin until it is completely soaked, which may take 8 wk or more. Liquid petrolatum appears to be the best preservative for iodine-stained amyloid containing tissues.
2. Congo red stain *(21)*. The specimen is fixed in Kaiserling I solution (*see* above) and subsequently immersed for 1 h in 1% Congo red. It then is transferred to a saturated solution of lithium carbonate for 2 min and differentiated in 80% alcohol. Normal arteries and veins tend to retain their color. The specimen is mounted in Kaiserling III solution (glycerin 300 mL, sodium acetate 100 g, 0.5% formalin solution to a final volume of 1,000 mL; adjust to pH 8.0; if necessary, filter to clear the solution). In this instance, sodium hydrosulfite should not be added before sealing the jar.

Calcium Stains *(18)*

1. Silver nitrate method. Wash the formalin-fixed specimen under running water for 24 h and then in several changes of distilled water for 24 h. In a darkroom, immerse the specimen in a 1% solution of silver nitrate in distilled water and stain for 6–15 h. Rinse it in distilled water and then place it in 5% sodium hydrosulfite solution for 24 h. The specimen can now be exposed to light, washed, and mounted in 50% alcohol or Kaiserling solution,
2. Alizarin method. Immerse the specimen for 12 h in a 1:10,000 solution of alizarin red S with just enough potassium hydroxide to render the solution basic. For differentiation, transfer the specimen to a solution of equal parts of alcohol and glycerin and expose the jar to sunlight. Alizarin dyes stain calcium pink. After several days, mount the specimen in Kaiserling solution that is made alkaline by adding a small amount (1:1,000) of potassium hydroxide.

Specimens With Gouty Changes For the demonstration of deposits in gout or pseudogout, the *murexide test* is used. A sample of finely dispersed tissue fragments is heated with an equal volume of 25% nitric acid until the acid has evaporated. To the dry residue add 2–3 drops of 25% ammonium hydroxide solution and then the same amount of 20% sodium hydroxide solution. In the presence of urates, the dry residue will be bright red or orange, purple after addition of ammonium hydroxide, and blue-violet after addition of sodium hydroxide. For the preparation of museum specimens, the sample is dehydrated over 2 wk in several changes of absolute alcohol. Transfer into mounting fluid (*see* below). Deposits also can be displayed in their native state.

1. Procedure. Fix specimen, preferably in an anhydrous fixative such as alcohol. Although urate crystals are freely soluble in water, crystalline deposits are usually identifiable in the center of the specimens even after aqueous formalin fixation. The crystals often also resist the dehydration and staining procedure.
2. Mounting. Mount in plastic jar with undiluted glycerin. Seal without leaving air under the lid.

Gallbladder If the gallbladder can be obtained within a few hours after death, the oxidative greenish discoloration will not yet have occurred and can be prevented by the following procedure *(23)*.

1. Procedure. Place specimen in 3% solution of sodium sulfite for 20 min. Rinse for a few minutes in running water. Place in 10% formalin solution for 12–24 h. Wash thoroughly and mount.

   If the greenish color of biliverdin has already formed, a 5% sodium sulfite solution is used, to which 1% formalin is added. The specimen is left in this solution for 12 h. The subsequent steps remain the same.
2. Mounting fluid: 10 g potassium acetate, 5 g chloral hydrate, 10 mL glycerin, 90 mL tap water.

Instead of the sodium sulfite-formalin mixture, a saturated solution of calcium chloride can be used. The specimen should be soaked in this solution for 24–48 h *(21)*.

TUMORS

Chloroma

1. Procedure *(22)*. The specimen should be fixed without previous washing and then placed for 24 h in methyl alcohol. Transfer for the following 24 h to the following solution: 0.5 g sodium hydrosulfite ($Na_2S_2O_4$), 1 g sodium hydroxide (NaHO), 100 mL tap water.

   The container with this fluid should be filled to the brim, and the lid should be sealed with petroleum jelly.
2. Mounting fluid: 0.1 g sodium hydrosulfite ($Na_2S_2O_4$), 30 mL glycerin, 10 g sodium acetate, 0.5 mL formalin, 70 mL tap water.

Melanoma and Melanotic Tissue

1. Procedure. This slices (about 6 mm) of fixed tissue are kept in methyl alcohol for 12 h. Transfer into acetone for another 12–18 h and then into xylol for about 2 h. Remove when shrinkage begins and put into mounting fluid.
2. Mounting fluid. Mount in liquid paraffin.

Pheochromocytoma

1. Procedure. Place a few drops of Zenker's fixative stock solution (*see* page 131), without glacial or formic acid, on a slice of fresh tumor tissue. A pheochromocytoma containing adrenaline or noradrenaline or both will turn brown in less than 20 min. Light of a photolamp will accelerate the reaction. Tissue is subsequently fixed in 10% buffered neutral formalin solution. For histologic demonstration of chromaffin granules in these tumors, the tissue should be fixed in Orth's solution. (*See* above under "Fixation for Light Microscopy."

SHIPPING OF AUTOPSY MATERIAL

CONTAINERS FOR DRY MATERIAL Most commonly, slides and paraffin blocks are sent. *Paraffin Blocks* should be sealed with paraffin after microtomy to prevent tissue from drying out. Blocks can be wrapped in paper or plastic, but cotton should not be used because cotton fibers may stick to the paraffin and cause knife lines and abrasions. *Glass slides* should be shipped in unbreakable slide containers cushioned with cotton or other material. The packages should be sealed with tape because staples may injure personnel in the accessioning areas.

CONTAINERS FOR WET MATERIAL Two containers should be used, one within the other. Absorbent material (*see* below) is placed between the two containers. Paper, plastic, glass, or metal jars are used. Ordinarily, plastic jars are most convenient for shipping autopsy tissues. However, for toxicologic examinations, the inner container should be of glass, particularly when the tissues or body fluids are to be analyzed for volatile substances. Plastics may be permeable to gases, and corrosion of metal containers may interfere with toxicological studies. Stoppers, corks, and lids should be taped in place.

For use as an absorbent, cotton can be soaked with 10% formalin solution and wrapped around the tissues. Towels and gauze cause marks on tissue surfaces and should not be used for wrapping or covering of tissues. Fixatives should not be used if the material is sent for toxicologic or microbiologic examination. Enough cotton or paper should be placed between the inner container (or plastic bag) and the outer container to take up all liquid in case of breakage or leakage. The absorbent material is also useful for cushioning the inner container.

Shipping of frozen material is recommended for submission for toxicologic and biochemical examinations. Ordinary ice is sufficient if the specimen is transported by a messenger who will replenish the ice if necessary. Dry ice will be effective for about 24 h. For longer periods, refilling is required, or the specimen has to be sent in dry ice with ether or acetone in a thermos bottle of appropriate size. The dry ice is put around and on top of the specimen and on the inside of the absorbent material. The mailing container should be insulated.

As mailing containers, durable shipping cartons, wooden boxes, or metal containers are used. For frozen material, the mailing container should be insulated e.g., with styrofoam. Shipping cartons are sealed with strips of gummed paper.

Inside the mailing container, a tag or letter should be placed, giving: 1) name and address of the submitter; 2) name and address of receiver of the shipment; 3) name, clinic number or other alphanumeric identifier, and autopsy number and year of the patient from whom the material came; and 4) type of examination requested, together with pertinent data. If a separate letter has been sent, a copy should always be put into the mailing container. This may help to avoid much confusion and delay. It is a continuing problem for many institutions to receive slides, blocks, or tissues without any further information, and a frustrating search follows for a misfiled or lost letter to match the shipment. If a clinician or person other than the submitting pathologist has requested the consultation, that address should be supplied also. The pathologist does not always know why the request for the shipment had been made.

Letters and addresses in the shipping container should be protected from leaking fluids by sealing them in plastic.

Mailing containers should be marked on the outside with appropriate warnings such as "Biohazard," "Glass, Handle With Care," and "Perishable Material." Additional labels are recommended for medicolegal or microbiologic material (*see* below).

SHIPPING AND LABELING FOR MEDICOLEGAL MATERIAL Medicolegal material is sent by messenger, registered mail, or air express. Care must be taken that the chain of custody remains uninterrupted (*see* Chapter 2). Medicolegal material will often be passed through local police authorities to the state bureau of criminal identification or investigation laboratory. The address for shipments to the laboratories of the FBI is:

Director, Federal Bureau of Investigation
US Department of Justice
Washington, DC 20012
Attention: FBI Laboratory

Specimen labels should contain: 1) name and address of the submitter; 2) name and address of the receiver of the shipment; 3) description of the container and of the source and nature of its contents; 4) a tag describing the shipment as "evidence;" and 5) if applicable, a request for specific examination.

Containers with medicolegal material should be sealed before shipping so that the contents cannot be tampered with. Sealing wax imprinted with the thumb of the submitter may serve this purpose.

The mailing container should show: 1) the name and address of the submitter; 2) the name and address of the receiver; and 3) warning tags such as a red "Biohazard" label, "Glass, Handle With Care," "Perishable Material," or "Fragile, Rush, Specimen for Toxicological Study."

SHIPPING OF BLOOD AND TISSUES FOR CARBON MONOXIDE DETERMINATION For blood, 10 mL is placed over 10 mg of lithium oxalate in a screwcap test tube. The blood is covered with mineral oil, and the cap or stopper is sealed with hot paraffin or plastic tape. Tissues can be packed in plastic and shipped in dry ice in an insulated mailing container.

SHIPPING OF TISSUES AND BODY FLUIDS FOR MICROBIOLOGIC STUDY (BY BRENDA WATERS) Three goals should be met when shipping specimens taken from a patient at autopsy: 1) preservation of the specimen during transit, 2) supplying sufficient clinical information for proper handling and interpretation, and 3) providing adequate protection of postal and other mail handlers. The United States Postal Service publishes regulations for the proper shipping of such materials in their publication, "Domestic Mail Manual," which undergoes revision every one to two years. The autopsy service may find it prudent to review this manual from time to time to ensure that federal requirements are met. The postal recommendations are paraphrased below.

> *"All clinical specimens destined for shipping must be placed in a securely sealed, break-resistant inner container which must be surrounded by sufficient cushioning to withstand the shocks of normal handling. If the specimen is liquid, the cushioning material must have enough absorbent capacity to completely absorb the liquid. In addition, liquid materials must be placed in a container with sufficient extra volume to accommodate expansion in low pressure environments, such as during air travel. The inner container and cushioning material must then be placed in a larger outer container, which will carry the labels and mailing addresses. This larger container must also be break-resistant and have a surface to which labels will firmly affix. Clinical specimens exceeding 50 mL must be packaged in fiberboard or other material of equivalent strength. Single containers must not contain more than 1 L of material. No more than 4 L of specimen may be enclosed in any single outer container."*

Any information for the receiving laboratory, such as requisitions, patient information, and accompanying letters from the sender should be placed in the outer container. In some situations, it may be advisable to send a separate letter to the medical director or chief technologist of the receiving laboratory. Telephoning the receiving laboratory at the time of shipment may also facilitate proper and timely handling of the specimen upon arrival.

REFERENCES

1. Prophet EB, Mills B, Arrington JB, Sobin LH, eds. Laboratory Methods in Histotechnology. Armed Forces Institute of Pathology. American Registry of Pathology, Washington, DC, 1992.
2. Luna LG. Histopathologic Methods and Color Atlas of Special Stains and Tissue Artifacts. Johnson Printers, Downer's Grove, IL, 1992.
3. Rosen Y, Ahuja SC. Ice crystal distorsion of formalin-fixed tissues following freezing. Am J Surg Pathol 1977;1:179–181.
4. Meyer R, Niedobitek F, Wenzelides K. Erfahrungen mit der Formalinersatzlösung NoToX. Pathologe 1996;17:130–132.
5. Leong AS, Daymon ME, Milios J. Microwave irradiation as a form of fixation for light and electron microscopy. J Pathol 1985;146:313–321.
6. Lundquist R. A proposed modification of the Kaiserling method for preserving gross specimens. Int Assoc Med Mus Bull 1925;11:16–18.
7. Meiller FH. A method for preserving gross specimens in color. J Tech Methods 1938;18:57–58.
8. Legault JM, Huang S. Color preservation of gross specimens for teaching and medical illustration. Arch Pathol Lab Med 1979;103: 300–301.
9. Robertson HE, Lundquist R. Experiences with the carbon monoxide method of preparing museum specimens. J Tech Methods 1934;13: 33–35.
10. Baker PB. Electron microscopy. In: Hutchins GM, ed. Autopsy, Performance and Reporting. College of American Pathologists, Northfield, IL, 1990, pp. 138–140.
11. McDowell EM, Trump BF. Histologic fixatives suitable for diagnostic light and electron microscopy. Arch Pathol Lab Med 1976;100: 405–414.
12. Robards AW, Wilson AJ (principal eds.). Procedures in Electron Microscopy. Centre for Cell & Tissue Research, The University, York, UK, John Wiley & Sons, New York, 1993.
13. Baker PB. Special autopsy studies. In: Hutchins GM, ed. Autopsy, Performance and Reporting. College of American Pathologists, Northfield, IL, 1990, pp. 142–146.
14. Landas S, Turner JW, Moore KC, Mitros FA. Demonstration of iron and thorium in autopsy tissues by X-ray microanalysis. Arch Pathol Lab Med 1984;108:231–233.
15. Sigee DC, Morgan AJ, Sumner AT, Warley A, eds. X-ray Microanalysis in Biology: Experimental Techniques and Applications. Cambridge University Press, Cambridge, UK, 1993.
16. Loehry CA, Creamer B. Post-mortem study of small-intestinal mucosa. BMJ 1966;I:827–829.
17. Dymock IW, Gray B. Staining method for the examination of the small intestinal villous pattern in necropsy material. J Clin Pathol 1968;21:748–749.
18. Kramer FM. Macroscopic staining of anatomic and pathologic specimens. J Tech Methods 1939;19:72–78.
19. Dukes C, Bussey HJR. Preparation and mounting of museum specimens of intestinal tumours. J Tech Methods 1936;15:44–48.
20. Tompsett DH. Anatomical Techniques. E & S Livingstone, Edinburgh, 1956.
21. Pulvertaft RJV. Museum techniques: a review. J Clin Pathol 1950;3: 1–23.
22. Edwards JJ, Edwards MJ. Medical Museum Technology. Oxford University Press, London, 1959.
23. Mentzer SH. Methods of preparing gall-bladders and calculi for study and museum display. Int Assoc Med Mus Bull 1925;11:37–40.

15 Museum Techniques and Autopsy Photography

JURGEN LUDWIG AND WILLIAM D. EDWARDS

THE PATHOLOGY MUSEUM

The role of the pathology museum has declined. The costs of space, maintenance, and administration of specimen collections and displays are difficult to justify in the current economic environment, particularly because color photography, printed atlases, CD-ROM libraries, and commercially available organ models represent excellent alternatives, at least for teaching purposes. However, temporary preparation, storage, and display of specimens still is important for photographic documentation or use of actual samples in clinicopathologic conferences and other activities (*see* "Autopsy Photography"). In this chapter, only a few basic techniques are discussed. For comprehensive reviews of classic museum techniques, *see* refs. *1–3*.

PREPARATION OF SPECIMENS

AVAILABLE METHODS The most frequent approach is perfusion fixation (Chapter 4), gross staining, and use of color-preserving fluids (Chapter 14). In rare instances, injection and corrosion techniques still are used for scientific studies and for teaching purposes. Paraffin infiltration of organs and mummification may be useful as methods to prepare dry, low-cost teaching specimens that require almost no maintenance. These and other methods are described below.

REHYDRATION OF MUMMIFIED TISSUES If mummified tissues are found in a museum, they can be rehydrated with modified Ruffer's solution (*see* ref. *4*): 3 parts ethyl alcohol, 5 parts aqueous formalin, 2%, 2 parts aqueous sodium carbonate, 5%.

For rejuventaion of old, formalin-fixed specimens, *see* Chapter 14.

MOUNTING OF SPECIMENS

USE OF JARS AND PLASTIC BAGS In the past, only thick-walled glass jars were used and these still can be recommended. They are inert to fixatives and aggressive mounting fluids such as oil of wintergreen (used for cleared specimens), which dissolves plastics. However, glass jars are heavy and not always available in the desired shape and size; they also break easily.

Currently, acrylic resins are the material of choice. Excellent optical properties, low weight, minimal breakability, and chemical stability to most mounting fluids are the outstanding characteristics of this material. Museum jars can be prepared in many sizes and shapes. The material is easy to cut, machine, and assemble. Fusion of the plates is accomplished with WELD•ON 4™ (IPS Corporation, Box 379, 17109 S. Main Street, Gardena, CA 90248). There are a few disadvantages. Plastics of this type are easily scratched and may have to be repolished on occasion. As stated, oil of wintergreen but also benzyl benzoate cannot be used as mounting fluid because they dissolve plastics. Instead of alcohol, which crazes the surface of plastic containers, mounting media with Prague solution should be used as described below.

An alternative to acrylic museum jars are plastic bags. They are suitable for many purposes because they are light, tough, inexpensive, and easy to prepare. Their pliability permits palpation of the specimen. The preservation fluid can be replaced repeatedly if cloudiness develops. Plastic bags are now used for teaching, examinations, and storage. Plastic bag materials and sealing procedures are described in Chapter 16.

MOUNTING MEDIA We fill our plastic museum jars with *Prague solution*: 128 g Prague powder*, 25 g erythorbic acid (*L*-ascorbic acid), 10,000 mL distilled water, 1,000 mL concentrated formalin, 4,000 mL solution A (*see* below), 4,000 mL solution B (*see* below).

*Milwaukee Seasonings, N113W18900 Carnegie Drive, Germantown, WI 53022.

Solution A: 47 g sodium phosphate (Na_2HPO_4), formalin solution, 10%, to make 5,000 mL.

Solution B: 45 g potassium phosphate (K_2HPO_4), formalin solution, 10%, to make 5,000 mL.

Solutions A and B must be stored in separate containers.

For mounting fluids used with grossly stained specimens, *see* Chapter 14.

PLASTINATION This method may replace many of the traditional museum techniques because one can not only mount the samples in the traditional manner but tissues also can be merely infiltrated (without mounting them) and then be palpated and viewed more directly than organs and tissues mounted in jars *(5–7)*. We had much success with a commercially available material *(8)* (Plastination Biodur™ Products Program, Dr. von Hagens, Rathausstrasse 18, Heidelberg, Germany). Specimens such as aortas can be infiltrated and in many respects resemble

From: *Handbook of Autopsy Practice*, 3rd Ed. Edited by: J. Ludwig © Humana Press Inc., Totowa, NJ

the fresh tissue. Other samples such as slices of brain can be embedded in solid blocks. The materials used for the plastination procedure vary, depending on the intended end product. Company directions must be followed closely.

MOUNTING IN SOLID PLASTIC If successful, embedding of specimens in solid blocks of plastic compounds yields excellent museum specimens. Materials are commercially available and may give satisfactory results (Wards Natural Science Establishment, Inc., P.O.Box 92912, 5100 West Henrietta Road, Rochester, NY, 14692-9012).

Unfortunately, the embedding techniques are complicated because the samples must be carefully dehydrated, a procedure that will distort most autopsy tissues. Cracks, incomplete hardening, or clouding of the polymer may occur, and specimens may shrink or become spongy. Artifacts may also be created by the heat of the exothermic polymerization of the monomer. Best results are usually achieved with specimens such as bullets, concrements, or casts. Again, the instructions of the suppliers must be followed closely, and one must heed the warnings as to the danger of explosions and the need to protect eyes and hands. Specimens embedded in solid blocks are difficult or impossible to retrieve for further study.

LABELS To identify and describe museum specimens, labels can be glued to the jar or inserted between an outer and an inner plastic bag. Labels on the outside of a container can accidentally be torn off; an identifying tag should always be attached to the actual specimen inside the jar or plastic bag. Identifying tags or labels enclosed with the specimen must be made of material capable of resisting the chemical action of the mounting fluid.

INJECTION, CORROSION, AND CLEARING TECHNIQUES

Blood vessels, airways, hollow viscera, and cavities can be injected with a great variety of materials. If injection is combined with corrosion, excellent casts may be prepared but little or no material will be available for histologic study. The reader is referred to the descriptions of techniques for various organs and organ systems in Chapters 3–7. Indications and techniques of injecting placental vessels with milk are described in Chapter 5.

INJECTABLE MEDIA

Barium Sulfate Mixtures These are probably the most widely used radiopaque media for vascular injection. Some dry-powder preparations are commercially available (Sigma B-3758, Sigma, P.O. Box 14508, St. Louis, MO). The barium sulfate usually is diluted with 10% formalin solution. In most instances, 5% gelatin is added to cause the mass to solidify after injection. The viscosity of the solution can be decreased by decreasing the amount of gelatin added or by adding more saline. Vessels as small as 30–60 μm in luminal width can be filled. The actual viscosity of the medium within the specimen depends on many variables, including the speed of injection and the temperature of the injected tissues. Therefore, each laboratory will have to standardize its own techniques. The injection often is done by quite elaborate methods, but, in our experience, injection by hand with a large glass syringe will give excellent results for routine examination and most qualitative studies.

We have used barium sulfate-gelatin mixtures to inject most organ-related vascular systems, the vessels of the lower extremities, the aorta and its branches, and the inferior vena cava system (*see* Chapters 3–6). For postmortem coronary angiography (*see* Chapter 12), we use gelatine mixtures, either with barium sulfate or with iothalamate-meglumine, as shown here:

Barium sulfate mixture		*Iothalamate-meglumine mixture*
500 mL distilled water		500 mL distilled water
650 g barium sulfate[a]	OR	100 mL iothalamate meglumine (Conray®)[b]
15 g gelatine[c]		15 g gelatine[c]
3 g thymol[d]		3 g thymol[d]

[a]Barosperse® (Cat. no. 130108; NDC 59081-621-13), Lafayette Pharmaceutical, Inc., Lafayette, IN 47904.

[b]Conray® (iothalamate meglumine injection U.S.P. 60%), Mallinckrodt Medical, Inc., St. Louis, MO 63042.

[c]Gelatin (laboratory grade, 275 bloom), Fisher Scientific, Fair Lawn, NJ 07410.

[d]Thymol (Cat. no. T185-100), Fisher Scientific, Fair Lawn, NJ 07410.

For the preparation of these mixtures, heat the distilled water to about 45°C in a beaker on a magnetic stir plate. Add the gelatine and let it stir until completely dissolved. Then add the contrast agent (barium sulfate or Conray), with thymol as a preservative to retard bacterial or fungal growth. Stir for approx 30 min until the solution is smooth. Divide the mixture into aliquots of 50–60 mL. These may be stored unrefrigerated in capped bottles for up to 1 yr.

In rare instances, staining of the injection mass may be required —for example, for differential display of the right and left coronary artery systems. For a setup of pressure- controlled injection in such a setting, *see* Chapter 12, Fig. 12-5. Barium sulfate with various pigment colors is commercially available (Sigma, *see* above). We have occasionally stained barium sulfate-gelatine mixtures with carmine, Berlin blue, naphthol green, or acridine yellow.

Media Containing Heavy Metals The media often contained lead or mercuric salts *(9,10)*. Because of the toxic hazard, their use is no longer recommended.

Clinical Contrast Media These media (e.g., Ethiodol®, Savage Laboratories, 60 Baylis Road, Melville, NY 11747, or Sodium Diatrizoate from SIGMA, P.O. Box 14508, St. Louis, MO 63178-9916) are expensive and, when pure, are lost for histologic identification during processing. However, they are readily available in most hospitals and can be recommended for pathologists who do injection work only on occasion. As described earlier, we use an iothalamate-meglumine mixture for coronary arteriography. Coloring agents can be added to these media for macroscopic and microscopic identification.

India Ink This material is used primarily for microscopic study of the microvasculature. The black pigment stands out readily before and after histologic processing. India ink can be mixed with gelatine and water. Thick sections usually are studied. If these are to be studied microradiographically, a radiopaque mass such as diluted Chromopaque neutral medium is required.

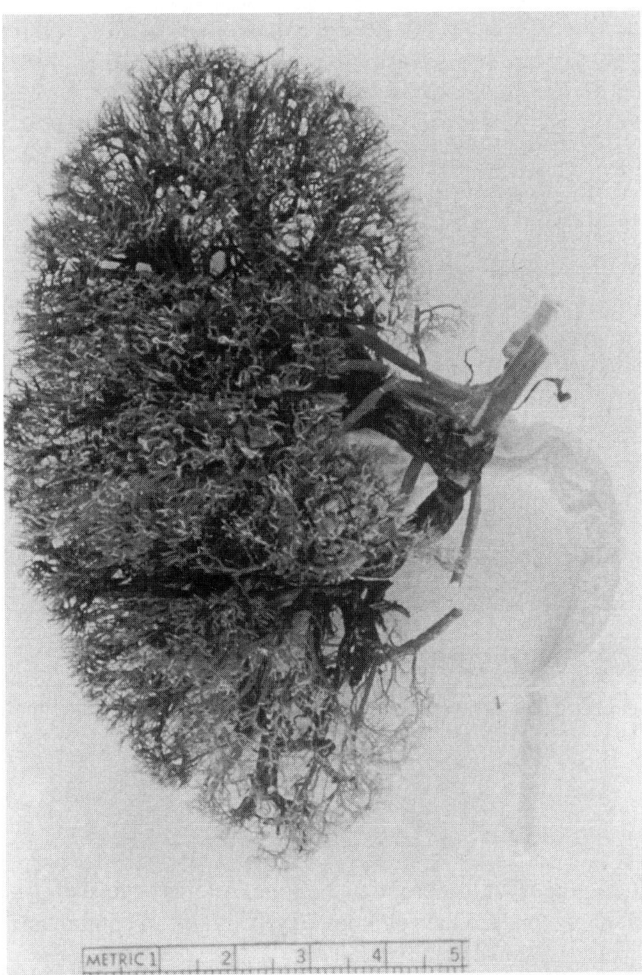

Fig. 15-1. Vinyl plastic cast of normal kidney. Red, blue, and yellow plastic was used so that in the corrosion cast, arteries were red, veins blue, and pelvis with ureter, yellow.

Plastics Excellent casts of vessels and cavities can be prepared with vinyl-acetate plastic mixtures (Aldrich Chemical Co., Inc., 1001 West Saint Paul Ave., Milwaukee, WI, 53233), as shown in Fig. 15-1. Some of these have also been made radiopaque.

Metal Casts These are made of alloys with very low melting points such as Wood's metal. Bronchograms or casts of hydronephroses or cystic tumors can easily be prepared with this method. For tissue maceration, antiformin is suggested (*see* Chapter 8).

CORROSION METHODS

Vascular or other casts of plastic or metal can be viewed in roentgenograms or after corrosion of the organ (Fig. 15-1) or tissue that was injected. Concentrated hydrochloric acid or 40% potassium hydroxide are used for this purpose. The duration of the process depends on the size of the specimen but may last several days. An alternative to the use of aggressive chemicals are prolonged cooking, followed by repeated rinsing in a strong jet stream of water. Placing the untreated specimen in an ant hill probably gives good results but the logistics of such an undertaking may be a major obstacle.

CLEARING TECHNIQUES

Clearing techniques are used to demonstrate bones or injected blood vessels without destroying the outline of the surrounding tissue. The clearing medium is benzene (*see* Chapter 5, Fig. 5-2) or oil of Wintergreen, which is a skin irritant, has an unpleasant smell, and dissolves plastic and most sealants. This disadvantage and the availability of computed tomography and related methods have made the techniques *(2,3)* largely obsolete. Only one method shall be described here.

CLEARING METHOD AFTER SPALTEHOLZ

- Fix specimen in 10% formalin or Kaiserling I solution.
- Wash in tap water.
- Dehydrate in changes of 80 and 95% ethyl alcohol for 24 h at each change and in absolute alcohol for 48 h.
- Soak in benzene for 24 h.
- Mount in a glass jar with oil of Wintergreen.
- Seal with the following mixture: Cabinetmakers' glue sticks 80 g; powdered arabic gum 20 g; glycerin 10 g; tap water 150 mL; acetic acid 5 mL; and thymol crystals 0.05 g.

Fixation and clearing of intact fetuses has been accomplished with a mixture of alcohol, potassium carbonate, and potassium hydroxide *(3)*; staining of skeletal structures in the cleared specimen was done with an alizarin solution (*see* Chapter 14) *(3)*.

INFILTRATION AND MUMMIFICATION TECHNIQUES

INFILTRATION TECHNIQUES Plastination (*see* above) can be used as an infiltration method which provides excellent specimens. This is the method of choice if one wants to prepare dry samples that can be handled similar to fresh specimens, without the need of gloves or risk of infection.

Infiltration of organs with paraffin and other substances can be accomplished without special commercial additives; the techniques permit permanent preservation of dry specimens *(11)*. The infiltration methods are quite time-consuming but the paraffinized organs, e.g., hearts with chronic valvular disease, are very instructive and pleasant to handle. However, with the possible exception of plastination, little need appears to remain for such specimens and therefore, the technical aspects of paraffin infiltration that were illustrated in the last edition, shall not be described here again.

MUMMIFICATION TECHNIQUES Mummification of organs is the simplest and oldest preservation technique. Mummification of whole bodies is described by Evans *(12)*. Shrinkage and loss of material for histologic study are the main disadvantages of organ mummification. This type of dry preservation is best applied to lungs (*see* Chapter 4) and intestines (*see* Chapter 5).

ORGAN MODELS

Organ models are of great didactic value, primarily for the presentation of normal anatomic structures. An enormous number of such models are now commercially available and previously described methods *(1)* for model preparation are now largely obsolete. Computer-generated models that can be

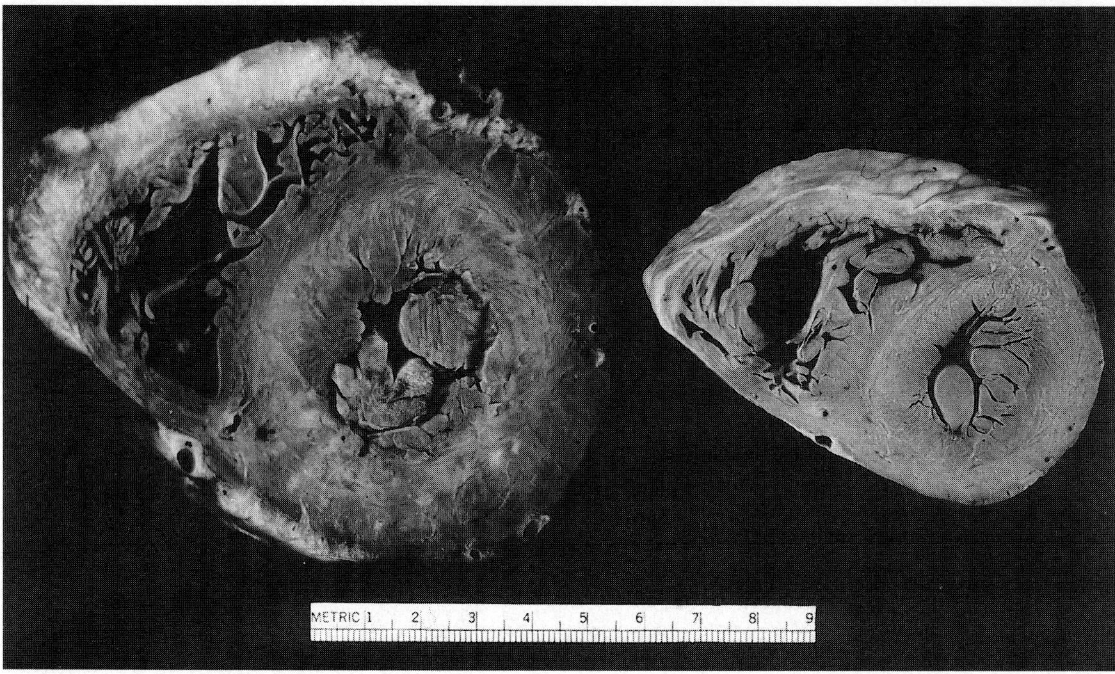

Fig. 15-2. Comparison of specimens in autopsy photography. Concentric left ventricular hypertrophy (left), with normal heart (right) for comparison.

viewed on the screen in three dimensions are becoming another readily available learning tool.

PHOTOGRAPHY (WITH WILLIAM D. EDWARDS)

Color photographs, prepared with a 35-millimeter single-ens-reflex (SLR) camera or a digital camera, have become an integral part of autopsy records and the main tool of presenting findings at clinical conferences, in the classroom, and in court. These advantages have led to the decline of the pathology museum. Because most autopsy pathologists are sufficiently familiar with photographic equipment and the indications for its use, only a brief overview shall be provided here.

INDICATIONS Four main reasons exist to request autopsy photography:

- Documentation of autopsy findings to supplement the protocol;
- Documentation of autopsy findings for use in clinicopathologic conferences, classroom teaching, and related activities;
- For the development of teaching files and scientific registries to supplement collections of actual (museum) specimens or, if necessary, to substitute for such specimens;
- For medicolegal purposes, such as crime scene investigation, identification of bodies (e.g., face, tattoos, or scars), and documentation of findings (e.g., photography of sequential *in situ* dissection).

TECHNICAL ASPECTS Generally, one camera unit should be available to prepare, while the autopsy is in progress, *in situ* photographs with appropriate lighting. Another unit should be available for specimen photography. This type of equipment is readily available commercially.

SPECIMEN PREPARATION Before pictures are taken, specimens should be prepared as if they were intended for display in the museum. This may involve restoration of color with 80% ethanol, additional trimming and dissection, support of lesions with pins or other devices, drying of light-reflecting surfaces and use of a black matte background with rulers. For the use of labels in photographs for medicolegal purposes, *see* Chapter 2. Comparison with a corresponding normal sample can be most instructive (for example, a normal left ventricle side by side with the left ventricle of a heart with chronic hypertension; *see* Fig. 3-3B in Chapter 3 and Fig. 15-2).

High-quality *in situ* pictures are much more difficult to prepare than specimen photographs. Light reflections should be reduced as much as possible, and a probe or other instrument not fingers) may be used to point to the lesion in question. Most important, a clear description of the findings should be provided on the label for the photograph or digital image.

PHOTOGRAPHIC FILES An enormous number of photographs tend to accumulate, not only in institutional files but also in the personal files of pathologists, particularly when they teach and publish. The principles of filing photographs are essentially the same as those for filing other autopsy documents. This is discussed in Chapter 16. Before photographs are filed, the following steps are necessary.

- Slides or digital images (and prints) should be scrutinized to determine whether they are worth keeping. Restraint in this regard may help to reduce an otherwise unmanageable volume of photographs.

- Each picture should be properly identified (e.g., name and identifying number of patient or autopsy, and diagnosis or description of whatever the photograph is supposed to show).
- A retrieval system must be in place that allows users to access the file successfully. Information in such a data carrier (usually a card file or a computer file) should readily locate the actual slide by the patient's name or number and by the subject of the photograph. For example, the identifying data of a photograph showing hepatic metastases from a malignant melanoma might appear in the files under the key words (or SNOMED codes) "liver," "metastases," and "malignant melanoma." Of course, the list of key words can be extended, for example, if a file for pigmented lesions is kept.
- A note should be entered into the autopsy records, stating that photographs are on file, what they show, and how they can be located.

REFERENCES

1. Tompsett DH. Anatomical Techniques. E & S Livingstone, Edinburgh, 1956.
2. Pulvertaft RJV. Museum techniques: a review. J Clin Pathol 1950;3: 1–23.
3. Edwards JJ, Edwards MJ. Medical Museum Technology. Oxford University Press, London, 1959.
4. Allison MJ, Gerszten. Paleopathology in Peruvian Mummies: Application of Modern Techniques. Virginia Commonwealth University, Medical College of Virginia, Richmond, 1975, p. 17.
5. Sloka K, Schilt G. Utilization of the postmortem examination with emphasis on audiovisual aids. Arch Pathol Lab Med 1987;111:883–884.
6. Ruschoff J, Thomas C. Plastination in der Pathologie. Methodische und didaktische Erfahrungen mit der Biodur-S 10-Standardtechnik. Pathologe 1991;12:35–39.
7. Bickley HC, Townsend FM. Preserving biological material by plastination. Curator (American Museum of Natural History) 1984;27: 65–73.
8. Bickley HC, Walker AN, Jackson RL, Donner RS. Preservation of pathology specimens by silicone plastination. An innovative adjunct to pathology education. Am J Clin Pathol 1987;88:220–223.
9. Prinzmetal M, Kayland S, Margoles C, Tragerman LJ. A quantitative method for determining collateral coronary circulation: preliminary report on normal human hearts. J Mount Sinai Hosp NY 1942;8:933–945.
10. Schlesinger MJ. An injection plus dissection study of coronary artery occlusions and anastomoses. Am Heart J 1938;15:528–568.
11. Kramer FM. Dry preservation of museum specimens: a review with introduction of simplified technique. J Tech Methods 1938;18:42–50.
12. Evans WED. The Chemistry of Death. Charles C. Thomas, Springfield, IL, 1963.
13. Edwards WD. Photography of Medical Specimens: experiences from teaching cardiovascular pathology. Mayo Clin Proc 1988;63:42–57.
14. Vetter, JP, ed. Biomedical Photography. Butterworth-Heinemann, Boston, MA, 1992.
15. McGavin MD, Thompson SW. Specimen Dissection and Photography for the Pathologist, Anatomist and Biologist. Charles C. Thomas, Springfield, IL, 1988.
16. Hansell P, ed. A Guide to Medical Photography. MTP Press Limited, Ipswich, UK, 1979.

16 Organization, Maintenance, and Safety Concerns of the Autopsy Service; Tissue Registries; Interviews With the Next of Kin

JURGEN LUDWIG

THE FLOW OF SPECIMENS AND DOCUMENTS

At the time of autopsy, the pathologist selects the gross specimens for preliminary storage. On the back of our preliminary autopsy diagnosis forms, instructions are given for further processing of the specimens, including requests for refrigeration, fixation, preparation for organ review, mounting for museum display (*see* Chapter 15), photography, roentgenography, and gross staining. Xerox copies of these diagnosis and instruction sheets are prepared for the staff and resident pathologists, the autopsy technicians, and the institutional files. Material for deep freezing and for microbiologic, chemical, or other studies is labeled and sent directly from the autopsy room, together with the appropriate request forms.

When a gross specimen is to be saved, it is immediately identified with a plastic tag that shows the autopsy number and, for paired organs, the side (we identify sides with one punched-out notch for right and two, for left). In the autopsy laboratory, gross specimens are processed as indicated by the written instructions. As a rule, they are stored in plastic containers until the histologic slides have been reviewed by a pathologist. Thus, additional material can be retrieved if the need arises.

Additional clinical information, unsuspected microbiologic test results, histologic findings, or other information may create a need for further study of stored organs, tissues, or body fluids. However, after that has been accomplished, some or all wet specimens can be discarded. If an institutional tissue registry is available, organs intended for permanent storage are entered into the record book or computer file of the autopsy gross tissue laboratory. On completion of the final autopsy diagnosis, designated gross specimens are sent to the tissue registry for permanent storage.

We keep specimens for microscopic examination in "stock bottles" with formalin solution. These bottles contain fragments of all organs, tissues, and lesions. The case number is inscribed on a plastic tag inside the jar and on a label on the outside. Tissues requiring special identification or fixatives are kept in separate jars. After material for histologic study has been selected, the remaining tissues in the stock bottles are trimmed and transferred to Sealac bags with fresh formalin solution (*see* below: "The Institutional Tissue Registry: Storage Methods"). In institutions with appropriate recording and storage facilities (tissue registries), bottles or bags with fixed tissue samples can be saved permanently. If, in such a setting, a pathologist desires to review an old specimen or needs old blocks or slides, a request card, fax, or E-mail message is sent to the autopsy tissue laboratory where the records are kept. A computerized list will reveal whether the specimen is still available. In institutions with a properly run tissue registry, the list will state where stored specimens, blocks, or slides can be found. After the review is completed, the material is returned and the computer records are updated.

For further details about autopsy documents, *see* Chapters 17 and 18.

MINIMAL STORAGE REQUIREMENTS

Most institutions have only minimal storage space for slides, blocks, wet specimens, and even documents. They will be interested in the minimal storage times that are compatible with practical and legal requirements. One recommendation *(1)* is shown in Table 16-1. Undoubtedly, the time periods in this table represent minimum saving times. If documents are saved as microfiches or on computer disks, the space needed for data storage can be greatly reduced and saving times increased.

MAINTENANCE OF AUTOPSY FACILITIES

Maintenance, cleaning, waste disposal, and related activities in the autopsy facilities are now rather strictly regulated because of the increased risk of infections.

CLEANING OF AUTOPSY ROOM AND EQUIPMENT The walls and floors of the autopsy facilities are washed regularly with soft brushes and disinfectant such as 10% solution of sodium hypochlorite (household bleach—1 part bleach to 9 parts water). We use Hi-lex solution. For the floors, we use

From: *Handbook of Autopsy Practice,* 3rd Ed. Edited by: J. Ludwig © Humana Press Inc., Totowa, NJ

Table 16-1
Recommended
Minimal Storage Requirements[a]

Wet tissues	6 mo
Accession records	1 yr
Quality assurance documents	2 yr
Paraffin blocks and photographs	5 yr
Autopsy authorization forms	7 yr[b]
Autopsy reports and slides	20 yr

[a]Data from ref. *(1)*.
[b]In ref. *(1)*, 1 yr is considered sufficient.

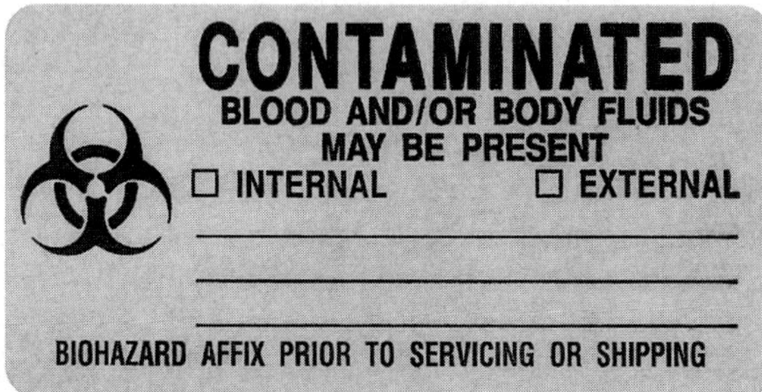

Fig. 16-1. Warning label. Such a label must be affixed to potentially contaminated equipment.

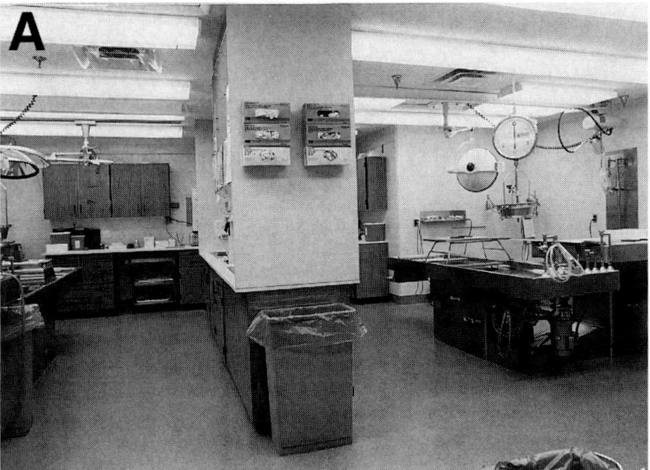

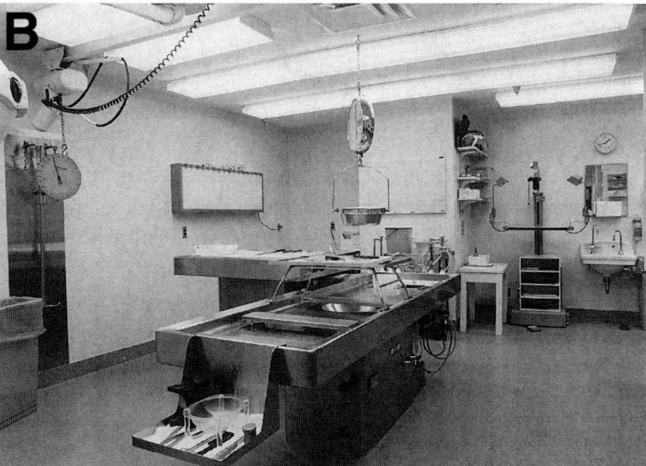

Fig. 16-2. Safety features of an autopsy room. *Upper*, This facility has two autopsy tables. The room is partially divided by supply cabinets, which also can be seen in the background. Note bright lighting throughout the room. Containers (in foreground) with biohazard plastic bags are for contaminated material (see text). *Lower*, Autopsy table that can be pneumatically adjusted to the height of the prosector. Two scales are visible; the one on the very left is part of a crane system for lifting and weighing deceased on a metal rack, and the one in the center, suspended over the table from the ceiling, is for weighing organs. A separate table for dissecting organs is in the background, adjacent to the autopsy table.

Wesodyne (95 mL in 20 L of water). The solutions should be made up daily with tap water to prevent loss of germicidal action during storage. The autopsy tables are rinsed after each autopsy with water, Hi-lex, and Haemosol. During cleaning, personnel should don protective gear (*see* below). Paper towels, gauze, and gloves used for cleaning should be disposed in biohazard bags, as described in the next paragraph. If contamination with radioactive material may have occurred, follow recommendations in Chapter 13.

If *large spills* occur, the cleaning crew, during clean-up, must wear face shields or safety glasses, in addition to the usual protective garments. Absorb spill with paper towels. Broken glass and other sharp objects must be removed with mechanical devices such as dust pan and cardboard pusher, *never by hand*. For safe disposal of these objects, *see* below.

Equipment used for diagnosis, research, and other applications must be decontaminated with 10% bleach (*see* above). It is particularly important that this is done before any equipment leaves the autopsy laboratory area. If reliable decontamination cannot be achieved, a warning label "CONTAMINATED" should be affixed to the equipment. The label should state which part of the equipment remains contaminated (Fig. 16-1).

WASTE DISPOSAL Proper organization of waste disposal may decrease the hazards as well as the costs of the autopsy service *(2)*. Containers used to discard material should be clearly marked so that items that should be incinerated are not inadvertently placed in containers that might be intended for the laundry, for example. Thus, we collect dressings, cotton wool swabs, hair, and other loose material from deceased persons in red biohazard bags (Fig. 16-2) for immediate incineration. Sharp objects are disposed in "sharps" containers, which are especially designed for this purpose. Infectious waste disposal containers are used to transport the biohazard plastic bags. These containers also must be cleaned regularly (at least every 6 mo) because leakage from the bags may occur.

In most autopsy facilities, paper-type protective garments, plastic aprons, surgical gloves, plastic face shields, and hair covers can be discarded after each autopsy (or series of autopsies if they were done in sequence). These items should be considered contaminated and they should be placed, together with other possibly contaminated articles in a separate bag that is labeled with a warning tag and sent for disposal in an approved incinerator.

CLEANING OF REUSABLE ITEMS Heavy rubber autopsy gloves are washed with detergent, autoclaved, and checked for leaks before they are used again. It is recommended to wear double surgical gloves underneath the heavy autopsy gloves. Pants, garments made of cloth, and towels are first washed in cold water to remove blood, then soaked in a detergent for several hours, and finally autoclaved or sent to the laundry, again in a bag with a warning tag.

Metal instruments are washed to remove all particulate matter and then are soaked in a detergent—for example, a 1:40 Hilex solution or Haemosol, 15 g/3.8 L of water. Metal instruments also should be autoclaved. They should be transported in covered stainless-steel containers. Plastic syringes and needles are placed in disposal containers designed for this purpose. These containers are discarded in the aforementioned incinerator bags when they are filled to about 3/4 their capacity.

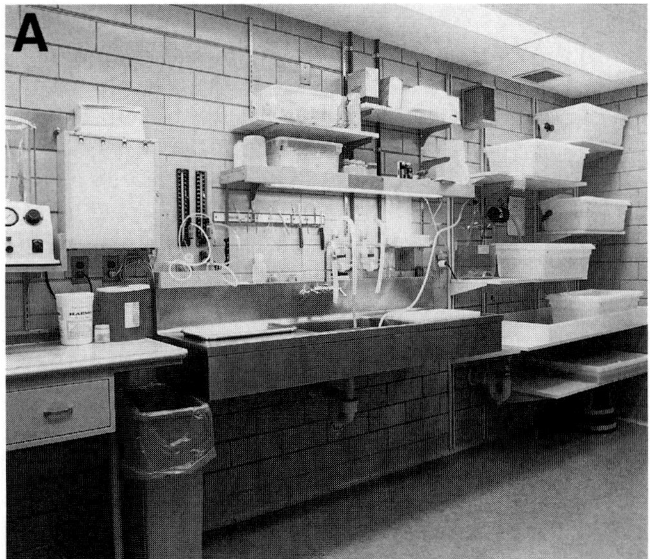

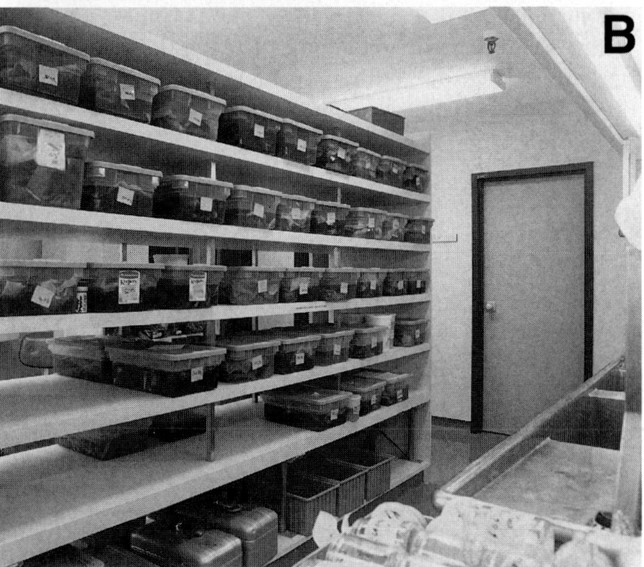

Fig. 16-3. The autopsy laboratory. Upper, Working space with manometers and other equipment for vascular injections and related procedures. Note organ perfusion apparatus in the background (also shown in Fig. 4-4). Lower, Shelves for plastic containers with specimens in formalin solution.

SAFETY CONCERNS OF THE AUTOPSY SERVICE

GENERAL PRECAUTIONS Autopsy rooms should be clean, spacious, properly ventilated *(3)* and well lit. Safety-oriented design of the autopsy undoubtedly is part of the general precautions. For example, the level of the autopsy tables should be adjustable to the height of the prosector. It is preferred to have dissecting tables separate from the autopsy table. The autopsy laboratory also should have a safety-oriented design. These and other features are illustrated in Figs. 16-2 and 16-3. Morgue and other laboratory personnel at risk should receive annual instructions in infection precautions and receive appropriate immunizations and tests for the agents handled or potentially present in the autopsy area (e.g., hepatitis B vaccine and skin testing to detect tuberculosis).

Access to the Autopsy Area The morgue area and all adjacent laboratories and storage facilities should be locked at all times so that only authorized persons can enter—for example, with a card key. Other persons would have to ring and use an intercom to gain access. Most important, the morgue area should be off limits for *all* persons who have not donned proper protective gear (*see* above, "Maintenance of Autopsy Facilities"). Appropriate warning signs should be posted. Also, in the autopsy laboratory, warning signs should be posted for toxic hazards such as formalin fumes.

Protective Garments Although the chance of nontraumatic infection is minimal, any contact between skin and body fluids should be avoided as much as possible. Therefore, appropriate gear should be donned for all autopsies. Caps or hoods are part of these garments; they should completely cover the hair. Disposable space suits and forearm guards should be worn and discarded after each high-risk autopsy. Waterproof disposable plastic aprons and disposable water-impermeable shoe covers are needed also.

Face Protection Plastic face shields covering the entire face and neck region should be worn. Alternatively, surgical masks can be used with safety goggles that have a cushion that seals the skin around the eyes. During autopsies of patients with tuberculosis or other highly infectious conditions, morgue personnel now carry powered-air purifying respirators or HePa respirators (the latter must be individually fitted and training for using this equipment must be provided). Face protection is particularly important when aerolization hazards are great as during the opening of the cranial vault. For additional protection, this latter procedure should be performed with the saw inside a plastic bag as discussed in Chapter 6.

Gloves Powdered or powder-free latex gloves are most commonly used. During the actual autopsy, double gloves (one on top of the other) should be used. The inner glove may be a surgical glove and the outer, a heavy rubber autopsy glove. Steel-mesh cloves may provide the most effective protection, particularly in high-risk autopsy cases. Unfortunately, they greatly reduce the "feel" that is needed to dissect properly and to evaluate the texture of organs and lesions. If a rubber or latex glove gets torn, it should be replaced immediately. If both gloves are torn, the hand should be washed and inspected carefully in order to detect wounds, particularly puncture wounds (*see* below). Disposable gloves, once removed, should not be reused.

Instruments Proper care of autopsy instruments reduces the risk of accidents. Knives and saw blades should be kept sharp (blunt knives require undue force during cutting and thus are more prone to slip). In our opinion, scalpels should only be used if absolutely necessary. Cleaning should be done after each autopsy session; the methods are described above. *See* also Chapter 8 under "Autopsy Saws."

Only needle-locking syringes or disposable syringe-needle units should be used for aspiration of body fluids and infectious material. Used disposable needles must not in any way be manipulated by hand but placed in a nearby puncture-resistant container used for "sharps" disposal. Nondisposable sharps must be placed in a plastic or metal container for transport to the decontamination process, generally autoclaving.

Protection From Toxic Fumes In the autopsy laboratories, this involves primarily formalin fumes. Their concentration in the air must be monitored intermittently, as described earlier under "The Institutional Tissue Registry."

Protection From Irradiation The risk most commonly comes from exposure to radioactive isotopes. This is discussed in detail in Chapter 13.

Shipping This is discussed in Chapter 14. Tissues and body fluids should be placed in containers that will not leak during collection, handling, processing, storage, transport, and shipping.

Injuries Each autopsy facility should have clearly posted or otherwise accessible outlines of the procedures that must be followed after an injury has occurred. Most injuries involve the hands. In these cases, remove gloves immediately, allow wound to bleed while flushing it for several minutes under running water. Some authors *(4)* suggest to treat injuries immediately with iodine or phenol-containing preparations, O.5 *M* NaOH or 1:3000 potassium permanganate. If potentially contaminated material made contact with the eye, it should be flushed immediately, preferably under a properly installed eye flush device. Flushing should be continued for 15 min. In most instances of injury, persons are sent to the Employee Health Service for further advice, observation (e.g., repeated testing for HIV), or treatment. Also, a detailed Employee Incident—Injury/Illness Investigation Report is filed (in triplicate) in each case because all accidents of this type must be documented in permanent records. Workmen's compensation and other proceedings may rely on such records.

POLICIES FOR HIGH-RISK AUTOPSIES Of course, all autopsies are potentially high-risk procedures and thus, the work routine in the autopsy room should provide reasonable protection, whether or not a special risk had been identified. Nevertheless, careful review of the clinical charts may reveal warning signs that a patient might have had a disease in the high-risk category, such as tuberculosis, the acquired immunodeficiency syndrome, or Creutzfeldt-Jakob disease. (*See* also under these entries in Part II.) Although most of these conditions do not appear to be very contagious *(5,6)*, needle-stick injuries and comparable trauma *(7)* or other forms of exposure *(8,9)* can lead to clinically manifest infections or even fatalities. Risks and safety precautions have been discussed in numerous publications, particularly for HIV *(6,7,10–14)*, tuberculosis *(5,8,9,15)*, and Creutzfeldt-Jakob disease *(4,14,16)*. However, hepatitis viruses and bacteria causing septicemia, meningitis, or gastrointestinal diseases also may fall into this category *(17)*.

We recommend in these cases to limit the number of persons in the autopsy room to: 1) the prosector, 2) a technician who assists the prosector on the autopsy table, and 3) a "clean" assistant who completes paper work and all other assignments that do not require contact with body fluids, tissues, instruments, or other potentially contaminated surfaces. It is important that the prosector and the assistant *work apart* so that they cannot injure each other. Proper face protection, gloves, and garments, cleaning procedures, and waste disposal are discussed above.

THE INSTITUTIONAL TISSUE REGISTRY

A well-organized tissue registry is the most valuable source of material for service and research work in pathology. Unfortunately, only few tissue registries worth their name have survived. The costs of space and personnel are considerable; there are also security issues and workplace hazards, particularly because of the large volumes of formalin that must be used. No outside funding can be expected.

The Mayo Clinic Tissue Registry keeps on file: 1) all histologic slides (an estimated 370,000/yr) and paraffin blocks (approx 160,000/yr) prepared in the pathology laboratories; 2) gross specimens from the surgical and autopsy service; as well as 3) the concentrated stock bottles (*see* above under "The Flow of Specimens and Documents"), which allow access to wet tissue and which are kept for at least 15 yr.

TISSUE REGISTRY FILE Elaborate card files had been used in the past and are now replaced by SNOMED-based or other computer files. We use the Co-Path Computer System for our inventory and to track storage and retrieval of slides, blocks, and wet tissues.

STORAGE METHODS Wet tissue is saved in plastic bags (Searle & Kapak). Ten percent formalin solution is the only fixative still in use for permanent storage. All stored material is identified by plastic tags with the autopsy number inside the bags or containers, and by labels on the outside. Warning labels are used to alert personnel to the hazards of formalin fumes. The plastic bags are sealed with a heat sealer (CLAMCO Heat Sealing & Packaging Co., Cleveland Detroit Corporation, Cleveland, OH) (Fig. 16-4).

MONITORING FOR TOXIC FUMES The concentration of formalin fumes in the air must be monitored intermittently, as directed by Occupational Safety and Health Administration (OSHA) formaldehyde standard (29CFR1910.1048) and required by the College of American Pathologists (CAP) *(18)*. Good ventilation, safety-oriented working methods, and properly designed containers allow to reduce the exposure to toxic fumes to acceptable levels.

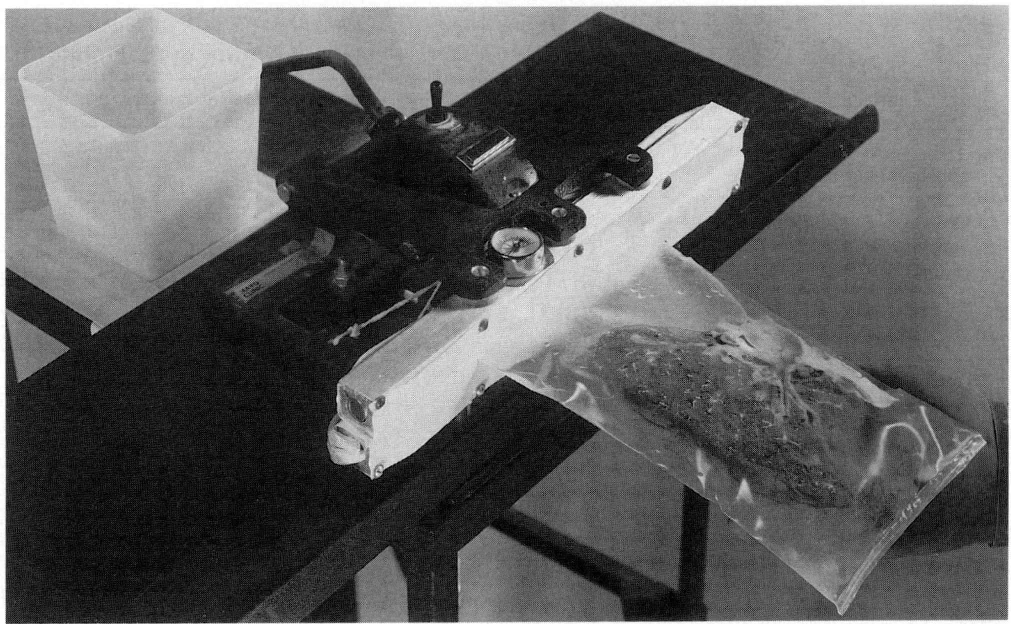

Fig. 16-4. Heat sealing for storage of slice of lung in plastic bag containing formalin solution.

THE NATIONAL REGISTRIES

The Armed Forces Institute of Pathology (AFIP) has as one of its objectives the running of numerous separate registries of pathology that are co-sponsored by national medical, dental, veterinary, or other organizations. These registries co-operate under the name "American Registry of Pathology" and may be consulted if diagnostic problems arise. The registries are depositories for both common and unusual specimens and data and as such serve as resources for and collecting points of other pertinent information. The organization of the American Registry of Pathology and the names of registrars are shown in Table 16-2. Address correspondence to:

American Registry of Pathology
Armed Forces Institute of Pathology
14th St & Alaska Ave NW
Washington DC 20306-6000
Phone: 202-782-2143; Fax: 202-782-4567

Many additional national and international registries have been organized that are not members of the American Registry of Pathology. All of these registries collect material for scientific purposes but also provide scientific consultations. The names and addresses of these registries generally can be obtained from the appropriate scientific societies. A comprehensive, alphabetical directory of these organizations has been published in the Journal of the American Medical Association 1999;282:390–396.

INTERVIEW WITH NEXT OF KIN

In most institutions, the attending physician will explain the cause of death to the family of the deceased. However, after autopsy permission has been granted, the next of kin may want detailed information about the autopsy findings. In this instance, the attending physician should discuss the matter with the pathologist and either personally convey the preliminary autopsy findings to the family or schedule an interview with the pathologist. Letters describing the autopsy findings are often delayed, and as a rule, they are a poor alternative for an interview—letters cannot respond to unexpected problems and questions, and their preparation may be just as time-consuming as an interview. The granting of permission for an autopsy is a favor, and failure to inform the family speedily about the autopsy findings understandably causes anger and frustration.

Most hospitals have a "Quiet Room," often close to the religious center and chapel, for relatives of the deceased who wish privacy. This is also a proper place for the attending physician or the pathologist to meet after an autopsy had been done. It does not take much more than tact, compassion, and understanding to adjust to the emotional needs of the bereaved family members. Another important and often overlooked aspect of the interview with the next of kin is its role as a source of additional data. A patient with hepatic cirrhosis may have denied chronic alcoholism, but at the time of the interview the family may readily volunteer the information. An unexpected amebic abscess of the liver will prompt diligent inquiry about former residencies. A suicide may come to light.

An interview may serve to relieve feelings of hostility against the attending physicians, surgeons, or paramedical personnel. Many lawsuits originate from misunderstanding, misinformation, and lack of communication. The pathologist, at the time of the interview, may be the first one to sense such feelings. He may be able to provide the needed explanations, to correct misconceptions, or to realize the need for the attending physician to talk to the family about their concerns. The benefits of

Table 16-2
The American Registry of Pathology at the Armed Forces Institute of Pathology[a]

Name of registry	*Names of registrars*
Acquired Immunodeficiency Syndrome (AIDS)	*See* "Infectious and Parasitic Disease."
Breast Pathology	*See* "Gynecologic/Breast Pathology"
Cardiovascular Pathology	Dr. Renu Virmani, M.D.
Cellular Pathology	Timothy J. O'Leary, M.D., Ph.D., Chair. Cytopathology Division (Miguel Tellado, M.D., Chief); Quantitative Division (Robert L. Becker, M.D., Chief); Molecular Division (Jeffery Taubenberger, M.D., Ph.D., Chief); and Biophysics Division (Jeffrey Mason, Ph.D., Chief).
Dental & Oral Pathology	*See* "Oral and Maxillofacial Pathology."
Dermatopathology	George O. Lupton, M.D., Chair
Developmental Anatomy Human Developmental Anatomy Center	Adrianne Noe, Ph.D.
DNA Registry	Vern Armbrustmacher, M.D.
Environmental and Toxicologic Pathology	Florabel K. Mullick, M.D., Chair. Division of Biochemistry (William Fishbein, Ph.D., Chief); Division of Chemical Pathology (Frank Johnson, M.D., Chief); Division of Environmental Pathology (Victor Kalasinsky, Ph.D., Chief); Radiation Division (David Busch, Ph.D., M.D., Chief) and Biophysical Toxicology Branch (Jose Centeno, Ph.D., Chief).
Gastrointestinal Pathology	*See* "Hepatic and Gastrointestinal Pathology."
Genitourinary Pathology	Fathollah K. Mostofi, M.D., Chair. Division of Urologic Pathology (Charles J. Davis, Jr., Chief); Division of Medical Nephropathology (Sharada G. Sabins, M.D., Chief); Division of Urogenital Research (Isabell Sesterhenn, M.D., Chief).
Gerontology	William Fishbein, M.D., Ph.D.
Gynecologic and Breast Pathology	Fattaneh A. Tavassoli, M.D., Chair.
Hematologic and Lymphatic Pathology	Susan L. Abbondanzo, M.D., Chair.
Hepatic and Gastrointestinal Pathology	Kamal G. Ishak, M.D., Ph.D., Chair. Division of Hepatic Pathology (Zachary D. Goodman, M.D., Ph.D., Chief) and Division of Gastrointestinal Pathology (Leslie H. Sobin, M.D., Chief).
Infectious and Parasitic Disease	Douglas Wear, M.D., Chair. Division of AIDS Pathology and Emerging Infectious Diseases (Ann M. Nelson, M.D., Chief) and Division of Microbiology (Ted Hadfield, LTC, Chief).
Lymphatic Pathology	*See* "Hematologic and Lymphatic Pathology."
Mediastinal Pathology	*See* "Pulmonary & Mediastinal Pathology."
Medical Museum	Adrianne Noe, Ph.D. (acting chair)
Nephropathology	*See* "Genitourinary Pathology"
Neuropathology	Hernando Mena, M.D., Chair.
Ophthalmic Pathology	Ian W. McLean, M.D., Chair.
Oral and Maxillofacial Pathology	Charles W. Pemble III, Chair.
Orthopedic Pathology	Donald E. Sweet, M.D., Chair.
Otolaryngic and Endocrine Pathology	Dennis K. Heffner, M.D., Chair. Division of Otolaryngic Pathology (Bruce M. Wenig, M.D., Chief) and Division of Endocrine Pathology (Clara S. Heffess, M.D., Chief).
Pediatric Pathology	Eric S. Suarez, M.D. (acting chief)
Pulmonary & Mediastinal Pathology	Michael N. Koss, M.D. and William D. Travis, M.D., Co-chairs.
Radiologic Pathology	Kelly K. Koeller, M.D., CAPT (Select), MC, USN
Soft Tissue Pathology	Markku Miettinen, M.D., Chair.
Telepathology	Bruce Williams, D.V.M., Director.
Toxicologic Pathology	*See* "Environmental and Toxicologic Pathology."
Urologic Pathology	*See* "Genitourinary Pathology."
Veterinary Pathology	William Inskeep, D.V.M., Chair.

[a]For the mailing address and phone/fax numbers of the American Registry of Pathology at the Armed Forces Institute of Pathology, *see* previous page.

interacting with the families as a matter of policy have recently been reconfirmed *(19)*.

SUGGESTIONS FOR CONDUCTING INTERVIEWS

1. Before you go to an interview, familiarize yourself with the history of the deceased, and discuss the case with the attending physician. As a minimum, the attending physician should be made aware of the interview and thus can provide the needed information.
2. Do not wear your hospital attire. Your attitude should be unhurried and adapted to the emotional needs of the family.
3. At the time of the interview, introduce yourself, present a card with your name and address, and ask for the names of the persons present and their kinship to the deceased. Failing to do this, pathologists may find themselves talking to newspaper reporters, private investigators, or curious neighbors. The possible legal consequences are obvious.
4. Report your findings in appropriate lay terms that the family members can comprehend. Omit unimportant findings. Be sure that your report is understood, and encourage the family to ask questions. The risk of the same fatal disease afflicting other members of the family often needs to be discussed, and in some cases arrangements must be made for genetic counseling at a later date.
5. Occasionally, the emotional shock to the next of kin may make an interview futile. In such a case it is better to postpone the interview or, if agreeable to the family, talk to their closest friend or clergyman. If the results of histologic, microbiologic, or chemical studies must be awaited, explain this to the next of kin and give a date when a final report can be expected. Point out that the attending and referring physicians also will receive such a report. Allow ample time for your workup. It is easier to explain the difficulties of laboratory procedures and to point out to the next of kin that they may have to wait for 6 wk than to promise an earlier date that cannot be kept. Delays of more than 6 wk should be considered unacceptable; at least telephone contact should be made by that time to explain why still more time is needed.
6. Express your appreciation for the permission to perform an autopsy and point out that others may be helped with the insights that were gained from the procedure. If organs or tissues had been donated for transplantation or other purposes, this should be especially acknowledged. However, the pathologist must remember that no information may be provided about the recipients of such donations. It is easiest to refer such questions to the transplant coordinator.
7. After the interview, dictate and sign a report of what was said. This should also include the time and place of the interview, the names and addresses of the persons present, and their kinship to the deceased. Bring to the attention of the attending physician all grievances or other important points that might have been mentioned during the interview. Sometimes, the clinical abstract that typically is part of the autopsy documents must be supplemented with details that were revealed during the interview.

ACKNOWLEDGMENT

Darrell M. Ottman, former supervisor of the Mayo Clinic Autopsy Laboratories and of the Mayo Clinic Tissue Registry, has graciously shared his expertise with the author.

REFERENCES

1. Geller AS. Retention of autopsy materials. In: Hutchins GM, ed. Autopsy—Performance and Reporting. College of American Pathologists, Northfield, IL, 1990, pp. 148–149.
2. Hamann W, Kadegis A. "Abfälle" in der Pathologie. Recycling, Entsorgung—Kosteneinsparung. Pathologe 1991;12:123–125.
3. al-Wali W, Kibbler CC, McLaughlin JE. Bacteriological evaluation of a down-draught necropsy table ventilating system. J Clin Pathol 1993;46:746–749.
4. Uysal A, Kaaden OR. Zum Umgang mit unkonventionellen Erregern. Pathologe 1993;14:351–354.
5. Kappel TJ, Reinartz JJ, Schmid JL, Holter JJ, Azar MM. The viability of mycobacterium tuberculosis in formalin-fixed pulmonary autopsy tissue: review of the literature and brief report. [Review]. Hum Pathol 1996;27:1361–1364.
6. Geller AS. The autopsy in acquired immunodeficiency syndrome. How and why. Arch Pathol Lab Med 1990;114:324–329.
7. Johnson MD, Schaffner W, Atkinson J, Pierce MA. Autopsy risk and acquisition of human immunodeficiency virus infection: a case report and reappraisal. Arch Pathol Lab Med 1997;121:64–66.
8. Wilkins D, Woolcock AJ, Cossart YE. Tuberculosis: medical students at risk. Med J Austral 1994;160:395–397.
9. Ussery XT, Bierman JA, Valway SE, Seitz TA, DiFerdinando GT Jr, Ostroff SM. Transmission of multidrug-resistant Mycobacterium tuberculosis among persons exposed in a medical examiner's office, New York. Inf Contr & Hosp Epidemiol 1995;16:160–165.
10. Karhunen PJ, Brummer-Korvenkontio H, Leinikki P, Nyberg M. Stability of human immunodeficiency virus (HIV) antibodies in postmortem samples. J Forensic Sci 1994;39:129–135.
11. McCaskie AW, Roberts M, Gregg PJ. Human tissue retrieval at postmortem for musculoskeletal research. Br J Biomed Sci 1995;52:222–224.
12. Claydon SM. The high risk autopsy. Recognition and protection. Am J Forensic Med Pathol 1993;14:253–256.
13. Douceron H, Deforges L, Gherardi R, Sobel A, Chariot P. Long-lasting postmortem viability of human immunodeficiency virus: a potential risk in forensic medicine practice. Forensic Sci Int 1993;60:61–66.
14. Ironside JW, Bell JE. The 'high-risk' neuropathological autopsy in AIDS and Creutzfeldt-Jakob disease: principles and practice. [Review] Neuropathol Appl Neurobiol 1996;22:388–393.
15. Lundgren R, Norrman E, Asberg I. Tuberculosis infection transmitted at autopsy. Tubercle 1987;68:147–150.
16. Budka H, Aguzzi A, Brown P, Brucher JM, Bugiani O, Collinge J, Diringer H, et al. Consensus report: tissue handling in suspected Creutzfeldt-Jakob disease (CJD) and other spongiform encephalopathies (prion diseases) in the human. Brain Pathol 1995:5:319–322.
17. Healing TD, Hoffman PN, Young SE. The infection hazards of human cadavers. Commun Dis Rep. CRD Review. 1995;5:R61–R68.
18. CAP Commission on Laboratory Accreditation inspection checklist. Anatomic Pathology (Section: 8): Formaldehyde vapor concentrations. Northfield, IL.
19. Hague AK, Patterson RC, Grafe MR. High autopsy rates at a university medical center. What has gone right? Arch Pathol Lab Med 1996;120:727–732.

17 Autopsy Documents, Data Processing, and Quality Assurance

JURGEN LUDWIG

AUTOPSY DIAGNOSES

Autopsy diagnosis represents an interpretation of objective, primarily morphologic, findings. For the next of kin, attending physicians, insurance companies, and public health authorities, these diagnosis sheets are important documents, but they may become meaningless in the future. Interpretations change, names of syndromes and diseases change, and so do autopsy diagnoses. This is one of the reasons why protocols should include objective descriptions.

Autopsy diagnoses can be reported and listed: 1) in a standard sequence (for example, cardiovascular system, respiratory system, digestive system, and so forth) to facilitate anatomic orientation, statistical analysis, and coding; 2) in order of causal relationships and relative importance (for example, chronic alcoholism, alcoholic cirrhosis, ruptured esophageal varices, and gastrointestinal hemorrhage); or 3) in a problem-oriented fashion. The first method is preferred by statisticians and those charged with coding, whereas the latter two methods appeal most to the clinician because more interpretative information is provided. Problem-oriented autopsy diagnoses and protocols (*see* below) are essential wherever problem-oriented medical records are used *(1,2)*.

PRELIMINARY DIAGNOSIS Forms that we fill out in the autopsy room contain:

- Name, age, weight, length, clinic number, and autopsy number of the patient;
- Date and time of death;
- Date and time of autopsy;
- Names of resident and staff pathologists;
- Preliminary autopsy diagnosis, primarily in the order of causal relationships;
- Directions as to which organs and lesions to photograph, to prepare for organ review, or to save permanently; and
- Directions for histologic sectioning and staining.

Space for the last two items is provided on the back of the preliminary autopsy form.

From: *Handbook of Autopsy Practice,* 3rd Ed. Edited by: J. Ludwig © Humana Press Inc., Totowa, NJ

FINAL AUTOPSY DIAGNOSIS Forms contain the identifying data as listed with the preliminary form, and the actual findings in three main categories: 1) main cause of death; 2) other major diseases and findings; and 3) additional findings. Major surgical procedures or other important diagnostic and therapeutic interventions that may have been carried out are listed as a fourth category. Thus, if a patients died during an attempt to clamp a leaking cerebral artery aneurysm, the diagnosis would state under "Immediate Cause of Death" (*see* below), "Leaking cerebral artery aneurysm (for attempted surgical repair, *see* below under "Surgeries")." The actual procedure would then be listed under "Surgeries." Procedures such as surgery or other interventions should *not* be listed under "Causes of Death" or under "Contributing Conditions" unless that is indeed the intended meaning that the pathologist wants to convey. Copies of the final diagnosis, typically with an explanatory cover letter, are encoded and filed, mailed to the clinicians who cared for the patient, and forwarded to the appropriate quality assurance officers or committees.

THE DEATH CERTIFICATE

Death certificates are required by law. They are needed for burial permits, life insurance claims, settlement of estates, and claims for survivorship benefits. The death certificate requirement also serves crime detection. The public interest in medical certification of the cause of death reflects the demand for reliable morbidity data that rarely are available in any other way. Death certificates help to locate cases for clinical investigators and aid in follow-up studies. Proper completion of death certificates requires a clear understanding of the organization of these documents and the differences—as defined in Chapter 2 and below—between causes of death, mechanism of death (mode of dying), and manner of death *(3)*.

The determination of the cause of death may be an extremely difficult task. Certain rules and regulations must be observed to secure reasonable and comparable data. The mechanisms causing a death may be so complex that the provisions of the death certificate may be insufficient for adequate documentation, in proper relationship, of the events that led to death. Nevertheless, the law must be satisfied. The physician, the biostatistician, and the judge each may accept as correct a different cause of death and thus, three types of causes of death could be distinguished: scientific, statistical, and legal *(4)*.

The death certificates in the United States are based on the "International Form of Medical Certificate of Cause of Death." The following entries are used:

1. *Immediate Cause of Death*, defined as the disease, injury of complication that directly led to death. This may be the only entry, for example, if death occurred immediately after a gunshot injury;
2. *Due to....*This entry was provided for the *intervening causes of death*, defined as conditions that contributed to death and were the result of the underlying cause. An example would be venous thromboses caused by a carcinoma of the pancreas (underlying cause) and leading to massive pulmonary embolism (immediate cause);
3. *Due to....*This entry is provided for the underlying cause of death, defined as the disease or injury that initiated the train of morbid events resulting in death, or the circumstances or violence that produced the fatal injury (for an example, see #2);
4. *Other significant conditions*. Diseases and conditions are recorded here that appear important for statistical and other purposes but that do not fit into the chain defined under #1 to #3. An example would be "carcinoma of breast with metastases" in a women who died of multiple injuries in an automobile accident.

It should be noted that the death certificate is not primarily designed for entries describing the *mechanism of death*, as defined in Chapter 2. Thus, "cardiorespiratory arrest" or "renal failure" represent mechanisms of death. Although terms describing mechanisms of death are found more frequently in death certificates than any other diagnosis, they should not be entered routinely. These diagnoses are acceptable, however, if they are reported together with an etiologically specific underlying cause or if some other criteria are met *(5)*. Generally, the mechanism of death will simply be ignored by the health authorities, as long as it is entered in conjunction with a valid entry, for example, "Cardiac arrest *due to* rheumatic mitral valvular stenosis."

In contradistinction to the mechanism of death, the death certificate provides space for the *manner of death*, defined as natural, accident, suicide, and homicide. Deaths as a result of suicide and homicide always are under the jurisdiction of the medical examiner or a comparable official. If a crucial investigation is pending or if the cause of death could not be determined, that also should be noted in this part of the death certificate. The designation "pending" should be used only in very rare situations, as described below under "Delayed Certification."

DEATH CERTIFICATE PROCEDURES Instructions for physicians who must determine and ascribe natural causes of death have been published by the College of American Pathologists *(6)*. The proper use of United States death certificates had been described earlier in a Public Health Service publication *(7)*. Every physician in the United States who is charged with certifying deaths should have the 1994 publication (ref. *6*) on hand.

Death Certificates in Medicolegal Cases A United States Standard Certificate of Death is filled out. A form for medical examiners or coroners and a combined form for physicians, medical examiners, or coroners are available. The medical examiner or coroner or equivalent official is charged with filling out and signing the death certificate, or the appropriate section of it, in deaths caused by violence (homicide, suicide, or accident) and in other cases if so defined by state law. Pathologists must be familiar with the appropriate laws in the states where they practice. The correct use of medicolegal death certificates is described in a special publication of the Public Health Service *(8)*.

Proper Completion of Death Certificates U.S. Public Health Service publications *(7,8)* contain the following general instructions:

- Use the current form designated by the state.
- Type all entries whenever possible. Do not use worn typewriter ribbons. If a typewriter is not used, print legibly in dark, unfading ink. Black ink gives the best copies.
- Complete all items or attach a note explaining any omissions.
- Do not make alterations or erasures.
- All signatures must be written. Rubber stamp or other facsimile signatures are not acceptable.
- Do not submit carbon copies, reproductions, or duplicates for filing. The registrar will accept originals only.
- Avoid abbreviations.
- Spell entries correctly. Verify names that sound the same, but have different spellings (Smith vs Smyth, Gail vs Gayle, Wolf vs Wolfe, etc.)
- Refer problems not covered in specific instructions to the state vital statistics office, or local registrar.

Classification and Terminology Entries should be based on "International Classification of Disease, Clinical Modification 1998" *(9)*. Another valuable source is the American Medical Association's "Physicians' Current Procedural Terminology (cpt 98), Standard Edition" *(10)*.

Delayed Certification Occasionally, the cause of death can be established only after further, and often time-consuming, microbiologic, chemical, or other studies. The legal requirements in such cases vary somewhat throughout the United States, but the statement on the death certificate "Pending further investigations" will be accepted in most if not all places. Local laws, customs, or arrangements determine how long a delay will be acceptable. The following guidelines were recommended by the Public Health Service *(8)* for delay of a definitive statement as to the cause of death:

- The term "pending" is intended to apply only to cases in which there is a reasonable expectation that an autopsy, other diagnostic procedure, or investigation may significantly change the diagnosis.
- Certification of cause of death should not be deferred merely because "all details" of a case are not available. Thus, for example, if it is clear that a patient died of "carcinoma of the stomach," reporting of the cause should not

be deferred while a determination of the histologic type is being carried out. Similarly, if a death is from "influenza," there is no justification for delaying the certification because a virological test is being carried out.

- In cases where death is known to be from an injury, but the circumstances surrounding the death are not yet established, the injury should be reported immediately. The circumstances of the injury should be noted as "deferred," and a supplemental report filed.
- Lastly, the term "pending" is not intended to apply to cases in which the cause of death is in doubt, but for which no further diagnostic procedures can be carried out. In this case, the "probable" cause should be entered on the basis of the facts available and the certification made in accordance with the best judgment of the certifier.

Daylight Saving Time "Daylight Saving Time" has to be recorded on death certificates during the entire period in which daylight saving time is in effect.

WHAT HAPPENS TO THE DEATH CERTIFICATE? After the physician has completed and signed the death certificate, he turns the document over to the funeral director or local registrar. Fig. 17-1 shows the way data of the death certificate are passed on and how they are used.

CERTIFICATION PROBLEMS All problems not answered by the *Physicians' Handbook on Medical Certification (7)* or the *Medical Examiners' and Coroners' Handbook on Death and Fetal Death Registration (8)* should be referred to the vital statistics office of the state or to the local registrar. One option is to send the incomplete death certificate with a separate autopsy diagnosis and an explanatory note.

Incorrect certification of cause of death is frequent. Numerous studies have confirmed that educational efforts in this regard have had little effect. This must be considered when studies are evaluated that rely primarily on death certificate diagnoses. Even if an autopsy had been done, the death certificate often fails to reveal the most important diagnosis, for example, when a patient had carcinoma of the ovary with metastases but the death certificate states only "Heart failure due to bronchopneumonia and recurrent pulmonary embolism."

AUTOPSY PROTOCOLS

PURPOSE AND PRINCIPLES OF PREPARATION The autopsy protocol represents a permanent record of objective, primarily morphologic findings, with little interpretation. Organs and lesions are described by: 1) location and relationship to other organs and structures, 2) size, 3) weight, 4) shape, 5) color, 6) consistency, 7) odor, and 8) other special features such as texture of cut surfaces. Thus, the protocol describes the characteristics, extent, and severity of a lesion or condition interpreted in the diagnosis.

Numerous forms with the correct case identification must be filled out for each autopsy, such as diagnosis sheets, protocol forms, weight sheets, and requests for histologic, microbiologic, or chemical studies. Computerized forms with the same identifying data on each sheet have made this task much easier.

There is no ideal format for protocols because the requirements that have to be satisfied are to some extent mutually exclusive. Autopsy protocols should contain complete, detailed, yet concise and well-organized descriptions of abnormal findings. To describe a normal appearing organ as "normal," without any further specifications, appears acceptable in principle but often puts too much trust in the experience of the pathologist. Narrative parts of the protocol must be entered in the computer, proofread, and signed. Autopsy protocols should require little time to complete by pathologists and secretaries. Protocol forms should be self-explanatory so that the resident pathologist is in some way guided by the protocol. And, finally, protocol forms should be inexpensive.

Each institution has to compromise. Experience of personnel may be limited and manpower may be in short supply, while the need persists for optimal protocols for service, training, research, and record-keeping. Autopsy protocol writing is an art. Descriptions should be brief yet complete. There should be no interpretations and no descriptions of the mechanics of dissection ("The left atrium of the heart is opened, and the mitral valve is found to be..."). The statement that a nodule is yellow will not become more informative by adding, "in color."

Sizes should be stated in centimeters, and comparisons with fruits or other objects should be avoided. Weights should be stated in grams and kilograms, and volumes in liters and milliliters.

For autopsy protocols in *medicolegal cases*, Chapter 2 should be consulted.

NARRATIVE PROTOCOLS This time-honored type of protocol is inexpensive and may be most instructive. Virchow's protocols *(11)* are classic examples.

The narrative protocol permits detailed description of complicated findings and, at the same time, utmost brevity in describing the normal. There are no space limitations, and yet no space is wasted by printed provisions for abnormalities that do not apply. Unfortunately, good narrative protocols can be expected only from experienced pathologists whose style is lucid and whose descriptions are fitting. An established narrative pattern must be maintained. Those not fluent in the language in which the protocol is written may have additional difficulties with this type of protocol.

PROTOCOLS BASED ON SENTENCE COMPLETION AND MULTIPLE CHOICE SELECTION The protocols can be completed with ease and speed. Even the inexperienced can be expected to provide the most important information in most instances. These protocols can be tailored to specific types of autopsies, such as sudden infant death cases *(12)*. In paper forms, space limitations often make addenda on separate sheets necessary, and at the same time much paper is wasted by printed provisions for abnormalities that do not apply. In computer-based forms, many of these disadvantages can be avoided. Computers can generate programmed text *(13)* when key descriptive phrases or words are spoken but whether this will be useful in practice remains to be seen.

PICTORIAL PROTOCOLS Hand-drawings, photographs, or computer-generated outlines of organs may be part of any protocol but protocols in which pictures are the main form of documentation have not stood the test of time.

Responsible person or agency	Birth certificate	Death certificate	Fetal death certificate (stillbirth)
Physician, other professional attendant, or hospital authority	1. Completes entire certificate in consultation with parent(s); physician's signature required 2. Files certificate with local office of district in which birth occurred	1. Completes medical certification and signs certificate 2. Returns certificate to funeral director	1. Completes or reviews medical items on certificate 2. Certifies to the cause of fetal death and signs certificate 3. Returns certificate to funeral director 4. In absence of funeral director, files certificate
Funeral director	⇩	1. Obtains personal facts about deceased 2. Takes certificate to physician for medical certification 3. Delivers completed certificate to local office of district where death occurred and obtains burial permit	1. Obtains the facts about fetal death 2. Takes certificate to physician for entry of causes of fetal death 3. Delivers completed certificate to local office of district where delivery occurred and obtains burial permit
Local office (may be local registrar or city or county health department)	1. Verifies completeness and accuracy of certificate 2. Makes copy, legdger entry, or index for local use 3. Sends certificates to state registrar	1. Verifies completeness and accuracy of certificate 2. Makes copy, ledger entry, or index for local use 3. Issues burial permit to funeral director and verifies return of permit from cemetery attendant 4. Sends certificates to state registrar	
City and county health departments use certificates in allocating medical and nursing services, follow-ups on infectious diseases, planning programs, measuring effectiveness of services, and conducting research studies			
State registrar, Bureau of Vital Statistics	1. Queries incomplete or inconsistent information 2. Maintains files for permanent reference and as the source of certified copies 3. Develops vital statistics for use in planning, evaluation, and administering state and local health activities and for research studies 4. Compiles health-related statistics for state and civil divisions of state for use of the health department and other agencies and groups interested in the fields of medical science, public health, demography, and social welfare 5. Prepares copies of birth, death, and fetal death certificates or records for transmission to the National Center for Health Statistics		
Public Health Service and National Center for Health Statistics	1. Prepares and publishes national statistics of births, deaths, and fetal deaths; and constructs the official U.S. life tables and related actuarial tables 3. Conducts health and social-research studies based on vital records and on sampling surveys linked to records 4. Conducts research and methodological studies in vital statistics including the technical, administrative, and legal aspects of vital records registration and administration 2. Maintains a continuing technical assistance program to improve the quality and usefulness of vital statistics		

CA-858902B-01

Fig. 17-1. The vital statistics registration system in the United States. Adapted with permission from ref. *(7)*.

PROBLEM-ORIENTED PROTOCOLS Protocols of this type are designed to supplement the Problem-Oriented Medical Record System and may combine information that otherwise would be found in either the autopsy diagnosis or the conventional autopsy protocol. Pertinent examples can be found in various original publications *(1,2)*.

METHODS OF DATA RETRIEVAL

INSTITUTIONAL AUTOSPY RECORDS The files containing autopsy documents tend to become quite voluminous. Traditionally, cases are numbered consecutively and filed by year. If no further provisions are made, information retrieval is possible only by manually searching each individual record. This may be quite acceptable if autopsy records are kept only for legal reasons and otherwise are used only in rare family studies. In these instances, only names, clinic number, and other essential identifiers must be kept in a master file. However, for scientific studies based on diagnoses or findings, more elaborate filing and retrieval systems are needed.

PLANNING OF DATA PROCESSING For all practical purposes, data processing has become a computer-based activity. With this in mind, a decision must be made as to the expected use of the autopsy data-processing system. These expectations must be reconciled with the investments they would require in terms of time, personnel, hardware, software, computer time, and related issues. Experience shows that this is rarely done in a realistic manner. Typically, a powerful computerized system has been purchased and a paramedical operator is available who has been trained to run the system, but the physicians who must make the decisions of what should be encoded and how, fall more and more behind with this work, sometimes until the endeavor must be pronounced dead. Only experienced record librarians can achieve satisfactory results without the aid of physicians with expertise in coding.

Typically, autopsy pathologists, surgical pathologists, cytologists, and often, clinical pathologists want or need to use the same database. This usually requires an integrated data-processing system within the medical center, often with linkage to satellite centers or other institutions. Unfortunately, the costs of such large systems are enormous, system breakdowns possible, and issues of privacy protection difficult to solve. Application of such systems *(14–16)* has not been studied widely.

How elaborate the autopsy data-processing system will be depends on whether all or only a portion of relevant autopsy data should be retrievable. Most general pathologists are principally interested in: 1) a basic documentation of major pathologic findings and 2) data that can be used for workload recording and other administrative functions. The system should also contain information about photographs and other material germane to the specific question.

CODING MANUALS Only few major coding manuals currently are in general use.

1. *International Classification of Diseases, Fifth Edition (ICD×9×CM) (9).* This classification is required for billing purposes and many other tasks. Unfortunately, it is based on the concept that each condition should have one number; such a monoaxial system is of very limited scientific value if one compares it with SNOMED (*see* below). Also, disease designations are often obsolete. The international classification of tumors (ICD-O) is part of the ICD (**I**nternational **C**lassification of **D**iseases for **O**ncology) but of greater scientific usefulness because tumors are more suitable for this type of classification.
2. *SNOMED International (17).* The volumes contain eleven modules (topography; morphology; function; living organisms; chemicals, drugs and biologic products; physical agents, forces, and activities; occupation and social context; procedures; and general linkage modifiers). The codes from the International Classification of Diseases (ICD-9-CM) are included also. The tumor codes in SNOMED International are the same as in ICD-O. Systematized nomenclature of medicine (SNOMED) coding can be done manually or in an automated fashion; it appears that automated coding yields almost the same results as manual coding *(18).*
3. *Physicians' Current Procedural Terminology.* This is an important supplemental tool for the encoding of autopsy documents *(10).*

SNOMED International is available from the American College of Pathologists in Chicago, IL. The other coding manuals, together with CD-ROM versions, teaching material, and related publications can be purchased from several companies such as Medicode, Inc., 5225 Wiley Post Way, Suite 500, Salt Lake City, UT 84116-2889 and PMIC 4727 Wilshire Boulevard, Los Angeles, CA 90010.

Some computer programs provide codes automatically if a diagnosis is entered. In addition, natural language could be stored and retrieved without the use of codes. However, much confusion may arise if these capabilities are applied indiscriminately because of our often undisciplined use of medical terminology. Thus, the same term often is used for different conditions or one condition may have different names. Worse yet, diagnoses often are entirely descriptive ("swollen kidneys") and the proper diagnostic term ("acute renal allograft rejection") is not mentioned at all. In any event, encoded diagnoses should be reviewed by a physician knowledgeable in this field. Because this is rarely possible, it is probably best if the paramedical personnel charged with these duties encodes only familiar diagnoses, avoids the encoding of minutiae, and obtains consultations in doubtful cases.

It should be noted that encoding of well-defined diagnoses is valuable not just for data retrieval but also for ongoing clinical communication because the need to code enforces uniformity in the use of diagnostic designations, and exposes or even prevents the use of ambiguous language. This allows institutions to maintain an up-to-date terminology in all fields and, at the same time, prevent the use of obsolete names. Unfortunately, this added benefit of coding is seldom appreciated. Because it is unrealistic to expect detailed knowledge of the changing terminologies in all fields of pathology, coding manuals and computer programs are needed that suggest current names whenever an obsolete term is typed into the system.

QUALITY ASSURANCE

The Joint Commission of Accreditation of Health Care Organizations (JCAHO) and the College of American Pathologists (CAP) use the term *quality assurance* in a broader sense than the name *quality control*; the former refers to a professional activity of the supervising pathologists, whereas the latter refers to the specific mechanisms by which the concepts of quality assurance (QA) are put into effect *(19).* A review of the inspection checklists reflects these concepts. The lists cover questions related to the running and maintenance of the morgue and the autopsy and histopathology laboratories; they also refer to safety issues, record keeping, the interactions between staff and technicians, the quality of autopsy documents, and the timeliness of reporting. In short, the questions in the checklists that must be answered and evaluated before an autopsy service is accredited reflect the expectations of excellence as described in the CAP manual *(20)*.

Accreditation also requires that each service has an *intradepartmental* quality assurance program. Educational activities such as organ reviews and clinicopathologic conferences are part of such a program but also quality control of the autopsy itself *(21–26)*. This typically consists of a review of all autopsy documents and slides pertaining to a specified, randomly selected number of cases—for example, 5% of all autopsies. The review generally is the responsibility of another staff pathologists. A review form is filled out and filed. The reviewing pathologist states as a minimum whether he or she agrees with the diagnoses and the written communications such as letters to the clinician and next of kin, that were based on these diagnoses. Also evaluated are the histologic findings, the quality and number of slides, and the adequacy of microbiologic and other laboratory studies, and photographs. Finally, the reviewer evaluates whether protocol descriptions and clinical abstracts are complete and clear and whether documentation and reporting had been completed within the agreed-upon time limits *(27)*. Subspecialties such as neuropathology *(28)* and pediatric pathology *(29)* are developing their own QA programs.

Preliminary studies suggest that in general, a good agreement exists between pathologists in the diagnosis of the main diseases but that the agreement was less in the establishment of the immediate cause of death and in the diagnosis of minor diseases *(30)*. As one would expect, discrepancies between antemortem and postmortem diagnoses also tended to increase with the age of the patient *(31)*.

In addition to these intradepartmental QA activities, the autopsy findings also become an important part of *extradepartmental* quality assurance programs *(21,22,32)*, primarily in the departments of internal medicine and surgery. Because of sample-selection bias, this method must be applied with caution *(32)*. In institutions that use autopsies in this manner, the final autopsy diagnosis and a cover letter are sent to the clinicians who took care of the patient but also to the colleague who acts as clinical QA officer; that physician also receives a form that specifically addresses clinical QA issues, for example, if a major disease or condition had not been recognized. Timeliness of reporting is exceedingly important in this context *(27)*.

Review of autopsy services for accreditation purposes concentrates primarily on activities within the service. The reporting to clinical departments for external QA programs is also evaluated but the usage of the information by these departments is evaluated by their own accreditation procedures.

It should be noted that quality control needs to be applied not only to the original autopsy documents but also to the codes (generally ICD and SNOMED codes) that are generated from these documents.

REFERENCES

1. Saladino AJ, Dailey ML. The problem-oriented postmortem examination. Am J Pathol 1978;69:253–257.
2. Gravanis MB, Rietz CW. The problem-oriented postmortem examination and record: an educational challenge. Am J Clin Pathol 1973; 60:522–535.
3. Kircher T, Anderson RE. Cause of Death. Proper completion of the death certificate. JAMA 1987;258:349–352.
4. Orth J. Was ist Todesursache? Berl Klin Wochenschr 1908;45:485–490.
5. Hanzlick R. Principles for including or excluding ‘mechanisms’ of death when writing cause of death statements. Arch Pathol Lab Med 1997;121:377–380.
6. The Medical Cause of Death Manual: Instructions for Writing Cause of Death Statements for Deaths due to Natural Causes (Hanzlick K, ed.). College of American Pathologists, Northfield, IL, 1994.
7. U.S. National Center for Health Statistics, Public Health Service: Physicians’ Handbook on Medical Certification: Death, Fetal Death, Birth. (Publication No. 593-B). U.S. Government Printing Office, Washington, DC, 1967.
8. U.S. National Center for Health Statistics, Public Health Service: Medical Examiners’ and Coroners’ Handbook on Death and Fetal Death Registration. (Publication No. 593-D.) U.S. Government Printing Office, Washington, DC, 1967.
9. International Classification of Diseases. 9th Revision. Clinical Modification, 5th ed., vols. 1 & 2. Medicode, Inc. Salt Lake City, UT, 1998.
10. Physicians’ Current Procedural Terminology (cpt 98). Professional edition or Standard edition (Kirschner CG, ed.). American Medical Association. Practice Management Information Corporation, Los Angeles, CA, 1998.
11. Virchow R. Post-Mortem Examinations With Especial Reference to Medico-Legal Practice. Fourth German edition. (English translation by TP Smith.) P. Blakiston, Son & Co., Philadelphia, PA, 1885.
12. Helweg-Larsen K. Post-mortem protocol. Acta Paediatr 1993:389: 77–79.
13. Klatt EC. Voice-activated dictation for autopsy pathology. Computers Pathol Med 1991;21:429–433.
14. Matturi L, Barbolini G, Bauer D, Buffa D, Campesi G, Fante R, et al. A computer network-based system for local storage and nationwide processing of autopsy diagnoses. Int J Epidemiol 1989;18:720–722.
15. Ohtsubo K, Shibasaki K, Kawamura N, Shimada H. A pathology database system for autopsy diagnoses using free-text method. Med Informat 1992;17:47–52.
16. Moore GW, Berman JJ, Hanzlick RL, Buchino JJ, Hutchins GM. A prototype Internet autopsy database. 1625 consecutive fetal and neonatal autopsy face sheets spanning 20 years. Arch Pathol Lab Med 1996;120:782–785.
17. Coté RA, Rothwell DJ, Polotay JL, Beckett RS, eds. SNOMED International (Systematized Nomenclature of Human and Veterinary Medicine), 3rd ed, vol. I and II, Numeric Indices, vol. III and IV, Alphabetic Indices. College of American Pathologists, Chicago, 1993.
18. Moore WG, Berman JJ. Performance analysis of manual and automated systematized nomenclature of medicine (SNOMED) coding. Am J Clin Pathol 1994;101:253–256.
19. Peters HJ, Chandler AB. Quality control and assurance of the autopsy. In: Autopsy: performance and practice (Hutchins, ed.). College of American Pathologists, Northfield, IL, 1990.
20. College of American Pathologists. Inspection Checklist VIII: Anatomic Pathology and Cytology. Northfield, IL, 1988.
21. Anonymous. Recommendations on quality control and quality assurance in surgical pathology and autopsy pathology. The Association of Directors of Anatomic and Surgical Pathology. Mod Pathol 1992; 5:567–568.
22. Anderson RE, Hill RB, Gorstein F. A model for the autopsy-based quality assessment of medical diagnostics. Arch Pathol Lab Med 1990; 114:1163.

23. Kolmann E-W. Qualitätssicherung in der Pathologie. Pathologe 1991; 12:120–122. (Review)
24. Harrison M, Hourihane DO. Quality assurance programme for necropsies. J Clin Pathol 1989;42:1190–1193.
25. Deppich LM, ed. Surgical Pathology/Cytopathology Quality Assurance Manual. College of American Pathologists. Skokie, IL, 1988, p. 80.
26. Joint Commission of Accreditation of Healthcare Organizations. Quality Assurance and Risk Management in Hospital, Clinical, and Support Services. Chicago: The Commission, 2002.
27. Zarbo RJ, Baker PB, Howanitz PJ. Quality assurance of autopsy permit form information, timeliness of performance, and issuance of preliminary report. A College of American Pathologists Q-probes study of 5434 autopsies from 452 institutions. Arch Lab Med 1996; 120:346–352.
28. Pearl GS, Nelson JS. Continuous quality improvement (CQI) in neuropathology. J Neuropathol Exp Neurol 1996;55:875–879.
29. Rutledge JC. Quality assurance in pediatric anatomic pathology: the Society for Pediatric Pathology slide survey program. Pediatr Pathol Lab Med 1995;15:957–965.
30. Veress B, Gadaleanu V, Nennesmo I, Wikstrom BM. The reliability of autopsy diagnostics: inter-observer variation between pathologists, a preliminary report. Qual Assurance Health Care 1993;5:333–337.
31. Mitchell ML. Interdepartmental quality assurance using coded autopsy results. Mod Pathol 1993;6:48–52.
32. Saracci R. Problems with the use of autopsy results as a yardstick in medical audit and epidemiology. Qual Assurance Health Care 1993; 5:339–344.

18 Autopsy Law

VERNARD I. ADAMS AND JURGEN LUDWIG

In this chapter, general legal principles are discussed pertaining to autopsies in the United States. Pathologists should familiarize themselves with the laws that govern the performance of autopsies in the states in which they practice. Laws governing autopsies in other nations vary widely *(1)*, and are beyond the scope of this chapter.

AUTOPSIES BY STATUTE

AUTHORIZATION In most states, autopsies in cases of suspicious death are authorized by medical examiners or coroners. Many states also invest this authority in county physicians; coroners' physicians; coroners' juries; justices of the peace; local magistrates; attorneys general; and district, state, and prosecuting attorneys. In a few instances, autopsies may be ordered by the sheriff or county manager.

Outside the military services, no federal law exists that supersedes state authority to order autopsies or move bodies. Within the United States, military law, not state law, applies on military bases with exclusive federal jurisdiction. Some installations have concurrent jurisdiction or partial legislative jurisdiction. Medical examiners or coroners who have military bases within their areas of jurisdiction can contact the Directorate of Engineering and Housing and the legal office at the military base to determine the style of jurisdiction *(2)*.

The Federal Bureau of Investigation (FBI) is charged by federal law with the investigation of the death of a President or other specified dignitaries, and as such displaces the sheriff or police department who would ordinarily conduct a criminal death investigation. Although this law has no provision that overrides the authority of the local medical examiner or coroner to move or autopsy the body, it has been so interpreted.

A statutory autopsy may be performed without the consent or even against the expressed will of the surviving spouse or next of kin, but there should be reasonable grounds, usually specified by statute, for a medical examiner or coroner to authorize such an autopsy.

OBJECTIONS TO STATUTORY AUTOPSIES Objections based on religious views must be handled with sensitivity. In Miami, FL, the Orthodox Rabbinical Council has rabbis who are specifically delegated to attend autopsies; they discuss the procedures to keep them to the minimum needed to serve the public interest *(3)*. This usually entails the use of *in situ* dissection as much as possible. The State of New York now has a statute that requires a hearing before a judge if there is a religious objection to statutory autopsy. In these cases, the judge decides if there will be an autopsy *(4)*. California, Louisiana, New Jersey, New York State, Ohio, and Rhode Island have restricted the discretion of medical examiners to order autopsies in the face of religious objections *(5)*. Sensitivity in these situations can mean delaying the autopsy until the family members had time to discuss the matter and consult with an attorney, or it can mean omitting the autopsy when the public interest is outweighed by the religious objection, as in the case of a fractured femoral neck from a fall at home.

WHO MAY PERFORM AN AUTOPSY? In most states, autopsies conducted pursuant to statute may be performed by medical examiners and their deputies, coroners (if they are physicians), and coroners' physicians, county physicians and their deputies, or other designated physicians. Autopsies performed outside the purview of medical examiner or coroner statutes are conducted by permission of the person who claims the remains for burial (*see* below).

WHEN AND WHERE STATUTORY AUTOPSIES MAY BE PERFORMED In most instances, statutes authorize autopsies when the medical examiner or coroner deems them necessary as part of the statutory duty to determine the cause of death. This duty generally arises when death has resulted from violence (homicide, suicide, or accident) or from unlawful or criminal means. Some state laws require the medical examiner to determine the cause of death when death has occurred in a penal institution, has been caused by criminal abortion, or involves a possible threat to the public health, or when cremation is intended. In some states, statute or administrative code requires autopsies in certain types of deaths, such as the sudden infant death syndrome.

Statutes in some states also authorize an autopsy when the death took place without an eyewitness, when the decedent was not attended by a physician at the time of death, when death was sudden and unexplained, or when the death was of unknown cause.

SOURCE MATERIAL The laws governing medicolegal autopsies vary greatly from state to state. An excellent compi-

From: *Handbook of Autopsy Practice,* 3rd Ed. Edited by: J. Ludwig © Humana Press Inc., Totowa, NJ

lation of the medicolegal autopsy laws of the 50 states, the District of Columbia, and the territories of the United States has been published by the Centers for Disease Control (CDC) *(6)*. This publication also lists addresses, and telephone numbers of medical examiners and coroners.

AUTOPSIES BY PERMISSION

PERSONS WHO REQUEST AUTOPSY PERMISSION

Typically, clinical residents or staff physicians will ask the next of kin to authorize an autopsy. In some institutions, specially trained technicians from the autopsy service or transplant-service coordinators assume this task *(7)*. Although autopsy permission usually must be requested at what appears to be the most inappropriate time for the next of kin, a tactful explanation of the benefits for the family of the deceased and for other patients will usually be successful in securing permission. In institutions without such persons, a physician should seek permission for autopsy.

WHEN IS AN AUTOPSY INDICATED? Ideally, autopsy permission should be obtained in all deaths because: 1) for reliable data analysis, number of cases should be large and the selection as random as possible; and 2) the most interesting and important findings may be totally unexpected and thus are often missed if authorization is requested only for defined groups of deceased patients. However, despite these compelling reasons to request autopsy permission in every case, financial, legal, and other constraints often cause institutions to seek autopsy permission only under specific circumstances. Thus, the College of American Pathologists *(8)* recommends including in such a list: 1) unknown or unanticipated complications; 2) unknown causes of death; 3) special concerns of the next of kin or the public; 4) deaths following diagnostic procedures and therapeutic interventions; 5) deaths of patients who have participated in clinical trials; 6) natural deaths that were under the jurisdiction of the medical examiner or some equivalent official who then decided not to do the autopsy; 7) deaths that may have resulted from environmental or occupational hazards; 8) deaths resulting from high-risk infectious and contagious diseases; 9) all obstetric deaths; 10) all neonatal and pediatric deaths; and 11) deaths in which it is believed that autopsy would disclose a known or suspected illness that may have a bearing on survivors or recipients of transplant organs. It should be noted that deaths in some of these examples may fall under the jurisdiction of the medical examiner.

PERSONS WHO MAY AUTHORIZE AUTOPSY The right to grant, restrict, or withhold authorization for an autopsy rests with the surviving spouse or, if there is no surviving spouse, the next of kin. In the absence of known kin, autopsy permission may often be granted by the person who has custody of the body. Although a dead human body is not property in the commercial sense and may not be bargained for, bartered, or sold, there is a right, protected by law, to possess the body for the purpose of burying it *(9–11)*. Authorization of an autopsy should be documented on an appropriate form (Fig. 18-1).

Surviving Spouse The wishes of the surviving spouse clearly override those of the next of kin *(10)*. However, divorce terminates the spouse's authority. Separated couples are considered legally married; a separated surviving spouse has the same right to claim the remains as does a cohabiting spouse. In other words, "separated" is a living arrangement, not a civil status.

Next of Kin The order of priority may or may not be specified by statute in any given state, either under autopsy law or under the funeral directing act or the probate act. The following order often applies:

1. Children of the deceased, if they are of age;
2. Grandchildren of the deceased, if they are of age;
3. Parents;
4. Brothers and sisters;
5. Cousins, nieces, nephews, grandparents, uncles, and aunts (local law should be consulted with regard to right to consent and priority). Of course, if the next of kin are that far removed in degree, competing claims would be unusual.
6. Friends or any person of legal age who assumes responsibility for the burial. The institution or person obtaining permission may ask for an affidavit stating the facts of the friendship or other relation, and stating that the person in question will assume the costs of the burial.

Persons Entitled by Statute Autopsy authorization in medicolegal cases and under related circumstances is discussed in the beginning of this chapter. In addition, statutes in some states provide that hospitals or physicians may give permission for an autopsy on a body if it is to be buried at public expense when no one is known who would be legally entitled to take custody of the body for burial *(12)*. Autopsies may be done on such bodies or they may be surrendered to established medical or dental schools for scientific studies. In all these instances, reasonable efforts must be made over a specified period to communicate with relatives or friends who might want to assume custody of the body and the costs of burial. Most hospitals are reluctant to exercise this option and will refer such cases to the medical examiner.

Authorization by institutional officers may be contested unless the procedures outlined in the statute are followed carefully. Some state workmen's compensation laws provide statutory immunity for autopsies performed by order of the Industrial Commission. However, unless so provided by statute, courts have held that the economic interest of the insurance carrier involved in a workmen's compensation claim is not sufficient to override the refusal of the next of kin to grant autopsy permission *(13)*. Another authority states that policies giving a life insurer the right to have an autopsy performed are valid in the absence of a statute to the contrary; and that refusal by the next of kin to permit an autopsy constitutes breach of policy *(14)*.

In most states, a decision made by the person having the *highest priority* is binding and may not be overruled by persons with lower priority. If several persons have an equal degree of kinship, some statutes state that permission of only one such person is required *(15)*. When acting on the authority of such a person, it would be wise to obtain a statement that this person is acting on behalf of all members of the group.

Permission for Postmortem Examination

Postmortem Examination: (Read to or have next of kin, guardian, conservator or health care agent or proxy read) study of the cause of death and the interrelations between the various organs of the body is useful in furthering medical science. Future generations may be helped by scientific discoveries made from postmortem examinations. An examination will not delay funeral arrangements or cause additional expenses to the family.

Marital Status (circle correct status): Married Divorced Widowed Never married

☐ Postmortem examination is authorized by advance directive dated: ______________
(But if next of kin, guardian, conservator or health care agent or proxy decline postmortem examination, it must be documented below.)

☐ Permission is granted for **postmortem examination** on the remains of the deceased, including removal and retention of such organs or body parts and organ/tissue as may be used for appropriate diagnostic, educational, and scientific purposes (subject to restrictions listed below).

Are there any restrictions? ______________

____

____

______________ ______________ ______________
Signature of relative or guardian Relationship to deceased Date

☐ Permission granted by telephone recording ______________
Name of family member contacted

☐ Permission refused

If permission is refused or not requested, (e.g., medical contraindication, family refused, coroner case, other)

____

____

______________ ______________
Signature of physician or health care professional requesting permission **Date**

Letter regarding autopsy results to be sent to: **Name** ______________

Address ______________

Fig. 18-1. Mayo Clinic Autopsy Authorization Form. This form is part of a larger document that also contains: 1) the clinician's summary of the clinical course; 2) check boxes to indicate the manner of death—for example, "natural" or "suicide"; 3) a statement that federal law requires all deaths to be reported to a donation agency and how to contact such an agency; 4) provisions concerning funeral arrangements; and 5) detailed instructions for proper completion of the document.

Permission From Decedent In many states, a person may authorize an autopsy on himself or herself but in some of these states, co-consent of the surviving spouse is required. Persons may, under the Uniform Anatomical Gift Act, donate their remains to an institution for the sole purpose of performing an autopsy *(16)*. In the absence of state law permitting kin to override such a consent, the permission is binding on the surviving kin. However, we would recommend not to rely on such a permission in the face of objections from the next of kin who are claiming the remains.

CUSTODY ISSUES In general, it seems prudent to delay an autopsy whenever the right to custody of a body seems questionable and a risk of litigation exists. In the authors' experience, custody issues sort themselves out with time. Commonly, the claimant with the best legal claim lacks funds to bury the body and yields to a claimant with lower priority but greater financial resources. Unfortunately, such delays decrease the likelihood that permission for an autopsy can be obtained.

PERMISSION FOR SPECIAL PROCEDURES Authorization for an autopsy without specified restrictions is given with the understanding that the autopsy will be carried out in the usual manner—that is, the chest and abdomen may be examined and the brain and the neck organs may be removed. For any procedures requiring additional incisions, particularly of the face, neck, or hands (*see* Chapter 1), or that may interfere with proper reconstruction, such as total removal of the spinal column (*see* Chapter 6), it seems prudent to secure a special permission specifying the nature of the intended maneuver. This also holds true for removal of the eyes (*see* Chapter 7). A medical examiner or coroner who intends to perform these extended procedures must be sure that they serve the public interest and are not conducted solely for research or educational purposes.

AUTOPSY TECHNIQUES AND THE WORK OF THE FUNERAL DIRECTOR In order to maintain good professional relationships, extended autopsy procedures should be discussed with the funeral director first and every effort should be made to avoid interfering with the embalming. Funeral directors who understand and support the objectives of the autopsy may be expected to make their skills available when defects from extended autopsies must be reconstructed or when an occasional technical mishap must be repaired. Such goodwill requires that prosectors help the funeral director by identifying the vessels needed for arterial embalming. As described in Chapter 1, this can be accomplished by placing clearly visible ligatures around the carotid, axillary, and femoral arteries. If it is necessary to remove these arteries for examination or if there is a risk that they might be damaged during dissection on an extremity, the dissection procedure should be done in the funeral home, after embalming. Proper procedures for removal of the brain, dissection at the base of the skull, and removal of the eyes are described in Chapters 6 and 7, respectively. It is obvious that technical mishaps in the head area are particularly distressing. Finally, prosectors should be reminded to make complete slices through liver, lungs, and other solid organs so that slices are not connected by narrow bridges that can break and cause specimens to drop and spatter.

In areas with vigorous organ- and tissue-procurement agencies, complaints by funeral directors related to organ donation generally are limited to genuine grievances. Preparing a body for viewing after harvesting of long bones is considered more challenging than preparing a body that has been autopsied.

RESTRICTED AUTHORIZATION FOR AUTOPSY The place, manner, and extent of the autopsy may be restricted, for any reason, by the person who has the right to refuse an autopsy *(17)*. Restrictions regarding the place of autopsy generally are intended to secure privacy which is discussed in the next section. The *extent* of the autopsy may be restricted to the abdominal or chest cavity, to exploration through an operative incision, or to inspection of organs without permission to remove samples for histologic study, to name only a few examples. Whether an autopsy should be done at all under such circumstances must be carefully considered by the pathologist because restricted examinations may lead to highly misleading results—for example, if potentially fatal coronary artery disease is found but a ruptured berry aneurysm is not detected because no permission had been obtained to inspect the cranial cavity.

WHO MAY WATCH AN AUTOPSY? Privacy issues must be considered if persons other than physicians are allowed to view an autopsy. Policies in this regard vary widely. In some institutions, only physicians and medical students are allowed to view autopsies because of unwelcome experiences with curiosity seekers and the resulting gossip. Others consider the educational value worthwhile and will admit nurses, law enforcement officers, or other persons who have a plausible professional relationship. Such sessions should be scheduled and the professional relationships of all attendees should be scrutinized in each instances. A compromise between the opposing views in this matter is to admit nurses and other qualified persons in the medical field to organ reviews rather than the autopsy itself.

UNAUTHORIZED AUTOPSIES AND INSURANCE ISSUES The performance of an unauthorized autopsy or the violation of an autopsy restriction may be construed as mutilation of the dead body. The survivors may claim that this has caused them mental anguish *(18)*. Damages are collectible without proof of physical injury to the claimant. The proper party claimant, and the person to recover for the mutilation of the dead body, generally would be the one who had rightful custody of the body and therefore had the right to restrict or withhold authorization for the autopsy.

Many insurance policies providing indemnity of accidental death contain clauses that give the insurer the right to demand an autopsy. However, as mentioned in the context of workmen's compensation claims, the economic interest of the insurance carrier does not override the right of the surviving spouse or the next of kin to control the disposition of the body *(13)*. The pathologist should insist on proper authorization from the next of kin. In many instances, the cases can be referred to the medical examiner or coroner because almost all medical examiner enabling statutes include deaths by accident.

RETENTION OF ORGANS AND TISSUES FOR STUDY Temporary removal of organs and tissues for histologic study is accepted as a normal part of the autopsy *(13)*. It appears reasonable to include here related procedures such as organ angiography. Permanent retention of entire organs may not be contemplated by the next of kin and thus, the authorization that has been obtained should be broad enough to permit the procedure. Most permission forms used by hospitals have a specific clause that grants permission to retain tissues for the purposes of education and research. In the absence of such a clause, the organs should be returned to the body; permanent retention of organs without permission is actionable *(19)*. After autopsies performed pursuant to statute, tissues may only be retained if this is in the public interest—for example, for cause of death determination, for identification purposes, and as evidence for testing by defense experts.

AUTOPSY CONSENT FORM Permission forms must be consistent with local law and should be reviewed or developed with counsel. Inclusion of the following provisions has been recommended *(20)*:

1. The adjective "complete" modifying the word autopsy to establish consent for procedures not specifically excluded.
2. The nature and number of attendees to be left to the discretion of the physician.
3. The discretion to retain organs and tissues for study or research and to dispose of them in an appropriate and lawful way.
4. A section affording the opportunity to restrict the autopsy or add special instructions.
5. A statement that the grantor of consent has been afforded the opportunity to ask questions, and that the questions have been answered satisfactorily.
6. Name, address, and signature of grantor of consent, date of signature, and relationship to decedent.
7. Signatures of the person obtaining the consent and of a witness.
8. Other provisions to meet the requirements of local statutes.

DONATION OF BODY, ORGANS, AND TISSUES A number of states have enacted laws permitting the donation of dead bodies or parts of them by will. Authorization forms for the use of tissues and organs, including eyes, are available from regional organ procurement organizations, such as "Life Source," the Upper Midwest Organ Procurement Organization and the Minnesota Lions Eye Bank. Anatomical bequest forms vary from institution to institution but generally follow the terms of the Uniform Anatomical Gift Act. Under these terms, an institution also may reject a body, for example, if it is decomposed and thus not suitable for anatomic study. All states now have adopted the Uniform Anatomical Gift Act in some form *(21)*. Under the provisions of this act, a small card, signed by the deceased and two witnesses, is a legal document providing for the donation of organs for transplantation purposes or for the donation of the body for anatomical study, or for both. The card also has a space in which limitations of its provisions or special wishes may be entered. A driver's license also may indicate that the owner agrees to be an organ donor. The Anatomical Gift Act clarifies priorities of persons who may consent to the donation of a body for educational or research purposes or for the donation of specific organs and tissues for transplantation. Information on related topics is provided in refs. *(22–26)*. In reality, the organ- and tissue-procurement agencies always obtain permission from the next of kin and use the donor cards only as evidence of the intentions of the decedent during discussion with the next of kin.

If deaths come under the jurisdiction of the medical examiner or coroner, the organ-procurement agency must obtain permission from these officials, in addition to the permission from the next of kin. In the department of the first author (V.I.A.), it is rare for the medical examiner to deny permission for organ harvest. Flexibility of both parties makes this possible. Thus, the organ-procurement team will do studies such as coronary angiography if they are requested by the medical examiner. The medical examiner will sometimes perform an external inspection at the hospital or attend the subsequent surgical harvesting. Fortunately, the likelihood of a murder prosecution failing because organ harvesting has been permitted is minimal if the medical examiner is an experienced witness. To help a pathologist with little court experience, the prosecutor, at the expense of his office, may bring in another expert.

Some states have a provision in law that permits a medical examiner or coroner to donate *corneas* if the next of kin cannot be located after reasonable efforts to do so. However, medical records must be reviewed in such instances to ascertain that they do not contain objections to such a donation. If this is not done, the official may be liable *(5)*.

PREVENTION OF WRONGFUL AUTOPSY

The following three steps should be taken by the pathologist and not delegated to other personnel.

1. Contact the medical examiner or coroner if the jurisdiction of a case is in doubt.
2. Review all name tags and identification bracelets to ascertain that the body is in fact the one for which an autopsy permission has been granted. The apparent age, sex, wounds, and therapeutic apparatuses should be consistent with the information available in the medical history. A pathologist may be found liable for an unauthorized autopsy unless it can be proven that the actions did not result from negligence *(13)*.
3. If a body is released from a hospital to the medical examiner or coroner, it appears advisable to notify the next of kin that the office has custody of the body, particularly if review of the records indicates any objections to an autopsy. The medical examiner or coroner also must be informed about such an objection, otherwise the hospital might be held liable *(5)*. The possibility that the medical examiner or coroner would have done the autopsy anyway does not change the need for such communication.
4. Ascertain that the autopsy authorization form is properly completed and signed. Possible restrictions must be noted and conveyed to technicians, residents, or other persons who might help with the autopsy. If a signed authorization form is not used, a form containing all pertinent information should, nevertheless, be used to avoid errors and misunderstandings.

DEATH CERTIFICATES AND AUTOPSY PROTOCOLS: ADMISSIBILITY AS EVIDENCE

The death certificate is a public record. In almost all states a certified copy is admissible in court as evidence that death in fact occurred. In some but not all states, the cause of death opinion on the certificate is similarly admitted. Autopsy protocols and diagnoses may or may not be admitted into evidence, depending on the state concerned. In most states, the protocols and diagnoses are not admissible by themselves as evidence. Rather, an expert who may or may not be the autopsy pathologist who signed the report, must give opinions under oath. This allows for cross examination, which is a right of the defendant in the USA in criminal cases. Hospital records, including autopsy records, may be treated as business records, that is, the physician may rely on this material as foundation for opinions and the hearsay rule does not apply. In medical malpractice suits, the testimony of the autopsy pathologist may be taken in deposition but if there is a trial, the courtroom testimony will be provided by hired experts for the plaintiff and the defense. If no deposition was given, the hospital pathologist may never be aware that the autopsy played a role in a lawsuit. Autopsy pathologists, like other expert witnesses, are allowed to refer to their file notes and reports when testifying *(27,28)*.

CONFIDENTIALITY OF AUTOPSY RECORDS In most jurisdictions, information gained at autopsy is not privileged because a dead body is not considered a patient. Under common law, no rights of confidentiality relate to a dead body but codified law (statute) may change this rule. Restrictions to the release of autopsy records may exist. For example, in the State of New York, medical examiner autopsy reports are available only to the district attorney, the next of kin, and anyone with a court order. In any event, a physician who discloses autopsy findings must be careful not to reveal facts that he or she learned during the patient's life while a professional relationship existed between the patient and the physician *(27,29)*.

Diagnoses or opinions concerning autopsy findings frequently are sought by private insurance carriers. Generally, such information should be released only after a signed authorization has been obtained from the person who had custody of the body and who gave permission for the autopsy. However, if the autopsy was performed pursuant to statute in a state with a "sunshine" public records law, the autopsy report is considered a public record unless it concerns an active criminal investigation or related exceptions *(30)*.

The foremost reason for the surviving spouses or the next of kin to authorize autopsies is their desire to have the findings explained to them, either in an interview or in writing. Recommendations for such interviews have been described in detail in Chapter 16. As stated, care must be taken that the findings are disclosed primarily to the individual who had custody of the body and therefore, interviews should be conducted in person rather than by phone. With consent from the custodian of the body, an interview may be held with a friend of the family or their clergyman. Letters with autopsy findings must be addressed to the surviving spouse or the next of kin who had custody of the body.

Medical examiners or coroners sometimes receive requests from the spouse or next of kin to do an autopsy because of some suspicion of malpractice and the fear that the hospital pathologist might not render an independent opinion. An example would be the request to do an autopsy to determine if a decedent received an overdose of a particular drug 2 wk prior to death. Although the autopsy may not answer the posed question, it still makes the requestors feel that they obtained information concerning the medical care.

Statutory autopsies also may be explained to relatives of the deceased. If such autopsies involve criminal cases, the prosecuting attorney or lead detective should be consulted first. Interviews concerning autopsies in criminal cases should be limited to the cause of death opinion as it appears on the death certificate. In suicide or accident cases it seems humane not to elaborate on suffering that the deceased may have endured. In homicide cases, that opinion is best reserved for trial. Testimony that pain and suffering occurred may affect the penalty.

TRANSPORTATION OF BODIES

Autopsy pathologists should be familiar with the laws concerning the transportation of bodies in or from their state by motor vehicle, aircraft or other means. In Minnesota, regulations specify that the remains of the dead must be properly embalmed if they are shipped by public transportation *(31)*. Transportation permits must be issued for each body by local or state registrars. The signatures of the embalmer, the registrar, and the person in charge of the conveyance are required on the transportation permit. Burial and transportation permits are delivered with the body to the person in charge of the cemetery or to the health officer in cities that have local ordinances requiring burial permits by this official.

In Florida, the business of transporting dead bodies is regulated by the Health Department but the transporters are not required to have funeral director licenses, as they are in Massachusetts, to name an example. Relatives can convey remains of loved ones from a Florida hospital or medical examiners morgue. There is no requirement to embalm before transportation. Death certificates are not required for transportation to the site of disposition, but burial permits are required. Any subregistrar of the vital records office may issue burial permits. Most licensed funeral directors are also subregistrars, and all medical examiners offices have one person who is a subregistrar.

If a body is to be shipped out of the country, the pathologist is often asked by the funeral director to supply a letter stating that the autopsy showed no evidence of any infectious or communicable diseases. The letter should have enough identifying information such as name and date of death to match it to the death certificate or transit permit, but need not offer any cause of death opinion. The following letter represents a useful sample.

"To Whom it may Concern:
[Name of deceased] died on [month, day, year]. The autopsy revealed no evidence of any communicable or infectious disease. The remains may be transported out of the country.
[Name of physician], M.D.
[Function of physician, such as "Associate Medical Examiner"]"

Each state has regulations concerning embalming, caskets, containers, transportation, and disinterment. These regulations are the province of the funeral director.

Final disposition of the body is by burial, cremation, and, uncommonly, burial at sea or donation for anatomic dissection. Removal of a body from the state is considered a form of disposition as far as state health departments are concerned. The bone fragments left after cremation are ground into small pieces to help perpetuate the illusion of ashes; this material, known as cremains, is not subject to state rules pertaining to disposition of human bodies. However, some municipalities have enacted ordinances to regulate and reduce the numbers of bone fragments strewn from airplanes, bridges, and water craft.

EMBALMING

In the United States, embalming is a widely practiced procedure. An important exception involves the burial practices of Orthodox Judaism *(32)* which forbids embalming and application of cosmetics. For the transportation of bodies, embalming sometimes is required by state law. For example, in Minnesota, embalming is required unless the person dead of a noncommunicable disease is buried within 72 h after death. In Florida, embalming is not required at all.

Embalming consists of arterial infusion of embalming fluid and trocar perforation of the viscera. In bodies without extensive postmortem clotting, the arterial infusion is typically through a right subclavian skin incision, with access to the right common carotid artery after division of the sternocleidomastoid muscle. If bodies do not perfuse well, the brachial arteries may be accessed through axillary incisions, or the femoral arteries may be accessed through incisions below the inguinal ligaments. After autopsy, the aortic arch vessels and the external iliac arteries can be accessed directly.

In the second stage of embalming, a trocar is used to perforate the left side of the abdomen, and then to aspirate any liquids from the chest, abdomen, and pelvis, followed by infusion of embalming fluid. Arterial embalming fluid contains methanol, formalin, and orange dye. Trocar work is not necessary after autopsy.

EXHUMATION

Exhumation requests most often come from surviving relatives who want to move the remains to another burial site or who want to cremate long-buried remains. In criminal investigations, exhumation is unusual, and in the absence of permission from the surviving spouse or next of kin requires a court order. Such an order must be based on the reasonable expectation that the examination will yield important evidence for the prosecution or the defense of a criminal charge. In areas with competent medicolegal systems, the majority of such exhumations will be for suspected poisoning. A policy of retaining toxicology specimens on all deaths that come under medical examiner or coroner jurisdiction can reduce the number of exhumations. Of course, this policy does not address the cases that were never referred to these officials.

In areas with low rates of medicolegal autopsies, exhumation may be for the purpose of performing a primary autopsy to detect a homicide that may have been masquerading as an accident or a suicide. Or, exhumation may be to identify the decedent, to develop evidence in a medical malpractice case, or to search for lost objects. In one instance, a body was exhumed to complete an autopsy in which neck organs or cranial contents had not been removed *(33)*. Thus, autopsies on exhumed bodies may be done both in criminal and in civil court cases.

State laws define who may authorize disinterment and under what circumstances this may be done. If the exhumation is pursuant to court order, the prosecuting attorney or civil attorney with the interest in the exhumation will draw up the order, and make application to a court. If the judge approves, he merely signs the order prepared by the attorney. The interested parties, including the pathologist, will normally be informed about date, time, and other particulars before the order is signed. After the autopsy, the remains are re-interred, the pathologist prepares a report, and makes copies as he would for a routine autopsy.

The principal participants in an exhumation are the petitioner, the cemetery director, the funeral director, and the pathologist. For the pathologist, the procedures differ little from those used in any other autopsy. The pathologist's assistant usually has to remove the remains from the casket, undress them, and redress them after the autopsy. The funeral director arranges with the cemetery director for the timely arrival of the back hoe operator and the diggers, both for disinterment and re-interment.

REFERENCES

1. Svendsen E, Hill RB. Autopsy legislation and practice in various countries. Arch Pathol Lab Med 1987;111:846–850.
2. Shemonsky NK, Reiber KB, Williams LD, Froede RC. Jurisdiction on military installations. Am J Forens Med Pathol 1993;14:39–42.
3. Mittleman RE, Davis JH, Kasztl W, Graves WM Jr. Practical approach to investigative ethics and religious objections to the autopsy. J Forens Sci 1992;37:824–829.
4. McKinney's Consolidated Laws of New York, Annotated, Book 44, Public Health Law, Section 4210-C. West Publishing Co., St. Paul, MN, 1998.
5. Bierig JR. A potpourri of legal issues relating to the autopsy. Arch Pathol Lab Med 1996;120:759–762.
6. Combs DL, Parrish RG, Ing R. Death Investigation in the United States and Canada, 1990. Department of Health and Human Services, Public Health Service, Centers for Disease Control, Atlanta, GA, August 1990.
7. Haque AK. Decedent affairs office. In: Hutchins GM, ed. Autopsy. Performance & Reporting. College of American Pathologists, Northfield, IL, 1990, pp. 46–49.
8. CAP Board of Governors. Criteria for autopsies. In: Hutchins GM, ed. Autopsy. Performance & Reporting. College of American Pathologists, Northfield, IL, 1990, p. 24.
9. Waldman MJ. Dead bodies. In: VanKnapp DP, ed. American Jurisprudence, 2nd ed., vol. 22A, The Lawyers Cooperative Publishing Co., Rochester, NY, and Bancroft Whitney, San Francisco. 1988.
10. Waldman MJ. 22A Am Jur 2d, § 86.
11. MacDonald MG, Meyer KC, Essig B. Health Care Law: A Practical Guide. §20.06 [2] [a] Matthew Bender, New York, 1985.
12. MacDonald MG, Meyer KC, Essig B. Health Care Law: A Practical Guide. §20.06 [2] [b][v] Matthew Bender, New York, 1985.
13. Holder AR. Unauthorized autopsies. JAMA 1970;214:967–968.
14. Johnson SL, Linden DA, Miller MD, Sakamoto CD, Wishaud B. 44 Am Jur 2d, § 1367, 1368.
15. MacDonald MG, Meyer KC, Essig B. Health Care Law: A Practical Guide. §20.06 [2] [b] [iv]. Matthew Bender, New York, 1985.
16. MacDonald MG, Meyer KC, Essig B. Health Care Law: A Practical Guide. §20.06 [2] [b] [ii]. Matthew Bender, New York, 1985.
17. Waldman MJ. 22A Am Jur 2d, §64.
18. Waldman MJ. 22A Am Jur 2d, §152.
19. MacDonald MG, Meyer KC, Essig B. Health Care Law: A Practical Guide. §20.06 [2] [b] [vi]. Matthew Bender, New York, 1985.
20. MacDonald MG, Meyer KC, Essig B. Health Care Law: A Practical Guide. §20.06 [2] [d]. Matthew Bender, New York, 1985.
21. Waldman MJ. 22A Am Jur 2d, §119.
22. Taylor RJ, Engelsgjerd JS. Contemporary criteria for cadaveric organ donation in renal transplantation: the need for better selection parameters. World J Urol 1996;14:225–229.
23. Arnold RM, Yougner SJ. Time is of the essence: the pressing need for comprehensive non-heart-beating cadaveric donation policies. Transpl Proc 1995;27:2913–2917.
24. Cutler JA, David SD, Kress CJ, Stocks LM, Lewino DM, Fellows GL, et al. Increasing the availability of cadaveric organs for transplantation maximizing the consent rate. Transplantation 1993;56: 225–228.
25. Anaise D, Rapaport FT. Use of non-heart-beating cadaver donors in clinical organ transplantation: logistics, ethics, and legal considerations. Transpl Proc 1993;25:2153–2155.
26. Mohacsi PJ, Thompson JF. The organisation of cadaver multiple organ donation: a critical issue for establishing and maintaining successful transplantation programs. Transpl Proc 1992;24:2046.
27. Chayet NL. Autopsy protocols: confidentiality and admissibility. N Engl J Med 1964;271:728–729.
28. Sagall EL, Reed BC. Documentary evidence; autopsy reports. In: The Heart and the Law: A Practical Guide to Medicolegal Cardiology. Macmillan, New York, 1968, pp. 256–262.
29. Rose EF. Pathology reports and autopsy protocols: confidentiality, privilege, and accessibility. Am J Clin Pathol 1972;57:144–155.
30. Chapter 119, Florida Statutes.
31. Statute 149A, Ruke 4610, State of Minnesota law and rule governing mortuary science (149A.93, Subd. 9). 1997.
32. Hershey N. Who may authorize an autopsy? Am J Nursing 1963;63: 103–105.
33. Eckert WG, Katchis GS, James S. Disinterments: their value and associated problems. Am J Forens Med Pathol 1990;11:9–16.

19 The State of Autopsy Practice

An Annotated Bibliography

Many articles, workshop proceedings, editorials, and letters have been published that bemoan the continued decline of autopsy rates. A detailed review of these issues is beyond the scope of this book. However, a condensed annotated bibliography, presented in the next paragraphs, should provide readers with easy access to important publications revolving around the past and future roles of autopsies.

HISTORY OF THE AUTOPSY

1. Hill RL, Anderson RE. The recent history of the autopsy. Arch Pathol Lab Med 1996;120:702–712. *(A condensed description of the evolution of autopsy pathology during the last 400 years.)*

DOCUMENTING THE VALUE OF AUTOPSIES

1. Hill RL, Anderson RE. The recent history of the autopsy. Arch Pathol Lab Med 1996;120:702–712. *(Contains a detailed tabulation of diseases discovered or critically clarified through autopsy since 1950.)*
2. Cartlidge PH, Dawson AT, Stewart JH, Vujanic GM. Value and quality of perinatal and infant postmortem examinations: cohort analysis of 400 consecutive deaths. BMJ 1995; 310:155–158. *(The clinicopathological classification was altered by necropsy in 13% of the cases and new information was obtained in 60%.)*
3. Hagerstrand I, Lundberg LM. The importance of post-mortem examinations of abortions and perinatal deaths. Qual Assurance Health Care 1993;5:295–297. *(Major diseases and cause of death were identified at autopsy in 25% of the cases.)*
4. Hill RB. The current status of autopsies in medical care in the USA. Qual Assurance Health Care 1993;5:309–313. *(Review of values and initiatives to improve autopsy rates.)*
5. Stambouly JJ, Kahn E, Boxer RA. Correlation between clinical diagnoses and autopsy findings in critically ill children. Pediatrics 1993;92:248–251. *(Unexpected autopsy findings in 10% of the cases which, if known prior to death, would have altered clinical management and might have improved survival.)*
6. Kay MH, Moodie DS, Sterba R, Murphy DJ Jr, Rosenkranz E, Ratliff N, Homa A. The value of the autopsy in congenital heart disease. Clin Pediatr 1991;30:450–454. *(Eight percent of the patients had one missed major diagnosis but this would not have affected survival.)*
7. Nemetz PN, Ludwig J, Kurland AT. Assessing the autopsy. Am J Pathol 1987;128:362–379. *(Review of benefits provided by autopsies, including epidemiologic research.)*
8. Goldman L, Sayson R, Robbins S, Cohn LH, Bettmann M, Weisberg M. The value of the autopsy in three medical eras. N Engl J Med 1983;308:1000–1005. *(Advances in diagnostic technology have not reduced the value of the autopsy.)*
9. Welsh TSA, Kaplan J. The role of postmortem examination in medical education. Mayo Clin Proc 1998;73:802–805. *(Recommendations for an autopsy curriculum in postgraduate training are presented.)*

DOCUMENTATION OF DECLINING AUTOPSY RATES

1. Landers S, MacPherson T. Prevalence of the neonatal autopsy: a report of the study group for complications of perinatal Care. Pediatr Pathol Lab Med 1995;15:539–545. *(Low autopsy rate was not influenced by the type of medical center.)*
2. Stolman CJ, Castello F, Yorio M, Mautone S. Attitudes of pediatricians and pediatric residents toward obtaining permission for autopsy. Arch Pediatr Adolesc Med 1994;148: 843–847. *(Failure to obtain autopsy permission related to lack of exposure to autopsies during training, the fear that families might become upset, and the conviction that the autopsy will yield little useful information.)*
3. Favara BE, Cottreau C, McIntyre L, Valdes-Dapena M. Pediatric pathology and the autopsy. Pediatr Pathol 1989;9: 109–116. *(Autopsy rate in 25 childrens' hospitals was about 25%. Strategies for improvement are discussed.)*

AUTOPSY COSTS

1. Jason DR, Lantz PE, Preisser JS. A national survey of autopsy costs and workload. J Forensic Sci 1997;42:270–275. *(The average fee for medicolegal autopsies was $518. Overall, no major premium was paid* for Board qualification of the pathologists conducting the autopsy.)

2. O'Leary DS. Relating autopsy requirements to the contemporary accreditation process. 1996;120:763–766. *(A plea to provide more funds for autopsy services.)*
3. Chernof D. The role of managed health care organizations in autopsy reimbursement. Arch Pathol Lab Med 1996;120: 771–772. *(Major public and commercial managed care and fee-for-service payers in California failed to provide autopsy reimbursement.)*
4. Trelstad RL, Amenta PS, Foran DJ, Smilow PC. The role of regional autopsy centers in the evaluation of covered deaths. Survey of opinions of US and Canadian chairs of pathology and major health insurers in the United States. Arch Pathol Lab Med 1996;120:753–758. *(Most health insurers were disinterested in the autopsy as a measure of outcome and unwilling to provide support.)*
5. Reid WA. Cost effectiveness of routine postmortem histology. J Clin Pathol 1987;40:459–461. *(Suggests that unselected postmortem histology is, for diagnostic purposes, not cost-effective.)*
6. McCarthy EF, Gebhardt F, Bhagavan BS. The frozen-section autopsy. Arch Pathol Lab Med 1981;105:494–496. *(Use of frozen sections with the occasional supplementation with paraffin sections decreases costs and improves turnaround times.)*

IMPROVING THE AUTOPSY SERVICE

1. Adickes ED, Sims KL. Enhancing autopsy performance and reporting. A system for a 5-day completion time. Arch Pathol Lab Med 1996;120:249–253. *(A method to improve turnaround time.)*
2. McManus BM, Wood SM. The autopsy. Simple thoughts about the public needs and how to address them. Am J Clin Pathol 1996;106:S11–S14. *(Emphasizes need to better integrate autopsy and other services, improve follow-up with families, make better use of research opportunities, and enhance public awareness of the role of autopsies.)*
3. Start RD, Sherwood SJ, Kent G, Angel CA. Audit study of next of kin satisfaction with special necropsy service. BMJ 1996; 312:1516. *(Communication improves satisfaction.)*
4. McPhee SJ. Maximizing the benefits of autopsy for clinicians and families. What needs to be done. Arch Pathol Lab Med 1996;120:743–748. *(Advocates shorter turnaround times and improved communication with clinicians and families.)*
5. Setlow VP. The need for a national autopsy policy. Arch Pathol Lab Med 1996;120:773–777. *(Describes efforts of the Institute of Medicine, a branch of the National Academy of Sciences, to evaluate the need for a national autopsy policy.)*
6. Haque AK, Patterson RC, Grafe MR. High autopsy rates at a university medical center. What has gone right? Arch Pathol Lab Med 1996;120:727–732. *(Describes the 'Decedent Affairs Office,' quality control, improved communication with clinicians, and support by the hospital administration.)*
7. Diamond I. New approach needed to revive autopsy. Arch Pathol Lab Med 1996;120:713. *(Avoid "routine," increase use of ancillary methods, improve communication, improve art of narrative description.)*
8. Hutchins GM. Whither the autopsy?...To regional autopsy centers. Arch Pathol Lab Med 1996;120:718. *(Advocates regional autopsy centers.* See *also ref. [11].)*
9. Hill RB. College of American Pathologists Conference XXIX on restructuring autopsy practice for health care reform: summary. Arch Pathol Lab Med 1996;120:778–781. *(Review of use of autopsy in medical care, research, and education; reimbursement issues; need for a national autopsy policy.)*
10. Kleiner DE, Emmert-Buck MR, Liotta LA. Necropsy as a research method in the age of molecular pathology. Lancet 1995;346:945–948. *(Describes possible applications of molecular biology techniques in the autopsy setting.)*
11. Mitchell EK, Prior JT. Where have all the autopsies gone? A proposal for a centralized autopsy service. J Commun Health 1995;20:441–446. *(Proposes central off-hospital site facilities that perform hospital autopsies.* See *also ref. [8].)*
12. Emson HE. Notes on necropsy. J Clin Pathol 1992;45:85–86. *(The dead body must be treated with dignity but it is not the person who used the body during life. If this is understood by the next of kin, autopsy permissions might be given more readily.)*
13. Hill RB, Anderson RE. The autopsy and health statistics. Legal Med 1990:57–69. *(More and better autopsies and proper completion of death certificates are needed to improve health statistics.)*
14. AMA Council on Scientific Affairs. Autopsy. A comprehensive review of current issues. JAMA 1987;258:364–369. *(Urges integration of new technologies and reimbursement for autopsies as instruments of quality assurance.)*
15. Bellwald M. Autopsien mit unbefriedigenden Resultaten. Schweiz Med Wochenschr 1982;112:75–82. *(In 3.7% of 3,076 cases, the autopsy did not provide the needed answers. Use of more sophisticated diagnostic techniques and better communication with clinicians might improve these negative results.)*

VERBAL AUTOPSIES

The reader should note that "verbal autopsies" are not autopsies in a technical sense; the name was coined to describe attempts to diagnose diseases and causes of death by interviewing the next of kin and thus to come reasonably close to what might have been found at autopsy. Of course, the meaning of the term autopsy—"a seeing for oneself" —makes the name "verbal autopsies" an oxymoron. "Verbal autopsies" are practiced primarily in tropical countries. Two references are listed here because the effort is laudable if no autopsy permission can be obtained.

1. Quigley MA, Armstrong Schellenberg Jr, Snow RW. Algorithms for verbal autopsies: a validation study in Kenyan children. Bull World Health Org 1996;74:147–154.
2. Chandramohan D, Maude GH, Rodrigues LC, Hayes RJ. Verbal autopsies for adult deaths: issues in their development and validation. Int J Epidemiol 1994;23:213–222.

II

Alphabetic List of Diseases and Conditions, with Recommendations for Case-Specific Autopsy Procedures

Organization of Part II

Some general remarks about objectives for the preparation of Part II can be found in the preface of this third edition. The following paragraphs explain the format in which diseases and conditions are listed in Part II.

Diseases and Conditions. All main entries are arranged in alphabetic order of the noun. Thus, "Viral hepatitis" will be found under "Hepatitis, viral" and "Lung abscess" under "Abscess, lung." In general, the organization of the entries corresponds to that used in *Dorland's Illustrated Medical Dictionary*, 28th ed., W. B. Saunders, Philadelphia, PA, 1994. Findings related to operative procedures are listed under the alphabetized entry of "Surgery,... " or "Transplantation,...." Diseases or conditions that are not included in the alphabetic list may still be found in the index.

"See..." Such a reference to another disease or condition indicates that the autopsy procedures are the same for both but not necessarily that the two diseases or conditions are the same.

Diseases and Conditions, followed by a Table. If diseases or conditions (in bold print) are listed in both the right and left column of text preceding a table, the table always belongs to the bold entry in the right column.

Synonyms and Related Terms. This subtitle has been modified to either "Synonym(s)" or "Related Term(s)" whenever the entries seemed to fit definitely into one of these categories. An **asterisk** indicates a disease or condition that is included in the alphabetic list in Part II.

Note. Suggestions pertaining to the entire autopsy procedure are made under this heading. For instance, a warning will be given here whenever special precautions are indicated in the presence of certain infectious diseases or whenever a disease or condition must be reported to the authorities.

Possible Associated Conditions. Diseases or conditions listed under this heading are generally assumed to be linked to the main entry by a common pathogenetic mechanism. An example is the association of malformations, such as coarctation of the aorta and congenital mitral stenosis.

Organs and Tissues. These are listed in the order in which they are generally handled during an autopsy.

Procedures. Ample reference is made to the appropriate page numbers in Part I. We have assumed that routine hematoxylin and eosin sections will be prepared in all instances. Most special stains that are listed below represent but one of several available methods; many pathologist undoubtedly will have other preferences.

From: *Handbook of Autopsy Practice,* 3rd Ed. Edited by: J. Ludwig © Humana Press Inc., Totowa, NJ

Special Histological Stains[a]

Name of Stain (as used in text)	*Complete Designation and/or Purpose of Stain*	*Source and Comments*
Alcian blue stain	For demonstration of sulfated mucosubstances (at pH 1.0) or acid mucopoly-saccharides (at pH 2.5).	Ref. *(1)* Also used with periodic acid Schiff stain (Alcian blue/PAS).
Alcian blue and phloxine-tartrazine stain of Lendrum	For demonstration of mucus and squamous epithelial cells in one section.	Ref. *(2)* See also below under Lendrum's stain.
Aldehyde-Fuchsin stain	For staining of beta cells of pancreatic islets, of elastic fibers, and of cells of adenohypophysis.	Ref. *(3)* Aldehyde fuchsin also stains sulfated mucosubstances and hepatitis B surface antigen.
Aldehyde-thionin stain	For staining of cells of adenohypophysis.	Ref. *(3)* Can be combined with periodic acid Schiff stain (PAS) and with Luxol fast blue (LFB).
Auramine-rhodamine	Truant's fluorescent method for tubercle and Leprae bacilli.	Ref. *(2)*
Azure-eosin stain	Routine stain (can be substituted for the hematoxylin and eosin methods).	Ref. *(3)* The Giemsa stain and the Wright stain for blood cells also are azure-eosin stains.
Best's carmine stain	Best's carmine method for glycogen.	Ref. *(2)*
Bielschowsky stain	Bielschowsky's method for axis cylinders and dendrites.	Ref. *(2)*
Bodian stain	Bodian's method for nerve fibers and nerve endings.	Ref. *(2)*
Congo red stain	Bennhold's method for amyloid.	Ref. *(2)*
Cresyl echt violet stain		See Luxol fast blue stain.
Crystal violet stain	Lieb's method for amyloid (crystal violet).	Ref. *(2)*
Cyanuric chloride stain	Cyanuric chloride method of Yoshiki for osteoid.	Ref. *(4)*
Ferric ferricyanide reduction test	Schmorl's ferric ferricyanide reduction test for the demonstration of melanin and other reducing substances.	Ref. *(3)* See also Fontana-Masson silver stain.
Fluorochrome stain for acid fast bacteria	Truant's fluorescent method for acid fast organisms	Ref. *(2)*
Fontana-Masson silver stain	Fontana-Masson silver method for demonstration of argentaffin granules and melanin.	Ref. *(2)* See also Ferric ferricyanide reduction test and Grimelius silver stain.
Giemsa stain	May-Grünwald Giemsa method for hematologic and nuclear elements.	Ref. *(2)* Several modifications of this methods are in use.
Gomori's chromium hematoxylin phloxine stain	Gomori's method for pancreatic islet cells.	Ref. *(2)*
Gomori's iron stain	Gomori's method for iron.	Ref. *(2)*
Gram stain	Brown and Benn, Brown-Hopps, Maccallum-Goodpasture, or Taylor's method for demonstration of Gram positive and Gram negative bacteria.	Ref. *(2)* As shown in the middle column, several modifications of this method are in use. The Gram-Weigert stain (ref. *[3]*) also stains fungi and *Pneumocystis carinii.*
Grimelius silver stain (Grimelius' argyrophil stain)	For demonstration of argyrophil neurosecretory granules (e.g., in pancreatic islets).	Ref. *(1)* The Fontana-Masson stain for melanin and argentaffin granules can also be used.
Grocott's methenamine silver stain (GMS stain)	Grocott's method for fungi.	Ref. *(2)* Also stains *Pneumocystis carinii.*
Hale's colloidal iron stain	The Hale colloidal ferric oxide procedure for acid mucopolysaccharides.	Ref. *(5)* The alcian blue stain at pH. 2.5 (see above) also can be used.
Jones' silver stain	Jones' method for reticulum and basement membranes.	Ref. *(3)* See also methenamine silver stain.
Kinyoun's stain	Kinyoun's method for acid-fast bacteria.	Ref. *(2)*
Lendrum's stain	Lendrum's method for inclusion bodies.	Ref. *(2)* For use with alcian blue, see above.
Levaditi's stain	Levaditi-Manovelian method for spirochetes.	Ref. *(2)*
Luxol fast blue stain (LFB stain)	Klüver-Barrera method for myelin and nerve cells.	Ref. *(2)* Also used with periodic acid Schiff stain (LFB/PAS) or with cresyl echt violet stain (ref. *[1]*).

Name of Stain (as used in text)	*Complete Designation and/or Purpose of Stain*	*Source and Comments*
Masson's trichrome stain	Masson's trichrome method.	Ref. *(2)* Used to distinguish between collagen (blue) and smooth muscle fibers (red).
Methenamine silver stain	Chromotrope silver methenamine stain of glomerular lesions.	Ref. *(6)* See also Jones' silver stain.
Methyl violet stain	Highman's method for amyloid (methyl violet).	Ref. *(2)*
Mucicarmine stain	Mayer's mucicarmine method for mucin and *Cryptococcus.*	Ref. *(1)*
Periodic acid-Schiff stain (PAS stain)	The periodic acid, Schiff Reagent (PAS) for demonstration of polysaccharides, neutral mucosubstances, and basement membranes.	Ref. *(1)* Also used with diastase digestion (diastase digests glycogen, e.g., in liver tissue). For use with alcian blue, see under that heading.
PAS-alcian blue stain (PAS/alcian blue)	PAS-alcian blue method for mucosubstances.	See above under "Alcian blue stain."
Perl's stain for iron	Perl's method for iron.	Ref. *(2)*
Peroxidase reaction	Immunoenzymic staining methods for the detection of antigens or antibodies.	Ref. *(3)* Direct and indirect staining methods can be applied, usually with horseradish peroxidase (HPR).
Phosphotungstic acid hematoxylin stain (PTAH stain)	Mallory's phosphotungstic acid hematoxylin method.	Ref. *(2)* Stains skeletal muscle with cross striations (blue), collagen (red), nuclei, and fibrin (both blue).
Reticulum stain	Gomori's method for reticulum.	Ref. *(2)*
Rhodanine stain	Rhodanine method for copper.	Ref. *(3)* Rhodanine should not be confused with rhoda*m*ine, which is a fluorochrome, e.g., for the detection of mycobacteria.
Shikata's orcein stain	Orcein method for demonstration of hepatitis B surface antigen in paraffin sections of liver biopsy specimens.	Ref. *(3)* Orcein also is an excellent stain for elastic fibers.
Sirius red stain	Sweat-Puchtler method for amyloid (Sirius red).	Ref. *(2)*
Sudan stain	Sudan black B method for fat (in frozen sections). For other Sudan stains, see right-hand column.	Ref. *(2)* Oil red O solution also can be used; it gives better results than either Sudan III or Sudan IV (ref. *[5]*).
Sulfated alcian blue	Sodium sulfate alcian blue (SAB) method for amyloid.	Ref. *(8)*
Thioflavine S	Fluorochrome technics for acid fast bacteria and protozoa.	Ref. *(7)*
Thioflavine T stain	Vassar-Culling method for amyloid (thioflavine T).	Ref. *(2)*
Toluidine blue O stain	Toluidine blue O nuclear stain.	Ref. *(3)* Toloidin blue can be used for mast cells, mucin, nerve cells and glia.
Trichrome stain		See Masson's trichrome stain.
Van Gieson's stain	Van Gieson's method for collagen fibers.	Ref. *(2)* See also Verhoeff-van Gieson stain.
Verhoeff-van Gieson stain	Verhoeff-van Gieson technic.	Ref. *(3)* Stains elastic fibers black, collagen red, nuclei blue to black, and other tissue elements yellow. See also Shikata's orcein stain.
Von Braunmühl's stain	Von Braunmühl's stain for senile plaques.	Ref. *(9)*
Von Kossa's stain	Von Kossa's silver test for calcium.	Ref. *(3)*
Warthin-Starry stain	Warthin-Starry method for spirochetes and Donovan bodies.	Ref. *(2)* Also stains *H. pylori.*
Wright stain	Wright stain for blood smears.	Ref. *(3)* Also used with Giemsa stain.
Ziehl-Neelsen stain	Ziehl-Neelsen method for acid-fast bacteria.	Ref. *(2)*

[a]Most of these stains are recommended with appropriate entries in Part II. Some of them can be used for more purposes than stated in the middle column. For alternative stains and recommended fixatives, see current staining manuals.

Possible or Expected Findings. Listed under this heading are manifestations of the disease or condition in the alphabetic title. Also included in this column are many causes and complications, provided they can be identified at autopsy. Occasionally, some overlap will be found with "Possible Associated Conditions" (*see* above).

Removal of Formalin Pigment from Histological Sections *(2)*

1. Deparaffinize sections through two changes each of xylene, absolute alcohol, and 95% alcohol.
2. Rinse well in distilled water.
3. Place slides for 5–10 min in *freshly made up* bleaching solution, consisting of 25 mL hydrogen peroxide 3%, 25 mL acetone, and 1 drop ammonium hydroxide.
4. Wash well in running tap water and distilled water.
5. Stain as desired.

References

1. Carson FL. Histotechnology. A Self-Instructional Text. ASCP Press, American Society of Clinical Pathology, Chicago, IL, 1990.
2. Luna LG. Histopathologic Methods and Color Atlas of Special Stains and Tissue Artifacts. Johnson Printers, Downer's Grove, IL, 1992.
3. Sheehan DC, Hrapchak BB. Theory and Practice of Histotechnology, 2nd ed. CV Mosby Company, St. Louis, MO, 1980.
4. Clark WE. Osteomalacia, histopathologic diagnosis made simple (letter to the editor). Am J Clin Pathol 1976;66:1025–1026.
5. Lillie RD. Histopathologic Technic and Practical Histochemistry, 3rd ed. McGraw-Hill, New York, 1965.
6. Ehrenreich T, Espinosa T. Chromotrope silver methenamine stain of glomerular lesions. Am J Clin Pathol 1971;56:448–451.
7. Bancroft JD, Stevens A. Theory and practice of histological techniques. Churchill Livingstone, New York, 1982.
8. Thompson SW, Hunt RD. Selected Histochemical and Histopathological Methods. Charles C. Thomas, Springfield, IL, 1966.
9. Putt FA. Manual of Histopathological Staining Methods. John Wiley & Sons, New York, 1972.

A

Abetalipoproteinemia

Synonyms and Related Terms: Acanthocytosis; Bassen-Kornzweig syndrome.

NOTE: Autopsies on patients with this rare genetic disease *(1,2)* should be considered research procedures.

Possible Associated Conditions: Hemolytic anemia;* malabsorption syndrome.*

Organs and Tissues	*Procedures*	*Possible or Expected Findings*
External examination	Record body weight and length. Prepare chest roentgenogram (frontal and lateral view).	Below-normal weight in infants. Kyphoskoliosis.
Blood	Submit for serum lipid analysis.	Very low concentrations of cholesterol and triglycerides; serum β-lipoprotein decreased or absent; α-lipoproteins present.
	Prepare smears of undiluted blood.	Acanthocytosis (spiny red cells).
Small bowel	For preservation of small intestinal mucosa and for preparation for study under dissecting microscope, see Part I, Chapter 5. Submit sample for histologic study.	Abnormal shape of villi; vacuolation of epithelial cells.
Large bowel	Submit stool for chemical analysis.	Fatty stools
Liver	Record weight and submit sample for histologic study.	Fatty changes.
Other organs		Systemic manifestations of malabsorption syndrome* and of vitamin A deficiency.*
Spine	Record appearance of spine (see also chest roentgenogram).	Kyphoscoliosis.
Brain, spinal cord, peripheral nerves	For removal and specimen preparation, see pp. 65, 67, and 79, respectively. Request Luxol fast blue stain (p. 172).	Axonal degeneration of the spinocerebellar tracts; demyelination of the fasciculus cuneatus and gracilis *(2)*. Possible involvement of posterior columns, pyramidal tracts, and peripheral nerves.
Eyes	For removal and specimen preparation, see p. 85.	Atypical retinitis pigmentosa *(2)* with involvement of macula. Angioid streaks *(3)*.

References

1. Case records of the Massachussetts General Hospital. Case 35-1992. N Engl J Med 1992;327:628–635.
2. Rader DJ, Brewer HB Jr. Abetalipoproteinemia. New insights into lipoprotein assembly and vitamin E metabolism from a rare genetic disease [clinical conference]. JAMA 1993;270:865–869.
3. Gorin MB, Paul TO, Rader DJ. Angioid streaks associated with abetalipoproteinemia. Ophthalmic Genet 1994;15:151–159.

Abortion

NOTE: If a fetus is present, follow procedures described under "Stillbirth." If no recognizable fetal tissue is found, an indication might exist to submit material for chromosome study as decribed in Chapter 10. If attempts to induce abortion appear to have caused the death of the mother, see "Death, abortion-associated."

From: *Handbook of Autopsy Practice,* 3rd Ed. Edited by: J. Ludwig © Humana Press Inc., Totowa, NJ

Abscess, Brain

Synonym: Cerebral abscess.

NOTE: For microbiologic study of tissues and abscesses, see Part I, Chapter 9. Include samples for anaerobic culture. It is best to study the brain after fixation but if specimen is examined fresh, aspirate and prepare smears of abscess content. Photograph surface and coronal slices of brain. Request Giemsa stain, Gram stain, PAS stain, and Grocott's methenamine silver stain for fungi (p. 172, 173).

Organs and Tissues	*Procedures*	*Possible or Expected Findings*
External examination	Record presence or absence of features listed in right-hand column.	Skin infections in upper half of face. Edema of forehead, eyelids, and base of nose, proptosis, and chemosis indicate cerebral venous sinus thrombosis.* Trauma; craniotomy wounds.
	If there is evidence of trauma, see also under "Injury, head." Prepare roentgenograms of chest and skull.	Skull fracture and other traumatic lesions. For possible intrathoracic lesions, see below under "Other organs."
Cerebrospinal fluid	Submit for microbiologic study (p. 104).	
Brain and spinal cord	For removal and specimen preparation, see pp. 65 and 67, respectively. For microbiologic study, photography, and special stains, see under "Note."	Traumatic lesions of brain. Foreign body.
Base of skull with sinuses and middle ears	For exposure of venous sinuses, see p. 71. Sample walls of sinuses for histologic study.	Cerebral venous sinus thrombosis* or thrombophlebitis.
	For exposure of paranasal sinuses, mastoid cells, and middle ears, see p. 71–73.	Paranasal sinusitis and mastoiditis. Subacute and chronic otitis media.* Osteomyelitis* and fractures of base of skull may be present.
Eyes	For removal and specimen preparation, see p. 85.	Thrombosis of angular and superior ophthalmic veins, associated with cavernous sinus thrombosis.*
Other organs	Procedures depend on suspected lesions as listed in right-hand column.	Congenital heart disease with right-to-left shunt; infective endocarditis.* Bronchiectasis;* lung abscess;* pleural empyema.* *Entamoeba histolytica* abscesses in liver and lung.

Abscess, Epidural

Synonym: Epidural Empyema.

NOTE: Procedures are the same as those suggested under "Empyema, epidural."

Abscess, Lung

Synonym: Pulmonary abscess.

NOTE: For microbiologic procedures and related suggestions, see also under "Pneumonia."

Organs and Tissues	*Procedures*	*Possible or Expected Findings*
External examination	Prepare chest roentgenogram.	Pulmonary cavities and infiltrates; foreign body.
	Record appearance of oral cavity.	Periodontal infection.
	If peripheral veins contain potentially infected catheters, see below under "Central veins."	Infected intravenous catheter.
Chest cavity	Before chest is opened, puncture pleural cavity and submit exudate for microbiologic study (p. 102).	Empyema;* pleural effusion or exudate.*
	Prepare smears of exudate and request Gram, Kinyoun, and Grocott methenamine silver stains (p. 172).	Bacteria or fungi in exudate.

Organs and Tissues	*Procedures*	*Possible or Expected Findings*
Central veins	If a metastatic abscess from an infected intravenous catheter is suspected, ligate appropriate vein proximal and distal to catheter tip and submit for microbiologic study.	Infected intravenous catheter.
Heart	See "Endocarditis, infective."	Infective endocarditis* of tricuspid or pulmonary valve.
Lungs	For bronchography and pulmonary arteriography, see Part I, Chapter 5. If abscess contents are aspirated or microbiologic studies are not crucial, perfuse intact lung with formalin (p. 47).	Tumor of lung,* foreign body, or other obstructive bronchial lesion.
Other organs	Procedures depend on expected sources of infection.	Manifestations of possible underlying conditions such as acquired immunodeficiency syndrome.*

Abscess, Subdural (See "Empyema, epidural.")

Abscess, Subphrenic (See "Empyema, subphrenic.")

Abuse, Child (See "Infanticide.")

Abuse, Drugs or Other Chemicals (See "Abuse, hallucinogen(s)," "Abuse, marihuana," "Dependence,..." "Poisoning,..." See also "Alcoholism and alcohol intoxication.")

Abuse, Hallucinogen(s)

Related Terms: Diethyltryptamine (DET); dimethyltryptamine (DMT); lysergic acid diethylamide (see "Poisoning, LSD"); marihuana;* mescaline; psilocin; psilocybin ("magic mushrooms"); psychedelics; psychotomimetics; and others *(1)*.

NOTE: See also under "Dependence, drug(s), all types or type unspecified." For routine toxicologic sampling, see p. 16. There are no specific morphologic findings related to hallucinogen intake.

Reference

1. Baselt RC, Cravey RH. Disposition of Toxic Drugs and Chemicals in Man, 4th ed. Chemical Toxicology Institute, Foster City, CA, 1995.

Abuse, Marihuana

Synonyms: Cannabis; hashish.

NOTE: The tissues at autopsy show no specific changes. Tetrahydrocannabinol is routinely detected by the EMIT screening procedure (*see* Part I, Chapter 2) in urine, and is confirmed and quantitated by specific assays on a variety of body fluids, including blood. However, these latter procedures are rarely needed. If abuse of other drugs is suspected, see under "Dependence, drug(s), all types or type unspecified."

Accident, Aircraft

In the event of a major catastrophic air carrier accident, the local police should be called and then The Federal Aviation Administration (FAA) in Washington, DC.* The FAA will notify the National Transportation Safety Board (NTSB). Most fatal air crashes are investigated by the NTSB.** The FAA investigates crashes in which the gross weight of the craft is less than 12,500 pounds *(1)*. The investigations are conducted by a team of federal and other specialists. Local police, firemen, or other officials will seal off the area of the crash, and no one should be allowed to approach the bodies or any objects until the identification teams and the medical examiner or coroner have taken charge.

Several medical examiner and coroner offices have published accounts detailing their approaches to managing mass fatality disasters *(2–6)*. The sudden influx of bodies after a commercial air carrier accident and the request for speedy identification of the victims and for detailed autopsy reports of the crew members would overburden almost any institution. Managing such a disaster requires an efficient organization, and it seems advisable to devise a plan before the necessity arises. Temporary morgue facilities may have to be established near the scene of the crash. Refrigerated trucks may serve as storage space. A practical approach is to deal first with those bodies that seem to be the easiest to identify, in order to narrow the field for the more difficult cases.

If bodies are scattered, the exact locations should be identified by stakes in the ground or spray paint on pavement; only then should these bodies (or remaining parts) and all objects that might belong to them be collected. For this, plastic bags with paired tags are generally used. One tag is used as a marker for the stake; the other stays with the bag. Or, if the stakes are numbered, one tag can be used and the stake number is put on the tag, in addition to the bag number. Proper records and diagrams of the relative positions of victims are prepared during this phase. If the victims are still within the airplane, their exact positions within the wreckage must also be recorded, and appropriate photographs should be taken.

For the identification of the victims, the airline will provide a list of the passengers and the Federal Bureau of Investigation (FBI) disaster team will take fingerprints and aid in the acquisition of other identifying data such as age, race, weight, height, and hair color and style. If dental records can be obtained, this provides one of the most certain methods of identification. A medical history indicating amputations, internal prostheses, or other characteristic surgical interventions or the presence of nephrolithiasis, gallstones, and the like will be helpful. Fingerprints (and footprints of babies) should be taken in all instances. Wallets with identification cards, jewelry, name tags in clothing, or other personal belongings may provide the fastest tentative identification.

The medical examiner may elect to autopsy only the flight crew but not the passengers of an aircraft crash. However, the grossly identifiable fatal injuries should be described, photographed, and x-rayed. This may reveal identifying body changes. If comparison of somatic radiographs, dental records, fingerprints, or photographs do not identify the victim, DNA comparison must be considered. Burned or fragmented bodies of passengers and the bodies of crew members, and particularly the pilots, must have a complete autopsy, including roentgenographic and toxicologic examinations, which must always include alcohol and carbon monoxide determinations. Internal examination might reveal a coronary occlusion, or roentgenograms may disclose a bullet as evidence that violence preceded the crash. In some airplane crashes, particularly in light airplane accidents, suicide must be considered and a suicide note should be sought. Some authors recommend performing autopsies on all deceased occupants of aircraft crashes, including passengers, and cite the need to distinguish among blunt impact trauma, smoke inhalation, and flash fires as causes of death, in order to answer future questions concerning pain and suffering, intoxication, and sequence of survivorship.

After a crash victim has been identified, the coroner or medical examiner will issue a death certificate. If remains of a decedent cannot be found, a judge can, upon petition, declare a passenger dead and sign a death certificate prepared by a medical examiner.

*Phone # of FAA Command Center: 202-267-3333

**Phone # of NTSB Command Center: 202-314-6290.

References

1. Wagner GN, Froede CH. Medicolegal investigation of mass disaster. In: Medicolegal Investigation of Death, 3rd ed. Spitz WU, ed. Charles C. Thomas, 1993.
2. Clark MA, Hawley DA, McClain JL, Pless JE, Marlin DC, Standish SM. Investigation of the 1987 Indianapolis Airport Ramada Inn incident. J Forens Sci 1994;39:644–649.
3. Clark MA, Clark SR, Perkins DG. Mass fatality aircraft disaster processing. Aviation Space Environm Med 1989;60:A64–A73.
4. McCarty VO, Sohn AP, Ritzlin RS, Gauthier JH. Scene investigation and victim examination following the accident of Galaxy 203: disaster preplanning does work. J Forens Sci 1987;32:983–987.
5. Randall B. Body retrieval and morgue operations at the crash of United Flight 232. J Forens Sci 1001;36:403–409.
6. Wagner GN. Aerospace pathology. In: Handbook of Forensic Pathology. Froede RC, ed. College of American Pathologists, Northfield, IL, 1990.

Accident, Automobile (See “Accident, vehicular.”)

Accident, Diving (Skin or Scuba)

NOTE: *Skin* diving fatalities are usually caused by drowning,* and autopsy procedures described under that entry should be followed. Usually, the circumstances that led to drowning are not apparent from the autopsy findings but can be reconstructed from reports of witnesses and the police. Because the reflex drive to seek air is triggered by hypercarbia, not hypoxia, loss of consciousness and drowning can ensue after hyperventilation and breath-holding by experienced swimmers who then drown without a struggle. There are no specific autopsy findings. A search for trauma, including a posterior neck dissection (see p. 67), should be made in all instances. Head and cervical injuries may be responsible for loss of consciousness and drowning, usually in individuals diving into shallow water with the head striking the bottom. Toxicologic examination as described below for scuba diving accidents is always indicated.

With *scuba* diving fatalities, investigation of the equipment and circumstances is far more important than the autopsy. Scuba fatalities should be studied by or with the aid of diving experts—for instance, members of the nearest diving club or the U.S. Navy. Careful investigation of the scene and study of reports of witnesses and the police are essential. Records should state the site of diving (currents and other underwater hazards), the estimated depth, the water temperature (exposure to cold), and a description of water clarity. Water of the area should be sampled, particularly if it seems heavily polluted. Records should also state whether there were electric underwater cables (if electrocution might have occurred, see “Injury, electric”) and whether explosives had been used in the vicinity (blast injury). The method of recovery of the body (injuries by grappling hooks) and the type of resuscitation efforts should be noted. The medical history of the diving victim should be reviewed (for example, evidence of seizure disorders or drug use).

The most frequent cause of death ascribed to scuba diving accidents is drowning. Although drowning may be the terminal event in many scuba deaths, the investigation should be focused on the adverse environmental and equipment factors that place a capable swimmer at risk of drowning (see “Embolism, air” and “Sickness, decompression”). If exhaustion, panic, or cardioinhibitory reflexes were responsible for loss of consciousness, autopsy findings will only be those of drowning. Gas bubbles should be documented at autopsy, but their interpretation is problematic. Bodies recovered immediately are subjected to resuscitation efforts, which can by themselves produce extraalveolar air artifacts. Bodies not recovered immediately tend to be found in a putrified condition, full of postmortem gas. In the remaining cases, the pathologist must consider the potential of introducing artifactual gas bubbles by the forcible retraction of the chest plate and by sawing the calvarium. The following procedures apply primarily to scuba diving accidents *(1–4)*.

Organs and Tissues	*Procedures*	*Possible or Expected Findings*
External examination	Photograph victim as recovered and after removal of wet suit and other diving gear. Record condition of clothing and gear. Impound all diving equipment for study by experts, particularly scuba tank, breathing hoses, and regulators. Residual air in tank should be analyzed.	Mask, fins, weight belt, life vest, scuba tank and regulator, watch, depth gauge, or other gear may be missing. Clothing may be torn. Quick-release mechanisms of scuba tank or of weight belt may have been improperly adjusted and may not work. Mask, mouthpiece, regulator, or exhalation hose may contain vomitus. Air supply may be contaminated.
	Record color of skin (including face, back, soles, palms, and scalp).	Cyanosis after hypoxia,* cherry-red color after CO poisoning,* or marbling after air embolism.*
	Palpate skin and record presence or absence of crepitation.	Crepitation from subcutaneous emphysema.
	Record extent and character of wounds. Prepare histologic specimens.	Antemortem and postmortem abrasions, lacerations, contusions, bites, or puncture wounds (marine life—for instance, coelenterate stings). Electrocution marks, blast injuries.
	Record appearance of face (including oral and nasal cavities) and of ears.	Froth on mouth and nares. Facial edema and edema of pinnae. ("Facial squeeze" and "external ear squeeze" occur during descent.) Vomitus in mouth and nose.
	Prepare roentgenograms. If air embolism must be expected, as in the presence of pneumomediastinum, follow procedures described under "Embolism, air." For evaluation of findings, see also above under "Note."	Fractures—for example, of cervical spine in skin diving accidents (see above); bone necroses (see below); foreign bodies. Pneumothorax,* pneumoperitoneum, pneumopericardium, and mediastinal and subcutaneous emphysema (all indicating rapid ascent).
Eyes and ears	Otoscopic examination.	Otitis externa. Rupture of tympanic membrane.
	Funduscopic examination. Save vitreous (p. 85) for possible toxicologic and other studies.	Gas in retinal vessels after air embolism. For interpretation of other studies, see p. 115.
Head (skull and brain)	For removal of brain, see pp. 65 and 71. Record contents of arteries of the circle of Willis and its major branches and basilar artery.	Gas bubbles in cerebral arteries after air embolism* (after rapid ascent). Nitrogen bubbles in cerebral vessels are found in victims who had "staggers." Subdural and subarachnoid hemorrhages. Cerebral edema, with ischemic necroses and focal hemorrhages, after air embolism.
	Strip dura from base of skull and from calvarium.	Skull fracture.
Middle ears	For removal and specimen preparation, see p. 72.	Edema and hemorrhage. ("Middle ear squeeze" occurs during descent; hemorrhage occurs in drowning.) Ruptured tympanic membranes.
Chest	For demonstration of pneumothorax, see p. 430.	Pneumothorax; pneumomediastinum. Petechial hemorrhages of serosal surfaces.
Blood (from heart and peripheral vessels)	If gas is visible in coronary arteries, photograph. Photograph and aspirate gas in heart chambers. (For procedures, see p. 290.)	Air embolism.*

Organs and Tissues	*Procedures*	*Possible or Expected Findings*
Blood (from heart and peripheral vessels) *(continued)*	Submit samples of heart blood and peripheral blood for toxicologic study and drug screen (p. 16).	Alcohol intoxication (see "Alcoholism and alcohol intoxication"); carbon monoxide poisoning.*
Heart		Ischemic heart disease;* patent oval foramen.
Tracheobronchial tree and lungs	Examine lungs *in situ*. Save bronchial washings for analysis of debris. Fresh dissection is recommended.	Foam, aspirated vomitus, or other aspirated material in tracheobronchial tree. Pulmonary lacerations, bullae, and atelectases. Pulmonary edema and hemorrhage. "Pulmonary squeeze" develops during descent; nitrogen bubbles in precapillary pulmonary arteries develop during rapid ascent ("chokes").
Other organs	Complete toxicologic sampling should be carried out (p. 16). Record nature of gastric contents.	
Neck organs and tongue	Remove neck organs toward end of autopsy. For posterior neck dissection, see p. 67. Incise tongue.	Interstitial emphysema. Aspiration (see above). Trauma to cervical spine. Mottled pallor of tongue after air embolism. Contusion of tongue after convulsive chewing.
Spinal cord	For removal and specimen preparation, see p. 67.	Nitrogen bubbles in spinal cord arteries may occur after rapid ascent.
Bones and joints	For removal, prosthetic repair, and specimen preparation, see p. 95. Consult roentgenograms.	Aseptic necroses (infarcts, "dysbaric osteonecrosis"), most often in head of femur, distal femur, and proximal tibia. Infarcts indicate repeated hyperbaric exposures. Nitrogen bubbles in and about joints and in periosteal vessels ("bends") occur during rapid ascent.

References

1. Gallagher TJ. Scuba diving accidents: decompression sickness, air embolism. J Florida Med Assoc 1997;84:446–451.
2. Blanksby BA, Wearne FK, Elliott BC, Blitvich JD. Aetiology and occurrence of diving injuries. A review of diving safety. Sports Med 1997;23:228–246.
3. Arness MK. Scuba decompression illness and diving fatalities in an overseas military community. Aviation Space Environm Med 1997; 68:325–333.
4. Hardy KR. Diving-related emergencies. Emerg Med Clin North Am 1997;15:223–240.

Accident, Vehicular

Related Terms: Automobile accident; motorcycle accident.

NOTE: A visit to the *scene* can make the interpretation of the autopsy findings easier. The vehicle can also be inspected in a more leisurely fashion at the impound lot. This is particularly useful for correlating patterned injuries with objects in the vehicle. Most vehicular crashes occur as intersection crashes or because a vehicle with excessive speed left a curved road.

The *medical examiner or coroner* should gain a basic understanding of the crash mechanism so that informed descriptions can be rendered, e.g., "Impact to the B pillar of the decedent's automobile by the front of a pickup truck which failed to stop for a stop sign at an intersection, resulting in a 2-feet intrusion into the cabin; restraint belts not employed; air bag deployed; extrication required which took 15 minutes."

Police are responsible for determining mechanical and environmental risk factors for the crash and for determining some human risk factors such as suicidal or homicidal intent. The *pathologist* determines other risk factors for crashes such as heart disease, a history of epilepsy, and intoxication by carbon monoxide, drugs, and alcohol.

Suicide as a manner of death should be considered when a single-occupant vehicle strikes a bridge abutment or a large tree head-on, with no evidence of evasive action or braking. In such a situation, the standard police traffic investigation should be supplemented of interviews of the victim's family and friends.

The *ambulance run sheet* is an invaluable source of observations that often are not available from the police. This document should be acquired in all instances, even if the paramedics determined that death occurred and did not transport.

The basic *autopsy* procedures are listed below. Most traffic victims who die at the scene or who are dead on arrival at the hospital died from neurogenic shock caused by wounds of the head or vertebral column, or from exsanguination from a torn vessel or heart. As such, they have little lividity, and little blood is found in the vehicles. Presence of intense lividity may indicate suffocation or heart disease as a cause of death.

If postural *asphyxia* is suspected, the first responders to the scene should be interviewed to determine the position of the decedent in the vehicle, and the vital signs, if any, of the decedent from the time of the crash to the time of extrication. Posterior neck dissection (p. 67) is indicated in these instances.

If manifestations of heart disease, intense lividity, and absence of lethal wounds suggest that a *crash occurred because the driver was dead*, other drivers on the road may have observed that the victim was slumped at the wheel before the crash. The determination of heart attack at the wheel is usually simple, because most such victims realize that something is wrong, and bring the vehicle to a stop at the side of the road, or coast gently into a fixed object. In such instances, damage to the vehicle is minor, and wounds to the decedent are usually trivial.

While *patterned wounds* can often be matched to objects (see below), patternless wounds usually cannot be visually matched to specific objects, although an opinion can sometimes be given as to what object was struck, based on the direction of motion and position of the body with respect to the vehicle. Impacts with the A-pillar produce narrow vertical zones of facial laceration and fractures extending from forehead to jaw. Tempered glass shatters into small cubes on impact, and leaves so-called "dicing" wounds, which are abraded cuts arranged in a somewhat rectilinear pattern. Windshield glass leaves shallow, abraded, vertically oriented cuts on the face or scalp.

With *pedestrians*, the lower extremities are of particular forensic interest, to determine the height and direction of impact from vehicles that left the scene. Scalp hair and blood should be collected from such "hit and run" victims and from occupants of a suspect car if police have a question as to which occupant was the driver; these exemplars can be compared to fibers and tissue recovered from the vehicle in question. Likewise, foreign material in wounds can sometimes be matched to suspect vehicles, and should be sought and retained as evidence. For pedestrians, the distance between the impact point on the lower extremities and the soles of the feet should be recorded. The legs should be opened to inspect tibial fractures; cortical fractures initiate propagation opposite to the side of impact, where they usually have a pulled-apart appearance, and then splinter the cortex at the side of impact. Abrasions are better impact markers than contusions, because subcutaneous blood extravasation can be caused not only by impact to the skin, but also from blood extravasating from underlying fractures. If no cutaneous abrasions or fractures of the leg bones are found, the skin of the legs should be incised to expose contusions.

Fracture descriptions should include location in the bone (e.g., proximal metaphysis or shaft), whether the fracture is complete or incomplete, and whether the fracture is displaced or distracted. Lacerations of intervertebral disks, facet joint capsules, and ligamenta flava should not be loosely termed "fractures." The presence or absence of blood extravasation in soft tissue adjacent to the fractures should be recorded, and its volume estimated if it appears severe enough.

Venous air embolism from torn dural sinuses cannot be diagnosed without a pre-autopsy chest radiograph or an *in situ* bubble test. If an X-ray machine is readily available, an anterior-posterior chest radiograph should be obtained in every traffic victim who dies at the scene or after a failed resuscitation attempt.

If a *hemothorax* is shown by the pleural window technique (p. 13), the rib cuts should be placed further lateral and the chest plate reflected so that the internal mammary vessels can be inspected before the chest plate is removed. After measuring and removing the bloody effusion, the underlying serosal surfaces should be inspected for defects. Lacerations of the heart and aorta will be obvious. Tamponaded lacerations of the aorta, around which the adventitia still holds, must be noted as such. If no lacerations are found at the usual sites, lacerations of the azygous veins must be considered, especially in association with fracture dislocations of the thoracic vertebral column; other sites are the internal mammary arteries, especially with fractures of ribs 1 and 2 or of the sternum, and intercostal arteries with displaced rib fractures. Only after the serosal defect is identified should the organs be removed, because that procedure creates many more holes in the serosa. For that reason, as much information as possible should be gained by *in situ* observation.

The only evidence of *concussion of the heart* may be a cardiac contusion or a sternal fracture. The usual clinical history suggests cardiovascular instability that is not associated with craniocerebral trauma and which does not respond to the infusion of intravenous volume agents.

The autopsy assistant may saw but should not retract the skull cap and remove the brain. The pathologist should observe *in situ* whether shallow lacerations of the pontomedullary junction with stretching of the midbrain are present; these lesions cannot be distinguished from artifact by examining the brain later. Thus, only after appropriate *in situ* inspection should the pathologist remove the brain.

A *posterior neck dissection* is required if no lethal craniocerebral or cardiovascular trauma can be found, or if suffocation is suspected; neck trauma must be ruled out to diagnose suffocation in a traffic fatality. Sudden death in a patient with seemingly trivial wounds may be caused by undiagnosed trauma of the craniocervical articulation. A posterior neck dissection (p. 67) is required in these instances.

The diagnosis of diffuse axonal injury of the brain in victims with no appreciable survival interval requires that suffocation was ruled out and that no resuscitaion from a cardiac arrest had been attempted. Clinicians are quick to apply the label "*closed head injury*" when a victim of a traffic crash has cerebral edema on a computerized axial tomogram of the head, even if no cerebral contusions, scalp contusions, or skull fractures are evident. This may be a misinterpretation, because cerebral edema can be caused by hypoxic encephalopathy made evident after resuscitation from a cardiac arrest, or by hypoxia caused by suffocation.

Organs and Tissues	*Procedures*	*Possible or Expected Findings*
External examination	Record presence of lividity.	Intense lividity and absence of lethal wounds may indicate that the crash occurred because the driver was dead from heart disease.
	Photograph all external wounds; measure all lacerations.	Small, medium, or large patternless abrasions and contusions.
	Photograph and measure all patterned abrasions and patterned contusions.	Patterned injuries often can be matched to objects in or about the vehicle.
	Record cuts from windshield glass.	Tempered glass injuries (see above under "Note").
	Determine impact injuries in pedestrians. Collect scalp hair and blood (see below) from victims of hit and run accidents. Collect foreign material in wounds.	Impact injuries in pedestrians may help to reconstruct the accident. Hair and blood of the victim may identify the vehicle involved in a hit and run accident.
	Prepare roentgenograms if venous air embolism is supected.	Venous air embolism.*
Blood, urine, and vitreous	Collect sample for toxicologic study (p. 16) from all victims, including passengers.	Evidence of alcohol or drug intoxication.
Chest cavities	Create pleural window to detect pneumothorax. If blood is seen, examine internal mammary vessels (see under "Note"). Measure volume of blood.	Pneumothorax, hemothorax, e.g., after laceration of internal mammary vessels.
Heart and great vessels	Record evidence of cardiac contusion.	Cardiac contusion after concussion of the heart.
	Laceration of heart or great vessels (measure volume of blood).	Evidence of exsanguination.
	Follow routine procedures for dissection of heart and great vessels (see Chapter 3).	Evidence of coronary occlusion or other major cardiovascular disease that may have been the cause of the accident.
	In situ bubble test may reveal venous air embolism.	Air embolism.*
Abdomen	Record evidence of trauma and volume of blood in peritoneal cavity; estimated volume of blood in retroperitoneal soft tissues.	Laceration of solid organs; rupture of hollow viscera or vessels, other evidence of trauma and hemorrhage into the abdominal cavity or soft tissues.
Skull and brain	Autopsy assistant may saw the skull but pathologist should inspect brain *in situ* and remove it personally. For removal and specimen preparation of brain, see p. 65. Record brain weight.	Cerebral lacerations at the pontomedullary junction. Cerebral edema.
Neck	Posterior neck dissection is indicated (p. 67) if there is no craniocerebral or cardio-vascular trauma, or if suffocation is suspected.	Trauma to the craniocervical articulation.
Soft tissue compartments at any location	Record evidence of trauma and estimate volume of blood.	

Achalasia, Esophageal

Synonyms and Related Terms: Cardiospasm; diffuse esophageal spasm; primary symptomatic achalasia; secondary achalasia.

Possible Associated Conditions: Chagas disease;* gastric malignancies; irradiation; lymphoma.*

Organs and Tissues	*Procedures*	*Possible or Expected Findings*
Larynx, trachea, bronchi, and lungs		Airway obstruction;* aspiration bronchopneumonia.

Organs and Tissues	Procedures	Possible or Expected Findings
Esophagus	Remove esophagus together with stomach. Photograph esophagus and record diameter of lumen at various levels.	Segmental dilatation and hypertrophy of esophagus. Accumulation of ingested food and esophagitis. Squamous cell carcinoma is a possible complication *(1)*.
	Prepare histologic sections (cut on edge) of narrow and dilated segments.	Barrett's esophagus* with or without adenocarcinoma may be found *(2)*.
	Request Bodian stains and Verhoeff–van Gieson (p. 172).	Loss of myenteric ganglion cells; partial replacement of myenteric nerves.

References

1. Streitz JM Jr, Ellis FH Jr, Gibb SP, Heatley GM. Achalasia and squamous cell carcinoma of the esophagus: analysis of 241 patients. Ann Thorac Surg 1995;59:1604–1609.
2. Ellis FH Jr, Gibb SP, Balogh K, Schwaber JR. Esophageal achalasia and adenocarcinoma in Barrett's esophagus: a report of two cases and a review of the literature. Dis Esophagus 1997;10:55–60.

Achondroplasia

Synonyms: Chondrodystrophia fetalis; Parrot syndrome.

NOTE: The appropriate resource is the International Skeletal Dysplasia Registry

(Cedars-Sinai Medical Center, 444 S. San Vincente Blvd, Ste. 1001, Los Angeles, CA 90048. Phone #310-855-7488).

Organs and Tissues	Procedures	Possible or Expected Findings
External examination	Record body length, head circumference, length of extremities, and abnormal features. Prepare skeletal roentgenograms. Photograph head, thorax, hands, and all abnormalities. Radiographs should be reviewed by a pediatric radiologist.	Dwarfism;* micromelia with pudgy fingers; frontal bossing; depressed nasal bridge. Bowing of legs; kyphosis; short pelvis; broad iliac wings; horizontal acetabular roofs; narrowed vertebral interpedicular distance; shortened tubular bones of hands and feet; precocious ossification centers of epiphyses.
Base of skull and spinal canal; brain and spinal cord; pituitary gland	For removal and specimen preparation of brain and spinal cord, see pp. 65 and 67, respectively. For removal of pituitary gland, see p. 71. Record appearance and photograph base of skull; record diameter of foramen magnum *(1)*. Submit sections of spinal cord at sites of compression.	Growth retardation of base of skull with compression of foramen magnum. Internal hydrocephalus.* Narrow spinal canal with compression of spinal cord (and clinical symptoms of paraplegia). Atrophy of pituitary gland.
Bones	For removal, prosthetic repair, and specimen preparation, see p. 95.	Dorsolumbar kyphosis and lumbosacral lordosis; short iliac wings; short and thick tubular bones; excessive size of epiphysis in long bones; elongated costal cartilage.
	Submit samples (especially of epiphyses) for histologic study. Snap-freeze tissue for molecular analysis.	Decreased cartilage cell proliferation at costochondral junction and at epiphyses of long bones.

Reference

1. Knisely AS, Singer DB. A technique for necropsy evaluation of stenosis of the foramen magnum and rostral spinal canal in osteochondrodysplasia. Hum Pathol 1988;19:1372–1375.

Acidosis

NOTE: Acidosis cannot be diagnosed from postmortem blood pH values. Ketone values remain fairly constant in blood and vitreous and may thus support the diagnosis—for instance, of diabetic acidosis. See also under "Disorder, electrolyte(s)" and p. 115.

Acromegaly

Synonyms and Related Terms: Familial acromegaly; hyperpituitary gigantism.

Possible Associated Condition: Multiple endocrine neoplasia 1 (MEN 1)* *(1)*. See also below under "Other organs."

Organs and Tissues	*Procedures*	*Possible or Expected Findings*
External examination, skin and subcutaneous tissue	Record body length and weight, length of extremities, and abnormal features.	Gigantism in younger persons; coarse facial features with prominent eyebrows and prognathism; maloccluded, wide-spaced teeth. Large, furrowed tongue with tooth marks. Parotid enlargement. Narrow ear canal.
	Prepare sections of skin and subcutaneous tissue.	Increased subcutaneous tissue; thickened skin; hypertrichosis; acanthosis nigricans.
	Prepare skeletal roentgenograms, including skull.	Osteoporosis;* kyphosis. See also below under "Bones and joints."
Breast	Incise and prepare sections.	Lactating breast tissue.
Blood	Submit sample for calcium analysis and radioimmunoassay of plasma growth hormone.	Hypercalcemia in MEN 1 syndrome. Growth hormone excess.
Other organs	Record organ sizes and weights.	Splanchnomegaly, involving heart ("acromegalic heart disease"), liver, spleen, intestine, kidneys, and prostate.
	Sample all endocrine glands for histologic study. See also below under "Pituitary gland."	Endocrine organs may be enlarged (diffuse or nodular goiter; adrenal cortical hyperplasia; enlarged gonads; and parathyroid hyperplasia or adenoma).
	Other procedures depend on expected findings or grossly identified abnormalities as listed in right-hand column.	Pulmonary infections. Nephrolithiasis.* Manifestations of congestive heart failure,* diabetes mellitus,* hyperparathyroidism,* hypertension,* and pituitary insufficiency.* Tumors of breast, colon, thyroid gland, and other organs *(1–4)*.
Pituitary gland	For *in situ* cerebral arteriography, see p. 80. For removal and of pituitary gland, see p. 71. Weigh and photograph gland (include scale). Snap-freeze tumor tissue for histochemical study and hormone assay. For preparation for electron microscopic study, see p. 132.	Usually, pituitary adenoma with predominantly eosinophilic or with mixed eosinophilic-chromophobe cells. Enlargement or destruction of pituitary fossa. Tumor growth (see also "Tumor, pituitary") or hemorrhage may be the cause of death. Tumors may be ectopic (sphenoid sinus or parapharyngeal).
Skeletal muscles	For sampling and specimen preparation, see p. 80.	Proximal myopathy.
Bones and joints	For removal, prosthetic repair, and specimen preparation, see p. 95.	Overgrowth of facial bones and enlarged sinuses (best seen in roentgenogram); thickening of long bones and of clavicles. Periosteal growth of metacarpal and metatarsal bones. Osteoporosis* (primarily of spine). Hypertrophy of costal cartilages. Acromegalic arthritis.

References

1. The BT, Kytola S, Farnebo F, Bergman L, Wong FK, Weber G, et al. Mutation analysis of the MEN 1 gene in multiple endocrine neoplasia type 1, familial acromegaly and familial isolated hyperparathyroidism. J Clin Endocrinol Metabol 1998;83:2621–2626.
2. Melmed S. Acromegaly. N Engl J Med 1990;322:966–971.
3. Cheung NW, Boyages SC. Increased incidence of neoplasia in females with acromegaly. Clin Endocrinol 1997;47:323–327.
4. Barzilay J, Heatley GJ, Cushing GW. Benign and malignant tumors in patients with acromegaly. Arch Intern Med 1991;151:1629–1632.

Actinomycosis

Synonym: *Actinomyces* infection.

NOTE: (1) Collect all tissues that appear to be infected. (2) Request anaerobic cultures for *Actinomyces*. (3) Request Gram stain (p. 172). (4) No special precautions are indicated. (5) Serologic studies are not reliable at present. (6) This is not a reportable disease.

Organs and Tissues	Procedures	Possible or Expected Findings
External examination	Prepare roentgenograms (p. 117) and photographs of fistulas.	Fistulas to skin of face, neck, and other sites. Periostitis or osteomyelitis of mandible. Extension of fistulas into orbits or paranasal sinuses. Mixed infections (microaerophilic streptococci, *Bacteroides* spp.).
	Submit samples of infected tissue for histologic study. For culturing fistules, see p. 104.	Suppurative fibrosing reaction with "sulfur granules" or gram-positive filaments of bacteria.
Chest organs	Submit samples of infected tissue for histologic study.	Chronic cavitary pneumonia; empyema; fistulas through chest wall, pericardium, or diaphragm or into thoracic vertebrae.
Gastrointestinal tract	Submit samples of infected tissue for histologic study. For proper tracing of fistulas, *in situ* dissection is recommended.	Inflammatory masses. Fistulas through abdominal wall, to kidneys or pelvic organs (rare), or ileocecal and anorectal fistulas.
Other organs	Procedures depend on expected findings or grossly identified abnormalities as listed in right-hand column.	Rare manifestations include cerebral, renal, or hepatic abscess, abscesses in other organs or tissues, endocarditis,* or periostitis and osteomyelitis* with fistulas to skin.

Addiction (See "Abuse, hallucinogen(s)," "Abuse, marihuana," "Dependence,..." and "Poisoning,..." See also "Alcoholism and alcohol intoxication.")

Adenoma (See "Neoplasia, multiple endocrine" and "Tumor...")

Adenomatosis, Multiple Endocrine (See "Neoplasia, multiple endocrine.")

Afibrinogenemia (See "Dysfibrinogenemia.")

Agammaglobulinemia (See "Syndrome, primary immunodeficiency.")

Agenesis, Renal

Synonym: Renal aplasia.

Organs and Tissues	Procedures	Possible and Expected Findings
External examination	Photograph infant. Record anomalies.	Evidence of oligohydramnios: flattened nose; prominent palpebral folds; flattened low set ears; flattened hands; recessed chin; joint contractures.
Lungs	Weigh lungs; calculate ratio of lung weight to body weight. (For expected weights, see Part III.)	Pulmonary hypoplasia. Normal LW/BW ratio is greater than 0.015, less than 28 wk gestation and 0.012, older than 28 wk gestation.
Abdominal cavity	Record presence or absence of renal arteries and veins, as well as of ureters, urinary bladder, and internal genital organs. Ascertain patency of the lower urinary tract.	Absence of kidneys and associated malformations (see middle column).
Placenta	Weigh and photograph fetal surface.	Amnion nodosum.

Agranulocytosis (See "Pancytopenia")

AIDS (See "Syndrome, acquired immunodeficiency.")

Alcohol, Ethyl (Ethanol) (See "Alcoholism and alcohol intoxication.")

Alcohol, Isopropyl (See "Poisoning, isopropyl alcohol.")

Alcohol, Methyl (See "Poisoning, methanol (methyl alcohol).")

Alcohol, Rubbing or Wood (See "Poisoning, isopropyl alcohol.")

Alcoholism and Alcohol Intoxication

Synonyms and Related Terms: Alcoholic cirrhosis; alcoholic liver disease;* ethanol intoxication; ethyl alcohol intoxication; fetal alcoholic syndrome;* Wernicke-Korsakoff syndrome.*

NOTE: No reliable interpretation of alcohol concentrations can be problematic if body has been embalmed or is putrefied.

Organs and Tissues	*Procedures*	*Possible or Expected Findings*
External examination		Malnutrition; signs of exposure, injuries, needle marks.
Blood from femoral, subclavian, or brachial veins	Use heart blood only if peripheral blood is unavailable. In this instance, massage heart gently for good mixing. If the blood is not analyzed immediately, add sodium fluoride (10 mg/mL of blood). Fill container to just under the lid so that evaporation remains minimal. Shake thoroughly. Record time of sampling and refrigerate. Request determination of alcohol concentration and drug screen and carbon monoxide determination.	See below under "Can Postmortem Changes and Specimen Storage Affect Blood Alcohol (Ethanol) Concentrations?"
Hematoma	If there are subdural or other hematomas, submit blood for alcohol determination.	Hematoma may show alcohol concentration at time of injury *(1)*.
Vitreous	Submit (pp. 16 and 85) for alcohol determination, particularly if blood is not available. Process like blood. Request determination of potassium, sodium, and chloride concentrations.	See below under "Interpretation of Laboratory Reports" and p. 113.
Cerebrospinal fluid	Submit with or instead of vitreous (p. 104). (Vitreous is probably preferable.)	
Urine	Submit for alcohol determination (p. 16). Process like blood. Record volume.	See below, "How Can One Estimate Blood Alcohol (Ethanol) Concentrations From Vitreous, Urine, or Tissue Alcohol Levels and From Alcohol in Stomach Contents?
Stomach	Record character and volume of contents. Submit samples for histologic study.	Gastritis. See also note above under "Urine."
Bile	Store for possible drug screen.	
Heart	Record weight. Submit samples for histologic study.	Alcoholic cardiomyopathy.*
Lungs	Submit for microbiologic study (p. 103).	Aspiration of vomitus. Lobar pneumonia. Tuberculosis.*
Liver	Record weight and submit samples for histologic study.	Alcoholic liver disease.*
Pancreas		Acute or chronic pancreatitis.*
Brain	For removal, see p. 65. Submit for determination of alcohol concentration (p. 16). Submit samples for histologic study (p. 79).	See below under "Interpretation of Laboratory Reports." Cerebellar cortical degeneration;* Marchiafava-Bignami disease;* Wernicke-Korsakoff syndrome.*
Peripheral nerves and skeletal muscles	For sampling and specimen preparation, see p. 79.	Alcoholic neuropathy or alcoholic myopathy (or both).
Bones		Osteonecrosis* ("aseptic necrosis of bone").

INTERPRETATION OF LABORATORY REPORTS IN ALCOHOL INTOXICATION

How Are Alcohol (Ethanol) Concentrations in Body Fluids Expressed?

In European countries, the concentration is expressed in promille (grams per liter). In the United States, it has become customary to refer to concentration by percentage (grams per deciliter), and values in these units have been written into legislation and included in the uniform vehicle codes. Unless qualified, the use of promille or percentage does not indicate whether the result of the analysis is weight/weight, weight/volume, or volume/volume. Another common way of expressing concentration, milligrams per deciliter, has also been used to indicate alcohol concentrations. The method of expressing concentration must be clearly specified whenever the alcohol level is mentioned. The desired expression can be derived from the toxicologic report by using the following equation:

$$1{,}000\ \mu g/mL = 100\ mg/dL = 21.74\ mmol/L = 1.0\ \text{promille} = 0.10\%$$

What Are the Effects of Alcohol (Ethanol) Intoxication?
Physiologic Effects:*

Blood-Alcohol Concentration g/100 mL	*Stage of Alcoholic Influence*	*Clinical Signs/Symptoms*
0.01–0.05	Subclinical	No apparent influence. Behavior nearly normal by ordinary observation. Slight changes detectable by special tests.
0.03–0.12	Euphoria	Decreased inhibitions. Increased self-confidence. Diminution of attention, judgment, and control. Beginning of sensory-motor impairment. Slowed information processing. Loss of efficiency in finer performance tests.
0.09–0.25	Excitement	Emotional instability; loss of critical judgement. Impairment of perception, memory, and comprehension. Decreased sensory response; increased reaction time. Reduced visual acuity, peripheral vision, and glare recovery. Sensory-motor incoordination; impaired balance. Drowsiness.
0.18–0.30	Confusion	Disorientation, mental confusion; dizziness. Exaggerated emotional states (e.g., fear, rage, sorrow). Disturbances of vision (e.g., diplopia) and of perception of color, form, motions, dimensions. Increased pain threshold. Increased muscular incoordination; staggering gait; slurred speech. Apathy; lethargy.
0.25–0.40	Stupor	General inertia; approaching loss of motor function. Markedly decreased response to stimuli. Marked muscular incoordination; inability to stand or walk. Vomiting; incontinence of urine and feces. Impaired consciousness; sleep or stupor.
0.35-0.50	Coma	Complete unconsciousness; coma; anesthesia. Depressed or abolished reflexes. Subnormal temperature. Incontinence of urine and feces. Impairment of circulation and respiration. Possible death.
0.45+	Death	Death from respiratory arrest.

*Reprinted by permission from KM Dubowsky. Copyright 1987, *(2)*.

Biochemical effects:

Hyponatremia and hypochloremia are common in the chronic alcoholic *(3)*. Hyperlipidemia also may be found.

What is the Legal Interpretation of Alcohol (Ethanol) Intoxication?

Objective impairment of driving ability is observed at threshold blood alcohol concentrations of 35–40 mg/dL. However, values less than 50 mg/dL are considered evidence of "not under the influence" by courts in most states. Values greater than 150 mg/dL are prima facie evidence of "under the influence"; most persons are obviously intoxicated in this range. In 1971 the National Safety Council Committee of Alcohol and Drugs released the following statement: "The National Safety Council Committee on Alcohol and Drugs takes the position that a concentration of 80 milligrams of ethanol per 100 milliliters of whole blood (0.08% w/v) in any driver of a motor vehicle is indicative of impairment in his driving performance."

Can Postmortem Changes and Specimen Storage Affect Blood Alcohol (Ethanol) Concentrations?

Blood alcohol concentrations obtained at autopsy are valid until putrefaction begins. This may vary from several hours to a few days, depending on the environment. Sodium fluoride in a concentration of 10 mg/mL of blood should be added to the sample, and the specimen should be stored in the refrigerator. If the blood is analyzed soon after withdrawal or if the blood is kept in the refrigerator, results are usually reliable even if no sodium fluoride has been added. If the air space above the blood samples in the container is large, alcohol can evaporate and a falsely low blood alcohol level can result. Putrefactive changes before autopsy or during storage may cause a falsely high blood alcohol concentration. Ethanol can be produced in the specimen container; this is more like in the absence of a preservative. Because fluoride inhibits bacteria far more than fungi, higher fluoride concentrations are required for the inhibition of fungal growth *(4)*.

Can the Sites Where Blood Was Withdrawn Affect Alcohol (Ethanol) Concentrations?

Although there is no major difference in the alcohol concentrations of blood samples from the intact heart chambers and the femoral vessels *(5)*, autopsy samples from pooled blood in the pericardial sac or pleural cavity are unsatisfactory. We therefore recommend that blood be withdrawn from peripheral vessels.

Is There Normal "Endogenous" Blood Alcohol (Ethanol) in a Living Person?

Blood alcohol concentrations are generally believed to be negligible in the absence of ingested alcohol. "Endogenous" ethanol in human blood exists at a concentration of about 0.0002 g/dL, which is below the limit of detection for most methods *(6)*.

Which Conditions or Factors May Lower the Tolerance to Alcohol (Ethanol) So That Death May Occur at Levels That Are Not Usually Fatal?

First in such a list would be postural asphyxia, for example, in drunks who fall asleep face down. Also, depressant drugs in the tricyclic, analgesic, barbiturate, and benzodiazepine classes all potentiate the effect of alcohol *(7)*. Also included in such a list would be infancy and childhood; ischemic heart disease;* chronic bronchitis and emphysema;* other chronic debilitating diseases; poisoning with carbon tetrachloride* or carbon monoxide;* and other causes of hypoxia.*

How Can One Estimate Blood Alcohol (Ethanol) Concentrations From Vitreous, Urine, or Tissue Alcohol Levels and From Alcohol in Stomach Contents?

The ratio of serum, plasma, urine, vitreous, and various tissues has been compiled by Garriot *(8)*. The values may vary considerably. For vitreous, the ratios varied from 0.46–1.40. These variations may depend on whether blood alcohol concentrations were increasing or decreasing at the time of death. Most other body fluids and tissues showed ranges closer to 1. Most urine values were above the blood alcohol concentrations. In another study *(9)*, the blood/vitreous (B/V) ratio in the early absorption phase was 1.29 (range, 0.71–3.71; SD 0.57) and in the late absorption and elimination phase, the B/V ratio was 0.89 (range, 0.32–1.28; SD 0.19). Blood ethanol concentrations probably can be estimated using B = 1.29V for early absorption and B = 0.89V for later phases. A urine/blood ethanol ratio of 1.20 or less indicates that the diceased was in the early absorption phase.

How Can One Use Alcohol (Ethanol) Concentrations in Postmortem Specimens To Estimate the Blood Alcohol Concentration at Various Times Before Death?

With certain limitations, one can base calculations of this kind on the assumption that the blood alcohol level decreases from its peak at a fairly constant rate of 0.015–0.018/h until death *(10)*. If blood is not available, conversion factors (see above) must be used. Alcoholics have been reported to metabolize at a rate of up to 0.043%/h *(6)*.

Example: The driver of an automobile had been drinking at a party until midnight. He had left his host at about 1:30 a.m. and was involved in a head-on collision at 2:15 a.m. He died in the emergency room of the hospital at 6:35 a.m. There were multiple injuries and the patient had exsanguinated. The autopsy was done at 1:30 p.m. Although this appears quite unlikely, let us assume that no satisfactory blood sample was obtained and that no blood or plasma expanders were given. If under such circumstances the alcohol concentration in the vitreous was found to be 157 mg/dL, what was the alcohol concentration in the blood at the time of the accident?

Vitreous and blood alcohol concentrations may be assumed to have remained unchanged after death. Therefore, the blood alcohol level at the time of death must have been approx 157 (vitreous humor alcohol) × 0.89 (conversion factor, see above) = 140 mg/dl. The time interval between the accident (2:15 a.m.) and death (6:35 a.m.) was 4 h and 20 min or 4 1/3 h. If we assume that the decedent was not an alcoholic and that the blood alcohol concentration was decreasing from its peak at a constant rate of 15 mg/dL/h, then the concentration at the time of the accident is estimated to have been 140 (concentration at time of death) + (4 1/3 x 15) = 140 + 65 = 205 mg/dL or 0.2%.

The blood alcohol concentration at the time of the accident could have been lower if the victim stopped drinking later than 1 h or 1 1/2 h before the accident. In the latter case, the peak alcohol level would have occurred after the accident, reflecting the time to absorb the latest drink.

The blood alcohol concentration at the time of the accident could have been lower or higher if the time when the patient stopped drinking, the time of the accident, or the time of the death is uncertain.

The blood alcohol concentration at the time of the accident could have been higher if the victim was a chronic alcoholic (based on the history or the presence of alcoholic hepatitis or alcoholic cirrhosis). The elimination rate in such persons may be as high as 40 mg/dL, which would change the figures in our example above to 140 + (4 1/3 × 40) = 140 + 173 = 313 mg/dl or 0.3%.

How Can One Use Alcohol (Ethanol) Concentrations in Postmortem Specimens To Estimate How Much the Victim Had Been Drinking?

Only rough estimates are possible. First, the peak blood alcohol level must be determined or calculated, as described in the previous paragraphs. Tables (see below) are available that relate blood alcohol level to the minimal amounts of whiskey, wine, or beer that must have been consumed *(10)*. However, tables of this type are often based on the minimum amount of alcohol circulating in the body after specific numbers of drinks; such tables do not yield reliable results if used conversely. Furthermore, inasmuch as drinking and elimination of alcohol may take place concomitantly, over a longer period the total amount of alcohol consumed may have been much greater than the tables would indicate. It cannot be lower. According to these tables, 6 pints of ordinary beer or 8 fl oz of whiskey would be the minimal amounts needed to produce a blood alcohol level of about 200 mg/dL in a person weighing 140–180 pounds. The total body alcohol can be calculated from the blood alcohol level by using Widmark's formula:

$$\frac{\text{Average concentration of alcohol in entire body} = .68}{\text{Concentration of alcohol in the blood}}$$

In a person weighing 70 kg, the blood alcohol concentration would be increased 50 mg/dL (0.05%) by the absorption of 1 oz of ethanol (2 oz of 100-proof whiskey).

What Is the Alcohol (Ethanol) Content of Various Beverages?

Strength of alcohol is measured in "proof"; absolute alcohol is 200 proof. Therefore, in the United States, alcohol content as volume percent is half the proof (for example, 100-proof whiskey contains 50% alcohol by volume). The alcohol content of various beverages is shown in the following table.

Approximate Alcohol Content in Various Beverages†

Beverage	*Ethanol Content in %*
Whiskey and gin	40
Brandy	45.5–48.5
Sherry and port wines	16–20
Liqueurs	34–59
Rum	50–69.5
Beers (Lager)	2–6
Light wines	10–15

†Data from Glaister, Rentoul E. Medical Jurisprudence and Toxicology, 12th ed. E & S Livingstone, Edinburgh, 1966 with permission.

What Blood Alcohol (Ethanol) Concentrations Can Be Predicted From a Known Amount and Type of Alcoholic Beverage?

Number of Drinks and Predicted Blood Alcohol Concentrations†

Drinks (no.)‡	*Predicted Blood Alcohol Level (mg/dL)*
1	10–30
2	30–50
3	50–80
4	80–100
5	100–130
6	130–160
8	160–200
10	190–230
12	250–320

†Within 1 h after consumption of diluted alcohol (approx 15%) on an empty stomach, assuming body weight of 140–180 pounds (63.6–81.7 kg) reproduced from *(11)* with permission.

‡One ounce (about 30 mL) of whiskey or 12 oz (about 355 mL) of beer.

What Is the Toxicity of Alcohol Other Than Ethanol?

In general, the toxicity increases as the number of carbon atoms in the alcohol increases. Thus, butyl alcohol is two times as toxic as ethyl alcohol,* but isopropyl alcohol is only two-thirds as toxic as isobutyl alcohol and one-half as toxic as amyl alcohol. Primary alcohols are more toxic than the corresponding secondary isomers *(10)*.

References

1. Hirsch CS, Adelson L. Ethanol in sequestered hematomas. Am J Clin Pathol 1973;59:429–433.
2. Dubowsky KM. Stages of acute alcoholic influence/intoxication. In: Medicolegal Aspects of Alcohol. Garriott JC, ed. Lawyers & Judges Publishing Co., Phoenix AZ, 1997, p. 40.
3. Sturner WQ, Coe JI. Electrolyte imbalance in alcoholic liver disease. J Forensic Sci 1973;18:344–350.
4. Harper DR, Corry JEL. Collection and storage of specimens for alcohol analysis. In: Medicolegal Aspects of Alcohol. Garriott JC, ed. Lawyers & Judges Publishing Co., Phoenix, AZ, 1997, pp. 145–169.
5. Garriott JC. Analysis for alcohol in postmortem specimens. In: Medicolegal Aspects of Alcohol. Garriott JC, ed. Lawyers & Judges Publishing Co., Phoenix, AZ, 1997, pp. 87–100.
6. Baselt RC, Danhof IE. Disposition of alcohol in man. In: Medicolegal Aspects of Alcohol. Garriott JC, ed. Lawyers & Judges Publishing Co., Tuscon, AZ, 1993, pp. 55–74.
7. Garriott JC. Pharmacology of ethyl alcohol. In: Medicolegal Aspects of Alcohol. Garriott JC, ed. Lawyers & Judges Publishing Co., Phoenix, AZ, 1997, pp. 36–54.
8. Caplan YH. Blood, urine and other tissue specimens for alcohol analysis. In: Medicolegal Aspects of Alcohol. Garriott JC, ed. Lawyers & Judges Publishing Co., Phoenix, AZ, 1997, pp. 74–86.
9. Chao TC, Lo DS. Relationship between postmortem blood and vitreous humor ethanol levels. Am J Forens Med Pathol 1993;14:303–308.
10. Larson CP. Alcohol: fact and fallacy. In: Legal Medicine Annual 1969. Wecht CH, ed. Appleton-Century-Crofts, New York, 1969, pp. 241–268.
11. Camps FE. Gradwohl's Legal Medicine, 2nd ed. Williams & Wilkins Company, Baltimore, MD, 1968, p. 554.

Aldosteronism

Synonyms and Related Terms: Bartter's syndrome; Conn's syndrome; hyperaldosteronism; idiopathic aldosteronism; primary aldosteronism; secondary aldosteronism.

Organs and Tissues	*Procedures*	*Possible or Expected Findings*
External examination	Record presence or absence of edema.	Edema of lower extremities (absent in most uncomplicated cases).
Vitreous	Submit for sodium and potassium determination (pp. 16 and 33).	Changes reflecting high sodium and low potassium concentrations in the blood.
Heart	Weigh heart and measure thickness of ventricles.	Prominent left ventricular hypertrophy *(1)*.
Adrenals	Dissect, weigh, and photograph both adrenal glands. Place portion (including tumor, if present) of gland in deep freeze for hormone assay.	Aldosterone-secreting adrenal cortical adenoma (Conn's syndrome), adrenal cortical nodular hyperplasia, or, rarely, adrenal carcinoma. Primary aldosteronism may be present in all these instances.
	Submit samples for light and electron microscopic (p. 132) study.	Idiopathic aldosteronism is characterized by normal adrenal glands.

Organs and Tissues	*Procedures*	*Possible or Expected Findings*
Kidneys	Weigh, measure, photograph. Submit samples for histologic and electron microscopic (p. 132) study. If there is a renal tumor, place portion in a deep freeze for hormone assay.	Vacuolar (osmotic) nephropathy due to hypokalemia. Various renal diseases may be associated with secondary hyperaldosteronism; features of juxtaglomerular cell hyperplasia may be present.
Other organs	Procedures in secondary aldosteronism depend on expected cause.	Manifestations of hypertension.* Cirrhosis,* nephrotic syndrome,* toxemia of pregnancy,* and many other conditions that may be associated with secondary aldosteronism.
Brain	For removal and specimen preparation, see p. 65. For cerebral angiography, see p. 80.	Ruptured intracranial aneurysm* and hemorrhagic stroke *(2)*.

References

1. Tanabe A, Naruse M, Naruse K, Hase M, Yoshimoto T, Tanaka M, et al. Left ventricular hypertrophy is more prominent in patients with primary aldosteronism than in patients with other types of secondary hypertension. Hypertension Res 1997;20:85–90.
2. Litchfield WR, Anderson BF, Weiss RJ, Lifton RP, Dluhy RG. Intracranial aneurysm and hemorrhagic stroke in glucocorticoid-remediable aldosteronism. Hypertension 1998;31:445–450.

Alkalosis

NOTE: There are no diagnostic findings. Postmortem chemical analysis is of limited value in these instances. See also under "Disorder, electrolyte(s)" and p. 115.

Alkaptonuria

Synonyms and Related Terms: Alkaptonuric ochronosis *(1)*; familial (hereditary) ochronosis *(2)*.

Organs and Tissues	*Procedures*	*Possible or Expected Findings*
External examination and skin	Record extent of discoloration of skin and eyes. Photograph these features. Prepare histologic sections of pigmented areas.	Brown-black pigment in skin, eyes (conjunctivas, corneas, scleras), and external ears. Pigment in dermal sweat glands.
	Record appearance of joint deformities.	Deformities of knees and other joints.
	Prepare skeletal roentgenograms.	Ochronotic arthropathy, particularly of knee joints; spondylosis and disk calcification with fusion of vertebrae.
Urine	Submit sample for biochemical study.	Hemogentisic aciduria.
Heart and large arteries	Prepare histologic sections of pigmented areas. If electron microscopic study is intended, see p. 132.	Pigmentation of heart valves (e.g., with stenosis *[2]*), endocardium, and intima of large arteries.
Larynx and trachea	Prepare histologic sections of pigmented cartilage.	Pigmentation of laryngotracheal cartilage.
Kidneys and prostate	Submit samples for histologic study.	Nephrolithiasis;* prostatitis; ochronotic pigmentation.
Other organs and tissues	Submit samples for histologic study.	Pigmentation in islets of Langerhans, pituitary gland, and other endocrine organs; pigment in reticuloendothelial system.
Middle ears	For removal and specimen preparation, see p. 72.	Pigmentation of tympanic membranes and ossicles of middle ears.
Eyes	For removal and specimen preparation, see p. 85.	See under "External examination and skin."
Bones and joints	For removal, prosthetic repair, and specimen preparation, see p. 95. Submit samples of cartilage of diarthrodial joints and from adjacent tendons for histologic study. Prepare frontal section through spine.	Ochronotic arthropathy (see above under "External examination and skin"). Fragments of pigmented cartilage may be found in the synovia.

References

1. Gaines JJ Jr. The pathology of alkaptonuric ochronosis. Hum Pathol 1989;20:40–46.
2. Cortina R, Moris C, Astudillo A, Gosalbez F, Cortina A. Familial ochronosis. Eur Heart J 1995;16:285–286.

Aluminosis (See "Pneumoconiosis.")

Alveolitis, Extrinsic Allergic (See "Pneumoconiosis" and "Pneumonia, interstitial.")

Amaurosis Fugax

Organs and Tissues	*Procedures*	*Possible or Expected Findings*
Eyes	For removal and specimen preparation, see p. 85.	Papilledema.
Brain	For removal and specimen preparation, see p. 65. Other procedures depend on expected findings or grossly identified abnormalities as listed in right-hand column.	Tumor of the brain or other cause of intracranial hypertension, including benign intracranial hypertension (pseudotumor cerebri*).

Amblyopia, Nutritional

Related Terms: Alcohol amblyopia; retrobulbar neuropathy; tobacco amblyopia.

NOTE: If chronic malnutrition is associated with corneal degeneration, glossitis, stomatitis, and genital dermatitis, the condition is referred to as Strachan's syndrome.

Organs and Tissues	*Procedures*	*Possible or Expected Findings*
Brain	For removal and specimen preparation, see p. 65. Leave optic nerve attached (see below).	See below under "Eyes with optic nerves."
Eyes with optic nerves	For removal and specimen preparation, see p. 85. Request Luxol fast blue stain of optic nerves (p. 172).	Bilateral symmetric loss of myelinated fibers in central parts of optic nerves. Ganglion cells in macula may be lost.
Other organs	Procedures depend on expected findings or grossly identified abnormalities as listed in right-hand column.	Manifestations of alcoholism,* diabetes mellitus,* malnutrition,* megaloblastic anemia,* tobacco dependence, and tuberculosis* (isoniazid treatment may cause the optic nerve damage).

Amebiasis

Synonym: *Entamoeba histolytica* infection.

NOTE: (1) Collect all tissues that appear to be infected. (2) Request parasitologic examination as well as aerobic and anaerobic cultures. Bacterial infections may be associated with amebiasis. (3) Request Gram and Giemsa stains (p. 172). (4) No special precautions are indicated. (5) Serologic studies are available in many local and state health department laboratories (p. 135). (6) This is a **reportable** disease.

Possible Associated Conditions: Acquired immunodeficiency syndrome (AIDS)* *(1)*.

Organs and Tissues	*Procedures*	*Possible or Expected Findings*
External examination and skin	Photograph and prepare sections of cutaneous or mucosal lesions.	Perianal and perineal ulcers after extension of amebic colitis; rarely, destruction of external genitalia. Cutaneous amebiasis from fistulas after hepatic abscess, laparotomy, or, rarely, distant spread.
Chest organs, abdominal cavity, retroperitoneal space, and pelvic organs	Record presence and course of fistulas before removal of organs. Material for parasitologic study and bacterial cultures is best removed at this time.	Amebic pneumonia, often associated with hepatic abscess (see below). Pleuropulmonary amebiasis, with or without empyema. Amebic pericarditis or amebic peritonitis is rare. Intestinal perforation into peritoneal cavity, retroperitoneal space, or other hollow viscera.

Organs and Tissues	Procedures	Possible or Expected Findings
Intestine	Examine as soon as possible so as to reduce the effects of autolysis.	
	Photograph ulcers and collect samples for smears and histologic study. Specimens should include cecum; ascending, sigmoid, transverse, and descending colon; appendix; and ileum.	Buttonhole or flask-shaped mucosal ulcers are always present, in an order of involvement as listed in the middle column.
Liver	If there is a hepatic abscess with fistulas, record their course before removal of liver. Use Letulle technique (p. 3) for organ removal, and open inferior vena cava along posterior midline.	Hepatic abscess(es) with or without perforation and fistula(s). Hepatic fibrosis and necroses. Portal vein thrombosis can occur. Abscess may communicate with inferior vena cava, gallbladder, bile ducts, and other structures.
	Aspirate abscess contents and submit for microbiologic study. Prepare smears and sections from periphery of abscess.	Amebae are difficult to demonstrate in amebic hepatic abscesses.
Urinary tract	If urinary tract system appears involved, incise kidneys *in situ*, in frontal plane from periphery toward pelvis (leave vessels attached); open renal pelves, ureters, and urinary bladder *in situ*.	Rarely, ascending amebic infection associated with amebic colitis and perianal spread.
Other organs	Procedures depend on expected findings or grossly identified abnormalities as listed in right-hand column.	Rarely, spread to spleen, aorta, or larynx. Other sites may be affected by systemic hematogenous dissemination.
Brain	For removal and specimen preparation, see p. 65.	Cerebral abscess* almost always associated with hepatic abscess and pulmonary amebiasis.

Reference

1. Fatkenheuer G, Arnold G, Steffen HM, Franzen C, Schrappe M, Diehl V, Salzberger B. Invasive amebiasis in two patients with AIDS and cytomegalovirus colitis. J Clin Microbiol 1997;35:2168–2169.

Aminoaciduria

Related Terms: Proprionic acidemia; methyl malonic acidemia; isovaleric acidemia; cystinuria; homocystinuria;* maple syrup urine disease;* urea cycle disorders; tyrosinemia; phenylketonuria.*

NOTE: Aminoaciduria is a collective name for all the conditions mentioned under "Related Terms." Because few autopsy studies of aminoaciduria have been done, each case should be considered a potential source of new, unpublished information. Multiple abnormalities of virtually all organ systems are possible.

Organs and Tissues	Procedures	Possible or Expected Findings
Blood, cerebrospinal fluid, and urine	For removal of cerebrospinal fluid, see p. 104. Freeze samples for biochemical study.	Many abnormalities may be present. For specific enzyme defects, see ref. *(1)*.
Fascia lata, liver, spleen, or blood	These specimens should be collected using aseptic technique for tissue culture for chromosome analysis and biochemical studies (see Chapter 10).	Rare translocations are described *(2)*.
Other organs	See above under "Note."	Multiple organs and tissues may be involved. Frequently affected is the central nervous system, eyes, liver, kidneys, and skeletal system (rickets).

References

1. Chalmers RA, Lawson AM. Organic Acids in Man: The Analytical Chemistry, Biochemistry and Diagnosis of the Organic Acidurias. Chapman and Hall, London, 1982.
2. Hodgson SV, Heckmatt JZ, Hughes E, Crolla JA, Dubowitz V, Bobrow M. A balanced de novo X/autosome translocation in a girl with manifestations of Lowe syndrome. Am J Med Gen 1986;23:837–847.

Ammonia (See "Poisoning, gas" and "Bronchitis, acute chemical.")

Amphetamine(s) (See "Dependence, amphetamine(s).")

Amyloidosis

Related Terms: Familial amyloidosis (multiple forms, including familial Mediterranean fever and familial amyloid nephropathy with urticaria and deafness; hereditary cerebral angiopathies); idiopathic or primary amyloidosis (AL protein) *(1)*; localized or isolated amyloidosis (amyloid in islets of Langerhans and insulinoma; congophil cerebral angiopathy;* isolated atrial amyloid; medullary carcinoma of thyroid); reactive or secondary amyloidosis (AA protein); systemic senile amyloidosis.

Possible Associated Conditions: Alzheimer's disease;* Behçet's disease;* bronchiectasis;* chronic dialysis;* Creutzfeldt-Jakob disease;* Crohn's disease;* diabetes mellitus type II; Down's syndrome;* leprosy;* malignant lymphoma, Hodgkin's type; macroglobulinemia; multiple myeloma;* osteomyelitis;* paraplegia; Reiter's syndrome;* rheumatoid arthritis* and other immune connective tissue diseases (all types); syphilis;* tuberculosis;* Whipple's disease.*

NOTE: Stain 15-micron tissue sections with Congo red and examine under polarized light for green birefringence. In AA-type amyloid but not in AL amyloid, pretreatment of tissue with permanganate, followed by routine staining with Congo red, will abolish the green birefringence. An immunohistochemistry panel is available to differentiate the subtypes of amyloidosis. Crystal violet, methyl violet, Sirius red, sodium sulfate alcian blue, and thioflavin T also stain amyloid in many instances. Electron microscopic studies *(2)* are particularly useful if routine stains are negative or controversial. For macroscopic staining of amyloid, e.g., in the heart, see p. 133.

Organs and Tissues	*Procedures*	*Possible or Expected Findings*
External examination and skin	Submit grossly involved and uninvolved skin for histologic study (look for amyloid in subcutaneous fat). For special stains, see above under "Note."	Papules or plaques, particularly around eyes, ears, axillae, inguinal regions, and anus. Papules may be tumorous or pigmented. Periorbital ecchymoses may be present.
Mouth	Submit gingiva, palate, and tongue for histologic study.	Amyloid infiltrates; macroglossia.
Blood and urine	In unsuspected cases, submit samples for immunoelectrophoresis and immunofixation.	Presence of monoclonal light chain.
Heart	Submit tissue from atria and myocardium of ventricles. Photograph endocardial lesions. For gross and microscopic staining, see above under "Note."	Amyloid deposits may be identifiable under endocardium of left atrium. Nonischemic congestive heart failure *(1)*.
Liver	Record size and weight. For gross and microscopic staining, see above under "Note."	Hepatomegaly with amyloid infiltrates.
Gastrointestinal tract	Take sections of all segments of the gastrointestinal tract.	Amyloid infiltrates with ulcerations and hemorrhages.
Other organs	Microscopic samples should include respiratory system with larynx, gallbladder, pancreas, spleen, all portions of urogenital system, including prostate, seminal vesicles, and vasa deferentia, and all endrocrine glands, blood vessels, lymph nodes, and other tissues, such as omentum. For gross and microscopic staining methods, see above under "Note."	Almost all organs and tissues may be involved. Diffuse, nodular, or primary vascular deposits may predominate. Evidence of portal hypertension* may be found but splenomegaly also may be caused by amyloid infiltrates. Nephrotic syndrome;* renal involvement also may be associated with renal vein thrombosis.* See also above under "Possible Associated Conditions."
Eyes	For removal and specimen preparation, see p. 85.	Ocular amyloidosis *(3)*.
Brain, spinal cord, and peripheral nerves	For removal and specimen preparation, see pp. 65, 67, and 79, respectively.	Amyloid associated with senile plaques or neurofibrillary tangles; congophilic angiopathy *(4)*. Spinal cord compression *(5)*. Peripheral amyloid neuropathy.
Bones and bone marrow, joints, tendons	For removal, prosthetic repair of bones and joints, and specimen preparation, see p. 95.	Amyloid in bone marrow, synovium, and carpal tunnel. Bone may contain osteolytic tumor (multiple myeloma*).

References

1. Gertz MA, Lacy MQ, Dispenzieri A. Amyloidosis: recognition, confirmation, prognosis, and therapy. Mayo Clin Proc 1999;74:490–494.
2. Lin CS, Wong CK. Electron microscopy of primary and secondary cutaneous amyloidosis and systemic amyloidosis. Clin Dermatol 1990; 8:36–45.
3. Gorevic PD, Rodrigues NM. Ocular amyloidosis. Am J Ophthalmol 1994;117:529–532.
4. Duchen LW. Current status review: cerebral amyloid. Intern J Exp Pathol 1992;73:535–550.
5. Villarejo F, Perez Diaz C, Perla C, Sanz J, Escalona J, Goyenechea F. Spinal cord compression by amyloid deposits. Spine 1994;19:1178–1181.

Amyotonia Congenita

NOTE: Amyotonia congenita encompasses several different neuromuscular disorders. See under "Disease, motor neuron."

Anaphylaxis (See "Death, anaphylactic.")

Ancylostomiasis

Synonyms: Hookworm disease; miners' anemia; uncinariasis.

NOTE: (1) Collect all tissues that appear to be infected. (2) Cultures are usually not necessary, only parasitologic examination. (3) Request azure-eosin stains (p. 172). (4) No special precautions are indicated. (5) Serologic studies are available at the state health department laboratories (p. 135). (6) This is not a reportable disease.

Organs and Tissues	*Procedures*	*Possible or Expected Findings*
Small intestine	For *in situ* fixation and preparation for study by dissecting microscopy, see p. 54. Request PAS with diastase treatment, azure-eosin, Perl's (or Gomori's) stain for iron, and Verhoeff–van Gieson stains (p. 172).	Erosions; hemorrhages *(1)*; mucus in lumen; thickening of wall. Sprue-like mucosal changes (atrophy of villi) with deposition of hemosiderin, necrosis of mucosa, eosinophils in wall, and fibrosis of submucosa. Worms in second and third portions of jejunum.
Mesentery	Submit lymph nodes for histologic study.	Mesenteric lymphadenitis.
Liver and spleen	Submit tissue samples for histologic study.	Myeloid metaplasia.
Other organs	Procedures depend on expected findings or grossly identified abnormalities as listed in right-hand column.	Manifestations of iron deficiency anemia,* hypoproteinemia, and congestive heart failure.*

Reference

1. Kuo YC, Chen PC, Wu CS. Massive intestinal bleeding in an adult with hookworm infection. J Clin Gastroenterol 1995;20:348–350.

Anemia (See under specific designations.)

Anemia, Aplastic (See "Anemia, Fanconi's" or "pancytopenia.")

Anemia Associated With Chronic Systemic Diseases

Related Term: Normochromic normocytic anemia.

NOTE: This type of anemia occurs with chronic inflammatory conditions such as endocarditis,* osteomyelitis,* or tuberculosis* but may also be associated with connective tissue disorders such as lupus erythematosus* or rheumatoid arthritis.* Malignancies, uremia, chronic liver disease, endocrine disorders (e.g., Adrenal insufficiency,* hypothyroidism,* or pituitary insufficiency*), or poisoning with chemicals or drugs and radiation injury may also be involved.* The anemia in some of these conditions may be slightly microcytic or macrocytic.

Organs and Tissues	*Procedures*	*Possible or Expected Findings*
All organs	Request iron stain.	See above under "Note." Extramedullary hematopoiesis and hemosiderosis, particularly of liver and spleen.
Bone marrow	For preparation of sections and smears, see p. 96.	Frequently hyperplastic. Hypoplastic in bone marrow failure (pancytopenia*).

Anemia, Fanconi's

Synonyms: Congenital aplastic anemia; congenital pancytopenia; constitutional infantile panmyelopathy; familial panmyelophthisis; Fanconi's pancytopenia; Fanconi's syndrome (see also under "NOTE"); pancytopenia-dysmelia syndrome.

NOTE: Another disease group, also named "Fanconi's syndrome," is marked by proximal renal tubular transport defect; this latter syndrome is unrelated to Fanconi's anemia.

Organs and Tissues	*Procedures*	*Possible or Expected Findings*
External examination	Record and photograph abnormalities. Request radiographs of skeleton.	Short stature; microcephaly; café au lait spots; dyskeratosis congenita; absent/ hypoplastic thumbs; hyperpigmentation; nail dystrophy; hypogonadism; microphthalmia.
Blood, fascia lata, or liver (liver obtained by percutaneous biopsy)	These specimens should be collected using aseptic technique for tissue culture for chromosome analysis (see Chapter 10).	Chromosomal breaks.
Other organs	Culture any sites suggestive of infection. Record and photograph sites of bleeding. Record weight of spleen. Request iron stains.	Hemosiderosis. Small spleen. Small pituitary gland. Evidence of infection or hemorrhage at various sites. Solid tumors *(1)* (liver and other organs or tissues, including eyes and bones).
Bone marrow	For preparations of sections and smears, see p. 96. If the patient underwent bone marrow transplantation, follow procedures under that heading also.	Pancytopenia;* myelodysplastic syndromes and leukemia* *(1)*.
Eyes	For removal and specimen preparation, see p. 85.	Epiphoria, blepharitis, cataracts.

Reference

1. Alter BP. Fanconi's anemia and malignancies. Am J Hematol 1996; 53:99–110.

Anemia, Hemolytic

Synonyms and Related Terms: Acquired hemolytic anemia; extracorpuscular hemolytic anemia; hereditary hemolytic anemia (hereditary elliptocytosis, pyropoikilocytosis, stomatocytosis. spherocytosis); immunohemolytic anemia; intracorpuscular hemolytic anemia; microangiopathic hemolytic anemia; spur cell anemia.

Possible Associated Conditions: Disseminated intravascular coagulation;* eclampsia;* glucose-6-phosphatase deficiency (G6PD); hemolytic uremic syndrome;* malignant hypertension; lymphoma* and other malignancies; paroxysmal nocturnal hemoglobinuria; sickle cell disease;* thalassemia;* thrombotic thrombocytopenic purpura.* (See also below under "NOTE.")

NOTE: Hemolysis also may be caused by conditions such as poisoning with chemicals or drugs, heat injury, snake bite,* or infections or may develop as a transfusion reaction* or be secondary to adenocarcinoma, heart valve prostheses (see below), liver disease (see below), renal disease, or congenital erythropoietic porphyria.*

Organs and Tissues	*Procedures*	*Possible or Expected Findings*
External examination	Prepare skeletal roentgenograms.	Jaundice; skin ulcers over malleoli. In young patients: thickening of frontal and parietal bones with loss of outer table ("hair-on-end" appearance); paravertebral masses caused by extramedullary hematopoiesis; deformities of metacarpals, metatarsals, and phalanges. Osteonecrosis* of femoral heads. Osteoporosis.*
Blood	In the absence of in vivo studies, submit samples for bacterial and viral cultures, or toxicologic, immunologic, or other laboratory studies, depending on the expected cause.	Bacteremia or septicemia. Viremia (e.g., parvovirus infection in hereditary spherocytosis). Chemical poisons or drugs. Beta-lipoprotein deficiency (abetalipoproteinemia*). Abnormal antibodies. Hyperbilirubinemia.
	For hemoglobin electrophoresis, autolyzed blood can be used; one can also use blood that was drained from tissues.	Abnormal hemoglobins.

Organs and Tissues	Procedures	Possible or Expected Findings
Urine	See above under "Blood."	Hemoglobinuria.
Heart	Record weight. Request iron stain (p. 172).	Hemosiderosis and cardiomegaly. Valvular heart disease with or without inserted prosthesis may be cause of hemolytic anemia.
Lungs	Perfuse one lung with formalin (p. 47).	Infarcts in sickle cell disease.*
Liver	Record weight. Request iron stain (p. 172).	Hemosiderosis and hepatomegaly. Extramedullary hematopoiesis. Liver diseases such as viral hepatitis* and acute fatty change may cause hemolytic anemia.
Gallbladder and common bile duct	Describe appearance of stones or request chemical analysis.	Cholelithiasis,* cholecystitis,* or choledocholithiasis associated with pigment stones (particularly in hereditary hemolytic anemia such as spherocytosis).
Spleen	See above under "Liver" and below under "Kidneys." Request iron stain.	Hemosiderosis and splenomegaly. Extramedullary hematopoiesis. Infarctions in sickle cell disease.*
Kidneys	If abnormalities are present, photograph cut sections.	Infarcts and papillary necrosis in sickle cell disease.* Renal diseases may also be cause of hemolytic anemia.
Other organs and tissues	Extensive histologic sampling is indicated, particularly if the cause of the hemolysis is not known.	See above under "Possible Associated Conditions" and under "Note." Search for fibrin deposits in microvasculature as seen in thrombotic thrombocytopenic purpura.*
Bones and bone marrow	For preparation of sections and smears, see p. 96. Request Giemsa stains and Gomori's or Perl's iron stains (p. 172). Consult roentgenograms for proper sampling.	Erythroid hyperplasia or, rarely, hypoplasia or normal marrow; hemosiderosis of bone marrow. Osteonecrosis* in sickle cell disease.*

Anemia, Hypochromic (See "Anemia, iron deficiency.")

Anemia, Iron Deficiency

Possible Associated Conditions: Conditions associated with blood loss (e.g., Crohn's disease;* diaphragmatic hernia,* diverticula,* malabsorption syndrome,* tumor,* ulcer of stomach or duodenum,* or ulcerative colitis); lead poisoning* in children.

Organs and Tissues	Procedures	Possible or Expected Findings
External examination	Record body weight and height. Photograph finger nails.	Manifestations of malnutrition.* Angular stomatitis; spoon nails (koilonychia).
Blood	Prepare smears.	Hypochromic and microcytic erythrocytes.
Heart		Dilatation of chambers.
Esophagus and neck organs with tongue	Remove as one specimen. Photograph web or stricture from above. Submit tissue samples of all segments for histologic study.	Glossitis; postcricoid esophageal web or stricture (Plummer-Vinson syndrome*).
Gastrointestinal tract with anus	Search for possible source of chronic hemorrhage.	See above under "Possible Associated Conditions." Hemorrhoids.
Spleen	Record weight.	Splenomegaly.
Genitourinary system	Search for possible source of chronic hemorrhage.	Tumors or inflammatory conditions.
Other organs		Manifestations of congestive heart failure.*
Bone marrow	For preparation of sections and smears, see p. 96. Request iron stain.	Hyperplasia. Reduced or absent iron in macrophages.

Anemia, Megaloblastic

Related Terms: Pernicious anemia; vitamin B_{12} deficiency.

NOTE: The condition can be caused by many disorders associated with cobalamin or folic acid deficiency (e.g., malabsorption-related); other causes include adverse drug effects, alcoholism, and rare metabolic disorders. The condition may occur in infancy or during pregnancy. Hemolytic anemia,* hypoparathyroidism,* adrenal cortical insufficiency* (Addison's disease), or scurvy may be present.

Organs and Tissues	*Procedures*	*Possible or Expected Findings*
External examination and oral cavity	Record body weight, color of skin and sclerae, and presence or absence of conditions listed in right-hand colum.	Jaundice. Manifestations of malnutrition.* Stomatitis with cheilosis and perianal ulcerations due to folic acid deficiency. Chronic exfoliative skin disorders. Vitiligo.
Blood	Prepare smears.	Macrocytosis; poikilocytosis; macroovalocytes; hypersegmentation of leukocytes; abnormal platelets.
Esophagus and neck organs with tongue	Submit tissue samples of tongue.	Atrophic glossitis with ulcers. Pharyngoesophagitis (folic acid deficiency).
Stomach	Remove and place in fixative as early as possible in order to minimize autolysis (alternatively, formalin can be injected *in situ*; see below).	Previous total or subtotal gastrectomy. Carcinoma of stomach.
	Samples should include oxyntic corpus and fundus mucosa.	Autoimmune gastritis (diffuse corporal atrophic gastritis) with intestinal metaplasia.
Intestinal tract	For *in situ* fixation and preparation for study by dissecting microscopy, see p. 54. For preservation of jejunal diverticula by air drying, see p. 55.	Crohn's disease;* sprue;* other chronic inflammatory disorders; jejunal diverticula; intestinal malignancies; fish tapeworm infestation; previous intestinal resection or blind intestinal loop; enteric fistulas.
Liver and spleen	Record weights.	Hepatosplenomegaly. Alcoholic liver disease.*
Vagina	Submit tissue samples for histologic study.	Giant epithelial cells.
Thyroid gland	Record weight of thyroid gland.	Hyperthyroid goiter; thyroiditis.
Brain, spinal cord, and peripheral nerves	For removal and specimen preparation, see pp. 65, and 67, respectively. Request Luxol fast blue stain (p. 172).	Demyelination of cerebral white matter (in advanced cases). Demyelination in posterior and lateral columns of spinal cord, most frequently in thoracic and cervical segments. Demyelination of peripheral nerves.
Eyes with optic nerves	For removal and specimen preparation, see p. 85. If there is a clinical diagnosis of anemia-related amblyopia, follow procedures described under "Amblyopia, nutritional."	Retinal hemorrhages; demyelination of optic nerves.
Bone marrow	For preparation of sections and smears, see p. 96.	Hypercellular; megaloblastic. Myeloproliferative disorder.

Anemia, Pernicious (See "Anemia, megaloblastic.")

Anemia, Sickle Cell (See "Anemia, hemolytic" and "Disease, sickle cell.")

Anencephaly

Organs and Tissues	*Procedures*	*Possible or Expected Findings*
External examination	Photograph all abnormalities.	Absence of calvarial bones; protrusion of orbits; area cerebrovasculosa (disorganized hypervascular neuroglial tissue at the base of the skull).
	Prepare full-body skeletal roentgenograms.	Delay in development of ossification centers.

Organs and Tissues	Procedures	Possible or Expected Findings
Eyes	For removal and specimen preparation, see p. 85.	Absence of ganglion cells in retina; absence or hypoplasia of optic nerves.
Thymus, adrenals, gonads, and thyroid	Record weights. Submit tissue samples for histologic study.	Thymic and thyroid enlargement. Small adrenal glands with rudimentary fetal cortex after 20 wk gestation; small gonads.
Base of skull	Identify and record structures at base of skull.	Shallow sella turcica; small pituitary gland; hypoplastic medulla oblongata.
Lungs	Prepare histologic sections.	Aspiration of brain tissue.

Anesthesia (See "Death, anesthesia-associated.")

Aneurysm, Aortic Sinus

NOTE: For general dissection techniques, see Part I, Chapter 3. Prepare sections of aorta and request Verhoeff–van Gieson stain (p. 173). Rupture of aneurysm usually causes a fistula to the right ventricle or right atrium.

Possible Associated Conditions: Cystic medial degeneration of aorta; infective endocarditis;* ventricular septal defect.*

Aneurysm, Ascending Aorta

Possible Associated Conditions: History of polymyalgia rheumatica;* see also below under "Possible or Expected Findings."

Organs and Tissues	Procedures	Possible or Expected Findings
Aorta	Collect 5–6 specimens for microscopic study. Request Verhoeff–van Gieson stain (p. 173).	Cystic medial degeneration; active arteritis (often giant cell type), or healed arteritis.
Muscular arteries	Collect specimens for microscopic study. Request Verhoeff–van Gieson stain.	Temporal arteritis; systemic giant cell arteritis.*

Aneurysm, Atherosclerotic Aortic

Organs and Tissues	Procedures	Possible or Expected Findings
Aorta	If aneurysm was perforated, identify location of rupture *in situ*. Record location and volume of blood in peritoneum and retroperitoneum. Transverse or longitudinal sections of aneurysms are instructive. Request Verhoeff–van Gieson stain (p. 173). Decalcification may be required (p. 97).	Saccular aneurysm, often inferior to origin of renal arteries. Mural thrombosis in aneurysm. Rupture into peritoneal cavity, retroperitoneum, or hollow viscus.
Kidneys	Major arteries and kidneys may be left attached to aorta.	Arterial and arteriolar nephrosclerosis. Atheromatous emboli and microinfarcts of kidneys.

Aneurysm, Atrial Septum of Heart

Synonyms: Aneurysm of valve of fossa ovalis; fossa ovalis aneurysm.

NOTE: For general dissection techniques, see Part I, Chapter 3.

Possible Associated Conditions: Patent oval foramen (patent foramen ovale).

Aneurysm, Berry (See "Aneurysm, cerebral artery.")

Aneurysm, Cerebral Artery

Related Terms: Berry aneurysm; congenital cerebral artery aneurysm.

Organs and Tissues	Procedures	Possible or Expected Findings
Brain	If mycotic aneurysms are expected and microbiologic studies are intended, follow procedures described below under "Aneurysm, mycotic aortic." Request Verhoeff–van Gieson, Gram, and Grocott's methenamine silver stains (p. 172). For cerebral arteriography, see p. 80.	Mycotic aneurysms are often multiple and deep in brain substance.
	If arteriography cannot be carried out, rinse fresh blood gently from base of brain until aneurysm can be identified. Record site of rupture and estimated amount of extravascular blood. For paraffin embedding of aneurysms, careful positioning is required.	Berry aneurysms are the most frequent types and often are multiple. Most frequent sites are the bifurcations and trifurcations of the circle of Willis. Saccular atherosclerotic aneurysms are more common than dissecting aneurysms, which are very rare.
Other organs	Expected findings depend on type of aneurysm.	With congenital cerebral artery aneurysm: coarctation of aorta;* manifestations of hypertension;* and polycystic renal disease. With mycotic aneurysm: infective endocarditis;* pulmonary suppurative processes; and pyemia.

Aneurysm, Dissecting Aortic (See "Dissection, aortic.")

Aneurysm, Membranous Septum of Heart

NOTE: For general dissection techniques, see Part I, Chapter 3. Most aneurysms of the membranous septum probably represent spontaneous closure of a membranous ventricular septal defect by the septal leaflet of the tricuspid valve.

Aneurysm, Mycotic Aortic

NOTE: (1) Collect all tissues that appear to be infected. (2) Request aerobic, anaerobic, and fungal cultures. (3) Request Gram and Grocott methenamine silver stains (p. 172). (4) No special precautions are indicated. (5) No serologic studies are available. (6) This is not a reportable disease.

Organs and Tissues	Procedures	Possible or Expected Findings
Chest and abdominal organs	Submit blood samples for bacterial culture (p. 102). En masse removal of adjacent organs is recommended (p. 3).	Septicemia and infective endocarditis.*
Aorta	Photograph all grossly identifiable lesions. Aspirate material from aneurysm or para-aortic abscess and submit for culture. Prepare sections and smears of wall of aneurysm and of aorta distant from aneurysm. Request Verhoeff–van Gieson and Gram stains (p. 172).	Streptococcus, staphylococcus, spirochetes, and salmonella can be found in mycotic aneurysm. Para-aortic abscess.
Other organs		Septic emboli with infarction or abscess formation.

Aneurysm, Syphilitic Aortic

Organs and Tissues	Procedures	Possible or Expected Findings
Heart and aorta	En masse removal of organs is recommended (p. 3). For coronary arteriography, see p. 118.	Aneurysm usually in ascending aorta. May erode adjacent bone (sternum). Syphilitic aortitis may cause intimal wrinkling, narrowing of coronary ostia, and shortening of aortic cusps.
	Request Verhoeff–van Gieson stain from sections at different levels of aorta, adjacent great vessels, and coronary arteries (p. 173).	Disruption of medial elastic fibrils.

Organs and Tissues	Procedures	Possible or Expected Findings
Other organs	See also under "Syphilis."	Aortic valvulitis and insufficiency;* syphilitic coronary arteritis; syphilitic myocarditis.

Aneurysm, Traumatic Aortic

Organs and Tissues	Procedures	Possible or Expected Findings
External examination	Penetrating or blunt trauma with wounds, abrasions, hematomas, and other traumatic lesions.	
	Prepare chest and abdominal roentgenograms.	Fractures of ribs.
Aorta	Open aorta along line of blood flow, or bisect into anterior and posterior halves. Photograph tear(s). Measure or estimate amount of blood in mediastinum.	Hemorrhage into mediastinum.
	Request Verhoeff–van Gieson stain (p. 173).	Microscopy may show transmural rupture, false aneurysm, or localized dissection.

Angiitis (See "Arteritis, all types or type unspecified.")

Angina Pectoris

NOTE: See under "Disease, ischemic heart" and Table 3-2 (p. 32) in Part I, Chapter 3.

Angiokeratoma Corporis Diffusum (See "Disease, Fabry's.")

Angiomatosis, Encephalotrigeminal (See "Disease, Sturge-Weber-Dimitri.")

Angiopathy, Congophilic Cerebral

Synonyms and Related Terms: Beta amyloid angiopathy due to β-amyloid peptide deposition (β A4) (associated with Alzheimer's disease; hereditary cerebral hemorrhage with amyloid angiopathy of Dutch type; or sporadic beta amyloid angiopathy); hereditary cerebral amyloid angiopathy, due to deposition of other amyloidogenic proteins such as cystatin C (Icelandic type) and others (e.g., transthyretin, gelsolin) *(1)*.

Organs and Tissues	Procedures	Possible or Expected Findings
Brain	For removal and specimen preparation, see p. 65.	Multiple recent cerebral cortical infarctions or small cortical hemorrhages, or both, or massive hemispheric hemorrhages, both recent and old.
	Request stains for amyloid, particularly Congo red (p. 172), and thioflavine S (examine with polarized and ultraviolet light, respectively). Request immunostain for β A4. Some tissue should be kept frozen for biochemical studies.	Amyloid deposition in leptomeninges and cortical blood vessels. Senile plaques are usually present. In some cases, angiopathy is part of Alzheimer's disease.*
	Prepare material for electron microscopy (p. 132).	Electron microscopic study permits definite confirmation of diagnosis.
Other organs		Organs and tissues may be minimally affected by amyloidosis.

Reference

1. Kalimo H, Kaste M, Haltia M. Vascular diseases. In: Greenfield's Neuropathology, vol. 1. Graham BI, Lantos PL, eds. Arnold, London, 1997, pp. 315–396.

Anomaly, Coronary Artery

Possible Associated Conditions: With double outlet right ventricle; persistent truncal artery; tetralogy of Fallot;* and transposition of the great arteries.*

NOTE: Coronary artery between aorta and pulmonary artery, often with flap-valve angulated coronary ostium. Coronary artery may communicate with cardiac chamber, coronary sinus, or other cardiac veins, or with mediastinal vessel through pericardial vessel. Saccular aneurysm of coronary artery with abnormal flow, infective endarteritis of arteriovenous fistula, and myocardial infarction may be present. If one or both coronary arteries originate from pulmonary trunk, myocardial infarction may be present.

Organs and Tissues	Procedures	Possible or Expected Findings
Heart	For coronary angiography, see p. 118.	Ectopic origin of coronary arteries or single coronary artery.
	If infective endarteritis is suspected, submit blood sample for microbiologic study (p. 102).	Sudden death. For a detailed description of possible additional findings, see above under "Note."

Anomaly, Ebstein's (See "Malformation, Ebstein's")

Anorexia Nervosa

NOTE: Sudden death from tachyarrhythmias may occur in advanced cases and thus, autopsy findings may not reveal the immediate cause of death.

Organs and Tissues	Procedures	Possible or Expected Findings
External examination	Record height and weight, and prepare photographs to show cachectic features. Record abnormalities as listed in right-hand column.	Cachexia, often with preserved breast tissue; hirsutism; dry, scaly, and yellow skin (carotenemia). Mild edema may be present. Parotid glands may be enlarged.
All organs	Follow procedures described under "Starvation." Record weight of endocrine organs and submit samples for histologic study.	Manifestations of starvation.* Ovaries tend to be atrophic; other endocrine organs should not show abnormalities.

Anthrax

Synonyms: Cutaneous anthrax; gastrointestinal anthrax; pulmonary (inhalational) anthrax.

NOTE: (1) Collect all tissues that appear to be infected. (2) Request aerobic cultures. (3) Request Gram stain (p. 172). For the study of archival tissue samples, polymerase chain reaction (PCR) analysis can be attempted *(1)*. (4) Special **precautions** are indicated because the infection can be transmitted by aerosolization (see Part I, Chapter 16). (5) Serologic studies are available at the Center for Disease Control and Prevention, Atlanta, GA. (6) This is a **reportable** disease. Bioterrorism must be considered in current cases.

Organs and Tissues	Procedures	Possible or Expected Findings
External examination and skin	Photograph cutaneous papules, vesicles, and pustules. Prepare smears and histologic sections. Submit samples for bacteriologic study.	Disseminated anthrax infection may occur without skin lesions. Edema of neck and anterior chest in nasopharyngeal anthrax.
Blood	Submit sample for serologic study.	Anthrax septicemia. See above under "Note."
Lungs	Record character and volume of effusions. After sampling for bacteriologic study (see above under "Note") perfuse one or both lungs with formalin (p. 47). Extensive sampling for histologic study is indicated.	Pleural effusions;* hemorrhagic mediastinitis; anthrax pneumonia (inhalational anthrax; Woolsorter's disease). Histologic sections reveal hemorrhagic necrosis, often with minimal inflammation and gram-positive, spore-forming, encapsulated bacilli.
Gastrointestinal tracts and mesentery	For *in situ* fixation of intestines, see p. 54. Extensive sampling for histologic study is indicated.	Gastrointestinal anthrax with mucosal edema and ulcerations. Hemorrhagic mesenteric lymphadenitis.
Neck organs		Tongue, nasopharynx, and tonsils may be involved.
Brain	For removal and specimen preparation, see p. 65. Photograph meningeal hemorrhage *in situ*.	Hemorrhagic meningitis (hemorrhage tends to predominate).

Reference

1. Jackson PJ, Hugh-Jones ME, Adair DM, Green G, Hill KK, Kuske CR, et al. PCR analysis of tissue samples from the 1979 Sverdlovsk anthrax victims: the presence of multiple Bacillus anthracis strains in different victims. Proc Natl Acad Sci USA 1998;95:1224–1229.

Antifreeze (See "Poisoning, ethylene glycol.")

Antimony (See "Poisoning, antimony.")

Anus, Imperforate

Related Terms: Anorectal malformation; ectopic anus.

Possible Associated Conditions: Abnormalities of sacrococcygeal vertebrae; cardiovascular malformations; esophageal and intestinal atresias,* including rectal stenosis or atresia; malformations of the urinary tract.

Organs and Tissues	*Procedures*	*Possible or Expected Findings*
External examination	Photograph perineum. Measure depth of anal pit, if any.	Absence of normally located anus; anal dimple.
Distal colon and rectum	Dissect distal colon, rectum, and perirectal pelvic organs *in situ* (as much as possible). Search for opening of fistulous tracts from lumen; inject tract with stained contrast medium (see Part I, Chapter 12). Use roentgenologic study or dissection, or both, to determine course of tract.	Abnormal termination of the bowel into the trigone of the urinary bladder, the urethra distal to the verumontanum, the posterior wall of the vagina, the vulva, or the perineum.

Aortitis

NOTE: See also under "Arteritis" and "Aneurysm, ascending aortic."

Organs and Tissues	*Procedures*	*Possible or Expected Findings*
Heart and aorta	Remove heart with whole length of aorta and adjacent major arteries. Record width and circumference of aorta at different levels. Describe and photograph appearance of intima and of orifices of coronary arteries and other aortic branches.	Secondary aortic atherosclerosis or intimal fibroplasia. Widening of aorta; syphilitic aneurysm.*
	Submit multiple samples for histologic study and request Verhoeff–van Gieson stain (p. 173).	Giant cell aortitis; rheumatoid aortitis; syphilitic aortitis; Takayasu's arteritis.*
Other organs and tissues	Procedures depend on expected findings or grossly identified abnormalities as listed in right-hand column.	Manifestations of rheumatoid arthritis,* syphilis,* systemic sclerosis,* Hodgkin's lymphoma, and many other diseases associated with vasculitis.

Aplasia, Thymic (See "Syndrome, primary immunodeficiency.")

Arachnoiditis, Spinal

Synonym: Chronic spinal arachnoiditis.

Organs and Tissues	*Procedures*	*Possible or Expected Findings*
External examination	Prepare roentgenogram of spine.	Signs of previous spinal surgery or lumbar puncture (myelography). Evidence of previous trauma or previous myelography.
Brain	For removal and specimen preparation, see p. 65.	Cerebral arachnoiditis.
Spine and spinal cord	For removal of spinal cord and specimen preparation, see p. 67. Expose nerve roots. Record appearance and photograph spinal cord *in situ*.	Fibrous arachnoidal adhesions and loculated cysts.
	Submit samples of spinal cord and inflamed tissue for histologic study. Request Gram, Gomori's iron, and Grocott's methenamine silver stains (p. 172).	Tuberculosis;* syphilis;* fungal or parasitic infection.

Organs and Tissues	Procedures	Possible or Expected Findings
Other organs	Procedures depend on expected findings or grossly identified abnormalities as listed in right-hand column.	Systemic infection (see above). Ascending urinary infection or other manifestations of paraplegia.

Arch, Aortic, Interrupted

Synonym: Severe coarctation.

NOTE: The basic anomaly is a discrete imperforate region in the aortic arch, with a patent ductal artery joining the descending thoracic aorta. Type A interruption is between the left subclavian and ductal arteries; type B between the left subclavian and left common carotid arteries; and type C (rare) between the left common carotid and brachiocephalic (innominate) arteries. For general dissection techniques, see Part I, Chapter 3.

Possible Associated Conditions: Bicuspid aortic valve (with type A); di George syndrome* with thymic and parathyroid aplasia (with type B); hypoplasia of ascending aorta (with all types); persistent truncal artery (truncus arteriosus); ventricular septal defect.

Arrhythmia, Cardiac

NOTE: See also under "Death, sudden cardiac." Toxicologic studies may be indicated, for instance, if digitalis toxicity (see "Poisoning, digitalis") is suspected. If a cardiac pacemaker had been implanted, the instrument should be tested for malfunction.

Organs and Tissues	Procedures	Possible or Expected Findings
Heart	For coronary arteriography, see p. 118. Dissection techniques depend on nature of expected underlying disease. Submit samples for histologic study (p. 30). For study of conduction system, see p. 26.	Coronary arteriosclerosis. Congenital heart disease. Valvular heart disease. Myocardial infarction. Myocarditis.* Cardiomyopathy.*

Arsenic (See "Poisoning, arsenic.")

Arteriosclerosis (See "Atherosclerosis.")

Arteritis, All Types or Type Unspecified

Synonyms and Related Terms: Allergic angiitis and granulomatosis (Churg-Strauss);* allergic vasculitis; anaphylactoid purpura* and its synonyms; angiitis; Buerger's disease;* cranial arteritis; giant cell arteritis;* granulomatous arteritis (angiitis); hypersensitivity angiitis; infectious angiitis; necrotizing arteritis; polyarteritis nodosa;* rheumatic arteritis; rheumatoid arteritis, syphilitic arteritis; Takayasu's arteritis;* temporal arteritis; thromboangiitis obliterans; and others (see also below under "Note").

NOTE: Autopsy procedures depend on (1) the expected type of arteritis, such as giant cell arteritis,* polyarteritis nodosa,* or thromboangiitis obliterans (Buerger's disease*); and (2) the nature of suspected associated or underlying disease, such as aortic arch syndrome,* Behçet's syndrome,* Cogan's syndrome, Degos' disease,* dermatomyositis,* erythema nodosum and multiforme,* Goodpasture's syndrome,* polymyositis, rheumatic fever,* rheumatoid arthritis,* syphilis,* and other nonspecific infectious diseases, systemic lupus erythematosus,* systemic sclerosis (scleroderma),* or Takayasu's disease. For histologic study of blood vessels, Verhoeff–van Gieson stain or a similar stain is recommended (p. 172).

Arteritis, Giant Cell

Synonyms and Related Terms: Cranial arteritis; giant cell aortitis; juvenile temporal arteritis; systemic giant cell arteritis; temporal arteritis.

Possible Associated Conditions: Polymyalgia rheumatica.

Organs and Tissues	Procedures	Possible or Expected Findings
External examination and skin	Prepare sections of skin lesions.	Skin nodules; scalp necroses.
	Record appearance of oral cavity; submit tissue samples of tongue.	Gangrene of tongue.
	Probe nasal cavity and record appearance of septum.	Perforation of nasal septum.
Heart	For coronary arteriography, see p. 118.	Coronary arteritis; myocardial infarction. Pericardial infiltrates.

Organs and Tissues	Procedures	Possible or Expected Findings
Aorta and other elastic arteries	For angiographic procedures, see p. 118 and below, under "Arteritis, Takayasus." Request Verhoeff–van Gieson stain (p. 172).	Aortic dissection;* spontaneous rupture of aorta. Arteritis of aorta, aortic arch branches (carotid arteries, subclavian arteries, vertebral arteries, brachiocephalic artery) and celiac, mesenteric, renal, iliac, and femoral arteries. Arteries may show aneurysms.
Lungs		Pulmonary arteritis.
Other organs		Giant cell arteritis may occur in many organs and tissues.
Brain and spinal cord	For removal and specimen preparation, see pp. 65 and 67, respectively.	Cerebral infarctions.
Temporal and ophthalmic arteries	Expose temporal and ophthalmic arteries; prepare histologic sections.	Temporal and ophthalmic arteritis.
Eyes	For removal and specimen preparation, see p. 85.	Arteritis of ciliary and retinal vessels.
Skeletal muscles	For sampling and specimen preparation, see p. 80.	Clinically, polymyalgia.
Bone marrow	For preparation of sections and smears, see p. 96.	Anemia.

Arteritis, Takayasu's

Synonyms: Aortic arch syndrome; pulseless disease.

Organs and Tissues	Procedures	Possible or Expected Findings
External examination		Facial muscular atrophy and pigmentation.
Heart, aorta, and adjacent great vessels	For *in situ* aortography, clamp distal descending thoracic aorta and neck vessels as distal as possible from takeoff at aortic arch.	Narrowing at origin of brachiocephalic arteries.
	Remove heart together with aorta and long sleeves of neck vessels. For coronary arteriography, see p. 118 (method designed to show coronary ostia).	Dilated ascending aorta. Narrowing of coronary arteries at origins. Myocardial infarction.
	Test competence of aortic valve.	Aortic insufficiency.*
	Open aortic arch anteriorly and measure (with calipers) lumen at origin of great neck vessels.	
	Photograph aorta and neck vessels and submit samples for histologic study. Request Verhoeff–van Gieson stain (p. 173).	Aortic atherosclerosis. Thromboses of brachiocephalic arteries. Giant cell arteritis.*
Eyes and optic nerve	For removal and specimen preparation, see p. 85.	Atrophy of optic nerve, retina, and iris; cataracts; retinal pigmentation.
Brain	For removal and specimen preparation, see p. 65.	Ischemic lesions.

Artery, Patent Ductal

Synonym: Patent ductus arteriosus.

NOTE: The basic anomaly is persistent postnatal patency of the ductal artery, usually as an isolated finding (in 75% of cases in infants, and in 95% in adults). It is more common in premature than full-term infants and at high altitudes than at sea level. Possible complications in unoperated cases include congestive heart failure,* plexogenic pulmonary hypertension,* ductal artery aneurysm or rupture, fatal pulmonary embolism,* or sudden death. In some conditions, such as aortic atresia* or transposition with an intact ventricular septum,* ductal patency may be necessary for survival. For general dissection techniques, see p. 33.

Possible Associated Conditions: Atrial or ventricular septal defect;* coarctation of the aorta;* conotruncal anomalies; necrotizing enterocolitis in premature infants; postrubella syndrome; and valvular or vascular obstructions.

Artery, Persistent Truncal

Synonym and Related Terms: Type 1, pulmonary arteries arise from single pulmonary trunk (in 55%); type 2, pulmonary arteries arise separately but close-by (in 35%); type 3, pulmonary arteries arise separately but distal from one another (in 10%).

NOTE: The basic anomaly is a common truncal artery, with truncal valve, giving rise to aorta, pulmonary arteries, and coronary arteries, usually with a ventricular septal defect. Interventions include complete Rastelli-type repair, with closure of ventricular septal defect, and insertion of valved extracardiac conduit between right ventricle and detached pulmonary arteries. For general dissection techniques, see p. 33.

Possible Associated Conditions: Absent pulmonary artery (in 15%); atrial septal defect (in 15%); absent ductal artery (in 50%); coronary ostial anomalies (in 40%); Di George syndrome;* double aortic arch; extracardiac anomalies (in 25%); interrupted aortic arch* (in 15%); right aortic arch (in 30%); truncal valve insufficiency (uncommon) or stenosis (rare); truncal valve with three (in 70%), four (in 20%), or two (in 10%) cusps.

Organs and Tissues	*Procedures*	*Possible or Expected Findings*
Heart and great vessels	If infective endocarditis is suspected, follow procedures described on p. 103.	Infective endocarditis,* usually of truncal valve. Late postoperative conduit obstruction. Postoperative late progressive truncal artery dilation with truncal valve insufficiency.
Lungs	Request Verhoeff–van Gieson stain (p. 173).	Hypertensive pulmonary vascular disease.
Brain		Cerebral abscess,* if right-to-left-shunt was present.

Arthritis, All Types or Type Unspecified

NOTE: For extra-articular changes, see under the name of the suspected underlying conditions. Infectious diseases that may be associated with arthritis include bacillary dysentery,* brucellosis,* gonorrhea, rubella,* syphilis,* tuberculosis,* typhoid fever,* and varicella.* Noninfectious diseases in this category include acromegaly,* Behçet's syndrome,* Felty's syndrome,* gout,* rheumatoid arthritis,* and many others, too numerous to mention.

Organs and Tissues	*Procedures*	*Possible or Expected Findings*
Joints	Remove synovial fluid and prepare smears. Submit synovial fluid for microbiologic and chemical (p. 96) study. For removal of joints, prosthetic repair, and specimen preparation, see p. 96.	In suppurative arthritis, organisms most frequently involved are *Streptococcus hemolyticus*, *Staphylococcus aureus*, *Pneumococcus*, and *Meningococcus*.

Arthritis, Juvenile Rheumatoid

Synonym: Juvenile chronic arthritis; Still's disease.

NOTE: Involvement of more than five joints defines the polyarticular variant of the disease.

Possible Associated Condition: Amyloidosis.*

Organs and Tissues	*Procedures*	*Possible or Expected Findings*
External examination and skin	Submit samples of skin or subcutaneous lesions.	Rheumatoid nodules.
	Prepare skeletal roentgenograms.	Monarthritis or polyarthritis; abnormalities of bone, cartilage, and periosteal growth adjacent to inflamed joint(s). Osteoporosis.* In the polyarticular variant, facial asymmetry may be noted.
Blood	Submit samples for serologic study and for microbiologic study (p. 102).	Rheumatoid factor positive in some cases.
Heart		Pericarditis.*
Lungs	Perfuse one lung with formalin (p. 47); submit one lobe for microbiologic study.	Interstitial pneumonitis; pleuritis. (See also under "Arthritis, rheumatoid.")
Lymph nodes	Submit samples for histologic study; record average size.	Lymphadenopathy.
Spleen	Record size and weight; submit samples for histologic study.	Splenomegaly.
Bones and joints	For removal, prosthetic repair, and specimen preparation, see p. 95. Include joints of cervical spine and sacroiliac joints.	Monarthritis or severe, erosive polyarthritis; see also under "Arthritis, rheumatoid" and above under "External examination and skin." Ankylosing spondylitis* may be present.

Organs and Tissues	Procedures	Possible or Expected Findings
Eyes	For removal and specimen preparation, see p. 85.	Chronic iridocyclitis.
Other organs and tissues		See "Arthritis, rheumatoid."

Arthritis, Rheumatoid

Synonyms and Related Terms: Ankylosing spondylitis;* Felty's syndrome;* juvenile rheumatoid arthritis* (Still's disease); rheumatoid disease; and others.

Possible Associated Conditions: Amyloidosis;* polymyositis (dermatomyositis*); psoriasis;* Sjögren's syndrome;* systemic lupus erythematosus;* systemic vasculitis, and others.

Organs and Tissues	Procedures	Possible or Expected Findings
External examination and skin	Record character and extent of skin and nail changes. Prepare sections of normal and abnormal skin and of subcutaneous nodules.	Subcutaneous rheumatoid nodules on elbows, back, areas overlying ischial and femoral tuberosities, heads of phalangeal and metacarpal bones, and occiput.
	Prepare skeletal roentgenograms.	Deformities and subluxation of peripheral joints (see also below under "Joints"). Subaxial dislocation of cervical spine may be cause of sudden death.
Pleural cavities	Prepare chest roentgenogram.	Pneumothorax;* pleural empyema.*
Thymus	Record weight. Submit samples for histologic study.	T-cell abnormalities *(1)*.
Blood	Submit samples for microbiologic study (p. 102).	Bacteremia.
	Keep frozen sample for serologic or immunologic study.	Positive rheumatoid factor.
Heart and blood vessels	For coronary arteriography, see p. 118. Open heart in direction of blood flow. For histologic sampling, see p. 30. Submit specimens with blood vessels from all organs and tissues.	Rheumatoid granulomas in myocardium (septum), pericardium, and at base of aortic and mitral valves; constrictive pericarditis;* aortic stenosis;* coronary arteritis. Systemic vasculitis (arteritis*).
Lungs	Record weights. Submit one lobe for microbiologic study (p. 103). For pulmonary arteriography and bronchography, see p. 50. For perfusion-fixation, see p. 47.	Rheumatoid granulomas in pleura and lung (with pneumoconiosis*); bronchopleural fistula; rheumatoid pneumonia with interstitial pulmonary fibrosis and honeycombing; bronchiectasis;* bronchiolitis with cystic changes; pulmonary arteritis. Pneumoconiosis* in Caplan's syndrome.*
Esophagus	Record width of lumen.	Dilatation.
Stomach	Submit samples for histologic study.	Mucosal atrophy in Sjögren's syndrome.*
Mesentery and intestine	For mesenteric angiography, see p. 55. Submit samples from mesenteric vessels for histologic study.	Mesenteric vasculitis (acute necrotizing arteritis; subacute arteritis; arterial thrombosis; venulitis) and intestinal infarctions.
Spleen	Record weight.	Splenomegaly; rupture of spleen *(2)*.
Adrenals		Cortical atrophy.
Lymph nodes	Submit samples of axillary, cervical, mediastinal, and retroperitoneal lymph nodes for histologic study.	Lymphadenopathy.
Neck organs	In patients with suspected Sjögren's syndrome,* snap-freeze sample of salivary (submaxillary) gland for immunofluorescent study.	Atrophic sialadenitis with salivary gland atrophy and atrophy of taste buds in Sjögren's syndrome.*
	Search for evidence of upper airway obstruction. Submit samples of base of tongue, thyroid gland, cricoarytenoid joints (see p. 96), and paralaryngeal soft tissues for histologic study.	Hashimoto's struma; cricoarytenoid arthritis. Rheumatoid granulomas in paralaryngeal soft tissues.

Organs and Tissues	Procedures	Possible or Expected Findings
Brain, spinal cord, and pituitary gland	For removal and specimen preparation, see pp. 65, 67, and 71, respectively. For cerebral arteriography, see p. 80.	Rheumatoid granulomas in dura mater and in leptomeninges of brain and spinal canal. Cerebral vasculitis and microinfarcts. Spinal cord compression after cervical subluxation (see above under "External examination and skin").
Eyes and lacrimal glands	For removal and specimen preparation, see pp. 85 and 87, respectively.	Uveitis and scleritis. Dacryosial adenitis.
Middle ears	For removal and specimen preparation, see p. 72. If patient had a hearing problem, prepare sections of incudomalleal joints.	Rheumatoid arthritis of joints of middle ear ossicles.
Joints	Remove synovial fluid from affected joints for microbiologic study (p. 96).	Bacterial arthritis.
	For removal, prosthetic repair, and specimen preparation, see p. 96. Remove peripheral diarthroidial joints together with synovia, adjacent tendons, adjacent bones, and bursae. Snap-freeze synovial tissue for fluorescent microscopic and histochemical study.	Destructive rheumatoid arthritis; rheumatoid tenosynovitis (particularly tendon of flexor digitorum profundus muscle); synovial outpouchings; subluxations; osteoporosis* with pseudocysts; bursitis with "rice bodies."
Skeletal muscles	For sampling and specimen and specimen preparation, see p. 80.	Lymphorrhagias; perivascular nodular myositis; vasculitis.
Bone marrow	For preparation of sections and smears, see p. 96.	Megaloblastic changes; normoblastic hypoplasia; relative plasmacytosis; hemosiderosis.

References

1. Weyand CM, Goronzy JJ. Pathogenesis of rheumatoid arthritis. Med Clin North Am 1997;81:29–55.
2. Fishman D, Isenberg DA. Splenic involvement in rheumatic diseases. Semin Arthr Rheum 1997;27:141–155.

Arthrogryposis Multiplex Congenita

Synonyms and Related Terms: Congenital contractures; amyoplasia *(1)*; congenital muscular dystrophy; fetal akinesia/hypokinesia sequence.

NOTE:

Arthrogryposis *(2)* may be a primary muscle disease, or it may involve abnormalities of the brain, spinal cord, and/or peripheral nerves. Etiologies are numerous, as are the modes of inheritance. Critical to making the appropriate diagnosis is the collection of muscles from various sites for routine histology, muscle histochemistry, and electron microscopy. Portions of peripheral motor nerves must also be prepared for histology and electron microscopy.

Organs and Tissues	Procedures	Possible and Expected Findings
External examination	Record and photograph all contractures. Obtain routine external measurements and body weight. Prepare full body radiographs.	Contractures. Facial anomalies, such as hypertelorism, telecanthus, epicanthal folds, malformed ears, small mouth, micrognathia.
Lungs	Record weights; perfuse one or both lungs with formalin (see p. 47) and submit samples for histologic study.	Pulmonary hypoplasia.
Muscles	Snap freeze at –70°C at least four muscle groups (e.g., quadriceps, biceps, psoas, diaphragm) for histochemical study. Submit sections in glutaraldehyde and formalin for electron microscopy and histologic study, respectively. For specimen preparation see also p. 80.	Fiber type disproportion; myofiber hypoplasia; fatty replacement; fibrosis.
Nerves	Submit segments of peripheral motor nerves for electron microscopy and histologic study (see pp. 79 and 132). Request Luxol fast blue stain for myelin.	Hypomyelination of nerves.

Organs and Tissues	*Procedures*	*Possible and Expected Findings*
Brain and spinal cord	For removal and specimen preparation, see pp. 65 and 67, respectively. Prepare for histologic study.	Polymicrogyria, cortical white matter dysplasia, variable decrease of anterior horn cells; increased numbers of abnormally small anterior horn cells.
Placenta		Short umbilical cord.

References

1. Sawark JF, MacEwen GD, Scott CI. Amyoplasia (A common form of arthrogryposis). J Bone Joint S 1990;72:465–469.
2. Banker BQ. Arthrogryposis multiplex congenita: spectrum of pathologic changes. Hum Path 1986;17:656–672.

Asbestosis (See "Pneumoconiosis.")

Ascites, Chylous

Organs and Tissue	*Procedures*	*Possible or Expected Findings*
Abdominal cavity	Puncture abdominal cavity and submit fluid for microbiologic study (p. 102).	
	Record volume of exudate or transudate and submit sample for determination of fat and cholesterol content.	For interpretation of chemical analysis, see "Chylothorax."
	Prior to routine dissection, lymphangiography (see below) may be indicated.	Lymphoma and other retroperitoneal neoplasms; surgical trauma; intestinal obstruction.
Intra-abdominal lymphatic system	For lymphangiography, see p. 34. Cannulate lymphatics as distally as possible.	Ruptured chylous cyst; intestinal lymphangiectasia and other malformations of lymph vessels. See also above under "Abdominal cavity."

Aspergillosis

Related Term: Allergic bronchopulmonary aspergillosis.

NOTE: (1) Collect all tissues that appear to be infected. (2) Request fungal cultures. (3) Request Grocott's methenamine silver stain (p. 172). (4) No special precautions are indicated. (5) Serologic studies are available in local and state health department laboratories (p. 135). (6) This is not a reportable disease.

Possible Associated Conditions: With pulmonary aspergillosis—bronchiectasis;* bronchocentric granulomatosis;* sarcoidosis;* tuberculosis.* With systemic aspergillosis—leukemia;* lymphoma;* and other conditions complicated by immunosuppression *(1,2)*.

Organs and Tissues	*Procedures*	*Possible or Expected Findings*
Lungs	Carefully make multiple parasagittal sections through the unperfused lungs. Culture areas of consolidation. If diagnosis was confirmed, perfuse lungs with formalin (p. 47). Prepare histologic sections from walls of cavities, cavity contents, and pneumonic infiltrates.	Bronchiectasis;* tumor cavities; cysts. Fungus ball may be present in any of these.
Other organs	Procedures depend on expected findings or grossly identified abnormalities as listed in right-hand column.	Suppuration and necrotic lesions from disseminated aspergillosis in heart *(3)*, brain *(1)*, bones *(1,2)*, and other organs *(3)*.

References

1. The W, Matti BS, Marisiddaiah H, Minamoto GY. Aspergillus sinusitis in patients with AIDS: report of three cases and review. Clin Infect Dis 1995;21:529–535.
2. Gonzales-Crespo MR, Gomes-Reino JJ. Invasive aspergillosis in systemic lupus erythematosus. Semin Arthritis Rheum 1995;24:304–314.
3. Sergi C, Weitz J, Hofmann WJ, Sinn P, Eckart A, Otto G, et al. Aspergillus endocarditis, myocarditis and pericarditis complicating necrotizing fasciitis. Case report and subject review. Virchows Arch 1996;429:177–180.

Asphyxia (See "Hypoxia.")

Aspiration (See "Obstruction, acute airway.")

Assault

NOTE: All procedures described under "Homicide" must be followed.

Asthma

NOTE: Spray death* may occur in asthma sufferers from pressurized aerosol bronchodilators.

Organs and Tissues	*Procedures*	*Possible or Expected Findings*
External examination and skin	Record appearance of skin and conjunctivae. Palpate subcutaneous tissue to detect evidence of crepitation.	Eczema. Conjunctival hemorrhages and subcutaneous emphysema may be present after fatal attack.
Chest	Prepare chest roentgenogram. For tests for pneumothorax, see under that heading.	Pneumothorax;* mediastinal emphysema. Low diaphragm (see below).
Blood	Submit sample for biochemical study.	Increased IgE concentrations in fatal asthma; postmortem tryptase determination is of doubtful value in this regard *(1)*.
Diaphragm	Record thickness and position.	Hypertrophy. Low position of diaphragm.
Lungs	Perfuse one lung with formalin (p. 47).	Hyperinflated lungs.
	Because mucous plugs may block bronchial tree, attach perfusion apparatus to pulmonary artery or to bronchus and pulmonary artery. Monitor perfusion to ensure proper inflation.	Thick-walled bronchi with prominent viscid mucous plugs.
	Prepare photograph of fixed cut section.	
	Submit samples of pulmonary parenchyma and bronchi for histologic study. Request azure-eosin and Verhoeff–van Gieson stains (p. 172).	Typical microscopic inflammatory changes *(2)*. Asthmatic bronchitis with eosinophilic infiltrates. Bronchocentric granulomatosis.* Pulmonary atherosclerosis with breakup of elastic fibers.
Heart	Record weight and thickness of walls.	Cor pulmonale.
Esophagus	Leave attached to stomach.	Reflux esophagitis *(3)*.
Stomach and duodenum		Peptic ulcer.*
Intestine	Photograph and submit samples for histologic study.	Pneumatosis of small intestine; emphysema of colon.
Liver		Centrilobular congestion and necrosis.
Kidneys	Record weights. Submit samples of both kidneys for histologic study.	Kidneys and glomeruli may be enlarged.
Neck organs	Submit samples of larynx and trachea for histologic study. Request azure-eosin stains (p. 172).	Laryngitis and tracheitis.
Brain and spinal cord	For removal and specimen preparation, see pp. 65 and 67, respectively.	Petechial hemorrhages in hypothalamus; necrosis of cerebellar folia; anoxic changes in cortex, globus pallidus, thalamus, Sommer's sector of hippocampus, and Purkinje cells of cerebellum. Suspected changes in anterior horn cells of spinal cord in patients with asthma-associated poliomyelitis-like illness (Hopkins syndrome) *(4)*.
Nasal cavities	For exposure, see p. 71. Submit samples of mucosa and polyps for histologic study. Request azure-eosin stains (p. 172).	Allergic polyps and other allergic inflammatory changes *(5)*.
Bone marrow	For preparation of sections and smears, see p. 96.	Increased erythropoiesis.

References

1. Salkie ML, Mitchell I, Revers CW, Karkhanis A, Butt J, Tough S, Green FH. Postmortem serum levels of tryptase and total and specific IgE in fatal asthma. Allergy Asthma Proc 1998;19:131–133.
2. Hogg JC. The pathology of asthma. APMIS 1997;105:735–745.
3. Sontag SJ. Gastroesophageal reflux and asthma. Am J Med 1997;103: 84S–90S.
4. Mizuno Y, Komori S, Shigetomo R, Kurihara E, Tamagawa K, Komiya K. Polyomyelitis-like illness after acute asthma (Hopkins syndrome): a histological study of biopsied muscle in a case. Brain Dev 1995; 17:126–129.
5. Glovsky MM. Upper airway involvement in bronchial asthma. Curr Opin Pulm Med 1998;4:54–58.

Ataxia, Friedreich's (See "Degeneration, spinocerebellar.")

Atherosclerosis

Synonyms and Related Terms: Arteriosclerosis obliterans.

Organs and Tissues	*Procedures*	*Possible or Expected Findings*
Arteries	For grading of atherosclerotic lesions, see p. 34. For angiographic techniques, see under affected organ or p. 118.	Atherosclerotic aneurysm.*
Other organs		Manifestations of vascular occlusions, such as infarctions and gangrene. Manifestations of diabetes mellitus.*

Atresia, Anal and Rectal (See "Anus, imperforate.")

Atresia, Aortic Valvular

Synonym: Aortic atresia; aortic atresia with intact ventricular septum; hypoplastic left heart syndrome.

NOTE: The basic anomaly is an imperforate aortic valve, with secondary hypoplasia of left-sided chambers and ascending aorta. For possible surgical interventions, see two-stage Norwood and modified Fontan procedures in Chapter 3 Appendices 3 and 4, p. 41. For general dissection techniques, see p. 33.

Possible Associated Conditions: Atrial septal defect* (or patent foramen ovale, usually restrictive); dilatation of myocardial sinusoids that communicate with coronary vessels; dilatation of right atrium, right ventricle, and pulmonary trunk; fibroelastosis of left atrial and left ventricular endocardium; hypertrophy of ventricular and atrial walls; hypoplastic left atrium, mitral valve, left ventricle, and ascending aorta; mitral atresia* with minute left ventricle; patent ductal artery (ductus arteriosus); small left ventricle with hypertrophic wall; tubular hypoplasia of aortic arch, with or without discrete coarctation.

Atresia, Biliary

Synonyms and Related Terms: Congenital biliary atresia; extrahepatic biliary atresia; infantile obstructive cholangiopathy; syndromic (Alagille's syndrome) or nonsyndromic paucity of intrahepatic bile ducts ("intrahepatic" biliary atresia).

Possible Associated Conditions: Alpha$_1$-antitrypsin deficiency;* choledochal cyst;* congenital rubella syndrome;* polysplenia syndrome* *(1)*; small bowel atresia; trisomy 17–18; trisomy 21; Turner's syndrome;* viral infections (cytomegalovirus infection;* rubella*).

Organs and Tissues	*Procedures*	*Possible or Expected Findings*
External examination		Jaundice.
Blood	Submit samples for serologic or microbiologic study (p. 102).	Congenital rubella and other viral infections.
	Submit sample of serum for determination of alpha$_1$-antitrypsin concentrations. Submit sample for chromosomal analysis (p. 108).	Alpha$_1$-Antitrypsin deficiency;* defects in bile acid synthesis. Chromosomal abnormalities.
Extrahepatic bile ducts and liver	After removal of small and large bowel, open duodenum anteriorly. Squeeze gallbladder and record whether bile appeared at papilla. For cholangiography, see p. 56.	In atresia of the hepatic duct, the gallbladder will be empty. In isolated atresia of the common bile duct, the gallbladder contains bile but it cannot be squeezed into the duodenum.
	Dissect extrahepatic bile ducts *in situ* or leave hepatoduodenal ligament intact for later fixation and sectioning (see below). Record appearance and contents of gallbladder and course of cystic duct.	Atresia or hypoplasia of bile duct(s); choledochal cyst(s).
	In postoperative cases, submit sample of anastomosed hepatic hilar tissue for demonstration of microscopic bile ducts.	Biliary drainage created by Kasai operation.

Organs and Tissues	Procedures	Possible or Expected Findings
Extrahepatic bile ducts and liver *(continued)*	Remove liver with hepatoduodenal ligament. Prepare horizontal sections through ligament and submit for histologic identification of ducts or duct remnants.	Obliterative cholangiopathy *(2)*.
	Prepare frontal slices of liver and sample for histologic study. Request PAS stain with diastase digestion (p. 173).	Intrahepatic cholelithiasis; postoperative ascending cholangitis; secondary biliary cirrhosis; giant cell transformation; paucity of intrahepatic bile ducts. PAS-positive inclusions in alpha$_1$-antitrypsin deficiency.*
Other organs	Procedures depend on expected findings or grossly identified abnormalities as listed in right-hand column.	Polysplenia syndrome* *(1)* with malrotation, situs inversus, preduodenal portal vein, absent inferior vena cava, anomalous hepatic artery supply, and cardiac defects. For other abnormalities outside the biliary tree, see under "Possible Associated Conditions"). Nephromegaly *(3)*.

References

1. Vazquez J, Lopex Gutierrez JC, Gamez M, Lopez-Santamaria M, Murcia J, Larrauri J, et al. Biliary atresia and the polysplenia syndrome: its impact on final outcome. J Pediatr Surg 1995;30:485–487.
2. Lefkowitch JH. Biliary atresia. Mayo Clin Proc 1998;73:90–95.
3. Tsau YK, Chen CH, Chang MH, Teng RJ, Lu MY, Lee PI. Nephromegaly and elevated hepatocyte growth factor in children with biliary atresia. Am J Kidney Dis 1997;29:188–192.

Atresia, Cardiac Valves (See "Atresia, aortic valvular," "Atresia, mitral valvular," "Atresia pulmonary valvular, with intact ventricular septum," "Atresia, pulmonary valvular, with ventricular septal defect," and "Atresia, tricuspid valvular.")

Atresia, Duodenal

Possible Associated Conditions: With membranous obstruction of the duodenum—annular pancreas; atresia of esophagus* with tracheoesophageal fistula; congenital heart disease; cystic fibrosis;* Down's syndrome;* Hirschsprung's disease; imperforate anus* or other congenital obstructions of the intestinal tract *(1)*; intestinal malrotation; lumbosacral, rib-, and digit/limb anomalies; single umbilical artery; spinal defects; undescended testis *(1)*.

NOTE:
See also under "Atresia, small intestinal."

Organs and Tissues	Procedures	Possible or Expected Findings
Fascia lata, blood, or liver	Obtain cells for tissue culture for karyotype analysis (see p. 108).	Trisomy 21 and other aneuploidies.
Duodenum	Photograph and dissect organ *in situ*. Inflate duodenum with formalin; open only after fixation. For air-drying techniques and for mesenteric angiography, see p. 55, respectively.	Fibrous membrane across lumen of intact duodenum. Septum may have orifice so that duodenal stenosis results. Rarely, fusiform narrowing.
Other organs		See above under "Possible Associated Findings."

Reference

1. Kimble RM, Harding J, Kolbe A. Additional congenital anomalies in babies with gut atresia or stenosis: when to investigate, and which investigation. Pediatr Surg Intl 1997;12:565–570.

Atresia, Esophageal

Possible Associated Condition: Congenital rubella syndrome;* VACTERL syndrome (Vertebral anomalies, Anal atresia, Cardiovascular anomalies, Tracheo-Esophageal fistula, Rib anomalies, Limb anomalies) *(1)*.

Organs and Tissues	Procedures	Possible or Expected Findings
External examination		Limb anomalies.
Chest organs	Photograph the atresia prior to opening the esophagus. Open the esophagus posteriorly or the trachea anteriorly for best visualization (see Chapter 4, Fig. 4-1 in Part I).	Tracheoesophageal fistula or tracheoesophageal atresia; cardiac, rib, and vertebral anomalies.

Organs and Tissues	*Procedures*	*Possible or Expected Findings*
Abdominal organs	Photograph all anomalies. Procedures depend on expected findings or grossly identified abnormalities as listed in right-hand column.	Renal agenesis or dysplasia; anal atresia; duodenal or other small intestinal atresia;* lumbosacral anomalies; undescended testis *(2)*.

References

1. Perel Y, Butenandt O, Carrere A, Saura R, Fayon M, Lamireau T, Vergnes P. Oesophageal atresia, VACTERL association: Fanconi's anemia related spectrum of anomalies. Arch Dis Child 1998;78:375–376.
2. Kimble RM, Harding J, Kolbe A. Additional congenital anomalies in babies with gut atresia or stenosis: when to investigate, and which investigation. Pediatr Surg Intl 1997;12:565–570.

Atresia, Mitral Valvular

Synonym: Congenital mitral atresia.

NOTE: For general dissection techniques, see p. 33.

Possible Associated Conditions: Aortic valvular hypoplasia or atresia;* closed foramen ovale with anomalous venous channel (levoatriocardinal vein) connecting left atrium with left innominate vein; patent foramen ovale; transposition of great arteries associated with single functional ventricle;* ventricular septal defect(s).*

Atresia, Pulmonary Valvular, With Intact Ventricular Septum

NOTE: The basic anomaly is an imperforate pulmonary valve, with a hypoplastic right ventricle. In unoperated cases, ductal closure is the most common cause of death. For possible surgical interventions, see modified Blalock-Taussig shunt, modified Fontan procedure, and pulmonary valvulotomy in Chapter 3 Appendix 3-4, p. 41. For general dissection techniques, see p. 33.

Possible Associated Conditions: Dilated myocardial sinusoids that may communicate with epicardial coronary arteries or veins; patent ductal artery (ductus arteriosus); patent oval foramen (foramen orale); tricuspid atresia with minute right ventricle; tricuspid stenosis with hypoplastic right ventricle (in 95%); tricuspid insufficiency with dilated right ventricle (in 5%).

Atresia, Pulmonary Valvular, With Ventricular Septal Defect

Synonym: Tetralogy of Fallot with pulmonary atresia.

NOTE: The basic anomaly is atresia of the pulmonary valve and of variable length of pulmonary artery, and ventricular septal defect (membranous or outlet type), with overriding aorta, and with pulmonary blood supply from ductal or systemic collateral arteries. For possible surgical interventions, see Rastelli-type repair and unifocalization of multiple collateral arteries in Chapter 3 Appendix 3-4, p. 41. For general dissection techniques, see p. 33.

Possible Associated Conditions: Right ventricular outflow tract a short blind-ended pouch (70%) or absent (30%); atresia of pulmonary artery bifurcation, with nonconfluent pulmonary arteries; right aortic arch (40%); atrial septal defect (50%); persistent left superior vena cava; anomalous pulmonary venous connection; tricuspid stenosis or atresia; complete atrioventricular septal defect; transposed great arteries; double inlet left ventricle; asplenia, polysplenia, or velocardiofacial syndromes; dilated ascending aorta, with aortic insufficiency.

Atresia, Small Intestinal

Related Term: Jejuno-ileal atresia.

Possible Associated Findings: Esophageal atresia* with tracheoesophageal fistula; lumbosacral, rib-, or digit/limb anomalies; undescended testes *(1)*.

NOTE: See also under "Atresia, duodenal."

Organs and Tissues	*Procedures*	*Possible or Expected Findings*
Fascia lata, blood, or liver	These specimens should be collected using aseptic technique for tissue culture for chromosome analysis (see Chapter 10).	Trisomy 21.
Intestinal tract	For mesenteric angiography, see p. 55. Leave mesentery attached to small bowel, particularly to the atretic portion.	Multiple atresias; proximal dilatation; volvulus; malrotation; meconium impaction; other evidence of cystic fibrosis. Anorectal malformation *(1)*.
Pancreas		Annular pancreas *(1)*.

Reference

1. Kimble RM, Harding J, Kolbe A. Additional congenital anomalies in babies with gut atresia or stenosis: when to investigate, and which investigation. Pediatr Surg Intl 1997;12:565–570.

Atresia, Tricuspid Valvular

NOTE: The basic anomaly is an absent right atrioventricular connection (85%) or imperforate tricuspid valve (15%), with a hypoplastic right ventricle (100%), muscular ventricular septal defect (90%) that is restrictive (85%), and a patent oval foramen (80%) or secundum atrial septal defect (20%). For possible surgical interventions, see modified Fontan or Glenn procedures in Chapter 3 Appendix 3-4, p. 41. For general dissection techniques, see p. 33.

Possible Associated Conditions: Juxtaposed atrial appendages; large left ventricular valvular orifice; large left ventricular chamber; persistent left superior vena cava; pulmonary atresia; transposition of the great arteries (25%), with aortic co-arctation (35% of those); anomalies of musculoskeletal or digestive systems (20%); Down's,* asplenia, or other syndromes.

Atresia, Urethral

Organs and Tissues	*Procedures*	*Possible or Expected Findings*
Pelvic organs	Prepare urogram (see pp. 59 and 62). For removal and dissection of pelvic organs, see p. 59. Leave ureters and kidneys attached to bladder. Open penile urethra (see Figs. 5-12; p. 63). Search for fistulas. If there is evidence of drainage via the urachus, demonstrate this before removal of pelvic organs.	Posterior urethral valves; strictures; absence of canalization of penile urethra; dilated bladder; hypoplastic prostate; hydroureters and hydronephrosis;* renal cystic dysplasia; fistulas to rectum or via urachus to umbilicus. Ascites with attenuation of anterior abdominal wall; cryptorchidism.

Atrial Septal Defect (See "Defect, atrial septal.")

Atrium, Common (See "Defect, atrial septal.")

Atrophy, Multiple System

Synonyms and Related Terms: Olivopontocerebellar atrophy, Shy-Drager syndrome, striatonigral degeneration.

Organs and Tissues	*Procedures*	*Possible or Expected Findings*
Brain, spinal cord, and paraspinal sympathetic chain	For removal and specimen preparation of brain and spinal cord, see pp. 65 and 67, respectively. Modified Bielschowsky, Bodian or Gallyas silver stains are necessary to highlight the characteristic glial cytoplasmic inclusions (see p. 172). Record pallor of white matter tracts related to neuronal loss in affected areas. This can be seen especially in external capsule, striatopallidal fibers, cerebellar white matter, cerebellar peduncles and transverse pontine fibers. Immunostain for synuclein is positive in inclusions.	Cell loss and gliosis with characteristic cytoplasmic and nuclear glial and neuronal inclusions and neuropil threads in affected areas. Clinical subtype and duration of illness influence distribution of lesions. Involved areas include: putamen, especially dorso-lateral, substantia nigra, locus coeruleus, cerebellar cortex (Purkinje's cells), basis pontis, inferior olive, dorsal motor nucleus of vagus, intermediolateral column of spinal cord.

Atrophy, Pick's Lobar (See "Disease, Pick's.")

Atrophy, Progressive Spinal Muscular (See "Disease, motor neuron.")

Atropine (See "Poisoning, atropine.")

Attack, Transient Cerebral Ischemic

Synonyms and Related Terms: Cerebrovascular disease; transient cerebral ischemia; transient stroke.

Organs and Tissues	*Procedures*	*Possible or Expected Findings*
Heart	If infective endocarditis* is suspected, follow procedures described on p. 102.	Vegetative endocarditis; mural cardiac thromboses.
Aorta and cervical arteries	For dissection of carotid and vertebral arteries, see p. 82.	Aortic, carotid, and vertebral atherosclerosis (see also under "Infarction, cerebral"). Atherosclerotic or other type of stenosis of subclavian artery proximal to takeoff of vertebral artery (subclavian steal syndrome).
Brain	For removal and specimen preparation, see p. 65. For cerebral arteriography, see p. 80.	Basilar atherosclerosis.

Avitaminosis (See "Deficiency, vitamin...")

B

Bagassosis (See "Pneumoconiosis.")

Barbiturate(s) (See "Poisoning, barbiturate(s).")

Baritosis (See "Pneumoconiosis.")

Bartonellosis

Synonyms and Related Terms: Bacillary angiomatosis *(1)*; *Bartonella bacilliformis, henselae*, or *quintana* infection; Carrión's disease; cat scratch disease *(1)*;* Oroya fever; Peruvian anemia; verruga peruana.

NOTE: (1) Collect all tissues that appear to be infected. (2) Organisms are usually demonstrated by direct stains rather than by culture. Detection by polymerase chain reaction (PCR) is possible *(2)*. (3) Request Giemsa stains (p. 172). (4) No special precautions are indicated. (5) Serologic studies are available from the Center for Disease Control and Prevention, Atlanta GA (p. 135). (6) This is a **reportable** disease.

Possible Associated Conditions: Acquired immunodeficiency syndrome (AIDS)* and other immunodeficiency states *(3)*; hemolytic anemia;* *Salmonella* infection.

Organs and Tissues	*Procedures*	*Possible or Expected Findings*
External examination and skin	Prepare sections of skin lesions. Request Giemsa stain (p. 172).	Jaundice. Miliary and nodular skin lesions with or without ulceration. Histologically, pigmented (hemosiderin) vascular granulomas. Bacillary angiomatosis *(1)*.
Blood	Prepare smears. Request Giemsa stain (p. 172).	*Bartonella* in erythrocytes.
Blood and lymphatic vessels (all organs and lesions)	Request Giemsa stain (p. 172).	*Bartonella bacilliformis* in swollen reticuloendothelial cells lining blood and lymphatic vessels. Thromboses. Erythrophagocytosis.
Heart	For demonstration of fat, prepare frozen section of myocardium with Sudan IV stain.	Fatty changes of myocardium in anemic patients.
Liver and spleen	Record weights. Submit samples for histologic study and request Giemsa and Gomori iron stains (p. 172).	Centrilobular hepatic necrosis; bacillary peliosis hepatis and bacillary splenitis; granulomatous hepatitis *(3)*; hemosiderosis of liver and spleen. Erythrophagocytosis; thromboses; necrosis *(3)*; and infarcts of spleen.
Lymph nodes	See above under "Liver and Spleen."	Lymphadenopathy (see above under "Blood and lymphatic vessels").
Bone marrow	See above under "Liver and Spleen."	Erythroid hyperplasia.

References

1. Wong R, Tappero J, Cockerell CJ. Bacillary angiomatosis and other Bartonella species infections. Semin Cutan Med Surg 1997;16:188–199.
2. Goldenberger D, Zbinden R, Perschil I, Altwegg M. Nachweis von Bartonella (Rochalimaea) henselae/B. quintana mittels Polymerase-Kettenreaktion (PCR). Schweiz Med Wschr 1996;126:207–213.
3. Liston TE, Koehler JE. Granulomatous hepatitis and necrotizing splenitis due to Bartonella henselae in a patient with cancer: case report and review of hepatosplenic manifestations of bartonella infections. Clin Infect Dis 1996;22:951–957.

From: *Handbook of Autopsy Practice,* 3rd Ed. Edited by: J. Ludwig © Humana Press Inc., Totowa, NJ

Beriberi

Synonyms and Related Terms: Thiamine deficiency; Wernicke encephalopathy (cerebral beriberi).

Possible Associated Conditions: Chronic alcoholism; chronic peritoneal dialysis; hemodialysis; Wernicke disease; Wernicke-Korsakoff syndrome.*

Organs and Tissues	*Procedures*	*Possible or Expected Findings*
External examination and oral cavity		Evidence of malnutrition;* edema. Glossitis.
Heart	Record weight and submit samples for histologic study (p. 30).	Alcoholic cardiomyopathy;* cardiac hypertrophy.*
Brain and spinal cord with dorsal-root ganglia	For removal and specimen preparation, see pp. 65, 67, and 69, respectively. Request Luxol fast blue and Bielschowsky stains (p. 172).	For cerebral changes, see "Syndrome, Wernicke-Korsakoff."
Cerebral, spinal, and peripheral nerves	For sampling and specimen preparation of peripheral nerves, see p. 79.	Axonal degeneration with relative sparing of small myelinated and unmyelinated fibers. Proximal segmental demyelination is considered a secondary phenomenon *(1)*. Degeneration may also occur in terminal branches of vagus and phrenic nerves.

Reference

1. Windebank AJ. Polyneuropathy due to nutritional deficiency and alcoholism. In: Peripheral Neuropathy, vol. 2. Dyck PJ, Thomas PK, eds., W.B. Saunders, Philadelphia, PA, 1993, pp. 1310–1321.

Berylliosis

NOTE: Close similarities exist between berylliosis and sarcoidosis *(1)**.

Organs and Tissues	*Procedures*	*Possible or Expected Findings*
Skin	Prepare sections from various sites.	Granulomas.
Vitreous	For removal and specimen preparation, see p. 85.	Increased calcium concentration (associated with hypercalcemia *[1]*).
Lungs	Perfuse one lung with formalin (p. 47). Freeze one lobe for possible chemical study. See also under "Pneumoconiosis."	Chronic interstitial and granulomatous pneumonia.
Other organs	Procedures depend on expected findings or grossly identified abnormalities as listed in right-hand column.	Noncaseating tuberculoid granulomas with giant cells and calcific inclusions in liver, spleen, lymph nodes, and other organs. Nephrolithiasis *(1)*.

Reference

1. Rossman MD. Chronic beryllium disease: diagnosis and management. Environm Health Perspect 1996;104:945–947.

Bilharziasis (See "Schistosomiasis.")

Bismuth (See "Poisoning, bismuth.")

Blastomycosis, European (See "Cryptococcosis.")

Blastomycosis, North American

Synonym: *Blastomyces dermatitidis* infection.

NOTE: (1) Collect all tissues that appear to be infected. (2) Request fungal cultures. (3) Request Grocott's methenamine silver stain (p. 172). (4) No special precautions are indicated. (5) Serologic studies are available from the state health department laboratories (p. 135). (6) This is not a reportable disease.

Organs and Tissues	Procedures	Possible or Expected Findings
External examination and skin	Prepare sections of skin and of subcutaneous lesions. Submit scrapings of skin lesion for fungal cultures.	Weeping and crusted elevated skin lesions, predominantly of face and hands. Abscesses, fistulas, and ulcers with central healing and scarring may be present.
	Request mucicarmine stain (p. 173).	Organisms should *not* be stainable with mucicarmine.
	Prepare chest roentgenogram and roentgenographic survey of bones.	Pulmonary infiltrates; osteomyelitis* and periostitis of thoracic, lumbar, and sacral spine, long bones of lower extremities, pelvic bones, and ribs (in this order of frequency).
Lungs	Perfuse one lung with formalin (p. 47). Photograph cut surface. For histologic staining, see above under "External examination and skin."	Chronic pneumonia; possibly, suppurative and granulomatous lesions; rarely, cavitation and calcification.
Other organs and tissues	Prepare cultures of grossly affected organs and tissues. Other procedures depend on expected findings or grossly identified abnormalities as listed in right-hand column.	Involvement probably secondary to hematogenous dissemination; cerebral abscess;* meningitis;* adrenalitis; endocarditis;* pericarditis;* thyroiditis.* Other organs, such as eyes and larynx may also be affected.
Genital organs	For dissection techniques, see Part I, Chapter 5.	Inflammatory infiltrates—rarely with fistulas—of prostate, epididymis, and seminal vesicles.
Bones	For removal, prosthetic repair, and specimen preparation, see p. 95.	Osteomyelitis* or periostitis (see above under "External examination and skin"). Psoas abscess may be present.

Blastomycosis, South American (See "Paracoccidioidomycosis.")

Block (Heart) (See "Arrhythmia, cardiac.")

Bodies, Foreign

If a foreign body is discovered during a medicolegal autopsy or if the discovery of a foreign body may have medicolegal implications (e.g., presence of a surgical instrument in the abdominal cavity), the rules of the chain of custody apply (p. 17). For the handling of bullets or bullet fragments, see "Injury, firearm." For museum display of foreign bodies, see p. 137. Metallic foreign objects are particularly suitable for embedding in plastic for display (p. 138). If analysis of foreign material is required, commercial laboratories may be helpful.

Bolus (See "Obstruction, acute airway.")

Botulism

Synonym: *Clostridium botulinum* infection.

NOTE: (1) Submit sample of feces *(1)*. Best confirmation of diagnosis is demonstration of toxin in the same food that the victim ingested. (2) Cultures are usually not indicated. (3) Special stains are usually not indicated. (4) No special precautions are indicated. (5) Serologic studies and toxin assays are available from the state health department laboratories (p. 135). (6) This is a **reportable** disease.

Organs and Tissues	Procedures	Possible or Expected Findings
Blood	Refrigerate a specimen until toxicologic study of serum can be done.	Toxin lethal to mice. Can be neutralized by specific antitoxin.
Other organs and tissues		No diagnostic morphologic findings. Aspiration;* bronchopneumonia; manifestations of hypoxia.*
Serum, gastric, or intestinal contents; stool return form sterile water enema; exudate from wound	Submit for toxicologic study.	*Clostridium botulinum* and its toxins may be found in feces.

Reference

1. Dezfulian M, Hatheway CL, Yolken RH, Bartlett JG. Enzyme-linked immunosorbent assay for detection of *Clostridium botulinum* type A and type B toxins in stool samples of infants with botulism. J Clin Microbiol 1984;20(3):379–383.

Bromide (See "Poisoning, bromide.")

Bronchiectasis

Possible Associated Conditions: Abnormalities of airway cartilage (Williams-Campbell syndrome; Mounier-Kahn syndrome); allergic bronchopulmonary fungal disease; alpha$_1$-antitrypsin deficiency;* amyloidosis;* cystic fibrosis;* IgA deficiency with or without deficiency of IgG subclasses; Kartagener's syndrome (situs inversus, chronic sinusitis, and bronchiectasis) and other primary ciliary dyskinesias; obstructive azoospermia (Young syndrome); panhypogammaglobulinemia; ulcerative colitis; rheumatoid arthritis;* yellow nail syndrome (hypoplastic lymphatics).

Organs and Tissues	*Procedures*	*Possible or Expected Findings*
External examination		Clubbing of fingers and toes.
	Prepare chest roentgenogram.	Pneumothorax;* pulmonary infiltrates; pleural effusion or exudate.*
Chest cavity	For tests for pneumothorax, see under that heading.	Pneumothorax;* pleural empyema.* Situs inversus in Kartagener's syndrome.
Blood	Submit sample for microbiologic study (p. 102).	Septicemia.
Heart	Record weight and thickness of right and left ventricles.	Cor pulmonale.
Lungs	Submit one lobe for bacterial and fungal cultures. If only one lobe contains bronchiectases, aspirate contents for microbiologic study.	Bronchiectasis, usually in lower lobes. In cystic fibrosis,* upper lobes are more severely affected. Purulent bronchitis.* Peribronchiectatic pneumonia or abscess. Allergic bronchopulmonary aspergillosis; tuberculosis.*
	For bronchography, see p. 50.	Fungus ball in cavity (aspergillosis*).
	For bronchial arteriography, see p. 50.	Dilatation of bronchial arteries. Bronchopulmomary anastomoses.
	Slice perfused lung along probes introduced into bronchiectases for guidance.	Saccular, tubular, or varicose bronchiectases.
	Request Gram, Grocott's methenamine silver, and —if indicated because of suspected tuberculosis —Kinyoun's stains (p. 172).	Evidence of bacterial *(P. aeruginosa; Staphylococcus aureus; H. influenzae; Escherichia coli),* mycobacterial, or fungal (aspergillus sp.) infection.
	Prepare sections of tracheobronchial cartilage.	Abnormal cartilage; see above under "Possible Associated Conditions."
Kidneys		Amyloidosis;* glomerular enlargement.
Other organs	If amyloidosis is suspected, request Congo red, crystal violet, methyl violet, Sirius red, and thioflavine T stains (p. 172).	Amyloidosis.*
	If cystic fibrosis is present, follow procedures described under that heading.	Cystic fibrosis.*
Brain and spinal cord; nasal cavity and sinuses	For removal and specimen preparation, see pp. 65, 67, and 71, respectively.	Cerebral abscess.* Nasal polyps; sinusitis.

Bronchitis, Acute Chemical

NOTE: This occurs after inhalation of toxic gases, such as sulfurous acid (H_2SO_3), sulfur dioxide (SO_2), chlorine (Cl_2), and ammonia (NH_3). See also under "Poisoning, gas" and under "Edema, chemical pulmonary."

Organs and Tissues	*Procedures*	*Possible or Expected Findings*
Upper airways and lungs	Remove lungs together with pharynx, larynx, and trachea. Open airways in posterior midline.	Acute chemical laryngotracheitis.
	Perfuse one lung with formalin under low pressure (tissue may be viable) (p. 47).	Necrotizing bronchitis; aspiration of acid vomitus; chemical pulmonary edema.*

Bronchitis, Chronic

Synonyms and Related Terms: Chronic asthmatic bronchitis; chronic bronchitis with obstruction; chronic chemical bronchitis; chronic mucopurulent bronchitis; infectious bronchitis.

Organs and Tissues	*Procedures*	*Possible or Expected Findings*
Heart	Record weight and thickness of right and left ventricles.	Cor pulmonale. See also under "Failure, congestive heart."
Lungs	Submit one lobe for microbiologic study (p. 103). Slice fresh lung in sagittal plane. After submitting samples of cross-sections of bronchi for histologic study, open remainder of bronchi longitudinally. For bronchography, see p. 50.	Bronchopneumonia. Bronchiectasis.* Emphysema.*
	For bronchial arteriography, see p. 50.	Dilatation of bronchial arteries; bronchopulmonary anastomoses.
	Perfuse one lung with formalin (p. 47). For semiquantitative determination of severity of bronchitis, use the Reid index or related morphologic methods *(1)*.	Most methods of wet inflation tend to distend bronchi and to overinflate lungs. Hyperplasia of submucosal bronchial glands and smooth muscle tends to parallel severity of chronic bronchitis.
	Request Gram and Grocott's methenamine silver stains (p. 172).	Bacterial or fungal infection.
Diaphragm	Record size and thickness of muscular diaphragm.	Decrease in surface area and thickness in chronic bronchitis.
Stomach and duodenum		Peptic ulcers.*
Kidneys		Glomerular enlargement.
Brain and spinal cord	For removal and specimen preparation, see pp. 65 and 67, respectively.	Hypoxic changes.

Reference

1. Thurlbeck WM. Pathology of chronic airflow obstruction. In: Chronic Obstructive Pulmonary Disease, Chernack NS, ed. W.B. Saunders, Philadelphia, PA, 1991.

Bronchopneumonia (See "Pneumonia, all types or type unspecified.")

Brucellosis

Synonyms: *Brucella* spp. infection; undulant fever; Mediterranean fever; Malta fever.

NOTE: (1) Collect all tissues that appear to be infected. (2) Request aerobic cultures for *Brucella.* (3) Request Gram stains (p. 172). (4) Special **precautions** are indicated (p. 146). (5) Serologic studies are available from local or state health department laboratories (p. 135). (6) This is a **reportable** disease.

Organs and Tissues	*Procedures*	*Possible or Expected Findings*
External examination	For exposure of joints and microbiologic specimen preparation, see p. 96.	Subcutaneous abscesses. Purulent arthritis (sacroiliac and hip joints) and periarticular bursitis.
	Prepare roentgenograms of skeletal system.	Osteomyelitis* of long bones and of spine.
Blood	Submit samples for culture and serum agglutination tests. See also above under "Note."	
Lymph nodes		Generalized lymphadenopathy.
Heart	If endocarditis is suspected, follow procedures described on p. 103.	Infective endocarditis* (particularly with pre-existing aortic stenosis); myocarditis;* pericardial effusions.
Arteries and veins	For angiography, see under specific site or organ. Submit samples for histologic study. Request Verhoeff–van Gieson stain (p. 173).	Arterial aneurysms; arteriovenous fistulas. Granulomatous endophlebitis.

Organs and Tissues	Procedures	Possible or Expected Findings
Lungs	Submit sample for culture (see above under "Note" and p. 103).	Pleural effusions;* granulomas that may be associated with abscesses and calcification. Embolism secondary to granulomatous endophlebitis.
Liver	Record weight. Submit sample for culture (see above under "Note" and p. 102).	Hepatomegaly; granulomatous hepatitis; nonspecific reactive changes.
Gallbladder		Acute cholecystitis.*
Spleen	Record weight. Submit sample for culture (p. 102).	Splenomegaly with granulomas.
Kidneys and ureters	Submit samples of renal tissue for histologic study. Record appearance of renal pelvic and ureteral mucosa.	Granulomas; ulceration of mucosa of renal pelvis. See also above under "Lungs."
Urinary bladder	Photograph ulceration; submit for histologic study.	Ulceration of mucosa.
Ovaries, prostate, epididymides, and testes	Submit samples for culture (see also above under "Note.")	Abscesses.
Bones and joints	For removal, prosthetic repair, and specimen preparation, see p. 95.	Osteomyelitis* of long bones and of spine; arthritis *(1)*.
Brain	For removal and specimen preparation, see p. 65. Submit for culture (see p. 102). See also above under "Note." For cerebral arteriography, see p. 80.	Meningoencephalitis; mycotic intracerebral aneurysm* with rupture and hemorrhage.
Eyes	For removal and specimen preparation, see p. 85.	Iritis; choroiditis; keratitis.

Reference

1. Colmenero JD, Reguera JM, Martos F, Sanchez-De-Mora D, Delgado M, Causse M, et al. Complications associated with Brucella melitensis infection: a study of 530 cases. Medicine 1996;75:195–211.

Burns

NOTE: Fatal burns should be reported to the medical examiner's or coroner's office. The questions to be answered by the pathologist depend on whether the incident was accidental, suicidal, or homicidal, and whether the victim survivied to be treated in the hospital. A pending death certificate should be issued if the fire and police investigators are not sure of the circumstances at the time of the autopsy. For electrical burns, see under "Injury, electrical."

For victims who were treated at the hospital, autopsy procedures should be directed toward the discovery or confirmation of the mechanism of death, such as sepsis or pulmonary embolism.* Death can be caused primarily by heart disease, with otherwise minor burns and smoke inhalation serving as the trigger that leads to lethal ventricular arrhythmia. Because carbon monoxide concentrations are halved approx every 30 min with 100% oxygen therapy, the pathologist must obtain the first clinical laboratory test results for CO-hemoglobin. Soot can be detected with the naked eye 2 or 3 d after inhalation of smoke. Ambulance records should be examined to determine whether a persistent coma might have been caused by hypoxic encephalopathy following resuscitation from cardiac arrest at the scene.

Admission blood samples should be acquired to test for CO-hemoglobin and alcohol. This may not have been done in the emergency room. Persons suffering from chronic alcoholism succumb to fire deaths more often than persons who do not drink. A very high initial serum alcohol concentration suggests a risk factor for the fire and presence of chronic alcoholism. Patients with chronic alcoholism typically are deprived of alcohol when they are in the burn unit and this can cause sudden, presumably cardiac, death, just as it occurs under similar circumstances, not complicated by burns. Under these circumstances, the heart fails to show major abnormalities. This mode of dying seems to have no relationship to the presence or absence of liver disease.

Organs and Tissues	Procedures	Possible or Expected Findings
External examination and skin	If the body is found dead and charred at the scene, prepare whole body roentgenograms, before and after removal of remnants of clothing. See also under "Identification of the body" (p. 11) and under "External examination" (p. 13). One or two fingerpads may yield sufficient ridge detail for identification. If this is not possible, ante- and postmortem somatic and dental radiographs must be compared for identification, or DNA comparison must be used.	Roentgenograms may detect bullets in cases where arson was used to mask murder. Bullets or knife blades must be secured as evidence. Objects such as hairpins, keys, jewelry, dentures, or other evidence, and demonstration of old fractures may help provisionally identify the victim. Fractures of bones and lacerations of soft tissue can all occur as heat artifacts and must be identified as such. See also above under "Note."

Organs and Tissues	*Procedures*	*Possible or Expected Findings*
External examination and skin *(continued)*	Photograph burnt body and make diagrams of wounds.	
	Prepare histologic sections of blisters and of surrounding skin.	Inflammatory changes in the skin indicate a vital reaction.
Blood	If victim was found burnt, submit samples for carbon monoxide determination and toxicologic study, primarily for alcohol and illicit drugs.	Increased carbon monoxide concentration (saturation of >15–20%) is strong evidence that the victim was alive and breathing for some time during burning. CO-concentrations may not be elevated in flash-fire victims.
	If victim survived for some time, submit samples for bacterial and fungal culture (p. 102).	Septicemia and bacteremia.
Vitreous	Submit sample for alcohol and other toxicologic studies (p. 85), particularly if no blood is available, and also for electrolyte determination.	Water and electrolyte loss in patients who had survived burns for some time.
Serosal surfaces	Record volume and character of exudate or transudate.	Exudate indicates vital reaction. Watery transudate may develop with rigorous infusions of crystalloid during fruitless resuscitation efforts.
Neck organs and tracheobronchial tree	Remove carefully. Inspect hyoid bone; search for hemorrhages in soft tissues of neck.	Strangulation effect (fractured hyoid bone).
	Record appearance and photograph mucosal surfaces of larynx and trachea. If patient had survived for some time and had been intubated, search for intubation trauma.	Soot particles and other heat injuries indicate that the patient was breathing in fire. Absence of soot particles does not prove that the patient was already dead when fire started unless there is reasonable evidence that the fire was not a flash fire.
	Inspect supraglottic area.	Supraglottic edema may cause sudden death in patients who had survived burns—particularly of face—for some time.
	Submit samples of tracheobronchial mucosa for histologic study.	Herpes virus inclusions in tracheobronchial ulcerations of victims who had survived burns for some time.
Other organs	Follow routine autopsy procedures.	Bronchopneumonia; pulmonary emboli; heart disease in victims who survive for some time. See also above under "Note."
Pelvic organs	Examination of pelvic organs may permit sex determination in severely burnt bodies.	Sex determination.
	In female victims whose burns are less severe, a search should be made for evidence of rape.	Evidence of rape.*
Durae and brain		Epidural hematomas may occur as heat artifacts.

Bypass, aortocoronary (See "Surgery, aortocoronary bypass.")

Byssinosis (See "Pneumoconiosis.")

C

Cadmium (See "Poisoning, cadmium.")

Calcinosis, Mönckeberg's Medial

Synonyms: Medial sclerosis of arteries; Mönckeberg's arteriosclerosis.

NOTE: This is generally considered an age-related phenomenon that is usually of little clinical consequence, with calcification of the internal elastic membrane and subjacent media. It commonly involves femoral and thyroid arteries.

Calcium (See "Disorder, electrolyte(s).")

Calculi, Renal (See "Nephrolithiasis.")

Canal, Complete Atrioventricular (See "Defect, complete atrioventricular septal.")

Candidiasis

Synonyms and Related Terms: Candidosis, moniliasis, thrush.

NOTE: Candidiasis may follow or complicate antibacterial or corticosteroid therapy, cardiac surgery,* dehydration,* diabetes mellitus,* drug (heroin) dependence,* leukemia* or other systemic malignant diseases, tuberculosis,* and other debilitating diseases.

(1) Collect all tissues that appear to be infected. (2) Request fungal cultures. (3) Request Grocott's methenamine silver or PAS stain, or both (p. 172). (4) No special precautions are indicated. (5) Serologic studies are available from many reference laboratories (p. 135). (6) This is not a reportable disease.

Organs and Tissues	*Procedures*	*Possible or Expected Findings*
External examination and skin	Prepare sections of skin. For special stains, see above under "Note."	Intertrigo. Nail destruction may occur without skin involvement.
Oral cavity		Creamy patches.
Blood	Submit sample for fungal culture (p. 102).	*Candida* septicemia.
Heart	If endocarditis is suspected, for instance, in drug addicts or after cardiac surgery, follow procedures described on p. 103.	*Candida* endocarditis.
Lungs	Submit one lobe for bacterial and fungal culture. For special stains, see above under "Note."	*Candida* bronchopneumonia, often in association with other processes.
Pharynx, esophagus, and gastrointestinal tract with rectum; vagina, and cervix	Photograph all lesions. Submit samples for histologic study. For special stains, see above under "Note."	*Candida* infection with membranes, erosions, and ulcers.
Other organs	Submit samples of liver, pancreas, kidneys, adrenal glands, thyroid, and joints for histologic study. If available, sample umbilical cord.	Systemic candidiasis; multiple abscesses due to septic embolization. In the umbilical cord, necrotizing inflammation (funisitis) may be found.
Cerebrospinal fluid	Submit sample for fungal culture (p. 104).	Meningitis.
Brain	For removal and specimen preparation, see p. 65. For special stains, see above under "Note."	Meningitis.

Carbon Monoxide (See "Poisoning, carbon monoxide.")

Carbon Tetrachloride (See "Poisoning, carbon tetrachloride.")

From: *Handbook of Autopsy Practice,* 3rd Ed. Edited by: J. Ludwig © Humana Press Inc., Totowa, NJ

Carcinoma (See "Tumor...")

Cardiomegaly (See "Cardiomyopathy,... and "Hypertrophy, cardiac.")

Cardiomyopathy, Alcoholic

NOTE: For general dissection techniques, see p. 22.

Organs and Tissues	*Procedures*	*Possible or Expected Findings*
External examination, heart and lungs	See below under "Cardiomyopathy, dilated."	See below under "Cardiomyopathy, dilated."
Abdominal cavity and liver	Record volume of ascites. Record actual and expected weight of liver. Request iron stain (p. 172).	Alcoholic cirrhosis and alcoholic cardiomyopathy rarely coexist. However, in genetic hemochromatosis,* cirrhosis and heart failure are common findings.

Cardiomyopathy, Dilated (Idiopathic, Familial, and Secondary Types)

NOTE: For general dissection techniques, see p. 22.

Organs and Tissues	*Procedures*	*Possible or Expected Findings*
External examination	Prepare chest roentgenogram.	Cardiomegaly; pleural or pericardial effusions;* pacemaker.
Chest cavity	Record volume of pleural and pericardial effusions.	Hydrothorax; hydropericardium.
Heart	Record actual and expected heart weights. Measure and record maximum internal short-axis diameter of left ventricular chamber. Record ventricular thicknesses and valvular circumferences. Note location and size of mural thrombus. Request iron stain (p. 172).	Cardiomegaly; biventricular hypertrophy; four-chamber dilatation; focal left ventricular fibrosis; dilated valve annuli; relatively mild coronary atherosclerosis; possible iron in cardiac myocytes; microfocal interstitial fibrosis, particularly subendocardial; myocarditis (idiopathic or drug-related).
Lungs	Record actual and expected weights. Request Verhoeff–van Gieson and iron stains from one lower lobe (p. 172).	Pulmonary congestion; pulmonary edema; changes of chronic pulmonary venous hypertension; pulmonary emboli; pulmonary infarcts; bronchopneumonia.
Abdominal cavity	Record volume of ascites.	Ascites.
Liver	Record actual and expected weights.	Chronic congestive hepatomegaly; centrilobular (zone 3) steatosis, fibrosis, or necrosis (not true cirrhosis).

Cardiomyopathy, Hypertrophic (Idiopathic, Familial, and Secondary Types)

Synonyms: Idiopathic hypertrophic subaortic stenosis (IHSS); hypertrophic obstructive cardiomyopathy (HOCM); and many others.

NOTE: For general dissection techniques, see p. 22.

Possible Associated Conditions: See below under "Possible or Expected Findings."

Organs and Tissues	*Procedures*	*Possible or Expected Findings*
External examination	Sample skin lesions for histologic study. Prepare chest roentgenogram.	Lentiginosis (part of LEOPARD syndrome). Mild cardiomegaly.
Heart	Record actual and expected weights. Record ventricular thicknesses and valvular circumferences. Determine ratio between left ventricular septal and free wall thicknesses (normal, <1.3) at basal, midventricular, and apical levels. Request amyloid stain (Congo red or sulfated alcian blue) (p. 172).	Biventricular hypertrophy; disproportionate septal hypertrophy (>1.3 in 90%); gross and microscopic fibrosis; thickened anterior mitral leaflet; subaortic septal endocardial fibrotic patch (contact lesion from mitral valve); left atrial dilatation; focal septal myofiber disarray microscopically.
Brain and spinal cord	For removal and specimen preparation, see pp. 65 and 67, respectively.	Friedreich's ataxia.*

Cardiomyopathy, Restrictive (Non-eosinophilic and Secondary Types)

NOTE: For general dissection techniques, see p. 22.

Organs and Tissues	*Procedures*	*Possible or Expected Findings*
Heart	Record actual and expected weights. Record ventricular thicknesses and valvular circumferences. Evaluate atrial size, compared to ventricular chamber size. Request amyloid stain (Congo red or sulfated alcian blue) (p. 172).	Prominent biatrial dilatation. Relatively normal ventricular size. Prominent biventricular interstitial fibrosis or amyloidosis, microscopically.

Cardiomyopathy, Restrictive (With Eosinophilia)

Synonyms: Eosinophilic endomyocardial disease; hypereosinophilic syndromes; Löffler's eosinophilic endomyocarditis; Davies' endomyocardial fibrosis.

NOTE: For general dissection techniques, see p. 22.

Organs and Tissues	*Procedures*	*Possible or Expected Findings*
Heart	Record actual and expected weights. Record ventricular thicknesses and valvular circumferences. Evaluate relative atrial and ventricular chamber sizes.	Mural thrombus along apex and inflow tract of one or both ventricles, with extensive intact or degranulated eosinophils microscopically. Ventricular dilatation only if mitral or tricuspid valve or both are regurgitant.
Other organs and tissues	Procedures depend on expected findings or grossly identified abnormalities as listed in right-hand column.	Conditions associated with eosinophilia, such as asthmatic bronchiolitis or Churg-Strauss syndrome (see also under "Syndrome, hypereosinophilic"); malignancies; parasitic disease; vasculitis.

Cardiomyopathy, Arrhythmogenic Right Ventricular

Synonyms: Arrhythmogenic right ventricular dysplasia; right ventricular cardiomyopathy.

NOTE: For general dissection techniques, see p. 22.

Organs and Tissues	*Procedures*	*Possible or Expected Findings*
Heart	Record actual and expected weights. Record ventricular thicknesses and valvular circumferences. Evaluate pattern and extent of epicardial fat, especially over right ventricle. Take multiple samples from right ventricle for microscopic study.	Prominent right ventricular dilatation, grossly; right ventricular hypertrophy, fibrosis, and adiposity, by microscopy (excessive for patient's age and body size). Occasional left ventricular involvement. Microfocal myocarditis or epicarditis.

Carditis (See "Myocarditis.")

Chickenpox (See "Varicella.")

Chloride (See "Disorder, electrolyte(s)" and p. 114.)

Chloroma

NOTE: Follow procedures described under "Leukemia, all types or type unspecified." For gross staining of chloroma, see p. 134.

Cholangiopathy, Infantile Obstructive (See "Atresia, biliary" and "Hepatitis, neonatal.")

Cholangitis, Chronic Nonsuppurative Destructive

Synonym: Primary bilary cirrhosis.

NOTE: Follow procedures described under "Cirrhosis, liver."

Cholangitis, Sclerosing

Synonyms: Idiopathic sclerosing cholangitis; primary sclerosing cholangitis; secondary sclerosing cholangitis.

Possible Associated Conditions: Acquired immunodeficiency syndrome;* acute or chronic pancreatitis;* ankylosing spondylitis;* autoimmune hemolytic anemia;* autoimmune hepatitis; bronchiectasis;* chronic ulcerative colitis;* celiac disease; Crohn's disease;* eosinophilia; glomerulonephritis;* immune thrombocytopenic purpura; Peyronie's disease; pseudotumor of the orbit; retroperitoneal fibrosis;* rheumatoid arthritis;* Riedel's struma; sclerosing mediastinitis;* Sjogren's syndrome;* systemic lupus erythematosus;* systemic sclerosis;* vasculitis; and many others (the associations are not equally well documented) *(1)*.

Organs and Tissues	Procedures	Possible or Expected Findings
External examination	Record presence or absence of laparotomy scars and drains.	Jaundice.
Intestinal tract and pancreas		See above under "Possible Associated Conditions."
Hepatoduodenal ligament	For cholangiography, see p. 56. Open duodenum anteriorly and insert catheter into papilla of Vater. After removal of liver and hepatodudenal ligament, prepare cholangiograms. Record diameter of lumens and thickness of walls at various levels of common bile duct, hepatic duct, cystic duct, and gallbladder.	Sclerosis and narrowing of extrahepatic bile ducts. Choledocholithiasis; cholelithiasis; adenocarcinoma of bile ducts or gallbladder.
	Record appearance of portal veins and hepatic arteries.	Occlusion or narrowing of hepatic artery or its branches may cause ischemic cholangitis, which closely resembles primary sclerosing cholangitis *(2)*.
	Prepare histologic sections of extrahepatic bile ducts and hepatoduodenal lymph nodes.	Intraductal carcinoma may imitate primary sclerosing cholangitis. Lymph nodes may contain metastatic carcinoma. For possible infections, see below under "Liver."
Liver	Photograph before and after slicing. Submit samples for histologic study; include sections of perihilar intrahepatic bile ducts.	Intrahepatic sclerosing cholangitis; cholestasis; ascending cholangitis; biliary cirrhosis. Cholangiocarcinoma. Evidence of cytomegalovirus or cryptosporidium infection.
Other organs and tissues		See above under "Possible Associated Conditions."

References

1. Lazarides KN, Wiesner RH, Porayko MK, Ludwig J, LaRusso NF. Primary sclerosing cholangitis. In: Diseases of the Liver, 8th ed. Schiff ER, Sorrell MF, Maddray WC, eds. Lippincott-Raven, Philadelphia, PA, 1999.
2. Batts KP. Ischemic cholangitis. Mayo Clin Proc 1998;73:380–385.

Cholangitis, Suppurative

Related Terms: Ascending cholangitis; obstructive suppurative cholangitis; (oriental) recurrent pyogenic cholangitis.

Organs and Tissues	Procedures	Possible or Expected Findings
External examination		Jaundice.
Blood	Submit sample for microbiologic study (p. 102).	Septicemia.
Heart	If infective endocarditis is suspected, follow procedures described on p. 103.	Infective endocarditis.*
Hepatoduodenal ligament	For cholangiography, see p. 56. Dissect common bile duct, hepatic duct, and portal vein *in situ*.	Stricture; tumor, stones. Portal vein thrombosis; pylephlebitis.
Liver and gallbladder	Record weight of liver and photograph it. Submit portion of liver for aerobic and anaerobic bacterial culture. Submit samples for histologic study and request Gram stain (p. 172).	Cholangitic abscesses; cholecystitis,* cholelithiasis.* Carcinoma or other conditions causing obstruction or compression of bile ducts.

Cholecystitis

Related Terms: Acute acalculous cholecystitis; chronic cholecystitis; gallstone cholecystitis.

Possible Associated Conditions: Brucellosis;* major trauma or operation unrelated to biliary system; polyarteritis nodosa;* *Salmonella typhosa* infection (typhoid fever*).

Organs and Tissues	Procedures	Possible or Expected Findings
External examination	Prepare roentgenogram of upper abdomen.	Jaundice. Air in biliary tract indicates biliary fistula. Gallstones
Abdominal cavity	Submit peritoneal exudate and aspirated contents of gallbladder for aerobic and anaerobic culture. Also submit exudate from subphrenic empyema* or other intraperitoneal empyemas (abscesses).	Peritonitis;* intraperitoneal empyemas (abscesses).
Blood	Submit sample for bacterial culture (p. 102).	Septicemia.
Heart	If endocarditis is suspected, follow procedures described on p. 103.	Infective endocarditis.*
Intestine	If biliary fistula is suspected, open stomach, duodenum, and hepatic flexure of colon *in situ*. Record location and size of fistula.	Biliary fistula, with or without gallstone ileus.
Gallbladder; hepatoduodenal ligament with extrahepatic bile ducts	For cholangiography, see p. 56. Open all extrahepatic bile ducts, portal vein, and hepatic artery *in situ*. Remove liver and gallbladder. For specimen preparation, see p. 57. Describe appearance, position, and contents of gallbladder. Record number and character of stones. For preservation of gallbladder and stones, see pp. 134 and 137.	Acute or chronic cholecystitis; cholelithiasis;* cholangitis;* choledocholithiasis. Ulcers, abscesses, empyema, gangrene, or perforation of gallbladder; emphysematous cholecystitis; fistula. Hydrops or porcelain gallbladder; limey bile. Torsion of gallbladder. Portal vein thrombosis; pylephlebitis. Polyarteritis nodosa* of gallbladder. Hepatoduodenal lymphadenitis.
Liver	Record size and weight. Submit samples for histologic study.	Suppurative cholangitis;* cholangitic abscesses; pylephlebitis; pylephlebitic abscesses; venous thromboses.
Pancreas	If pancreatitis is present, record whether common bile duct and pancreatic duct have a common entry.	Pancreatitis.*

Choledocholithiasis

NOTE: Follow procedures described under "Cholecystitis."

Cholelithiasis

NOTE: Follow procedures described under "Cholecystitis." Cholelithiasis may be associated with all types of cholecystitis, with cholesterosis of the gallbladder, and with polyps of the gallbladder. The presence of "white bile" (limey bile) indicates obstruction of the cystic duct. Record number and character of stones. To prevent the green discoloration of gallbladder mucosa, see Chapter 14, p. 134.

Cholera

Synonym: *Vibrio cholerae* infection; asiatic cholera.

NOTE: The disease may complicate anemia,* chronic atrophic gastritis, vagotomy, gastrectomy, chronic intestinal disease, and malnutrition.

(1) Collect all tissues that appear to be infected. (2) Request cultures of intestinal contents for cholera. (3) Request Gram stain (p. 172). (4) Special **precautions** are indicated (p. 146). (5) For serologic studies, see below under "Blood." (6) This is a **reportable** disease.

Organs and Tissues	Procedures	Possible or Expected Findings
External examination	Record body weight and length and extent of rigor.	Early onset and prolongation of rigor mortis. Shriveled fingers ("washer-woman's hands") and toes.
Vitreous	Submit sample for sodium, chloride, and urea nitrogen determination (p. 85).	Dehydration.* (See also p. 115).
Blood	Prepare serum for tube agglutination or enzyme-linked immunosorbent assay (ELISA) test for retrospective diagnosis or epidemiologic purposes.	

Organs and Tissues	*Procedures*	*Possible or Expected Findings*
Intestinal tract	Record volume and appearance of intestinal contents. Submit samples of feces and other intestinal contents for culture and for determination of sodium, potassium, and chloride content.	Blood-stained or "rice-water type" intestinal contents. The organism may be present in pure culture.
	Submit samples of all portions of the intestinal tract for histologic study.	Intact mucosa with edema of lamina propria; dilatation of capillaries and lymphatics; mononuclear infiltrates and goblet cell hyperplasia. All changes confined to small bowel. Bacteria situated on or between epithelial cells.
Kidneys	Submit samples for histologic study.	Tubular necrosis;* focal cortical necrosis.
Adrenal glands		Lipid depletion.
Urine	Record volume and specific gravity.	Absence or minimal amount of urine suggests dehydration.*
Other organs and tissues		All tissues appear abnormally dry. Lungs are usually pale and shrunken, less frequently congested.

Chondrocalcinosis (See "Pseudogout.")

Chondrodysplasia

Synonyms and Related Terms: Achondroplasia; chondrodystrophia fetalis; Ellis-van Creveld syndrome.*

Organs and Tissues	*Procedures*	*Possible or Expected Findings*
External examination	Record body length, length of extremities, and abnormal features. Measure head, chest, and abdominal circumferences.	Dwarfism;* micromelia with pudgy fingers; bulging head with saddle nose.
	Prepare skeletal roentgenograms. All radiographs should be reviewed by a radiologist.	Chest deformities; separation of spinal ossification centers; abnormal pelvis and, in infants, ossification centers in metaphyseal ends of long bones.
Thyroid gland	Record weight and submit sample for histologic study.	Atrophy.
Other organs	Perfuse at least one lung with formalin (p. 47).	Restrictive and obstructive lung disease *(1)*.
Base of skull, pituitary gland, brain, and spinal canal with cord	For removal and specimen preparation of brain and spinal cord, see pp. 65 and 67, respectively. For removal of pituitary gland, see p. 71. Record appearance and photograph base of skull; record size of foramen magnum. Remove middle ears (see p. 72).	Growth retardation of base of skull with compression of foramen magnum. Internal hydrocephalus.* Narrow spinal canal with compression of spinal cord. (Clinically: paraplegia.) Atrophy of pituitary gland. Otitis media* *(2)*.
Bones	For removal, prosthetic repair, and specimen preparation, see p. 95.	Dorsolumbar kyphosis and lumbosacral lordosis; short iliac wings; short and thick tubular bones; excessive size of epiphysis in long bones; elongated costal cartilage; tibial bowing.
	Submit samples (especially epiphyses, if present) for histologic study.	Decreased cartilage cell proliferation at costochondral junction and at epiphysis-diaphysis junction of long bones.

References

1. Hunter AG, Bankier A, Rogers JC, Sillence D, Scott CL Jr. Medical complications of achondroplasia: a multicenter patient review. J Med Genet 1998;35:705–712.
2. Erdincler P, Dashti R, Kaynar MY, Canbaz B, Ciplak N, Kuday C. Hydrocephalus and chronically increased intracranial pressure in achondroplasia. Childs Nerv System 1997;13:345–348.

Chondrosarcoma (See "Tumor of bone or cartilage.")

Chordoma (See "Tumor of bone or cartilage.")

Chorea, Acute

Related Terms: Infectious chorea (poststreptococcal; often part of rheumatic fever); St. Vitus' dance; Sydenham's chorea.

Organs and Tissues	*Procedures*	*Possible or Expected Findings*
Brain and spinal cord	For removal and specimen preparation, see pp. 65 and 67, respectively. Submit sample of cerebral tissue for microbiologic study (p. 102).	Morphologic changes largely unknown. Degenerative processes of basal ganglia.
Other organs	Procedures depend on expected findings or grossly identified abnormalities as listed in right-hand column.	Manifestations of carbon monoxide poisoning;* diphtheria;* hyperthyroidism;* idiopathic hypocalcemia; pertussis;* pregnancy; rheumatic fever;* systemic lupus erythematosus.*

Chorea, Hereditary

Synonyms: Chronic progressive chorea; Huntington's chorea; Huntington's disease.

NOTE: Huntington's disease maps to the short arm of chromosome 4. The gene is widely expressed but of unknown function; it contains a CAG repeat sequence, which is expanded (range, 37 to 86) in patients with Huntington's disease. A sensitive diagnostic test is based on the determination of this CAG sequence, which can be done on fresh-frozen tissue or blood *(1)*. In the absence of genetic confirmation, sampling of organs and tissues cannot be excessive because a complex differential diagnosis must be resolved.

Organs and Tissues	*Procedures*	*Possible or Expected Findings*
Brain and spinal cord	For removal and specimen preparation, see pp. 65 and 67, respectively. Place fresh cerebral tissue in deep freeze for further study.	Mild to severe cerebral atrophy. Atrophy of head of caudate nucleus, putamen, and globus pallidus (due to neuronal loss and gliosis).
Other organs	Samples should include peripheral nerves (p. 79), adrenal glands, skeletal muscle (p. 80), and bone marrow (p. 96). (See also above under "Note").	Respiratory and other intercurrent infections.

Reference

1. Lowe J, Lennox G, Leigh PN. Disorders of movement and system degenerations. In: Greenfield's Neuropathology, vol. 2. Graham BI, Lantos PL, eds. Arnold, London, 1997, pp. 281–366.

Choriomeningitis, Lymphocytic (See "Meningitis.")

Chylothorax

Related Terms: Congenital chylothorax.

Organs and Tissues	*Procedures*	*Possible or Expected Findings*
External examination	Prepare chest roentgenogram. Puncture pleural cavity and submit fluid for microbiologic study (p. 102).	Pleural effusion.*
Chest cavity	Record volume of exudate or transudate and submit sample for determination of fat and cholesterol content. If infection is suspected (extremely rare in true chylothorax), submit sample for microbiologic study.	Chylous pleural effusions have high fat content. Nonchylous milky effusions—for instance, in tuberculosis* and rheumatoid arthritis*—have high cholesterol and low fat content. Tumor of pleura, lung, or chest wall; lymphangiomatosis *(1)*.

Organs and Tissues	Procedures	Possible or Expected Findings
Thoracic duct	For lymphangiography and for dissection of the thoracic duct, see p. 34.	Surgical or other traumatic lesions of thoracic duct. Tumor in posterior mediastinum.
Skeletal system	Prepare skeletal roentgenogram and, if abnormalities are present, sample bone for histologic study.	Massive osteolysis in Gorham's syndrome *(2)*.

References

1. Moerman P, van Geet C, Devlieger H. Lymphangiomatosis of the body wall: a report of two cases associated with chylothorax and fatal outcome. Pediatr Pathol Lab Med 1997;17:617–624.
2. Riantawan P, Tansupasawasdikul S, Subhannachart P. Bilateral chylothorax complicating massive osteolysis (Gorham's syndrome). Thorax 1996;51:1277–1278.

Cirrhosis, Liver

NOTE: All types of cirrhosis are included here (alcoholic, autoimmune, biliary, cryptogenic, pigment [hemochromatosis], cirrhosis with viral hepatitis, and other types).

If the cause or underlying condition is known, see also under the appropriate heading, such as alcoholic liver disease, a_1-antitrypsin deficiency, sclerosing cholangitis, or viral hepatitis. If the patient had undergone liver transplantation, see also under that heading.

Organs and Tissues	Procedures	Possible or Expected Findings
External examination	Record body weight and length, nutritional state, distribution of hair, type of skin pigmentation, appearance of breasts and hands, and abdominal circumference. Prepare sections of skin and breast tissue.	Jaundice; spider nevi; pectoral alopecia and loss or abnormal distribution of pubic hair; gynecomastia; white nail beds; clubbing of fingers. Diffuse or nodular (e.g., cervical) lipomatosis (Madelung collar) in alcoholism. Xanthelasmas and vitiligo in primary biliary cirrhosis. Skin pigmentation of hemochromatosis.* Bruises and hemorrhages.
	Prepare skeletal roentgenograms	Hypertrophic osteoarthropathy* of tibia and fibula; osteomalacia;* osteoporosis.*
Blood	Submit samples for bacterial culture (p. 102) and for biochemical or immunologic study, depending on expected underlying disease (see above under "Note").	Septicemia; hyperbilirubinemia. Viral antigens and/or antibodies.
Abdominal and chest cavity	Record volume and character of ascites. Culture exudate.	Ascites; spontaneous bacterial peritonitis.
	Record volume and character of pleural effusions.	Hydrothorax.
	For lymphangiography, see p. 34. For arteriography and for cholangiography, see p. 56. Record appearance and contents of extrahepatic bile ducts. If liver transplantation had taken place, see also under that heading.	Dilatation of abdominal lymphatics and thoracic duct. Strictures, stones, or tumors in secondary biliary cirrhosis; portal or splenic vein thrombosis; thrombosis of surgical anastomosis. A peritoneovenous shunt may be in place.
	Remove esophagus together with stomach. Clamp midportion of stomach and remove together with esophagus for demonstration of varices (p. 53). Record appearance of varices and preserve specimen, particularly in cases where attempts had been made to sclerose the varices.	Esophageal* or gastric varices, or both, with or without evidence of rupture and hemorrhage. Gastroesophageal mucosal tears in Mallory-Weiss syndrome. (See also below under "Gastrointestinal tract.")
Lungs	Perfuse one lung with formalin (p. 47).	Manifestations of portopulmonary hypertension.
Diaphragm	Record defects and presence of dilated lymphatics.	
Gastrointestinal tract	Record estimated volume of blood in gastrointestinal tract.	Gastrointestinal hemorrhage.* Gastric varices.
	Submit samples of abnormal lesions for histologic study	Peptic ulcers.* Crohn's disease* or chronic ulcerative colitis in primary sclerosing cholangitis.* Portal hypertensive gastropathy.

Organs and Tissues	Procedures	Possible or Expected Findings
Liver and gallbladder	Record size and weight of liver and average size of regenerative nodules of liver. Describe appearance and contents of gallbladder. Prepare frontal or horizontal slices of liver (p. 56). If there is evidence of tumor(s), see under "Tumor of the liver." For macroscopic iron stain, see p. 133.	Cirrhosis. Cholelithiasis.* Hepatocellular carcinoma. Hemosiderosis. An intrahepatic portal-caval shunt may be in place.
	Freeze hepatic tissue for possible biochemical or histochemical study. Request van Gieson's stain, PAS stain with diastase digestion, and Gomori's iron stain (p. 172). If hepatitis B virus infection is suspected, request immunostains for B antigens. For preparation for electron microscopic study, see p. 132.	Hepatitis B or other viral antigens.
Spleen	Record size and weight.	Congestive splenomegaly.
Pancreas	Prepare pancreatogram (p. 57) and dissect pancreatic ducts.	Chronic pancreatitis, particularly with alcoholic cirrhosis.
Urine	Chemical study is feasible.	Urobilinuria; aminoaciduria.
Testes and prostate	Record weights of testes. Submit samples of testes and prostate for histologic study.	Atrophy of testes and prostate.
Brain	For removal and specimen preparation, see p. 65.	Hepatic encephalopathy. Histologic changes, primarily in cerebral cortex, putamen, globus pallidus, and cerebellum.
Eyes	For removal and specimen preparation, see p. 85.	Yellow sclerae. Cataracts in galactosemia.*

Clonorchiasis

Synonyms: *Clonorchis sinensis* infection; Chinese or oriental liver fluke infection; *Opisthorchis sinensis* infection *(1)*.

NOTE: (1) Collect all tissues that appear to be infected. (2) Culture methods are not generally available. However, aerobic and anaerobic cultures may be indicated in patients who die of superimposed sepsis. (3) Request Gram stain (p. 172); parasites can be identified with hematoxylin and eosin stain. (4) No special precautions are indicated. (5) Serologic studies are not available. (6) This is not a reportable disease.

Organs and Tissues	Procedures	Possible or Expected Findings
Blood	Submit sample for anaerobic and aerobic culture (p. 102).	Septicemia.
Stool	Submit sample for study of eggs.	
Liver and extrahepatic biliary system	For postmortem cholangiography, see p. 56. Leave extrahepatic bile ducts and gallbladder attached to liver. Dissect and fix as shown in Chapter 5, Figs. 5-5 and 5-6, pp. 57 and 58. Submit samples of liver, gallbladder, and extrahepatic bile ducts for histologic study. Request Verhoeff–van Gieson stain (p. 173).	Hyperplasia of bile duct epithelium; periductal chronic inflammation; severe portal fibrosis; cirrhosis. Acute or recurrent suppurative cholangitis;* Cholangiocarcinoma.
Abdominal organs	Weigh liver, spleen. Examine veins around esophagus and rectum carefully.	Evidence of portal hypertension.
Pancreas	Submit samples for histologic study. If roentgenographic study is intended, see p. 57.	Acute pancreatitis.* Parasitic invasion of pancreatic duct with fibrosis and dilatation.

Reference

1. Case Records of Massachusetts. General Hospital. Clonorchis sinensis [Opisthorchis sinensis] infection of biliary tract. N Engl J Med 1990;323: 467–475.

Coagulation (See "Coagulation, disseminated intravascular," "Disease, Christmas," "Disease, von Willebrand's," "Hemophilia," and "Purpura,...")

Coagulation, Disseminated Intravascular

Synonyms and Related Terms: Consumption coagulopathy; hypofibrinogenemia; intravascular coagulation and fibrinolysis syndrome (ICF).

NOTE: Disseminated intravascular coagulation (DIC) often is a complication of obstetrical mishaps such as abruptio placentae or amniotic fluid embolism,* or it complicates malignancies (such as adenocarcinomas or leukemia*) or bacterial, viral, and other infections. Other conditions such as aortic aneurysm* or hemolytic uremic syndrome* are known causes also. If the nature of the underlying disease is known, follow the procedures under the appropriate heading also.

Organs and Tissues	*Procedures*	*Possible or Expected Findings*
External examination and skin	Prepare sections of skin of grossly involved and of uninvolved areas.	Petechiae, purpura, hemorrhagic bullae, gangrene, and other skin lesions.
Heart		Nonbacterial thrombotic endocarditis.*
Large blood vessels		Thromboses, predominantly around indwelling catheters.
Other organs	Submit tissue samples from grossly involved and uninvolved areas. Organs involved include brain, heart, kidneys, lungs, adrenal glands, spleen, gastrointestinal tract, pancreas, and liver, approximately in this order. Skin, testes, and choroid plexus also are frequently involved.	Fibrin or hyaline thrombi in capillaries, venules, or arterioles, and occasionally in larger vessels. Hemorrhages and ischemic infarcts may occur.
	Special stains such as phosphotungstic acid hematoxylin (p. 173) are not particularly helpful. Postmortem determination of fibrin split products is not helpful either.	For common underlying diseases or conditions, see above under "Note."

Coarctation, Aortic

Related Term: Aortic isthmus stenosis.

Possible Associated Conditions: Anomalous origin of right subclavian artery; atresia or stenosis of left subclavian artery; biscuspid aortic valve;* congenital mitral stenosis;* double aortic arch with stenosis of the right arch and coarctation of the left; stenosis of right subclavian artery; Turner's syndrome;* ventricular septal defect;* Shone's syndrome.

Organs and Tissues	*Procedures*	*Possible or Expected Findings*
External examination	Prepare chest roentgenogram.	Pressure atrophy of ribs with enlargement of costal grooves or focal erosions at inferior and ventral aspects of main body of ribs (rib notching).
Blood	Submit sample for microbiologic study (p. 102).	Septicemia associated with endocarditis* or endarteritis (see below).
Heart	If endocarditis is suspected, follow procedures described on p. 103. For general dissection techniques, see p. 33.	Infective endocarditis* (of bicuspid aortic valve); endocardial fibroelastosis. For associated malformations, see above under "Possible Associated Conditions."
	For coronary angiography, see p. 118.	Premature coronary atherosclerosis.
Aorta and adjacent arteries	Record size and location of coarctation (relation to ductal artery and great vessels).	Preductal coarctation (isthmus stenosis) is often classified as "infantile type of coarctation." "Adult type" is at insertion of duct or distal to it. Rarely, coarctation occurs proximal to left subclavian artery, in lower thoracic aorta, or at multiple sites.
	If bacterial aortitis is suspected, obtain sample for microbiologic study through sterilized window in wall of aorta.	Bacterial aortitis. For ductal artery, see below.
	For arteriography, clamp proximal and distal thoracic aorta before injecting contrast medium.	Dilatation of subclavian, internal mammary, intercostal, scapular, and anterior spinal arteries. Among the intercostal arteries, the fourth through seventh pairs are predominantly affected.

Organs and Tissues	Procedures	Possible or Expected Findings
Aorta and adjacent arteries *(continued)*	Record width of left subclavian artery and compare with contralateral vessel; record width of aorta and of vessels proximal and distal to coarctation. Verhoeff–van Gieson stain (p. 173).	Subclavian artery is considerably dilated if proximal to coarctation. Other complications include poststenotic dilatation of aorta, mycotic or noninfectious saccular aneurysm distal to coarctation (with or without rupture), and dissecting hematoma of aorta* (with or without rupture).
Ductal artery	Probe duct and record width of lumen.	Ductal artery may be patent or closed.
Abdominal arteries		Dilatation of epigastric and lumbar arteries. Rarely, coarctation of abdominal aorta.
	After surgical correction of coarctation, search for infarcts and sample arteries for histologic study.	Abdominal hypertensive arteritis and visceral infarctions after correction of coarctation.
Other organs		Manifestation of congestive heart failure.*
Brain	For removal and specimen preparation, see p. 65. For cerebral arteriography, see p. 80.	Rupture of aneurysm, circle of Willis.

Cocaine (See "Dependence, cocaine.")

Coccidioidomycosis

Synonyms and Related Terms: *Coccidioides immitis* infection; San Joaquin fever; valley fever.

NOTE: (1) Collect all tissues that appear to be infected. (2) Request fungal cultures. (3) Request Grocott methenamine silver stain (p. 172). (4) Special **precautions** are indicated (p. 146). (5) Serologic studies are available from many reference and state health department laboratories (p. 135). (6) This is a **reportable** disease in some states.

Organs and Tissues	Procedures	Possible or Expected Findings
External examination and skin	Prepare chest roentgenogram.	Pulmonary infiltrates; pulmonary cavitations; hilar lymphadenopathy.
	Prepare histologic sections of skin lesions. For a special stain, see above under "Note."	Erythema nodosum or multiforme,* various types of skin rashes; skin ulcers.
Blood	Submit sample for serologic study.	
Lungs	Prior to sectioning lungs, culture for fungi and bacteria any areas of consolidation (p. 103). Prepare smears from fresh, grossly infected pulmonary tissue. For special stain, see above under "Note."	Chronic pulmonary cavitation; pulmonary fibrosis.
	Perfuse one lung with formalin (p. 47). Submit samples of hilar lymph nodes for histologic study.	Bronchiectasis.*
Other organs	Submit samples of material for culture and histologic study wherever extrapulmonary lesions are suspected.	Lymphogenous and hematogenous dissemination to almost all organs may occur, causing abscesses and sinuses of skin, subcutaneous tissue, bones, and joints.
	If involvement of central nervous system is suspected, submit sample of cerebrospinal fluid for culture and serologic study (p. 104).	Meningitis* and encephalitis.*

Codeine (See "Dependence, drug[s], all types or type unspecified.")

Cold (See "Exposure, cold.")

Colitis, All Types or Type Unspecified (See "Enterocolitis, Other Types or Type Undetermined.")

Colitis, Chronic Ulcerative (See "Disease, inflammatory bowel.")

Colitis, Collagenous

Related Terms: Lymphocytic colitis; microscopic colitis.

NOTE: This is a cause of diarrhea. The colon is grossly normal but microscopically, increased lymphocytes in the lamina propria and a subepithelial band of collagen is found. If only the lymphocytic infiltrate is found, the term "lymphocytic colitis" or "microscopic colitis" should be applied. A trichrome stain should be ordered in all instances, because the collagen band may be difficult to see without the special stain.

Coma, Hepatic

NOTE: See under name of suspected underlying hepatic disease, such as "Cirrhosis, liver" or "Hepatitis, viral."

Complex, Eisenmenger's (See "Defect, ventricular septal.")

Complex, Taussig-Bing (See "Ventricle, double outlet, right.")

Craniopharyngioma (See "Tumor of the pituitary gland.")

Cretinism (See "Hypothyroidism.")

Crisis, Sickle Cell (See "Disease, sickle cell.")

Croup (See "Laryngitis.")

Cryptococcosis

Synonyms: European Blastomycosis; torulosis.

NOTE: Cryptococcosis may follow or complicate AIDS *(1)* and other immunodeficient states, bronchiectasis,* bronchitis,* diabetes mellitus,* leukemia,* lymphoma,* sarcoidosis,* and tuberculosis.* (1) Collect all tissues that appear to be infected. (2) Request fungal cultures. (3) Request Grocott's methenamine silver, periodic acid Schiff, and mucicarmine stains (p. 172). (4) No special precautions are indicated. (5) Serologic studies are available from many reference laboratories and from state health department laboratories (p. 135). (6) This is not a reportable disease.

Organs and Tissues	*Procedures*	*Possible or Expected Findings*
Cerebrospinal fluid	Submit sample for fungal culture (p. 104). Use India ink or a nigrosin preparation for direct examination.	
Brain and spinal cord	For removal and specimen preparation, see pp. 65 and 67, respectively. Submit material for Gram stain and fungal culture. For special stains, see above under "Note."	Meningitis;* meningoencephalitis; hydrocephalus;* cysts in cortical gray matter and basal ganglia. Note that inflammation may be minimal.
Eyes	For removal and specimen preparation, see p. 85.	Endophthalmitis; optic neuritis.
Other organs	See above under "Note." Procedures depend on expected findings or grossly identified abnormalities as listed in right-hand column.	Infiltrates and abscesses in skin, endocardium, pericardium, liver, kidneys, adrenal glands, prostate, bones, and joints. Other infections may coexist *(2)*. Hypereosinophilia may be noted *(3)*.

References

1. Kanjanavirojkul N, Sripa C, Puapairoj A. Cytologic diagnosis of Cryptococcus neoformans in HIV-positive patients. Acta Cytol 1997;41: 493–496.
2. Benard G, Gryschek RC, Duarte AJ, Shikanai-Yasuda MA. Cryptococcosis as an opportunistic infection in immunodeficiency secondary to paracoccidioidomycosis. Mycopathologia 1996;133:65–69.
3. Marwaha RK, Trehan A, Jayashree K, Vasishta RK. Hypereosinophilia in disseminated cryptococcal disease. Pediatr Inf Dis J 1995;14: 1102–1103.

Cryptosporidiosis

Synonym: *Cryptosporidium parvum* infection.

Possible Associated Conditions: AIDS *(1)* and other immunodeficient states.

NOTE: (1) Collect feces, intestinal wall tissue, bile ducts, and pancreas. (2) Cultures are not available. (3) Request Kinyoun stain (p. 172). (4) No special precautions are indicated. (5) Serologic studies are unreliable. (6) This is not a reportable disease.

Organs and Tissues	*Procedures*	*Possible or Expected Findings*
External examination	Record body weight and length and extent of rigor.	Evidence of dehydration following chronic diarrhea in immunosuppressed hosts.
Vitreous	Submit sample for sodium, chloride, and urea nitrogen determination (pp. 85 and 115).	Dehydration.* (See p. 247).
Lungs	Perfuse one lung with formalin (p. 47) and submit samples of bronchi and lung for histologic study.	Bronchopulmonary cryptosporidiosis in HIV *(2)*.

Organs and Tissues	Procedures	Possible or Expected Findings
Intestinal tract	Record volume and appearance of intestinal contents. Submit samples of feces prepared with saline or iodine solution. Submit samples for determination of sodium, potassium, and chloride content.	Cryptosporidiosis may complicate inflammatory bowel disease *(3)*.*
	Submit samples of small bowel for histologic and electron microscopic study.	Parasites attached to mucosa.
Bile ducts, gallbladder, and pancreas	For cholangiography, see p. 56.	Changes resembling sclerosing cholangitis in patients with AIDS or other immunodeficiency states complicated by cryptosporidiosis *(4)*.
	Submit samples for histologic study and electron microscopic study.	*Cryptosporidium parvum* may be found on mucosal surfaces.

References

1. Ramratnam B, Flanigan TP. Cryptosporidiosis in persons with HIV infection. Postgrad Med J 1997;73:713–716.
2. Poirot JL, Deluol AM, Antoine M, Heyer F, Cadranel J, Meynard JL, et al. Broncho-pulmonary cryptosporidiosis in four HIV-infected patients. J Eukaryotic Microbiol 1996;43:78S–78S.
3. Manthey MW, Ross AB, Soergel KH. Cryptosporidiosis and inflammatory bowel disease. Dig Dis Sci 1997;42:1580–1586.
4. Davis JJ, Heyman MB, Ferrell L, Kerner J, Kerlan R Jr, Thaler MM. Sclerosing cholangitis associated with chronic cryptosporidiosis in a child with a congenital immunodeficiency disorder. Am J Gastroenterol 1987;82:1196–1202.

Cyanide (See "Poisoning, cyanide.")

Cyst(s), Choledochal

Synonyms and Related Terms: Choledochocyst; congenital cystic dilatation of the common bile duct; idiopathic dilatation of the common bile duct.

Possible Associated Conditions: Biliary atresia;* Caroli's disease;* congenital hepatic fibrosis.*

Organs and Tissues	Procedures	Possible or Expected Findings
External examination and skin	Prepare sections of skin lesions.	Jaundice; xanthomas.
Abdominal cavity	Submit peritoneal exudate for culture.	Bile peritonitis.
Gallbladder and extrahepatic bile ducts	Follow procedures described under "Cholecystitis." Record size and location of cyst(s) and relationship to surrounding organs, particularly to the portal vein. Puncture cyst(s) and submit contents for aerobic and anaerobic bacterial cultures. Dissect and photograph *in situ*.	Cyst may displace stomach, duodenum, and colon. Portal vein may be compressed, which may cause portal hypertension.* Cyst may perforate or contain stones or a carcinoma. Congenital anomalies such as double gallbladder, double common bile ducts, absence of gallbladder, biliary atresia, or annular pancreas may co-exist.
Liver	Record size and weight. Submit samples for histologic study.	Abscesses. Fibropolycystic disease of the liver.* See also above under "Possible Associated Conditions."

Reference

1. Crittenden SI, McKinley MJ. Choledochal cyst—clinical features and classification. Am J Gastroenterol 1985;80:643–647.

Cyst(s), Liver (See "Disease, fibropolycystic, of the liver and biliary tract.")

Cyst(s), Pulmonary

Related Terms: Congenital cystic adenomatoid malformation; congenital pulmonary lymphangiectasis; intralobular bronchopulmonary sequestration.

Possible Associated Conditions: Polycystic kidney disease;* renal cysts* or cysts of other organs.

Organs and Tissues	*Procedures*	*Possible or Expected Findings*
External examination	Prepare chest roentgenogram.	Cyst(s) with air, fluid, or both.
Chest organs	Search—*in situ* or after en bloc removal of chest organs—for anomalous arterial supply from aorta. Prepare pulmonary (see below) and thoracic aortic arteriograms. If infection of cyst is suspected, submit cyst contents or portions of the lung for bacterial culture (p. 103). For bronchial and pulmonary arteriography, see p. 50. Perfuse lung with formalin (p. 47).	Congenital cysts in lower lobes may have anomalous arterial supply ("intralobular bronchopulmonary sequestration"). Perifocal bronchopneumonia; hemorrhage. Cysts may represent lymphangiectasias (see above under "Related Terms").
Other organs		In rare instances, cysts may co-exist in other organs, e.g. the kidneys.

Cyst(s), Renal

Related Terms: Acquired cystic renal disease; autosomal dominant (adult) polycystic renal disease *(1)*; autosomal recessive (infantile and childhood form) polycystic renal disease *(1)*; cystic renal lymphangiectasis; familial juvenile nephronophthisis; glomerulocystic disease; medullary cystic disease; multicystic dysplasia.

NOTE: Bilateral cystic disease of the kidneys may be acquired after long-term hemodialysis.

Possible Associated Conditions: Alagille's syndrome; Caroli's disease;* cerebral artery aneurysm* (with adult polycystic disease) *(2)*; congenital hepatic fibrosis;* congenital pyloric stenosis; cysts of liver, pancreas, spleen, lungs,* and testes; Ehlers-Danlos syndrome;* hemihypertrophy.

Organs and Tissues	*Procedures*	*Possible or Expected Findings*
Kidneys	For renal arteriography, venography, or urography, see p. 59. If infection of cysts is suspected, submit cyst contents or portions of the kidney for bacteriologic study (p. 102). For demonstration of cysts by injection of plastics, see p. 139. Formalin-gelatin mixtures are usually preferred.	Infection or calcification of cysts; pyelonephritis;* perinephric abscess. Obstructive uropathy;* nephrolithiasis;* carcinoma *(3)* (see "Tumor of the kidneys"); hemorrhages, and related complications *(4)*.
Liver	Prepare photographs and sample for histologic study.	In recessive polycystic renal disease, diffuse biliary dysgenesis may be present but the bile ducts are normal in dominant cases.
Other organs	See above under "Possible Associated Conditions." Other procedures depend on expected findings or grossly identified abnormalities as listed in right-hand column.	See above under "Possible Associated Conditions." Manifestations of portal or systemic hypertension* and kidney failure;* polycythemia.*

References

1. Rapola J, Kaariainen H. Polycystic kidney disease. Morphological diagnosis of recessive and dominant polycystic kidney disease in infancy and childhood. APMIS 1988;96:68–76.
2. Chapman AB, Rubinstein D, Hughes R, Stears JC, Earnest MP, Johnson AM, et al. Intracranial aneurysm in autosomal dominant polycystic kidney disease. N Engl J Med 1992;327:916–920.
3. Banyai-Falger S, Susani M, Maier U. Renal cell carcinoma in acquired renal cystic disease 3 years after successful kidney transplantation. Two case reports and review of the literature. Eur Urol 1995;28:77–80.
4. Wilson PD, Falkenstein D. The pathology of human renal cystic disease. Curr Topics Pathol 1995;88:1–50.

Cystinosis

Synonyms and Related Terms: Cystine storage disease; de Toni-Debré-Fanconi syndrome;* infantile Fanconi syndrome.

Organs and Tissues	*Procedures*	*Possible or Expected Findings*
External examination	Record body weight and length.	Growth retardation.
Kidneys	Freeze tissue samples or fix them in absolute alcohol or Carnoy's fixative (p. 130) for preservation of cystine crystals. See also under "Glomerulonephritis." For preparation for electron microscopy, see p. 132. (See also under "Other organs.)	Cystine crystals in tubular epithelial cells *(1)* and foam cells in the interstitium. "Swan's neck" deformity of nephrons (not specific). Atrophy with interstitial scarring and tubular degeneration.

Organs and Tissues	Procedures	Possible or Expected Findings
Urine	Submit sample for chemical analysis.	Glycosuria; generalized aminoaciduria.
Other organs	Submit samples of lymph nodes for histologic study (see above under "Kidneys"). For removal and specimen preparation of eyes, see p. 85. Excellent views of crystals can be provided in scanning electron microscopic preparations.	Cystine crystals occur throughout the reticuloendothelial system and in many other tissues, such as liver *(2)* or corneae and conjunctivae. Diagnostic doubly refractive brick- or needle-shaped cystine crystals in frozen sections or in smears from spleen, liver, lymph nodes, and bone marrow.
Bone and bone marrow	For removal, prosthetic repair, and specimen preparation of bones, see p. 95.	Cystine crystals in bone marrow.
	For preparation of sections and smears of bone marrow, see p. 96. See also above under "Kidneys."	Hypophosphatemic rickets.

References

1. Thoene JG. Cystinosis. J Inherited Metabolic Dis 1995;18(4):380–386.
2. Klenn PJ, Rubin R. Hepatic fibrosis associated with hereditary cystinosis: a novel form of noncirrhotic portal hypertension. Modern Pathol 1994; 7:879–882.

Cytomegalovirus (See "Infection, cytomegalovirus.")

D

Damage, Diffuse Alveolar (See "Syndrome, Adult Respiratory Distress [ARDS].")

Death, Abortion-Associated

Related Terms: Criminal abortion; stillbirth.*

NOTE: Anesthesia-associated death* must be considered in some of these cases. If criminal abortion is suspected, notify coroner or medical examiner.

Organs and Tissues	*Procedures*	*Possible or Expected Findings*
External examination and breasts	Prepare roentgenograms of chest and abdomen. Describe appearance of breasts and sample glandular tissue for histologic study.	Pulmonary air embolism.* Pregnancy changes.
	Record appearance of external genitalia.	Instrument marks on vulva.
Peritoneal cavity	Submit exudate for bacteriologic study (p. 102).	Peritonitis.*
Blood vessels and heart	Inspect and puncture right atrium and right ventricle of heart under water, also retroperitoneal and pelvic veins.	Pulmonary air embolism.* Abdominal and pelvic veins may also contain air.
Blood	Submit for bacteriologic (p. 102) and toxicologic study (p. 16).	Septicemia. Absorption of intrauterine corrosives or other chemicals.
Lungs	Submit portion for bacteriologic study (p. 103). Prepare sample for electron microscopy (p. 132).	Abscesses; bacterial pneumonia. Thromboembolism; embolism of soap and other chemicals.
Pelvic organs	If there are vascular lacerations, identify vessel. Submit samples of placenta and fetal parts for histologic study. Submit liquid intrauterine contents for toxicologic study. Sample ovaries for histologic study.	Lacerated blood vessels; pelvic hemorrhages. Instrument marks; foreign bodies;* perforation(s). Placenta, fetus, and fetal parts. Soap or other toxic foreign intrauterine materials. Corpus luteum of pregnancy.
Fetus	Determine weight and length, and estimate age (pp. 557 and 560).	Malformations. See also under "Stillbirth."

Death, Anaphylactic

Synonym: Generalized anaphylaxis.

NOTE: Autopsy should be done as soon as possible after death. Neck organs should be removed before embalming. If death is believed to be caused by drug anaphylaxis, inquire about type of drug(s), drug dose, and route of administration (intravenous, intramuscular, and oral or other). This will determine proper sampling procedures—for instance, after penicillin anaphylaxis. Allergy to bee stings, wasp stings, fire ants, and certain plants may also be responsible for anaphylaxis. However, envenomation also can be fatal in the absence of anaphylaxis.

Organs and Tissues	*Procedures*	*Possible or Expected Findings*
External examination	Search for injection sites or sting marks. If such lesions are present, photograph and excise with 5-cm margin.	Foam in front of mouth and nostrils. Swelling of involved tissue.
	Freeze excised tissue at –70°C for possible analysis. Prepare chest roentgenogram.	Antigen-antibody reaction in involved tissues.

From: *Handbook of Autopsy Practice,* 3rd Ed. Edited by: J. Ludwig © Humana Press Inc., Totowa, NJ

Organs and Tissues	*Procedures*	*Possible or Expected Findings*
Blood	Submit sample for immunologic study and study of drug levels. For serum IgE testing (Mayo Medical Laboratories), sample must be kept refrigerated (frozen or refrigerated coolant).	Antibodies against suspected antigen.
Neck organs	Remove as soon as possible after death. Photograph rima of glottis from above, together with epiglottis. For histologic study, fix larynx and epiglottis in Zenker's (p. 131) or Bouin's (p. 129) solution.	Laryngeal edema may recede soon after death.
Tracheobronchial tree and lungs	Record character of contents of tracheobronchial tree. Photograph lungs and record weights. In order to avoid artificial distention, do not perfuse with fixative. For proper fixation, see above under "Neck organs." Request Giemsa stain (p. 172).	Foamy edema in trachea and bronchi; diffuse or focal pulmonary distention ("acute emphysema") alternating with collapse; pulmonary edema and congestion; accumulation of eosinophilic leukocytes.
Spleen		Eosinophilic leukocytes in red pulp.

Death, Anesthesia-Associated

NOTE: There are many possible causes of anesthesia-associated death that are not drug-related, such as acute airway obstruction* by external compression, aspiration, tumor, or an inflammatory process. Some of the complications are characteristically linked to a specific phase of the anesthesia, and many cannot be proved morphologically.

The most important step in these autopsies is to obtain the anesthesia-associated records and to secure the consulting services of an independent anesthesiologist. When information is gathered about drugs and chemical agents that had been administered or to which the victim may have had access, pathologists must keep in mind that some nonmedical chemicals and many drugs are known to affect anesthesia. Drugs and their metabolic products, additives, stabilizers, impurities, and deterioration products may be present and can be identified in portmortem tissues. Therefore, all appropriate body fluids, particularly bile, and organs (see p. 16) should be submitted for toxicologic examination. If the anesthetic agent had been injected into or near the spinal canal, spinal fluid should be withdrawn from above the injected site, preferably from the suboccipital cisterna; 250 mg of sodium fluoride should be added per 30 mL of fluid. If the anesthetic agent was injected locally, tissue should be excised around needle puncture marks, at a radius of 2–4 cm. Serial postmortem analysis of specimens may permit extrapolation to tissue concentration at the time of death. The time interval between drug administration and death sometimes can be calculated from the distribution and ratio of administered drugs and their metabolic products. For a review of anesthetic death investigation, see ref. *(1)*.

Halothane anesthesia and some other anesthetic agents may cause fulminant hepatitis and hepatic failure. The autopsy procedures suggested under "Hepatitis, viral" should be followed.

Reference

1. Ward RJ, Reay DT. Anesthetic death investigation. Legal Med 1989; 39-58.

Death, Bolus (See "Obstruction, acute airway.")

Death, Crib (See "Death, sudden unexpected, of infant.")

Death due to Child Abuse or Neglect (See "Infanticide.")

Death, Intrauterine (See "Stillbirth.")

Death, Postoperative

NOTE: For special autopsy procedures, see p. 4. In some instances, procedures described under "Death, anesthesia-associated" may be indicated. For a thorough review of investigational procedures and autopsy techniques in operating-room-associated deaths, see ref. *(1)*. In patients who developed a cerebral infarct after open heart surgery, arterial air embolism should be considered as a possible cause. The diagnosis often must be based on excluding other causes because the air has been absorbed prior to death. If a patient bled to death despite attempted repair, e.g., of hepatic lacerations, hospital records may not suffice to reach competent opinions but personal accounts from the surgeon and anesthesiologist may be needed.

Reference

1. Start RD, Cross SS. Pathological investigations of deaths following surgery, anaesthesia and medical procedures. J Clin Pathol 1999;52: 640–652.

Death, Restaurant (See "Obstruction, acute airway.")

Death, Sniffing and Spray

Related Terms: Glue sniffing; sudden sniffing death syndrome.

NOTE: No anatomic abnormalities will be noted at autopsy. Sudden death may occur after cardiac dysrhythmia or respiratory arrest.

Organs and Tissues	Procedures	Possible or Expected Findings
Lungs	If poison had been inhaled at the time when death occurred, tie main bronchi. Submit lungs in glass container for gas analysis.	Trichloroethane, fluorinated refrigerants, and other volatile hydrocarbons are most often involved in the "sudden sniffing death syndrome."
	Submit samples of small bronchi for histologic study.	Spray death may occur in asthma sufferers using pressurized aerosol bronchodilators. Freons and related propellants may also be responsible for sudden death.
Brain	For removal and specimen preparation, see p. 65. Submit samples of fresh or frozen brain for toxicologic study.	Toxic components of glue—such as toluene—accumulate in the brain of glue sniffers. Also present in various glues are acetone, aliphatic acetates, cyclohexane, hexane, isopropanol, methylethyl ketone, and methylisobutyl ketone.
Other organs	Submit samples in glass containers (not plastic) for toxicologic study.	Aerosols may occlude the airway by freezing the larynx. Carbon tetrachloride sniffing may cause hepatorenal syndrome (see also under "Poisoning, carbon tetrachloride").

Death, Sudden Unexpected, of Adult

NOTE: Medicolegal autopsies are usually indicated, and appropriate procedures should be followed (p. 8). If anaphylactic death is suspected, see also under that heading. A history of recent drinking (e.g., among college students) or of chronic alcoholism may be an important clue. The list of "Possible or Expected Findings" below is not complete. For general toxicologic sampling, see p. 16.

Organs and Tissues	Procedures	Possible or Expected Findings
Abdomen	Submit sample of blood or exudate.	Hemoperitoneum; peritonitis.*
Chest cavity	Record volume and character of contents of pleural and pericardial cavities.	Hemothorax may occur—for instance, after rupture of aortic aneurysm. Hemopericardium usually occurs after rupture of myocardial infarction or of aortic dissection.*
Blood	Submit samples for microbiologic (p. 102) and toxicologic (p. 16) study.	Meningococcal disease* or streptococcal septicemia may cause sudden death.
Heart	Submit samples of myocardium (p. 30) with the conduction system (p. 26) for histologic study. For coronary arteriography, see p. 118.	Coronary atherosclerosis, thrombosis, or arteritis; myocardial infarction, with or without perforation; myocarditis;* valvular heart disease, such as aortic stenosis or ballooning posterior leaflet syndrome.* Anatomic conduction system defects may indicate presence of arrhythmia (p. 34).
Lungs	Dissect all pulmonary arteries (p. 45). Submit samples for histologic study.	Pulmonary thromboembolism; tumor embolism. Pulmonary intravascular (arterial and arteriolar) platelet aggregates may be cause of sudden death.
Aorta	Procedures depend on grossly identified abnormalities as listed in right-hand column.	Ruptured aneurysm;* aortic dissection.*
Pancreas		Islet cell tumor.
Adrenal glands	Photograph adrenals if hemorrhages are noted.	Hemorrhage may indicate presence of meningococcal disease.*
Neck organs	Remove carefully to avoid dislodging food or other objects from larynx.	Occlusion of larynx by bolus (see "Obstruction, acute airway"). Laryngeal edema may be cause of anaphylactic death.*

Organs and Tissues	*Procedures*	*Possible or Expected Findings*
Brain and spinal cord	For removal and specimen preparation, see pp. 65 and 67, respectively. For cerebral arteriography, see p. 80.	Intracranial hemorrhage after trauma or rupture of aneurysm or—occasionally—with no apparent reason. Changes suggestive of epilepsy* may be present.
Vitreous	Submit samples for possible chemical and toxicologic study (pp. 85 and 113).	Increased glucose concentrations may indicate the presence of hyperglycemia in undetected diabetes mellitus.*

Death, Sudden Unexpected, of Infant

Synonyms and Related Terms: Sudden infant death syndrome; SIDS; cot death; crib death.

NOTE: The autopsy alone does not suffice as an adequate investigation of sudden death of an infant. A thorough medical history, as well as complete information regarding the scene and circumstances of death must also be conducted. It should be recorded whether the infant was found in a prone position. Photographs of the scene should be taken. The environmental and the infant's body temperature should be recorded as close to the time of death as possible. Cases of infanticide have been disguised as SIDS; a high level of suspicion should be maintained, particularly if more than one SIDS case reportedly occurred in the same family. Thus, while some of the "Possible or Expected Findings" in the table refer to typical cases of SIDS *(1)*, other refer to possible infanticide *(2)*.

Organs and Tissues	*Procedures*	*Possible or Expected Findings*
External examination	Record weight of infant; measure crown-rump and crown-heel length and head, chest and abdominal circumference. For expected values, see p. 554. Test skin turgor and look for "sunken eyes" (signs of deydration). Prepare skeletal roentgenograms.	Growth retardation. Signs of dehydration. Crusts or frothy fluid around nose and mouth. Emaciation indicates organic disease or neglect. Bruises or burns indicative of child abuse. Jaundice; edema. Old or recent fractures due to child abuse.
Eyes	Ophthalmic examination.	Retinal hemorrhages indicative of "shaken baby syndrome." Conjunctival petechiae may be a sign of strangulation *(2)*.
Cerebrospinal fluid	If there is clinical or pathologic evidence of infection, submit sample for bacterial and viral cultures (p. 104). Prepare smear.	
Vitreous	Submit sample for possible electrolyte studies and urea nitrogen and glucose determination (pp. 85 and 113). In suspected child abuse, photograph fundus (see p. 85) before considering an aspiration.	Increased glucose concentrations may indicate undiagnosed diabetes mellitus.* Manifestations of dehydration.*
Chest cavity		Petechial serosal hemorrhages.
Thymus	Record weight and submit samples for histologic study.	Accelerated involution indicates stress and/or disease, of prolonged duration. Thymic petechiae.
Blood	Submit for culture (p. 102). Submit blood drops dried on filter paper for tests for inborn errors of metabolism. Refrigerate blood samples for toxicologic study (p. 16).	In SIDS, blood in heart chambers tends to remain fluid.
Heart and great vessels; ductus arteriosus	Check venous return and origin and course of coronary arteries and great vessels. Submit samples for histologic study (p. 30).	In rare instances, congenital heart disease, myocarditis, coronary artery aneurysm, or coronary artery arising from the pulmonary artery may explain the sudden death.
Lungs	Record weights; culture and Gram-stain areas of consolidation. Submit samples for histologic study.	Congestion; hemorrhage; edema; pleural petechiae; atelectasis. Acute pulmonary emphysema may indicate strangulation *(2)*.

Organs and Tissues	Procedures	Possible or Expected Findings
Neck organs and trachea	Photograph and culture sites of infection. Samples submitted for histologic study should include trachea, larynx, epiglottis, pharyngeal wall, tonsils, submaxillary glands, parathyroid glands, and cervical lymph nodes.	Laryngitis;* tracheitis. Epiglottitis. Infection affecting other neck organs and tissues.
	Dissect, weigh, and section carotid bodies.	Hypoplasia of carotid bodies (few are hyperplastic).
Stomach	Record character and amount of contents.	This may be pertinent to allegations of starvation.
Intestinal tract	Record appearance of serosal surface (exudate? discoloration?). Assess attachment of the mesenteric root, which normally runs obliquely from the left upper quadrant (ligament of Treitz) to the right lower quadrant near the inferior pole of the right kidney.	Contusions; malrotation; volvulus; infarction.
Pancreas	Submit samples for histologic study.	Degeneration of islets may indicate presence of undetected diabetes mellitus.*
Urine	Obtain two samples; one saved in preservative and the other frozen or refrigerated for toxicologic assays (p. 16).	Drug intoxication, increased organic acids with medium chain acyl-coenzyme A dehyrogenase deficiency *(3)*.
Other organs	Submit portions of spleen, for culture as a double check for the blood culture. Carefully examine, weigh, and submit samples of organs, including endocrine organs, for histologic study.	Extramedullary hematopoiesis in the liver. Congenital adrenal hypoplasia.
Brain and spinal cord	For removal and specimen preparation, see pp. 66 and 70, respectively. Submit portion of brain for microbiologic study if indicated by clinical history or pathologic findings.	Head trauma in abused child. Birth injuries; encephalitis. Astroglial proliferations in brain stem. Retarded myelination of brain stem.
Middle ears	Open middle ears and mastoid cells (pp. 71–73). Submit exudate for microbiologic study. Prepare Gram-stained smears of exudate and histologic sections of middle ears.	Otitis media.*
Bones and bone marrow	Submit samples from costochondral junctions. For removal and specimen preparation of bone, see p. 95. For preparation of sections and smears of bone marrow, see p. 96.	Bone changes of vitamin D deficiency* (rickets). Normoblastic hyperplasia of bone marrow. Retardation of the rate of enchondral ossification such that hematopoiesis abuts the transition zone.

References

1. Valdez-Dapena M, McFeeley PA, Hoffman HJ, et al., eds. Histopathology Atlas for the Sudden Infant Death Syndrome. Armed Forces Institute of Pathology Washington, DC, 1993. (Order from American Registry of Pathology Sales Office, AFIP, Room 1077, Washington, DC 20,306–26,000.)
2. Becroft DM, Lockett BK. Intra-alveolar pulmonary siderophages in sudden infant death: a marker for previous imposed suffocation. Pathology 1997;29:60–63.
3. Betz P, Hausmann R, Eisenmenger W. A contribution to a possible differentiation between SIDS and asphyxiation. For Sci Intl 1998;91: 147–152.

Decompression (See "Sickness, decompression.")

Defect, Aortopulmonary Septal

Synonyms: Aortopulmony window; aorticopulmonary window or septal defect.

NOTE: The basic anomaly is a defect between ascending aorta and main pulmonary artery. For general dissection techniques, see p. 33.

Possible Associated Conditions: Atrial septal defect;* bicuspid aortic valve;* coarctation,* hypoplasia, or interruption (type A) of aortic arch; coronary artery from main pulmonary artery; right atrial arch; patent ductal artery;* right pulmonary artery from ascending aorta; subaortic stenosis;* tetralogy of Fallot;* ventricular septal defect.* (In approx 50% of the cases, one or more of these associated conditions are found.)

Defect, Atrial Septal

NOTE: The basic anomaly is a defect of the atrial septum, usually at the oval fossa (in 85%). Possible complications in unoperated cases include atrial arrhythmias, congestive heart failure; paradoxic embolism; plexogenic pulmonary hypertension (<10%), and pulmonary artery aneurysm. Possible surgical interventions include surgical and transcatheter closure of defect. For general dissection techniques, see p. 33.

Possible Associated Conditions: *With secundum type:* Often isolated; may occur with conotruncal anomalies, patent ductal artery,* valvular atresia,* and ventricular septal defect.* *With primum type:* Cleft in anterior mitral leaflet. *With sinus venosus type*: Anomalous connection of right pulmonary veins. *With coronary sinus type* (unroofed coronary sinus): Left atrial connection of a persistent left superior vena cava. *With absent atrial septum or multiple large defects* (common atrium): Complete atrioventricular defect;* asplenia syndrome.*

Defect, Complete Atrioventricular Septal

Synonyms and Related Terms: Complete atrioventricular canal; complete AV canal; endocardial cushion defect.

NOTE: The basic anomaly is a large combined atrioventricular septal defect and a common atrioventricular valve, with displacement of the atrioventricular conduction tissues. For possible surgical interventions, see complete repair, "mitral" valve replacement in Chapter 3 Appendix 3-4, p. 41. For general dissection techniques, see p. 33.

Possible Associated Conditions: Aortic coarctation; (35%); asplenia or polysplenia syndrome;* atrial septal defect;* common atrium; discrete subaortic stenosis;* double outlet right ventricle;* Down's syndrome;* patent ductal artery;* persistent left superior vena cava; pulmonary stenosis;* tetralogy of Fallot.*

Defect, Partial Atrioventricular Septal

Synonyms and Related Terms: Endocardial cushion defect; primum atrial septal defect with cleft mitral valve.

NOTE: The basic anomaly is a primum atrial septal defect and a cleft in the anterior mitral leaflet. Possible surgical interventions consist of surgical repair of both malformations. For general dissection techniques, see p. 33.

Possible Associated Conditions: Mitral regurgitation.

Defect, Ventricular Septal

Synonyms: Inlet (subtricuspid, AV canal type); membranous (paramembranous, perimembranous, infracristal); muscular (persistent bulboventricular foramen); and outlet (subarterial, supracristal, conal, doubly committed juxta-arterial).

NOTE: The basic anomaly is a defect of the ventricular septum, usually at the membranous septum (in 75%). Possible surgical intervention consists of surgical closure of the defect. Late postoperative death may be sudden and related to residual pulmonary hypertension or ventricular arrhythmias. For general dissection techniques, see p. 33. If hypertensive pulmonary artery disease is suspected, perfuse one lung with formalin (p. 47) and request Verhoeff–van Gieson stain (p. 173).

Possible Associated Conditions: With membranous type: Often isolated; may occur with atrial septal defect,* conotruncal anomalies, or patent ductal artery.* With outlet type: Conotruncal anomalies such as double outlet right ventricle,* persistent truncal artery,* or tetralogy of Fallot.* With inlet type: Atrioventricular septal defect* or atrioventricular discordance. With muscular type: Isolated or with tricuspid atresia* or double inlet left ventricle.

Deficiency, alpha$_1$-Antitrypsin

Possible Associated Conditions: See below under "Possible or Expected Findings."

Organs and Tissues	*Procedures*	*Possible or Expected Findings*
Skin and subcutaneous tissue	Sample normal and abnormal appearing areas for histologic study.	Panniculitis *(1)*.
Blood (serum)	Submit frozen sample for determination of alpha$_1$-antitrypsin concentrations (1 mL is required).	Decreased a$_1$-antitrypsin values. Many genetic alleles can be determined by starch-gel electrophoresis.
Lungs	Perfuse lungs with formalin (p. 47). See also under "Emphysema."	Panlobular pulmonary emphysema,* primarily of lower lobes; chronic bronchitis and, rarely, brochiectases; interstitial pulmonary fibrosis.
Liver	If cirrhosis or tumor is present, follow procedures described under those headings. Request PAS stain, with diastase digestion (p. 56).	Cirrhosis in infants and adults; cholangiocellular or hepatocellular carcinoma; paucity of intrahepatic bile ducts; neonatal (giant cell) hepatitis; periportal hepatitis or cirrhosis and hepatocellular carcinoma in adults *(2,3)*.
	Characteristic accumulations of alpha$_1$-antitrypsin can be shown in routine paraffin sections with PAS-D or immunostains.	PAS-positive, diastase-resistant globular inclusions, primarily in periportal hepatocytes or in the periphery of regenerative nodules.

Organs and Tissues	Procedures	Possible or Expected Findings
Small and large intestine		Inflammatory bowel disease (rare) *(3)*.
Extrahepatic bile ducts	For cholangiography, see p. 56. Dissect bile ducts *in situ*.	Biliary atresia.* Generally no abnormalities in adults.
Pancreas		Chronic pancreatitis; fibrosis of pancreas.
Kidneys	See under "Glomerulonephritis."	Membranoproliferative glomerulonephritis* in childhood *(4)*.

References

1. O'Riordan K, Blei A, Rao MS, Abecassis M. Alpha 1-antitrypsin deficiency-associated panniculitis: resolution with intravenous alpha 1-antitrypsin administration and liver transplantation. Transplantation 1997;63:480–482.
2. Perlmutter DH. Clinical manifestations of alpha 1-antitrypsin deficiency. Gastroenterol Clin North Am 1995;24:27–43.
3. Elzouki AN, Eriksson S. Risk of hepatobiliary disease in adults with severe alpha 1-antitrypsin deficiency (PiZZ): is chronic viral hepatitis B or C an additional risk factor for cirrhosis and hepatocellular carcinoma? Eur J Gastroenterol 1996;8:989–994.
4. Yang P, Tremaine WJ, Meyer RL, Prakash UB. Alpha 1-antitrypsin deficiency and inflammatory bowel disease. Mayo Clin Proc 2000;75: 450–455.
5. Elzouki AN, Lindgren S, Nilsson S, Veress B, Erisksson S. Severe alpha1-antitrypsin deficiency (PiZ homozygosity) with membranoproliferative glomerulonephritis and nephrotic syndrome, reversible after orthotopic liver transplantation. J Hepatol 1997;26:1403–1407.

Deficiency, alpha-Lipoprotein (See "Disease, Tangier's.")

Deficiency, beta-Lipoprotein (See "Abetalipoproteinemia.")

Deficiency, Congenital Transferrin (See "Hemochromatosis.")

Deficiency, Folic Acid (See "Anemia, megaloblastic.")

Deficiency, Myeloperoxidase (See "Disorder, inherited, of phagocyte function.")

Deficiency, Vitamin A

Synonyms and Related Terms: Hypovitaminosis A; keratomalacia; xerophthalmia.

Organs and Tissues	Procedures	Possible or Expected Findings
External examination	Record extend and character of skin lesions and appearance of eyes; prepare sections of skin.	Sebaceous glands covered with keratin; keratomalacia; enlarged meibomian glands of eyelids.
Other organs		For conditions that may produce vitamin A deficiency, see under "Syndrome, malabsorption."
Eyes	For removal and specimen preparation, see p. 85.	Bitot's spots (keratinized epithelium and air bubbles at corneal rim); keratomalacia.

Deficiency, Vitamin B_1 (Thiamine) (See "Syndrome, Wernicke-Korsakoff.")

Deficiency, Vitamin B_6 (See "Beriberi.")

Deficiency, Vitamin B_{12} (See "Anemia, megaloblastic.")

Deficiency, Vitamin C

Synonyms: Hypovitaminosis C; scurvy.

Organs and Tissues	Procedures	Possible or Expected Findings
External examination and skin	Record extent and character of skin lesions; prepare sections of skin.	Hyperkeratotic hair follicles with perifollicular hemorrhages (posterior thighs, anterior forearms, abdomen); petechiae and ecchymoses (inner and posterior thighs); subcutaneous hemorrhages.
	Describe appearance of gums, and prepare sections.	Gingivitis.

Organs and Tissues	Procedures	Possible or Expected Findings
Other organs	Record evidence of bleeding.	In rare instances, gastrointestinal or genitourinary hemorrhages.
Bones, joints, and soft tissues	For removal, prosthetic repair, and specimen preparation of bones and joints, see p. 95.	Hemorrhages into muscles and joints. Subperiosteal hemorrhages occur primarily in distal femora, proximal humeri, tibiae, and costochondral junctions (scorbutic rosary).

Deficiency, Vitamin D

Synonyms: Hypovitaminosis D; rickets.

NOTE: Features or rickets may be found in familial hypophosphatemia (vitamin D-resistent rickets; Fanconi syndrome).

Organs and Tissues	Procedures	Possible or Expected Findings
External examination	Prepare skeletal roentgenograms.	In infants, rachitic changes at costochondral junctions; in adults, osteoporosis* and osteomalacia*—with or without pseudofractures (Milkman's syndrome).
	In infants with suspected rickets, record size of anterior fontanelle and shape of head; state of dentition; and shape of costochondral junctions, wrists, long bones, and spine.	Craniotabes; delayed dentition and enamel defects; protrusion of sternum; rachitic rosary; swelling of costochondral junctions and of wrists.
Vitreous or blood (serum)	Submit samples for calcium, magnesium, and phosphate determination (p. 85).	Hypocalcemia, hypomagnesemia, hypophosphatemia.
Other organs	Procedures depend on expected findings or grossly identified abnormalities as listed in right-hand column.	Possible causes of vitamin D deficiency include diseases associated with malabsorption syndrome,* biliary atresia,* and primary biliary cirrhosis.
	Weigh parathyroid glands and submit samples for histologic study.	Parathyroid hyperplasia (hyperparathyroidism*) secondary to hypocalcemia and impaired absorption of vitamin D.
	Submit samples of intestine for histologic study.	Conditions causing malabsorption.
Bones	For removal, prosthetic repair, and specimen preparation, see p. 95.	Osteomalacia.*
	In infantile rickets, diagnostic sites for histologic sampling are costochondral junctions, distal ends of radius and ulna, and proximal ends of tibia and humerus. For adults, see under "Osteomalacia."	Characteristic abnormalities of osteochondral growth plates in infants. Abundant osteoid in osteomalacia.*

Deformity, Klippel-Feil

Synonym: Congenital fusion of cervical vertebrae.

Organs and Tissues	Procedures	Possible or Expected Findings
External examination		Short neck; low posterior hairline. Disorders with dysraphia (see below).
	Prepare roentgenograms of chest, neck (lateral view), and head.	Fusion of cervical vertebrae. Congenital elevation of the scapula (Sprengel's deformity).
Neck organs		Malformed larynx *(1)*.
Skull, spine, brain,	For removal and specimen preparation of brain and spinal cord, see pp. 65 and 67, respectively.	Arnold-Chiari malformation;* basilar impression; meningomyelocele; platybasia; spinal cord compression; syringomyelia.* Intracranial or spinal cord tumors *(2)*.

References

1. Clarke RA, Davis PJ, Tonkin J. Klippel-Feil syndrome associated with malformed larynx. Case report. Ann Otol Rhinol Laryngol 1994; 103:201–207.
2. Diekmann-Guiroy B, Huang PS. Klippel-Feil syndrome in association with a craniocervical dermoid cyst presenting as aseptic meningitis in an adult: case report. Neurosurgery 1989;25:652–655.

Degeneration, Cerebellar Cortical

Synonyms and Related Terms: Alcoholic cerebellar degeneration; parenchymatous cerebellar degeneration.

Organs and Tissues	*Procedures*	*Possible or Expected Findings*
Brain and spinal cord	For removal and specimen preparation, see pp. 65 and 67, respectively.	Cortical atrophy (predominantly loss of Purkinje cells) of dorsal vermis of cerebellum and adjacent anterior lobe.
Other organs	Procedures depend on expected findings or grossly identified abnormalities as listed in right-hand column.	Manifestations of chronic alcoholism,* amebiasis,* cirrhosis,* malnutrition, or pellagra.*

Degeneration, Cerebello-Olivary (See "Degeneration, spinocerebellar.")

Degeneration, Hepatolenticular (See "Disease, Wilson's.")

Degeneration, Spinocerebellar

Related Terms: Familial cortical cerebellar atrophy; Friedreich's ataxia; hereditary ataxia; Machado-Joseph disease; olivopontocerebellar atrophy.

NOTE: The term spinocerebellar degeneration encompasses a variety of lesions whose classification is controversial. A new approach has come from linkage analysis and molecular biology. For instance, Friedreich's ataxia, the classic form of hereditary ataxia, is due to an intronic expansion of a GAA trinucleotide repeat. Other forms are also identified by their specific gene loci. Neuropathologic examination still is important and ample sampling is suggested, which should include cerebral cortex, basal ganglia (caudate nucleus, putamen, and globus pallidus), thalamus, subthalamic nucleus, midbrain (red nucleus and substantia nigra), pons (pontine nuclei), spinal cord (at cervical, thoracic, and lumbar levels), optic tract, optic nerves with lateral geniculate nucleus, and sensory and motor peripheral nerves.

Organs and Tissues	*Procedures*	*Possible or Expected Findings*
Brain and spinal cord	For removal and specimen preparation, see pp. 65 and 67, respectively.	Symmetric neuronal loss with reactive astrocytosis in the affected areas. See also above under "Note."
Peripheral nerves	For removal and specimen preparation, see p. 79.	

Reference

1. Koeppen AH. The hereditary ataxias. J Neuropathol Exp Neurol 1998;57:531–543.

Degeneration, Spongy, of White Matter

Synonyms and Related Terms: Bertrand-van Bogaert disease; Canavan's disease; familial leukodystrophy.

NOTE: The disease is caused by defective asparto acylase activity. The gene has been cloned and mutations found.

Organs and Tissues	*Procedures*	*Possible or Expected Findings*
External examination	Record head circumference. Prepare roentgenograms of skull.	Enlargement of head.
Brain and spinal cord	For removal and specimen preparation, see pp. 66 and 70, respectively. Request Luxol fast blue stain (p. 72).	Poor demarcation between cortex and gelatinous white matter. Extensive demyelination and vacuolation of white matter, particularly subcortically.
Eyes and optic nerves	For removal and specimen preparation, see p. 85.	Optic atrophy.

Degeneration, Striatonigral (See "Atrophy, multiple system.")

Dehydration

Related Term: Thirst.

NOTE: Possible underlying conditions not related to inaccessibility of water include burns, exposure to heat, gastrointestinal diseases, recent paracentesis, renal diseases, and use of diuretic drugs. See also under "Disorder, electrolyte(s)."

Organs and Tissues	*Procedures*	*Possible or Expected Findings*
External examination		Skin turgor may be decreased and eyes may be sunken.
	Prepare histologic sections of blisters, ulcers, or skin abrasions.	Microscopic changes help to decide whether skin lesions are antemortem or postmortem.
Vitreous	Submit sample for sodium, chloride, and urea nitrogen determination (p. 85).	Sodium concentrations more than 155 meq/L, chloride concentrations more than 130 meq/ and urea nitrogen concentrations between 40 and 100 meq/dL indicate dehydration.
Urine	Record volume and specific gravity	Absence or minimal amount of urine (p. 115).

Dementia (See "Disease, Alzheimer's.")

Dependence, Amphetamine(s)

NOTE: There are no diagnostic autopsy findings. Follow procedures described under "Dependence, drug(s)."

Dependence, Cocaine

NOTE: Cocaine is spontaneously hydrolyzed by blood esterases, even after death. However, its major metabolite, benzoylecgonine, is routinely identifiable by EMIT and ELISA screening tests (see p. 17). When cocaine is abused concurrently with heroin or other drugs, it may be difficult to ascribe death to a single agent.

Organs and Tissues	*Procedures*	*Possible or Expected Findings*
External examination	Record condition of nasal septum.	Chronic inflammation and perforation of nasal septum after prolonged sniffing of cocaine.
	Submit nasal swab for toxicologic study.	Remnant of cocaine.
Blood	Submit sample with NaF added for toxicologic study (see Chapter 2); request drug screen (p. 14).	See above under "Note."
Heart	Record heart weight and thickness of ventricles. For dissection of the heart and coronary arteries, and for histologic sampling, see also Chapter 3.	Left ventricular hypertrophy caused by hypertension complicating or aggravated by cocainism. Cardiotoxicity with focal myocarditis and myocyte necrosis *(2)*, contraction bands *(3)*, and coronary occlusion.
Stomach and colon	Save gastric contents for toxicologic study.	
	Sample stomach and colon for histologic study.	Ischemia of gastric mucosa after ingestion of cocaine. Ischemic colitis *(4)*.
Liver and gallbladder	Save liver tissue and bile for toxicologic study.	
	Sample liver for histologic study.	Zonal hepatic necrosis *(5)*.
Other body fluids and organs	Save vitreous (p. 16), urine, kidneys, and brain for toxicologic study.	See above under "Note."

References

1. Brody SL, Slovis CM, Wrenn KD. Cocain-related medical problems. Consecutive series of 233 cases. Am J Med 1990;88:325–331.
2. Peng SK, French WJ, Pelikan PCD. Direct cocaine cardiotoxicity demonstrated by endomyocardial biopsy. Arch Pathol Lab Med 1989; 113:842–845.
3. Karch SB, Billingham ME. The pathology and etiology of cocaine-induced heart disease. Arch Pathol Lab Med 1988;112:225–230.
4. Brown DN, Rosenholtz MJ, Marshall JB. Ischemic colitis related to cocaine abuse. Gastroenterology 1994;89:1558–1561.
5. Silva MO, Roth D, Reddy KR, Fernandez JA, Albores-Saavedra J, Schiff ER. Hepatic dysfunction accompanying acute cocaine intoxication. J Hepatol 1991;12:312–315.

Dependence, Drug(s), all Types or Type Unspecified

Related Terms: Cocaine dependence;* crack dependence; heroin dependence; intravenous narcotism; morphinism.

NOTE: If narcotic paraphernalia and samples of the drug itself are found at the scene of the death, they should be submitted for analysis. Helpful information about the nature of a drug may be obtained from witnesses. State crime laboratories may provide much assistance. If name of drug is known, see also under "Poisoning,..." The slang name of a drug may be insufficient for identification because these names often are used for different compounds at different times of places.

Opoid narcotics can be injected intravenously, or subcutaneously, or snorted. Death may occur with such speed that the bodies may be found with needles and syringes in the veins or clenched in the hands. Drug dependence may be associated with a multitude of local (see below) or systemic complications, including malaria* and tetanus.*

For general toxicologic study, see p. 14. As stated in Chapter 2, for a growing number of analytes, most notably tricyclic antidepressants, peripheral blood is preferred over central blood. Peripheral blood is aspirated by percutaneous puncture before autopsy, from the femoral vein or the subclavian vein. The authors prefer the femoral approach in order to avoid any question of artifact in the diagnosis of venous air embolism. It may be prudent to add NaF to some of the samples.

Possible Associated Conditions: Acquired immunodeficiency syndrome (AIDS) and many other acute and chronic infections; malnutrition.*

Organs and Tissues	*Procedures*	*Possible or Expected Findings*
External examination and skin	In suspected homicides or other unusual circumstances, excise fresh needle marks with surrounding skin and underlying tissues and submit for toxicologic analysis. (In routine accidental drug-related deaths, this is not necessary.) Submit samples with needle marks for histologic study under polarized light. If victim has not been identified, follow procedures described on p. 11. Photograph changes that indicate addiction.	Foam may exude from nostrils. Erosions of the nasal septum occur in heroin sniffers. Needle marks may be found at any accessible site. Scars, "track hyperpigmentation," ulcers, skin abscesses, and subcutaneous hemorrhages may be abundant. Other complications are ischemic crush injuries with acute rhabdomyolysis, myositis ossificans (brachial muscle), and thrombophlebitis.
Blood	For toxicologic sampling, see above under "Note." Submit samples for bacterial, fungal, and viral cultures, study of viral antibodies (hepatitis B and C), and blood alcohol determination.	Septicemia; evidence of acute or chronic viral infection; alcohol intoxication.
Heart	If endocarditis is suspected, follow procedures described under that heading (p. 103).	Infective endocarditis* that is often on the right side. Expected organisms include *Acinebacter* spp., *Staphylococcus aureus, Staphylococcus albus, Salmonella* spp., enterococci, and *Staphylococcus epidermidis.*
Lungs	Submit portions for toxicologic and microbiologic study (p. 103). Submit multiple samples for histologic study. Request Verhoeff–van Gieson stain (p. 173). Study sections under polarized light.	Pulmonary edema; aspiration; diffuse lobular pneumonia. Septic pulmonary abscesses. Perivascular pulmonary talc granulomas; foreign body emboli; pulmonary necrotizing angiitis; atelectases and fibrosis.
Gallbladder	Submit sample of bile for toxicologic study (p. 16).	Heroin is metabolized to morphine. Morphine accumulates in bile, where it is sometimes easier to detect than in blood.
Liver	Submit samples for toxicologic and histologic study.	Nonspecific portal hepatitis; acute or chronic viral hepatitis;* alcoholic liver disease.* Foreign body granulomas may be present in the liver.
Perihilar lymph nodes		Chronic lymphadenitis.
Spleen	Record weight.	Splenomegaly with follicular hyperplasia.
Urine	Submit sample for toxicologic study.	Detects monoacetylmorphine to distinguish heroin from morphine poisoning.
Brain and spinal cord	For removal and specimen preparation, see pp. 65 and 67, respectively.	Bilateral symmetric necrosis of globus pallidus; cerebral abscess;* meningitis;* transverse myelitis; mycotic aneurysms; subdural or epidural empyema.* Acute cerebral falciparum malaria.*
Bones and joints	Submit samples of grossly abnormal areas for histologic study.	Infectious spondylitis and sacroiliitis.

Depressant(s) (See "Dependence, drug(s),...")

Dermatomyositis

Related Term: Childhood dermatomyositis (or polymyositis) associated with vasculitis; dermatomyositis (or polymyositis) associated with neoplasia or collagen vascular disease; primary idiopathic dermatomyositis; primary idiopathic polymyositis.

Possible Associated Conditions: Carcinoma (lung, stomach, intestine, and prostate in males; breast, ovary, and uterus in females; miscellaneous sites in both sexes); lymphoma* (rare) and other malignancies *(1)*; lupus erythematosus;* mixed connective tissue disease; progressive systemic sclerosis;* rheumatoid arthritis;* Sjögren's syndrome;* and others. Vasculitis of childhood polymyositis (dermatomyositis).

Organs and Tissues	*Procedures*	*Possible or Expected Findings*
External examination and skin	Photograph grossly involved skin.	Erythema; maculopapular eruption; eczematoid or exfoliative dermatitis; ulcerations; calcification.
	Prepare sections of involved (anterior chest, knuckles, knees) and grossly uninvolved skin and subcutaneous tissue.	Microscopically, dermatitis and panniculitis with edema and fibrinoid necroses are found. Vasculitis in childhood cases. Lipodystrophy *(2)*.
	Prepare roentgenograms.	Pneumomediastinum and subcutaneous emphysema *(3)*.
Heart	Submit samples from myocardium for histologic study (p. 30).	Mycarditis* (rare). Microscopic changes similar to those in skeletal muscles (see below).
Lungs	Perfuse one lung with formalin (p. 47).	Lymphocytic pneumonitis; obliterating bronchiolitis; edema; interstitial pulmonary fibrosis (see "Pneumonia, interstitial").
Esophagus and gastrointestinal tract	Submit samples from all segments for histologic study.	Vasculitis; myositis, rarely with rupture *(4)*. Features of inflammatory bowel disease may be present.
Kidneys		Arteritis* and phlebitis* with thrombosis, fibrosis, and infarctions.
Other organs	Submit samples of liver for histologic study. For sampling in diabetes mellitus, see under that heading.	Steatohepatitis and manifestations of diabetes mellitus* may be found *(2)*.
Skeletal muscles	Submit samples from deltoid, biceps, cervical, gluteal, and femoral muscles, and also from other muscles that may have been involved clinically (pharynx, tongue), for histologic study. Photograph abnormal gross specimens. For specimen preparation, see p. 80.	Myositis with muscular atrophy and fibrosis; vasculitis in childhood cases.
Peripheral nerves	For removal and specimen preparation, see p. 79.	Polyneuropathy (rare) *(5)*.
Joints	For removal, prosthetic repair, and specimen preparation, see p. 95.	Arthritis.

References

1. Maoz CR, Langevitz P, Livneh A, Blumstein Z, Sadeh M, Bank I, et al. High incidence of malignancies in patients with dermatomyositis and polymyositis: an 11-year analysis. Semin Arthritis Rheum 1998; 27:319–324.
2. Quecedo E, Febrer I, Serrano G, Martinez-Aparicio A, Aliaga A. Partial lipodystrophy associated with juvenile dermatomyositis: report of two cases. Pediatr Dermatol 1996;13:477–482.
3. de Toro-Santos FJ, Verea-Hernando H, Montero C, Blanco-Aparicio M, Torres Lanzas J, Pombo Felipe F. Chronic pneumomediastinum and subcutaneous emphysema: association with dermatomyositis. Respiration 1995;62:53–56.
4. Dougenis D, Papathanasopoulos PG, Paschalis C, Papapetropoulos T. Spontaneous esophageal rupture in adult dermatomyositis. Eur J Cardio-Thor Surg 1996;10:1021–1023.
5. Vogelsang AS, Gutierrez J, Klipple GL, Katona IM. Polyneuropathy in juvenile dermatomyositis. J Rheumatol 1995;22:1369–1372.

Diabetes Insipidus

Organs and Tissues	*Procedures*	*Possible or Expected Findings*
Brain and pituitary gland	For cerebral arteriography, see p. 80. For removal and specimen preparation of brain and pituitary gland, see pp. 65 and 71, respectively. If infection is suspected, follow procedures described on p. 102. Submit samples from brain and pituitary gland for histologic study.	Head injury* (including birth trauma); Langerhans cell (eosinophilic) granulomatosis;* local infection; metastatic tumor (frequently from carcinoma of breast); neurosurgical procedures; primary neoplasm involving neurohypophyseal system; sarcoidosis.*
Vitreous	Submit sample for sodium, chloride, and urea nitrogen determination (p. 85).	Changes associated with dehydration.*
Other organs	Procedures depend on expected findings or grossly identified abnormalities as listed in right-hand column.	No diagnostic findings. Nephrogenic diabetes insipidus is caused by renal tubular defect. Manifestations of histiocytosis,* sarcoidosis,* and other possible underlying conditions.

Diabetes Mellitus

Synonyms: Type I (insulin-dependent or juvenile-onset) diabetes mellitus; type II (insulin-independent or adult onset) diabetes mellitus; secondary diabetes mellitus (e.g., due to drugs or pancreatic disease).

NOTE: In infants of diabetic mothers, megasoma and congenital malformations of the cardiovascular and central nervous systems must be expected. Record size and weight of placenta and total weight and length, crown to rump length, and crown to heel length of infant. Compare with expected measurements (pp. 555 and 561). Expected histologic finding include hyperplasia with relative increase of B cells of the islands of Langerhans with interstitial and peri-insular eosinophilic infiltrates, decidual changes of the endometrium, enhanced follicle growth in the ovaries, and Leydig cell hyperplasia.

Possible Associated Conditions: Acanthosis nigricans; acromegaly;* amyotrophic lateral sclerosis;* ataxia telangiectasia;* Fanconi's anemia;* Friedreich's ataxia;* gout;* hemochromatosis;*hyperlipoproteinemia;* hyperthroidism;* obesity;* Turner's syndrome;* and many others, too numerous to mention.

Organs and Tissues	*Procedures*	*Possible or Expected Findings*
External examination and skin		Gangrene of lower extremities and other ischemic changes.
	Prepare sections of skin lesions, of grossly unaffected skin, and of subcutaneous tissue.	Xanthelasmas of eyelids. Diabetic xanthomas on forearms. Diabetic lipoatrophy. Subcutaneous atrophy at former sites of insulin injection.
	If there is evidence of mastopathy, sample tissue for histologic study.	Diabetic mastopathy.
	Prepare sections and smears of intertriginous and other skin infections. Request Gram and Grocott's methenamine silver stains (p. 172).	Fungal vulvitis.
	Prepare whole-body roentgenograms.	Subcutaneous and vascular calcifications. Joint deformities (see below under "Joints").
	Submit samples of skin tissue for electron microscopic study (p. 132).	Diabetic microangiopathy.
Blood	Submit sample for bacterial and fungal cultures (p. 102). If diabetic coma must be ruled out or if disease is only suspected, submit samples of blood and vitreous (see below) for biochemical study. For interpretation, see p. 114.	Septicemia. Increased concentrations of blood glucose (unreliable for diagnosis) and serum ketones and lipids. Postmortem insulin determination may permit the diagnosis of insulin poisoning.
Heart	Record weight and thickness of walls. For coronary arteriography, see p. 118. For histologic sampling, see p. 30.	Cardiac hypertrophy;* coronary atherosclerosis;* myocardial infarction.

Organs and Tissues	*Procedures*	*Possible or Expected Findings*
Heart *(continued)*	If glycogen content is to be evaluated, place specimens in alcohol (p. 129) or Carnoy's fixative (p. 130) or—preferably—prepare for electron microscopic study (p. 132).	
Lungs	Submit one lobe for bacterial and fungal cultures (p. 103). Request Gram and Grocott's methenamine silver stain (p. 172).	Bacterial or fungal (aspergillosis,* candidiasis,* cryptococcosis*) pneumonia.
Esophagus	Sample for histologic study. For special stains, see "Lungs."	Intramural pseudodiverticulosis (dilatation of submucosal gland ducts). Fungal esophagitis.
Liver	Record weight and sample for histologic study.	Hepatomegaly; fatty changes; diabetic steatohepatitis or steatohepatitic cirrhosis. Other types of cirrhosis may be a cause of secondary diabetes (Naunyn's diabetes).
Gallbladder	Record appearance of concrements.	Cholelithiasis.*
Spleen	Submit sample for histologic study.	Lipoid histiocytosis.
Stomach	Record size and shape of stomach and appearance of mucosa.	Gastric dilatation; mucosal hemorrhages.
Pancreas	Prepare soft tissue roentgenogram. Dissect pancreas and record weight. Slice organ in 2-mm sagittal sections. Place one slice in alcohol or Carnoy's fixative (p. 130). Request Best's carmine, Masson's trichrome, Congo red, and Gomori's chromium hematoxylin phloxine stains (p. 172). For the last stain, formalin-fixed organs should be refixed for 12–24 h in Bouin's solution (p. 129). Whenever granules are to be demonstrated in beta cells, a slice of fresh tissue should be placed in Bouin's or Helly's fixative (p. 131).	Glycogenosis of beta cells in prolonged hyperglycemia (in type II diabetes); degranulation of islets of Langerhans; lymphocytic or eosinophilic infiltration around islets (in type I diabetes); amyloidosis or fibrosis of islets. Lesions that may have caused secondary diabetes include pancreatitis, tumors of the pancreas,* cystic fibrosis,* and hemochromatosis.* Focal or diffuse nesidioblastosis in infants of diabetic mothers (may be a cause of hyperinsulinemic hypoglycemia).
Adrenal glands	Record weights. If abnormalities are noted, sample for histologic study.	Adrenocortical nodules or tumor or pheochromocytoma (see also under "Syndrome, Cushing's" and "Tumor of the, adrenal glands").
Kidneys	Record weights of both organs. For renal arteriography, see p. 59. Submit samples for histologic and electron microscopic study (p. 132). Request PAS-alcian blue and Grocott's methenamine silver stains (p. 172). All sections should include papillae.	Diabetic nephropathy and microangiopathy. Arteriolonephrosclerosis; diabetic intercapillary glomerulosclerosis; tubular atrophy and interstitial fibrosis; pyelonephritis* and necrotizing papillitis.
	Submit fresh material for immunofluorescence study.	Glomerular capillary and tubular basement membranes stain for IgG and albumin.
Urine	Prepare sediment and submit sample for protein, glucose, and acetone determination.	Abnormal sediment. Proteinuria, glycosuria, and acetonuria.
Urinary bladder		Urocystitis.
Seminal vesicles, spermatic cords, and testes	Submit samples for histologic study.	Submucosal granular deposits in seminal vesicles; calcification of vas deferens; tubular atrophy of testes.
Ovaries	Submit samples for histologic study.	Stromal hyperthecosis.
Lower extremities	For arteriography, see p. 120. Submit samples from smaller arteries for histologic study. For decalcification procedures, see p. 97.	Gangrene. Obliterating arteriosclerosis of anterior and posterior tibial arteries, peronealarteries, and dorsal artery of the foot.
	Request von Kossa's and Verhoeff–van Gieson stains (p. 172).	Mönckeberg's sclerosis* of muscular arteries.

Organs and Tissues	Procedures	Possible or Expected Findings
Calvarium	Record color of bone.	Calvarium often strikingly yellow (carotene deposition).
Brain and spinal cord	For removal and specimen preparation, see pp. 65 and 67, respectively.	Degeneration of spinal tracts and microinfarctions.
	If cerebral infection is suspected, submit sample for bacterial and fungal cultures (p. 102).	Cerebral mucormycosis.*
	For cerebral arteriography, see p. 80.	Cerebral infarctions.*
Pituitary gland	For removal and specimen preparation, see p. 71.	Infarctions.
Eyes	For removal and specimen preparation, see p. 85.	Diabetic retinopathy with capillary microaneurysms; cataracts; microaneurysms of conjunctival vessels. Nutritional amblyopia.*
Vitreous	If diabetic coma or ketoacidosis must be ruled out, submit sample of vitreous (p. 85) from one eye for determination of glucose and ketone concentrations (see p. 115).	Glucose values less than 2 h after death or combined glucose and lactate values several days after death can be used for the diagnosis of hyperglycemia *(1)*.
Peripheral nerves	For sampling and specimen preparation, see p. 79. Include anterior tibial and sciatic nerves. Request Luxol fast blue stain for myelin (p. 172).	Diabetic neuropathy. Patchy demyelinization.
Skeletal muscles	For sampling and specimen preparation, see p. 80.	Diabetic myopathy.
Breast tissue	Submit sample for histologic study.	Hyalinization around mammary ducts.
Joints	For removal, prosthetic repair, and specimen preparation, see p. 96.	Deformation (Charcot joints) of tarsal and metatarsal joints or—less commonly—of ankle and knee joints. Such deformations occur after diabetic neuropathy.

Reference

1. Sippel H, Möttönen M. Combined glucose and lactate values in vitreous humor for postmortem diagnosis of diabetes mellitus. Forens Sci Internat 1982;19:217–222.

Dialysis (for Chronic Renal Failure)

NOTE: Body fluids and tissues may be infectious (e.g., hepatitis C).

Organs and Tissues	Procedures	Possible or Expected Findings
External examination	Expose intraperitoneal catheters or arteriovenous shunts with as little contamination as possible. Submit material for aerobic and anaerobic bacterial and fungal cultures. Remove vessel from shunt site for histologic study.	Infection of catheters and shunts. Infectious vasculitis.
Blood	Submit sample for aerobic and anaerobic bacterial and for fungal cultures (p. 102).	Septicemia.
Heart	If endocarditis is suspected, follow procedures described under that heading (p. 103).	Infective endocarditis.*
Peritoneal cavity	If peritoneal dialysis had been used, culture contents of peritoneal cavity (see above under "Blood"). Submit samples of peritoneum for histologic study.	Peritonitis.*
Liver	Submit samples for histologic study.	Chronic hepatitis B or C.* Hepatic granulomas *(1)*.
Kidneys and other organs	Procedures depend on expected findings or grossly identified abnormalities as listed in right-hand column.	Chronic renal disease (e.g., glomerulonephritis) and systemic manifestations of kidney failure.*

Reference

1. Kurumaya H, Kono N, Nakanuma Y, Tomoda F, Takazahura E. Hepatic granulomata in long-term hemodialysis patients with hyperalbuminemia. Arch Pathol Lab Med 1989;113:1132–1134.

Diathesis, Bleeding (See "Coagulation, disseminated intravascular," "Disease, Christmas," "Disease, von Willebrand's," and "Hemophilia."

Digitalis (See "Poisoning, digitalis.")

Diphtheria

Synonyms: *Corynebacterium diphtheriae* infection; diphtheric fever.

NOTE: The disease has been nearly eliminated in the USA but not in many other countries.

(1) Collect all tissues that appear to be infected. (2) Request aerobic bacterial cultures. (3) Request Gram stain (p. 172). (4) Special **precautions** are indicated (p. 146). (5) Serologic studies are not helpful, but the organism may be typed for epidemiologic purposes. Toxin assays are also available. (6) This is a **reportable** disease.

Organs and Tissues	*Procedures*	*Possible or Expected Findings*
Head and neck	Remove neck organs with oropharynx, tongue, tonsils, soft palate, and uvula. Record degree of laryngeal obstruction. Photograph larynx and pharynx before and after opening.	Diphtheric pharyngitis.
	Submit sample of pharyngeal pseudomembranes for culture; prepare smears of membranes.	Gram-positive pleomorphic bacilli.
Heart	Photograph. Record weight and submit samples for histologic study (see p. 30).	Diphtheric myocarditis.
Kidneys	Submit samples for histologic study.	Nonsuppurative interstitial nephritis. Renal tubular necrosis.*
Brain and peripheral nerves	For removal and specimen preparation, see pp. 66 and 70, respectively. Request Luxol fast blue stain (p. 172).	Myelin degeneration and destruction of myelin sheaths.
Nasal cavities, sinuses, and middle ears	For exposure of epipharynx, nasal cavities, sinuses, and middle ears, see pp. 71–73. Prepare smears and swab cultures of these spaces. Photograph, prepare histologic sections, and request Gram stain (p. 172).	Diphtheritic pseudomembranes.

Disease,... (See subsequent entries and under "Sickness,..." and "Syndrome,...")

Disease, Addison's (See "Insufficiency, adrenal.")

Disease, Albers-Schönberg (See "Osteopetrosis.")

Disease, Alcoholic Liver

Related Terms: Alcoholic cirrhosis; alcoholic fatty liver; alcoholic hepatitis.

NOTE: Several conditions such as obesity-related steatohepatitis may be histologically indistinguishable from alcoholic liver disease *(1)*. Thus, the diagnosis should not be based on liver histology alone.

Organs and Tissues	*Procedures*	*Possible or Expected Findings*
External examination	Record presence or absence of features listed in right-hand column.	Jaundice; clubbing of fingers; Dupuytren's contractures; decreased body hair and gynecomastia in men.
Serosal cavities	Record volume of effusions.	Ascites; pleural effusions.*
Blood and urine	Submit samples for alcohol determination and other toxicologic studies.	Alcoholic cardiomyopathy* *(2)*.
Heart		Record weight.
Lungs	Prepare frozen sections for fat stains.	Fat embolism* (if severe, systemic circulation may be involved—for instance, kidneys and brain).
Esophagus	For demonstration of varices, see p. 53.	Esophageal varices.
Liver	Record weight and sample for histologic study.	Micro- or macronodular alcoholic cirrhosis; alcoholic hepatitis (steatohepatitis); alcoholic fatty liver. Hepatocellular carcinoma. Typical groundglass changes in some patients who were treated with disulfiram or cyanamide *(3)*.

Organs and Tissues	Procedures	Possible or Expected Findings
Portal vein system		See "Hypertension, portal."
Spleen	Record weight.	Congestive splenomegaly.
Pancreas		Alcoholic pancreatitis.*
Brain, peripheral nerves, skeletal muscles, and other organs	For removal of muscles, peripheral nerves, and brain, see pp. 65, 67, and 85, respectively.	Myopathy; neuropathy;* see also under "Alcoholism and alcohol intoxication" and "Syndrome, Wernicke-Korsakoff."
	For removal of lacrimal glands, see p. 87. Remove parotid tissue from scalp incision (p. 65) with biopsy needle.	Parotid and lacrimal gland enlargement with increased glandular secretions.
Testes	Record weights.	Testicular atrophy.

References

1. Kanel GC. Hepatic lesions resembling alcoholic liver disease. Pathology 1994;3:77–104.
2. Estruch R, Fernandez-Sola J, Sacanella E, Pare C, Rubin E, Urbano-Marquez A. Relationship between cardiomyopathy and liver disease in chronic alcoholism. Hepatology 1995;22:532–538.
3. Yokoyama A, Sato S, Maruyama K, Nakano M, Takahashi H, Okuyama K, et al. Cyanamide-associated alcoholic liver disease: a sequential histologic evaluation. Alcohol Clin Exp Res 1995;19:1307–1311.

Disease, alpha-Chain (See "Disease, heavy-chain.")

Disease, Alzheimer's

Synonyms and Related Terms: Alzheimer's dementia; presbyophrenic dementia; presenile dementia syndrome.

NOTE: For pathogenesis and criteria for staging, see refs. *(1–3)*.

Organs and Tissues	Procedures	Possible or Expected Findings
Brain and spinal cord	For removal and specimen preparation, see pp. 65 and 67, respectively. Record brain weight. Histologic sections should include frontal, temporal, occipital, cingulate, enthorinal, and amygdala, hippocampus, deep nuclei and thalamus, substantia nigra, and occipital cortex and hippocampus. For silver impregnation of paraffin sections, request Bielchowsky silver stain (p. 172). Immunostain for βA4 and tau protein are available for plaques and tangles. Some tissue samples should be kept frozen for biochemical studies.	Cortical atrophy, particularly of frontal and temporal lobes, with dilatation of ventricles. Neuronal loss and reactive astrocytosis; characteristic senile plaques (argentophilic neuritic plaques) and Alzheimer's neurofibrillary tangles. In some cases, cerebral meningeal and cortical blood vessels show amyloid angiopathy.

References

1. Esiri MM, Hyman BT, Beyreuther K, Masters CL. Aging and dementia in Greenfield's Neuropathology, vol. 2. Graham BI, Lantos PL, eds. Arnold, London, 1997, pp. 153–233.
2. The National Institute on Aging, and Reagan Institute Working Group on Diagnostic Criteria for the Neuropathological Assessment of Alzheimer's Disease. Consensus recommendations for the postmortem diagnosis of Alzheimer's disease. Neurobiol Aging 1997;Jul-Aug;18(4 Suppl): S1-2.
3. The Ronald and Nancy Reagan Research Institute of the Alzheimer's Association and the National Institute on Aging Working Group. Consensus report of the Working Group on: Molecular and Biochemical Markers of Alzheimer's Disease. Neurobiol Aging 1998;Mar-Apr;19 (2):109–116. (Published erratum appears in Neurobiol Aging 1998; May-Jun;19(3):285.)

Disease, Atherosclerotic Heart (See "Disease, ischemic heart.")

Disease, Bornholm (See "Pleurodynia, epidemic.")

Disease, Bourneville's (See "Sclerosis, tuberous.")

Disease, Buerger's

Synonyms: Thromboangitis obliterans; Winiwater-Buerger syndrome.

Organs and Tissues	Procedures	Possible or Expected Findings
External examination	Record presence or absence of abnormalities listed in right-hand column.	Ischemic ulcers of digits; gangrene; amputations; elevated skin lesions accompanying thrombophlebitis.*
Extremities	If permitted, submit samples from dorsal artery of the foot, and tibial, anterior fibular, popliteal, and femoral arteries. Include specimens of accompanying veins (p. 34).	Arterial lesions are often segmental. Digital arteries are involved more often than are ulnar and radial arteries. Thrombophlebitis* is part of the disease.
	Section arteries and veins crosswise at different levels. Request Verhoeff–van Gieson stain (p. 173). Section veins that have gross evidence of thrombosis* or thrombophlebitis.*	Thrombi in small and medium-sized vessels contain mixed inflammatory cells, giant cells, and sterile microabscesses. Later stages of the process are characterized by hypercellular intraluminal granulation tissues without medial scarring.
Abdominal and visceral vasculature	Dissect abdominal aorta with iliac, mesenteric, and renal arteries. Dissect coronary arteries. Submit samples for histologic study, including Verhoeff–van Gieson stain (p. 173).	Thromboses in mesenteric, renal, and coronary arteries are rare. Aortoiliac disease is also rare. Manifestations of the Budd-Chiari syndrome* may be present.
Brain	For removal and specimen preparation, see p. 65. For cerebral arteriography, see p. 80.	Cerebral artery involvement may be present and may be associated with cortical ischemic lesions.

Disease, Caisson (See "Sickness, decompression.")

Disease, Canavan's (See "Degeneration, spongy, of white matter.")

Disease, Caroli's

Synonyms and Related Terms: Caroli's syndrome; fibropolycystic liver disease; idiopathic dilatation of intrahepatic bile ducts.

NOTE: The term "Caroli's syndrome" often is used for cases that also show histologic features of congenital hepatic fibrosis or other manifestations of fibropolycystic liver disease,* whereas the name "Caroli's disease" refers to idiopathic dilatation of intrahepatic bile ducts, without associated abnormalities.

Possible Associated Conditions: Choledochal cyst* and related extrahepatic biliary abnormalities *(1)*; congenital hepatic fibrosis;* cysts of kidneys (renal tubular ectasia or medullary sponge kidney; autosomal-recessive polycystic kidney disease, and rarely, autosomal-dominant polycystic kidney disease *[2]*)* and of pancreas.

Organs and Tissues	Procedures	Possible or Expected Findings
Blood	Submit samples for aerobic and anaerobic bacterial cultures (p. 102).	Septicemia.
Liver and extrahepatic bile ducts	If there are superficial abscesses or easily accessible cysts, sterilize capsule of liver and aspirate contents for aerobic and anaerobic cultures. Remove small and large bowel, and open duodenum *in situ*. Aspirate bile from gallbladder or dilated ducts for bacterial culture. For cholangiography, see p. 56. Open extrahepatic bile ducts *in situ* and record width. Slice liver in frontal or horizontal plane and submit samples for histologic study.	Dilatation of the hepatic and common bile ducts (may not involve entire liver *[1]*); choledochal-type cyst;* hepatolithiasis; cholelithiasis;* choledocholithiasis; rupture of bile duct *(3)*; suppurative cholangitis;* hepatic abscesses. Adenocarcinoma of bile ducts.
Kidneys	If abnormalities are present, prepare photographs prior to histologic sampling.	See above under "Possible Associated Conditions."
Other organs		Manifestations of portal hypertension.*

References

1. Dagli U, Atalay F, Sasmaz N, Bostanoglu S, Temucin G, Sahin B. Caroli's disease: 1977–1995 experiences. Eur J Gastroenterol Hepatol 1998;10: 109–112.
2. Mousson C, Rabec M, Cercueil JP, Virot JS, Hillon P, Rifle G. Caroli's disease and autosomal dominant polycystic kidney disease: a rare association? Nephrol Dialysis Transplant 1997;12:1481–1483.
3. Chalasani N, Nguyen CC, Gitlin N. Spontaneous rupture of a bile duct and its endoscopic management in a patient with Caroli's syndrome. Am J Gastroenterol 1997;92:1062–1063.

Disease, Cat Scratch

Possible Associated Conditions: AIDS and other immunodeficient conditions.

Organs and Tissues	*Procedures*	*Possible or Expected Findings*
External examination and skin		Cat-scratch mark and lymphadenopathy.
Heart	If endocarditis is suspected, follow procedures described under that heading (p. 103).	Endocarditis *(1)*.
Liver	Sample for histologic study.	Granulomatous hepatitis; bacillary peliosis hepatis *(2)* (see also below under "Other organs").
Other organs	Photograph lesions that might have been caused by the infection. Sample material for microbiologic and histologic study; prepare Gram stains (p. 172).	Infection caused by *Bartonella hensleae* or *Afipia felis.* In patients with AIDS, bacillary (epithelioid) angiomatosis and bacillary peliosis hepatis are associated with *B. hensleae (1)* infection.
Skeletal system	If osteomyelitis is suspected, follow procedures described under that heading.	Osteomyelitis.*
Brain and spinal cord	For removal and specimen preparation, see pp. 65 and 67, respectively.	Encephalitis; meningitis; transverse myelitis.

References

1. Holmes AH, Greenough TC, Balady GJ, Regnery RL, Anderson BE, O'Keane JC, et al. Bartonella henselae endocarditis in an immunocompetent adult. Clin Inf Dis 1995;21:1004–1007.
2. Chomel BB. Cat-scratch disease and bacillary angiomatosis. Rev Scientifique Technique 1996;15:1061–1073.

Disease, Celiac (See "Sprue, celiac.")

Disease, Cerebrovascular (See "Attack, transient cerebral ischemic" and "Infarction, cerebral.")

Disease, Chagas'

Synonyms and Related Terms: American trypanosomiasis; Chagas' syndrome; *Trypanosoma cruzi* infection.

NOTE: (1) Collect all tissues that appear to be infected. (2) Request cultures for trypanosomiasis. (3) Request Giemsa stain (p. 172). (4) Special **precautions** are indicated (p. 146). (5) Serologic studies are available from the Centers for Disease Control and Prevention, Atlanta, GA (p. 135). (6) Usually, this is not a reportable disease.

Possible Associated Conditions: AIDS *(1)* and other conditions associated with immunosuppression.

Organs and Tissues	*Procedures*	*Possible or Expected Findings*
External examination and skin	Record and photograph the findings listed in right-hand column. Prepare sections of skin lesions.	In acute disease, unilateral bipalpebral edema, chemosis, and swelling of preauricular lymph nodes (Romaña's sign); skin nodules showing histiocytic and granulomatous inflammation; regional lymphadenitis, primarily in uncovered regions (chagoma), and subcutaneous edema. Hypopigmentation.
Body cavities	Record volume of effusions.	Effusions in congestive cardiac failure.*
Blood	Prepare smears of fresh blood or of buffy coat, or make thick-drop preparation. Submit sample for xenodiagnosis or animal inoculation and for serologic study (p. 102).	In acute Chagas' disease, trypanosomes in blood. In acute cases, positive hemagglutination and precipitin tests; in chronic cases, positive complement-fixation tests.
Heart	Record weight. In chronic Chagas' disease, perfuse intact heart with formalin (p. 28) and slice fixed heart in a frontal plane so as to create anterior and posterior halves. Prepare photographs. Histologic samples should include conduction system (p. 26).	In chronic Chagas' disease, cardiac hypertrophy and dilatation; fibrous epicarditis, myocardial cell hypertrophy; apical aneurysm; endomyocardial fibrosis, and atrial and apical ventricular mural thrombi. Valves and coronary arteries are normal.

Organs and Tissues	Procedures	Possible or Expected Findings
Heart *(continued)*	Include several sections of atrial (auricular) walls for histologic study of autonomous ganglia.	There may be parasitic pseudocysts or granulomas, fibrosis, myocytolysis, and degeneration and fibrous replacement of ganglion cells. In acute Chagas' disease, heart shows acute or subacute myocarditis* with dilatation. Intracellular parasites (i.e., pseudocysts with amastigote forms); necrosis of ganglion cells in atrial walls.
Lungs	Perfuse one lung with formalin (p. 47).	In chronic Chagas' disease, emboli with infarctions, bronchiectasis,* fibrosis, hemosiderosis, and, rarely, acute hemorrhage.
Esophagus and gastrointestinal tract	Leave affected hollow viscera intact and fill with formalin. Cut fixed organs in half, photograph, and cut histologic sections on edge.	Megaesophagus is frequent, with or without carcinoma. Stomach, duodenum, colon *(2)*, and appendix (rarely) may be enlarged; diminution in number of ganglion cells in Auerbach plexus.
Liver and biliary system	Record liver weight and submit samples for histologic study.	In acute Chagas' disease, hepatomegaly may be present. Rarely, in chronic cases, the gallbladder and bile ducts may be enlarged.
Spleen	Record weight.	Infarctions. In acute Chagas' disease, splenomegaly.
Kidneys, ureters, and urinary bladder	Prepare photographs of abnormalities.	Renal infarctions. Rarely, in chronic Chagas' disease, the ureters and urinary bladder may be enlarged.
Placenta	Weigh and examine. Prepare histologic sections.	Pale, enlarged placenta; chronic villitis; increased perivillous fibrin; amastigotes in Hofbauer cells, amniotic epithelium and syncytiotrophoblasts.*
Brain and spinal cord	For removal and specimen preparation, see pp. 65 and 67, respectively.	Cerebral infarctions.* Meningoencephalitis (particularly in reactivated forms in immunodeficient patients *[3]*) with or without involvement of spinal cord; cerebral atrophy with pressure atrophy of frontal gyri. Histologically, ruptured pseudocysts with spread of amastigote forms.
Skeletal muscles, peripheral nerves, and other tissues	For sampling of skeletal muscles, see p. 80. For sampling of peripheral nerves, see p. 79.	There is a predilection for muscle and nerve tissue, but all organs and tissues can be involved.

References

1. Sartori AM, Shikanai-Yasuda MA, Amato Neto V, Lopes MH. Follow-up of 18 patients with human immunodeficiency virus infection and chronic Chagas' disease, with reactivation of Chagas' disease causing cardiac disease in three patients. Clin Inf Dis 1998;26: 177–179.
2. Oliveira EC, Lette MS, Ostermayer AL, Almeida AC, Moreira H. Chagasic megacolon associated with colon cancer. Am J Trop Med Hyg 1997;56:596–598.
3. Chimelli L, Scaravilli F. Trypanosomiasis. Brain Pathol 1997;7:599–611.

Disease, Cholesteryl Ester Storage

Related Terms: Lysosomal acid lipase deficiency; Wolman's disease.*

Organs and Tissues	Procedures	Possible or Expected Findings
Fascia lata	Specimens should be collected using aseptic technique for tissue culture for biochemical studies (see Chapter 10).	The lysosomal acid lipase deficiency can be demonstrated in cultured fibroblasts.
Blood		Hyperbetalipoproteinemia; hypercholesterolemia.

Organs and Tissues	Procedures	Possible or Expected Findings
Liver and spleen	Accumulation of cholesteryl esters may be demonstrated by thin-layer chromatography of lipid extracts of liver tissue. Lipid is PAS and aldehyde-fuchsin positive.	Hepatosplenomegaly. Hepatic fibrosis or cirrhosis with fatty changes in hepatocytes, cholangiocytes, portal macrophages, and Kupffer cells; deposition of cholesteryl crystals and triglycerides in Kupffer cells *(1)*.
Other organs and tissues		Atherosclerosis and its manifestations may be more severe than expected for the age of the patient *(2)*.

References

1. Di Bisceglie AM, Ishak KG, Rabin L, Hoeg JM. Cholesteryl ester storage disease: Hepatopathology and effects of therapy with lovestatin. Hepatology 1990;11:764–772.
2. Tylki-Szymanska A, Rujner J, Lugowska A, Sawnor-Korsznska D, Wozniewicz B, Czarnowska E. Clinical, biochemical and histological analysis of seven patients with cholesterol ester storage disease. Acta Paediatr Japan 1997;39:643–646.

Disease, Christmas

Synonyms: Christmas factor deficiency; Factor IX deficiency.

NOTE: Follow procedures described under "Hemophilia." The expected findings are the same as for hemophilia.

Disease, Chronic Granulomatous

Synonyms and Related Terms: Autosomal recessive chronic granulomatous disease; chronic granulomatous disease of childhood; X-linked chronic granulomatous disease.

NOTE: The condition occurs not only in children but also in adults. Infections with catalase-positive microorganisms such as *S. aureus, Pseudomonas sp.* or *Aspergillus sp.*, predominate. The disease is part of a family of inherited disorders of phagocyte function (neutrophil dysfunction syndrome); other disorders in this family include the Chediak-Higashi syndrome,* myeloperoxidase deficiency, and other rare disorders.

Organs and Tissues	Procedures	Possible or Expected Findings
External examination, skin, and oral cavity	Record extend and character of skin lesions, particularly those around body orifices. Photograph skin lesions and prepare sections.	Seborrheic dermatitis, mainly around eyes (with conjunctivitis), around mouth (with stomatitis), and around nose and anus. Aphthous ulcers; gingivitis. Bacterial or fungal perianal and perineal abscesses and fistulas; wound infections. Skin granulomas with pigmented macrophages *(1)*.
	Prepare chest and skeletal roentgenograms.	Pulmonary infiltrates. Osteomyelitis,* particularly of hands and feet.
Abdominal cavity	Submit sample of exudate for microbiologic study (see below under "Lymph nodes").	Subphrenic empyema.*
Chest cavity	Submit sample of exudate for microbiologic study (see below under "Lymph nodes"). Record volume of contents.	Pleural effusions;* empyema.
Blood	Submit sample for bacterial and fungal cultures (p. 102).	Septicemia (staphylococci, gram-negative organisms, or fungi, such as *Aspergillus* and *Candida*).
Lymph nodes	Submit samples of inguinal, axillary, mediastinal, mesenteric, and other grossly involved lymph nodes for microbiologic (p. 102) and histologic study. Request Gram and Grocott methenamine silver stains for fungi and Sudan black-stained frozen sections for lipid (p. 172).	Lymphadenitis with abscesses and lipid-filled macrophages; granulomas with central necrosis. For suspected organisms, see above under "Blood."
Heart	If pericarditis or endocarditis are suspected, follow procedures described under these headings (p. 103).	Pericarditis and, rarely, endocarditis* *(2)*.

Organs and Tissues	Procedures	Possible or Expected Findings
Lungs	Submit one lobe for microbiologic study (p. 103); perfuse one lung with formalin (p. 47).	Bacterial and fungal bronchopneumonia and abscesses; hilar lymphadenitis.
Esophagus and gastrointestinal tract	Prepare photographs of abnormal lesions. Submit samples of normal and abnormal appearing areas for histologic study.	Involvement by granulomatous disease may occur from mouth to anus. Colon lesions may resemble chronic ulcerative colitis *(3)*.
Liver and spleen	Record weights; photograph. Submit samples for microbiologic and histologic study (see above under "Lymph nodes").	Hepatosplenomegaly with bacterial and fungal abscesses and granulomas.
Other organs	Submit samples of abnormal appearing areas for histologic study.	Abscesses and granulomas may occur in all organs and tissues.
Brain, spinal cord, and eyes	For removal and specimen preparation, see pp. 65, 67, and 85.	Granulomatous lesions in central nervous system *(4)* and eyes *(5)*.
Bones and bone marrow	For removal, prosthetic repair, and specimen preparation of bones, see p. 95. For microbiologic sampling, see p. 102. For preparation of sections and smears of bone marrow, see p. 96.	Fungal osteomyelitis* that may be multifocal, including sites such as metacarpals and metatarsals.

References

1. Dohil M, Prendiville JS, Crawford RI, Speert DP. Cutaneous manifestations of chronic granulomatous disease. A report of four cases and review of the literature. J Am Acad Dermatol 1997;36:899–907.
2. Casson DH, Riordan FA, Ladusens EJ. Aspergillus endocarditis in chronic granulomatous disease. Acta Pediatr 1996;85:758–759.
3. Sloan JM, Cameron CH, Maxwell RJ, McCluskey DR, Collins JS. Colitis complicating chronic granulomatous disease. A clinicopathological case report. Gut 1996;38:619–622.
4. Adachi M, Hayashi A, Ohkoshi N, Nagata H, Mizusawa H, Shoji S, et al. Hypertrophic cranial pachymeningitis with spinal epidural granulomatous lesion. Intern Med 1995;34:806–810.
5. Valluri S, Chu FC, Smith ME. Ocular pathologic findings of chronic granulomatous disease of childhood. Am J Ophthalmol 1995;120: 120–123.

Disease, Chronic Obstructive Pulmonary (See "Bronchitis, chronic" and "Emphysema.")

Disease, Collagen

Synonym: Connective tissue disease.

NOTE: See under specific name, such as "Arthritis, rheumatoid," "Dermatomyositis," "Lupus erythematosus, systemic," "Polyarteritis nodosa," "Sclerosis, systemic," and "Syndrome, Sjögren's."

Disease, Congenital Heart (See under specific name of malformation.)

Disease, Creutzfeldt-Jakob

Synonyms and Related Terms: Creutzfeldt-Jakob disease (CJD), "new variant"; iatrogenic Creutzfeldt-Jakob disease; familial Creutzfeldt-Jakob disease; fatal familial insomnia; Gerstmann-Straussler-Scheinker syndrome; Kuru; Prion disease; sporadic spongiforme encephalopathy; subacute spongiforme encephalopathy; transmissible spongiforme encephalopathy; variant Creutzfeldt-Jakob disease.

NOTE:

Autopsy is desirable in suspected cases because the diagnosis can only be firmly established after neuropathologic examination. Serologic studies are not available. Unfortunately, all tissues (not just the brain and spinal cord) may remain infectious even after prolonged fixation and histologic processing. Thus, the autopsy recommendations for most other infectious diseases do not apply here. This is a **reportable** disease in some states. Special **precautions** are indicated and therefore, the procedures described here should be followed strictly *(1–4)*:

All persons in the autopsy room must wear disposable long-sleeved gowns, gloves, and masks. Contamination of the autopsy table should be prevented by covering it with a disposable, non-permeable plastic sheet. Autopsy generally should be restricted to the brain. If organs in the chest or abdomen need to be examined, this is best done *in situ*. To prevent aerosolization of potentially infectious bone dust, a hood or other protective device (see p. 67) should be used while opening the skull with a Stryker saw. After completing the autopsy, instruments and other potentially contaminated objects should be autoclaved in a steam autoclave (1 h at 134ºC). Porous load is considered more effective than gravity displacement autoclaves. Immerse autopsy instruments in distilled water before and during autoclaving, in order to protect them from corrosion. If no autoclave is available, chemical disinfection (see below) is a satisfactory alternative. Disposable items should be put in a container for infectious hospital waste and ultimately incinerated. Contaminated objects not suitable for autoclaving (such as the Stryker saw) should be soaked with a 2 *N* NaOH solution for 1 h (alternatively, 1 *N* NaOH may be used for 2 h). Contaminated surfaces should be thoroughly washed with the same solution. Aluminum should be treated for 2 h with a fresh 5% NaOCl (sodium hypochlorite) solution with at least 20,000 ppm free chloride. Wash waters should be collected; if no autoclave is available, 2 *N* NaOH or >4 volumes of 5% sodium hypochlorite bleach should be added to the water and left for a minimum of 2 h before being discarded. Before removing the body from the autopsy room, it should be sponged with 5% sodium hypochlorite.

To deactivate CJD infectivity, tissue blocks, 5 mm or less in thickness, should be fixed in formalin in a formalin-to-tissue ratio of at least 20:1 for at least 48 h and then soaked in concentrated formic acid (95–100%) for 1 h, followed by another 48 h of formalin fixation. The fixation fluid should be collected and decontaminated, as described earlier for wash water. Glassware and tissue carriers should also be decontaminated as previously described. After this deactivation, the tissue blocks can be processed in a routine fashion. At any stage of these procedures, special care must be taken to avoid cuts with potentially contaminated glassware, blades, or other objects. Parenteral exposure to potentially contaminated material also should be avoided.

Remains of patients who have died of the disease should not be accepted for anatomy teaching for students. If specimens are prepared for pathology collections, they should be handled with great caution. Morticians and mortuary workers should be warned of possible hazards posed by tissues of patients with transmissible spongiforme encephalopathies; they should be advised about proper use of disinfectants. Clinical laboratories that receive autopsy tissues or fluids must be warned about the infectious nature of the material. If possible, decontamination should be done at the site where the autopsy was done. For the shipping of potentially infected material, see p. 135.

Organs and Tissues	*Procedures*	*Organs and Tissues*
Cerebrospinal fluid	Submit sample (p. 104) for neuron-specific enolase (NSE).	Increased concentrations of NSE *(5)*.
Brain	For removal and specimen preparation, see p. 65 and above under "Note." Submit fresh-frozen material for confirmation of diagnosis by histoblot technique on protease K-digested frozen tissue or Western blot preparations on brain homogenates. Immunohistochemical localization of PrPres protein on paraffin-embedded tissue is possible.	Spongiforme changes, astrocytosis, neuronal loss, and amyloid plaque formation are the typical findings.

References

1. Ironside JW. Review: Creutzfeldt-Jakob disease. Brain Pathol 1996;6: 379–388.
2. Gajdusek DC, Gibbs CJ Jr. Survival of Creutzfeldt-Jakob disease virus in formol-fixed brain tissue. N Engl J Med 1976;294:553.
3. Brown P. Guidelines for high risk autopsy cases: special precautions for Creutzfeldt-Jakob disease. In: (Hutchins GM, ed.) Autopsy Performance and Reporting. College of American Pathologists, Northfield, IL, 1990, pp. 68–74.
4. Budka H, Aguzzi A, Brown P, Brucher JM, Bugiani O, Collinge J, et al. Tissue handling in suspected Creutzfeldt-Jakob disease and other human spongiforme encephalopathies (prion diseases). Brain Pathol 1995;5:319–322.
5. Zerr I, Bodemer M, Racker S, Grosche S, Poser S, Kretzschmar HA, Weber T. Cerebrospinal fluid concentration of neuron-specific enolase in diagnosis of Creutzfeldt-Jakob disease. Lancet 1995;345: 1609–1610.

Disease, Crohn's

Synonyms and Related Terms: Inflammatory bowel disease;* regional enteritis.

NOTE: If the distinction between Crohn's disease and chronic ulcerative colitis cannot be made clearly, see under "Disease, inflammatory bowel."

Possible Associated Conditions: Amyloidosis;* ankylosing spondylitis;* polyarthritis; Sjögren's syndrome.*

Organs and Tissues	*Procedures*	*Possible or Expected Findings*
External examination and skin	Record character and extent of skin lesions. Submit samples for histologic study.	Orbital edema and lid edema; ulcerative oral lesions; cutaneous fistulas after laparotomies; clubbing of fingers; perianal fistulas; vulval abscesses; cutaneous polyarteritis nodosa; erythema multiforme; erythema nodosum; pyoderma gangrenosum. Granulomatous inflammatory changes in mucosal/skin lesions *(1)*.
	Prepare skeletal roentgenograms.	See below under "Bones and joints."
Vitreous	If dehydration or other electrolyte disturbances are expected, request determination of sodium, chloride, potassium, and urea nitrogen concentrations (pp. 85 and 115).	Dehydration;* electrolyte disorders.*

Organs and Tissues	*Procedures*	*Possible or Expected Findings*
Blood	Submit sample for culture and for determination of immunoglobulin concentrations (p. 102).	Septicemia; selective IgA deficiency.
Heart	See "Stenosis, acquired valvular aortic."	Aortic stenosis.*
Lung	Submit at least one sample from each lobe for histologic study.	Noncaseating granulomas in rare instances *(2)*.
Esophagus	Leave specimen attached to stomach; submit tissue samples for histologic study.	Esophagus may be affected by the disease.
Gastrointestinal tract	For *in situ* fixation and preparation for study under the dissecting microscope, see p. 54. In some instances, adhesions may be so severe that the intestines must be removed and sliced en bloc. Dissect fistulas *in situ*, or inject for roentgenographic study.	All segments of the gastrointestinal tract (appendix included) may be affected. Complications include adenocarcinoma, lymphoma,* or other tumors (rare), pneumatosis coli, fistulas (enterovaginal, perirectal, and others), and perirectal abscess. Acute toxic dilatation of the colon may be present.
	Submit samples of stomach and of all portions of intestinal tract for histologic study.	Mucosal abnormalities also may be present in grossly normal portions of colon and rectum.
Mesentery	Submit lymph nodes for histologic study.	Granulomatous lymphadenitis. Mesenteric fibromatosis *(3)*.
Liver	Record weight. For postmortem cholangiography, see p. 56. Submit multiple samples for histologic study.	Primary sclerosing cholangitis,* with or without cholangiocarcinoma* *(4)*; biliary cirrhosis;* fatty changes; granulomas.
Gallbladder	Record nature of concrements.	Cholelithiasis.*
Retroperitoneal tissues with pancreas	Submit abscess contents for microbiologic study (p. 102).	Psoas abscess; para-aortic lymphadenopathy. Granulomatous pancreatitis *(5)*.
Kidneys with ureters	Submit stones for chemical analysis. Photograph kidneys with renal pelves and ureters. Sample for histologic study.	Nephrolithiasis* (uric acid and calcium stones); hydronephrosis.* Hydroureters; periureteral fibrosis and ureteral obstruction.
Internal genital organs	Submit purulent material for microbiologic study.	Pyosalpinx.
Eyes	For removal and specimen preparation, see p. 85.	Conjunctivitis; marginal corneal ulcers; keratitis; scleritis; episcleritis; retinitis; neuroretinitis; optic neuritis.
Skeletal muscles	For sampling and specimen preparation, see p. 80.	Myositis; in rare instances, dermatomyositis* *(6)*.
Bones and joints	For removal, prosthetic repair, and specimen preparation, see p. 95.	Aseptic necrosis of bone; ossifying periostitis; granulomatous bone disease; ankylosing spondylitis;* polyarthritis; nonspecific or granulomatous synovitis.
Brain and spinal cord	For removal and specimen preparation, see pp. 65 and 67, respectively.	Manifestations of disseminated intravascular coagulation.*

References

1. Kafity A, Pellegrini A, Fromkes J. Metastatic Crohn's disease: a rare cutaneous manifestation. J Clin Gastroenterol 1993;17:300–303.
2. Calder CJ, Lacy D, Raafat F, Weller PH, Booth IW. Crohn's disease with pulmonary involvement in a 3 year old boy. Gut 1993;34:1636–1638.
3. DiGiacomo JC, Lasenby AJ, Salloum LJ. Mesenteric fibromatosis associated with Crohn's disease. Am J Gastroenterol 1994;89:1103–1105.
4. Choi PM, Nugent FW, Zelig MP, Munson JL, Schoetz DJ Jr. Cholangiocarcinoma and Crohn's disease. Dig Dis Sci 1994;39:667–670.
5. Gschwantler M, Kogelbauer G, Klose W, Bibus B, Tscholakoff D, Weiss W. The pancreas as a site of granulomatous inflammation in Crohn's disease. Gastroenterology 1995;108:1246–1249.
6. Leibowitz G, Eliakim R, Amir G, Rachmilewitz D. Dermatomyositis associated with Crohn's disease 1994;18:48–52.

Disease, Cushing's (See "Syndrome, Cushing's.")

Disease, Cytomegalic Inclusion (See "Infection, cytomegalovirus.")

Disease, Demyelinating
(See "Degeneration, spongy, of white matter," "Encephalomyelitis, all types or type unspecified," "Leukodystrophy, globoid cell," "Leukodystrophy, sudanophilic," "Sclerosis, multiple," and "Sclerosis, Schilder's cerebral.")

Disease, Diffuse Alveolar

Synonym: Diffuse pulmonary disease.

NOTE: Autopsy procedures are listed under the more specific diagnoses, such as "Hemosiderosis, idiopathic pulmonary," "Lipoproteinosis, pulmonary alveolar," "Microlithiasis, pulmonary alveolar," "Pneumonia, lipoid," and "Syndrome, Goodpasture's."

Disease, Eosinophilic Endomyocardial
(See "Cardiomyopathy, restrictive [eosinophilic type].")

Disease, Fabry's

Synonyms: Alpha-galactosidase deficiency; Anderson-Fabry disease; angiokeratoma corporis diffusum; glycosphingolipid lipidosis.

Organs and Tissues	*Procedures*	*Possible or Expected Findings*
External examination and skin	Prepare skin sections from multiple sites. Request Sudan black, PAS, and toluidine blue O stains (p. 173).	Telangiectatic lesions. Glycolipid storage (PAS-positive, Sudan black-positive, metachromatic, and double refractile with toluidine blue) in arrectores pilorum muscles, vascular endothelium, and sweat glands.
Blood		Leukocyte alpha-galactosidase deficiency.
Heart	For recommended special stains, see above under "External examination and skin."	Glycolipid storage with nonobstructive hypertrophic cardiomyopathy* (this may be the only manifestation *[1,2]*). Myocardial infarction.
Lungs	For recommended special stains, see above under "External examination and skin."	Narrowing of airways by glycosphingolipid in patients with clinical features of obstructive lung disease *(3)*.
Urine	Examine sediment.	"Mulberry cells" in sediment.
Kidneys	For recommended special stains, see above under "External examination and skin."	Glycosphingolipids in glomeruli and distal convoluted tubules. If applicable, see also under "Failure, kidney."
Other organs	Procedures depend on expected findings or grossly identified abnormalities as listed in right-hand column.	Glycosphingolipid storage in liver, spleen, small and large bowel, lymph nodes, and bone marrow.
Brain and spinal cord	For removal and specimen preparation, see pp. 65 and 67. For cerebral angiography and dissection of vertebral arteries, see pp. 80 and 82. For recommended special stains, see above under "External examination and skin."	Elongated tortuous and ectatic vertebral and basilar arteries *(4)*, sometimes with thrombosis *(5)*. Glycosphingolipid storage. Cerebral infarction(s)* or hemorrhages.
Eyes	For removal and specimen preparation, see p. 85. For recommended special stains, see above under "External examination and skin."	Glycosphingolipid storage in cornea; lens opacities; dilated vessels in conjunctiva and lens; thrombi in blood vessels *(5)*.

References

1. Elleder M, Bradová V, Smid F, Budesinsky M, Harzer K, Kustermann-Kuhn B, et al. Cardiocyte storage and hypertrophy as a sole manifestation of Fabry's disease. Report on a case simulating hypertrophic non-obstructive cardiomyopathy. Virchows Arch [Pathol Anat] 1990;417:449–455.
2. Von Scheidt W, Eng CM, Fitzmaurice TF, Erdmann E, Hubner G, Olsen EG, et al. An atypical variant of Fabry's disease with manifestations confined to the myocardium. N Engl J Med 1991;324:395–399.
3. Brown LK, Miller A, Bhuptani A, Sloane MF, Zimmerman MI, Schilero G, et al. Pulmonary involvement in Fabry disease. Am J Respir Crit Care Med 1997;155:1004–1110.
4. Mitsias P, Levine SR. Cerebrovascular complications of Fabry's disease. Ann Neurol 1996;40:8–17.
5. Utsumi K, Yamamoto N, Kase R, Takata T, Okumiya T, Saito H, et al. High incidence of thrombosis in Fabry's disease. Intern Med 1997;36:327–329.

Disease, Fibropolycystic, of the Liver and Biliary Tract

NOTE: "Fibropolycystic disease of the liver and biliary tract" comprises a group of well defined conditions, which, however, may overlap or occur together and hence need a collective designation. The conditions include autosomal-recessive (infantile) and autosomal dominant (adult) polycystic disease of the liver; Caroli's disease or syndrome;* choledochal cyst,* congenital hepatic fibrosis,* multiple biliary microhamartomas, and related disorders. For autopsy procedures, see also under more specific designations.

Organs and Tissues	*Procedures*	*Possible or Expected Findings*
External examination	Record and photograph abnormalities.	Polydactyly; spina bifida.
Lungs	If cysts can be identified, prepare arteriograms (p. 50) and perfuse with formalin (p. 47). See also below under "Liver and hepatoduodenal ligament."	Cysts of lungs.*
Esophagus	For demonstration of esophageal varices, see p. 53.	Esophageal varices.*
Gastrointestinal tract	Estimate and record volume of blood in lumen.	Gastrointestinal hemorrhage* after rupture of varices.
Spleen	Record weight.	Splenomegaly in presence of portal hypertension.*
Liver and hepatoduodenal ligament	Dissect common bile duct *in situ* (see also under "Cyst(s), choledochal"). Record weight of liver; photograph surface of liver. For cholangiography, venography, or arteriography, see p. 56. Aspirate contents of infected cysts or abscesses and submit samples for microbiologic study (p. 102). Prepare smears of exudate. Inject large cysts with warm, freshly prepared, 5% gelatin solution dissolved in 10% formalin. Slice with large knife (p. 57) after solution has hardened. Photograph cut surface; record size and distribution of cysts; submit tissue samples for histologic study.	Microcysts associated with ductal plate malformations as in autosomal-recessive polycystic liver disease, may not be noticeable macroscopically. Large intra-hepatic cysts may be calcified *(1)*. Choledochal cyst.* Hepatomegaly. Abscesses.
Other organs	Procedures depend on expected findings or grossly identified abnormalities as listed in right-hand column.	Cysts of kidneys,* pancreas, and ovaries. Polycystic kidney disease (autosomal-recessive or autosomal-dominant) may be the main finding at autopsy.

Reference

1. Coffin B, Hadengue A, Degos F, Benhamou JP. Calcified hepatic and renal cysts in adult dominant polycystic kidney disease. Dig Dis Sci 1990; 35:1172–1175.

Disease, Gaucher's

Synonyms and Related Terms: Adult, infantile, or juvenile Gaucher's disease; glucosylceramide lipidosis; acute neuronopathic (infantile) Gaucher's disease; chronic non-neuronopathic (adult) Gaucher's disease.

Possible Associated Conditions: Leukemia,* lymphoma,* and other malignant neoplasms.

Organs and Tissues	*Procedures*	*Possible or Expected Findings*
External examination and skin	Record and photograph skin changes. Prepare histologic sections of skin. Request Gomori's iron stain (p. 172).	Yellowish brown skin pigmentation; pingueculae near cornea. Sinus tracts.
	Prepare skeletal roentgenograms.	Lytic defects and osteonecrosis may occur in long bones, phalanges, ribs, spine, pelvis, and skull. Aseptic necrosis of femoral head. Fractures of long bones may be present.
Blood	Submit sample for biochemical study.	Increased plasma glucosylceramide concentrations.
Heart		Cor pulmonale.
Lungs	Perfuse one lung with formalin (p. 47). Submit one fresh lobe for bacterial culture (p. 103).	Pulmonary involvement in severe cases of Gaucher's disease *(1)*; manifestations of pulmonary hypertension* in adults. Pulmonary infections in children.

Organs and Tissues	Procedures	Possible or Expected Findings
Spleen	Record weight. Photograph cut surface. Submit samples of fresh material for biochemical study, and snap-freeze specimens for histochemical analysis. Prepare unstained smears for phase-contrast microscopy. Request PAS and Masson's trichrome stains (p. 173). Prepare material for electron microscopy (p. 132).	Splenomegaly caused by accumulation of glucocerebroside-containing Gaucher cells. Increased acid phosphatase in Gaucher cells.
Other organs	Submit tissue samples of liver, pancreas, kidneys, gastrointestinal tract, intrathoracic and intra-abdominal lymph nodes, thymus, tonsils, thyroid, and adrenal glands. For processing, see above under "Spleen."	Hepatomegaly; manifestations of portal hypertension; lymphadenopathy. Infiltration of organs (listed in middle column) by Gaucher cells; hemosiderosis.
Brain and spinal cord	For removal and specimen preparation, see pp. 65 and 67, respectively. See also above under "Spleen."	Acute nerve cell degeneration. Accumulation of glucocerebrosides and—in children with acute neuronopathic disease—gangliosides. See above under "External examination and skin."
Bones and bone marrow	Submit specimens of involved bones, as indicated on skeletal roentgenograms; include femur in all instances. Photograph saw section of femur. For prosthetic repair and for decalcification, see p. 97; for specimen preparation, see p. 95. For preparation of bone marrow sections and smears, see p. 96.	

Reference

1. Cox TM, Schofield JP. Gaucher's disease: clinical features and natural history. Baillieres Clin Haematol 1997;10:657–689.

Disease, Glycogen Storage

Synonyms: Andersen's disease or brancher deficiency (glycogenosis, type IV); Cori's or Forbes' disease (glycogenosis, type III); cyclic AMP dependent kinase (type X); glycogen synthetase deficiency (type O); Hers' disease (glycogenosis, type VI); McArdle's disease (glycogenosis type V); phosphorylase B kinase deficiency (types IXa, b, and c); Pompe's disease (glycogenosis, type II); Tarui disease (glycogenosis type VII); von Gierke's disease (glycogenosis, type Ia); X-linked glycogenosis (type VIII).

NOTE: If the diagnosis had not been confirmed prior to death, samples of liver, skeletal muscle, blood, and fascia (for fibroblast culture, see below) should be snap-frozen for enzyme assay, which will determine the specific deficiency. Types Ia and b, III, VI, and hepatic phosphorylase B kinase deficiency (types IXa, b and c) are hepatic-hypoglycemic disorders, whereas types V and VII affect muscle energy processes. Type II also affects the musculature, whereas type IV may cause cirrhosis and death in infancy from extreme hypotonia.

Determination of type of glycogenosis usually can be based on (1) pattern of glycogen storage in liver, (2) presence or absence of nuclear hyperglycogenation in liver, (3) cytoplasmic lipid in liver, (4) presence or absence of liver cirrhosis, and (5) presence or absence of glycogen and basophilic deposits in skeletal muscles.

Possible Associated Conditions: Fanconi syndrome* or gout* with type Ia glycogenosis; neutropenia, recurrent infections, and Crohn's disease with types Ib or Ic.

Organs and Tissues	Procedures	Possible or Expected Findings
External examination and skin	Record body weight and length. Submit tissue samples of skin lesions. Record size of tongue and submit specimens for histologic study (may be easier to do after removal with neck organs). For specimen preparation, see below under "Heart...."	Growth retardation. Xanthomas in von Gierke's disease. Macroglossia.
Blood	Submit sample for uric acid and ketone determination. If blood is to be used for tissue culture, follow procedures described in Chapter 10 (see also "Fascia lata" below).	Hyperuricemia in gout.* Ketoacidosis may be associated with sudden death. Hypoglycemia* and hyperlipidemia occur in von Gierke's disease.

Organs and Tissues	*Procedures*	*Possible or Expected Findings*
Fascia lata	Specimens should be collected using aseptic technique for tissue culture for biochemical studies (see Chapter 10).	For enzyme deficiencies, see above under "Note."
Liver	For recommended fixatives and special stains, see below. Frozen sections protected with celloidin and then stained with PAS allows an accurate determination of the glycogen content.	Enlarged hepatocytes with glycogen storage in types I, III, and IV. Fatty changes most common in types 0, I and III. Periportal fibrosis in types III and IV and, rarely, cirrhosis in type IV.
	Prepare samples for electron microscopic study (p. 132), particularly in glycogenosis types II and IV.	Adenomas and, rarely, hepatocellular carcinomas may be found in type Ia. No abnormalities in types V and VII. See also above under "Note."
Heart, blood vessels, lungs, skeletal muscles, esophagus, intestine, pancreas, spleen, kidneys, adrenal glands, urinary bladder, lymph nodes, bone marrow.	Photograph enlarged or discolored organs and obtain samples for histologic study. Recommended fixatives for glycogen include alcohol, Bouin's (p. 129) or Carnoy's fixative and formalin alcohol (p. 130). Glycogen may still be dissolved during exposure to watery staining solutions. Request van Gieson's stain, PAS stain with and without diastase digestion, and Best's stain for glycogen (p. 172). Request Sudan-stained frozen sections of myocardium, liver, and skeletal muscles. For use of frozen sections for study of glycogen, see above under "Liver." Embed tissue samples for electron microscopic study.	Uric acid nephropathy and glomerulo-sclerosis in type Ia. Distribution of glycogen storage and other abnormalities varies with subtype of disease. Glycogen depositis may be found in myocardium (cardiomegaly), small and large arteries, skeletal muscle (for instance, of diaphragm, neck, trunk, and extremities), bronchial mucosa, and all other organs listed in left-hand column. See also above under "Note."
Eyes	For removal and specimen preparation, see p. 85. Use Zenker's solution for fixation (p. 131). Other fixatives and procedures are listed above.	Glycogen primarily in retinal ganglion cells and ciliary muscle.
Brain and spinal cord	For removal and specimen preparation, see pp. 65 and 67, respectively. Submit specimens of sympathetic nerve ganglia for histologic study.	Glycogen in sympathetic nerve ganglia and neurons of cranial nerves in type VII.
Joints	For removal, prosthetic repair, and specimen preparation, see p. 95.	Gouty arthritis.

Disease, Graft-Versus-Host

NOTE: This disease occurs most commonly after bone marrow transplantation. The disease has also occurred after transfusion of viable lymphocytes, for example, to patients with cancer or leukemia.*

In patients with graft-versus-host disease (GVHD), autopsy also may reveal recurrence of the underlying disease such as leukemia.

Organs and Tissues	*Procedures*	*Possible or Expected Findings*
External examination and skin; oral cavity	Record and photograph skin lesions and prepare histologic sections of normal and abnormal skin.	Generalized erythroderma and jaundice. Microscopic examination shows irregular epidermal-dermal junctions with basal cell vacuolation, spongiosis, and eosinophilic bodies associated with infiltrates of aggressor lymphocytes.
	Small biopsies of labial salivary glands and buccal mucosa may be useful to evaluate chronic GVHD *(1)*.	Buccal mucositis; lichenoid lesions in chronic GVHD *(1)*.

Organs and Tissues	Procedures	Possible or Expected Findings
Heart	Record volume of pericardial fluid.	Pericardial effusion (in rare cases with features of polyserositis in chronic GVHD) *(2)*.
Lungs	Perfuse on lung with formalin (p. 47). Submit samples from other lung for microbiologic study (p. 103).	Diffuse alveolar damage; lymphocytic bronchitis/bronchiolitis obliterans; organizing pneumonia *(3)*. Bronchiectases in rare instances *(4)*.
Liver	Record weight. Submit samples for histologic study.	Hepatomegaly. Portal and periportal hepatitis with destruction of interlobular ducts; oncocytic metaplasia of bile duct epithelium *(5)*; endotheliitis; cholestasis.
Esophagus	Prepare photographs of mucosa and sample for histologic study.	Infectious esophagitis or chronic GVHD with vesicobullous lesions or, in late stages, strictures.
Small and large intestine	For *in situ* fixation of small intestinal mucosa, see p. 54. Submit samples for histologic study.	Enteritis with cellular debris in crypts, atypical epithelial lining of crypts, and inflammatory infiltrates.
Other organs	Procedures depend on expected findings or grossly identified abnormalities as listed in right-hand column.	Inflammatory infiltrates. Hemorrhagic necroses in lymph nodes and spleen. Immune-mediated myelopathy *(6)*.
Eyes	For removal and specimen preparation, see p. 85.	Keratoconjunctivitis. Optic neuropathy *(6)*.
Bone marrow	For preparation of sections and smears, see p. 96.	Evidence of proliferating graft cells.

References

1. Nakamura S, Hiroki A, Shinohara M, Gondo H, Ohyama Y, Mouri T, et al. Oral involvement in chronic graft versus host disease after allogenic bone marrow transplantation. Oral Surg Oral Med Oral Pathol 1996;82:556–563.
2. Toren A, Nagler A. Massive pericardial effusion complicating the course of chronic graft-versus-host disease (cGVHD) in a child with acute lymphoblastic leukemia following allogeneic bone marrow transplantation. Bone Marrow Transplant 1997;20:805–807.
3. Yousem AS. The histological spectrum of pulmonary graft-versus-host disease in bone marrow transplant recipients. Hum Pathol 1995; 26:668–675.
4. Morehead RS. Bronchiectasis in bone marow transplantation. Thorax 1997;52:392–393.
5. Bligh J, Morton J, Durrant S, Walker N. Oncocytic metaplasia of bile duct epithelium in hepatic GVHD. Bone Marrow Transplant 1995; 16:317–319.
6. Openshaw H, Slatkin NE, Parker PM, Forman SJ. Immune-mediated myelopathy after allogeneic marrow transplantation. Bone Marrow Transplant 1995;15:633–636.

Disease, Graves' (See "Hyperthyroidism.")

Disease, Günther's (See "Porphyria, congenital erythropoietic.")

Disease, Heavy-Chain

Synonyms and Related Terms: Gamma heavy-chain disease (Franklin's disease); alpha heavy-chain disease (Seligmann's disease); μ heavy-chain disease.

NOTE: Alpha heavy-chain disease is related to Mediterranean lymphoma and μ heavy-chain disease occurs in rare patients with chronic lymphocytic leukemia.* Infections generally are the cause of death in gamma heavy-chain disease. Evidence of malabsorption* may be observed in alpha heavy-chain disease.

Organs and Tissues	Procedures	Possible or Expected Findings
External examination and oral cavity	Record body weight and length.	Profound wasting in alpha-chain disease. For oral changes, see under "Neck organs."
Blood	Submit samples for microbiologic study and for protein electrophoresis (p. 102).	Septicemia. See also above under "Note." Anomalous serum M component in gamma heavy-chain disease.
Lungs	Submit one lobe for microbiologic study. (p. 103).	Pneumonia in gamma heavy-chain disease. Rarely lymphoplasmacytoid infiltrates in alpha heavy-chain disease.
Urine	Submit sample for protein electrophoresis.	Anomalous serum M component in gamma heavy-chain disease.

Organs and Tissues	Procedures	Possible or Expected Findings
Lymph nodes	Prepare Wright stains of touch preparations (p. 173). Fix tissue in Zenker's or Helly's solution (p. 131).	Mesenteric and para-aortic lymphadenopathy with infiltrates of lymphocytes and plasma cells.
Small bowel and mesentery	For *in situ* fixation and preparation for study under dissecting microscope, see p. 54. For microscopic study, submit samples of all segments of gastrointestinal tract and portions of mesentery with lymph nodes.	Infiltrates of lymphocytes and plasma cells in lamina propria of small bowel in alpha heavy-chain disease. See also under "Syndrome, malabsorption."
Neck organs	Remove together with pharynx.	Palatal edema (Waldeyer ring lymphadenopathy) in gamma heavy-chain disease.
Bone marrow	For preparation of sections and smears, see p. 96.	Infiltrates of lymphocytes and plasma cells; eosinophilia.
Bones	For removal, prosthetic repair, and specimen preparations, see p. 95.	Osteoporosis* in alpha heavy-chain disease.

Disease, Hippel-Lindau (See "Disease, von Hippel-Lindau.")

Disease, Hirschsprung's (See "Megacolon, congenital.")

Disease, Hodgkin's (See "Lymphoma.")

Disease, Hookworm (See "Ancylostomiasis.")

Disease, Huntington's (See "Chorea, hereditary.")

Disease, Hydatid (See "Echinococcosis.")

Disease, Inflammatory Bowel

Synonyms and Related Terms: Chronic ulcerative colitis; Crohn's disease;* idiopathic proctocolitis.

Possible Associated Conditions: Alpha$_1$-antitrypsin deficiency;* amyloidosis;* ankylosing spondylitis;* primary sclerosing cholangitis;* Sjögren's syndrome.* See also below under "Possible or Expected Findings."

NOTE: In many instances, either chronic ulcerative colitis or Crohn's disease* had been diagnosed clinically, but sometimes, the distinction is difficult to make, even at autopsy. Many features described below occur in chronic ulcerative colitis but some manifestations of Crohn's disease or conditions that may occur in all types of inflammatory bowel disease also are listed so that both positive and negative findings can be recorded properly.

Organs and Tissues	Procedures	Possible or Expected Findings
External examination, skin, and oral cavity	Record nature and extent of skin lesions, photograph, and submit specimens of accessible lesions for histologic study.	Aphthous stomatitis; pyoderma gangrenosum; erythema nodosum and multiforme; papular or pustular dermatitis; ulcerating erythematous plaques; neurodermatitis; herpes zoster; anal fissures.
	Record appearance of hands and feet.	Clubbing of fingers and toes. Emaciation.
	Prepare roentgenograms of fistulas after injection of contrast medium (p. 138).	Perianal abscesses and fistulas.
	Prepare skeletal roentgenograms.	See below under "Bones and joints."
Synovial fluid	If arthritis is suspected, submit sample of synovial fluid for microbiologic study, cell counts, and smears (p. 96).	Arthritis.*
Blood	Submit sample for microbiologic study (p. 102).	Septicemia.
Heart	If pericarditis or endocarditis are expected, follow procedures described under these headings (p. 103).	Endocarditis;* pericarditis.*
Lungs	Dissect pulmonary arteries; sample all lobes for histologic study. Request Verhoeff–van Gieson stain (p. 173).	Thromboemboli; pulmonary vasculitis.

Organs and Tissues	*Procedures*	*Possible or Expected Findings*
Abdominal cavity with retroperitoneum and pelvic organs	If peritonitis is present, submit exudate for aerobic and anaerobic bacteriologic study (p. 102). Aspirate contents of abscesses and record their size and location. Record volume of exudate and prepare smears.	Peritonitis.* Perianal, presacral, and ischiorectal abscesses; fistulas and anal fissures. Dilatation of colon ("toxic megacolon"). Fournier's gangrene (necrotizing fasciitis of the genitalia) in Crohn's disease.
Small and large intestine	For *in situ* fixation, see p. 54. If fistulas are present, dissect affected areas *in situ*. Opened colon and affected portions of small bowel should be pinned on corkboard and fixed with formalin. Submit samples of all types of lesions for histologic study.	Segmental (skip areas), transmural and granulomatous inflammation in Crohn's disease. Toxic megacolon more common in chronic ulcerative colitis. Retroperitoneal and rectovaginal fistulas; mucosal ulcers and pseudopolyps; multicentric lymphoma; dysplasia; carcinoma(s); hemorrhage. Rectal stricture. "Backwash ileitis." Colonic cytomegalovirus inclusions, associated with toxic dilatations. See also ref. *(1)*.
Bile ducts	For cholangiography, see p. 56. Dissect extrahepatic bile ducts *in situ* (see also under "Tumor of the bile ducts").	Sclerosing cholangitis;* adenocarcinoma of bile ducts.
Liver	Record weight; submit samples for histologic study.	Biliary cirrhosis.* Cholangiocarcinoma.
Stomach and duodenum		Ulcerative gastritis and duodenitis in Crohn's disease.
Pancreas	Submit samples for histologic study.	Pancreatitis.
Kidneys, ureters, and urinary bladder	Submit samples for histologic and bacteriologic study. If glomerulitis is suspected, follow procedures described under "Glomerulonephritis."	Glomerulonephritis;* pyelonephritis;* tubular degeneration; nephrocalcinosis. Renovascular disease *(2)*.
	Describe size and contents of urinary bladder, ureters, and renal pelves.	Cystopyelitis; urolithiasis; nephrolithiasis (oxalate stones).
Veins and arteries	For removal of femoral vessels, see p. 34.	Thrombophlebitis; arteritis *(2)* and arterial thromboses.
Eyes	For removal and specimen preparation, see p. 85. If there is evidence of Sjögren's syndrome,* remove lacrimal glands (p. 87).	Blepharitis; conjunctivitis; corneal ulcers; iritis; keratitis; neuroretinitis; retrobulbar neuritis; uveitis.
Brain and cerebral venous sinuses	For removal and specimen preparation, see pp. 65 and 67, respectively.	Cerebral venous sinus thrombosis* *(3)*.
Bones and joints	For removal, prosthetic repair, and specimen preparation, see p. 95.	Osteoporosis;* ankylosing spondylitis;* arthritis of peripheral joints; periarthritis; hypertrophic osteoarthropathy;* tendinitis (particularly of ankle and Achilles tendons).

References

1. Podolsky D. Inflammatory bowel disease (first of two parts). N Engl J Med 1991;325:928–937 (part 1) and 1008–1016 (part 2).
2. Sakhuja V, Gupta KL, Bhasin DK, Malik N, Chugh KS. Takayasu's arteritis associated with idiopathic ulcerative colitis. Gut 1990;31:831–833.
3. Johns D. Cerebrovascular complications of inflammatory bowel disease. Am J Gastroenterol 1991;86:367–370.

Disease, Iron Storage (See "Hemochromatosis.")

Disease, Ischemic Heart

Related Terms: Atherosclerotic heart disease.

NOTE: The most common anatomic finding at autopsy in subjects older than 30 yr is coronary atherosclerosis. Unusual underlying or associated conditions include chronic aortic stenosis or regurgitation; coronary artery anomalies; coronary artery dissection; coronary embolism; coronary ostial stenosis (due to calcification of aortic sinotubular junction or, rarely, to syphilitic aortitis);

Disease, Ischemic Heart *(continued)*

coronary vasculitis (for instance, in polyarteritis nodosa* or acute hypersensitivity arteritis); hyperthyroidism,* gastrointestinal hemorrhage;* hypothyroidism,* idiopathic arterial calcification of infancy; intramural coronary amyloidosis; pheochromocytoma, polycythemia vera;* pseudoxanthoma elasticum,* radiation-induced coronary stenosis; severe pulmonary hypertension (with *right* ventricular ischemia); sickle cell disease;* and others. If bypass surgery had been performed, see "Surgery, coronary bypass."

Organs and Tissues	*Procedures*	*Possible or Expected Findings*
External examination		Cyanosis; edema of legs; venous congestion. Gangrene of toes. Diabetic ulcers.
	Prepare chest roentgenogram.	Cardiomegaly; pleural effusions.*
Blood	If underlying metabolic disease is suspected, submit sample for biochemical study.	See above under "Note."
Heart	For coronary arteriography, see p. 118. For specimen preparation and grading of coronary arteries, see p. 21. Request Verhoeff–van Gieson stain (p. 172).	Coronary atherosclerosis; coronary thrombosis or embolism; congenital malformation(s) of coronary arteries; accidental operative coronary ligation; coronary arteritis (see above under "Note.")
	For dissection technique of the heart and for histologic sampling, see pp. 22 and 30. For detection of early myocardial infarction, see p. 32.	Myocardial infarction, old or acute. Mural thrombus. Ventricular aneurysm, true or false. Ventricular rupture (free wall, septum, or papillary muscles).
	For study of valvular cardiac lesions, see p. 32. Record actual and expected heart weight, ventricular wall thicknesses, and valvular annular circumferences. Record appearance, extent, and location of infarcts, mural thrombus, and aneurysms.	Aortic insufficiency;* aortic stenosis.*
Aorta		Acute aortic dissection.*
Other organs		Manifestations of congestive heart failure* and of possible underlying conditions (see above under "Note"), such as diabetes mellitus.*

Disease, Jakob-Creutzfeldt (See "Disease, Creutzfeldt-Jakob.")

Disease, Kawasaki (See "Syndrome, mucocutaneous lymph node.")

Disease, Krabbe's (See "Leukodystrophy, globoid cell.")

Disease, Legionnaires'

Synonyms and Related Terms: *Legionella pneumophila* infection; Pontiac fever.

NOTE: (1) Collect lung specimens, serum, and other tissues that appear to be infected. These should be inoculated on a nonselective medium, such as BCYE agar supplemented with α-ketoglutaric acid. A good selective agar is BCYE supplemented with antibiotics. (2) Request aerobic and anaerobic cultures for exclusion of other bacterial diseases. (3) Request Gram, Kinyoun, and Grocott's methenamine silver stains for exclusion of other bacterial or fungal diseases (p. 172). The Dieterle silver impregnation procedure is recommended for demonstration of the organism in paraffin-embedded sections *(1–3)*. (4) No special precautions are indicated. (5) Serologic immunofluorescent studies are available from the Centers for Disease Control and Prevention, Atlanta, GA (p. 135). (6) This is a **reportable** disease.

Organs and Tissues	*Procedures*	*Possible or Expected Findings*
Blood, pleural fluid	Submit sample for culture (p. 102).	
Lungs	Culture any areas of consolidation (p. 102). Perfuse one lung with formalin (see p. 47). Slice in the parasagittal plane. Submit affected areas for histological study.	Multifocal fibrinopurulent pneumonia with sparing of the bronchi and bronchioles. Exudate is rich in phagocytes, fibrin, and karyorrhectic debris.

References

1. Edelstein PH. Legionnaires' disease. Clin Infect Dis 1993;16(6):741–747.
2. Stout JE, Yu VL. Legionellosis. NEJM 1997;337(10):682–687.
3. Bhopal R. Source of infection for sporadic Legionnaires' disease: a review. J Infect 1995;30:9–12.

Disease, Lyme

Synonym: Lyme arthritis

NOTE: This infection is caused by the spirochete, *Borrelia burgdorferi*, which is transmitted from rodents to human by the hard deer ticks, *Ixodes dammini, I. ricinus*, and others.

Organs and Tissues	*Procedures*	*Possible and Expected Findings*
External examination and skin	Photograph skin lesions. Record presence of enlarged lymph nodes. Submit sections of affected skin for histologic study.	Erythema chronicum migrans; skin vesicles; annular skin lesions; lymphadenopathy; conjunctivitis.
Cerebrospinal fluid	For removal, see p. 104. Submit for IgG study and prepare smear.	Antispirochete IgG; lymphocytes and plasma cells *(1)*.
Blood	Obtain blood for chemical and serologic analysis.	Elevated liver enzymes; elevated IgM early in illness; normal or elevated C3 and C4; rheumatoid factor usually absent.
Joints	Aspirate fluid from joint effusions. Submit synovium of affected joints for histologic study.	Neutrophils in synovial fluid; synovitis resembling early rheumatoid arthritis with a distinctive arteritis with onionskin-like lesions; later in the disease, cartilage destruction.
Heart	Submit sections for histologic study (p. 30).	Myocarditis; spirochetes may be demonstrable.
Liver	Submit sections for histologic study.	Dense portal infiltrates.
Brain and spinal cord	For removal and specimen preparation, see pp. 65 and 67, respectively. Include meninges in histologic sections.	Mononuclear meningitis and meningoradiculitis.

Reference

1. Sindern E, Malin JP. Phenotypic analysis of cerebrospinal fluid cells over the course of Lyme meningoradiculitis. Acta Cytol 1995;39:73–75.

Disease, Lymphatic

NOTE: In all diseases of the thoracic duct and its major tributaries and also in cases of lymphedema or other peripheral lymphovascular diseases, postmortem lymphangiography (p. 34) may be an effective method of study.

Disease, Maple Syrup Urine

Synonyms and Related Terms: Branched-chain hyperaminoacidemia (various types); classic maple syrup urine disease; hyperleucinemia; hypervalinemia. See also aminoaciduria.*

NOTE: Collect all obtainable urine and freeze at –20°C; this should be done as soon as possible.

Organs and Tissues	*Procedures*	*Possible or Expected Findings*
Blood and urine	Submit samples for biochemical study.	Increased amino acids and urinary organic acids. The urine may have a "maple syrup" odor.
Fascia lata (or skin)	Submit sample for karyotype and biochemical analysis (p. 109).	Enzyme deficiency can be demonstrated in cultured fibroblasts, leukocytes, or amniocytes.
Other organs		Bronchopneumonia. Steatosis or increased glycogen deposition in liver.
Brain and spinal cord	For removal and specimen preparation, see p. 65 and 67, respectively.	Spongiosis; gliosis; edema; defective myelinization.

Disease, Marble Bone (See "Osteopetrosis.")

Disease, Marchiafava-Bignami

NOTE: Patients with this disease suffer from chronic alcoholism. Malnutrition, nutritional amblyopia,* and Wernicke-Korsakoff syndrome* may be present.

Organs and Tissues	*Procedures*	*Possible or Expected Findings*
Brain and spinal cord	For removal and specimen preparation, see pp. 65 and 67, respectively. Request Luxol fast blue stain for myelin (p. 172).	Symmetric and zonal demyelination in corpus callosum, anterior commissure, optic chiasm, optic tracts, and white matter of frontal lobes.

Disease, Mast Cell (See "Mastocytosis, systemic.")

Disease, Medullary Cystic Renal (See "Cyst(s), renal.")

Disease, Meningococcal

Synonyms: Meningococcemia; *Neisseria meningitidis* infection; Waterhouse-Friderichsen syndrome (fulminant meningococcemia).

NOTE: (1) Submit all tissues that appear to be infected (2). Request aerobic bacterial cultures. (3) Request Gram stain (p. 172). (4) Special **precautions** are indicated (p. 146). (5) Usually, serologic studies are not available. However, isolates should be segregated by seroagglutination into serogroups, i.e., A,B,C,D,X,Y,Z. (6) This is a **reportable** disease.

Possible Associated Conditions: Disseminated intravascular coagulation* is a common component of the disease.

Organs and Tissues	*Procedures*	*Possible or Expected Findings*
External examination and skin	Record extent of skin lesions and prepare photographs; submit tissue samples of skin for histologic study.	Cutaneous or subcutaneous hemorrhages (purpura fulminans, with or without skin loss and deep muscle damage *(1)*); herpes labialis; rarely, jaundice.
	Prepare skeletal roentgenograms if bone lesions are expected.	Osteomyelitis and osteonecrosis (see below) *(2)*.
Cerebrospinal fluid	Submit sample for aerobic bacterial culture (p. 104).	
Blood	Submit sample for microbiologic study (p. 102) and determination of serum cortisol concentration.	Meningococcal septicemia. Low serum cortisol level.
Heart and pericardial fluid	Submit samples of pericardium, pericardial fluid, and myocardium for aerobic bacterial cultures and Gram stain (p. 172). For procedures in infective endocarditis, see p. 103.	Pericarditis.* Infective endocarditis.*
Lungs	Submit consolidated areas for culture (p. 103).	Primary or secondary pneumonia; pleuritis.
Spleen	Record weight and submit tissue specimens for histologic study.	Splenitis.
Adrenal glands	Photograph; record weights; request Gram stain for histologic sections (p. 172).	Acute hemorrhage and necrosis.
Genital organs	Submit tissue samples for histologic study.	Urethritis; orchitis; epididymitis; endometritis.
Brain and spinal cord	Infectious material should be obtained as described on p. 104. For removal and specimen preparation of brain and spinal cord, see pp. 65 and 67, respectively. Request Bodian stain (p. 74).	Scant exudate with numerous bacteria in the hyperacute form; In the acute form, abundant pus surrounds the entire brain, vertex, and base and may extend to the ventricular system. In the chronic form, communicating hydrocephalus and cortical infarction are common complications.
Middle and inner ears	For removal and specimen preparation, see p. 72.	Otitis media.*

Organs and Tissues	Procedures	Possible or Expected Findings
Nasopharynx	For exposure, see p. 71. Prepare smears and submit tissue samples for histologic study.	Posterior nasopharyngeal meningococcal infection.
Eyes	For removal and specimen preparation, see p. 85.	Conjunctivitis; panophthalmitis.
Bones, joints, and soft tissues	Remove synovial fluid and submit sample for bacteriologic study (p. 96). For removal of bones and joints, prosthetic repair, and specimen preparation, see pp. 95–97, respectively. Prepare histologic sections of synovia and skeletal muscle.	Purulent arthritis; necrosis and hemorrhage of synovia. Osteonecrosis (rare in adults *[2]*) and osteomyelitis; rhabdomyolysis *(3)*.

References

1. Huang S, Clarke JA. Severe skin loss after meningococcal septicemia: complications in treatment. Acta Paediatr 1997;86:1263–1266.
2. Campbell WN, Joshi M, Sileo D. Osteonecrosis following meningococcemia and disseminated intravascular coagulation in an adult: case report and review. Clin Infect Dis 1997;24:452–455.
3. Van Deuren M, Neeleman C, Assmann KJ, Wetzels JF, van der Meer JW. Rhabdomyolysis during the subacute stage of meningococcal sepsis. Clin Infect Dis 1998;26:214–215.

Disease, Motor Neuron

Synonyms and Related Terms: Atrophy, progressive spinal muscular; infantile spinal muscular atrophy; Werdnig-Hoffman disease.

Organs and Tissues	Procedures	Possible or Expected Findings
External examination		Congenital fixation of multiple joints of extremities.
Brain and spinal cord	For removal and specimen preparation, see pp. 65 and 67, respectively.	Degeneration and loss of motor neurons from anterior horn and brainstem motor nuclei (particularly hypoglossal and facial) and thalamus (posteroventral nucleus).
Skeletal muscles	For sampling and specimen preparation, see p. 80.	Neurogenic atrophy.

Disease, Multicystic Renal (See "Cyst(s), renal.")

Disease, Niemann-Pick

Synonyms and Related Terms: Sphingomyelinase deficiency; sphingomyelin lipidosis; Niemann-Pick disease, types A, B, C, or D.

NOTE: For further details on specimen preparation, see ref. *(1)*.

Organs and Tissues	Procedures	Possible or Expected Findings
External examination and fascia lata	If diagnosis must be confirmed, prepare fibroblast culture for assay of sphingomyelinase (p. 109).	Growth retardation.
Skin and conjunctiva	Prepare samples for electron microscopic study (see p. 132).	Membrane-bound lamellar cytoplasmic inclusions.
Heart		Endocardial fibroelastosis.
Lungs	In infants, snap-freeze portion of fresh lung and perfuse one lung with formalin (p. 47). Submit consolidated areas for microbiologic study (p. 103).	Vacuolated histiocytes (foam cells) containing sphingomyelin, cholesterol, and ganglioside within alveoli and interstitium. Acute or organizing bronchopneumonia.
Liver and spleen	Record sizes and weights; snap-freeze tissue for biochemical sphingomyelin determination. Special stains of frozen sections for phospholipids and cholesterol are positive but not diagnostic.	Hepatosplenomegaly; foam cell transformation of Kupffer cells and hepatocytes; cholestasis; intra-acinar fibrosis and, rarely, cirrhosis. Hepatocellular giant cells may be present. Abundant foam cells in spleen.

Organs and Tissues	Procedures	Possible or Expected Findings
Liver and spleen *(continued)*	Submit sample for electron microscopic study (p. 132).	Laminated inclusions in the cytoplasm of affected cells.
Other organs		Transformation of reticuloendothelial cells to autofluorescent foam cells.
Bone marrow	For preparation of sections and smears, see p. 96. Prepare sample for electron microscopic study (p. 132). Prepare unstained smears for phase-contrast microscopy.	"Sea-blue" histiocytes may be present in variant forms of the disease. Lipid-laden cells have membrane-bound lamellar cytoplasmic inclusions.
Brain and spinal cord	For removal and specimen preparation, see pp. 65 and 67, respectively. See also under "Liver and spleen."	In the infantile form but not in the childhood form of the disease, neurons are distended with lipid. Eventually, neuronal loss, gliosis, and demyelination occur. Cerebral atrophy; neurons with inclusion; neuronal loss; gliosis and demyelination.
Eyes	For removal and specimen preparation, see p. 85.	In the infantile form of the disease, retinal degeneration.

Reference

1. Jevon GP, Dimmick JE. Histopathologic approach to metabolic liver disease. Persp Pediatr Pathol 1998;1:179–199.

Disease, Ollier's (See "Dyschondroplasia, Ollier's.")

Disease, Osler-Rendu-Weber

Synonyms: Hereditary familial angiomatosis; hereditary hemorrhagic telangiectasia.

Organs and Tissues	Procedures	Possible or Expected Findings
External examination and skin; oral cavity	Record distribution of skin lesions and submit tissue samples for histologic study.	Telangiectatic (often papular) lesions most commonly found in cheeks, scalp, nasal orifices, oral cavity, ears, neck, shoulders, fingers, toes, and nail beds. Cyanosis and clubbing may be prominent.
Lungs	For preparation of angiograms or corrosion casts of the pulmonary arterial and venous vasculature, see pp. 50 and 51, respectively.	Arteriovenous malformations/fistulas.
Aorta	If aneurysm or dissection is present, follow procedures described under those headings.	Aneurysm;* aortic dissection.*
Mesenteric vasculature	Prepare mesenteric angiograms (p. 55).	Mesenteric arteriovenous fistulas; aneurysms of the splenic and hepatic arteries; arteriovenous malformations of the colon.
Gastrointestinal tract	For demonstration of esophageal varices, see p. 53.	Telangiectasias in stomach and intestinal tract; see also above under "Mesenteric vasculature." Gastrointestinal hemorrhage.*
Liver	If cirrhosis is present, prepare angiograms of hepatic arteries and veins (p. 56). For preparation of corrosion casts of hepatic arteries, portal veins, and hepatic veins, see p. 57. Photograph and prepare sections of angiomatous lesions.	Hepatohepatic or hepatoportal arteriovenous malformations/fistulas with cirrhosis-like changes. Cavernous hemangiomas.
Urinary bladder and internal sex organs		Telangiectatic lesions.

Organs and Tissues	Procedures	Possible or Expected Findings
Brain and spinal cord	For removal and specimen preparation, see pp. 65 and 67, respectively. For preparation of cerebral arteriograms, see p. 80.	Arteriovenous malformations; aneurysms of cerebral arteries.* Brain abscess.*
Eyes	For removal and specimen preparation, see p. 85.	Retinal arteriovenous malformations.
Nasal cavities	For exposure, see p. 71.	Telangiectatic lesions.
Bone marrow		Hyperplasia (in patients with polycythemia).

Disease, Paget's, of Bone

Synonym: Osteitis deformans.

Organs and Tissues	Procedures	Possible or Expected Findings
External examination	Prepare skeletal roentgenograms.	Most commonly involved are sacrum, pelvic bones, tibia, and femur. Skull and other parts of the skeleton may also be affected.
Bones	For removal, prosthetic repair, and specimen preparation, see p. 95. If there was a history of cranial nerve palsies, measure diameter of corresponding bony apertures. If there were symptoms of paraplegia, expose and measure diameter of vertebral foramina. For maceration of bone, see p. 97.	Kyphosis; deformities of long bones; osteosarcomas and other malignant tumors *(1,2)*. See also under "Tumor of bone or cartilage." Thickening of calvarium (Fig. 8-1, p. 98). Accelerated osteoarthritis of joints in the vicinity of Paget's disease of bone *(3)*.
Heart		Cardiac hypertrophy.*
Other organs		Manifestations of congestive heart failure.*
Parathyroid glands	Record weights and submit samples for histologic study.	Normal size and histologic appearance.

References

1. Brandolini F, Bacchini P, Moscato M, Bertoni F. Chondrosarcoma as a complicating factor in Paget's disease of bone. Skeletal Radiol 1997;26:497–500.
2. Yu T, Squires F, Mammone J, DiMarcangelo M. Lymphoma arising in Paget's disease. Skeletal Radiol 1997;26:729–731.
3. Helliwell PS. Osteoarthritis and Paget's disease. Br J Rheumatol 1995; 34:1061–1063.

Disease, Parainfluenza Viral (See "Laryngitis.")

Disease, Parkinson's

Synonyms and Related Terms: Idiopathic Parkinson's disease; paralysis agitans.

NOTE: Parkinson's syndrome is caused by conditions that may simulate Parkinson's disease; these include carbon monoxide* and manganese poisoning, corticobasal degeneration, drug-induced parkinsonism, Huntington's disease, multiple system atrophy,* progressive supranuclear palsy* (Steele-Richardson-Olszewski syndrome), space-occupying lesions (rare), trauma (dementia pugilistica), and causes related to tumors and vascular diseases.

Organs and Tissues	Procedures	Possible or Expected Findings
Brain	For removal and specimen preparation, see p. 65. Histologic sections should include midbrain (substantia nigra), upper pons (locus ceruleus), medulla, nucleus basalis (substantia innominata), and basal ganglia. If Parkinsonian syndrome was diagnosed, follow procedures described under the name of the suspected underlying condition (see above under "Note").	Depigmentation of substantia nigra and locus coeruleus; neuronal loss and reactive gliosis; eosinophilic intracytoplasmic inclusion bodies (Lewy bodies) in some of the surviving neurons; no significant changes in basal ganglia.

Disease, Pelizaeus-Merzbacher

Synonyms: Sudanophilic (orthochromatic) leukodystrophy.

Organs and Tissues	Procedures	Possible or Expected Findings
Brain and spinal cord	For removal and specimen preparation, see pp. 66 and 70, respectively. Request Luxol fast blue/PAS stain for myelin and Bielschowsky's stain for axons (p. 172). Prepare frozen sections for Sudan stain.	Brain generally atrophic. Myelin loss in centrum ovale, cerebellum, and part of brain stem, with a tigroid pattern of residual myelin near vessels. Axons are preserved. Diffuse gliosis with relatively few lipoid-containing macrophages, compared to the myelin loss. Lipoid material stains with Sudan.

Disease, Periodic (See "Fever, familial Mediterranean.")

Disease, Perthes' (See "Osteonecrosis.")

Disease, Pick's

Synonym: Pick's lobar atrophy.

Organs and Tissues	Procedures	Possible or Expected Findings
Brain and spinal cord	For removal and specimen preparation, see pp. 65 and 67, respectively. Request silver stains (Bielchowsky or Bodian stain), (p. 172). Histochemical stains in Pick's cells and bodies reveal phosphorylated neurofilaments, ubiquitin, and tubulin. Some tissue should be kept frozen for biochemical studies.	Severe cerebral atrophy, involving primarily frontal and anterior temporal lobes (knife-blade atrophy; walnut brain). Microscopically, severe neuronal loss accompanied by astrocytosis. Characteristic argyrophilic, intracytoplasmic inclusions (Pick's bodies), particularly in hippocampus and swollen, distended "ballooned" neurons (Pick's cells). These changes are not always present.

Disease, Polycystic Kidney (See "Cyst(s), renal.")

Disease, Polycystic Liver (See "Disease, fibropolycystic, of the liver and biliary tract.")

Disease, Prion (See "Disease, Creutzfeldt-Jakob.")

Disease, Pulmonary Veno-Occlusive (See "Obstruction, pulmonary venous.")

Disease, Pulseless (See "Arteritis, Fahayasu's.")

Disease, Raynaud's

Related Term: Raynaud's phenomenon.

Organs and Tissues	Procedures	Possible or Expected Findings
External examination	Record extent of ischemic lesions.	Sclerodactyly; necrosis of fingertips; rarely, ischemic necroses on toes, ears, nose, cheeks, and chin.
Chest cavity and upper extremity	Dissect upper mediastinal, supraclavicular, and axillary soft tissues. Subclavian or axillar arteriograms can be prepared at this time. Tissue samples of brachial, ulnar, radial, and digital arteries can be submitted after embalming (consult with funeral director first).	Thoracic outlet compression by tumor or other lesions; thromboangiitis obliterans (Buerger's disease*); arteriosclerosis obliterans; arterial emboli; mural thrombosis of heart.
Abdominal cavity and lower extremity	Submit tissue samples for histologic study of aorta and other elastic arteries, muscular arteries, and veins. For angiography of lower extremities, see p. 120. For removal of femoral vessels, see p. 34.	Thromboangiitis and arteriosclerosis obliterans.

Organs and Tissues	Procedures	Possible or Expected Findings
Other organs		Systemic sclerosis* or other immune connective tissue diseases may be present.
Brain and spinal cord	For removal and specimen preparation, see pp. 65 and 67, respectively.	Poliomyelitis;* syringomyelia.*

Disease, Recklinghausen's (See "Hyperparathyroidism" and "Neurofibromatosis.")

Disease, Refsum

Synonym: Phytanoyl-coenzyme A hydroxylase deficiency.

NOTE: This peroxisomal disorder may occur in adults but also in an infantile form where it may be a cause of neonatal cholestatic jaundice. For a current review, see ref. *(1)*.

Organs and Tissues	Procedures	Possible or Expected Findings
External examination, skin, and adipose tissue		Ichthyosis. Phytanic acid accumulation in adipose tissues.
Blood	Submit sample for determinaion of phytanic acid concentration.	Phytanic acidemia.
Cerebrospinal fluid	For obtaining a sample, see p. 104.	Increased protein concentrations.
Heart		Cardiomyopathy.*
Liver and kidneys	Sample for histologic study.	Phytanic acid accumulation.
Brain, spinal cord, and peripheral nerves	For removal and specimen preparation, see pp. 65, 67, and 79, respectively.	Axonal neuropathy.
Eyes	For removal and specimen preparation, see p. 85.	Retinitis pigmentosa.

Reference

1. Hochner I, Blickle JF, Brogard JM. La maladie de Refsum. Revue Med Interne 1996; 17:391–398.

Disease, Schilder's (See "Sclerosis, Schilder's cerebral.")

Disease, Schüller-Christian (See "Histiocytosis, Langerhans cell.")

Disease, Sheehan's (See "Insufficiency, pituitary.")

Disease, Sickle Cell

Synonyms and Related Terms: Hemolytic anemia;* sickle cell anemia; sickle cell crisis.

NOTE: See also under "Anemia, hemolytic" and—if applicable—under "Exposure, cold," "Hypoxia," or the name of the infection that may have precipitated a fatal sickle cell crisis. Sickling of erythrocytes may be produced by formalin fixation, in the absence of sickle cell disease. If complications of transfusions or bone marrow transplantation *(1)* are expected, see under those headings.

Organs and Tissues	Procedures	Possible or Expected Findings
External examination	Record body weight, length, and habitus.	Asthenic habitus; jaundice; skin ulcers over malleoli.
	Prepare skeletal roentgenograms.	Abnormal trabeculations and infarctions of bone; osteonecrosis* of heads of femora or humeri; deformities of metacarpals, metatarsals, and phalanges; elevation of periosteum; widening of marrow cavities.
Blood	Submit sample for culture, toxicologic study, hemoglobin electrophoresis, and determination of bilirubin level. Prepare smears.	Bacteremia; septicemia; presence of hemoglobin S; hyperbilirubinemia.
Heart		Cardiomegaly; cor pulmonale.
Lungs	Submit one lobe for microbiologic study (p. 103).	Pneumonia (various types); embolism;* infarctions.
Liver	Record weight. Request Gomori's iron stain (p. 172).	Heptocellular ischemic necrosis caused by accumulation of erythrocytes in sinuses; sinusoidal dilatation *(2)*.
Gallbladder and common bile duct	Describe appearance of stones or request chemical analysis.	Cholelithiasis;* cholecystitis;* choledocholithiasis.

Organs and Tissues	Procedures	Possible or Expected Findings
Spleen	Record weight.	In infants, splenomegaly; in adults, infarctions and fibrosis.
Kidneys, renal veins, bladder ureters, and urinary bladder	Open renal veins *in situ*; section kidneys in frontal plane and prepare photographs.	Infarctions; papillary necroses; renal vein thrombosis;* renal failure;* urinary tract infection.
Penis	Submit tissue samples for histologic study of corpora cavernosa (p. 60).	Priapism.
Other organs		Manifestations of congestive heart failure* and of hemolytic anemia.*
Bones and bone marrow	For removal, prosthetic repair, and specimen preparation of bone, see p. 95. For preparation of sections and smears of bone marrow, see p. 96.	Hyperplastic bone marrow; megaloblastic changes.
	For microbiologic study of osteomyelitis, see p. 102. Consult roentgenograms for proper sampling.	*Salmonella* osteomyelitis.*
Eyes	For removal and specimen preparation, see p. 85.	Angioid streaks; anterior segment necrosis; inferior conjunctival capillary abnormalities; retinopathy; central vitreous hemorrhage.

References

1. Lane PA. Sickle cell disease. Pediatr Clin North Am 1996;43:639–664.
2. Charlotte F, Bachir D, Nenert M, et al. Vascular lesions of the liver in sickle cell disease. A clinicopathologic study in 26 living patients. Arch Pathol Lab Med 1995;119:46–52.

Disease, Silo-Filler's (See "Edema, chemical pulmonary.")

Disease, Still's (See "Arthritis, juvenile rheumatoid.")

Disease, Sturge-Weber-Dimitri

Synonym: Encephalotrigeminal angiomatosis; encephalofacial angiomatosis.

Organs and Tissues	Procedures	Possible or Expected Findings
External examination	Descibe extent of facial angioma, and photograph. Prepare roentgenogram of skull. Record appearance of limbs.	Facial angioma; unilateral exophthalmos; hemiatrophy of skull; linear cortical cerebral calcifications. Hypoplasia of limb.
Brain and spinal cord	For removal and specimen preparation, see pp. 65 and 67, respectively. Photograph surface and coronal slices of brain. Prepare roentgenograms of whole brain and of slices to demonstrate calcifications. Submit tissue samples for histologic study of vascular lesions.	Excessive unilateral capillary and venous-type vessels in leptomeninges; calcification within underlying cortex of one hemisphere that may be atrophic (ipsilateral to facial angioma) *(1)*.
Eyes	For removal and specimen preparation, see p. 85.	Choroidal hemangioma; manifestations of congenital glaucoma.

Reference

1. Harding B, Copp AJ. Pathology of Malformations. In: Greenfield's Neuropathology, vol. I. Graham BI, Lantos BL, eds. Arnold, London, 1997, pp. 397–507.

Disease, Takayasu's (See "Arteritis, Takayasu's.")

Disease, Tangier

Synonyms: Alpha-lipoprotein deficiency; familial high-density lipoprotein deficiency.

Organs and Tissues	Procedures	Possible or Expected Findings
Blood	Submit sample for electrophoretic and immunochemical analysis.	Hypoalphalipoproteinemia.
Lymph nodes	Submit samples for histologic study; snap-freeze samples for histochemical study and prepare specimens for electron microscopy (p. 132).	Lymphadenopathy with diffuse deposition of cholesterol esters.
Heart; elastic and muscular arteries		Premature atherosclerotic cardiovascular disease *(1)*.
Liver and spleen	Record weights. For preparation of specimens, see above under "Lymph nodes."	Hepatosplenomegaly with foam cells.
Neck organs and pharynx	If pharyngeal tonsils cannot be removed with neck organs, attempts should be made to take samples perorally. For preparation of specimens, see above under "Lymph nodes."	Enlarged tonsils with characteristic orange discoloration.
Peripheral nerves	For removal and specimen preparation, see p. 79.	Polyneuropathy *(2)*.
Eyes	For removal and specimen preparation, see p. 85.	In adults, corneal infiltrates.
Bone marrow	For preparation of sections and smears, see p. 95 and above under "Lymph nodes."	Foam cells.

References

1. Vega GL, Grundy SM. Hypoalphalipoproteinemia (low density lipoprotein) as a risk factor for coronary heart disease. Curr Opin Lipidol 1996;7:209–216.
2. Case Rec Mass Gen Hosp. Case 16-1996. A 36-year-old woman with bilateral facial and hand weakness and impaired truncal sensation [clinical conference]. N Engl J Med 1996;334:1389–1394.

Disease, Tay-Sachs (See "Gangliosidosis.")

Disease, Thomsen's (See "Myotonia congenita [Thomsen's disease].")

Disease, Valvular Heart (See "Insufficiency,..." and "Stenosis,..." For congenital valvular diseases, see also under "Valve, congenitally...and name of specific malformation.)

Disease, Veno-Occlusive, of Liver

NOTE: Follow procedures described under "Syndrome, Budd-Chiari." Most cases of fatal veno-occlusive disease in the USA are drug-induced *(1)*.

Reference

1. Culic S, de Kraker J, Kuljis D, Kuzmic I, Saraga M, Culic V, et al. Fatal hepatic veno-occlusive disease with fibrinolysis as the cause of death during preoperative chemotherapy for nephroblastoma. Med Pediatr Oncol 1998;31:175–176.

Disease, Veno-occlusive, of Lung (See "Hypertension, pulmonary.")

Disease, von Gierke's (See "Disease, glycogen storage.")

Disease, von Hippel-Lindau

NOTE: The gene for the disease has been identified. Type I VHL-disease without pheochromocytoma and type II VHL-disease with pheochromocytoma result from different mutations.

Organs and Tissues	Procedures	Possible or Expected Findings
Pancreas and kidneys; other organs		Cysts;* renal cell carcinoma; papillary cystadenoma of the epidydimis.
Adrenal glands	See "Tumor of the adrenal glands."	Pheochromocytoma.
Brain and spinal cord	For removal and specimen preparation, see p. 65 and p. 67, respectively. For cerebral arteriography, see p. 80.	Hemangioblastoma in cerebellum, medulla, and spinal cord, very rarely involving supratentorial area or peripheral nerve.
Eyes	For removal and specimen preparation, see p. 85.	Retinal angiomatosis.

Disease, von Recklinghausen's (See "Hyperparathyroidism" and "Neurofibromatosis.")

Disease, von Willebrand's

Synonyms: Factor VIII deficiency; vascular hemophilia.

NOTE: Follow procedures described under "Hemophilia." The expected findings are essentially the same as in classic hemophilia. However, hemarthrosis is rare in von Willebrand's disease.

Disease, Vrolik's (See "Osteogenesis imperfecta.")

Disease, Waldenström's (See "Macroglobulinemia, Waldenström's.")

Disease, Weber-Christian

NOTE: This probably is not a specific entity but represents panniculitis, which may be an incidental finding or part of a systemic disease. For further details, see under "Panniculitis."

Disease, Werdnig-Hoffmann (See "Disease, motor neuron.")

Disease, Whipple's

Organs and Tissues	*Procedures*	*Possible or Expected Findings*
External examination and skin	Record body weight and length and extent and character of pigmentation and edema. Submit skin samples for histologic study.	Emaciation. Hyperpigmentation, particularly of exposed skin and in scars. Hyperkeratosis.
Joints	If joints are swollen, remove synovial fluid for cell counts and smears. See also below under "Other organs and tissues."	Arthritis involving ankles, knees, shoulders, and wrists.
Abdominal cavity	Record character and volume of fluid, submit sample for microbiologic study, and prepare smears of sediment. Prepare sections of small intestinal serosa and of parietal peritoneum. Request PAS stain (p. 172). In granulomas, bacilli are not always PAS positive *(2)*.	Ascites; fibrinous peritonitis.* Nodules in peritoneum containing sickle-form particle-containing cells (SPC cells). For a classification of the bacillus, see ref. *(1) Tropheryma whippelii.*
Heart	For collection of histologic samples, see p. 30. Include all grossly involved tissues. For preparation for electron microscopy, see p. 132. Request PAS stain of paraffin sections (p. 173).	Pancarditis; SPC cells in cardiac valves, interstitium of ventricles and atria, and pericardium. Fibrous-adhesive pericarditis; myocardial fibrosis; endocarditis with valvular fibrosis.
Lungs	Perfuse one lung with formalin (p. 47).	SPC cells in parenchymal stroma and visceral pleura.
Intestine and mesentery	For *in situ* fixation and preparation for study in dissecting microscope, see p. 54. Submit tissue samples of various segments of intestinal wall; request PAS stain (p. 173). Submit portions of mucosa and of mesenteric lymph nodes for electron microscopy (p. 132). If immunofluorescent studies are intended, snap-freeze tissue samples.	SPC cells, primarily in lamina propria of villi; villous atrophy; thickening of intestinal wall. Rod-shaped bacillary bodies and serpiginous membranes in cytoplasm of SPC cells or extracellularly. Mesenteric lymphadenitis with SPC cells, granulomas, and giant cells.
Other organs and tissues	Submit tissue samples for histologic study of all gross lesions and—even in the absence of macroscopic changes—of esophagus, stomach, colon, spleen, pancreas, retroperitoneal soft tissues, kidneys, adrenal glands, urinary bladder, peripheral and other extramesenteric lymph nodes, brain, spinal cord, synovium with joint capsules, bone marrow, and skeletal muscles. For histologic techniques, see above under "Intestine and mesentery."	Characteristic SPC cells can occur in practically all organs and tissues, particularly in capsule and portal areas of spleen, interstitium of pancreas, stomach, retroperitoneal organs and tissues, lymph nodes, and central nervous system. Myopathy may occur.

References

1. Dutly F, Altwegg M. Whipple's disease and "Tropheryma whippelii." Clin Microbiol Rev 2001;14:561–583.
2. Wilcox GM, Tronic BS, Schecter DJ, Arron MJ, Righi DF, Weiner NJ. Periodic acid-Schiff-negative granulomatous lymphadenopathy in patient with Whipple's disease. Localization of the Whipple bacillus to noncaseating granulomas by electron microscopy. Am J Med 1987;83:165–170.

Disease, Willebrand's (See "Disease, von Willebrand's.")

Disease, Wilson's

Synonym: Hepatolenticular degeneration.
NOTE: For the gene defect, see ref. *(1)*.

Organs and Tissues	*Procedures*	*Possible or Expected Findings*
External examination and skin	Record character and extent of pigmentation; submit skin samples for histologic study.	Jaundice; hyperpigmentation of anterior aspects of lower legs; blue lunnulae of nails; increased fingerprint "whorl" pattern.
	Prepare skeletal roentgenograms.	See below under "Bones and joints."
Blood	Submit sample for biochemical study and for hemoglobin electrophoresis.	Low ceruloplasmin concentration (<20 mg/dL); normal or decreased serum copper concentrations. Hemolytic anemia and increase in hemoglobin A_2.
Urine		Increased copper (>100 µg Cu in 24 h) excretion, but single specimen of little use.
Lung		See below under "Kidneys."
Liver	Record weight and photograph. Tissue copper concentrations can be determined from sample in paraffin block *(2)*. Request rhodanine stain for copper (p. 173).	Fatty changes, periportal hepatitis or cirrhosis,* depending on stage of disease. Rarely massive hepatic necrosis. Stainable copper in many but not all specimens. Tissue copper concentrations >250 µg/g dry wt.
Kidneys	See above under "Liver."	Copper in proximal tubules; tubular fatty changes.
Other organs and tissues		Increased copper in skeletal muscles.
Brain and spinal cord	For removal and specimen preparation, see pp. 65 and 67, respectively. If biochemical copper determination is intended, see above under "Liver."	Symmetrical dilatation of lateral ventricles; discoloration of striatum, often with cavitation of putamen. Thalamic and cortical involvement is common. Microscopically, neuronal loss and gliosis, among other possible abnormalities *(3)*. Alzheimer's type 2 cells increased. Copper deposition primarily perivascular.
Eyes	For removal and specimen preparation, see p. 85. For copper staining, use rhodanine method (p. 173).	Copper of Kayser-Fleischer ring lies in Descemet's membrane. Copper-containing foreign bodies are found in posterior layer of lens capsule.
Bones and joints	For removal, prosthetic repair, and specimen preparation, see p. 95.	Osteoarthritis;* bone fragmentation; osteochrondritis of the vertebral column; osteochondritis dissecans of knees and ankles.

References

1. Bull PC, Thomas GR, Rommens JM, Forbes JR, Cox DW. The Wilson's disease gene is a putative copper transporting P-type ATPase similar to Menke's gene. Nature Genet 1993;5:327–337.
2. Ludwig J,, Moyer TP, Rakela J. The liver biopsy diagnosis of Wilson's disease. Methods in pathology. Am J Clin Pathol 1994;102:443–446.
3. Harper C, Butterworth R. Hepatolenticular degeneration (Wilson's disease). In: Greenfield's Neuropathology, vol. 1. Graham BI, Lantos PL, eds. Arnold, London, 1997, pp. 632–633.

Disorder, Coagulation (See "Coagulation, disseminated intravascular," "Disease, Christmas," "Disease, von Willebrand's," "Hemophilia," and "Purpura,...")

Disorder, Electrolyte(s)

Organs and Tissues	*Procedures*	*Possible or Expected Findings*
Vitreous	Submit sample for determination of sodium, potassium, chloride, glucose, urea nitrogen, and creatinine concentrations (p. 85). Calcium and phosphate concentrations can also be tested. If sample is small, indicate priority for testing.	Considerably increased or decreased values for sodium (more than 155 meq/L or less than 130 meq/L) and chloride (more than 135 meq/L or less than 105 meq/L) indicate that changes were present before death. For further interpretation, see p. 113.
Blood		Postmortem electrolyte concentrations are quite unreliable (see p. 113).
Urine	If indicated, submit sample for chemical study.	May be useful for calcium determination.
Kidneys	Submit tissue samples for histologic study.	Vacuolar nephropathy (vacuolar changes in proximal convoluted tubules) in potassium deficiency (may also occur after infusion of hypertonic solutions).

Disorder, Hemorrhagic
(See "Coagulation, disseminated intravascular," "Disease, Christmas," "Disease, von Willebrand's," "Hemophilia," and "Purpura,...")

Disorder, Inherited, of Phagocyte Function

NOTE: Several conditions represent phagocyte function disorders. Autopsy procedures for one of these disorders can be found under "Disease, chronic granulomatous." Consult this entry for other phagocyte function disorders.

Disorder, Lysosomal Storage

Synonyms and Related Terms: Fabry's disease* (angiokeratoma corporis diffusum); gangliosidosis;* Gaucher's disease;* glycogenosis,* type II; leukodystrophies (Krabbe's or globoid cell,* metachromatic leukoencephalopathy*); mucopolysaccharidoses* (Hunter, Hurler, Morquio, and Sanfilippo disease); mucolipidosis; Niemann Pick disease* (type A, B, C, or sphingomyelinase deficiency); neuraminidase deficiency; neuronal ceroid lipofuscinosis (Batten's disease or Kufs' disease).

Organs and Tissues	*Procedures*	*Possible or Expected Findings*
External examination	Obtain routine body measurements and weights. Photograph all abnormalities Prepare skeletal roentgenograms.	Coarse facial features are frequently present. Corneal clouding. Skeletal abnormalities may be present.
Fascia lata	Prepare specimen for fibroblast culture (see p. 109), for enzyme assay, and for electron microscopy.	See entries listed under "Synonyms and Related Terms."
Other organs and tissues (including bone marrow)	Record weights. See also below under "Brain and spinal cord."	Storage deposits in histiocytes ("sea-blue histiocytes" in Niemann-Pick disease); heart, liver, spleen (with hepatosplenomegaly), and kidneys may be involved.
Brain and spinal cord	For removal and specimen preparation, see pp. 66 and 70, respectively. Request LFB/PAS stain (p. 172). Submit samples for electron microscopy (p. 132). Store fresh/frozen tissue for enzyme assay or molecular genetic studies.	Atrophy. Cellular storage in neurons, histiocytes, and other cells. For possible storage sites, see under name of specific disorder.

Reference

1. Lake B. Lysosomal and peroxisomal disorders. In: Greenfield's Neuropathology, vol. 1. Graham BI, Lantos PL, eds. Arnold, London, 1997, pp. 658–753.

Disorder, Myeloproliferative (See "Leukemia, all types or type unspecified," "Myelofibrosis with myeloid metaplasia," and "Polycythemia.")

Disorder, Plasma Cell (See "Amyloidosis," "Disease, heavy chain," "Macroglobulinemia, Waldenström's," and "Myeloma, multiple.")

Dissection, Aortic

Synonym: Dissecting aortic aneurysm; dissecting aortic hematoma.

Organs and Tissues	*Procedures*	*Possible or Expected Findings*
External examination	Record and photograph abnormal features (see right-hand column). Prepare chest roentgenogram.	Features of Marfan's syndrome* or Turner's syndrome.* Widened aorta or mediastinum.
Pericardium	Record appearance and volume of contents.	Hemopericardium.
Aorta	Remove heart and major arteries attached to intact aorta. Open aorta along posterior midline. Photograph intimal tears and record their location and size. Record external rupture site, if possible, and extent of mediastinal or retroperitoneal hemorrhage. Record location and volume of blood in "false" lumen and presence or absence of intramural hematoma, not connected to lumen. Record location and size of re-entry tear, if present.	Coarctation of the aorta.* Dissection may involve major branches of aorta. Blood may be present in periaortic tissues and pericardium (see above). Intimal tear is most commonly located in ascending thoracic aorta. False lumen occurs with or without tear of reentry. The aorta may be atherosclerotic. In the descending thoracic or abdominal aorta, an intimal tear may involve an ulcerated plaque (penetrating ulcer).
	Request Verhoeff–van Gieson and PAS-alcian blue stains (p. 173).	Cystic medial degeneration of aorta. Rarely, giant cell aortitis.
	Sections should include grossly involved and uninvolved portions of aortic wall and of adjacent elastic arteries.	
Heart	Procedures depend on expected findings or grossly identified abnormalities as listed in right-hand column.	Congenitally bicuspid aortic valve.* Concentric left ventricular hypertrophy. Myxomatous mitral valve.
Other organs		Manifestations of hypertension* or of third-trimester pregnancy.
Brain and spinal cord	For removal and specimen preparation of brain and spinal cord, see pp. 65 and 67, respectively.	Ischemic lesions in brain and spinal cord and in other organs.

Diverticula

Related Terms: Diverticular disease; diverticulitis; diverticulosis; Meckel's diverticulum; pulsion diverticulum; traction diverticulum; Zenker's diverticulum.

Organs and Tissues	*Procedures*	*Possible or Expected Findings*
Esophagus	Dissect diverticulum *in situ* and photograph. Fix specimen in formalin before opening.	Hypopharyngeal pulsion diverticulum (Zenker's diverticulum) at lower margin of inferior constrictor muscle of pharynx. Traction diverticulum at midesophagus after an inflammatory process—for instance, tuberculous lymphadenitis. Epiphrenic diverticulum may also occur.
Stomach		Juxtacardiac or juxtapyloric diverticulum.
Small bowel	For preservation of jejunal diverticula by air drying, see p. 55. Prepare histologic sections of Meckel's diverticulum.	Heterotopic tissue in Meckel's diverticulum, with or without peptic ulceration.
Colon	Rinse carefully; openings of diverticula may be difficult to identify. Record thickness of colonic wall and extent, approximate number, and location of diverticula.	Colonic muscular hypertrophy and stenosis, usually in sigmoid colon. Diverticulitis with perforation, fistulas, or peritonitis.*

Diverticulitis (See "Diverticula.")

Diving (See "Accident, diving (skin or scuba).")

Drowning

Related Terms: Dry drowning; fresh-water drowning; near-drowning; salt (sea)-water drowning (see the following table).

Table II-1
Deaths from Drowning

Primary Drowning *("Immediate Drowning")*	*Secondary Drowning* *("Near-Drowning")*
Deaths occurring within minutes after immersion, before or without resuscitative measures	Deaths occurring from within 30 min to several weeks after resuscitation, because of metabolic acidosis, pulmonary edema, or infective or chemical pneumonitis
Type I *("Dry Drowning")*	*Type II* *("Wet Drowning")*
Deaths from hypoxia and acidosis caused by glottal spasm on breath holding. There may be no evidence of water entering stomach or lungs and no appreciable morphologic changes at autopsy.	Deaths from hypoxia and acidosis caused by obstruction of airway by water related to: Hypervolemia Hemolysis Hyponatremia Hypochloremia Hyperkalemia

NOTE: The diagnosis is one of exclusion. The pathologist should help the police to determine: 1) How did the person (or dead body) get in the water, and 2) why could that person not get out of the water? It is not enough to ask if a person could swim but investigators should find out how well (what strokes did the victim know?) and how far he or she could swim. The inquiry must include the depth of the water and must address hazards such as undertow or underwater debris, and the behavior of the victim immediately before submerging. Deaths of adults in bathtubs and swimming pools are usually from natural, cardiac causes, or they are suicides, unless the victim was drunk.

Diatom tests *(1)* have not proven useful in the United States but there is enthusiasm for such tests among European pathologists. The distinction between hyponatremic deaths in fresh water and hypernatremic deaths in salt water derives from experimental studies; in practice, one cannot reliably predict the salinity of the immersion medium from autopsy studies. Because many bodies of drowning victims are recovered only after the body floats to the surface, decomposition will often obscure even the nondiagnostic findings such as pleural effusions, which are often associated with drowning.

Organs and Tissues	*Procedures*	*Possible or Expected Findings*
External examination and skin (wounds)	If identity of drowning victim is not known, record identifying features as described on p. 11. Prepare dental and whole-body roentgenograms. Submit tissue samples for histologic study of wounds.	There may be wounds that were inflicted before drowning occurred—for instance, in shipwrecks or vehicular and diving accidents. Other wounds may be inflicted after death—for instance, from ship propellers or marine animals. Sometimes, premortem and postmortem wounds can be distinguished histologically.
	Inspect inside of hands.	Object (hair?) held by hands in cadaveric spasm. Cutis anserina and "washerwoman" changes of hands and feet are of no diagnostic help.
	Collect fingernail scrapings.	
	Record appearance and contents of body orifices.	Foreign bodies; semen (see also under "Rape").

Organs and Tissues	*Procedures*	*Possible or Expected Findings*
External examination and skin (wounds) *(continued)*	Record features indicative of drowning.	Foam cap over mouth and nose. In the autopsy room, water running from nose and mouth is usually pulmonary edema or water from the stomach.
	Photograph face from front and in profile. Take pictures of all injuries, with and without scale and autopsy number.	Identification (p. 11).
	Remove vitreous (p. 85).	High concentrations of alcohol indicate intoxication (see under "Alcoholism and alcohol intoxication").
	If diatom search is intended, clean body thoroughly before dissection to avoid contamination of organs and body fluids with algae and diatoms (see below).	
Blood	Submit sample for toxicologic study.	Evidence of alcohol intoxication may be found.
Organ samples for diatom search	Sample early during autopsy, before carrying out other dissections. Use fresh instruments for removal of specimens to avoid contamination. Submit subpleural portion of lung: subcapsular portions of liver, spleen, and kidneys; bone marrow; and brain. Store samples in clean glass jars. For technique of diatom detection, see below.	Diatoms may occur in the liver and in other organs of persons who have died from causes other than drowning. Comparison with diatoms in water sample from area of drowning may be helpful.
Serosal surfaces and cavities	Record volume of fluid in pleural spaces. Photograph petechial hemorrhages.	Penny-sized or smaller hemorrhages may indicate violent respiratory efforts or merely intense lividity. Presence of pleural fluid suggests drowning.
Neck organ and lungs	Photograph layerwise neck dissection if strangulation* is suspected.	
	Open airways posteriorly, and photograph, remove and save mud, algae, and any other material in tracheobronchial tree. Record size and weight of lungs.	Presence of "aqueous emphysema" indicates violent respiratory efforts.
	Request frozen sections for Sudan fat stain (p. 173).	Fat emboli and bone marrow emboli indicate fractures during life.
Heart	For coronary arteriography, see p. 118.	Coronary atherosclerosis and coronary thrombosis.*
Intestinal tract and stomach	Save stomach contents (p. 16) and record volume. Record character of intestinal contents and submit for toxicologic study. Record appearance of serosal and mesenteric lymphatics.	Gastric and intestinal contents indicate type and occasionally time of last meal. Intestinal lymphatics ("lacteals") dilated and quite conspicuous during resorptive state. Tablet residues may be present.
Other organs		Evidence of disseminated intravascular coagulation* may be found after fresh-water submersion.
Genital organs	Search for evidence of rape,* pregnancy,* or both.	
Brain	For removal and specimen preparation, see p. 65.	Anoxic changes.
Middle ears, paranasal sinuses, and mastoid spaces	Expose with chisel, and record presence or absence of hemorrhages; photograph hemorrhages; inspect eardrums for presence of perforation (p. 72). If perforated, prepare histologic sections.	Hemorrhages in middle ears or mastoid air spaces are strong evidence of drowning. Middle ear or mastoid hemorrhages can be documented histologically. Watery liquid in sphenoid sinuses.

Technique of Diatom Detection

For diatom detection *(1)*, boil 2–5 g of tissue for 10–15 min in 10 mL of concentrated nitric acid and 0.5 mL of concentrated sulfuric acid. Then, add sodium nitrate in small quantities until the black color of the charred organic matter has been dispelled. It may be necessary to warm the acid-digested material with weak sodium hydroxide, but the material must soon be washed free from alkali to avoid dissolving the diatoms. The diatoms should be washed, concentrated, and stored in distilled water. For examination, allow a drop of the concentrate to evaporate on a slide, and then mount it in a resin of high refractive index. All equipment must be well-cleaned, and distilled water must be used for all solutions. There are several variations and adaptations of this method.

Reference

1. Camps FE. Immersion in fluids. In: Recent Advances in Forensic Pathology. J & A Churchill, London, 1969, pp. 70–79.

Drugs (See "Abuse,...," "Dependence,...," and "Poisoning,...")

Ductus Arteriosus, Patent (See "Artery, patent ductal.")

Dwarfism

Synonyms and Related Terms. Achondroplastic dwarf; asexual dwarf; ateliotic dwarf; micromelic dwarf; normal dwarf; pituitary dwarf; true dwarf; and many other terms, too numerous to mention.

Organs and Tissues	*Procedures*	*Possible or Expected Findings*
External examination	Record lengths of extremities and length of rump (calculate ratio), head circumference, and other suspected abnormal dimensions. Prepare skeletal roentgenograms.	Short or deformed extremities, deformed head, and other deformities. Abnormalities of primary and secondary sex characteristics. Osseous and cartilaginous deformities; skeletal tumor (adamantinoma).
Endocrine organs	Record weights and prepare histologic sections of all endocrine organs. For removal and specimen preparation of pituitary gland, see p. 71.	Tumor; infection; posttraumatic lesions; infiltrates of Langerhans cell histiocytosis.*
Other organs	Follow procedures described under suspected underlying disease (see right-hand column). In true or primordial dwarfism, no associated abnormalities can be suspected.	Achondroplasia;* congenital heart disease;* Hurler's syndrome (see "Mucopolysaccharidosis"); hypothyroidism;* malabsorption syndrome;* pituitary insufficiency;* renal failure* (chronic); sexual precocity with premature fusion of epiphyses; other systemic diseases.

Dysbetalipoproteinemia, Familial (See "Hyperlipoproteinemia.")

Dyschondroplasia, Ollier's

Synonyms and Related Terms: Multiple enchondromatosis; Ollier's disease; osteochondrodysplasia.

Organs and Tissues	*Procedures*	*Possible or Expected Findings*
External examination	Record height and weight. Prepare skeletal roentgenograms.	Growth retardation. Abnormal growth of epiphyseal cartilage with enlargement of metaphysis. Long bones and pelvis most commonly affected.
Skin and soft tissues		Cavernous hemangiomas (Maffucci's syndrome).
Bones and joints	For removal, prosthetic repair, and specimen preparation, see p. 95.	See above under "External examination." Chondrosarcoma.

Dyscrasia, Plasma Cell

NOTE: These conditions are characterized by abnormally proliferated B-immunocytes that produce a monoclonal immunoglobulin. Multiple myeloma,* plasma cell leukemia, plasmacytoma, and Waldenström's macroglobulinemia* as well as heavy-chain diseases and monoclonal gammopathies of unknown type belong to this disease family. Amyloidosis* is closely related to these conditions. For autopsy procedures, see under "amyloidosis," "macroglobulinemia," or "multiple myeloma" and under name of condition that may have caused the plasma cell dyscrasia. Such conditions include carcinoma (colon, breast, or biliary tract), Gaucher's disease,* hyperlipoproteinemia,* infectious or noninfectious chronic inflammatory diseases, and previous cardiac surgery.

Dysentery, Bacillary

Synonym: *Shigella* dysentery.

NOTE: (1) Collect all tissues that appear to be infected. (2) Request aerobic bacterial cultures. (3) Request Gram stain (p. 172). (4) Special **precautions** are indicated (p. 146). (5) Serologic studies are available from local and state health department laboratories (p. 135). (6) This is a **reportable** disease.

Organs and Tissues	*Procedures*	*Possible or Expected Findings*
Blood	Submit sample for culture and for serologic study (p. 102).	*Escherichia coli* septicemia.
Bowel	Submit sample of feces or preferably blood-tinged mucus for culture. If bacteriologic diagnosis has already been confirmed, pin colon on corkboard, photograph, and fix in formalin for histologic study.	Colitis with microabscesses; transverse shallow ulcers and hemorrhages, most often in terminal ileum and colon.
Eyes	Submit sample of vitreous for study of sodium, potassium, chloride, and urea nitrogen concentrations (p. 85).	Dehydration* pattern of electrolytes and urea nitrogen (p. 115).
	For removal and specimen preparation of eyes, see p. 85.	Conjunctivitis, iritis.
Joints	For removal, prosthetic repair, and specimen preparation, see p. 96.	Serous arthritis* of knee joints is a late complication.

Dysfibrinogenemia

NOTE: Bleeding and thromboembolism* may be noted at autopsy. Clotting studies with postmortem blood are not indicated. AIDS,* liver disease, and lymphoproliferative disorders are possible underlying conditions.

Dysgenesis, Gonadal (Ovarian) (See "Syndrome, Turner's.")

Dysgenesis, Seminiferous Tubule (See "Syndrome, Klinefelter's.")

Dyskinesia, Ciliary

Synonyms and Related Terms: Immotile cilia syndrome; Kartagener's triad.

NOTE: Multiple conditions belong into this disease category, all characterized by a hereditary defect of the axoneme (the "motor" of the cilia).

Organs and Tissues	*Procedures*	*Possible or Expected Findings*
Chest cavity	If situs inversus is present, photograph chest organs *in situ*.	Situs inversus in Kartagener's triad (with sinusitis and bronchiectases—see below).
Lungs	Submit samples from one lung for microbiologic study (p. 103). Perfuse on lung with formalin (p. 47).	Bronchiectases and bronchopneumonia.
Nasal cavities, sinuses, and middle ears	For exposure and specimen preparation, see pp. 71 and 72.	Nasal polyps; sinusitis, and otitis media.*
	Prepare samples of mucosa for electron microscopic study of cilia (p. 132).	Missing dynein arms.

Dysphagia, Sideropenic (See "Syndrome, Plummer-Vinson.")

Dysplasia, Chrondroectodermal (See "Syndrome, Ellis-van Creveld.")

Dysplasia, Fibrous, of Bone

Related Term: McCune-Albright syndrome.

Possible Associated Conditions: Acromegaly;* Cushing's syndrome;* hyperthyroidism.*

Organs and Tissues	Procedures	Possible or Expected Findings
External examination	Record extent of pigmentation, facial features, and primary and secondary sex characteristics.	Unilateral skin pigmentation and precocious puberty in females (Albright's syndrome), less commonly in males. Abnormal facial features caused by distortion of facial bones.
	Prepare skeletal roentgenograms.	Cystlike lesions in metaphyses and shafts of bone; fractures; deformities.
Soft tissues		Myxomas.
Bones	For removal, prosthetic repair, and specimen preparation, see p. 95.	See above under "External examination."
	Record size of apertures of cranial nerves in base of skull.	Encroachment of cranial nerves.

Dysplasia, Renal (See "Cyst(s), renal.")

Dysplasia, Thymic (See "Syndrome, primary immunodeficiency.")

Dystonia, Torsion (See "Syndrome, Dystonia.")

Dystrophy, Duchenne's Progressive muscular (See "Dystrophy, muscular.")

Dystrophy, Muscular

Synonyms and Related Terms: Becker's muscular dystrophy; congenital muscular dystrophy; Duchenne's progressive muscular dystrophy; dystrophinopathy; Emery-Dreifuss mucular dystrophy; facioscapulohumeral dystrophy; limb girdle dystrophy; myotonic muscular dystrophy.

Organs and Tissues	Procedures	Possible or Expected Findings
External examination	Record pattern of scalp hair.	Frontal baldness (in myotonic muscular dystrophy).
	Record status of skeletal musculature.	Atrophy and wasting of muscles (generalized or local: predominantly distal in myotonic muscular dystrophy). Pseudohypertrophy of calf muscles in Duchenne's muscular dystrophy.
Skeletal muscle	For sampling and specimen preparation, see p. 80. Dystrophin staining of the sarcolemma is absent in Duchenne's muscular dystrophy and patchy in Becker's dystrophy.	Dystrophic changes include variations in fiber size, fiber degeneration and regeneration, peri- and endomysial fibrosis, and fatty replacement of muscle.

Reference

1. Engel AG, Yamamoto M, Fischbeck KH. Dystrophinopathies. In: Myology, 2nd ed., vol. 2. Engel AG, Franzini-Armstrong C, eds. MacGraw-Hill, New York, 1994, pp. 1130–1187.

Dystrophy, Myotonic Muscular (See "Dystrophy, muscular.")

E

Echinococcosis

Synonym: Hydatid disease.

NOTE: (1) Collect all tissues that appear to be infected. (2) Usually, cultures are not required, only direct examination for parasites. (3) Request Giemsa stain for parasites (p. 172). (4) Special **precautions** should be exercised in removing the cysts, as the contents are highly infectious (p. 146). (5) Serologic studies are available from the Center for Disease Control and Prevention, Atlanta, GA (p. 135). (6) This is not a reportable disease.

Organs and Tissues	*Procedures*	*Possible or Expected Findings*
Liver	If the liver is the site of involvement, prepare roentgenogram. Prepare cholangiogram if *Echinococcus multilocularis* organisms are present (p. 56). Photograph intact cysts and cut sections. Cysts should be placed in formalin before processing.	The liver, especially the right lobe, is the most common site of involvement. Secondary infection or calcification may be present.
Lungs	If the lung is the site of involvement, prepare roentgenogram. Photograph cysts. For further processing, the lung should be fixed in formalin (p. 47).	The lung is the second most common site of involvement. Fluid and air may be visible on the roentgenogram.
Other organs	Procedures depend on expected findings or grossly identified abnormalities as listed in right-hand column.	Cysts may be present in the abdominal cavity, muscles, kidneys, spleen, bones, heart, and brain.
Blood and bone marrow	For preparation of sections and smears, see p. 96. Request Giemsa stain (p. 172).	Eosinophilia.

Eclampsia (See "Toxemia of pregnancy.")

Edema, Angioneurotic

Synonym: Angioedema.

NOTE: Possible causes and suggested autopsy procedures are described under "Death, anaphylactic."

Edema, Chemical Pulmonary

Related Term: Silo-filler's disease.

NOTE: This condition is caused by inhalation of toxic gases, such as oxides of nitrogen (silo-filler's disease) and phosgene ($COCl_2$). See also "Bronchitis, acute chemical" and "Poisoning, gas."

Organs and Tissues	*Procedures*	*Possible or Expected Findings*
Upper airways and lungs	Remove lungs together with pharynx, larynx, and trachea. Open airways posteriorly. Record lung weights. Submit one lobe for microbiologic study (p. 103). Perfuse one lung with formalin (p. 47).	Acute chemical laryngotracheitis; acute pulmonary edema. Obliterating fibrous bronchiolitis and diffuse, progressive pulmonary fibrosis may be present after prolonged survival.

Effusion(s) and Exudate(s), Pleural

Organs and Tissues	*Procedures*	*Possible or Expected Findings*
External examination	Prepare chest roentgenogram.	300–500 mL of fluid must be present before it becomes visible.
Chest cavities and chest organs	Submit samples of pleural fluid for microbiologic study (p. 102). These samples should be obtained before the chest is opened because laceration of the subclavian veins renders clear exudates or transudates hemorrhagic. In true hemorrhagic exudates, determination of the hematocrit value may be useful. For cytologic study, spin down pleural fluid and prepare smears and histologic sections of pellet. Record volume of pleural fluid; remove fluid with vacuum suction apparatus. If the fluid is milky-white, dissect and record appearance of thoracic duct system (p. 34).	Myocardial infarction or other cardiac abnormalities that may have caused congestive heart failure;* pneumonia; pulmonary infarction; tumor(s); bacterial, fungal, or viral infection; immune connective tissue disease; amebiasis;* trauma to thoracic duct system; other causes.
Other organs		Pancreatitis;* subphrenic empyema;* other intra-abdominal disease, with or without ascites.

Electricity (See "Injury, electrical.")

Electrocution (See "Injury, electrical.")

Electrolyte(s) (See "Disorder, electrolyte(s).")

Elliptocytosis, Hereditary (See "Anemia, hemolytic.")

Embolism, Air

NOTE: Possible causes include: (1) blood transfusion when the bottle had emptied unnoticed (particularly when the pressure in the bottle had been artificially increased or when a pump had been used); (2) injury to large veins, particularly cranial sinuses (during neurosurgical procedures) and veins of the neck (knife wounds, surgery) or uterus (criminal abortion); (3) insufflation of fallopian tubes (particularly in pregnancy or during menstrual period); (4) malfunctioning of dialysis machine; (5) positive-pressure ventilation in newborn infants; (6) subclavian vein catheterization in the semi-Fowler position; and (7) fracture in the hub of a central venous catheter used for parenteral nutrition.

Autopsy Procedure and Diagnosis

If air embolism is suspected, the autopsy should be performed as soon after death as possible. Decomposition gases may be produced within a few hours. Roentgenography of the whole body may detect large quantities of air, and the roentgenograms may serve as a guide to the most advantageous way of dissection.

Air embolism can be diagnosed if one succeeds in demonstrating, with an ophthalmoscope, air bubbles in the retinal arteries. This should be done as a first step of the autopsy in all cases in which this diagnosis is entertained. The cornea must be moistened with isotonic saline so that the opaqueness of it does not interfere with this method of diagnosing air embolism *(1)*.

After the ophthalmoscopic examination, the prosector opens the thoracic cavity, lifts the bony chest plate, and clamps the internal mammary vessels below the sternoclavicular joints. (Particular care must be taken to clamp but not lacerate the upper thoracic or neck veins.) The prosector then cuts across the sternum distal to these clamped vessels so that the sternoclavicular joint area remains intact. The pericardial sac is carefully opened. Large fatal pulmonary air embolism is readily apparent. The right atrium and ventricle are distended with fine, frothy, bright-red blood, which also may distend the pulmonary arteries and large systemic veins. The blood is fluid throughout the body, the viscera are congested, and petechiae are present in the serous surfaces and in the white matter of the brain. Microbiologic examination of blood and pericardial sac contents (p. 102) will help to rule out the presence of gas-forming bacteria that may simulate air embolism (Fig. II-1). However, the differentiation between air and decomposition gases should be done at the autopsy table with the pyrogallol test.

A 2% pyrogallol solution is prepared (it should be water-clear). Two 10-mL syringes (syringe A and syringe B) are loaded with 4 mL of the pyrogallol solution in each, without permitting any air to enter the system. Immediately before the solution is used, 4 drops of 0.5 *N* NaOH is aspirated through the needle of syringe A to adjust the pH to about 8 (1 drop per 1 mL of solution); the mixture will turn faint yellow. Six mL of gas is then aspirated from the heart or blood vessels. The needle is immediately sealed with a cork or replaced by a cap, and the syringe is vigorously shaken for about 1 min. In the presence of air, the pyrogallol solution will turn brown. If the solution remains clear, decomposition gases were present. In the latter instance, 4 drops of 0.5 *N* NaOH and 6 mL of room air should be aspirated into syringe B, which is then also sealed and shaken for 1 min. The mixture should turn brown, thus serving as a control that the pyrogallol solution had been properly prepared. Syringe B may also serve as a reserve. If only one syringe is used, the

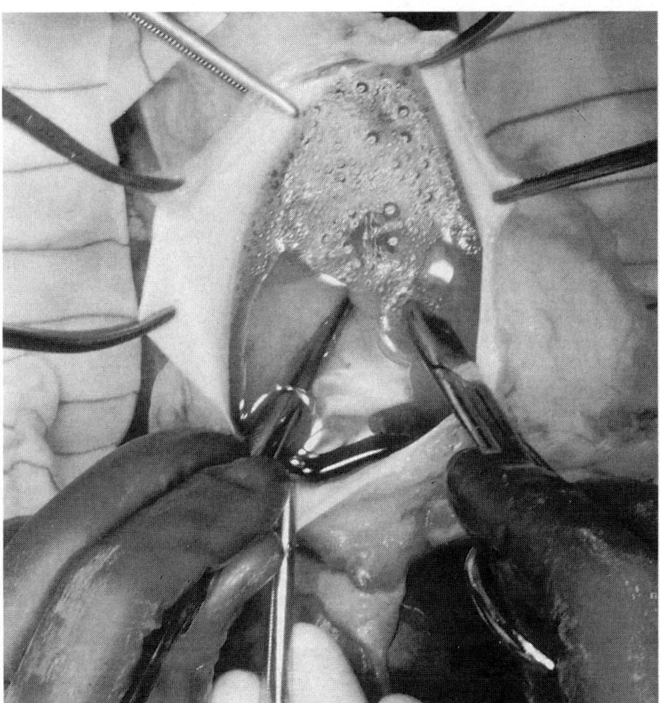

Fig. II-1. Gas-forming bacteria simulating air embolism. The pericardial sac is opened and filled with water. The heart is kept submerged with a pair of scissors. The coronary arteries have been incised with a scalpel. Note gas bubbles and foam on the water surface. No discoloration of 2% pyrogallol was noted. Blood cultures were positive for *Enterococcus* organisms. Microscopically, gram-negative rods were found in most tissues.

decomposition gas can be expelled and room air can be aspirated for the control test.

If only small amounts of gas can be aspirated, the volume of the pyrogallol solution should be decreased so that the gas-fluid volume ratio is at least 3:2.

If no bacterial gas formation is present, the edges of the pericardial incision are elevated and the pericardial sac is filled with water. Clamping of the ascending aorta and venae cavae prevents the escape of gas into these vessels. The heart is held under water while the coronary arteries are incised, and the escape of bubbles is recorded. When the right coronary artery is opened, care must be taken that the right atrium is not incised. Air in the coronary arteries indicates systemic embolism. The heart chambers are then incised.

When there is gas in any of the arteries or heart chambers, gas bubbles rise to the surface of the water in the pericardial sac ("bubble test"). Sometimes the vessels have to be somewhat compressed in order to cause the gas to escape. Because large amounts of air or other gases cause the heart to float, it must be kept submerged before the vessels and chambers are incised. Basically the same procedure is used for demonstrating the presence of gas in the superior or inferior vena cava and the pelvic veins (for example, in cases of criminal abortion). In this situation, the abdominal cavity is filled with water and the inferior vena cava and its tributaries are incised.

For the diagnosis of systemic air embolism, the skull vault should be removed without puncturing the meninges, so that the meningeal vessels can be inspected for gas bubbles. The demonstration of gas bubbles in the meningeal vessels and in the circle of Willis is meaningful only when the neck vessels are still intact and the internal carotid artery and basilar artery have been clamped before the brain is removed. In acute cases, gas bubbles will be visible within the cerebral vessels. They are released under water when the clamps are removed and the vessels are slightly compressed.

For the collection of gas from blood vessels or cavities, a system of little quantitative reliability is an air-tight, water-filled glass syringe with a needle. The needle is inserted into the vessel or cavity in question and gas is carefully aspirated.

A combined qualitative and quantitative method has been described by Kulka *(2)* (see Fig. II-2). He devised an apparatus for gas collection and described it as shown in Fig. II-2 and caption.

The entire system is filled with mineral oil so that, when the funnel is level with the upright bottle, the oil fills only about half of the funnel. In operation, the funnel is first raised to a position 30–40 cm above the level of the upright bottle. All the cocks are opened and the position is held until every trace of gas has been driven from the system through the needle, which is thereby coated on the inside by a film of oil. After all air has been expelled, the cocks are closed and the funnel is lowered to its original position.

As a precautionary measure and control, the air-tightness of the whole system should be tested before operation. This is done by inserting the needle into musculature or skin and attempting aspiration in the manner described in the next paragraph.

To make the test, the bottle is inverted and the needle is inserted into the cavity in question. When the needle is in position, all cocks are opened. The funnel is lowered about 70–90 cm, or until adequate suction is created. This aspirates the contents of the cavity, which may consist of air or other gases, either pure or mixed with blood or other liquid. Any gas or liquid entering this system may be observed through the wall of the short bent glass tubing. In a positive test, gas bubbles will collect in the bottle above the level of the oil. If desired, this gas can be saved for further examination by closing all the cocks and returning the bottle to its upright position *(4)*.

Interpretation of Findings

The volume of intravenous air needed to cause death in adults is probably in the range of 100 mL. Very small amounts entering the systemic circulation may cause death within minutes. Delayed air embolism with fatal outcome may also occur.

References

1. Kevorkian J. The fundus oculi and the determination of death. Am J Pathol 1956;32:1253–1269.
2. Kulka W. A practical device for demonstrating air embolism. J Forens Med 1965; 12:3–7.
3. Kulka W. Laboratory methods and technical notes: a practical device for demonstrating air embolism. Arch Pathol 1949; 48:366–369.
4. Bajanowski T, West A, Brinkmann B. Proof of fatal air embolism. Int J legal Med 1998;111:208–211.

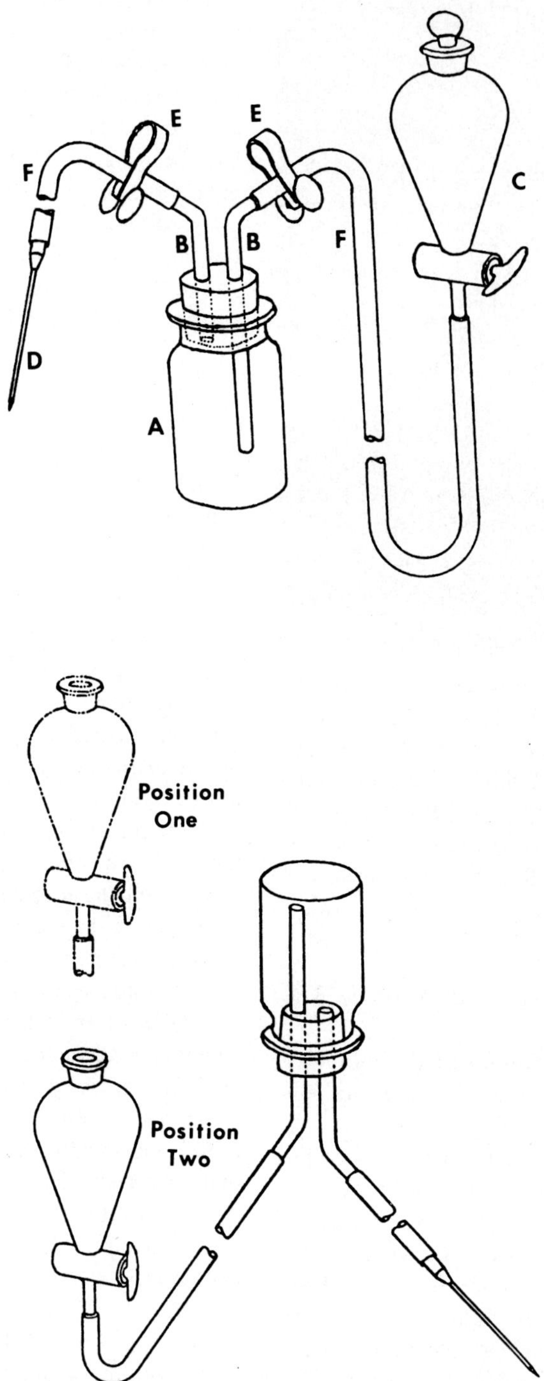

Fig. II-2. Apparatus for demonstration of air embolism. *Top*, Apparatus. *Bottom*, Position of separatory funnel during test. (**A**) One wide-mouth glass bottle (2–3 ounces; 60–90 mL) fitted tightly with a two-hole rubber stopper. (**B**) Two sections of glass tubing, approx 3 mm inside diameter, each bent at an angle of 120°. One of these sections should be longer than the other. The shorter one should reach just through and be even with the inner surface of the stopper. The longer one should reach to within 1 or 1.5 cm of the bottom of the bottle. Both tubes should fit tightly into the holes of the stopper. (**C**) One separatory funnel (60–100 mL, pear-shaped) connected to the longer section of bent glass tubing by rubber tubing 100 cm in length (**F**). An amber, pure gum rubber tubing, such as is used on blood-diluting pipets, has proved satisfactory. (**D**) One transfusion needle, 14- or 15-gauge and 4–5 cm long, connected to the shorter glass tube by a short (<5 cm) section of rubber tubing (F). (**E**) Two pinchcocks, one for each length of tubing. They may be of the spring type or of the household syringe type. The latter will prove advantageous if the gas collected is to be transported for analysis. Adapted with permission from ref. *(3)*.

Embolism, Amniotic Fluid

Organs and Tissues	*Procedures*	*Possible or Expected Findings*
External examination	If purpura is present, prepare photographs and record extent.	Skin purpura.
Blood	Submit sample (from right atrium) for microbiologic study (p. 102).	
	Collect blood from right atrium and right ventricle. After the heart has been removed, allow blood in pulmonary vessels to pool in the pericardial sac.	
	Centrifuge this blood and submit sample of flocculent layer above buffy coat for microscopic study *(1)*.	Vernix, lanugo hairs, and meconium can be found in pericardial blood pool.
Lungs	Submit one lobe for bacteriologic study (p. 103).	
	Dissect pulmonary arteries (p. 45); prepare histologic sections of all lobes; request mucicarmine stain and the alcian blue and phloxine-tartrazine stain of Lendrum (p. 172).	Meconium-type material in blood vessels. In histologic sections, squamous epithelium, meconium, and fat from vernix caseosa.
	Also request Sudan stain on frozen sections (p. 172).	
Uterus and placenta	For dissection techniques, see p. 60.	Complete or incomplete lower uterine tear; chorioamnionitis.
Other organs		Manifestations of disseminated intravascular coagulation* and fibrinolysis.
Lungs of stillborn		Intrauterine pneumonia.

Interpretation of Findings

Large amounts of debris in the blood vessels of all sections of the lungs may be considered to be lethal if there is no other cause of death. Small amounts in one or more blocks of pulmonary tissue are more likely incidental *(1)*. A small uterine tear is more likely followed by a fatal amniotic fluid embolization than is a large tear, which may result in fatal hemorrhage or fibrinogen depletion. Chorioamnionitis, intrauterine pneumonia, and positive lung cultures of the mother indicate infection of the amniotic fluid.

Reference

1. Attwood HD. Amniotic fluid embolism. In: Pathology Annual 1972. Sommers SC, Rosen PP, eds. Appleton-Century-Crofts, New York, 1972, pp. 145–172.

Embolism, Arterial

Synonyms and Related Terms: Arterial thromboembolism; atheroembolism; bone marrow embolism; embolic syndrome; foreign body embolism; paradoxic embolism; tumor embolism.

NOTE: A history of urinary eosinophilia may have been obtained in patients with renal atheroembolism.

Organs and Tissues	*Procedures*	*Possible or Expected Findings*
External examination		Gangrene of extremities.
Heart	Record patency and size of oval foramen, or presence of septal defect(s).*	In presence of intracardiac right-to-left communication, paradoxic embolism may occur.
	If infective endocarditis is suspected, follow procedures described on p. 103.	Infective endocarditis.*
	For general dissection techniques, see p. 22.	Myocardial infarction; mural or valvular thrombi in left atrium or in left ventricle; atrial dilatation in patients who had atrial fibrillation; mitral or aortic valve prostheses.
Aorta and elastic artery branches		Thrombi on atheromatous ulcers; thrombi in aneurysms.
	For celiac or mesenteric arteriography, see p. 55.	Embolism to celiac or mesenteric artery system.

Organs and Tissues	Procedures	Possible or Expected Findings
Other organs		Multiple infarctions may be present. See also above under "Note."
Peripheral arteries	For arteriography of the lower extremities, see p. 21. For removal of femoral vessels after embalming, see p. 34. Submit samples of arteries and veins for histologic study. Request Verhoeff–van Gieson stain (p. 173).	Localized arterial disease may simulate embolism. This includes infectious arteritis, such as bacterial arteritis after infective endocarditis* or syphilitic or tuberculous arteritis.

Embolism, Cerebral (See "Infarction, cerebral.")

Embolism, Fat

NOTE: Formalin-fixed tissues can be postfixed with osmium tetroxide, embedded in epoxy or paraffin, and stained with toluidine blue, hematoxylin, or Oil red O. Fat emboli are more easily recognized than in frozen tissue after Oil Red O staining *(1)*.

Organs and Tissues	Procedures	Possible or Expected Findings
External extermination		Petechial hemorrhages of skin (chest, neck, and face).
	Record evidence of trauma.	Wounds; other traumatic lesions.
	Prepare skeletal roentgenograms.	Bone fractures.
Eyes	For ophthalmoscopic examination, see p. 290.	Petechiae of conjunctivas and retinas.
Blood	Pool blood from pulmonary arteries.	Fat may accumulate on surface of blood pool. No useful technique is available for estimating the amount of fat globules in the blood.
Urine	Record presence of fat droplets.	
Lungs, myocardium, spleen, adrenal glands, kidneys	Record weights. Prepare frozen sections of fresh or formalin-fixed material. Request Sudan IV or oil red O stain (p. 173).	Fat emboli in lumen of small vessels and in pulmonary air spaces.
Liver	Record weight and sample for histologic study.	Severe fatty changes may be the cause of fat embolism.
Bones		Fractures are the most common cause of fat embolism.
Brain and spinal cord	For removal and specimen preparation, see p. 65 and 67, respectively. Photograph horizontal sections through brain, brain stem, and spinal cord.	Petechial hemorrhages.
	Prepare frozen sections and request Sudan stain (p. 173).	Fat emboli.
Pituitary gland	For removal and specimen preparation, see p. 71. Prepare frozen sections of one-half of gland and paraffin sections of the other half.	Fat emboli and hemorrhages are common in posterior lobe.

Reference

1. Davison PR, Cohle SD. Histologic detection of fat emboli. J Forensic Sci 1987;32:1426–1430.

Embolism, Pulmonary

Synonyms and Related Terms: Bone marrow embolism; foreign body embolism; pulmonary thromboembolism; tumor embolism.

NOTE: If air embolism, amniotic fluid embolism, or fat embolism is suspected, see under those headings. See also under "Phlebitis" and "Thrombosis, venous."

Organs and Tissues	Procedures	Possible or Expected Findings
External examination	Record circumference of legs, 20 cm above and below patella.	Leg edema accompanying venous thrombosis.
	For postmortem phlebography, see p. 121.	Thrombosis most common in deep leg veins.
	Prepare chest roentgenogram.	Infarction; pneumothorax* complicating perforated pulmonary infarction.
Pleural cavities	Record volume and character of pleural contents.	Effusion(s);* serofibrinous pleuritis; empyema.*
Heart	In the presence of systemic embolism, record patency of oval foramen or presence of septal defect(s).* Open pulmonary arteries *in situ*.	Paradoxic embolism. Mural thrombi in right atrium or right ventricle. Thrombi on pacing leads or indwelling central catheters.
Lungs	Inspect lumens of hilar pulmonary arteries to detect emboli. Perfuse lungs for a brief period during autopsy and then inspect slices to detect peripheral emboli.	Bland infarcts are more common in lower lobes; infarct abscesses are more common in upper lobes.
Veins	Remove and dissect femoral veins (after embalming) and pelvic veins (p. 34).	Phlebothrombosis or thrombophlebitis. See also above under "Note."

Emphysema

Synonyms and Related Terms: Chronic obstructive lung disease; pulmonary emphysema; vanishing lung disease.

Possible Associated Conditions: Alpha$_1$-antitrypsin deficiency; chronic bronchitis.*

Organs and Tissues	Procedures	Possible or Expected Findings
External examination		Cyanosis; clubbing of fingers.
	Prepare chest roentgenogram (roentgenograms are of limited value for detecting or assessing severity of emphysema).	Low diaphragm; pneumothorax.* Unilateral emphysema (congenital lobar emphysema) in infants. Incidental unilateral emphysema in adults (Macleod's syndrome).
Heart	Record weight of heart and thickness of ventricles. For separate weighing of right and left ventricles, see p. 26.	Cor pulmonale.
Pulmonary artery	Record width of artery and appearance of intima. For histologic sections, request Verhoeff–van Gieson stain (p. 173).	Pulmonary atherosclerosis; broken-up elastic membranes.
Lungs	For pulmonary arteriography and bronchography, see p. 50. For gaseous or perfusion fixation, slicing, barium impregnation, preparation of paper-mounted sections, see pp. 46 to 49.	Rarefaction of pulmonary artery tree. Chronic bronchitis;* bronchial obstruction; pneumoconiosis.* Emphysema may be centriacinar (centrilobular), focal, giant bullous, irregular, panacinar (panlobular), or paraseptal (distal acinar), or it may be related to scars (para-cicratical airspace enlargement).
	Submit one lobe for microbiologic study (p. 103).	*Haemophilus influenzae* and *Streptococcus pneumoniae* or other infections.
Diaphragm	Record thickness; submit specimens for histologic study.	Muscular hypertrophy.
Stomach and duodenum		Peptic ulcer(s).*
Liver	For histologic sections, request PAS stain with diastase digestion (p. 173).	Centrilobular congestion. In alpha$_1$-antitrypsin deficiency,* PAS-positive, diastase-resistant hepatocellular intracytoplasmic globules.
Kidneys		Glomerular enlargement.
Bone marrow	For preparation of sections and smears, see p. 96.	Increased erythropoiesis.

Organs and Tissues	*Procedures*	*Possible or Expected Findings*
Brain	For removal and specimen preparation, see p. 65.	Anoxic changes in cortex, corpus striatum, globus pallidus, thalamus, Sommer's sector of hippocampus, and Purkinje cells of cerebellum. Petechial hemorrhages of hypothalamus and necrosis of cerebellar folia may be present.

Empyema, Epidural

Synonym: Epidural abscess.

Organs and Tissues	*Procedures*	*Possible or Expected Findings*
External examination		Infected surgical wound(s).
	Prepare roentgenogram of skull.	Skull fracture(s).
Cerebrospinal fluid	Submit sample for microbiologic study (p. 104).	
Skull	In order to avoid contamination, aspirate infectious material for microbiologic study as soon as calvarium can be lifted (p. 65)—before complete removal of the calvarium. For exposure of sinuses, middle ears, and adjacent structures, see p. 71.	Mastoiditis; osteomyelitis* of parietal, mastoid, and other cranial bones; purulent sinusitis; skull fracture(s); postoperative state.

Empyema, Pleural

Synonym: Pyothorax.

Organs and Tissues	*Procedures*	*Possible or Expected Findings*
External examination	Prepare chest roentgenogram.	Pneumothorax.*
Pleural cavities	Record volume and appearance of empyema fluid. Submit sample of empyema fluid for microbiologic study (p. 102). Prepare smears and request Gram, Kinyoun's, and Grocott's methenamine silver stains (p. 172). Submit tissue samples of visceral and parietal pleura for histologic study.	Seropurulent or purulent empyema fluid with evidence of bacteria or fungi. Rarely other infectious agents.
Lungs	Submit any consolidated areas for microbiologic study (p. 103).	Emboli; infarcts; abscesses; pneumonia (various types); tuberculosis;* lung abscess;* tumor;* surgical or other trauma.
Other organs and tissues		Subphrenic empyema* and other intra-abdominal inflammatory diseases.

Empyema, Subdural

Synonym: Subdural abscess.

NOTE: Autopsy procedures and possible or expected findings are essentially the same as those described under "Empyema, epidural."

Empyema, Subphrenic

Synonyms: Subdiaphragmatic abscess; subphrenic abscess.

Organs and Tissues	*Procedures*	*Possible or Expected Findings*
Abdominal cavity	Submit sample of subphrenic exudate for aerobic and anaerobic cultures (p. 102). Record location and volume of subphrenic exudate.	Possible causes of subphrenic empyema include appendicitis, cholecystitis,* diverticulitis, intrahepatic abscess, pancreatitis,* ruptured viscus; penetrating abdominal wound(s), perforated ulcer of stomach or duodenum,* and other conditions.

Organs and Tissues	Procedures	Possible or Expected Findings
Pleural cavities and lungs	Record volume of effusion or exudate in pleural space.	Basal pleuritis and pneumonia, adjacent to empyema.

Encephalitis, All Types or Type Unspecified

Synonyms and Related Terms: Acute disseminated encephalomyelitis;* acute hemorrhagic encephalitis; acute infective encephalitis or encephalomyelitis; acute poliovirus encephalitis or encephalomyelitis; amoebic encephalitis; Arbovirus encephalitis (Japanese encephalitis; eastern encephalitis, western encephalitis, venezuelan equine encephalitis, St. Louis encephalitis); bulbar encephalitis;* brain stem encephalitis;* herpes encephalitis (cytomegalovirus encephalits, Epstein-Barr virus encephalitis, varicella-zoster encephalitis); herpes simplex encephalitis; HIV encephalitis; measles encephalitis; measles inclusion body encephalitis; postinfectious encephalitis; postvaccinal encephalitis; progressive multifocal leukoencephalitis or leukoencephalopathy; rabies* encephalitis; subacute encephalitis; subacute sclerosing panencephalitis; viral encephalitis, and many other terms *(1)*, too numerous to mention. See also under "Note" and under "Possible or expected findings."

NOTE: If the condition that caused the encephalitis is known, see also under that heading. If the cause of the encephalitis is unknown, submit samples of tissue for microbiologic and toxicologic study, particularly if there is a suspicion of lead poisoning.* See also under "Encephalitis, brain stem," "Encephalomyelitis,...," "Encephalopathy" and "Myelopathy, Myelitis."

Organs and Tissues	Procedures	Possible or Expected Findings
Cerebrospinal fluid	Submit sample for microbiologic study. Prepare cytospin.	
Blood	Submit sample for microbiologic or toxicologic study, or both. Freeze serum sample for possible serologic study.	
Brain and spinal cord; anterior and posterior spinal roots; sensory ganglia	For removal and specimen preparation, see pp. 65, 67, and 71, respectively. For microbiologic study, submit sample of fresh cerebral tissue. If infectious agent is known and need not be confirmed, fix intact brain in formalin. For toxicologic sampling, see Chapter 6.	Bacterial, fungal, rickettsial, viral, protozoal, or other infection, including amebiasis, cysticercosis, echinococcosis,* leptospirosis,* malaria* (falciparum), schistosomiasis,* syphilis,* toxoplasmosis,* trichinosis,* and trypanosomiasis.* Inclusion bodies may be present in various viral diseases or conditions.
Other organs	Microbiologic, toxicologic, and histologic studies may be indicated, depending on the expected underlying disease.	

References

1. Esiri MM, Kennedy PGE. Viral diseases. In: Greenfield's Neuropathology, vol. 2. Graham BI, Lantos PL, eds. Arnold, London, 1997, pp. 3–64.
2. Scaravilli F, Cook GC. Parasitic and fungal infections. In: Greenfield's Neuropathology, vol. 2. Graham BI, Lantos PL, eds. Arnold, London, 1997, pp. 65–112.
3. Gray F, Nordmann P. Bacterial infections. In: Greenfield's Neuropathology, vol. 2. Graham BI, Lantos PL, eds. Arnold, London, 1997, pp. 113–152.

Encephalitis, Brain Stem

Synonyms and Related Terms: Brain stem abscess; infectious brain stem encephalitis; Listeria monocytogenes brain stem encephalitis; viral brain stem encephalitis.

NOTE: See also under "Encephalitis, limbic."

Organs and Tissues	Procedures	Possible or Expected Findings
Brain	For removal and specimen preparation, see p. 65.	Necrotizing encephalitis, with or without abscess formation *(1)*.

Reference

1. Hall WA. Infectious lesions of the brain stem. Neurosurg Clin North Am 1993;4:543–551.

Encephalitis, Herpes Simplex (See "Infection, herpes simplex.")

Encephalitis, Limbic

Synonyms and Related Terms: Brain stem encephalitis; limbic encephalopathy; paraneoplastic encephalomyelitis; paraneoplastic sensory neuropathy.

Organs and Tissues	*Procedures*	*Possible or Expected Findings*
Blood and cerebrospinal fluid		Commonly high titers of antibodies anti-Hu (anti neuronal nuclear antibodies, type 1 or ANNA 1) *(1)*.
Brain, spinal cord, and dorsal root ganglia	For removal and specimen preparation, see pp. 65, 67, and 69, respectively.	Neuronal degeneration; neuronophagia; microglial nodules; gliosis in hippocampus, brain stem, and dorsal root ganglia; perivascular lymphoid infiltrates, especially in nerve roots.
Other organs	See also under "Tumor...," depending on expected primary site.	Carcinoma (bronchogenic small cell carcinoma in most instances; other primary tumors include non-small cell lung cancer or cancers of breast, ovary, uterus, and stomach).

Reference

1. Moll JWB, Vecht CH. Immune diagnosis of paraneoplastic neurological disease. Clin Neurol Neurosurg 1995;97:71–81.

Encephalomyelitis, Acute Disseminated

Synonyms and Related Terms: Acute hemorrhagic necrotizing encephalomyelitis; acute perivascular myelinoclasis; allergic encephalomyelitis; perivenous encephalomyelitis; postinfectious or parainfectious encephalomyelitis; postrabies vaccinal encephalomyelitis; postvaccinal encephalomyelitis.

Organs and Tissues	*Procedures*	*Possible or Expected Findings*
Brain and spinal cord; anterior and posterior spinal roots; sensory ganglia	For removal and specimen preparation, see pp. 65, 67, and 69, respectively. Microscopic findings vary and depend on the phase of the disease.	In acute phase, swelling and congestion of brain. Scattered perivenous demyelination with histiocytic and lymphocytic infiltrates, predominantly in white matter. Small perivascular hemorrhages may be present. In the hyperacute form of the condition (acute hemorrhagic necrotizing encephalopathy), swelling and congestion of the brain with signs of herniation. Petechial hemorrhages in the centrum semiovale white matter. Neutrophilic perivascular infiltrates with venule necrosis and fibrinous exudate.

Encephalomyelitis, All Types or Type Unspecified

Synonyms and Related Terms: Acute disseminated encephalomyelitis;* allergic encephalomyelitis; carcinomatous encephalomyelitis; hemorrhagic necrotizing encephalomyelitis; postinfectious or parainfectious encephalomyelitis; postrabies vaccinal encephalomyelitis; postvaccinal encephalomyelitis.

NOTE: For other related terms and for suggested procedures, see under "Encephalitis, ...," "Encephalomyelitis, acute disseminated," and "Myelopathy, Myelitis."

Encephalomyopathy (See "Myopathy.")

Encephalopathy, Hepatic

Synonyms and Related Terms: Acute hepatic encephalopathy; portal-systemic encephalopathy; Reye's syndrome.*

Organs and Tissues	Procedures	Possible or Expected Findings
Brain and spinal cord	For removal and specimen preparation, see pp. 65 and 67, respectively.	In fulminant hepatic failure, cytotoxic brain swelling with herniation and Duret's hemorrhages. In portal systemic encephalopathy, brain may be grossly normal. Alzheimer type 2 astrocytes, with pale watery nuclei (common in globus pallidus, thalamus, and deep layers of cortex).
Liver	Procedures depend on suspected underlying conditions as listed in right-hand column.	Alcoholic liver disease;* cirrhosis;* massive or submassive hepatic necrosis; microvesicular fatty changes in Reye's syndrome,* fatty liver of pregnancy, and other conditions; poisoning with hepatotoxic substances (e.g., mushroom poisoning with *Amanita phalloides*).

Encephalopathy, Hypertensive

Synonyms and Related Terms: Acute hypertensive encephalopathy; Binswanger's disease; progressive subcortical encephalopathy; subcortical dementia.

NOTE: See also under "Hypertension (systemic arterial), all types or type unspecified."

Organs and Tissues	Procedures	Possible or Expected Findings
Brain	For removal and specimen preparation, see p. 65. Request Luxol fast blue-PAS stains (p. 172).	Edema in sudden malignant hypertension. Focal ischemic changes; intracerebral hemorrhages. In Binswanger's disease, multiple small old infarctions or patchy or diffuse demyelination of the cerebral white matter is present, associated with sclerosis of small arteries. Demyelination and infarctions may occur together. Infarctions may be present in other portions of the brain.
Heart, kidneys, vascular system, and other organs		Causes (e.g., chronic renal disease) and manifestations of acute or chronic hypertension.

Encephalopathy, Type Unspecified

Related Term: Toxic encephalopathy.

NOTE: If a specific toxic exposure is expected—for example, lead poisoning, see under that heading.

Enchondromatosis, Multiple (See "Dyschondroplasia, Ollier's.")

Endocarditis, Infective

Synonyms and Related Terms: Acute endocarditis; bacterial endocarditis; prosthetic valve endocarditis; subacute endocarditis.

Possible Associated Conditions: See below under "Possible or Expected Findings."

Organs and Tissues	Procedures	Possible or Expected Findings
External examination and skin; peripheral veins	If jaundice is present, search for evidence of gonococcal infection. Record skin changes and prepare photographs.	Manifestations of malnutrition; jaundice; clubbing of fingers and toes; petechial hemorrhages of skin and mucous membranes; splinter hemorrhages of nail beds. Needle marks, furuncles, and other skin infections or scars may indicate dependence on intravenous drug(s).*

Organs and Tissues	*Procedures*	*Possible or Expected Findings*
External examination and skin; peripheral veins *(continued)*	If intravenous catheter is present, leave in place, tie vessel proximally and distally from tip, and submit for microbiologic study. If this is not possible, prepare smears and sections of thrombus at tip of catheter. Request Gram and Grocott's methenamine silver stains (p. 172). Submit tip for culture, even if it is contaminated.	Infected surgical arteriovenous shunts; infected intravenous catheters, including devices in surgically treated patients with hydrocephalus.*
	Record appearance of oral cavity.	Dental infection; petechial hemorrhages.
	Prepare chest roentgenogram.	
Eyes	For removal and specimen preparation, see p. 85.	Petechial hemorrhages of conjunctivas; Roth's spots.
Blood	If cultures had not been prepared antemortem, submit samples for bacterial and fungal cultures (p. 102). Request aerobic and anaerobic bacterial cultures. Freeze serum sample for serologic study.	Septicemia.
Heart	For sterile removal of infectious material, see p. 103. Photograph valvular lesions; prepare sections of vegetations; request Gram and Grocott's methenamine silver stains (p. 172).	Rheumatic valvulitis; congenital cardiac malformations; prosthetic valve(s) with valvular ring abscesses; mycotic aneurysms of ascending aorta; valvular perforations.
	For coronary arteriography, see p. 118.	Coronary arterial emboli.
	For collection of nonvalvular tissue for histologic study, see p. 30.	Myocardial infarction; myocardial abscesses.
Arteries and veins	For histologic sections, request Verhoeff–van Gieson stain (p. 173).	Mycotic aneurysms; septic thrombophlebitis.
Lungs		Metastatic abscesses—for instance, after right-sided endocarditis in heroin addicts.
Intestinal tract and mesentery	Dissect mesenteric arteries. Other procedures depend on expected findings or grossly identified abnormalities as listed in right-hand column.	Mesenteric emboli; intestinal infarction. Adenocarcinoma of colon may be associated with *Strep. bovis* endocarditis.
Spleen	Record size and weight.	Infarctions or abscesses, or both.
Liver		Alcoholic liver disease.
Kidneys	For histologic sections, request 4-μm sections, stained with PAS and with methenamine silver for glomerular lesions (p. 173).	Glomerulitis. Macroscopically, minute hemorrhages, infarctions, and abscesses may be present.
Internal genital organs		Complications of abortion;* gonococcal infection.
Bones	For removal; prosthetic repair, and specimen preparation, see p. 95.	Osteomyelitis.*
Brain	For removal and specimen preparation, see p. 65. If cerebral involvement is suspected, submit sample for microbiologic study (p. 102).	Infarctions, abscesses, or hemorrhages; mycotic aneurysms.

Endocarditis, Löffler's (See "Cardiomyopathy, restrictive [with eosinophilia].")

Endocarditis, Nonbacterial Thrombotic (NBTE)

Synonyms and Related Terms: Libman-Sacks verrucous nonbacterial endocarditis; marantic endocarditis; verrucous endocarditis.

NOTE: A history of multiple miscarriages may have been obtained.

Possible Associated Conditions: Disseminated intravascular coagulation;* antiphospholipid antibody syndrome; lupus anticoagulant.

Organs and Tissues	*Procedures*	*Possible or Expected Findings*
Heart	If the diagnosis is suspected, photograph and remove vegetations, as described for infective endocarditis, and submit portions for microbiologic (p. 103) and histologic study.	The mitral valve is usually affected, without other valvular abnormalities.

Organs and Tissues	Procedures	Possible or Expected Findings
Heart *(continued)*	Prepare histologic sections of vegetations and of affected valve(s). If microorganisms appear to be present, request Gram stain (p. 172).	
Other organs	Procedures depend on expected findings or grossly identified abnormalities as listed in right-hand column.	Emboli and infarctions. Possible underlying conditions include carcinoma of the lung, pancreas, stomach, and other, primarily mucus-producing adenocarcinomas, systemic systemic lupus erythematosus,* antiphospholipid syndrome, and chronic debilitating diseases.

Enteritis, All Types or Type Unspecified (See "Enterocolitis,...," "Enteropathy,...," "Gastroenteritis, eosinophilic," and names of specific infectious diseases, such as "Fever, typhoid," or possible noninfectious underlying conditions, such as "Shock.")

Enteritis, Eosinophilic (See "Gastroenteritis, eosinophilic.")

Enteritis, Granulomatous (See "Disease, Crohn's.")

Enteritis, Necrotizing

Synonyms and Related Terms: Clostridial gastroenteritis; Darmbrand; enteritis necroticans.

NOTE: Follow procedures described under "Enterocolitis, pseudomembranous." Clostridial enterotoxemia (*C. perfringens)* seems to be the cause of necrotizing enteritis. Hemorrhagic necrosis of the small bowel mucosa with pseudomembranes, ulcers, and peritonitis is the main finding at autopsy.

Enteritis, Other Types or Type Undetermined (See "Enterocolitis, Other types or Type Undetermined.)

Enteritis, Regional (See "Disease, Crohn's.")

Enterocolitis, Ischemic

Synonyms and Related Terms: Hemorrhagic enteropathy; hemorrhagic necrosis (gangrene; infarction) of intestine; intestinal ischemia; ischemic enteritis; ischemic colitis; pseudomembranous enterocolitis.*

NOTE: It is assumed here that the intestinal changes are clearly ischemic. If primary infection may be the cause of the condition, see below under "Enterocolitis, neutropenic," Enterocolitis, pseudomembranous," and "Enterocolitis, staphylococcal." In ischemic enterocolitis, superinfection should be ruled out and therefore, appropriate studies may be needed also: (1) Collect all tissues that appear to be infected. (2) Request aerobic and anaerobic bacterial cultures. (3) Request Gram stain (p. 172). (4) No special precautions are indicated. (5) Serologic studies are not available. (6) This is not a reportable disease.

Organs and Tissues	Procedures	Possible or Expected Findings
Intestinal tract and mesentery	For mesenteric arteriography, see p. 55. Dissect mesenteric vessels. If infection is expected as a cause, submit portions of intestine for aerobic and anaerobic cultures (p. 102). For *in situ* perfusion fixation of intestine, see p. 54.	Emboli, atherosclerosis, or other conditions that may cause obstruction of mesenteric arteries. Primary or secondary thrombosis of mesenteric veins. Fibrinous ischemic membranes or pseudomembranes and ulcers may be present in small and large intestine.
Other organs		Manifestations of hypotension and shock.*

Enterocolitis, Neutropenic

Synonyms and Related Terms: *C. septicum* enterocolitis; necrotizing cecitis or typhlitis.

NOTE: (1) Collect all tissues that appear to be infected. (2) Request aerobic and anaerobic bacterial cultures. (3) Request Gram stain (p. 172). (4) No special precautions are indicated. (5) Serologic studies are not available. (6) This is not a reportable disease.

Organs and Tissues	Procedures	Possible or Expected Findings
Intestinal tract	Collect material from lesions in cerum for aerobic and anaerobic culture. Sample for histologic study (p. 54).	*C. septicum* infection (or infection with other Clostridiae) with ulcers, hemorrhages, and pseudomembranes, primarily in cecum and ascending colon.
Other organs and tissues		Malignancies that required chemotherapy or other conditions associated with neutropenia and treatment with antibiotics.

Enterocolitis, Other Types or Type Undetermined

NOTE: A multitude of infectious and noninfectious agents may cause inflammation of the small bowel, large bowel, or both. If the condition is not listed under "Colitis," "Enteritis," or "Enterocolitis" or under another specific heading such as "Dysentery, bacillary," obtain sufficient material for microbiologic and histologic study to identify organisms such as *Clostridium, Chlamydia, Shigella, Salmonella, Yersinia, Helicobacter, verotoxic E. coli,* and others. If lymphogranuloma venereum,* or tuberculosis* are suspected, see also under these headings. See also under "Disease, inflammatory bowel" and "Disease, Crohn's."

Enterocolitis, Pseudomembranous

Synonyms and Related Terms: *C. difficile* colitis; Darmbrand; hemorrhagic necrosis (gangrene; infarction) of intestine; ischemic enteritis or enterocolitis;* neutropenic enterocolitis;* pseudomembranous colitis.

NOTE: The name "Pseudomembranous enterocolitis" is descriptive; the condition may be infectious, ischemic, or both. If the intestinal changes are clearly ischemic, see above under "Enterocolitis, ischemic." If the cause is in doubt and if pseudomembranes can be identified, follow the procedures described here.

(1) Collect all tissues that appear to be infected. (2) Request aerobic and anaerobic bacterial cultures. (3) Request Gram stain (p. 172). (4) No special precautions are indicated. (5) Serologic studies are not available. (6) This is not a reportable disease.

For other infectious intestinal diseases, see under specific names, such as "Enterocolitis, neutropenic" or "Enterocolitis, staphylococcal."

Organs and Tissues	*Procedures*	*Possible or Expected Findings*
Intestinal tract and mesentery	Collect material from pseudomembranes for aerobic and anaerobic culture (p. 102) and for *C. difficile* toxin assay.	Bacterial growth (*C. difficile* or verocytotoxin producing *E. coli* or other organisms such as *Shigella dysenteriae*). Generally, the condition is confined to the colon.
	Sample intestinal wall with pseudomembranes for histologic study.	Lamellated pseudomembranes with much mucin and layers of neutrophils and necrotic epithelial cells. Mucous glands distended with mucin. Gram-positive bacilli in exudate.
	If the condition is suspected to be caused by ischemia, follow procedures described above under "Enterocolitis, ischemic."	Occlusive vascular lesions or other conditions causing impaired intestinal perfusion.
Other organs	Procedures depend on expected findings as listed in right-hand column.	Manifestations of hypotension and shock.* Conditions that were treated with antibiotics (which in turn allowed the selective proliferation of the intestinal pathogens).

Enterocolitis, Staphylococcal

Related Term: Staphylococcal diarrhea.

NOTE: (1) Collect all tissues that appear to be infected. (2) Request aerobic bacterial cultures. (3) Request Gram stain (p. 172). (4) No special precautions are indicated. (5) Usually, serologic studies are not helpful. (6) This is not a reportable disease.

Organs and Tissues	*Procedures*	*Possible or Expected Findings*
External examination		Dehydration.*
Gastrointestinal tract	Culture contents of stomach, small intestine, and large intestine (p. 102). Prepare sections and Gram-stained smears of mucus on intestinal wall.	*Staphylococcus aureus.*
Other organs	Procedures depend on expected findings as listed in right-hand column.	Conditions that may have required administration of antibiotics. Previous surgery.

Enteropathy, Gluten-Sensitive (See "Sprue, celiac.")

Enteropathy, Hemorrhagic (See "Enterocolitis, pseudomembranous.")

Enteropathy, Protein-Losing

NOTE: This a collective name for a diverse group of diseases and conditions that cause gastrointestinal protein loss. Carcinoma of the esophagus, heart diseases,* nephrosis, and primary immunodeficiency syndrome also may be causes of this condition.

Organs and Tissues	Procedures	Possible or Expected Findings
Heart	Dissection procedures depend on the specific type of heart disease.	Atrial septal defect;* primary cardiomyopathy;* constrictive pericarditis.* Other conditions associated with congestive heart failure.*
Esophagus	If a carcinoma is present, see also under "Tumor, of the esophagus."	Carcinoma.*
Stomach	For fixation and specimen preparation, see p. 53. If a carcinoma is present, see also under "Tumor, of the stomach."	Allergic gastroenteropathy; carcinoma; giant hypertrophy of mucosa (Ménétrier's disease); atrophic gastritis. Status post gastrectomy.
Small intestine	For postmortem lymphangiography, see p. 34. For *in situ* fixation and for preparation of intestinal mucosa for study under the dissecting microscope, see p. 54. For histologic sections, request PAS and azure-eosin stains (p. 172). If infectious intestinal disease is suspected, submit portions of intestine for microbiologic study (p. 102).	Allergic gastroenteropathy; celiac* or tropical sprue;* Crohn's disease; intestinal lymphangiectasia; jejunal diverticulosis; lymphenteric fistula; lymphoma* and other malignancies; primary tuberculosis;* other infectious intestinal diseases (see also under "Enterocolitis,..."); Whipple's disease.*
Colon	Procedures depend on expected findings or grossly identified abnormalities as listed in right-hand column.	Carcinoma and other malignancies; chronic ulcerative colitis or Crohn's disease;* megacolon.
Other organs	Procedures depend on expected findings or grossly identified abnormalities as listed in right-hand column.	Manifestations of malabsorption syndrome* with osteomalacia;* manifestations of congestive heart failure.* Conditions associated with nephrotic syndrome;* systemic sclerosis* (sclerodema) in cases with involvement of small intestine.

Eosinophilia, Tropical Pulmonary (See "Syndrome, eosinophilic pulmonary.")

Epiglottiditis (See "Laryngitis.")

Epilepsy, Idiopathic (Cryptogenic)
Related Term: Status epilepticus.

Organs and Tissues	Procedures	Possible or Expected Findings
Brain	For removal and specimen preparation, see p. 65. Histologic sections should include (as a minimum) both hippocampi, cerebellar cortex, cerebral cortex, and thalami.	By definition, no gross changes or histologic lesions are demonstrable that could be responsible for seizures. In chronic epilepsy, secondary tissue changes, attributable to repeated anoxic episodes, are found. These include hippocampal sclerosis and Purkinje cell loss in cerebellum and changes attributable to closed head injury,* such as superficial contusions in frontal or temporal lobes.
Other organs		For possible side effects of therapy, see "Epilepsy, symptomatic."

Epilepsy, Myoclonus

Synonyms and Related Terms: Baltic myoclonus; Lafora's disease; Lafora body disease; progressive myoclonus epilepsy with Lafora bodies; progressive myoclonus epilepsy without Lafora bodies; Unverricht-Lundborg disease.

NOTE: Myoclonic seizures also have been described in a number of progressive encephalopathies with complex neurological symptoms, such as GM1 and GM2 gangliosidosis,* and Niemann-Pick* and Krabbe's disease but also acquired disorders, including

Epilepsy, Myoclonus *(continued)*

Alzheimer's disease,* Creutzfeldt-Jakob disease,* posthypoxic encephalopathy, and subacute sclerosing panencephalitis. Mitochondrial encephalomyopathy also can present with myoclonus epilepsy and a mitochondrial myopathy with ragged red fibers (MERRF syndrome) in skeletal muscles.

Organs and Tissues	*Procedures*	*Possible or Expected Findings*
Brain	For removal and specimen preparation, see p. 65. For histologic sections, request methyl violet or toluidine blue, Alcian blue, and PAS stains, with and without diastase digestion (p. 172).	Mild cortical atrophy. Diffuse neuronal loss with mild astrocytosis. In Lafora's disease, basophilic, metachromatic, PAS-positive, diastase-resistant, single or multiple (1–30 μm diameter) intracytoplasmic neuronal inclusion bodies (Lafora bodies), primarily in cerebral cortex (central region and prefrontal motor cortex), thalamus, globus pallidus, substantia nigra, cerebellar cortex, and dentate nuclei. Cerebellar atrophy (Dilantin).
Other organs and tissues, including eyes and peripheral nerves	For removal and specimen preparation of eyes, see p. 85. For sampling and specimen preparation of peripheral nerves, see p. 79. For histologic sections, request methyl violet or toluidine blue stain and PAS stain with and without diastase digestion (p. 173).	Lafora-body-type material in the heart, liver, retinas, peripheral nerves, skeletal muscles, and sweat gland ducts (especially axillary).
Skeletal muscles	For removal and specimen preparation, see p. 80. Request modified Gomori's trichrome stain.	Ragged red fibers in mitochondrial myopathies.

Epilepsy, Symptomatic

NOTE: Possible causes or underlying conditions include cerebrovascular diseases, congenital malformations of the brain, degenerative and demyelinating diseases of the brain, head injury,* intracranial and cerebral infections, toxic or metabolic disorders (alcoholism,* barbiturate,* carbon monoxide,* and lead poisoning,* hemodilution, hypocalcemia, or hypoglycemia),* and tumors of the brain.*

Organs and Tissues	*Procedures*	*Possible or Expected Findings*
External examination	If gum hypertrophy or hirsutism are present, record and prepare photographs. Record skin changes and presence or absence of lymphadenopathy.	Gum hypertrophy, hirsutism (in young women), and lymphadenopathy may be found in patients who received phenytoin (Dilantin); drug-related dermatitis may be found also.
Brain	For removal and specimen preparation, see p. 65. For histologic sampling, see also under "Epilepsy, idiopathic (cryptogenic)."	See above under "Note."
	For cerebral arteriography, see p. 80.	Cerebrovascular abnormalities.
	If intracranial infection is suspected, follow procedures described on p. 102.	Intracranial and cerebral infections.
Other organs	If a toxic or metabolic disorder is suspected, submit samples of body fluids and tissues for toxicologic study (p. 16).	Complications of anticonvulsive therapy: agranulocytosis (carbamazepine), megaloblastic anemia* (barbiturates) or liver damage (dilantin, valproic acid).

Erythema Multiforme

Synonyms and Related Terms: Erythema exudativum multiforme major; Stevens-Johnson syndrome; toxic epidermal necrolysis.

NOTE: The histologic changes of erythema multiforme, Stevens-Johnson syndrome, and toxic epidermal necrolysis may be quite similar *(1)*.

Organs and Tissues	Procedures	Possible or Expected Findings
External examination and skin	Record extent and character of skin lesions. Submit samples of affected and of unaffected skin for histologic study. Record extent and character of lesions in oral cavity.	Macules; papules; vesicles; bullae; hemorrhages. Vulvitis may be present. Ulcers, fissures, and hemorrhagic lesions of oral cavity.
Pleural cavities		Effusion(s).*
Lungs	Submit one lobe for microbiologic study (p. 103). Perfuse one lung with formalin (p. 47).	Bronchitis;* bronchopneumonia.
Heart		Pericarditis.*
Other organs	Record appearance of all mucosal surfaces. Submit samples for histologic study. Other procedures depend on expected findings or grossly identified abnormalities as listed in right-hand column.	Laryngitis;* pharyngitis; esophagitis; colitis; vaginitis; urethritis. Possible underlying diseases include nephritis, infectious disease, collagen disease, and malignant tumor. Radiation treatment may have been given also.
Eyes	For removal and specimen preparation, see p. 85.	Conjunctivitis; iritis, iridocyclitis; panophthalmitis.
Other organs and tissues		Lymphoma* (with erythema multiforme as paraneoplastic syndrome) *(2)*.

References

1. Rzany B, Hering O, Mockenhaupt M, Schroder W, Goerttler E, Ring J, Schopf E. Histopathological and epidemiological characteristics of patients with erythema exudativum multiforme major, Stevens Johnson syndrome and toxic epidermal necrolysis. Br J Dermatol 1996;135:6–11.
2. Kreutzer B, Stubiger N, Thiel HJ, Zierhut M. Oculomucocutaneous changes as paraneoplastic syndrome. Ger J Ophthalmol 1996;5:176–181.

Erythroblastosis Fetalis

Related Terms: Bilirubin encephalopathy; fetal hydrops; hemolytic anemia of the newborn; kernicterus.

NOTE: *Cytomegalovirus, Parvovirus,* syphilis, and *Toxoplasma* infections can cause erythroblastosis fetalis. These may be sought with routine histological as well as immunohistochemical methods on tissue sections. Immune-mediated destruction of fetal red cells or platelets, causing fetal hemorrhages and erythroblastosis. Serologic tests are also available.

Organs and Tissues	Procedures	Possible or Expected Findings
Blood (maternal and fetal)	Perform a direct Coomb's test on fetal cells and antibody screen on fetal or maternal cells. Determine the hematocrit on the fetal blood.	Alloantibody-mediated hemolysis; anemia.
External examination and oral cavity	Record body weight and length.	Generalized, severe edema (fetal hydrops); jaundice; purpuric rash. In long-term survivors, discolored deciduous teeth with hypoplastic enamel.
Thymus	Record weight.	Accelerated maturation.
Heart and lungs	Submit samples for histologic study.	Erythroblasts in vessels of myocardium and of lungs. Look for intranuclear inclusions typical of *Parvovirus*.
Liver	Record weight. Submit samples for histologic study. Request Gomori's stain for iron (p. 172). Use immunohistochemical stains to confirm the presence of *Parvovirus*.	Hepatomegaly with increased extramedullary hematopoiesis and hemosiderosis.
Spleen	Record weight. See also above under "Liver."	Splenomegaly with increased extramedullary hematopoiesis; hemosiderosis; small or absent Malpighian corpuscles.
Pancreas	Submit sample for histologic study.	Increased extramedullary hematopoiesis.
Retroperitoneal tissues with adrenal glands and kidneys	Submit samples for histologic study.	Extramedullary hematopoiesis in adrenal glands and in retroperitoneal (peripelvic and renal) soft tissues.
Lymph nodes		Hypoplasia with hemosiderosis.
Bone marrow	For preparation of sections and smears, see p. 96.	Erythroblastic hyperplasia.

Organs and Tissues	Procedures	Possible or Expected Findings
Brain and spinal cord	For removal and specimen preparation, see pp. 65 and 67, respectively. Prepare photographs of stained areas of brain.	Diffuse cerebral icterus or selective staining of subthalamic nuclei, globus pallidus, hippocampus, pontine nuclei, medullary nuclei in the floor of the fourth ventricle, thalamus, and cerebellar nuclei. Cortical and spinal gray matter is rarely involved.
Placenta	Weigh and submit samples for histologic study.	Villous edema; erythroblasts in vessels; inclusions consistent with *Cytomegalovirus* or *Parvovirus* infection; chronic plasma cell villitis.

Esophagus, Barrett's

Organs and Tissues	Procedures	Possible or Expected Findings
Lungs	Perfuse one lung with formalin (p. 47).	Aspiration (reflux) pneumonitis with fibrosis.
Diaphragm	Record size of diaphragmatic hernia.	Diaphragmatic hernia.*
Esophagus and stomach	Remove whole length of esophagus, together with stomach and portion of diaphragm with hiatus. Record diameter of esophageal stricture (a glass cone or wooden cone can be used) before opening narrowed portion of esophagus. After opening, pin esophagus and stomach on corkboard, photograph, and fix in formalin (in this position).	The esophagus (most commonly the distal portions) is lined by columnar epithelium that causes a brownish red discoloration of the mucosa. Chronic reflux esophagitis is present, and an ulcer and a stricture often are found at the squamocolumnar junction. Dysplasia and adenocarcinoma are common complications and arise in the areas of intestinal metaplasia.
Neck organs		Laryngitis and pharyngitis in cases of severe chronic reflux.

Ethanol (Ethyl Alcohol) (See "Alcoholism and alcohol intoxication," "Cardiomyopathy, alcoholic," "Disease, alcoholic liver," "Syndrome, fetal alcoholic," and "Syndrome, Wernicke-Korsakoff.")

Exposure, Cold

NOTE: In all instances, the blood alcohol level should be determined and a drug screen should be done. The tissues tend to be well preserved.

Possible Associated Conditions: Age-related increased susceptibility to cold (in infancy and senility); alcohol intoxication;* myxedema; pituitary insufficiency;* poisoning by depressants, narcotics, or other drugs; stroke.

Organs and Tissues	Procedures	Possible or Expected Findings
External examination, skin, and subcutaneous tissues	Prepare photographs of abnormalities, as listed in right-hand column.	Red discoloration of the face and extremities; generalized edema; erythematous patches on trunk and limbs.
	Submit samples of skin and of subcutaneous tissue for histologic study.	Frostbite; bullae; gangrene. Subcutaneous tissue usually contains little blood.
Blood and vitreous	Submit samples for toxicologic study. (See above under "Note" and p. 16).	Blood is fluid and bright red.
Lungs	Record weights and sample for histologic study.	Pulmonary hemorrhages.
Gastrointestinal tract	Record sites of lesions and submit samples for histologic study.	Small mucosal hemorrhages or—if patient had survived exposure for some time—ulcers. Rarely, perforation of ulcers.
Pancreas	Prepare photographs and sample for histologic study.	Peripancreatic fat tissue necroses, with or without pancreatitis.*
Other organs		Fatty changes of myocardium, liver, and kidneys; congestion of viscera; sludging of blood in small vessels.
Brain	For removal and specimen preparation, see p. 65.	Perivascular hemorrhages around third ventricle.

F

Failure, Congestive Heart

NOTE: Coronary atherosclerosis and manifestations of ischemic heart disease,* valvular heart disease, congenital cardiovascular diseases, and manifestations of systemic or pulmonary hypertension are the most frequent findings in patients dying of or with congestive cardiac failure. Other causes include cardiomyopathies* and secondary myocardial disease (such as amyloid or pericardial constriction). If the cause of the congestive cardiac failure is unknown or not immediately evident after dissection of the heart and of the great vessels, myocardium and other appropriate tissues may be submitted for microbiologic study—including viral cultures (p. 102)—and for electron microscopy (p. 132). Specimens can also be snap-frozen for possible immunofluorescent, biochemical, or histochemical studies, particularly of the myocardium.

Organs and Tissues	*Procedures*	*Possible or Expected Findings*
External examination	Record body weight and length. Prepare roentgenogram of chest.	Cyanosis; edema of legs; dilatation of veins. Cardiomegaly; pleural effusion(s).*
Chest and abdominal cavities	Record volume and character of effusion(s).	Hydrothorax; ascites.
Heart and great vessels	See above under "Note." Record weight of heart, valve circumferences, and ventricular wall thickness. Estimate extent of dilatation of each cardiac chamber. Note consistency of myocardium.	Possible causes of congestive cardiac failure are too numerous to mention. Dilatation of heart, with or without mural thrombosis. Myocardium may be soft, normal, or firm.
Other organs	Organs mentioned in right-hand column should be described and, if appropriate, weighed and measured. Submit samples for histologic study.	Pulmonary congestion, with or without hemosiderosis; congestion of viscera with organomegaly. Other organ manifestations include bowel edema or hemorrhagic enteropathy (without mechanical vascular occlusion) and zonal hepatic steatosis, fibrosis, or necrosis, with or without evidence of liver failure. Acute renal tubular necrosis may be present also.

Failure, Kidney

Synonyms and Related Terms: Acute kidney failure; chronic kidney failure; renal failure; uremia.

NOTE: If acute kidney failure had been diagnosed, the autopsy procedures will depend on the expected causes, such as poisoning with ethylene glycol,* lead,* mercury,* or methyl alcohol;* disseminated intravascular coagulation* and its various underlying conditions; glomerulonephritis* and its various underlying conditions; diabetes mellitus;* or multiple myeloma.* The procedures described below deal primarily with chronic renal failure. If the patient had had dialysis, see also under "Dialysis (for chronic renal failure)." If transplantation had been carried out, see also under "Transplantation, kidney."

Organs and Tissues	*Procedures*	*Possible or Expected Findings*
External examination and skin	Submit samples of skin for histologic study. Record position of shunts. Prepare skeletal roentgenograms and roentgenograms of soft tissues.	"Uremic frost." Uremic skin discoloration. Teflon-Silastic shunts. Bone deformities and fractures. (See also below under "Bones and joints.") Metastatic calcifications in soft tissues and bursae.

From: *Handbook of Autopsy Practice,* 3rd Ed. Edited by: J. Ludwig © Humana Press Inc., Totowa, NJ

Organs and Tissues	*Procedures*	*Possible or Expected Findings*
Vitreous	Submit sample for determination of urea nitrogen, creatinine, sodium, and chloride concentrations (p. 85).	For interpretation of findings (biochemical diagnosis of uremia), see p. 115.
Blood	Submit sample for microbiologic study (p. 102). Retain frozen serum for serologic or immunologic study. Submit sample for determination of urea nitrogen and creatinine concentrations.	For interpretation of findings, see p. 114.
Heart		Myocarditis;* pericarditis.*
Blood vessels	If infection or clotting of shunt is suspected, remove shunt together with ligated vessels and submit for culture.	Infected shunts; manifestations of hypertension;* metastatic calcification.
Lungs	Submit one lobe for bacterial, fungal, and viral cultures (p. 103); prepare smear of fresh cut section for the demonstration of *Pneumocystis carinii.** Collect fresh lung samples and freeze for possible immunofluorescent study. Perfuse one lung with formalin (p. 47).	Bacterial, fungal, viral, and/or uremic pneumonitis; pulmonary edema.
Esophagus		*Candida* esophagitis.
Gastrointestinal tract	Record character of contents; submit tissue samples for histologic study.	Hemorrhages; gastroenteritis.
Liver	For gross iron staining, see p. 133.	Transfusion hemosiderosis. Chronic hepatitis C.
Pancreas	Submit samples for histologic study.	Inspissation of pancreatic ducts.
Kidneys	For renal arteriography, renal venography, and retrograde urography, see p. 59. For other procedures, see under name of specific renal disease.	See under name of specific renal disease, such as "Glomerulonephritis." Acquired cystic disease may occur after long-term intermittent maintenance hemodialysis.
Urine	Collect and submit sample for urinalysis.	
Testes	Submit samples for histologic study or rete testis.	Cystic transformation of rete testis *(1)*.
Parathyroid glands	Record weights; submit samples for histologic study.	Hyperplasia, with or without adenoma(s).
Brain and spinal cord	For removal and specimen preparation, see pp. 65 and 67, respectively. If the choroid plexus is to be used for immunologic study, dissect fresh brain and snap-freeze plexus.	Edema and petechiae. Neuronal damage.
Eyes	For removal and specimen preparation, see p. 85.	Hypertensive retinopathy; steroid cataracts.
Skeletal muscles	For sampling and specimen preparation, see p. 80.	Myopathy.
Bones and joints	For removal, prosthetic repair, and specimen preparation, see p. 95.	Renal osteodystrophy (osteoporosis;* osteomalacia*). Gout.*

Reference

1. Nistal M, Santamaria L, Paniagua R. Acquired cystic transformation of the rete testis secondary to renal failure. Hum Pathol 1989;20:1065–1070.

Failure, Liver

NOTE: See under name of suspected underlying disease, such as "Cirrhosis, liver" or "Hepatitis, viral."

Failure, Lung

NOTE: See under name of suspected underlying conditions such as "Pneumonia,...," "Syndrome, adult respiratory distress (ARDS)," or "Syndrome, respiratory distress, of infant."

Fascioliasis (See "Clonorchiasis.")

Feminization, Testicular

Related Term: Hereditary male pseudohermaphroditism.

NOTE: This x-linked recessive condition is characterized by impairment of male phenotypic differentiation or virilization; it occurs in a complete and an incomplete (see below) form. Together with Reifenstein's syndrome* and the infertile male syndrome, these conditions represent androgen receptor disorders.

Organs and Tissues	Procedures	Possible or Expected Findings
External examination and breasts	Record body weight and length. Record appearance of breasts and submit samples of breast tissue for histologic study.	Female appearance with female external genitalia; sparse axillary and pubic hair.
Blood or fascia lata	Specimens should be collected using aseptic technique for tissue culture for chromosome analysis (see Chapter 10). Record presence of sex chromatin.	Karyotype is 46,XY.
Gonads and vagina	Record weights of testes and prepare histologic sections of both. Prepare histologic sections of vaginal mucosa.	Blind-ending vagina; absent internal genitalia except for testes, which may have descended to inguinae or labia. No spermatogenesis (but Leydig cells and seminiferous tubules are present). In incomplete testicular feminization, partial fusion of labioscrotal folds, clitoromegaly, and normal pubic hair are found.

Fever, Colorado Tick

Related Term: Orbivirus infection.

NOTE: (1) Collect all tissues that appear to be infected. (2) Request cultures for orbiviruses (*Reoviridae* family). This requires animal inoculation, and not all laboratories have the capability of isolating orbiviruses. (3) Special stains are not indicated. (4) Special **precautions** are indicated (p. 146). (5) Serologic studies are available from local or state health department laboratories (p. 135). The virus also can be detected by reverse transcription PCR of whole blood specimens *(1)*. (6) This is not a reportable disease.

Organs and Tissues	Procedures	Possible or Expected Findings
External examination		Skin rash; thrombocytopenic hemorrhages.
Cerebrospinal fluid	If meningitis or encephalitis is suspected, submit samples for viral culture and for cytologic study (p. 104).	Increased leukocyte counts and positive viral culture.
Blood	Submit samples for viral culture and for serologic study (p. 102) or study by PCR (see above under "Note.").	
Other organs and tissues		Thrombocytopenic hemorrhages; focal necrosis in multiple organs.
Brain and spinal cord	For removal and specimen preparation, see pp. 65 and 67, respectively. Submit fresh cerebral tissue for viral culture (p. 102).	Meningitis* and encephalitis.*

Reference

1. Johnson AJ, Karabatsos N, Lanciotti RS. Detection of Colorado tick fever virus by using reverse transcription PCR and application of the technique in laboratory diagnosis. J Clin Microbiol 1997;35:1203–1208.

Fever, Familial Mediterranean

Synonyms: Familial paroxysmal polyserositis; periodic fever; periodic polyserositis; recurrent polyserositis.

Organs and Tissues	Procedures	Possible or Expected Findings
Chest and abdomen	Record volume of pericardial, pleural, and peritoneal exudates. Submit samples for microbiologic study (p. 102). Prepare smears or sections of spun-down sediment. Submit samples of serosal surfaces for histologic study.	Exudate should be sterile, with many neutrophils. Acute serositis.

Organs and Tissues	Procedures	Possible or Expected Findings
Other organs	Request Congo red or other amyloid stains. For further details on staining procedures, see under "Amyloidosis." Other procedures depend on expected findings or grossly identified abnormalities as listed in right-hand column.	Amyloidosis* (common cause of death) involving arterioles, venules, glomeruli, and spleen. Heart and liver show only small-vessel amyloidosis. Acalculous cholecystitis* is a common complication. Acute orchitis *(1)*.
Joints	For removal, prosthetic repair, and specimen preparation, see p. 95. Submit samples of synovium for histologic study.	Arthritis,* mostly of large joints.

Reference

1. Moskovitz B, Bolkier M, Nativ O. Acute orchitis in recurrent polyserositis. J Pediatr Surg 1995;30:1517–1518.

Fever, Hemorrhagic, with Renal Syndrome

Related Terms: Balkan hemorrhagic fever with renal syndrome; Bunyaviridae infection; endemic or epidemic nephrosonephritis; Far Eastern hemorrhagic fever; Hantaan virus infection *(1)*; Korean hemorrhagic fever; Manchurian epidemic hemorrhagic fever; nephropathia epidemica.

NOTE: (1) Collect all tissues that appear to be infected. (2) Viral cultures are not available. (3) Special stains are not indicated. (4) Special **precautions** are indicated (p. 146). (5) Serologic studies are available from the Centers for Disease Control and Prevention, Atlanta, GA (p. 135). (6) This is a **reportable** disease. Bioterrorism must be considered in current cases.

Organs and Tissues	Procedures	Possible or Expected Findings
External examination	Record presence and location of petechiae.	Conjunctival petechiae; subconjunctival hemorrhages. Widespread petechiae.
Vitreous	For removal technique, see p. 85.	Increased potassium and phosphate concentrations, calcium concentrations decreased.
Blood	Submit sample for demonstration of specific IgM antibodies by ELISA and for determination of immune adherence hemagglutination titers.	See also above under "Note."
Gastrointestinal tract	Open bowel and fix samples of mucosa as early in the autopsy procedure as possible. Measure volume of blood in lumens. (If contents are fluid, one can attempt to obtain a hematocrit value.)	Intraluminal hemorrhages.
Liver	Submit samples for histologic study.	Midzonal necrosis *(2)*.
Kidneys, ureters and urinary bladder	Remove kidneys, ureters, and urinary bladder en block. Photograph cut surfaces of kidneys with renal pelves and ureters; submit samples for histologic study.	Parenchymal hemorrhages; tubular necrosis. Blood in renal pelves, ureters, and urinary bladder.
Other organs and tissues	Submit samples for histologic study.	Manifestations of hemorrhagic shock and hypotension;* retroperitoneal edema.
Brain and spinal cord	For removal and specimen preparation, see p. 65 and 67, respectively.	Hemorrhages.

References

1. Duchin JS, Koster FT, Peters CJ, Simpson GL, Tempest B, Zaki SR, et al. Hantavirus pulmonary syndrome: a clinical description of 17 patients with a newly recognized disease. N Engl J Med 1994;330: 949–955.
2. Elisaf M, Stefanaki S, Repanti M, Korakis H, Tsianos E, Siamopoulos KC. Liver involvement in hemorrhagic fever with renal syndrome. J Clin Gastroenterol 1993;17:33–37.

Fever, Lassa

Related Terms: Arenavirus infection; Argentine or Bolivian hemorrhagic fever.

NOTE:

Lassa fever is a **highly communicable** disease and **autopsy studies are not recommended** in the usually available surround-ings. If Lassa fever is suspected, contact the state health department and the Centers for Disease Control and Prevention, Atlanta, GA, for disposition and further studies *(1)*. If an autopsy is done, disinfection can be accomplished by washing instruments with 0.5% phenol in detergent (i.e., Lysol), 0.5% hypochlorite solution, formalin, or paracetic acid. (See also p. 143.) For shipping procedures, see p. 135. This is not a reportable disease.

Organs and Tissues	Procedures	Possible or Expected Findings
All organs	Experience is quite limited with cases of Lassa fever *(2)*. If an autopsy is done, it should be regarded as a research procedure. Prepare photographs. Submit samples of many organs and tissues for viral and other microbiologic studies and for histologic study. Prepare material for electron microscopic study (p. 132).	Gastrointestinal and cerebral hemorrhages; intercurrent infection; foci of necrosis.
Blood	Collect serum for serologic testing and for culture of the virus. An early diagnosis can be made from serum samples by reverse transcription PCR *(3)*.	Fourfold rise in antibody titer; high IgG titer or virus-specific IgM. Detection of Lassa virus RNA.
Other body fluids (e.g., urine, cerebrospinal fluid, breast milk, or joint fluid)	Freeze fluids at –70°C for arenavirus isolation.	

References

1. Holmes GP, McCormick JB, Trock SC, Chase RA, Lewis SM, Mason CA, et al. Lassa fever in the United States. Investigation of a case and new guidelines for management. N Engl J Med 1990;323:1120–1123.
2. Nzerue MC. Lassa fever: review of virology, immunopathogenesis, and algorithms for control and therapy. Centr Afr J Med 1992;38:247–252.
3. Demby AH, Chamberlain J, Brown DW, Clegg CS. Early diagnosis of Lassa fever by reverse transcription-PCR. J Clin Microbiol 1994; 32:2898–2903.

Fever, Periodic
(See "Fever, familial Mediterranian.")

Fever, Q

Synonyms: Acute Q fever; chronic Q fever; *Coxiella burnetii* infection.

NOTE: (1) Collect blood, urine, and all tissues that appear to be infected. (2) For the definite diagnosis of this rickettsial disease, inoculation into animals or embryonated eggs is required, which cannot be done safely in the usual clinical laboratory. (3) Special stains are not indicated. (4) This is a **highly communicable** disease, and special precautions are indicated (p. 146). (5) Serologic studies are available from local and state health department laboratories (p. 135). (6) This is a **reportable** disease.

Organs and Tissues	Procedures	Possible or Expected Findings
Blood	Submit blood sample for microbiologic study (p. 102) and serum for complement-fixation or agglutination tests.	
Heart	If endocarditis is suspected, follow procedures described on p. 103.	Bacterial suppurative vegetative endocarditis* may be present, and this is a likely cause of death. Pericarditis* and pericardial effusion.
Lungs	Submit consolidated areas for microbiologic study (p. 103). Perfuse at least one lung with formalin (p. 47).	Patchy hemorrhagic, necrotizing pneumonia; necrotizing bronchitis *(1)* and bronchiolitis.
Liver	Record weight and submit samples for histologic study.	Hepatomegaly; granulomas with fibrin ring and central lipid vacuole (not specific for the disease).
Spleen and bone marrow	Record weight and submit samples for histologic study.	Splenomegaly; splenitis with large granulomas.
Kidneys		Glomerulonephritis *(2)*.
Veins	For removal of femoral veins, see p. 34.	Thrombophlebitis.
Brain	For removal and specimen preparation, see p. 65.	Meningitis.*
Eyes	For removal and specimen preparation, see p. 85.	Uveitis; optic neuritis.
Bones, joints, and skeletal muscles	For removal and specimen preparation, see p. 95 and 80, respectively	Osteoarticular infection *(3)*; rhabdomyolysis *(4)*.

References

1. Kayser K, Wiebel M, Schulz V, Gabius HJ. Necrotizing bronchitis, angiitis, and amyloidosis associated with chronic Q fever. Respir 1995; 62:114–116.
2. Korman TM, Spelman DW, Perry GJ, Dowling JP. Acute glomerulonephritis associated with acute Q fever: case report and review of the renal complications of Coxiella burnetii infection. Clin Inf Dis 1998; 26:359–364.

3. Cottalorda J, Jouve JL, Bollini G, Touzet P, Poujol A, Kelberine F, Raoult D. Osteoarticular infection due to Coxiella burnetii in children. J Pediatr Orthopaed 1995;4:219–221.
4. Carrascosa M, Pascual F, Borobio MV, Gonzales Z, Napal J. Rhabdomyolysis associated with acute Q fever. Clin Inf Dis 1997;25:1243–1244.

Fever, Relapsing

Synonyms: Borreliosis; louseborne (epidemic) relapsing fever; tickborne (endemic) relapsing fever.

NOTE: (1) Collect all tissues that appear to be infected. (2) Rat/mouse inoculation with infected blood is the most sensitive method for the detection of the organism. Consult the state health department. (3) Before the autopsy, consultation with the microbiology laboratory is advised. (4) Request direct darkfield examination and Giemsa or Wright stain (p. 172). (4) No special precautions are indicated. (5) Serologic studies are of questionable value due to the antigenic variability of the organism. (6) This is not a reportable disease.

Organs and Tissues	*Procedures*	*Possible or Expected Findings*
Blood	Prepare smears and request Giemsa or Wright stain (p. 172).	Species of spirochetes of the genus *Borrelia*.
Spleen	Record weight. Stain touch preparations and paraffin sections with Giemsa or Wright stain (p. 172).	Organisms abundant in reticulum cells of white pulp.
Other organs	See above under "Note" and under "Spleen." Sample for histologic study as suggested in right-hand column.	Organisms in biliary epithelium, gastrointestinal tract, convoluted tubules of kidneys, brain, and meninges.

Fever, Rheumatic

NOTE: In young children, arthritis may be less conspicuous. Cardiac and other visceral manifestations may predominate in this age group.

Organs and Tissues	*Procedures*	*Possible or Expected Findings*
External examination, skin, and throat	Prepare histologic sections of subcutaneous nodules and other skin lesions and of grossly unaffected skin.	Rheumatic nodules (over bony prominences, such as elbow or occiput); erythema marginatum (annulare); cutaneous rheumatic arteritis.
	Submit swabs for throat culture.	Group A streptococci.
Pericardium	Submit fluid from pericardial sac for culture (p. 102). Record volume of pericardial contents.	Pericardial effusion or pericarditis.*
Blood	Submit samples for microbiologic and serologic studies (C-reactive protein, immunoglobulin, serum haptoglobin). For proper removal of microbiologic sample, see p. 102.	
Heart and ascending aorta	If infective endocarditis is suspected, follow procedures described on p. 102.	In chronic cases, infective endocarditis.*
	Record weight of heart; use inflow-outflow method for dissection (p. 21) and submit samples for histologic study (p. 30). Histologic samples should include posterior wall of the left atrium and chordae tendineae with papillary muscles. For histochemical and immunologic studies, freeze samples of epicardium and myocardium and of valves. Submit samples of coronary arteries and of ascending aorta for histologic study. Request Verhoeff–van Gieson stain (p. 173).	Rheumatic myocarditis; Aschoff bodies, predominantly beneath endocardium of left-sided heart chambers and within valves. Rheumatic valvular aseptic vegetative endocarditis. Coronary arteritis; intimal hyperplasia of ascending aorta, just above aortic valve.
Lungs	Submit one lobe for microbiologic study (p. 103). Perfuse one lung with formalin (p. 47). For pulmonary arteriography, see p. 50. Request Verhoeff–van Gieson stain (p. 173).	Rheumatic pneumonitis *(1)*; pulmonary vasculitis (arteritis). Chronic rheumatic mitral valvulitis may be complicated by hypertensive pulmonary vascular disease and—in rare instances—intra-alveolar ossification.

Organs and Tissues	Procedures	Possible or Expected Findings
Kidneys	Prepare thin (4-μm) paraffin sections; submit tissue samples for immunofluorescent study and for electron microscopy (p. 132).	Glomerulonephritis *(2)*; rheumatic arteritis.
Other organs	Prepare histologic sections of all organs and tissues, including skeletal muscles and cerebrospinal tissue. For immunofluorescent and electron microscopic study, see p.132. Request Verhoeff–van Gieson stain (p. 173).	Rheumatic arteritis with lesions distributed as in polyarteritis nodosa.* Thrombotic microangiopathy.
Eyes	For removal and specimen preparation, see p. 85.	Scleritis; uveitis *(3)*.
Brain		Sydenham's chorea.*
Joints	Submit samples of synovial fluid from swollen joints for microbiologic study and prepare smears for cytologic study (p. 96). For joint removal, prosthetic repair, and specimen preparation, see p. 95. Histologic samples should include synovia and periarticular tissue.	Rheumatic arthritis. Knees, ankles, hands, and wrists are primarily involved. In adults, large joints of lower extremities are usually affected.

References

1. Burgert SJ, Classen DC, Burke JP, Veasy LG. Rheumatic pneumonia: reappearance of a previously recognized complication of rheumatic fever. Clin Inf Dis 1995;21:1020–1022.
2. Imanaka H, Eto S, Takei S, Yoshinaga M, Hokonohara M, Miyata K. Acute rheumatic fever and poststreptococcal acute glomerulonephritis caused by T serotype 12 Streptococcus. Acta Paediatr Jap 1995;37: 381–383.
3. Ortiz JM, Kamerling JM, Fischer D, Baxter J. Scleritis, uveitis, and glaucoma in a patient with rheumatic fever. Am J Ophthalmol 1995; 120:538–539.

Fever, Rocky Mountain Spotted

Related Terms: *Rickettsia rickettsii* infection; tick typhus.

NOTE: (1) Collect all tissues that appear to be infected. (2) Request cultures for *Rickettsia.* This requires a special laboratory, and previous consultation with such a laboratory is recommended. Specimens for culture must be processed immediately or frozen at –60°C to ensure viability. (3) Request Giemsa stain for rickettsiae (p. 172). (4) Special **precautions** are indicated (p. 146). Laboratory infections have occurred *(1)*. Gloves should be worn when handling blood specimens. 5) Serologic studies are available from local and state health department laboratories (p. 135). Direct fluorescent antibody tests are available for formalin-fixed paraffin-embedded tissue *(2)*. (6) This is a **reportable** disease.

Organs and Tissues	Procedures	Possible or Expected Findings
External examination and skin	Submit samples of skin lesions.	Maculopapular and petechial skin lesions.
Blood	Collect serum for serologic diagnosis.	Indirect immunofluorescence positivity; ELISA positivity.
Lungs	Submit consolidated areas for microbiologic study (see p. 103 and above under "Note").	Bronchopneumonia.
Liver and spleen	Submit samples for microbiologic and histologic study (p. 102).	Hepatitis and splenitis.
Other organs and tissues	Submit tissue samples with hemorrhages and other gross lesions for microbiologic and histologic study.	Manifestations of disseminated intravascular coagulation* and of kidney failure.* (These conditions are the most frequent causes of death.) Arteriolar thromboses and necrosis with hemorrhage.
Brain and middle ears	For removal and specimen preparation, see pp. 65 and 72, respectively.	Otitis media.*
Skeletal muscles	For sampling and specimen preparation, see p. 80.	Necrosis.

References

1. Oster CN, Burke DS, Kenyon RH, Ascher MS, Harber P, Pedersen CE Jr. Laboratory-acquired Rocky Mountain spotted fever: the hazard of aerosol transmission. N Engl J Med 1977;297:859–863.
2. Walker DH, Cain BG. A method for specific diagnosis of Rocky Mountain Spotted Fever on fixed paraffin-embedded tissue by immunofluorescence. J Inf Dis 1978;137:206-209.

Fever, Scarlet

NOTE: Usually, this disease is a nonfatal group A streptococcal tonsillitis and pharyngitis with skin rash. Potentially fatal complications include suppurative otitis media,* mastoiditis, and pharyngeal abscess *(1)*, with or without septicemia.

(1) Collect all tissues that appear to be infected. (2) Request aerobic bacterial cultures. (3) Request Gram stain (p. 172). (4) Usually, no special precautions are indicated. (5) Serologic studies are available from local and state health department laboratories (p. 135). (6) This is not a reportable disease.

Reference

1. Chan TC, Hayden S. Early retropharyngeal abscess formation after treatment of scarlet fever. J Emerg Med 1996;14:377.

Fever, Tick

(See "Fever, relapsing" and "Fever, Rocky Mountain spotted.")

Fever, Typhoid

Synonym: *Salmonella typhi* infection.

NOTE: (1) Collect all tissues that appear to be infected. (2) Request aerobic bacterial cultures especially of blood. (3) Request Gram stain (p. 172). (4) Special **precautions** are indicated (p. 146). (5) Serologic studies are available from local and state health department laboratories (p. 135). (6) This is a **reportable** disease.

Organs and Tissues	*Procedures*	*Possible or Expected Findings*
External examination and skin	Prepare sections of skin lesions.	Maculopapular lesions; rose spots.
Cerebrospinal fluid	If meningitis or other intracranial abnormalities are suspected, submit sample of cerebrospinal fluid for culture and cell count (p. 104).	
Abdominal cavity	If peritonitis is present, record volume of exudate and submit sample for aerobic bacterial culture (p. 102); prepare sections of peritoneum.	Peritonitis* *(1)*.
Intestine	Inspect intestine *in situ* and record site(s) of perforation. For *in situ* fixation of small bowel, see p. 54. If intestinal hemorrhage is suspected, collect bowel contents and record volume of blood. Submit feces for aerobic bacterial culture (p. 102).	Perforation of ileum *(1)*; inflammation and ulceration of Peyer's plaques. Intestinal hemorrhage. Between third and fifth weeks of the disease, feces most often positive for *Salmonella typhi*.
Mesentery	Submit lymph nodes for histologic study.	Mesenteric lymphadenitis.
Blood	Submit samples for aerobic bacterial culture and for serologic study (p. 102).	See above under "Note."
Heart	If endocarditis is suspected, follow procedures described on p. 103. Submit sample of myocardium for aerobic bacterial culture (p. 102).	Endocarditis;* myocarditis.*
Lungs	Submit areas of consolidation for aerobic bacterial culture (p. 103).	Bronchitis and bronchopneumonia; diffuse alveolar damage *(1)*.
Liver and extrahepatic biliary system	Submit bile for aerobic bacterial culture. Submit samples of extrahepatic bile ducts, gallbladder, and liver for histologic study.	Cultures of bile may be positive for *Salmonella typhi*, particularly in chronic carriers. Acute acalculous cholecystitis;* cholelithiasis;* hepatitis *(2)* with focal necroses.
Spleen	Record weight. Submit sample for histologic study.	Splenitis; abscess.
Urine	Submit sample for aerobic bacterial culture (p. 102).	During third and fourth weeks of the disease, urine cultures most often positive for *Salmonella typhi*.
Veins	For removal of femoral veins, see p. 34.	Thrombophlebitis.
Brain and spinal cord	For removal and specimen preparation, see pp. 65 and 67, respectively.	Meningitis;* thrombosis of intracranial vessels; hydrocephalus.*
Bone, joints, and bone marrow	Submit samples of bone marrow for aerobic bacterial culture (p. 102). For removal, prosthetic repair, and specimen preparation of bones, see p. 95. For preparation of sections and smears of bone marrow, see p. 96. If osteomyelitis is present, submit sample for aerobic bacterial culture. Aspirate joint fluid at sites of joint effusion.	Bone marrow may still harbor *Salmonella typhi* when blood cultures have become negative. Megakaryocytosis may be present *(1)*. Osteomyelitis;* arthritis.

References

1. Azad AK, Islam R, Salam MA, Alam AN, Islam M, Butler T. Comparison of clinical features and pathologic findings in fatal cases of typhoid fever during the initial and later stages of the disease. Am J Trop Med Hyg 1997;56:490–493.
2. Khan M, Coovadia Y, Sturm AW. Typhoid fever complicated by acute renal failure and hepatitis: case reports and review. Am J Gastroenterol 1998;93:1001–1003.

Fever, Typhus

Synonyms and Related Terms: Brill-Zinsser disease; classic typhus; endemic typhus; louse-borne typhus; murine typhus; primary epidemic typhus; recrudescent typhus; *Rickettsia mooseri* infection; *Rickettsia prowazekii* infection.

NOTE: (1) Collect all tissues that appear to be infected. (2) Request cultures for *Rickettsia*. This requires a special laboratory, and previous consultation with such a laboratory is recommended. (3) Request Giemsa stain for rickettsiae (p. 172). (4) Special **precautions** are indicated (p. 146). (5) Serologic studies are available from local and state health department laboratories (p. 135). Indirect fluorescent antibody tests are available for use with formalin fixed paraffin-embedded tissue. (6) This is not a reportable disease.

Organs and Tissues	*Procedures*	*Possible or Expected Findings*
External examination and skin	Submit skin lesions for histologic study.	Macular and maculopapular rash; infectious vasculitis of small vessels. Rarely furunculosis.
	If gangrene of extremities is present, submit samples of necrotic tissues for histologic study.	Gangrene due to small vessel thrombosis.
Blood	See above under "Note." Specimens with viable organisms can be stored for a few days at 5°C.	Indirect immunofluorescence positivity; ELISA positivity.
Heart	Submit samples of myocardium for histologic study (p. 30).	Infectious vasculitis of small myocardial vessels; myocarditis.
Kidneys	Submit samples for histologic study.	Infectious vasculitis. Renal failure* may be the cause of death.
Veins	For removal of femoral veins, see p. 34.	Thrombophlebitis.
Brain and spinal cord	For removal and specimen preparation, see pp. 65 and 67, respectively.	Infectious vasculitis and meningitis;* inflammatory nodules within grey matter.
Middle ears	If otitis media is suspected, remove middle ears for histologic study (p. 72).	Otitis media.*

Fever, Yellow

Synonyms and Related Terms: Flavivirus (Group B arbovirus) infection; hemorrhagic fever syndrome; yellow fever virus infection.

NOTE: (1) Collect all tissues that appear to be infected. (2) After consultation with microbiology laboratory, request viral culture. (3) Usually, special stains are not helpful. (4) Special **precautions** are indicated (p. 146). (5) Serologic studies are available from the Center for Disease Control and Prevention, Atlanta, GA (p. 135). (6) This is a **reportable** disease.

Organs and Tissues	*Procedures*	*Possible or Expected Findings*
External examination		Jaundice; bleeding from nose and gums; rash; "black vomit."
Blood	Submit sample for serologic and microbiologic study (p. 102). Store blood at 4°C to maintain viral viability.	
Heart	Submit samples of myocardium for histologic study (p. 30). Request Sudan stain for frozen sections of myocardium (p. 173).	Myocardial degeneration.
Liver	Record weight and submit tissue for virologic study (p. 102). Submit samples for histologic study. Request Sudan stain for frozen sections.	Mild hepatitis with confluent focal and midzonal hepatic necrosis; Councilman bodies. Rarely, intranuclear Torres bodies. Fatty changes may be prominent.
Kidneys	See above under "Heart."	Fatty changes of renal tubular epithelium.
Other organs	Procedures depend on expected findings or grossly identified abnormalities as listed in right-hand column.	Disseminated intravascular coagulation* seems to be a frequent cause of death. Gastrointestinal hemorrhage* also may occur.
Brain	For removal and specimen preparation, see p. 65.	Focal hemorrhages.

Fibrillation and Flutter, Atrial (See "Arrhythmia, cardiac.")

Fibroelastosis, Endocardial (EFE)

NOTE: Most "primary" EFE is really secondary, associated with dilated cardiomyopathy* of infancy and childhood. EFE may also occur in hypoplastic ventricles due to congenital valvular atresia. EFE should not be confused with endomyocardial fibrosis (EMF), a condition associated with eosinophilic endomyocardial disease.

Fibrosis, Congenital Hepatic

Related Terms: Ductal plate malformation *(1)*; fibropolycystic disease of the liver and biliary tract.*

Possible Associated Conditions: Autosomal-recessive (rarely autosomal-dominant) polycystic liver disease.* Caroli's syndrome;* choledochal cyst(s);* medullary cystic renal disease (medullary tubular ectasia)* or nephronophthisis; multiple biliary microhamartomas.

Organs and Tissues	*Procedures*	*Possible or Expected Findings*
Portal vein system	For evaluation and display of portal vein, see p. 56. Record status of shunt if present.	Shunt for relief of portal hypertension.*
Liver	Record size and weight. For portal venous and hepatic arterial angiography and cholangiography, see p. 56. Photograph cut surface of liver.	Hepatomegaly; portal fibrosis; hypoplasia of portal veins. Cysts may be the site of hemorrhages. In rare instances, carcinoma of bile duct may occur.
Spleen	Record size and weight.	Congestive splenomegaly.
Esophagus and gastrointestinal tract	For demonstration of esophageal varices, see p. 53. Record volume of blood in lumen of gastrointestinal tract.	Esophageal varices.* Gastrointestinal hemorrhage.*
Kidneys	See under "Cyst(s), renal."	Cysts (see above under "Possible Associated Conditions").

Reference

1. Desmet VJ. Congenital diseases of intrahepatic bile ducts: variations on a theme "ductal plate malformation." Hepatology 1992;16:1069–1083.

Fibrosis, Cystic

Synonym: Mucoviscidosis.

Organs and Tissues	*Procedures*	*Possible or Expected Findings*
External examination	Record body weight and length.	Malnutrition *(1)* with growth retardation; clubbing of fingers.
	Prepare roentgenogram or do other tests for pneumothorax.*	Pneumothorax. Hypertrophic osteoarthropathy.
Mediastinum		Mediastinal emphysema.
Blood	Submit sample for microbiologic study (p. 102).	Septicemia (see also under "Lungs").
Heart	Record weight and thickness of ventricles.	Cor pulmonale.
Lungs	Submit one lobe for microbiologic study (p. 103).	Infections most frequently caused by *Hemophilus influenzae*, *Pseudomonas aeruginosa*, *Staphylococcus aureus*, and *Streptococcus pyogenes*.
	For postmortem bronchography and pulmonary angiography, see p. 50. If the bronchi are obstructed by tenacious secretions, formalin perfusion may be possible through pulmonary artery only. Photograph cut surface. Submit samples of bronchi and parenchyma of all lobes for microscopic study. Request Gram stain (p. 172).	Chronis bronchitis.* Bronchiectasis* and bronchiolectases; abscesses; bronchopneumonia; atelectases.
Esophagus and gastrointestinal tract	Submit samples of upper, middle, and lower esophagus; stomach, duodenum; jejunum; ileum; and colon for histologic study. If malabsorption was present, see under "Syndrome, malabsorption."	Esophageal varices (see below under "Liver"). Abnormal esophageal glands. Peptic esophagitis *(2)* and ulcers.* Meconium ileus* in small infants or meconium ileus equivalent in children and young adults. Fibrosing (submucosal) colonopathy *(2)*.

Organs and Tissues	Procedures	Possible or Expected Findings
Liver	Record weight, measure, and photograph cut section. Submit sample for histologic study.	Cirrhosis* ("focal or multilobular biliary cirrhosis"); fatty changes.
Gallbladder	Record volume and character of contents. Submit sample for histologic study. For preservation, see p. 134.	Cholecystitis;* cholelithiasis;* decreased amount of bile.
Pancreas	Record weight of dissected organ and photograph frontal section. Submit samples of head, body, and tail for histologic study.	Parenchymal atrophy with cystic fibrosis. Islets of Langerhans often preserved (manifestations of diabetes mellitus* increasingly prevalent with age *[3]*).
Male sex organs	Submit samples of testes, prostate, seminal vesicles, and spermatic ducts for histologic study.	Occlusion of vasa deferentia and associated changes, including absence or atrophy of body of epididymis.
Neck organs and skull	Remove submaxillary (with floor of mouth, p. 4) and lacrimal glands (p. 87). Expose frontal and sphenoid sinuses (p. 71), and prepare sections of mucosa. Inspect nasal cavities, and prepare sections of mucosa.	Glandular fibrosis and atrophy. Chronic sinusitis; nasal polyps.
Bones and joints	For removal, prosthetic repair, and specimen preparation, see p. 95.	Hypertrophic osteoarthropathy in adults. Joint abnormalities may be present also *(4)*.

References

1. Reilly JJ, Edwards CA, Weaver LT. Malnutrition in children with cystic fibrosis: the energy-balance equation. J Pediatr Gastroenterol Nutr 1997; 25:127–136.
2. Eggermont E. Gastrointestinal manifestations in cystic fibrosis. Eur J Gastroenterol Hepatol 1996;8:731–738.
3. Lanng S. Diabetes mellitus in cystic fibrosis. Eur J Gastroenterol Hepatol 1996;8:744–747.
4. Turner MA, Baildam E, Patel L, David TJ. Joint disorders in cystic fibrosis. J Roy Soc Med 1997;31:13–20.

Fibrosis, Endomyocardial (See "Cardiomyopathy restrictive [with eosinophilia].")

Fibrosis, Interstitial Pulmonary (See "Pneumonia, interstitial.")
Fibrosis, Mediastinal (See "Mediastinitis, chronic.")

Fibrosis, Pulmonary (See "Pneumonia, interstitial.")

Fibrosis, Retroperitoneal

Synonyms and Related Terms: Idiopathic retroperitoneal fibrosis; multifocal fibrosclerosis;* periureteral fibrosis; systemic idiopathic fibrosis.

Possible Associated Conditions: Immune complex glomerulonephritis; Peyronie's disease; pseudotumor of the orbit *(1)*; Riedel's fibrosing thyroiditis (Riedel's struma); sclerosing cholangitis;* sclerosing mediastinitis (mediastinal fibrosis).

Organs and Tissues	Procedures	Possible or Expected Findings
Retroperitoneal and pelvic tissues	For retrograde urography, see p. 59. Remove retroperitoneal and pelvic organs en bloc. Record character of dislocation and of obstruction of ureter(s), of inferior vena cava, and of other affected organs or tissues. This is best demonstrated in horizontal slices through the fibrosed areas. Submit samples for histologic study.	Hydronephrosis;* pyelonephritis;* renal amyloidosis. Fibrosis adjacent to kidneys, duodenum, descending colon, and urinary bladder or surrounding ureter(s), inferior vena cava, or pelvic organs. Lymphoma,* scirrhous adenocarcinoma, severe atherosclerosis of aorta *(2)* with or without abdominal aortic aneurysm,* or pelvic and retroperitoneal inflammatory diseases may imitate or be associated with retroperitoneal fibrosis.
Abdominal wall		Fibrosis of abdominal subcutaneous adipose tissue.
Other organs	See under "Failure, kidney" and above under "Possible Associated Conditions."	See above under "Possible Associated Conditions." Renal failure* is the most frequent cause of death.
Orbitae	For exposure, see p. 73 (Figs. 6–10).	Pseudotumor *(1)*.

References

1. Aylward GW, Sullivan TJ, Garner A, Moseley I, Wright JE. Orbital involvement in multifocal fibrosclerosis. Br J Ophthalmol 1995;79:246–249.
2. Gilkeson GS, Allen NB. Retroperitnoneal fibrosis. A true connective tissue disease. Rheum Dis Clin North Am 1996;22:23–38.

Fire (See "Burns.")

Fistula

NOTE:

For study of wound fistulas and related conditions, see p. 104. For study of cerebral arteriovenous fistula, see "Malformation, arteriovenous, cerebral or spinal (or both)." For demonstration of congenital coronary artriovenous fistula, prepare coronary arteriogram (p. 118). Such a fistula is usually found between the right coronary artery and the coronary sinus. Dissection of tracheoesophageal fistulas is discussed in Chapters 4 (Fig. 4-1) and 5.

Flukes, Hepatic (Biliary) (See "Clonorchiasis.")

Fluorosis

Organs and Tissues	*Procedures*	*Possible or Expected Findings*
External examination		Kyphosis; flexion contractures; enamel changes.
	Prepare skeletal roentgenograms.	Osteosclerosis; formation of osteophytes; ossification of tendons and ligaments.
Bones and teeth	For removal, prosthetic repair, and specimen preparation of bones, see p. 95. Snap-freeze fresh bone tissue for possible chemical analysis. Submit samples of tendons and ligaments for histologic study.	Osteomalacia* and osteosclerosis with periosteal new bone formation. Abnormal dental enamel. See also above under "External examination."
Spinal cord	For removal and specimen preparation, see p. 67.	Bone changes may have caused compression of spinal cord.

Fructose (See "Intolerance, fructose.")

Fusion, Congenital, of Cervical Vertebrae (See "Impression, basilar.")

G

Galactosemia

Organs and Tissues	*Procedures*	*Possible or Expected Findings*
External examination	Record body weight and length and head circumference.	Manifestations of malnutrition; dehydration;* jaundice; microcephaly.
Vitreous	Submit sample for determination of glucose; galactose, lactic acid, and ketone concentrations (p. 85).	
Blood	Submit sample for determination of galactose-1-phosphate uridyl transferase activity in erythrocytes. Compare with values in blood of controls.	Galactose-1-phosphate uridyl transferase deficiency.
Urine	Refrigerate immediately.	Reducing substances; glucosuria; aminoaciduria; phosphaturia.
Abdomen	Record volume of fluid.	Ascites.
Kidney	Submit sections for histologic study.	Tubular dilatation.
Liver	Record size and weight; photograph cut section; submit samples for histologic and electron microscopic study (p. 132). If histochemical study *(1)* is intended, snap-freeze tissue. Request frozen sections for Sudan stain (p. 173).	Giant cell transformation; ductular proliferation; acinar transformation of hepatocytes; cholestasis; regenerative nodules; macrovesicular steatosis; fibrosis; cirrhosis* *(2)*.
Pancreas	Submit samples of head, body, and tail for histologic study.	Hyperplasia of islets of Langerhans.
Brain and spinal cord	For removal and specimen preparation, see pp. 65 and 67, respectively.	Fibrillary astrocytosis of white matter; loss of Purkinje cells; lipofuscin overload in large neurons.
Eyes	For removal and specimen preparation, see p. 85.	Cataracts.

References

1. Landing BH, Ang SM, Villarreal-Engelhardt G, Donnell GN. Galactosemia: clinical and pathologic features, tissue staining patterns with labeled galactose- and galactosamine-binding lectins, and possible loci of nonenzymatic galactosylation. Persp Pediatr Pathol 1993;17:99–124.
2. Jevon GP, Dimmick JE. Histopathologic approach to metabolic liver disease: Part 2. Pediatr Dev Pathol 1998;1:261–269.

Ganglioneuroma (See "Tumor of the peripheral nerves.")

Gangliosidosis

Synonyms and Related Terms: Activator protein deficiency (type AB); beta galactosidase deficiency; GM_1 gangliosidosis, infantile, type 1 (with visceral involvement); late infantile, type 2; adult, type 3; GM2 gangliosidosis with infantile, late infantile, and adult forms; hexosaminidase A deficiency (type B); hexosamine A and B deficiency (type 0); lysosomal disorder *(1)*; Tay Sachs disease; Sandhoff's disease.

From: *Handbook of Autopsy Practice,* 3rd Ed. Edited by: J. Ludwig © Humana Press Inc., Totowa, NJ

Organs and Tissues	*Procedures*	*Possible or Expected Findings*
External examination	Obtain routine body measurements and weight. Photograph all abnormalities.	Hydrops fetalis; coarse facies; macroglossia; depressed, broad nose; large ears; frontal bossing; gingival hypertrophy; squat hands and feet; flexor contractures; ascites; hernias.
Fascia lata (see also "Liver and spleen")	Fascia lata should be collected using aseptic technique for tissue culture for biochemical studies (see Chapter 10) and electron microscopic examination (p. 132).	Cultured fibroblasts can be used for enzyme assay. "Empty" vacuoles in lymphocytes by EM.
Liver and spleen	Record weights. See also below under "Brain and spinal cord." Obtain tissue for tissue culture for assay of enzyme deficiency. Enzyme assay can be performed on fresh or frozen liver tissue.	Hepatosplenomegaly; accumulation of PAS and Sudan Black positive material (ganglioside) in histiocytes *(1)*.
Other organs	If evidence of other organ involvement (heart, kidney) is present, follow procedures described below under "Brain and spinal cord."	
Brain and spinal cord	For removal and specimen preparation, see pp. 66 and 70, respectively. Request LFB/PAS and/or Sudan Black (on frozen tissue) stains (p. 172). Submit samples for electron microscopic study (p. 132). Enzyme assay can be performed on fresh or frozen brain tissue. If analysis of lipids is intended, place fresh tissue in liquid nitrogen and store at –90ºC until lipids can be extracted and analyzed—for instance, by thin-layer chromatography.	Cerebral atrophy; neurons distended by lipid (ganglioside); disintegration of neurons and reactive phagocytosis and astrocytosis; fibrillogranular inclusions in fibroblasts and endothelial cells *(2–4)*.
Placenta	Weigh, snap-freeze a portion, and submit portion for histologic study.	Vacuolated syncytiotrophoblast.

References

1. Jevon GP, Dimmick JE. Histopathologic approach to metabolic liver disease: Part 2. Pediatr Dev Pathol 1998;1:261–269.
2. Lake B. Lysosomal and peroxisomal disorders. In: Greenfield's Neuropathology, vol. 1. Graham BI, Lantos PL, eds. Arnold, New York, 1997, pp. 658–668.
3. Rapola J, Lysosomal storage diseases in adults. Pathol Res Pract 1994; 190:759–766.
4. Suzuki K. Neuropathology of late onset gangliosidosis. A review. Dev Neurosci 1991;13:205–210.

Gangrene, Gas

Synonym: Clostridial infection.

NOTE: (1) Collect all tissues that appear to be infected. (2) Request aerobic and anaerobic bacterial cultures. (3) Request Gram stain (p. 172). Inflammation may be minimal or absent. (4) No special precautions are indicated. (5) Serologic studies are not indicated. (6) This is not a reportable disease.

Organs and Tissues	*Procedures*	*Possible or Expected Findings*
External examination	Record appearance of wounds or of other possibly infected lesions. If foreign bodies are present, record their nature and location (roentgenograms may be helpful). Prepare smears of wounds and request Gram stain (p. 172).	Edema surrounding wound; gas bubbles in a discharge; foul odor of the wound; loose blebs containing serosanguinous fluid.
Skeletal muscles	Prepare roentgenograms of suspected areas; palpate abnormal areas and record extent of crepitation; submit samples of grossly involved and of uninvolved skeletal muscle for bacteriologic and histologic study (see above under "Note").	Muscle necrosis (Clostridial myonecrosis) and accumulation of gas; little leukocytic infiltration.

Organs and Tissues	Procedures	Possible or Expected Findings
Other organs	Procedures depend on expected findings or grossly identified abnormalities as listed in right-hand column. See also above under "Note" and under "Skeletal muscles."	Pneumonia;* empyema;* cholecystitis;* uterine infection (postabortal or postpartum).

Gastroenteritis, Eosinophilic

Organs and Tissues	*Procedures*	*Possible or Expected Findings*
Abdomen	Record volume of peritoneal exudate and prepare smears of sediment.	Chronic peritonitis and ascites in cases with serosal involvement of the affected stomach or gut segments.
Esophagus and gastrointestinal tract	Record location of and photograph involved segments; state distance of these areas from anatomic landmarks. Leave esophagus attached to stomach. For *in situ* fixation of small bowel, see p. 54. Record thickness of wall, width of lumen, and length of involved segments. Submit samples of all grossly involved and of grossly uninvolved segments for histologic study. Request azure-eosin or Giemsa stain (p. 172).	Eosinophilic esophagitis may occur *(1)*. Presence of infiltrates most common in antrum of stomach with thickening of the pylorus. Ulcers may be found in antrum or duodenum. Various portions of small bowel also may be involved, with or without intestinal obstruction. Colonic involvement *(2)* is rare. Eosinophilic infiltrates may be found in all layers of the affected hollow viscera. There should be no evidence of parasite infestation.
Pancreas and bile ducts	Submit samples for histologic study. Request azure-eosin or Giemsa stain (p. 172).	Pancreatitis *(3)* and cholangitis *(2)* in rare instances.
Other organs	Procedures depend on expected findings or grossly identified abnormalities as listed in right-hand column.	Manifestations of malabsorption syndrome* and of protein-losing enteropathy.* There should be no evidence systemic eosinophilic disease.

References

1. Mahajan L, Wyllie R, Petras R, Steffen R, Kay M. Idiopathic eosinophilic esophagitis with stricture formation in a patient with long-standing eosinophilic gastroenteritis. Gastrointest Endosc 1997;46: 557–560.
2. Schoonbroodt D, Horsmans Y, Laka A, Geubel AP, Hoang P. Eosinophilic gastroenteritis presenting with colitis and cholangitis. Dig Dis Sci 1995; 40:308–314.
3. Maeshima A, Murakami H, Sadakata H, Saitoh T, Matsushima T, Tamura J, et al. Eosinophilic gastroenteritis presenting with acute pancreatitis. J Med 1997;28:265–272.

Gastroenteropathy, Hemorrhagic
(See "Enterocolitis, pseudomembranous" and "Shock.")

Gigantism, Hyperpituitary
(See "Acromegaly.")

Glomerulonephritis

Synonyms and Related Terms: Acute postinfectious glomerulonephritis (nonstreptococcal postinfectious glomerulonephritis;* minimal change disease; mesangial proliferative glomerulonephritis;* focal and segmental glomerulosclerosis with hyalinosis (focal sclerosis); poststreptococcal glomerulonephritis; idiopathic nephrotic syndrome; IgA nephropathy (Berger's disease); membranous glomerulonephritis; membranoproliferative glomerulonephritis; mesangial proliferative glomerulonephritis; rapidly progressive glomerulonephritis (associated with systemic infectious or immunologic multisystem diseases; drug idiosyncrasy; or as primary crescentic glomerulonephritis or superimposed on another primary glomerular disease).

Possible Associated Conditions: Acquired immunodeficiency syndrome (AIDS);* Alport's syndrome;* amyloidosis; anaphylactoid purpura; bee stings; chronic allograft rejection; dermatomyositis;* dermatitis herpetiformis; diabetes mellitus;* drug dependence;* Fabry's disease;* Goodpasture's syndrome;* Guillain-Barré syndrome;* Henoch-Schönlein purpura;* hemolytic uremic syndrome;* infective endocarditis;* leprosy;* malignancies; mixed connective tissue disease; myxedema; polyarteritis nodosa;* rheumatoid arthritis;* preeclamptic toxemia; renovascular hypertension; sarcoidosis;* serum sickness;* Sjögren's syndrome;* syphilis;* systemic lupus erythematosus;* systemic sclerosis;* thrombotic thrombocytopenic purpura;* thyroiditis;* vasculitis; viral hepatitis;* Wegener's granulomatosis;* and many other conditions.

Organs and Tissues	Procedures	Possible or Expected Findings
Blood	Refrigerate sample for possible serologic study —for instance, of basement membrane antibodies.	
Urine	Submit sample for urinalysis.	Cylindruria; hematuria; proteinuria.
Kidneys	Record weights; photograph surfaces and cut sections. Submit sample for immunofluorescent study. For electron microscopic study, see p. 132. Request 3-μm paraffin sections stained with PAS, methenamine silver, and Masson's trichrome stains (p. 173).	For specific types of glomerulonephritis, see above under "Synonyms and Related Terms." For further information, appropriate nephropathological texts should be consulted.
Other organs	Procedures depend on expected underlying, associated, or complicating conditions. If leg ulcers, wounds, or other acute infections are present, or if possibly nephritogenic chronic infections are found, submit material for appropriate bacterial cultures—for instance, from pharynx or middle ears.	See above under "Possible Associated Conditions." See also under "Failure, kidney" and, if applicable, under "Dialysis (for chronic renal failure)."
Eyes	For removal and specimen preparation, see p. 85.	Hypertensive retinopathy; in Alport's syndrome,* cataracts and other abnormalities.

Glycogenosis (See "Disease, glycogen storage.")

Gout

Related Term: Hyperuricemia.

Possible Associated Conditions: Alcoholism;* berylliosis;* chronic renal failure with long-term renal dialysis; diabetes insipidus;* Down's syndrome;* drug toxicity; glycogenosis (III, V, and VII); hemolysis; hyperparathyroidism;* hypertension;* hypothyroidism;* lead poisoning;* obesity;* Paget's disease; polycystic renal disease; polycythemia vera;* previous chemotherapy or radiation therapy of myeloproliferative disease; psoriasis;* pyelonephritis;* Reiter's syndrome;* rheumatoid arthritis;* sarcoidosis;* status post renal transplantation; toxemia of pregnancy,* and others.

Organs and Tissues	Procedures	Possible or Expected Findings
External examination and subcutaneous tissues	Photograph and record location of tophi. For fixation for histologic study, place tophi in alcohol (p. 129), formalin-alcohol (p. 130), or Carnoy's fixative (p. 130). For murexide test for the macroscopic diagnosis of urates, see p. 134. Prepare skeletal roentgenograms.	In tophaceous gout, tophi at helices of ears and on elbows, knees, hands, and feet. Acute or chronic gouty arthritis with punched-out bone lesions.
Blood	Submit sample for determination of uric acid concentration.	Hyperuricemia. For interpretation of postmortem findings, see p. 114.
Heart and blood vessels	Submit samples of myocardium and of elastic and muscular arteries for histologic study. For fixation procedures, see above under "External examination and subcutaneous tissues."	Sodium urate deposits (uncommon in heart but may be responsible for cardiac dysrhythmia*).
Trachea and major bronchi	Submit samples for histologic study.	
Kidneys	Prepare roentgenogram of soft tissues; photograph surfaces and cut sections. For fixation procedures, see above under "External examination and subcutaneous tissues."	Nephrolithiasis;* urate nephropathy; uric acid nephropathy.
Other organs	In cases of secondary gout, procedures depend on suspected underlying disease, as listed above under "Possible Associated Conditions."	See above under "Possible Associated Conditions."
Bones, joints, bursae, and tendons	For removal of synovial fluid and for identification of crystals in gout and pseudogout, see p. 96. For removal, prosthetic repair, and specimen preparation of bones and joints, see p. 95.	In rare instances, pseudogout* or pyarthrosis may occur. Monosodium urate in synovial neutrophils.

Organs and Tissues	Procedures	Possible or Expected Findings
Bones, joints, bursae, and tendons *(continued)*	Use brush to clean frontal saw section of spine, and photograph. Photograph joint surfaces and other synovial surfaces that show white deposits. Submit samples of all involved tissues for histologic study. For fixation procedures and murexide test, see above under "External examination and subcutaneous tissues." For proper sampling of joints, consult roentgenograms. For preparation of museum specimens, see p. 134.	Urate deposits in intervertebral disks and on synovial surfaces; gouty and tophaceous arthritis.
Eyes	For removal and specimen preparation, see p. 85. For fixation procedures, see above.	Urate deposits in scleras and corneas.

Granulocytopenia (See "Pancytopenia.")

Granuloma, All Types or Type Unspecified (See "Disease, chronic granulomatous," "Granuloma,...," "Granulomatosis,...," and "Pneumoconiosis." See also under name of specific granulomatous disease, such as "Sarcoidosis" and "Tuberculosis.")

Granuloma, Eosinophilic (See "Histiocytosis, Langerhans cell.")

Granuloma, Midline

Synonyms: Idiopathic midline granuloma; lethal midline granuloma; granuloma gangrenescens. (The last two names are obsolete.)

NOTE: Midline granulomas may belong to the angiocentric immunoproliferative lesions, which are related to lymphomatoid granulomatosis* and malignant lymphoma. The name "idiopathic midline granuloma" should be reserved for the few cases without evidence of malignant lymphoma or Wegener's granulomatosis* *(1)*. The diagnosis of *idiopathic* midline granuloma also can be ruled out if studies reveal fungal organisms or features of leishmaniasis;* leprosy,* rhinoscleroma, pseudotumor of the orbit or tuberculosis.* Complications of nasal cocaine abuse also may mimic midline granuloma *(2)*.

Organs and Tissues	Procedures	Possible or Expected Findings
External examination	Record extent of necrosis, and photograph facial lesions.	Necrosis of skin of nose and eyelids.
Nasal cavities and paranasal sinuses	For exposure of nasal cavities and sinuses, see p. 71. Submit material for bacterial and fungal cultures. Prepare smears and histologic sections of affected tissues. Request Verhoeff–van Gieson, Gram, and Grocott's methenamine silver stains (p. 172).	Necrosis with perforation of nasal septum, hard and soft palate, paranasal sinuses, and orbital cavities. Noncaseating granulomas with intense inflammatory reaction. Review material to rule out conditions mentioned under "Note."
Neck organs	Submit lymph nodes for microbiologic (p. 102) and histologic study.	See above under "Nasal cavities and paranasal sinuses."
Other organs		For manifestations of diseases that may produce features of midline granuloma, see above under "Note."

References

1. Barker TH, Hosni AA. Idiopathic midline destructive disease: does it exist? J Laryngol Otol 1998;112:307–309.
2. Sevinsky LD, Woscoff A, Jaimovich L, Terzian A. Nasal cocain abuse mimicking midline granuloma. J Am Acad Dermatol 1995;32:286–287.

Granulomatosis, Allergic, and Angiitis (Churg-Strauss Syndrome)

Related Term: Pulmonary granulomatous vasculitis *(1)*.

Possible Associated Condition: Asthma.*

Organs and Tissues	Procedures	Possible or Expected Findings
External examination	Record extent of skin lesions and prepare photographs.	Purpura; cutaneous and subcutaneous nodules (see below under "Other organs").

Organs and Tissues	Procedures	Possible or Expected Findings
Lungs	Perfuse lungs with formalin (p. 47) and sample for histologic study.	Eosinophilic pneumonitis (degenerating eosinophils with Charcot-Leyden crystals) and granulomas. Angiitis (mostly arteritis), typically with giant cells in tunica media *(1)*.
Other organs and soft tissues	Procedures depend on expected findings or grossly identified abnormalities as listed in right-hand column. Techniques are similar to those described under "Polyarteritis nodosa."	Findings resemble those in polyarteritis nodosa.* Heart *(2)*, grastrointestinal tract *(3)*, skin, muscles, and joints are commonly involved. However, renal disease is often (but not always) mild or absent.
	Histologic sampling should include cutaneous and subcutaneous nodules.	Necrotizing vasculitis of small arteries and veins is present, with extravascular granulomas and eosinophilic infiltration of vessels and perivascular tissues.
Eyes	For removal and specimen preparation, see p. 85.	Optic neuritis may be found *(4)*.
Brain, spinal cord, and peripheral nerves	For removal and specimen preparation, see pp. 65, 67, and 79, respectively.	May be affected by the vasculitis *(4)*.

References

1. Travis WD. Pathology of pulmonary granulomatous vasculitis. Sarcoid Vasculit Diff Lung Dis 1996;13:14–27.
2. Terasaki F, Hayashi T, Hirota Y, Okabe M, Suwa M, Deguchi H, et al. Evolution of dilated cardiomyopathy from acute eosinophilic pancarditis in Churg-Strauss syndrome. Heart Vessels 1997;12:43–48.
3. Matsuo K, Tomioka T, Tajima Y, Takayama K, Tamura H, Higami Y, et al. Allergic granulomatous angiitis (Churg-Strauss syndrome) with multiple intestinal fistulas. Am J Gastroenterol 1997;92:1937–1938.
4. Sehgal M, Swanson JW, DeRemmee RA, Colby TV. Neurologic manifestations of Churg-Straus syndrome. Mayo Clin Proc 1995;70:337–341.

Granulomatosis, Bronchocentric

Synonyms and Related Terms: Allergic bronchopulmonary aspergillosis *(1)*; eosinophilic pneumonia (eosinophilic pulmonary syndrome*); extrinsic allergic alveolitis; idiopathic bronchocentric granulomatosis; microgranulomatous hypersensitivity reaction of lungs; mucoid impaction of bronchi.

Possible Associated Conditions: Asthma;* cystic fibrosis.*

Organs and Tissues	Procedures	Possible or Expected Findings
Lungs	Submit one lobe for bacterial and fungal cultures (p. 103). Prepare smears of fresh cut sections. For pulmonary arteriography and bronchography, see p. 50. Perfuse one lung through bronchi and also through pulmonary arteries (plugged bronchi may prevent proper perfusion; see also p. 47).	*Aspergillus* (usually *Aspergillus fumigatus*) in dilated bronchi *(2)*, with or without inspissation of mucus or fungus ball; necrotizing granulomatous pneumonia or bronchitis *(2)* with bronchial chondritis; eosinophilic pneumonia; obstructive (cholesterol-type) pneumonia; atelectases; emphysema.* Secondary arteritis may be present.

References

1. Bosken C, Myers J, Greenberger P, Katzenstein A-L. Pathologic features of allergic bronchopulmonary aspergillosis. Am J Surg Pathol 1988;12: 216–222.
2. Yousem AS. The histological spectrum of chronic necrotizing forms of pulmonary aspergillosis. Hum Pathol 1997;28:650–656.

Granulomatosis, Lymphomatoid

Related Term: Angiocentric immunoproliferative lesion; angiocentric malignant lymphoma.

Possible Associated Conditions: AIDS* *(1)* and other immunodeficiency states such as Wiskott-Aldrich syndrome or post-transplant immunosuppression.

Organs and Tissues	Procedures	Possible or Expected Findings
External examination and skin	Record extent of skin lesions; photograph skin lesions; prepare histologic sections of involved skin and of grossly uninvolved skin.	Lymphoreticular infiltrates, primarily in dermis but also in subcutis. See also under "Lungs."

Organs and Tissues	Procedures	Possible or Expected Findings
External examination and skin *(continued)*	Prepare chest roentgenogram.	Multiple nodules, with or without cavitation; cavitation; rarely pneumothorax *(2)*.
Blood	Submit sample for bacterial, fungal, and viral cultures (p. 102). Snap-freeze sample for possible biochemical and immunologic study.	
Lungs	Record weights; submit samples of fresh tissue for B- and T-cell gene derangement studies, frozen-section immunostains, and other investigations (see refs. *3* and *4*). Submit one lobe for microbiologic study (p. 103). Touch preparations of cut surfaces of lungs for cytologic study may be helpful.	PCR studies on paraffin sections via RNA *in situ* hybridization may confirm presence of Epstein-Barr virus-positive B-cell proliferations combined with dense T-cell accumulations *(3–5)*. The condition closely resembles angiocentric T-/NK cell lymphoma *(3)*.
	For pulmonary arteriography, see p. 50. Perfuse one lung with formalin (p. 47). Photograph cut sections of lungs. Submit samples of all lobes and of hilar lymph nodes for histologic study. Request Verhoeff–van Gieson, Gram, and Gridley's fungal stains (p. 172). For preparation of specimens for electron microscopy, see p. 132.	Infiltration of lymphocytoid cells, plasma cells, and macrophages with necroses and granulomatous features, which are found primarily in the vicinity of blood vessels. Special stains may reveal evidence of infection.
Liver	Record weight and sample for histologic studies.	Lymphoreticular and granulomatous infiltrates (see "Lung").
Kidneys	Follow procedures described under "Glomerulonephritis."	Lymphoreticular and granulomatous infiltrates (see "Lung").
Other organs and tissues	Samples for histologic study should include heart, pancreas, spleen, adrenal glands, urinary bladder, prostate, neck organs (with nasopharynx and tongue), salivary glands, lymph nodes, thymus, bone marrow, and all other tissues with grossly identifiable lesions.	Characteristic infiltrates may be present in all organs and tissues. Involvement of spleen, lymph nodes, and bone marrow is uncommon. In rare instances, the disease is confined to the abdomen.
Brain and spinal cord	For removal and specimen preparation, see pp. 65 and 67, respectively.	In most instances, characteristic infiltrates are present.

References

1. Haque AK, Myers JL, Hudnall SD, Gelman BB, Lloyd RV, Payne D, et al. Pulmonary lymphomatoid granulomatosis in acquired immunodeficiency syndrome: lesions with Epstein-Barr virus infection. Mod Pathol 1998;11:347–356.
2. Morris MJ, Peacock MD, Lloyd WC III, Johnson JE. Recurrent bilateral spontaneous pneumothoraces associated with pulmonary angiocentric immunoproliferative lesion. South Med J 1995;88:771–775.
3. Jaffe ES, Wilson WH. Lymphomatoid granulomatosis: pathogenesis, pathology and clinical implications. Canc Surv 1997;30:233–248.
4. McNiff JM, Cooper D, Howe G, Crotty PL, Tallini G, Crouch J, et al. Lymphomatoid granulomatosis of the skin and lung. An angiocentric T-cell-rich B-cell lymphoproliferative disorder. Arch Dermatol 1996; 132:1464–1470.
5. Myers J, Kurtin P, Katzenstein A-L, Tazelaar H, Colby T, Strickler J, et al. Lymphomatoid granulomatosis. Evidence of immunophenotypic diversity and relationship to Epstein-Barr virus infection. Am J Surg Pathol 1995;19:1300–1312.

Granulomatosis, Wegener's

Related Terms: Angiocentric granulomatosis; granulomatous angiitis; pulmonary angiitis and granulomatosis *(1)*.

Organs and Tissues	Procedures	Possible or Expected Findings
External examination and skin; oral cavity; breasts	Prepare histologic sections of skin lesions and of grossly uninvolved skin.	Skin papules, vesicles, ulcers. Subcutaneous nodules (vasculitis and granulomas). Granulomatous infiltrates of breast *(2)*. Gangrene of digits *(2,3)*.
	Prepare histologic sections of accessible mucosal lesions in mouth.	Necrotizing and ulcerative stomatitis.

Organs and Tissues	*Procedures*	*Possible or Expected Findings*
Blood	Submit samples for microbiologic (p. 102) and for immunologic study.	Septicemia; circulating immunoglobulin complexes.
Lungs	Submit one lobe for microbiologic study (p. 103). For pulmonary arteriography, see p. 50. Perfuse one lung with formalin (p. 47). Request Verhoeff–van Gieson stain (p. 172).	Angiocentric granulomatosis *(4)*; necrotizing arteritis with infarctions; granulomatous bronchitis; pleuritis.
Spleen	Record weight; submit samples for histologic study.	Necrotizing arteritis. Infarctions *(5)*.
Kidneys	Follow procedures described under "Glomerulonephritis."	Focal necrotizing glomerulitis; necrotizing arteritis *(1)*.
Neck organs with larynx and trachea	Remove neck organs together with oropharynx and soft palate. Photograph lesions. For histologic study, submit samples with gross lesions and samples of grossly uninvolved tissue.	Necrotizing granulomatous inflammation and ulcers of soft palate, larynx, and trachea. Subglottic stenosis. Acute obstruction may be a cause of death *(6)*.
Other organs and tissues	Procedures depend on expected findings or grossly identified abnormalities as listed in right-hand column.	Necrotizing arteritis and granulomatous inflammation—for example in heart, gastrointestinal tract, and urogenital organs *(1)*.
Paranasal sinuses; ear, nose	For exposure of sinuses, see p. 71. Specimens should include surrounding bone; submit samples for histologic study (for decalcification procedures, see p. 97).	Necrotizing and ulcerative sinusitis with perifocal osteomyelitis. Necrotizing lesions in nasal cavities.
	For exposure of middle ear, see p. 72.	Otitis media.
Brain and spinal cord	For removal and specimen preparation, see pp. 65 and 67, respectively.	Angiocentric granulomatous lesions may be present *(1)*.
Eyes and orbitae	For removal and specimen preparation, see pp. 85 and 73, respectively.	Pseudotumor of the orbit; other ocular lesions *(1)*, such as conjunctivitis, dacryocystitis, scleritis, and episcleritis, granulomatous sclerouveitis; ciliary vasculitis.
Bones and joints		Arthritis.*

References

1. Lie JT. Wegener's granulomatosis: histological documentation of common and uncommon manifestations in 216 patients. VASA 1997; 26:261–270.
2. Trueb RM, Pericin M, Kohler E, Barandun J, Burg G. Necrotizing granulomatosis of the breast. Br J Dermatol 1997;137:799–803.
3. Handa R, Wali JP. Wegener's granulomatosis with gangrene of toes. Scand J Rheumatol 1996;25:103–104.
4. Travis WD. Pathology of pulmonary granulomatous vasculitis. Sarcoidosis, Vascul Diff Lung Dis 1996;13:14–27.
5. Fishman D, Isenberg DA. Splenic involvement in rheumatic diseases. Semin Arthritis Rheum 1997;27:141–155.
6. Matt BH. Wegener's granulomatosis, acute laryngotracheal airway obstruction and death in a 17-year-old female: case report and review of the literature. Int J Pediatr Otolaryngol 1996;37:163–172.

Gunshot (See "Injury, firearm.")

H

Hallucinogen(s) (See "Abuse, hallucinogen(s).")

Halothane (See "Death, anesthesia-associated.")

Hanging

NOTE: Most hangings in the United States are suicides with short drops producing no cervical derangements, in contrast to the now uncommon judical hangings. A few hanging deaths are industrial accidents, and a few are consequences of asphyxia, self-induced for the purpose of sexual pleasure. Clues to autoerotic asphyxia are nudity, cross dressing, bondage paraphernalia, pornography, remotely operated video cameras, escape mechanisms, and a history or evidence of prior such acts.

Organs and Tissues	*Procedures*	*Possible or Expected Findings*
External examination and skin	Photograph the neck and head with and without the ligature in place, from anterior, left, right, and posterior aspects, and the ligature after removal.	Corresponding patterns of ligature and furrow; presence or absence of cyanosis and factial petecchiae; protrusion of tongue.
	Record and photograph liver mortis.	Shift from lower extremities to back; Tardieau spots (petecchiae caused by pooling).
	Measure diameter of the ligature and the depth and width of the furrow.	Size and pattern of ligature should match size and pattern of furrow.
	Measure the circumference of both the ligature and the neck. Measure the vertical distance of the furrow from the ear lobe.	Circumference of ligature will be less than circumference of neck.
Neck organs	Use layerwise anterior dissection (p. 14).	Dessicated tan compressed subcutaneous facia; fractures of superior laryngeal cornua or hyoid in the elderly are consistent with hanging and can occur after prolonged suspension.

Hashish (See "Abuse, marihuana.")

Heart Disease, Congenital

NOTE: See under individual malformations, such as "Defect, ventricular septal." For a listing of Latin terms and their Anglicized equivalents, see Chapter 3, Appendix 3-3, p. 39. Synonyms for various forms of congenital heart disease are compiled in Chapter 3, Appendix 3-2, p. 39. For eponyms of various operations for congenital heart disease, see Chapter 3, Appendix 3-4, p. 41. Finally, a template for recording information at autopsy on patients with congenital heart disease is presented in Chapter 3, Appendix 3-5, p. 42.

Heat (See "Burns" and "Heatstroke.")

Heatstroke

Synonyms and Related Terms: Heat exhaustion; heat syncope; hyperthermia.

NOTE: Possible complications include disseminated intravascular coagulation* and fibrinolysis syndrome and Gram-negative septicemia.

From: *Handbook of Autopsy Practice,* 3rd Ed. Edited by: J. Ludwig © Humana Press Inc., Totowa, NJ

Organs and Tissues	Procedures	Possible or Expected Findings
External examination	Inquire about ambient and body temperature.	Hyperthermia when body was discovered.
Vitreous	Submit sample for determination of chloride, sodium, and urea nitrogen concentrations (p. 58).	Frequently, evidence of hypertonic dehydration.* See also p. 115.
Blood	Submit sample for toxicologic study, particularly for alcohol and drug screen (p 16).	
Urine	Record volume; determine specific gravity; record appearance of sediment.	High specific gravity; casts.
Thyroid gland	Sample for histologic study, particularly in unusual cases of heatstroke.	Thyroid disease such as Hashimoto's thyroiditis may predispose to heatstroke *(2)*.
Other organs	Submit samples for toxicologic (p. 16) and histologic study.	There may be no macroscopic changes *(2)*. Hemorrhages may be present, particularly in central nervous system, kidneys, and liver. Small parenchymal necroses with or without microthrombi may be found.

References

1. Donoghue ER, Graham MA, Jentzen JM, Lifschultz BD, Luke JL, Mirchandani HG. Criteria for the diagnosis of heat-related deaths: National Association of Medical Examiners. Position paper. National Association of Medical Examiners Ad Hoc Committee on the Definition of Heat-Related Fatalities. Am J Forens Med Pathol 1997;18:11–14.
2. Siegler RW. Fatal heatstroke in a young woman with previously undiagnosed Hashimoto's thyroiditis. J Forens Sci 1998;43:1237–1240.

Hematoma, Dissecting Aortic (See "Dissection, aortic.")

Hematoma, Spinal Epidural

Organs and Tissues	Procedures	Possible or Expected Findings
Spinal cord	For removal and specimen preparation, see p. 67.	Traumatic lesions; vascular malformations.
Other organs		Manifestations of hypertension.*

Hematoma, Subdural

Synonym: Subdural hemorrhage.

Organs and Tissues	Procedures	Possible or Expected Findings
External examination	Record evidence of trauma.	Abrasions; lacerations; subcutaneous hematomas.
	Prepare roentgenogram of skull.	Fractures.
Skull, meninges, and brain	For opening of skull and removal of calvarium, see p. 65.	Fractures may be identifiable only after stripping of dura.
	Record site and volume of subdural hematoma and relation of hematoma to burr holes (if present).	Compression of cerebral hemispheres, with or without edema, and secondary compression of rostral brain stem.
	Remove vitreous—particularly if subdural hematoma appears to be nontraumatic—and determine sodium, potassium, and chloride concentrations (p. 85).	Nontraumatic subdural hematoma rarely may be caused by hypernatremia and other hyperosmolar conditions. For interpretation of electrolyte values, see p. 113.

Hemochromatosis

Synonyms and Related Terms: Genetic hemochromatosis; pigment cirrhosis; primary hemochromatosis; secondary hemochromatosis.

NOTE: Secondary iron overload in other types of cirrhosis (e.g., alcoholic cirrhosis; alpha$_1$-antitrypsin deficiency, chronic viral hepatitis) may be severe enough to suggest genetic hemochromatosis. In such cases, quantitative iron studies (see below under "Liver") and calculation of the iron index are indicated *(1)*.

Organs and Tissues	*Procedures*	*Possible or Expected Findings*
External examination and skin and oral cavity	Record character and extent of pigmentation. Prepare histologic sections of pigmented areas and request Gomori's iron and Fontana-Masson silver stains (p. 172).	Melanin hyperpigmentation of skin in face, neck, dorsal aspect of forearms and hands, genital area and scars; pigmentation of oral mucosa in some instances. A positive Fontana-Masson stain is not specific for the presence of melanin. Some hemosiderin may be present also.
	Prepare skeletal roentgenograms, which should include major joints, wrists, and hands, as listed in right-hand column.	Osteoporosis* and osteoarthritis* of hands and wrists, with chondrocalcinosis, subarticular cysts (second and third metacarpophalangeal joints), or osteophytes; osteoarthritis of hip, knee, and other major joints. Calcification of synovium.
Heart	Record weight. For gross staining for iron, see p. 133. For dissection of the conduction system, see p. 26. Submit samples of myocardium for histologic study (p. 30) and request Gomori's iron stain (p. 172).	Cardiomyopathy with hemosiderosis and fibrosis of cardiac musculature.
Liver	Record weight and photograph. For gross staining for iron, see Chapter 14, p. 133. For microscopic sections, request Gomori's iron stain (p. 172). For quantitative iron studies, submit sample (this can be dug out from a paraffin block) for atomic absorption spectrophotometry *(1)*.	Pigment cirrhosis (see also above under "Note" and under "Cirrhosis, liver"). Hepatocellular carcinoma (see under "Tumor of the liver").
Pancreas	Record color and weight. Submit samples for histologic study, particularly of tail. See also above under "Liver."	Hemosiderosis of exocrine and endocrine parenchyma; interstitial fibrosis.
Other organs and tissues	Histologic samples should include oral mucosa, tongue, stomach, intestinal tract, spleen, adrenal glands, kidneys, thyroid gland, parathyroid glands, lymph nodes, pituitary gland, and bone marrow. For gross and microscopic staining procedures, see above under "Liver."	Manifestations of diabetes mellitus;* features of congestive heart failure,* particularly in patients with hemochromatotic cardiomyopathy. Generalized hemosiderosis with fibrosis of adrenal glands and pituitary gland. Secondary hemochromatosis may be caused by various conditions, such as spherocytosis, thalassemia,* and other types of anemia (see "Anemia, hemolytic"), treated or untreated by transfusions. See also above under "Note."
Testes	Record weights and submit samples for histologic study.	Tubular atrophy.
Bones and joints	For removal, prosthetic repair, and specimen preparation, see p. 95.	Osteoporosis* and osteoarthritis.* Hemosiderosis of joints and synovial membranes. Calcium pyrophosphate crystals in synovium. See also above under "External examination and skin and oral cavity."
Eyes	For removal and specimen preparation, see p. 85. Request Gomori's iron stain (p. 172).	Hemosiderosis of margin of retinal disk, ciliary body, and corneal epithelium.

Reference

1. Ludwig J, Hashimoto E, Porayko MK, Moyer T, Baldus WP. Hemosiderosis in cirrhosis: a study of 447 native livers. Gastroenterology 1997; 112: 882–888.

Hemoglobinuria, Paroxysmal Nocturnal (See "Anemia, hemolytic.")

Hemophilia

Synonyms: Hemophilia A (factor VIII coagulant protein deficiency); hemophilia B (Factor IX deficiency; Christmas disease).

NOTE: Rare hereditary deficiencies of other blood coagulation factors (II, V, VII, X, XI) may cause some symptoms of hemophilia. A reliable postmortem diagnosis is not possible; post-mortem blood coagulation studies do not yield useful results.

Possible Associated Conditions: Acquired immunodeficiency syndrome (AIDS)* *(1)*, chronic viral hepatitis* with or without cirrhosis, and other infections from contaminated plasma products.

Organs and Tissues	*Procedures*	*Possible or Expected Findings*
External examination	Record character and extent of skin changes.	Cutaneous ecchymoses; soft tissue hematoma; blood in body orifices.
	Prepare skeletal roentgenograms.	Joint deformities (ankle, knee, elbow); erosions of bones by pseudotumors; soft tissue calcifications.
Blood	If infectious complications are expected, submit samples for culture and serologic study (p. 102).	For common infections in hemophilic patients, see above under "Note."
Liver	Record weight and sample for histologic study.	Viral hepatitis C is very common but hepatitis B also may be encountered *(2)*. (See also under "Hepatitis, chronic.")
Other organs	Record sites and sizes of hematomas and hemorrhages, and photograph.	Hematomas and hemorrhages in soft tissues of floor of mouth, neck, subdural space, retroperitoneum, mesentery, renal pelves, gastrointestinal tract, and other sites.
Brain and spinal cord	For removal and specimen preparation, see pp. 65 and 67, respectively.	Hemorrhage *(1)*; microinfarctions, possibly related to treatment with large amounts of antihemophilic factor.
Joints	For removal, specimen preparation, and prosthetic repair, see p. 96. Photograph joint lesions.	Arthropathy with severe degenerative changes *(3)*; hemarthrosis.

References

1. Cahill MR, Colvin BT. Haemophilia. Postgrad Med J 1997;73:201–206.
2. Lee CA. Transfusion-transmitted disease. Baillieres Clin Haematol 1996;9:369–394.
3. Lan HH, Eustace SJ, Dorfman D. Hemophilic arthropathy. Radiol Clin North Am 1996;34:446–450.

Hemorrhage, Cerebral (See under name of suspected underlying condition, such as "Aneurysm, cerebral artery," "Infarction, cerebral," "Injury, head," and "Tumor of the brain." For removal of cerebrospinal fluid, see p. 104.)"

Hemorrhage, Gastrointestinal

Organs and Tissues	*Procedures*	*Possible or Expected Findings*
Abdomen		Diaphragmatic hernia.*
Esophagus and stomach	For demonstration of esophageal varices, see p. 53. Record appearance of mucosa; record volume of blood in lumen.	Reflux esophagitis; varices;* strictures with erosions; tumor;* mucosal erosions and peptic ulcer(s);* petechial mucosal hemorrhages.
Duodenum		Peptic ulcer(s).*
Small bowel and large bowel	If infectious enteritis is suspected, submit material for microbiologic study (p. 102). Submit samples of all segments for histologic study. If free blood is present, record volume.	Infectious—for instance, in typhoid fever*—and noninfectious enteritis; circulatory or neoplastic intestinal disease; other diseases, such as diverticulitis.
Other organs	Procedures depend on expected findings or grossly identified abnormalities as listed in right-hand column.	Cerebral space-occupying lesions; manifestations of coagulation disorder, including leukemia* or other neoplastic disease; pancreatitis;* manifestations of portal hypertension* or of kidney failure.*

Hemorrhage, Intracranial (See under "Hematoma, subdural" and under name of suspected underlying condition, such as "Aneurysm, cerebral artery," "Infarction, cerebral," "Injury, head," and "Tumor of the brain." For removal of cerebrospinal fluid, see p. 104.)

Hemorrhage, Subarachnoid (See under name of suspected underlying condition, such as "Aneurysm, cerebral artery," "Infarction, cerebral," "Injury, head," and "Tumor of the brain." For removal of cerebrospinal fluid, see p. 104.)"

Hemosiderosis, Idiopathic Pulmonary

NOTE: This diagnosis is made by exclusion; involvement of organs other than the lungs (see below under "Kidneys") suggests another disease.

Organs and Tissues	*Procedures*	*Possible or Expected Findings*
Heart		Cor pulmonale.
Lungs	Photograph fresh lungs (side by side with normal lung). Perfuse lungs with formalin (p. 47); for iron staining of gross specimens, see p. 133; for microscopic sections, request Gomori's iron stain (p. 172). For quantitation of iron in paraffin blocks, see "Hemochromatosis."	Hemorrhages into alveolar spaces. Hemosiderin in pulmonary septa and macrophages; interstitial pulmonary fibrosis; degeneration, shedding, and hyperplasia of alveolar epithelial cells.
	Immunofluorescent and electron microscopic studies (see below) also may be of value.	Goodpasture's syndrome and immune-complex mediated vasculitis need to be ruled out.
Kidneys	Prepare tissue for immunofluorescent study. Submit samples for electron microscopic study p. 132).	Kidneys should not be involved; if they are, Goodpasture's syndrome* must be considered as a cause.
Bone marrow	For preparation of sections and smears, see p. 96.	Secondary hyperplasia caused by anemia.

Hepatitis, Alcoholic (See "Disease, alcoholic liver.")

Hepatitis, Chronic

Synonyms and Related Terms: Autoimmune hepatitis; chronic viral hepatitis B (with or without D) and C.

NOTE: The term "chronic hepatitis" is not a complete etiologic diagnosis and related names such as chronic active (aggressive) hepatitis, chronic active liver disease, and chronic persistent hepatitis are obsolete. Most cases in these categories represent autoimmune hepatitis or chronic viral hepatitis B or C. Many other liver diseases, including drug-induced hepatitis, inborn errors of metabolism (e.g., alpha$_1$-antitrypsin deficiency* or Wilson's disease*), developmental disorders, and chronic biliary diseases such as primary biliary cirrhosis or primary sclerosing cholangitis also may present as chronic hepatitis.

If chronic hepatitis was the cause of death, submassive hepatic necrosis or cirrhosis* is usually present, often with manifestations of portal hypertension,* hepatic encephalopathy, hepatorenal syndrome,* and with ascites or spontaneous bacterial peritonitis.

Possible Associated Conditions: See also below under "Possible or Expected Findings." Conditions that may be associated with hepatitis C include *(1)*: autoimmune hepatitis; Behcet's disease; diabetes mellitus (type 2);* glomerulonephritis;* Guillain-Barré syndrome;* idiopathic pulmonary fibrosis; idiopathic thrombocytopenic purpura; IgA deficiency; lichen planus; mixed essential cryoglobulinemia; Mooren's corneal ulcers; polyarthritis; porphyria cutanea tarda;* thyroiditis.*

Organs and Tissues	*Procedures*	*Possible or Expected Findings*
External examination and skin	Record body weight and length, habitus, and extent and character of skin changes. Prepare histologic sections of skin lesions.	Hirsutism; cushingoid face; acne; maculopapular rash; erythema nodosum; lupus erythematosus-like changes in face; localized scleroderma; purpura; vitiligo; cutaneous small-vessel vasculitis and porphyria cutanea tarda in chronic hepatitis C *(2)*.
Blood	Submit sample for serologic studies if type of viral hepatitis (B, D, or C) or of autoimmune hepatitis is in question.	Viral antigens or antibodies; autoantibodies (ANA, SMA, and others) in autoimmune hepatitis. Essential mixed cryoglobulinemia in chronic hepatitis C *(2)*.
Heart	For histologic sampling, see p. 30.	Pericarditis.
Arteries		Polyarteritis nodosa*
Liver	Record weight and photograph surface and cut	Chronic viral or autoimmune hepatitis, with

Organs and Tissues	Procedures	Possible or Expected Findings
	sections. If chronic hepatitis B is suspected, order immunostains for B surface and core antigen.	or without cirrhosis;* hepatocellular carcinoma.
	Request PAS stain with diastase digestion, p. 173.	Alpha$_1$-antitrypsin deficiency.*
	If Wilson's disease must be ruled out, order rhodanine stain and quantitative copper study.	High hepatic tissue copper concentrations in Wilson's disease.*
	Request Gomori's iron stain (p. 172).	Hemosiderosis common in hepatitis C.
Gallbladder	Describe concrements.	Cholelithiasis
Pancreas	Submit samples for histologic study.	Changes associated with diabetes mellitus.*
Intestinal tract	Procedures depend on expected findings or grossly identified abnormalities as in conditions listed in right-hand column.	Crohn's disease* or chronic ulcerative colitis often associated with primary sclerosing cholangitis.* (See above under "Note.")
Kidneys	Follow procedures described under "Glomerulonephritis."	Membranous and membranoproliferative glomerulitis and nephrotic syndrome.
Thyroid gland	Record weight, photograph, and submit samples for histologic study.	Hashimoto's thyroiditis. Thyroid dysfunction in interferon-treated chronic hepatitis B and C *(3)*.
Brain and spinal cord	For removal and specimen preparation, see pp. 65 and 67, respectively.	Cerebritis and peripheral neuropathy in chronic hepatitis C *(2)*.
Eyes and lacrimal glands	For removal and specimen preparation, see pp. 85 and 87, respectively.	Keratoconjunctivitis; fibrosis and inflammation of lacrimal glands; manifestations of Sjögren's syndrome.*
Parotid and submandibular glands	Samples can be biopsied from scalp incision (p. 65) and removed with floor of the mouth (p. 41), respectively.	Fibrosis and inflammation.
Nose, pharynx, and larynx	Submit samples of mucosa for histologic study.	Atrophy of mucosal glands.
Bone, bone marrow, and joints	For removal, specimen preparation, and prosthetic repair of bones and joints, see p. 95. For preparation of sections and smears of bone marrow, see p. 96.	Osteoporosis* (particularly after steroid treatment); hypocellular bone marrow (aplastic anemia).

References

1. Gordon SC. Extrahepatic manifestations of Hepatitis C. Dig Dis 1996; 14:157–168.
2. Gross JB Jr. Clinician's guide to hepatitis C. Mayo Clinic Proc 1998; 73:355–361.
3. Deutsch M, Dourakis S, Manesis EK, Gioustozi A, Hess G, Horsch A, Hadziyannis S. Thyroid abnormalities in chronic viral hepatitis and their relationship to interferon alpha therapy. Hepatology 1997;26: 206–210.

Hepatitis, Fulminant (See "Hepatitis, viral.")

Hepatitis, Neonatal

Synonyms and Related Terms: Giant cell hepatitis; idiopathic neonatal hepatitis (familial or nonfamilial); infantile obstructive cholangiopathy; neonatal cholestasis.

NOTE: Neonatal hepatitis may have been a biopsy diagnosis in an earlier stage of paucity of intrahepatic bile ducts; at autopsy, biliary cirrhosis with ductopenia would be the main finding. For other conditions that may present clinically as neonatal hepatitis or jaundice, see below.

Organs and Tissues	Procedures	Possible or Expected Findings
External examination		Jaundice. Lymphedema in one form of hereditary neonatal hepatitis *(1)*.
Blood	Submit samples for microbiologic (p. 102) and serologic study. If chromosome abnormalities are suspected, submit sample for chromosome analysis (p. 108).	Hepatitis virus antigens or antibodies, including hepatitis B or C, cytomegalovirus, coxsackievirus, herpes simplex, rubeola, and varicella virus. Toxoplasmosis,* congenital syphilis,* and *Listeria monocytogenes* infection may also cause neonatal hepatitis.
Extrahepatic bile ducts	For postmortem cholangiography, see p. 56. If no roentgenologic studies can be carried out, open duodenum *in situ*, squeeze gallbladder, and record whether bile emerged from papilla.	Biliary atresia;* paucity of intrahepatic bile ducts (syndromic [Alagille's syndrome] or nonsyndromic); choledochal cyst.*

Organs and Tissues	Procedures	Possible or Expected Findings
Liver	Record size and weight; photograph surface and cut section; submit sample of fresh liver for viral culture (p. 102); submit samples for histologic study; request PAS stain with diastase digestion (p. 173).	Giant cell transformation of liver, with or without biliary atresia or paucity of intrahepatic bile ducts. Cholestasis and cirrhosis may be present. Alpha$_1$-antitrypsin deficiency. Fatty livers also may be found *(2)*.
Other organs and tissues	Procedures depend on expected findings or grossly identified abnormalities as listed in right-hand column.	Manifestations of conditions that may present clinically as neonatal hepatitis or jaundice, e.g., cystic fibrosis *(3)*;* erythroblastosis fetalis;* congenital rubella syndrome;* galactosemia;* Niemann-Pick disease;* trisomy 17-18; Turner's syndrome.*

References

1. Sharp HL, Krivit W. Hereditary lymphedema and obstructive jaundice. J Pediatr 1971;78:491–496.
2. Nishinomiya F, Abukawa D, Takada G, Tazawa Y. Relationships between clinical and histological profiles of non-familial idiopathic neonatal hepatitis. Acta Paediatr Japn 1996;38:242–247.
3. Lykavieris P, Bernard O, Hadchouel M. Neonatal cholestasis as the presenting feature in cystic fibrosis. Arch Dis Child 1996;75:67–70.

Hepatitis, Viral

Synonyms: Acute (or subacute) viral hepatitis; fulminant viral hepatitis; hepatitis virus hepatitis; viral hepatitis A, B, B with D, C, E, F, G, or type undetermined.

NOTE: Coinfection with other hepatitis viruses (e.g., C and G) and/or systemic viruses such as the immunodeficiency virus are common, particularly in drug addicts *(1,2)*. In many cases of fulminant hepatitis, tests for known hepatitis viruses are negative *(3,4)*. If the hepatitis was caused by a systemic virus, see under the specific disease name, for example, "Infection, cytomegalovirus." For chronic viral hepatitis, see under "Hepatitis, chronic." If the patients underwent liver transplantation *(3)* or bone marrow transplantation for complicating aplastic anemia *(4)*, see also under "Transplantation,..."

(1) Collect all tissues that appear to be infected. (2) Request viral cultures if systemic disease such as cytomegalovirus infection* is expected. (3) Stains for hepatitis B core and surface antigen may be helpful (p. 172). (4) Special **precautions** are indicated, particularly in suspected hepatitis B and D infection (p. 146). (5) Serologic studies are essential in undiagnosed cases and can be obtained from most clinical laboratories. (6) Hepatitis virus hepatitis is not a reportable disease.

Possible Associated Conditions: See "Hepatitis, chronic."

Organs and Tissues	Procedures	Possible or Expected Findings
External examination	If patient was on dialysis for chronic renal failure, see also under that heading.	Jaundice; skin rash or hemorrhages and other abnormalities. Needle marks may indicate intravenous substance abuse.
Blood	Submit sample for serologic studies for viral antigens or antibodies.	Viral antigens or antibodies may or may not be positive.
Heart	For histologic sampling, see p. 30.	Myocarditis;* necrosis of fibers in bundle of His.
Lungs	Perfuse one lung with formalin (p. 47). Sample for histologic study and request Verhoeff–van Gieson stain (p. 173).	Manifestations of pulmonary hypertension.*
Liver	Record weight and photograph surface and cut sections. If hepatitis B is suspected, order immunostains for B surface and core antigen. Immunostains for hepatitis D are also available.	Lobular inflammation with briding necrosis or multilobular collapse; massive necrosis with complete loss of parenchyma. Stains for viral antigens often are negative.
Gallbladder	Record appearance and volume of bile.	Bile may be absent.
Pancreas	Submit samples for histologic study.	Pancreatitis.*
Spleen	Record weight; request Gomori's stain for iron.	Pulpal hyperplasia; hemosiderosis; congestive splenomegaly.
Esophagus	Leave attached to stomach; submit sample for histologic study.	Ulcerations or erosions of distal esophagus; varices.
Stomach	Submit sample for histologic study.	Gastritis.

Organs and Tissues	Procedures	Possible or Expected Findings
Small intestine	For *in situ* fixation, see p. 54. Submit samples for histologic study.	Flattening, broadening, and possible fusion of villi. Phlegmonous inflammation and edema, mainly in ileocecal region.
Kidneys	Follow procedures described under "Glomerulonephritis."	Glomerular changes; bile casts in tubules; interstitial edema.
Lymph nodes	Submit cervical and mediatinal lymph nodes for histologic study.	Lymphadenitis.
Thyroid	Sample for histologic study.	See "Hepatitis, chronic."
Brain and spinal cord	For removal and specimen preparation, see pp. 65 and 67, respectively.	Encephalitis.*
Bone marrow	For preparation of sections and smears, see p. 96.	Leukopenia; thrombocytopenia; aplastic anemia *(4)* (pancytopenia*).
Joints	For removal, prosthetic repair, and specimen preparation, see p. 96. Submit samples of synovia for histologic study.	Synovitis (arthritis*).

References

1. Thiers V, Pol S, Persico T, Carnot F, Zylberberg H, Berthelot P, et al. Hepatitis G virus infection in hepatitis C virus-positive patients co-infected or not with hepatitis B virus and/or human immunodeficiency virus. J Viral Hep 1998;5:123–130.
2. Bortolotti F, Tagger A, Giacchino R, Zuccoti GV, Crivellaro C, Balli F, et al. Hepatitis G and C coinfection in children. J Pediatr 1997;131: 639–640.
3. Ferraz ML, Silva AE, Macdonald GA, Tsarev AS, Di Biscelgie AM, Lucey MR. Fulminant hepatitis in patients undergoing liver transplantation: evidence for a non-A, non-B, non-C, non-D, and non-E syndrome. Liv Transpl Surg 1996;2:60–66.
4. Kiem HP, McDonald GB, Myerson D, Spurgeon CL, Deeg HJ, Sanders JE, et al. Marrow transplantation for hepatitis-associated aplastic anemia: a follow up of long-term survivors. Biol Blood Bone Marrow Transpl 1996;2:93–99.

Hepatoma (See "Tumor of the liver.")

Hernia, Diaphragmatic

Related Terms: Congenital diaphragmatic hernia; hiatal hernia; sliding hiatus hernia.

NOTE: Congenital diaphragmatic hernia is right-sided or left-sided and may be associated with cardiac anomalies, such as the hypoplastic heart syndrome (with left-sided diaphragmatic hernia) *(1)* or anomalies of lungs or upper airways *(2)*.

Organs and Tissues	Procedures	Possible or Expected Findings
Thoracic and abdominal cavity	Record extent of hernia by palpation from abdominal cavity, before organ removal. Remove esophagus and stomach as one specimen; photograph opened esophagus and stomach, and pin on corkboard for fixation and histologic study.	Reflux esophagitis; esophageal ulcer(s) and stricture(s), Barrett's esophagus,* with or without adenocarcinoma.
	In infants, search for associated malformations in the chest cavity (see above under "Note"). In teenagers or adults with repaired congenital diaphragmatic hernias, prepare chest roentgenograms. Perfuse lungs with formalin (see p. 47).	In long-term survivors of repaired congenital diaphragmatic hernias, thoracic deformities, and restrictive or obstructive lung disease may be found *(3)*.

References

1. Losty PD, Vanamo K, Rintala RJ, Donahoe PK, Schnitzer JJ, Lloyd DA. Congenital diaphragmatic hernia: does the side of the defect in-fluence the incidence of associated malformations? J Pediatr Surg 1998;33:507–510.
2. Ryan CA, Finer NN, Etches PC, Tierney AJ, Peliowski A. Congenital diaphragmatic hernia: associated malformations: cystic adenomatoid malformation, extralobular sequestration, and laryngotracheoesophageal cleft: two case reports. J Pediatr Surg 1995;30:883–885.
3. Vanamo K, Rintala R, Sovijarvi A, Jaaskelainen J, Turpeinen M, Lindahl H, Louhimo I. Long-term pulmonary sequelae in survivors of congenital diaphragmatic defects. J Pediatr Surg 1996;31:1096–1099.

Heroin
(See "Dependence, drug(s), all types or type unspecified.")

Herpes Simplex
(See "Infection, herpes simplex.")

Herpes Zoster
(See "Infection, herpes zoster.")

Histiocytosis, Langerhans Cell

Synonym and Related Terms: Abt-Letterer-Siwe disease; eosinophilic granuloma of bone; Hand-Schüller-Christian disease; histiocytosis X (use of these names is no longer recommended *[1]*).

NOTE: Langerhans cell histiocytosis is a monoclonal disorder and thus a true neoplasm *(2)*. The disease most commonly is found in pediatric patients and is rare in adults *(3)*.

Possible Associated Conditions: Diabetes insipidus;* malignant lymphoma.*

Organs and Tissues	*Procedures*	*Possible or Expected Findings*
External examination, skin, and oral cavity	Prepare photograph of gross lesions as listed in right-hand column.	Exophthalmos ("Hand-Schüller-Christian disease." see below under "Eyes"). Nodules in scalp. Vulvar lesions. Hyperplasia and ulcerations of gums.
	Prepare skeletal roentgenograms.	Monostotic or polyostotic destructive bone lesions (lesions most common is skull); pathological fractures.
	Sample skin lesions for histologic study (see below under "Lymph nodes").	Papular, eczema-like eruptions; xanthomas; erythematous, purpuric, and ecchymotic lesions. Histiocytic and eosinophilic infiltrates (see lymph nodes).
Blood	Submit sample for microbiologic study (see p. 102).	Septicemia.
Lymph nodes	Sample grossly involved and uninvolved lymph nodes and set aside fresh material for the preparation of frozen sections (e.g., for CD1 stains).	Typical mononuclear cells and eosinophils in sinuses, with or without microabscess formation.
	Prepare material for electron microscopy (see p. 132).	Mononuclear cells with Langerhans' or Birbeck granules.
Heart	Record weight and thickness of walls.	Cor pulmonale.
Lungs	Dissect one fresh lung and sample for histologic study (see above under "Lymph nodes). Submit sample for microbiologic study (see p. 103). Perfuse one lung with formalin (see p. 47).	Destructive granulomas centered around distal bronchioles *(4)*. Pneumonia of various types.
Other organs and tissues	Sample grossly involved and uninvolved tissue for histologic study (see "Lymph nodes"), including liver, spleen, gastrointestinal tract, kidneys, and perirenal fat.	Histiocytosis with hepatosplenomegaly ("Letterer-Siwe disease"). Many other organs and tissues may be involved.
	Submit tissue samples for biochemical study (total cholesterol) and for electron microscopic study.	Increased tissue concentrations of total cholesterol.
Brain and spinal cord	For removal and specimen preparation, see p. 66 and 70, respectively. Histologic samples must include hypothalamus, pituitary gland, and cerebellum.	Langerhans cell infiltrates, most commonly in hypothalamic-pituitary area *(5)*; infiltrates arise from bone lesions, meninges, or choroid plexus.
Eyes	For removal and specimen preparation, see p. 85.	Orbital histiocytic infiltrates.
Middle ears	For removal and specimen preparation, see p. 72.	Otitis media* (in "Hand-Schüller-Christian disease").
Bones	Review roentgenograms. For removal and specimen preparation, see p. 95.	Monostotic lesions may be found ("eosinophilic granuloma").

References

1. Nezelof C, Basset F. Langerhans cell histiocytosis research. Past, present, and future. Hematol Oncol Clin North Am 1998;12:385–406.
2. Willman CL, McClain KL. An update on clonality, cytokines, and viral etiology in Langerhans cell histiocytosis. Hematol Oncol Clin North Am 1998;12:407–416.
3. Malpas JS. Langerhans cell histiocytosis in adults. Hematol Oncol Clin North Am 1998; 12:259–268.
4. Soler P, Tazi A, Hance AJ. Pulmonary Langerhans cell granulomatosis. Curr Opin Pulm Med 1995;1:406–416.
5. Grois NG, Favara BE, Mostbeck GH, Prayer D. Central nervous system disease in Langerhans cell histiocytosis. Hematol Oncol Clin North Am 1998;12:287–305.

Histoplasmosis

Synonyms: Darling's disease; *Histoplasma capsulatum* infection.

NOTE: (1) Collect all tissues that appear to be infected. (2) Request fungal cultures. (3) Request Grocott's stain for fungi (p. 172). (4) Usually, no special precautions are indicated. (5) Serologic studies are available from local and state health department laboratories (p. 135). (6) This is not a reportable disease.

Possible Associated Conditions: Histoplasmosis may be a complication of the acquired immunodeficiency syndrome* *(1)* and this possibility should be ruled out in all instances.

Organs and Tissues	*Procedures*	*Possible or Expected Findings*
Cerebrospinal fluid	If there is suspicion of cerebral involvement, submit for culture (p. 104).	
Oral cavity	Prepare histologic sections of ulcers. Submit specimens for fungal culture.	Ulcerations of tongue and palate.
Blood and urine	Submit samples for fungal culture (p. 102). Obtain sample for serologic study.	
Heart	If endocarditis is suspected, follow procedures described on p. 103.	Infective endocarditis;* pericarditis.*
Mediastinum and lungs (see also below under "Neck organs").	Perfuse one lung with formalin (p. 47). Brief decalcification may be necessary in chronic cases (p. 97).	Miliary granulomas, with or without calcification; cavitating pneumonia; mediastinal fibrosis; obstruction of bronchi by lymphadenopathy.
Esophagus	Leave esophagus attached to fundus of stomach.	Obstruction by enlarged mediastinal lymph nodes; traction diverticula of esophagus.
Liver	Record weight	Hepatomegaly; granulomatous hepatitis.
Spleen	Record weight; decalcification may be necessary.	Splenomegaly; granulomatous splenitis.
Adrenal glands	Dissect glands, record weights, and photograph (if there is evidence of involvement).	Severe destruction in systemic histoplasmosis; may be the cause of Adrenal insufficiency.*
Neck organs	After fixation, sample ulcers for histologic study.	Ulcers of epiglottis and larynx.
Lymph nodes		Granulomatous lymphadenopathy.
Eyes	For removal and specimen preparation, see p. 85.	Ocular histoplasmosis *(3)*.
Brain	For removal and specimen preparation, see p. 65. See also above under "Note"	*Histoplasma* meningitis.*
Bone marrow	For preparation of sections and smears, see p. 96.	*Histoplasma* granulomas. Hemophagocytic histiocytosis in patients with reactive hemophagocytic syndrome *(2)*.

References

1. Raza J, Harris MT, Bauer JJ. Gastrointestinal histoplasmosis in a patient with acquired immune deficiency syndrome. Mt Sinai J Med 1996;63: 136–140.
2. Koduri PR, Chundi V, DeMarais P, Mizock BA, Patel AR, Weinstein RA. Reactive hemophagocytic syndrome: a new presentation of disseminated histoplasmosis in patients with AIDS. Clin Inf Dis 1995;21:1463–1465.
3. Callanan D, Fish GE, Anand R. Reactivation of inflammatory lesions in ocular histoplasmosis. Arch Ophthalmol 1998;116:470–474.

Homicide

NOTE: The following procedures are listed in the order in which they are usually carried out. Of course, not all these procedures can be carried out or will be required in all cases, nor will this checklist be sufficient in all instances. Consult also the entries indicating the cause of death, such as "Injury, firearm" or "Injury, stabbing." If the victim is an infant, see also under "Infanticide."

Procedures Required Before the Body Arrives or Before Autopsy Is Begun:

1. Investigate the scene where the body was found and where the crime may have been committed (these may be two separate locations). If this is not possible, study the report and photographs submitted by the investigator or the police. Study all available information (p. 8). Request previous medical records and roentgenograms of the victim.

2. Emphasize to funeral director and other personnel that the body of the victim should not be undressed, washed, or otherwise disturbed. Embalming is not permitted before completion of the autopsy. Advise funeral director to put plastic bags over the hands of the victim. This will protect possible evidence, such as hair from the assailant.
3. Appoint a technician who will be in charge of the record sheet (for sample, see pp. 339–342) and of the chain of custody (p. 17). On that sheet, record the name, age, sex, and other information about the victim, the name of the technician, and the name of the pathologist who will perform the autopsy.
4. Prepare roentgenographic and photographic equipment.

Procedures Required After Body Arrives but Before Autopsy Is Begun:

1. The technician who is in charge of the record sheet should enter the time of arrival of the body. He/she should then stay with the body at all times. This technician will complete the record sheet that will also document the chain of custody. If the body must be left unguarded—for instance, overnight—a lock should be placed on the refrigerator or cool room where the deceased is kept, and the key should be retained by the technician.
2. Ask all persons other than the pathologist(s) and the technicians who are not immediately involved in the actual performance of the autopsy to leave the morgue. If detectives, police officers, police photographers, fingerprint experts, and other officials with legitimate assignments need access to the body of the victim, appropriate arrangements should be made. The technician in charge of the record sheet should ask these persons to identify themselves, and this should be entered on the record sheet, along with a statement about the arrival and departure times and what they were doing.
3. The body temperature of the victim can be recorded but this is rarely useful, particularly if the victim seems to have been dead for longer than a day or two or if the body had previously been stored in a refrigerator or cool room. Insert thermometer deep into the anus (about 7–8 cm). If this cannot be done, place thermometer in the axilla for about 3 min. Press arm of the victim to his chest. This will ensure close contact of the thermometer with the skin. Record temperature and manner and time of procedure.
4. Aspirate vitreous from one or both eyes and place the specimen in a tube (p. 16). Close the tube tightly and invert 12 times to ensure proper mixing; record the time of removal from the eye(s); store the tube in a refrigerator.
5. Prepare roentgenograms. In each case, a decision must be made whether roentgenograms should be made of the entire body or only of parts of it—or not at all—and whether they should be made before the victim is undressed, after the victim is undressed, or at both times.

Procedures During the Autopsy:

1. While performing the autopsy, the pathologist should dictate the protocol (p. 12). Height, weight, extent of rigor, and color and distribution of livor should be recorded, along with the state of preservation, nutrition, and hydration. Record appearance of hands, particularly of the volar surfaces.
2. Photograph frontal aspect and profile of the victim for identification purposes. Photograph all injuries and other forensically significant findings. This should be done during the various steps of undressing the victim and during the actual autopsy. Two photographs should be taken of each finding. One should include the autopsy number, a running identification number (to permit easy reference in the protocol), and a scale (because of possible subsequent use in court, the scale should be in inches and in centimeters). A second photograph should be taken without any extraneous objects. After gross features have been recorded and photographed, and after evidence (such as gunpowder flakes) has been collected, wash the victim carefully, especially if the skin is dirty. After cleaning the skin, all photographs should be retaken. Prepare diagrams of wounds; identify their location anteriorly, laterally, or posteriorly by stating the distance from the top of the head and from the soles of the feet, the distance from and the side (right or left) of the midline, and the distance from fixed anatomic landmarks, such as the acromion or the tuber ischii.
3. On the record sheet, note when victim was fingerprinted and when fingernail scrapings or clippings were collected. Hair should also be collected (p. 17), and its source should be identified (hair pulled from scalp, axillae, and pubis is identified as that of the victim; hair in hands or under fingernails or on clothing of victim may be from the assailant).
4. If the body is decomposed or mutilated or for any other reason has not been identified, prepare dental roentgenograms, preferably with the help of a dentist. Whole-body roentgenograms, including films of the sella turcica, may help the pathologist to identify the victim. Other items useful for identification include laundry marks in clothing, keys, and jewelry. All such objects should be put in labeled plastic bags.
5. In cases in which sexual assault may have been involved, collect pieces of clothing that may contain seminal fluid stains. Follow procedures described under "Rape."
6. Blood stains that may have come from the assailant should be scraped off or excised and submitted to the appropriate laboratories. Excise wounds or portions of wounds and submit for histologic study. This will help to distinguish antemortem from postmortem injuries. Specimens should be labeled individually. If maggots or pupas are present, preserve some in formalin. This may aid in determining the time of death (p. 11).

7. Preserve clothing or part of clothing as evidence. Wet clothing should be dried before it is stored in labeled and sealed plastic bags.
8. If air embolism is suspected, see p. 290. If pneumothorax is suspected, see p. 430. If there is evidence of strangulation or other neck injury, extend midline incision to tip of chin. This will ensure careful and complete removal of neck organs.
9. The record sheet should show when body fluids, tissues, and foreign bodies were collected, the volume and appearance of such specimens, and what was done with them. In all instances, the following items should be collected, as shown on p. 16: blood of victim for blood group determination and toxicologic study (determination of alcohol, carbon monoxide, and barbiturate concentrations will be requested most frequently); vitreous; cerebrospinal fluid; urine; gastric contents; tissues for toxicologic study; and bullets or other foreign bodies (touch only with smooth anatomic forceps; see also p. 137 and under "Bodies, foreign").

   For appropriate methods of sampling for toxicologic study, use of preservatives, methods of storage, type of containers, labeling, shipping, and chain of custody, see Chapters 2 and 14. Obtain receipts of specimens that were forwarded to the Forensic Physical Evidence Laboratory.

10. For general forensic autopsy protocols and procedures, see pp. 12 and 13, respectively. Retain appropriate gross organs that might be useful for further study or for demonstration in court.

Address of Pathology Department ____________________

(morgue): ____________________

Head of Department: ____________________

Name of pathologist(s) in charge of autopsy

____

____

Name of victim: ____________________

Address of victim: ____________________

____

Autopsy number: ____________________

Clinic number (if any): ____________________

Date: ____________________

Record Sheet for Suspected Homicide Cases

Name of autopsy technician: ____________________

Body arrived at ____ m.

Date: ____________________

Body was brought to morgue by: ____________________

Persons not from this department who had access to the victim's body:

Name	Occupation	Date	Time:	What did he/she do?

____

Body temperature (axillary/rectal)† was taken at _____ m. Temperature was _____ºC/_____ ºF.

Body of victim was/was not† stored in refrigerator/cool room before the temperature was recorded. Body was/was not† undressed during temperature measurements.

†Circle correct word or group of words.

Vitreous humor was aspirated at ____ m.

2 mL sent to chemistry laboratory for potassium determination: Yes[†] No[†]
____ mL labeled and stored in sterile tube in refrigerator: Yes[†] No[†]

Photographs

Site	Running identification number	What is the photograph supposed to show?
____	____	____
____	____	____
____	____	____
____	____	____
____	____	____
____	____	____
____	____	____
____	____	____
____	____	____
____	____	____
____	____	____
____	____	____
____	____	____
____	____	____
____	____	____

Roentgenograms

1. ____ 4. ____

2. ____ 5. ____

3. ____ 6. ____

[†]Circle correct word or group of words.

Fingernails

Scrapings/clippings† taken by ______________________________ from ____________________ finger(s) ______________ of hand(s). Clippings (or scrapings) sealed, labeled, and kept by /forwarded to ______________________________ .

Hair

From victim's head, axilla(e), and pubis taken by ______________________________ , labeled and kept by ____________________ /forwarded to ____________________ .

Seminal Fluid

Scrapings of seminal fluid/clothing with seminal fluid stains† sealed, labeled, and kept by ____________________ /forwarded to ____________________ . Other evidence (specify: ____________________) kept by /forwarded to ______________________________ .

Blood

______ mL blood without preservation/with ____ mg sodium fluoride†

kept by ____________________ /forwarded to ____________________ .

______ mL blood without preservation/with ____ mg sodium fluoride†

kept by ____________________ /forwarded to ____________________ .

______ mL blood for blood grouping forwarded to ______________________________ .

(Mix 40 mg sodium fluoride with 5 mL of blood. If the volumes are larger, increase amount of sodium fluoride appropriately.)

†Circle correct word or group of words.

Urine

______ mL urine without preservation/with ____ mg sodium fluoride†

kept by ______________________________ /forwarded to ______________________________ .

______ mL urine without preservation/with ____ mg sodium fluoride† ______________________________

kept by ______________________________ /forwarded to ______________________________ .

______ mL blood for blood grouping forwarded to ______________________________ .

(Mix 40 mg sodium fluoride with 5 mL of urine. If the volumes are larger, increase amount of sodium fluoride appropriately.)

Other Body Fluids or Tissues

______ mL cerebrospinal fluid,† ml bile,† other body fluids or tissues ______________________________

(Specify type of fluid or tissue, weight, and volume; state whether preservative was added and how much, and what type of examination was requested.)

kept by ______________________________ /forwarded to ______________________________ .

Clothing

Clothing put in plastic bag, labeled, and forwarded to ______________________________ .

(Specify articles: ______________________________

____

____

______________________________ .)

Body locked in refrigerator/cool room at ____ m. Date: ______________. Body removed from refrigerator/cool room at ____ m.

Date: ______________ . Body transmitted to funeral director ______________________________ (name) at ____ m.

Date: ______________ .

†Circle correct word or group of words.

Homocystinuria

Related Terms: Aminoaciduria;* cystathionine β synthase deficiency; cystathioninuria; sulfuraminoacidemia.

NOTE: For autopsy procedures and expected findings, see under "aminoaciduria*" and "Syndrome, Marfan's." Lax ligaments, lengthened extremities, and fine sparse hair may be present. Ocular abnormalities include dislocated lens, retracted zonular fibers, retinal degeneration with loss of pigmented epithelium and presence of pigment-laden macrophages, and cataracts. Ocular, vascular, and skeletal changes in older patients also may resemble those present in Marfan's syndrome.* Thromboembolism is a frequent cause of death. Submit sample of urine for determination of homocystine concentration (in homocystinuria, values should be increased).

Hydrocephalus

Synonyms and Related Terms: Active or progressive hydrocephalus; arrested hydrocephalus; communicating or malresorptive hydrocephalus; high pressure (or normal pressure or intermittent or occult) hydrocephalus; hydrocephalus ex vacuo; obstructive or noncommunicating hydrocephalus.

Organs and Tissues	*Procedures*	*Possible or Expected Findings*
External examination	If size or shape of head is abnormal, record head circumference. Prepare skull roentgenogram.	Enlarged head in presence of hydrocephalus that was acquired early. Enlargement of skull with distended sutures.
Head	If an extracerebral congenital malformation is suspected, follow procedures described under "Malformation, Arnold-Chiari." If cerebrospinal fluid is aspirated with a syringe, record volume.	Arnold-Chiari malformation* and related abnormalities; tentorial bleeding at time of birth; communicating or noncommunicating hydrocephalus.
Brain	For removal and specimen preparation, see p. 65. Record weight of brain; record size of brain in relation to inner dimensions of skull. Describe size of ventricles. For ventriculography or preparation of casts of the ventricular system, see p. 81 (rarely required).	In obstructive hydrocephalus, only one lateral ventricle may be enlarged or lateral and third ventricles may be involved (three-ventricular hydrocephalus); in communicating hydrocephalus, all ventricular cavities are enlarged.
	Other procedures depend on expected findings or grossly identified abnormalities as listed in right-hand column. If a surgical shunt is present, its location should be recorded and both ends of the implanted specimen that was used for shunting may be submitted for microbiologic study. If the shunt is not patent, record site and nature of obstruction.	Traumatic subarachnoid hemorrhage; rupture of congenital cerebral artery aneurysm;* adhesions after bacterial meningitis* or toxoplasmosis* in infancy or after tuberculosis,* mycotic basal meningitis, sarcoidosis,* or cysticercosis in adulthood; intracranial tumor of third and fourth ventricles; meningeal carcinomatosis.

Reference

1. Squier MV. Pathological approach to the diagnosis of hydrocephalus. J Clin Pathol 1997;50:181–186.

Hydronephrosis

Related Term: Obstructive uropathy.

Organs and Tissues	*Procedures*	*Possible or Expected Findings*
External examination	Prepare abdominal roentgenogram.	Stone; foreign bodies.
Blood	Submit sample for bacterial culture (p. 102).	Septicemia.
Retroperitoneal space	Record size of urinary bladder, width of ureters, and size of kidneys and renal pelves. Dissect *in situ*: ureters, abdominal aorta, and inferior vena cava and the major branches of these vessels. Prepare photographs of dissected retroperitoneal structures, showing the site of obstruction.	Tumor (lymphoma, carcinoma), cysts, fibrous band, or aberrant renal artery. Other possible causes include retroperitoneal fibrosis* and related extrinsic obstructive processes—for instance, radiation fibrosis, trauma, or accidental surgical ligation of ureter.

Organs and Tissues	*Procedures*	*Possible or Expected Findings*
Kidneys, ureters, and pelvic organs	Record volume of urine in the three compartments. For postmortem angiography and urography, see p. 59. Leave kidneys, abdominal aorta, ureters, urinary bladder, and—in male infants—entire urethra in one specimen (p. 60).	Pyelonephritis;* ureteritis; intraluminal tumor, clot, sloughed papillae, or foreign body; congenital narrowing or obstruction of ureterovesical junction, ureterocele, retrocaval ureter, and anterior or posterior urethral valves.
	Procedures depend on expected findings or grossly identified abnormalities as listed in right-hand column.	Meatal urethral stenosis or phimosis. Acquired strictures, tumors, calculi. Angulation or ptosis; diverticula; Endometriosis; malakoplakia; benign prostatic hyperplasia with median bar.
Spinal cord and peripheral nerves	For dissection and specimen preparation, see pp. 67 and 79.	Spinal cord disease; diabetic neuropathy, and other causes of neurogenic obstructive uropathy.

Hydrops Fetalis

Related Terms: Antibody-mediated hydrops fetalis; erythroblastosis fetalis;* nonimmune hydrops fetalis.

NOTE: The classic example of antibody mediated (Rh incompatibility) hydrops fetalis is hemolytic disease of the newborn (erythroblastosis fetalis*). However, nonimmune hydrops fetalis also may be caused by hematologic disorders, e.g., alpha-thalassemia* *(1)* or it may have no known cause. Infections, e.g., with human parvovirus B19 *(2)*, cytomegalovirus, or syphilis;* heart and vascular diseases *(3)* (cardiac tumors, cardiomyopathy,* myocarditis,* arterial calcification, and others); storage disease *(4)*; tumors (including neonatal leukemia*); and many other fetal (e.g., congenital chylothorax* or lymphatic dysplasia; pulmonary sequestration and cystic adenomatoid mal-formation) or maternal conditions, e.g., maternal thyrotoxicosis, also may cause nonimmune hydrops fetalis.

Organs and Tissues	*Procedures*	*Possible or Expected Findings*
Placenta	Record weight, size, and gross appearance. Sample for histologic study.	Placental hydrops; chorangioma and other vascular abnormalities; erythroblastosis.*
Blood	Submit sample if there is no autolysis.	Anemia; alpha-thalassemia.*
External examination	Record weight, size and gross appearance of neonate.	Fetal hydrops; sacrococcygeal teratoma; cystic hygroma.
	Photograph all external abnormalities.	
	Obtain Fascia lata or percutaneous liver biopsy; sample for karyotype analysis (see p. 109).	Monosomy X (Turner's syndrome*); Trisomy 21 (Down's syndrome*); Trisomy 18 (Edward's syndrome).
	Obtain radiograph of fetus.	Chondrodysplasia* (many types).
Chest and abdominal cavities	Record volume and color of effusions.	Pleural effusions that may be chylous; ascites. (Effusions become serosanguinous with intrauterine retention following fetal death.)
Heart and great vessels	Ascertain venous and arterial connections before separating the heart from the organ block.	Left or right ventricular hypoplasia;* atrioventricular septal defect;* rhabdomyoma.
Lungs	Note positioning of lungs *in situ.*	Right-sided diaphragmatic hernia with impingement on the inferior vena cava.
Genitourinary system	Ascertain patency of entire urinary system, from renal pelvis to urethra, including entire length of penis (p. 60).	Urethral obstruction due to urethral valves or lack of canalization of distal penile urethra; cloacal malformations. Cystic renal disease *(5)*.
Other organs and tissues	Conduct complete autopsy with extensive histologic sampling; procedures depend on suspected underlying conditions *(6)*.	See above under "Note" and also under the heading "Erythroblastosis fetalis."

References

1. Barron SD, Pass RF. Infectious causes of hydrops fetalis. Semin Perinatol 1995;19:493–501.
2. Cameron AD, Swain S, Patrick WJ. Human parvovirus B19 infection associated with hydrops fetalis. Aust NZ J Obstet Gynaecol 1997;37 :316–319.
3. Knilans TK. Cardiac abnormalities associated with hydrops fetalis. Semin Perinatol 1995;19:483–492.
4. Tasso MJ, Martinez-Gutierrez A, Carrascosa C, Vazquez S, Tebar R. GM1-gangliosidosis presenting as nonimmune hydrops fetalis: a case report. J Perinat Med 1996;24:445–449.
5. Kim CK, Kim SK, Yang YH, Lee MS, Yoon JH, Park CI. A case of recurrent infantile polycystic kidney associated with hydrops fetalis. Yonsei Med J 1989;30:95–103.
6. Knisely AS. The pathologist and the hydropic placenta, fetus, or infant. Semin Perinatol 1995;19:525–531.

Hyoscyamine (See "Poisoning, alkaloid" and "Poisoning, atropine.")

Hyperaminoaciduria (See "Aminoaciduria.")

Hyperbetalipoproteinemia (See "Hyperlipoproteinemia.")

Hypercalcemia (See "Disorder, electrolyte(s).")

Hypercholesterolemia (See "Hyperlipoproteinemia.")

Hypercorticism (See "Hyperplasia, congenital adrenal" and "Syndrome, Cushing's.")

Hyperglycemia (See "Diabetes mellitus" and p. 114.)

Hyperkalemia (See "Disorder, electrolyte(s)" and p. 114.)

Hyperlipemia (See "Hyperlipoproteinemia.")

Hyperlipoproteinemia

Synonyms and Related Terms: Primary hyperlipoproteinemia (familial forms of apoprotein CII deficiency, hyperalphalipoproteinemia; hypercholesterolemia, hypertriglyceridemia, lipoprotein lipase deficiency, multiple lipoprotein-type hyperlipidemia, and type 3 hyperlipoproteinemia; polygenic hypercholesterolemia).

Organs and Tissues	*Procedures*	*Possible or Expected Findings*
External examination and skin	Record body weight and length. Record extent and nature of skin changes, including evidence of gangrene. Prepare photographs and histologic sections of skin tumors and other cutaneous lesions.	Obesity* is a common finding. Eruptive xanthomas (palms, elbows, knees) in some but not all types of hyperlipoproteinemia. Most prominent in apoprotein CII deficiency. Xanthomas of tendons (knees, elbows, dorsum of hands), xanthelasmas, and arcus corneae in familial hypercholesterolemia. Gangrene of lower extremities (see below under "Arteries").
Blood	Submit sample of serum for biochemical study.	
Heart	Photograph valvular lesions; freeze involved tissue for biochemical and histochemical study. Submit samples of involved tissue for electron microscopic study (p. 132). If valvular leaflets contain calcific deposits, decalcification may be required (p. 97). Request Verhoeff–van Gieson stain and frozen sections for Sudan stain (p. 173). If coronary insufficiency or myocardial infarction is suspected, follow procedures described under "Disease, ischemic heart." For coronary arteriography, see p. 118.	Severe coronary atherosclerosis and myocardial infarcts in type 3 hyperlipoproteinemia and multiple lipoprotein-type hyperlipidemia.
Arteries	Record distribution of atherosclerotic lesions in aorta. Samples for histologic study should include aorta, coronary arteries, and peripheral arteries. See also above under "Heart."	Atherosclerosis of abdominal aorta and its branches and of carotid arteries. Coronary atherosclerosis (see above).
Pancreas	Submit samples of head, corpus, and tail for histologic study. If applicable, see also under "Diabetes mellitus."	Pancreatitis* in familial apoprotein CII deficiency.
Other organs	For special procedures and stains, see above under "Heart." Other procedures depend on expected findings or grossly identified abnormalities as listed in right-hand column.	Foam cells with triglycerides in liver, spleen, and bone marrow in familial lipoprotein lipase deficiency. Manifestations of diabetes mellitus* and hypothyroidism* in some cases of type 3 hyperlipoproteinemia.

Organs and Tissues	Procedures	Possible or Expected Findings
Brain	For removal and specimen preparation, see p. 65.	Cerebral infarct (stroke*) in type 3 hyperlipoproteinemia.

Hypernatremia (See "Disorder, electrolyte(s)" and p. 114.)

Hyperoxaluria

Synonyms and Related Terms: Oxalosis; primary hyperoxaluria type I (alanineglyoxylate aminotransferase deficiency); primary hyperoxaluria type II (D-glyceric acid dehydrogenase deficiency); secondary hyperoxaluria (see under "Note").

NOTE: In ethylene glycol poisoning,* oxalate crystals in media of small arteries, with associated ischemic lesions. Similar deposits may occur after long-term hemodialysis *(1)*. These conditions must be distinguished from the genetic disease. Also, oxalate nephropathy may be a complication of short bowel syndrome.

If patient with congenital hyperoxaluria underwent liver or combined liver/kidney transplantation *(2)*, see also under these headings.

Organs and Tissues	Procedures	Possible or Expected Findings
External examination and skin	Submit samples of skin for histologic study. Prepare skeletal roentgenograms.	Oxalates in skin. Osteosclerosis, periosteal changes; calcifications of vessels and soft tissues.
Liver	Record weight and submit samples for histologic study.	Grossly normal but site of peroxisomal enzyme deficiency in type I hyperoxaluria (see "Synonyms and Related Terms").
Kidneys	Record weights, photograph surfaces and cut surfaces with renal pelves. Submit samples for histologic study.	Calcium oxalate nephrolithiasis;* nephrocalcinosis.
Other organs and tissues	Procedures depend on expected findings or grossly identified abnormalities as listed in right-hand column.	Oxalosis. Manifestations of kidney failure (uremia).* For oxalate deposits unrelated to congenital hyperoxaluria, see above under "Note."
Urine	Submit sample for biochemical study (see right-hand column).	Excess oxalate and glycolate in type I hyperoxaluria. In type II disease, L-glyceric acid and oxalate are found in excess.
Peripheral nerves	For removal and specimen preparation, see p. 79.	Oxaluria-associated polyneuropathy *(3)*.
Bones	For removal and specimen preparation, see p. 95.	Osteosclerosis, periosteal changes.

References

1. Elmstahl B, Rausing A. A case of hyperoxaluria. Radiological aspects. Acta Radiol 1997;38:1031–1034.
2. Watts RWE, Morgan SH, Danpure CJ, Purkiss P, Calne RY, Rolles K, et al. Combined hepatic and renal transplantation in primary hyperoxaluria type I: clinical report of nine cases. Am J Med 1991;90:179–188.
3. Galloway G, Giuliani MJ, Burns DK, Lacomis D. Neuropathy associated with hyperoxaluria: improvement after combined renal and liver transplantation. Brain Pathol 1998;8:247–251.

Hyperparathyroidism

Synonyms and Related Terms: Primary hyperparathyroidism; secondary hyperparathyroidism (see below under "Kidneys").

Possible Associated Conditions: Multiple endocrine neoplasia, type 1 (Wermer's syndrome): Hyperparathyroidism, tumors of the pituitary gland* and tumors of pancreatic islet cells, often with peptic ulcers; Multiple endocrine neoplasia, type 2a (Sipple's syndrome): Hyperparathyroidism, pheochromocytoma, and medullary carcinoma of the thyroid.

Organs and Tissues	Procedures	Possible or Expected Findings
External examination and skin	Record location of scars of previous operations in neck area. If skin gangrene is present, prepare photographs and sample for histologic study. Prepare skeletal roentgenograms (include calvarium, distal clavicles, phalanges, and lamina dura of tooth sockets).	Cutaneous skin gangrene in hyperparathyroidism due to chronic renal failure *(1)*. In severe cases, generalized osteitis fibrosa cystica (osteoclastic osteoporosis) may be present.

Organs and Tissues	*Procedures*	*Possible or Expected Findings*
Vitreous	Submit specimen for calcium and phosphate determination (see p. 85).	Increased calcium concentrations.
Blood	Submit sample of serum for determination of calcium concentration.	Hypercalcemia occurs in primary hyperparathyroidism. Phosphate and phosphatase determinations are not reliable in postmortem blood. Calcium values may also increase after death.
Urine		Hypercalciuria.
Neck organs	Photograph neck organs with parathyroid glands or tumor(s) *in situ*. Dissect all 4 (or more) glands, trim carefully, and record weight of each gland. Snap-freeze adenomatous, hyperplastic, or carcinomatous parathyroid tissue for biochemical study. Prepare tissue sample for electron microscopic study (p. 132). Embed all glands in paraffin for histologic study.	Solitary adenoma; double or multiple adenomas; chief cell hyperplasia; carcinoma(s). Adenomas usually in the inferior glands. Aberrant glands in thymus, thyroid gland, pericardium, or behind esophagus.
	If metastases are suspected or identified, dissect all cervical lymph nodes and embed for histologic study. Dissect and record weight of thyroid gland. Prepare thin slices of gland and record presence and location of tumor(s) or intrathyroid parathyroid tissue.	Cervical lymph node metastases from thyroid (medullary carcinoma of the thyroid gland) or parathyroid carcinoma.
Lungs	Submit samples for histologic study and request von Kossa's stain (p. 173).	Metastatic calcification. Metastatic carcinoma.
Stomach and duodenum	Submit samples of stomach for histologic study.	Peptic ulcer(s);* metastatic calcification.
Gallbladder		Cholelithiasis.*
Pancreas	Submit samples of head, body, and tail for histologic study.	Pancreatitis* *(2)*, with or without calcifications.
Kidneys	Photograph cut surfaces with renal pelves. For histologic specimens, decalcification may be required (p. 97). Request von Kossa's stain (p. 173).	Nephrocalcinosis; nephrolithiasis* with calcium oxalate or calcium phosphate stones; pyelonephritis;* chronic glomerulonephritis* or other chronic renal disease causing secondary hyperparathyroidism.
Other endocrine glands	Dissect all endocrine glands. If endocrine tumors or other abnormalities are present, follow procedures described above under "Neck organs."	See above under "Possible Associated Conditions."
Bones	For removal, prosthetic repair, and specimen preparation, see p. 95; consult also roentgenograms.	Osteitis fibrosa generalisata (osteoclastic osteoporosis); osteoclastomas.
Joints	For study of synovial fluid, see under "Gout." For removal, prosthetic repair, and specimen preparation, see p. 96.	Chondrocalcinosis; pseudogout.*
Eyes	For removal and specimen preparation, see p. 85.	Band keratopathy; cataracts.

References

1. Torok L, Kozepessy L. Cutaneous gangrene due to hyperparathyroidism secondary to chronic renal failure (uremic gangrene syndrome). Clin Exp Dermatol 1996;21:75–77.
2. Inabnet WB, Baldwin D, Daniel RO, Staren ED. Hyperparathyroidism and pancreatitis during pregnancy. Surgery 1996;119:710–713.

Hyperpituitarism (See "Acromegaly.")

Hyperplasia, Congenital Adrenal

Synonyms and Related Terms: Adrenocortical hyperplasia; deficiency of 17α-hydroxylase, 20α-hydroxylase, or 11β-hydroxylase *(1)*; deficiency of 21-hydroxylase *(1,2)*; deficiency of 3β-hydroxysteroid dehydrogenase *(1)*; deficiency of 18-hydroxylase/hydroxysteroid dehydrogenase; deficiency of 20,22 desmolase; female pseudohermaphroditism.

Organs and Tissues	*Procedures*	*Possible or Expected Findings*
External examination	Record body weight and length. Describe and photograph primary and secondary sex characteristics.	Ambiguous, incompletely differentiated external genitalia; virilism in female infants and teenagers; precocious puberty in male patients; premature pubic hair *(3)*.
Adrenal glands	Record sizes and weights. Snap-freeze material for biochemical, DNA or histochemical study.	Cortical hyperplasia (for expected weights, see pp. 560, 561, and 571).
Gonads		Polycystic ovaries.
Other organs and body fluids, including urine	Submit samples for histologic study.	Manifestations of hypertension.*
	Submit urine sample for biochemical study.	Increased concentration of urinary pregnanetriol and 17-ketosteroids.
	For removal of vitreous, see p. 85.	Electrolyte abnormalities in vitreous, related to dehydration,* hyperkalemia, and hyponatremia. Hypoglycemia* may have been present but usually cannot be demonstrated after death.
	Submit tissue (i.e., fascia lata) for karyotype analysis (p. 109).	

References

1. Pang S. Congenital adrenal hyperplasia. Baillieres Clin Obstet Gynaecol 1997;11:281–306.
2. Cutler GB Jr, Lave L. Congenital adrenal hyperplasia due to 21-hydroxylase deficiency. N Engl J Med 1990;323:1806–1813.
3. Rosenfield RL. Hyperandrogenism in peripubertal girls. Ped Clin North Am 1990;37:1333–1358.

Hypertension (Systemic Arterial), All Types or Type Unspecified

Synonyms and Related Terms: Arterial hypertension; benign hypertension; essential hypertension; idiopathic hypertension; malignant hypertension; paroxysmal hypertension.

NOTE: If underlying disease is known—for instance, coarctation of the aorta, pheochromocytoma, or toxemia of pregnancy—see also under that entry.

Organs and Tissues	*Procedures*	*Possible or Expected Findings*
External examination	Record body weight and length. Prepare chest roentgenogram.	Obesity;* cushingoid features.
Blood and urine	Submit samples for biochemical and toxicologic study.	Lead poisoning;* porphyria.*
Heart	Record actual and expected weights (pp. 562 and 568). For coronary arteriography, see p. 118. For histologic sampling of myocardium, see p. 30.	Hypertrophy of the heart, primarily of the left ventricle; coronary atherosclerosis; ischemic myocardial changes; catecholamine cardiomyopathy (see below under "Adrenal glands").
Arteries	For carotid and cerebral arteriography, see p. 82. For arteriography of lower extremities, see p. 120. For renal arteriography, see p. 59. Request Verhoeff–van Gieson stain for histologic sections of elastic and muscular arteries (p. 173).	Atherosclerosis and arteriolosclerosis. Renal artery stenosis* or fibromuscular dysplasia. Coarctation of the aorta.* Polyarteritis nodosa.*
Pancreas	Submit samples for histologic study.	Arteriolar necrosis with hemorrhages and infarctions (in malignant hypertension).
Kidneys	Record appearance of renal ostia and arteries. If parenchymal renal disease is suspected, follow procedures described under "Glomerulonephritis."	Renal artery stenosis* or dysplasia. Diabetic nephropathy. Renal involvement in immune connective tissue disease; chronic or acute glomerulonephritis;* pyelonephritis.*
Adrenal glands	Freeze tissue for possible biochemical study (indicated only if a tumor is present or evidence is obtained of adrenocortical hyperfunction). "See also under "Tumor, of the adrenal glands."	Pheochromocytoma; congenital adrenal hyperplasia.* (See also under "Aldosteronism.")

Organs and Tissues	Procedures	Possible or Expected Findings
Ovaries	If a tumor is present, snap-freeze tissue for possible biochemical study.	Hypertension-producing ovarian tumor.
Parathyroid glands	See under "Hyperparathyroidism."	Hyperplasia or adenoma with hyperparathyroidism.*
Brain	For removal and specimen preparation, see p. 65.	Subarachnoid or intraparenchymal hemorrhage; infarction* or other condition causing increased intracranial pressure.
Eyes	For removal and specimen preparation, see p. 85.	Hypertensive retinopathy.

Hypertension, Intracranial (See "Pseudotumor cerebri.")

Hypertension, Portal

Related Terms: Idiopathic portal hypertension; postsinusoidal portal hypertension; presinusoidal portal hypertension.

Organs and Tissues	Procedures	Possible or Expected Findings
External examination	Record circumference of abdomen.	Periumbilical veins that were distended during life (caput medusae; Cruveilhier-Baumgarten syndrome) usually collapse after death.
Abdominal cavity	Submit fluid for bacterial culture (p. 102); record volume; submit samples of peritoneum for histologic study.	Ascites; peritonitis;* carcinomatosis.
Heart, inferior vena cava, and hepatic veins	If portal hypertension is suspected to have been caused by cardiac or other postsinusoidal venous disease, follow procedures described under "Syndrome, Budd-Chiari."	Manifestations of Budd-Chiari syndrome.*
Lungs	Submit samples for histologic evaluation of pulmonary vasculature. Request Verhoeff-van Gieson stain.	Coexistent pulmonary hypertension; hepatopulmonary syndrome.
Abdominal wall	If presence of portal vein thrombosis is suspected in a neonate, submit samples of umbilicus and umbilical vein for histologic study.	Umbilical sepsis in neonate.
	In adults with caput medusae, submit samples of ductus venosus and of umbilical vein for determination of luminal width.	Caput medusae.
Portal vein system	For portal venography, see p. 56. For hepatoduodenal lymphangiography, see p. 56. Open portal, splenic, and mesenteric veins *in situ* or after en bloc removal of abdominal organs (p. 56). If site of obstruction is unknown, prepare portal angiogram from splenic or mesenteric vein.	Portal vein thrombosis; pylephlebitis. Developmental obliteration or valve formation of portal vein is rare. Splenic arteriovenous fistula, tumor, or abscess may be present.
	If cavernous transformation of portal vein is suspected, prepare horizontal sections through hepatoduodenal ligament.	Cavernous transformation of portal vein.
Thoracic duct	For dissection of the thoracic duct, see p. 34.	Dilatation of thoracic duct.
Esophagus, stomach, and intestinal tract (with anus)	For demonstration of varices, see p. 53. Record volume of blood in lumen.	Esophageal varices;* gastric varices; gastrointestinal hemorrhage;* hemorrhoids.
Liver	Record weight and photograph. Slice liver in frontal planes and leave hepatoduodenal ligament attached to slice in hilar plane. Submit samples for histologic study. Other procedures depend on expected findings or grossly identified abnormalities as listed in right-hand column.	Cirrhosis;* tumor of the liver;* congenital hepatic fibrosis;* chronic alcoholic or nonalcoholic steatohepatitis; nodular regenerative hyperplasia, associated with conditions such as Felty's syndrome* or rheumatoid arthritis.* Schistosomiasis,* vascular malformation, and other hepatic conditions also may cause portal hypertension.

Organs and Tissues	Procedures	Possible or Expected Findings
Spleen	Record weight and size. Submit samples for histologic study.	Congestive splenomegaly; extramedullary hematopoiesis (see above under "Liver").
Pancreas		Pancreatitis.*
Other organs	If pylephlebitis is suspected, record site and character of suspected source of infection.	Appendicitis; other suppurative abdominal infection; malignant tumor; manifestations of polycythemia* or of other hematologic disorder. See also above under "Liver."
Brain	For removal and specimen preparation, see p. 65.	Hepatic encephalopathy.*

Hypertension, Pulmonary

Synonyms and Related Terms: Chronic pulmonary venous hypertension; coexistent portal and pulmonary hypertension; cor pulmonale; hypoxic pulmonary hypertension; neoplastic embolic pulmonary hypertension; primary pulmonary hypertension; plexogenic pulmonary hypertension; pulmonary heart disease; pulmonary veno-occlusive disease; thromboembolic pulmonary hypertension.

Organs and Tissues	Procedures	Possible or Expected Findings
External examination	Prepare chest roentgenogram.	Enlarged right atrium and pulmonary arteries.
Heart	Record heart weight and dimensions.	Hypertrophy and dilatation of right ventricle and right atrium. Straightened septum with D-shaped ventricles. Dilated tricuspid and pulmonary valves.
Lungs	Record weights of lungs. For pulmonary arteriography and venography, see p. 50. Perfuse lungs with formalin (p. 47). Prepare slides from each lobe, both centrally and peripherally. Request Verhoeff–van Gieson stain on all blocks (p. 173).	Obstructive pulmonary arterial and/or pulmonary venous lesions (most commonly plexogenic or thrombotic type). Interstitial pneumonia;* bronchiectases;* pulmonary emphysema;* pulmonary artery aneurysm; pulmonary artery rupture; pulmonary capillary hemangiomatosis. See also above under "Synonyms and Related Terms."
Abdominal viscera	Record actual and expected weights of liver and spleen.	Congestive hepatosplenomegaly. Pre-existing cirrhosis with portal and pulmonary hypertension.

Hyperthermia (See "Heatstroke.")

Hyperthyroidism

Synonyms and Related Terms: Basedow's disease; Graves' disease; thyrotoxicosis.

Organs and Tissues	Procedures	Possible or Expected Findings
External examination, skin, and breasts	Record body weight and length; photograph face and neck; record neck circumference. Prepare histologic sections of skin lesions and of breast tissue.	Emaciation; exophthalmos; hyperpigmen tation and vitiligo, particularly of hands and feet; fingernail (ring finger) abnormalities; pretibial myxedema above level of lateral malleolus; gynecomastia.
	Prepare skeletal roentgenograms.	Osteoporosis.*
Blood and urine	If hormone assay or preparation of a drug screen is intended, store samples in deepfreeze.	Postmortem concentrations of thyroxine or thyroid-stimulating hormone appear to reflect antemortem values.
	Determination of serum calcium concentration is unreliable (use vitreous).	Hypercalcemia may be present.
Thymus	Dissect and record weight. Submit samples for histologic study.	Hyperplasia of thymus.
Heart	Record weight of heart and size of heart chambers. For sampling for histologic study, see p. 30.	Atrial dilatation indicates previous episodes of atrial fibrillation *(1)*.

Organs and Tissues	Procedures	Possible or Expected Findings
Neck organs	Remove neck organs together with goiter and and tongue (p. 4); record weights of thyroid and parathyroid glands. If thyroid tumor is present, photograph together with scale. If carcinoma of the thyroid gland is suspected, dissect regional lymph nodes and submit for histologic study.	Nodular (colloid) goiter; diffuse thyroid hyperplasia; thyroid adenoma(s) or carcinoma(s); subacute thyroiditis.*
Lymph nodes; other endocrine glands	Record average size of lymph nodes. In addition to thyroid weight, record weights of all other endocrine glands and submit samples for histologic study. See also below under "Pituitary gland."	Lymphadenopathy.
Tumor with possible endocrine activity	Submit samples for hormone assay, light microscopic study, and electron microscopy (p. 132).	Choriocarcinoma of uterus or testis; hydatidiform mole may cause thyrotoxicosis without thyroid abnormalities. See also below under "Pituitary gland".
Other organs		Manifestations of congestive heart failure.*
Pituitary gland	For removal and specimen preparation, see p. 71. If a pituitary tumor is present, it should be weighed, measured, split in half, photographed, and one-half placed in deep-freeze for hormone assay. From the other half, a small sample should be prepared for electron microscopic study (p. 132) and the remainder for light microscopy.	Pituitary adenoma with secretion of thyroid-stimulating hormone may cause thyrotoxicosis without thyroid abnormalities. Acromegaly* (see above) may be present.
Vitreous	If electrolyte abnormalities are suspected, submit sample of vitreous (p. 85).	Manifestations of electrolyte disorder.*
Eyes and their adnexae	For removal and specimen preparation of eyes, see p. 85. Submit samples of retrobulbar tissue, extraocular muscles, and lacrimal glands (p. 87).	Exophthalmos with puffy lids, chemosis, and eye infection.
Skeletal muscles	For sampling and specimen preparation, see p. 80.	
Bones	For removal, prosthetic repair, and specimen preparation, see p. 95.	Osteoporosis.*

Reference

1. Aronow WS. The heart and thyroid disease. Clin Geriatr Med 1995;11:219–229.

Hypertrophy, Cardiac

Organs and Tissues	Procedures	Possible or Expected Findings
Heart	Record actual and expected weights. If determination of myocardial mass is needed, record specific gravity of heart (p. 569). For coronary arteriography, see p. 118. Record ventricular wall thicknesses and appearance and annular circumferences of valves. If cardiomyopathy is suspected, electron microscopic study may be indicated (p. 132).	Coronary atherosclerosis; myocardial infarction; pericarditis;* congenital or acquired valvular heart disease; other congenital heart disease. Most abnormal conditions of the heart are associated with hypertrophy (or increased mass), with or without chamber dilatation Cardiomyopathy.*
Other organs	Procedures depend on expected findings or grossly identified abnormalities as listed in right-hand column.	Manifestations of systemic hypertension;* pulmonary vascular disease with hypertension, including pulmonary embolism;* amyloidosis,* hemochromatosis,* Fabry's disease,* or glycogen storage disease.*

Hypervitaminosis A

Related Term: Vitamin A toxicity.

NOTE: The findings listed below refer to chronically increased vitamin A ingestion.

Organs and Tissues	*Procedures*	*Possible or Expected Findings*
External examination	Record extent and character of skin lesions; photograph skin lesions. Submit specimens of affected and unaffected skin for histologic study. Prepare skeletal roentgenograms.	Brittle hair; desquamation of skin, particularly of palms and soles; nail abnormalities. Clubbing of fingers (in children). Osteoporosis;* fractures; periosteal proliferation, particularly of ulnae, clavicles, and metatarsal bones; tumefaction of midshafts of long bones. Osteoarthritis *(1)*.
Liver	Record weight and size; photograph surface and cut section; submit fresh tissue for demonstration of vitamin A fluorescence in frozen sections or for chemical analysis. Request frozen sections for Sudan stain (p. 173). For paraffin sections, request van Gieson's stain (p. 173).	Fatty changes in liver with characteristic quick-fading green fluorescence. Hepatic fibrosis or cirrhosis.*
Other organs	Submit samples of spleen, kidneys, and parathyroid glands for histologic study.	
Brain	For removal and specimen preparation, see p. 65.	Pseudotumor cerebri;* hydrocephalus,* particularly in infants.
Bones and joints	For optimal sites for histologic study, see above under "External examination and skin." For removal, prosthetic repair, and specimen preparation, see p. 95.	Calcification of cartilage, broadening of osseous trabeculae, and periosteal proliferations. Hyperostotic and destructive osteoarthritis *(1)*. See also above under "External examination and skin."

Reference

1. Romero JB, Schreiber A, von Hochstetter AR, Wagenhauser FJ, Michel BA, Theiler R. Hyperostotic and destructive osteoarthritis in a patient with vitamin A intoxication syndrome: a case report. Bull Hosp Joint Dis 1996;54:169–174.

Hypervitaminosis D

Related Term: Vitamin D toxicity.

Organs and Tissues	*Procedures*	*Possible or Expected Findings*
External examination and skin	Prepare skeletal roentgenograms.	Osteoporosis;* para-articular calcifications; other metastatic calcifications. In infants, radiopacity may be found—primarily at epiphyseal ends of the shafts of long tubular bones.
	Submit specimens of skin and of subcutaneous tissue for histologic study.	Metastatic calcification.
Vitreous	Submit sample for determination of calcium and phosphate concentrations (p. 85). If histologic study of eyes is intended, remove vitreous from only one eye.	Increased calcium concentrations.
Blood	Postmortem calcium values are unreliable.	Hypercalcemia.
Lungs	Inflate one fresh lung with carbon dioxide and prepare roentgenogram for demonstration of calcium deposits. Then, perfuse lung with formalin (p. 47). For histologic sections, request von Kossa's stain for calcium (p. 173). Decalcification of tissue may be required (p. 97).	Metastatic calcification.

Organs and Tissues	Procedures	Possible or Expected Findings
Kidneys	Prepare soft tissue roentgenograms. Request von Kossa's stain (p. 173). Decalcification of tissue may be required (p. 97).	Metastatic calcification.
Parathyroid glands	Record weights of all parathyroid glands and submit samples for histologic study.	Normal parathyroid glands.
Other organs	Histologic samples should include heart, pancreas, fundus and body of stomach, elastic and muscular arteries, and lymph nodes. See also above under "Kidneys."	Metastatic calcification. If applicable, see also under "Failure, kidney."
Brain and spinal cord	For removal and specimen preparation, see pp. 65 and 67, respectively. Submit samples of tentorium and falx cerebri for histologic study.	Metastatic calcification of tentorium and falx cerebri.
Eyes	For removal and specimen preparation, see p. 85. See also above under "Vitreous."	Metastatic calcium deposits in corneas and conjunctivas.
Bones and joints	For removal, prosthetic repair, and specimen preparation, see p. 95. For optimal sampling, consult roentgenograms.	Metastatic calcification in synovial tissue and in bone marrow. See also above under "External examination and skin."

Hypnotic(s) (See "Dependence, drug(s), all types or type unspecified" and "Poisoning, barbiturate(s).")

Hypocalcemia (See "Disorder, electrolyte(s).")

Hypofibrinogenemia (See "Coagulation, disseminated intravascular.")

Hypogammaglobulinemia

Synonyms and Related Terms: Acquired hypogammaglobulinemia; agammaglobulinemia; congenital hypogammaglobulinemia; Good's syndrome (thymoma and hypogammaglobulinemia) *(1)*.

Possible Associated Conditions: Campylobacter, meningogoccal, pneumococcal and other infections, including infections by *S. pneumoniae* and *H. influenzae*. Malabsorption syndrome;* multiple myeloma,* and systemic amyloidosis* *(1)*. (See also under "Syndrome, primary immunodeficiency.")

Organs and Tissues	Procedures	Possible or Expected Findings
Chest cavity		Thymoma *(1)*.
Intestinal tract	For fixation and specimen preparation, see p. 54.	Sprue-type changes of intestinal mucosa with malabsorption syndrome.* *Giardia lamblia* infection.
Liver		Chronic hepatitis C *(3)*.
Brain and spinal cord	For removal and specimen preparation, see pp. 65 and 67, respectively.	Encephalomyelitis *(4)*.
Bones and joints	For removal, prosthetic repair, and specimen preparation, see p. 95.	Arthritis (with features of rheumatoid arthritis*)

References

1. Verne GN, Amann ST, Cosgrove C, Cerda JJ. Chronic diarrhea associated with thymoma and hypogammaglobulinemia (Good's syndrome). South Med J 1997;90:444–446.
2. Kotilainen P, Vuori K, Kainulainen L, Aho H, Saario R, Asola M, et al. Systemic amyloidosis in a patient with hypogammaglobulinemia. J Intern Med 1996;240:103–106.
3. Quinti I, Pandolfi F, Paganelli R, el Salman D, Giovannetti A, Rosso R, et al. HCV infection in patients with primary defects of immunoglobulin production. Clin Exp Immunol 1995;102:11–16.
4. Rudge P, Webster AD, Revesz T, Warner T, Espanol T, Cunningham-Rundles C, et al. Encepahomyelitis in primary hypogammaglobulinemia. Brain 1996;119:1–15.

Hypoglycemia

NOTE: Currently, no reliable diagnostic tests are available for the postmortem diagnosis of hypoglycemia.

Organs and Tissues	Procedures	Possible or Expected Findings
Vitreous	Usually, aspiration of vitreous is not indicated. If aspiration is desired, see p. 85.	Postmortem glycolysis in vitreous may be very rapid. Glucose may not be demonstrable within 3 h after death (tested in individuals who did not suffer from hypoglycemia).
Blood		Glucose concentrations are totally unreliable.
Urine	Submit sample for determination of glucose and ketone levels.	In presence of hypoglycemia, urine contains no glucose or ketone.
Cerebrospinal fluid		For interpretation of findings, see p. 115. Results may be unreliable.
Brain	For removal and specimen preparation, see p. 65. Request Luxol fast blue stain (p. 172).	Petechial or larger hemorrhages; ganglion cell degeneration, gliosis, and demyelinization.

Hypokalemia (See "Disorder, electrolyte(s)" and p. 114.)

Hypolipoproteinemia (See "Abetalipoproteinemia" and "Disease, Tangier's.")

Hyponatremia (See "Disorder, electrolyte(s)" and p. 114.)

Hypoparathyroidism

Synonyms: Acquired hypoparathyroidism; hereditary hypoparathyroidism; idiopathic hypoparathyroidism.

Possible Associated Conditions: Autoimmune polyglandular deficiency (often with alopecia, megaloblastic anemia;* mucocutaneous candidiasis, and vitiligo); DiGeorge syndrome* (defective development of thymus, parathyroid glands, and other organs).

Organs and Tissues	Procedures	Possible or Expected Findings
External examination and skin; teeth	Record location of scars of previous neck surgery and abnormalities of skin, hair, nails, and teeth. Submit samples of normal and abnormal skin for histologic study.	Scars of previous neck surgery; coarse skin, with or without subcutaneous calcifications; malformed nails; dysplasia of enamel; alopecia.
	Prepare skeletal roentgenograms.	Dense bones; thickening of calvarium.
Urine and vitreous	Submit samples (p. 85) for determination of calcium concentrations. Postmortem calcium values in blood are unreliable.	Hypocalcemia; hypocalciuria.
Parathyroid glands	Record weights of all parathyroid glands. Submit samples for histologic study.	Parathyroid glands may not be present (after intentional or unintentional surgical removal).
Other organs	Procedures depend on expected findings or grossly identified abnormalities as listed in right-hand column. If an infection is suspected, submit material for microbiologic study.	Cardiomyopathy* *(1)*; manifestations of Addison's disease; candidiasis;* ovarian failure, or megaloblastic anemia *(2)**. Malabsorption with steatorrhea and myopathy with muscular atrophy may occur.
Brain and spinal cord	For removal and specimen preparation, see pp. 65 and 67, respectively.	Calcification in basal ganglia.
Eyes	For removal and specimen preparation, see p. 85.	Cataracts.
Bones	For removal, prosthetic repair, and specimen preparation, see p. 95. Consult roentgenograms.	See above under "External examination and skin."

References

1. Suzuki T, Ikeda U, Fujikawa H, Saito K, Shimada K. Hypocalcemic heart failure: a reversible form of heart muscle disease. Clin Cardiol 1998;21: 227–228.

2. Abramowicz MJ, Cochaux P, Cohen LH, Vamos E. Pernicious anaemia and hypoparathyroidism in a patient with Kearns-Sayre syndrome with mitochondrial DNA duplication. J Inherit Metabol Dis 1996;19:109–111.

Hypophosphatasia (See "Deficiency, vitamin D" and "Osteomalacia.")

Hypophosphatemia, Familial (See "Syndrome, Fanconi.")

Hypopituitarism (See "Insufficiency, pituitary.")

Hypoplasia, Left Ventricular

NOTE: For general dissection techniques, see p. 33.

Possible Associated Conditions: Congenital aortic valvular stenosis* or atresia (hypoplastic left heart syndrome); coarctation of the aorta;* hypoplasia of ascending aorta; left ventricular endocardial fibroelastosis;* mitral atresia.*

Hypoplasia, Right Ventricular

NOTE: For general dissection techniques, see p. 33.

Possible Associated Conditions: Congenital pulmonary stenosis* or atresia with intact ventricular septum;* congenital tricuspid stenosis or atresia;* restrictive ventricular septal defect;* transposition of the great arteries.

Hypoplasia, Tubular, of Aortic Arch

NOTE: For general dissection techniques, see p. 33.

Possible Associated Conditions: Coarctation of the aorta;* malalignant ventricular septal defect; patent ductal artery;* sub-aortic stenosis.

Hypothermia (See "Exposure, cold.")

Hypothyroidism

Synonyms: Cretinism; goitrous hypothyroidism; myxedema; primary hypothyroidism; secondary hypothyroidism; supra-thyroidal (trophoprivic) hypothyroidism; thyroprivic hypothyroidism.

Organs and Tissues	*Procedures*	*Possible or Expected Findings*
External examination, skin, and breasts	Record body weight and length and facial features; record location of scars of previous neck surgery.	In cretinism, body is small for age and head is large with coarse facial features and protruding tongue. In adults, brittle hair, sparse eyebrows, and puffiness of face are present. Surgical scars of neck.
	Prepare histologic sections of skin and of breast tissue.	Perifollicular keratosis of skin; thickened nails; galactorrhea.
	Prepare roentgenograms of chest and of joints.	Pleural* and pericardial effusions; joint effusions; degenerative joint disease involving knees, hips, hands, and other joints *(1)*; thickening of joint capsules; bursitis.
Vitreous	Submit for determination of sodium concentration (p. 85).	Low sodium concentration.
Abdomen	Record volume of effusion.	Ascites.
Pleural and pericardial cavities	Record volume of effusion(s).	Hydrothorax and hydropericardium, with or without cardiac tamponade.
Blood	Submit sample for microbiologic study (p. 102). If hormone assay is intended, snap-freeze sample.	Septicemia; hypercholesterolemia.
Thymus	Record weight and submit samples for histologic study.	
Heart	Record weight; photograph; submit samples for histologic study (p. 30).	Dilatation of the heart.* See also under "Failure, congestive heart."
Arteries	Record degree of atherosclerosis of aorta, coronary arteries, cerebral arteries, and other muscular arteries.	Increased atherosclerosis.
Neck organs	Remove neck organ together with tongue (p. 4). Prepare histologic sections of tongue with papillae. Record weight of thyroid gland; photograph and submit samples for histologic study. Record weights of parathyroid glands. If patient was recently treated with radionuclides, see Chapter 13.	Macroglossia; Hashimoto's thyroiditis; Riedel's struma; subacute thyroiditis (see also under "Thyroiditis"); colloid goiter; tumor of the thyroid gland after treatment with radioactive iodine; surgically removed thyroid gland; thyroid aplasia (in cretinism).
Lymph nodes	Record average size and submit samples of histologic study.	
Intestinal tract	For *in situ* fixation, see p. 54.	Ileus; megacolon.
Urine	Submit sample for determination of glucose and ketone concentrations.	In presence of hypoglycemia,* urine contains no glucose or ketone.

Organs and Tissues	Procedures	Possible or Expected Findings
Other organs	Submit samples of adrenal glands, gonads, and tail of pancreas (for islets of Langerhans) for histologic study.	
Brain, spinal cord, and pituitary gland	For removal and specimen preparation, see pp. 65, 67, and 71, respectively.	Hypothalamic congenital defects, infections, tumor, or sarcoidosis* may cause trophoprivic hypothyroidsim. For other causes, see "Insufficiency, pituitary."
Skeletal muscles	For sampling and specimen preparation, see p. 80.	
Joints and bursae	For removal, prosthetic repair, and specimen preparation of joints, see p. 96.	See above under "External examination, skin, and breasts."

Reference

1. McLean RM, Podell DN. Bone and joint manifestations of hypothyroidism. Semin Arthritis Rheum 1995;24:282–290.

Hypovitaminosis A (See "Deficiency, vitamin A.")

Hypovitaminosis D (See "Deficiency, vitamin D.")

Hypoxemia (See "Hypoxia.")

Hypoxia

Related Terms: Asphyxia; hypoxemia; suffocation.

NOTE: There are no diagnostic autopsy findings for hypoxia. Possible causes of acute hypoxia include anesthesia-associated death,* diving accident,* exposure to toxic gas(es)—for instance, carbon monoxide poisoning;* mechanical failure of an oxygen supply system, as in an airplane; and sudden mechanical airway obstruction,* as in aspiration of a foreign body or strangulation. Causes of chronic asphyxia include prolonged exposure to high altitude and chronic pulmonary disease.

Organs and Tissues	Procedures	Possible or Expected Findings
External examination	Record appearance of head, oral cavity, and neck area.	Cyanosis; foreign body in mouth or pharynx; strangulation marks; scleral hemorrhages.
Blood	Submit sample for toxicologic study (p. 16), for instance, for determination of carbon monoxide concentration—and for determination of hemoglobin saturation.	Blood dark and liquid; oxygen saturation of hemoglobin may be less than 10%.
Pleura and pericardium		Petechial hemorrhages; Tardieu's spots.
Heart	Record weight.	Right ventricular hypertrophy.
Lungs	Record weights. Perfuse one lung with formalin (p. 47). Request Verhoeff–van Gieson stain (p. 173).	Profound medial hypertrophy of small pulmonary arteries and of pulmonary veins in patients who chronically were exposed to hypoxia. Acute pulmonary edema may also occur in chronic hypoxia.
Neck organs	Remove carefully to avoid dislodging foreign body.	
Brain	For removal and specimen preparation, see p. 65.	Cerebral edema in acute mountain sickness.
Middle ears	For removal and specimen preparation, see p. 72.	Mucosal hemorrhages.

I

Ileus, Meconium

Possible Associated Conditions: Congenital megacolon;* cystic fibrosis;* syphilis.* *(1)*.

Organs and Tissues	*Procedures*	*Possible or Expected Findings*
External examination	Record height, weight, and abdominal circumference.	Malnutrition.
Abdominal cavity and intestinal tract	Examine and sample the bowel early in the procedure to minimize autolysis. Record location and character of meconium and of liquid contents, and determine thickness of intestinal wall. Record location of stenosis, atresia, or dilatation. Submit samples of all portions of intestinal tract for histologic study.	Empty and collapsed colon; small amounts of gray and dry meconium in terminal ileum; meconium masses in dilated and hypertrophied mid-ileum; liquid contents in proximal intestine *(1)*; appendicitis; bowel perforation. Glandular inspissation and atrophy of intestinal mucosa. Volvulus, infarction, necrosis, perforation, peritonitis, and acquired intestinal atresia may be present. Absence of neural plexuses in congential megacolon* (Hirschsprung's disease).
Other organs	Procedures depend on expected findings or grossly identified abnormalities as listed in right-hand column.	Manifestations of cystic fibrosis, with or without cirrhosis;* biliary atresia* *(3)*.

References

1. Siplovich L, Davies MR, Kaschula RO, Cywes S. Intestinal obstruction in the newborn with congenital syphilis. J Pediatr Surg 1988;23:810–813.
2. Maurage C, Lenaerts C, Weber A, Brochu P, Yousef I, Roy CC. Meconium ileus and its equivalent as a risk factor for the development of cirrhosis: an autopsy study in cystic fibrosis. J Ped Gastroenterol Nutr 1989;9:17–20.
3. Adam G, Brereton RJ, Agrawal M, Lake BD. Biliary atresia and meconium ileus associated with Nieman-Pick disease. J Ped Gastroenterol Nutr 1988;7:128–131.

Immunodeficiency (See "Syndrome, acquired immunodeficiency" and "Syndrome, primary immunodeficiency.")

Impression, Basilar

NOTE: Basilar impression constitutes an upward bulging of the margins of the foramen magnum. When occipital condyles are displaced above the plane of the foramen magnum, basilar invagination is present.

Possible Associated Conditions: Klippel-Feil syndrome;* osteogenesis imperfecta;* osteomalacia;* Paget's disease of bone;* rheumatoid arthritis; rickets; syringobulbia; syringomylia.*

Organs and Tissues	*Procedures*	*Possible or Expected Findings*
External examination		Shortness of neck.
Skull and spine	Prepare roentgenograms. For dissection of cervical spine, see p. 71.	Arnold-Chiari malformation;* fusion of atlas to base of skull; malpositioning of odontoid process; platybasia.*

From: *Handbook of Autopsy Practice,* 3rd Ed. Edited by: J. Ludwig © Humana Press Inc., Totowa, NJ

Organs and Tissues	*Procedures*	*Possible or Expected Findings*
Brain and spinal cord	For removal and specimen preparation, see pp. 65 and 67, respectively.	Compression and secondary ischemic injury to lower brain stem and spinal cord. See also above under "Skull and spine" and under "Possible Associated Conditions."

Incompetence,... (See "Insufficiency,...")

Infanticide

Related Terms: Battered-child syndrome; child-abuse or child-neglect death.

NOTE: As stated on p. 85, vitreous should *not* be aspirated because there is a risk of artifactual damage to the retina. The retina that bears the brunt of the injury in child abuse and the assessment and position of retinal hemorrhages is of prime importance. Instead, prior to the removal of the eye, the fundus should be photographed.

Record appearance of clothing; undress body over plastic bag; dry clothing and then place in paper bags (each bag should be labeled separately). Record skin lesions after cleansing of body; record and photograph appearance of anus, genital, and oral frenula, if necessary. If sex-related crime is suspected, follow procedures described under "Rape." Collect hair from scalp and from wound sites (if hair present) for future comparison. Also follow other applicable procedures described under "Homicide."[a]

Organs and Tissues	*Procedures*	*Possible or Expected Findings*
External examination	Record body weight and height. Photograph body dressed and undressed; photograph and record extent of injuries and of other skin lesions. Collect any trace evidence. For additional procedures, see above under "Note." Prepare roentgenograms of entire body. Postmortem MRI is a valuable addition to autopsy findings in the investigation of child abuse *(1)*.	In the abused child, bruises, hematomas, burn marks, or other patterned injuries. In any child, diaper rash, Mongolian spots, self-inflicted fingernail scratches, skin infections, and emaciation. In the previously battered child, fractures in various states of healing.
Vitreous	For special considerations in suspected child abuse, see above under "Note." In other situations, or after study of the fundus (see above) submit sample of vitreous for chemical and possible toxicologic study (p. 16).	In hypertonic dehydration,* sodium concentrations more than 150 meq/L. This may be caused by organic disease, improper medical treatment, or physical neglect.
Umbilical cord attachment	Prepare histologic sections of umbilicus and end of umbilical cord.	If infant was born alive, inflammatory changes may be found, depending on survival interval.
Blood	Submit sample for toxicologic study (p. 16) and retain according to established schedule for possible additional testing (paternity testing may be required).	
Lungs	If there is a possibility that the cadaver represents a stillbirth, see p. 476.	For the hydrostatic lung test, see "Stillbirth." The test is unreliable. Extraneous material in air passages indicates that child was alive.
Gastrointestinal tract	If infant is thought to have died shortly after birth, determine the location of air in the intestinal tract; roentgenograms may be helpful.	Air reaches the stomach after 15 min, the small intestine after 1–2 h, the colon after 5–6 h, and the rectum after 12 h. There is no difference in the speed of gas propulsion between full-term and premature infants. Bacterial gas production and previous resuscitation attempts are potential sources of errors.
	Save stomach contents and record amount.	In questionable stillbirth, presence of milk proves that infant was alive and had been nursed.
Other organs	See also under "Homicide."	Traumatic lesions and signs of neglect may be present.

Reference

1. Hart BL, Dudley MH, Zumwalt RE. Postmortem cranial MRI and autopsy correlation in suspected child abuse. Am J Forens Med Pathol 1996;17: 217–224.

Infarction, Cerebral

Related Term: Stroke

Organs and Tissues	*Procedures*	*Possible or Expected Findings*
Heart	If infective endocarditis is suspected, follow procedures described on p. 103. Record presence or absence of patent oval foramen or other septal defects.	Myocardial infarction or other cardiac lesions that may cause systemic circulatory failure. Valvular vegetations and mural thrombi may be source of cerebral emboli; paradoxic embolism.
Aorta	Procedures depend on expected findings or grossly identified abnormalities as listed in right-hand column.	Aortic dissection. atherosclerosis with or without mural thrombi; atheromas.
Cervical arteries	For dissection and roentgenologic demonstration of carotid and vertebral arteries, see p. 82.	Dissecting hematoma of cervical arteries; atherosclerosis with or without thrombosis; atheromas of cervical arteries, particularly in carotid bulb.
Femoral and other systemic veins	For removal of femoral veins, see p. 34.	Thromboses as source of paradoxic cerebral embolism.
Brain	For cerebral arteriography, see p. 80. For removal and specimen preparation, see p. 65.	Atherosclerosis of intracranial arteries. Cerebral infarcts (white or red) of different size, age, and distribution. Watershed (boundary) zones are most frequently affected in global ischemia caused by systemic circulatory failure.
Cerebral venous sinuses	For exposure of venous sinuses, see p. 71.	Cerebral venous sinus thrombosis;* thrombosis of tributaries of venous sinuses. Parasagittal, bilateral, and hemorrhagic infarcts after sagittal sinus thrombosis.

Infarction, Myocardial (See "Disease, ischemic heart.")

Infarction, Pulmonary (See "Embolism, pulmonary.")

Infection, Cytomegalovirus

Synonyms: Cytomegalic inclusion disease; salivary gland virus disease.

NOTE: Cytomegalovirus infection may complicate any chronic debilitating disease, and may follow treatment with immunosuppressive and cytotoxic drugs. (1) Collect all tissues that appear to be infected. (2) Request viral cultures. (3) Immunohistochemical stains on paraffin-embedded sections are available in many laboratories. (4) No special precautions are indicated. (5) Serologic studies are available from many reference laboratories (p. 135), but these are not necessary to make the diagnosis. (6) This is not a reportable disease.

Possible Associated Conditions: *Pneumocystis carinii* infection.* Bacterial, fungal, protozoal, and other viral infections.

Organs and Tissues	*Procedures*	*Possible or Expected Findings*
Placenta	Record weight. For specimen preparation, see p. 60.	In congenital cytomegalovirus infection, mononuclear plasma cell villitis with villous edema and intranuclear and cytoplasmic inclusions.
External examination	Record changes as listed in right-hand column.	In congenital cytomegalovirus infection, microcephaly, jaundice, and a petechial rash may be found.
Urine	Submit sample for viral culture (p. 102). Prepare smears of sediment.	
Lungs	Culture consolidated areas of lung or random sites if the clinical suspicion is high.	Focal interstitial pneumonia. See also above under "Possible Associated Conditions."

Organs and Tissues	Procedures	Possible or Expected Findings
Esophagus and gastrointestinal tract	Submit samples for histologic study.	Ulcers or grossly normal mucosa with cytomegalic inclusions in epithelial and endothelial cells.
Liver	Record weight and submit samples for histologic study and viral culture.	Hepatitis with hepatomegaly.
Other organs	Submit samples of myocardium, pancreas, spleen, kidneys, adrenal glands, and eyes (p. 85) for histologic study and, if indicated, viral culture. For special stains, see above under "Note." If accessible, prepare sections of salivary glands [e.g., submandibular gland in flow of mouth (p. 4)].	Myocarditis; pancreatitis; splenitis; and adrenalitis. In adult and in congenital infections, focal necrotizing nephritis; chorioretinitis. Virtually all organs may be affected and have cytomegalic cells with viral inclusions.
Brain	For removal and specimen preparation, see p. 65.	Meningoencephalitis with subependymal calcifications of lateral ventricles.
Bone marrow		Fibrin ring granulomas in rare instances *(1)*.

Reference

1. Young J, Goulian M. Bone marrow fibrin ring granulomas and cytomegalovirus infection. Am J Clin Pathol 1993;99:65–68.

Infection, Hantavirus (See "Fever, hemorrhagic, with renal syndrome.")

Infection, Herpes simplex

Synonyms and Related Terms: Herpes simplex, type I; herpes simplex, type II; sporadic acute herpes simplex type I (rarely type II) encephalitis. For other names and manifestations, see below under "Possible or Expected Findings."

Organs and Tissues	Procedures	Possible or Expected Findings
Mouth, esophagus, distal colon, liver, adrenal glands, and other organs and tissues	Multiple organs and tissues may be involved, including oral cavity, esophagus, colon, liver, and adrenal glands. Sample tissue from these sites.	Herpetic gingivostomatitis, esophagitis, distal colitis, and proctitis (mostly type II infection); herpetic hepatitis with or without extensive necrosis, and adrenalitis with cortical necrosis.
Brain	For removal and specimen preparation, see pp. 65 and 67, respectively. Nuclear virus antigens can be identified immunohistochemically. Viral nucleic acid may persist years after the acute phase and be identified by *in situ* hybridization. In the acute phase, submit tissue for culture. For electron microscopic study, see p. 132.	In the acute phase, generalized swelling. Bilateral, often asymmetrical necrosis, involving particularly the temporal lobes. Neocortex, white matter, hippocampus, amygdaloid nucleus, and putamen may be involved and lesions may extend to the insular cortex. Typically, diffuse necrotizing herpetic meningoencephalitis; intranuclear inclusions may be difficult to detect. In the chronic phase, shrunken tissue with marked neuronal loss, gliosis, and frequently cystic degeneration.
Eyes	For removal and specimen preparation, see p. 85. Electron microscopy (p. 132), immunocytochemistry, *in situ* hybridization, and the polymerase chain reaction may be needed to confirm the diagnosis.	Herpes simplex keratitis and retinal necrosis. Corneal perforation.

Infection, Herpes Zoster

Synonyms and Related Terms: Herpes zoster oticus (Ramsay Hunt syndrome); postherpetic neuralgia; shingles; zona; zoster encephalomyelitis; zoster encephalopathy; zoster ophthalmicus.

NOTE: (1) Collect all tissues that appear to be infected. (2) Request viral cultures. (3) Stain for inclusion bodies (Lendrum's method; p. 172). Electron microscopy, labeled-antibody techniques, and *in situ* hybridization also can be useful in identifying viral particles. (4) Usually, no special precautions are indicated. (5) Serologic studies are available from the state health department laboratories (p. 135). (6) This is not a reportable disease.

Possible Associated Conditions: Heavy metal poisoning; leukemia;* lymphoma;* multiple myeloma;* other malignant tumors (particularly when the spine is involved or when the patient had been treated with immunosuppressive agents or irradiation); trauma; tuberculosis;* other chronic debilitating diseases.

Organs and Tissues	*Procedures*	*Possible or Expected Findings*
External examination	Record distribution of lesions. Prepare histologic sections of affected areas. For virus culture, aspirate vesicles aseptically.	Unilateral groups of skin vesicles, pustules, and crusts in thoracic, cervical, facial, lumbar, or sacral distribution. Eruptions may be bullous or gangrenous. Vesicles may be present on tip of nose. Generalized infections may occur. Granuloma annulare-like lesions following herpes zoster infection *(1)*.
Lymph nodes	Prepare histologic sections of lymph nodes that drained the region of the zoster lesions.	Lymphadenitis.
Blood	Submit sample for serologic study.	
Pleural and peritoneal cavities	Record appearance and volume of effusions	Effusions in presence of visceral herpes zoster.
Gastrointestinal tract	Submit samples from areas with gross lesions for histologic study.	Inflammatory lesions in visceral zoster.
Urinary bladder	Submit samples from areas with gross lesions for histologic study.	Unilateral ulcers in visceral zoster.
Brain and spinal cord	For removal and specimen preparation, see pp. 65 and 67, respectively. Submit fresh material for virologic study (p. 102).	In rare instances, diffuse meningo-encephalitis may occur. Limited necrotic and inflammatory lesions in the cord or brain stem at the level of the affected ganglion are common.
Sensory ganglia	For exposure of posterior root ganglia, see p. 69. If the face is involved, study trigeminal ganglia.	Ganglion cell necrosis; lymphocytic infiltration, hemorrhage, and, later, fibrosis. As a rule, only one ganglion is severely involved, but less severe lesions may occur in the ganglia that are immediately adjacent.
Peripheral nerves	For sampling and specimen preparation, see p. 79. Request Luxol fast blue stain (p. 172).	Diffuse lymphocytic infiltration; demyelination; axonal destruction; fibrosis.
Eyes	For removal and specimen preparation; see p. 85. Indicated only if there is clinical evidence of zoster ophthalmitis. If eye is affected, study also trigeminal nerve and ganglia.	Conjunctivitis; keratitis; iridocyclitis; retrobulbar neuritis; neuroretinitis; occlusion of retinal vessels.
Ears	Record appearance of pinna. If there was clinical evidence of herpes zoster oticus, remove tympanic membrane, middle ear, and inner ear (p. 72).	Herpes zoster oticus.
Other organs	Procedures depend on expected findings as listed in right-hand column and above under "Note."	Evidence of hematologic malignancies *(2)* or other conditions, as listed above under "Note."

References

1. Gibney MD, Nahass GT, Leonardi CL. Cutaneous reactions following herpes zoster infections: report of three cases and a review of the literature. Br J Dermatol 1996;134:504–509.
2. Smith JB, Fenske NA. Herpes zoster and internal malignancy. South Med J 1995;88:1089–1092.

Infection, Middle Ear (See "Otitis media.")

Infection, *Pneumocystis carinii*

Synonym: Pneumocystosis.

NOTE: (1) Collect all tissues that appear to be infected. (2) This organism cannot be cultured at present but is frequently associated with viral, bacterial, or fungal infections that can be diagnosed by culture. (3) For rapid staining of aspirates, use Gram-Weigert stain, which will stain cysts of *Pneumocystis carinii* and also fungi and bacteria. *Pneumocystis carinii* is best demonstrated

Infection, *Pneumocystis carinii (continued)*
with Grocott's methenamine silver stain (p. 172). (4) No special precautions are indicated. (5) Usually, no serologic studies are available. (6) This is not a reportable disease.

Organs and Tissues	*Procedures*	*Possible or Expected Findings*
Lungs	Prepare smears of fresh cut sections. For special stains for smears and paraffin sections, see above under "Note."	Pneumonia with foamy intra-alveolar exudate containing cysts of *Pneumocystis carinii.*
Other organs	Procedures depend on expected findings or grossly identified abnormalities as listed in right-hand column.	Manifestations of conditions requiring high-dose immunosuppressive therapy; AIDS;* hypogammaglobulinemia, leukemia,* lymphoma,* and prematurity.

Infection, Respiratory Syncytial Virus (See "Pneumonia, all types or type unspecified.")

Infection, Spinal Epidural

Organs and Tissues	*Procedures*	*Possible or Expected Findings*
External examination	If skin infections are presence, record character and extent; prepare photographs.	Pyogenic skin infections which may be trivial (*S. aureus*).
Cerebrospinal fluid	Submit sample for microbiologic study (p. 104); prepare smears.	Protein concentrations increased; WBC < 150/mm^3 (findings compatible with parameningeal infection).
Spinal canal and epidural space	For exposure of epidural space, see p. 65. Local removal of uncontaminated infectious material may not be possible. Prepare sections and smears. Prepare saw sections through be present. Tuberculous abscesses may also granulomas or from walls of abscesses for histologic study.	Trauma or osteomyelitis* (or both) of vertebrae. Occasionally, pleural, sub-diaphragmatic, or perirenal infections may adjacent bone. Submit samples of epidural occur.
Other organs	Procedures depend on expected findings or grossly identified abnormalities as listed in right-hand column.	Manifestations of cirrhosis;* diabetes mellitus;* intravenous drug abuse; malignancy; obstructive uropathy; or steroid-treated degenerative joint disease.

Influenza

Related Terms: Influenza A and B.

NOTE: (1) Collect all tissues that appear to be infected. (2) Request viral and aerobic bacterial cultures. (3) Request Gram stain (p. 172). (4) Special **precautions** are indicated (p. 146). (5) Serologic studies are available from the state health department laboratories (p. 135). (6) This is not a reportable disease.

Organs and Tissues	*Procedures*	*Possible or Expected Findings*
Larynx, trachea, and lungs	Remove en bloc; open extrapulmonary airways posteriorly and photograph mucosa.	Necrosis of respiratory tract epithelium.
	Submit samples of trachea for histologic study. Record weight of each lung. Submit consolidated or hemorrhagic/edematous areas for viral and bacterial culture (p. 103).	Primary influenzal pneumonia; super-infection with *Pneumococcus, Staphylococcus, Hemophilus influenzae,* and *Streptoccocus.*
	Perfuse one lung with formalin (p. 47).	Emphysema; interstitial pulmonary fibrosis; chronic bronchitis.
Nasal cavities and sinuses	For exposure, see p. 71.	Coryza.
Other organs	Procedures depend on expected findings or grossly identified abnormalities as listed in right-hand column.	Myositis; myocarditis;* Reye's syndrome;* transverse myelitis (rare).

Injury, Electrical

Synonyms and Related Terms: Electric burns; electric shock.

NOTE: Immediate scene investigation with an experienced electrical engineer may be crucial for reconstruction of the fatal events and for prevention of similar injuries to others (the expertise of electricians may not suffice; many erroneously believe that 110 volt alternating current cannot kill a human). Search for evidence of wetness that might have precipitated the fatal circuit through the victim. See also ref. *(1)*.

Organs and Tissues	*Procedures*	*Possible or Expected Findings*
External examination and skin	Record appearance of shoes and clothing, and retain burned areas with surrounding clothing for possible spectrographic and chemical tests. Photograph (with scale) suspected electrical burns. Record appearance and location of electrical burns; record appearance of hair around such lesions. Prepare histologic sections of electrical injuries.	Characteristic electric burns of shoes and clothing. Metal particles may be found near the burned areas. Small, multiple, craterlike defects or massive fourth-degree burns of hands or other areas of contact; arborescent skin markings; characteristic defects on surface of hair. Degeneration of epithelium and collagen with typical microblisters in epidermis. Gangrene (after electrically induced vascular thromboses) also may be present.
Blood	Record presence or absence of blood clots. Submit sample for alcohol determination. (Alcohol concentrations are important in compensation cases.)	Fluid blood.
Blood vessels	Submit portions for histologic study. Request Verhoeff–van Gieson stain (p. 173).	Intimal degeneration and tearing of elastic fibers, with or without thrombosis.
Heart	Record weight and sample for histologic study (p. 30).	Myocardial hemorrhagic necroses *(2)*.
Lungs	Record lung weights.	Pulmonary edema.
Kidneys	Prepare histologic sections.	Congestion; lower nephron nephrosis in cases with extensive muscle destruction.
Other viscera		Congestion.
Urine		Hemoglobinuria.
Skeletal muscles	Prepare histologic sections of traumatized portions.	Tears after tetanic convulsions.

References

1. Wright RK. Death or injury caused by electrocution. In: Clinics of Laboratory Medicine, vol. 3, No. 2. Symposium on Forensic Pathology, DiMaio JM, ed. W.B. Saunders, Philadelphia, PA, 1983, pp. 343–353.
2. Colonna M, Caruso G, Nardulli F, Altamura B. Myocardial hemorrhagic necrosis in delayed death from electrocution. Acta Medicinae Legalis et Socialis 1989;39:145–147.

Injury, Fire (See "Burns.")

Injury, Firearm

NOTE: Protect all drains of autopsy table, which will prevent accidental loss of bullets or bullet fragments. Recovery of bullet fragments and pellets can also be improved by passing tissue fragments, blood, and other appropriate materials through a fine nonmetallic sieve. Caution must be exercised because sharp edges and jagged projections of bullets and bullet fragments may cause injury *(1)*. This applies particularly to the Black Talon bullet. Bullets and bullet fragments should not be touched with forceps or other metal instruments that may produce artifactual markings; they must be placed in properly labeled evidence containers, and the chain of custody must be preserved (p. 17). From a birdshot wound, at least 10 pellets should be recovered. The firearms examiner will divide the total pellet weight by 10 and derive median pellet weight. From a buckshot wound, all pellets should be recovered. In many of these cases, procedures described under "Homicide" must also be followed.

Do not excise wounds before completion of autopsy (see below). As an academic exercise, excised firearm wounds may be used later for analysis of metal traces by neutron activation or for tests for carboxyhemoglobin. In practice, however, 35 mm photography is adequate to establish the presence or absence of gunpowder stippling or soot deposition toward the end of establishing the range of fire. The dimensions of the stippled areas and soot deposits should be recorded.

After completion of external examination, dry the wet clothing and keep as evidence. Clothing may also be used for possible test firing or for stain, powder, or particle analysis.

Organs and Tissues	*Procedures*	*Possible or Expected Findings*
External examination	If identity of victim is unknown, follow procedures described on p. 11.	
	Prepare roentgenograms of entire body, before and after disrobing of body, and then lateral films of body regions with bullets.	Systemic roentgenograms may reveal bullets from obscure entrance wounds, particularly in decomposed bodies, old bullets, or bullets external to the body in clothing.
	Record location and number of bullet holes in all layers of garments, indicating whether the involved area is bloodstained or shows gunpowder or soot.	Bullet(s) may have been arrested in hollow viscus or blood vessel and may have been transported to distant sites by peristalsis or bloodstream ("bullet embolus"). Bullets may be deflected in unexpected directions from bony surfaces.
	Study clothing with hand lens or dissecting microscope and record whether garment fibers were turned inward or outward. If there are several cutaneous perforations, number or letter each consecutively and refer to these numbers in all records. Location of bullet holes should be described by recording distance from soles of feet or top of head, and from midline of body. Prepare diagrams and photograph holes, with and without labels.	Soot ("smudging") and gunpowder strippling may occur around entrance wound, depending on the muzzle-to-skin distance. There may also be an impression from a recoiling handgun or from a power piston.
	Photographs should show surrounding garments and extent of blood stains. In hairy areas, shave around bullet wounds for better documentation. For evaluation of distance from where a shot had been fired, see Fig. II–3.	Wounds may be stellate, round, jagged, or slitlike, with or without wide margins of abrasion.
	Inspect hands for powder marks. Skin samples can be used for neutron activation analysis for antimony and bismuth.	Primer residues on hand of suicide victim after use of a handgun.
Internal examination	Describe wound track(s) in anatomic order and in complete separate paragraphs, with summarizing description of course of bullet with respect to the standard anatomical position (e.g., front to back, left to right, somewhat down). Avoid using numerical angular measurements.	Fatal secondary injuries, particularly hemorrhages.
	For toxicologic sampling of body fluids and tissues, see p. 16.	Alcohol intoxication is a frequent finding.

Reference

1. Russell MA, Atkinson RD, Klatt EC, Noguchi TT. Safety in bullet recovery procedures: a study of the Black Talon bullet. Am J Forens Med 1995;16:120–123.

Injury, Head

Synonyms and Related Terms: Contact injury; diffuse axonal damage; diffuse white matter shearing injury; head motion injury; inner cerebral trauma; shearing injury.

NOTE: The brain may show coup and contrecoup lesions, swelling, hematoma, with microscopic evidence of axonal swelling ("retraction balls") in cerebral white matter, corpus callosum, and upper brainstem. Hemorrhages in frontal white matter and corpus callosum, dorsolateral midbrain, and rostral pons. If patient survived days or weeks, macrophages infiltrate, later followed by microglial clusters and gliosis at the sites of injury.

In cases of gunshot injury to the head, see under that heading.

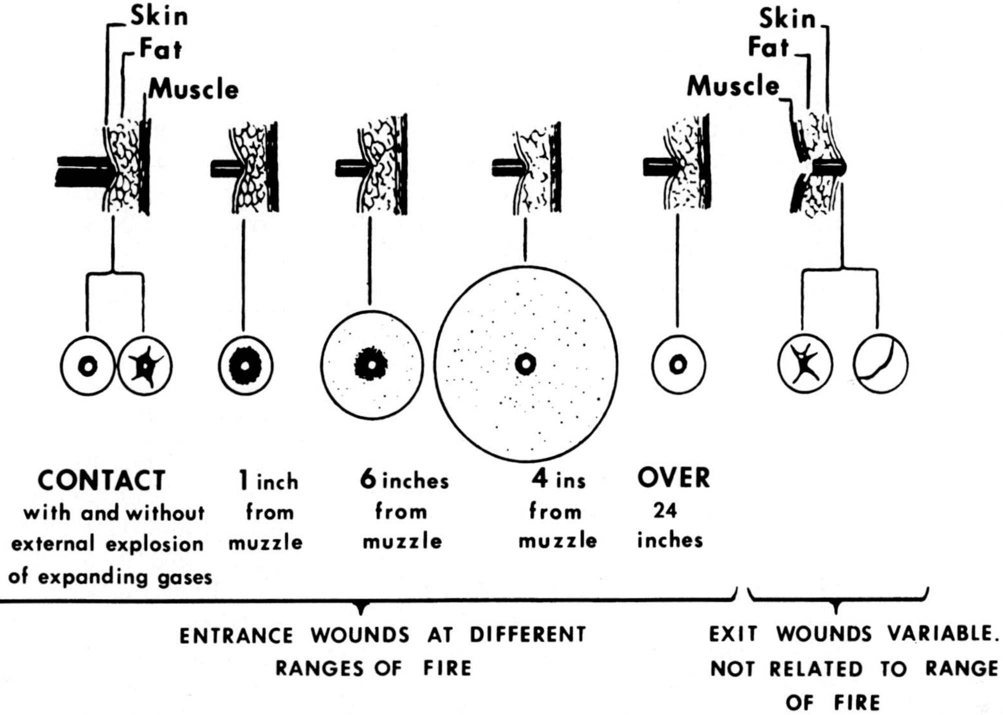

Fig. II-3. Bullet wounds. Differences in the appearance of cutaneous wounds of entrance and of exit and differences in wounds of entrance according to the distance between muzzle and skin at the moment of fire. Entrance wounds often differ from exit wounds in that the former are usually surrounded by a narrow zone of abrasion. If the muzzle of a gun is in close contact with the skin at the moment of fire, the combustion products will be blown into the wound and will not be visible on the surface. For close-range wounds, the stippling of the skin around the wound, produced by particles of burned and unburned powder, becomes progressively more dispersed as the range of fire increases and is ordinarily not perceptible if the range has been greater than 24 inches (61 cm) (with permission from Moritz AR, Morris CR. Handbook of Legal Medicine. Third edition, 1970. CV Mosby Company, St. Louis, MO.) Exit wounds usually have no marginal abrasion *(1)* and have no apparent tissue deficit.

Reference

1. DiMaio VJM. Gunshot Wounds: Practical Aspects of Firearms, Ballistics and Forensic Techniques. Elsevier Science Publishing Co., New York, 1985.

Injury, Head *(continued)*

Organs and Tissues	*Procedures*	*Possible or Expected Findings*
External examination	Record extent and character of soft tissue and scalp wounds. Prepare roentgenogram of skull and, in case of heart wound, roentgenogram of the chest.	Face and scalp ecchymoses, hematomas, lacerations. Firearm injury.* Linear, radiating, depressed, bursting, diastatic, and other skull fracture(s). Cardiac air embolism.*
Neck organs	Expose carotid arteries. For carotid arteriography, see p. 82.	Carotid artery thrombosis.
Skull (see also below under "Brain")	Record sites, appearance, and length of fractures. For detection of hairline fractures, strip dura from the base of skull and vault. Record separations or lacerations of dura. Open dural sinuses. Locate air embolus ingress. If osteomyelitis is suspected, submit material for bacterial culture and smears (p. 102).	Character of fractures may indicate site impact. Dural trauma indicates severe force. Superior longitudinal sinus thrombosis. Ingress of air embolus. Osteomyelitis* of skull bones.
Brain	For removal and specimen preparation of brain, see p. 65. Record site and amount of leptomeningeal hemorrhage.	For gross and microscopic findings, see above under "Note." Epidural or subdural hematomas;* subarachnoid hemorrhage. Cerebral abscess;* meningitis.*
Lungs	Prepare frozen, Sudan-stained sections.	Fat embolism.*

Injury, Intubation

Organs and Tissues	Procedures	Possible or Expected Findings
Extenal examination and neck organs	Intubation tube should be left in place until position is verified. Prepare roentgenograms. Remove neck organs with pharynx, and base of tongue (p. 4). Open trachea posteriorly or opposite perforation or fistula. Photograph lesions and submit samples for histologic study.	Intubation tube in wrong place; soft tissue emphysema. Ulcers; erosions; chondromalacia; perforation; fistula; herpetic infection.

Injury, Lightning

Organs and Tissues	Procedures	Possible or Expected Findings
External examination and skin		Electrical burns (head and legs) *(1)* or explosive tearing of clothing; mechanical damage from blast effects. See also under "Burns" and "Injury, electrical."
	Photograph erythema, electric burns, and injuries. Prepare histologic sections.	Fernlike distribution of electrically induced erythema is characteristic for lightning injury.
Other organs	For procedures involving the heart, see "Disease, ischemic heart."	See under "Injury, electrical." The most severe visceral manifestations of lightning injury generally affect the cardiovascular and central nervous system (see below) *(2)*. Sequelae of attempted resuscitation from cardiac or respiratory arrest are commonly noted.
Brain and spinal cord	For removal and specimen preparation, see pp. 65 and 67, respectively.	Cerebral edema with brain stem herniation; epidural hemorrhage.
Middle ear	For exposure of the middle ear, see p. 72.	Rupture of eardrums.
Eyes	For removal and specimen preparation, see p. 85.	Cataracts; interstitial keratitis; iridocyclitis; chorioretinal atrophy; hemorrhages *(2)*.
Skeletal muscle	Sample for histologic study (p. 80), particularly if myoglobinuria had been observed.	Muscle necroses.

References

1. Cooper MA. Lightning injuries: Prognostic signs of death. Ann Emerg Med 1980;9:134–138.
2. Tribble CG, Persing JA, Morgan RF, Kenney JG, Edlich RF. Lightning injuries. Comprehensive Ther 1985;11:32–40.

Injury, Radiation

Synonyms and Related Terms: Acute radiation syndrome; chronic (delayed) radiation injury; radiation enterocolitis; radiation nephritis; radiation pneumonitis.

NOTE: Procedures and expected findings depend on type of radiation damage, whether acute or chronic, localized or whole-body irradiation. If suspected radiation injury was associated with the administration of radionuclides such as ^{32}P, ^{131}I, or ^{198}Au, follow procedures suggested in Chapter 13 (p. 125). In fatal whole-body irradiation, findings are most likely related to bone marrow injury, and the suggested procedures and expected findings are those described under "Pancytopenia." Record extent of oropharyngeal and intestinal ulcerations and hemorrhages. Late complications include malignant tumors (carcinoma, leukemia,* lymphoma*), manifestations of hypothyroidism,* and cataracts. Organ changes in localized radiation injury depend on site of irradiation (lung, brain, kidney, intestine). The skin is involved in both acute (erythema) and chronic (atrophy, epilation) radiation injury.

Injury, Stabbing

Related Terms: Cutting injury; knife injury.

NOTE: In many of these cases, procedures described under "Homicide" must also be followed.

Organs and Tissues	Procedures	Possible or Expected Findings
External examination and skin (wounds)	Prepare diagrams and photographs of all wounds. Each wound can be labeled with identifying number or letter that can also appear on photographs and histologic sections.	Defense wounds occur on hands and arms.

Organs and Tissues	Procedures	Possible or Expected Findings
External examination and skin (wounds) *(continued)*	Examine edges of wounds on clothing and skin with hand lens, if necessary; record appearance of edges. Record location of wounds by stating distance from top of head or from sole of foot, distance from midline, location at front or back, and relation to fixed anatomic landmarks. Record the dimensions of the wounds and state whether the measurement is taken with the wound margins approximated (pushed together) or unapproximated. Keep clothing as evidence.	Serrations of skin tags along incised wound margins are caused by dragging action of knife. If contusions or abrasions are present, wounds are more likely caused by laceration. Undivided nerves, hair bulbs, and vessels in depth of wounds indicate laceration. (Knives or other sharp-edged instruments tend to cut these structures.)
	Submit samples from edges of wounds for histologic study, if necessary.	Inflammatory changes indicate vital response (absent in wounds received after death).
	Prepare roentgenograms of areas around wounds.	Metallic parts may have broken off weapon.
	If wounds were not immediately fatal or if tetanus* was present, cultures from wounds may be indicated.	Wound infection.
Wound tracks	Dissect layer by layer and follow tracks of cutting or stabbing instrument. Do not probe. Record lacerated vessels and organs penetrated.	
Body cavities	Record volume of accumulated blood.	Hematomas; hemothorax; hemoperitoneum.
Heart	Submit blood samples for alcohol determination and other toxicologic studies (p. 16).	
Lungs	Request Sudan stain of frozen sections (p. 173).	Pulmonary fat embolism.
Other organs	For toxicologic sampling, see p. 16.	

Insecticides (See "Poisoning, organophosphate(s).")

Insuffiency, Adrenal

Synonyms and Related Terms: Adrenocortical insufficiency; polyglandular autoimmune syndrome (type I, usually in childhood, with parathyroid insufficiency and chronic mucocutaneous moniliasis; type II, usually in adults, with two or more autoimmune endocrine disorders such as thyroiditis and diabetes mellitus*); primary adrenal insufficiency (Addison's disease); secondary adrenal insufficiency (in hypothalamic-pituitary disease or steroid induced); X-linked adrenal hypoplasia.

NOTE: Primary adrenal insufficiency (Addison's disease) is caused by anatomic changes (see below under "Adrenal glands"), drugs (enzyme inhibitors or cytotoxic drugs), or ACTH-blocking antibodies.

Possible Associated Conditions: AIDS with systemic infections *(1)*; antiphospholipid antibody syndrome *(2)*; autoimmune hepatitis; chronic lymphocytic thyroiditis; type I diabetes mellitus;* hypoparathyroidism;* hypothyroidism;* megaloblastic anemia;* surgical procedures, such as heart surgery or orthopedic procedures.

Organs and Tissues	Procedures	Possible or Expected Findings
External examination and skin	Prepare sections of pigmented areas of skin. Prepare photographs of pigmented abnormalities.	Decreased axillary and pubic hair in women; diffuse brown hyperpigmentation; bluish-black spots on mucous surfaces of lips and cheeks.
Vitreous	Submit sample for sodium, potassium, chloride, and urea nitrogen analysis (p. 85).	Electrolyte changes associated with dehydration.* Decreased sodium and chloride in primary adrenal insufficiency.
Blood	Submit sample for microbiologic (p. 102) and chemical study.	Septicemia, including systemic fungal infections. Low plasma cortisol concentration.
Adrenal glands	Record weights; photograph; prepare roentgenograms; submit portion for microbiologic study; submit samples for histologic study.	Idiopathic (autoimmune?) atrophy of adrenal cortex; tuberculosis* (also *Mycobacterium avium intracellulare* infection in AIDS);

Organs and Tissues	*Procedures*	*Possible or Expected Findings*
External examination and skin *(continued)*	Decalcification may be necessary (p. 97). Request acid fast, Gram, and Grocott's methenamine silver stains (p. 172).	coccidioidomycosis;* cryptococcosis* or nocardiosis* *(1)* (in AIDS); cytomegalovirus infection* (in AIDS); histoplasmosis;* rarely amyloidosis;* hemorrhages *(3)*; widespread lymphoma* *(4)* or metastases of malignant tumors.
Other endocrine glands	Describe and weigh all endocrine glands and sample for histologic study.	Abnormalities of pituitary gland (in secondary adrenal insufficiency), thyroid, parathroid glands, gonades, or islets of Langerhans (see under "Possible Associated Conditions.")
Other organs	Search for conditions that may have caused adrenal insufficiency.	See above under "Adrenal glands" and under "Possible Associated Conditions."

References

1. Arabi Y, Fairfax MR, Szuba MJ, Crane L, Schuman P. Adrenal insufficiency, recurrent bacteremia, and disseminated abscesses caused by Nocardia asteroides in a patient with acquired immunodficiency syndrome. Diagn Microbiol Inf Dis 1996;24:47–51.
2. Argento A, DiBenedetto RJ. ARDS and adrenal insufficiency associated with the antiphospholipid antibody syndrome. Chest 1998;113: 1136–1138.
3. Cozzolino D, Peerzada J, Heaney JA. Adrenal insufficiency from bilateral adrenal hemorrhage after total knee replacement surgery. Urology 1997;50:125–127.
4. Nasu M, Aruga M, Itami J, Fujimoto H, Matsubara O. Non-Hodgkin's lymphoma presenting with adrenal insufficiency and hypothyroidism: an autopsy case report. Pathol Internat 1998;48:138–143.

Insufficiency, Aortic

Synonyms: Aortic incompetence; aortic regurgitation.

NOTE: For general dissection techniques in valvular heart disease, see p. 23. For procedures in infective endocarditis, see p. 103.

Possible Associated Conditions: Acute aortic dissection* with or without Marfan's syndrome;* ankylosing spondylitis;* aortitis; congenitally bicuspid aortic valve;* cystic medial degeneration of aorta; giant cell aortitis;* hypertension;* late postoperative conotruncal anomalies (e.g., tetralogy); rheumatic aortic valve disease; syphilitic aortitis; Takayasu's arteritis;* trauma; ventricular septal defect.*

Organs and Tissues	*Procedures*	*Possible or Expected Findings*
External examination	Prepare chest roentgenogram.	Cardiomegaly; dilated ascending aorta.
Blood	If infective endocarditis is suspected, submit sample for microbiologic study (p. 102).	Septicemia.
Heart and great vessels	For general dissection techniques in congenital heart disease, see p. 33.	See above under "Possible Associated Conditions."
	If infective endocarditis is suspected, follow procedures described on p. 103.	Infective endocarditis.*
	Record weight and measurements of heart.	Cardiomegaly; acute or old myocardial infarction.
	For dissection, tests for valvular insufficiency, and measurement of valve size, see p. 29.	
Other organs		See above under "Possible Associated Conditions."

Insufficiency, Coronary (See "Disease, ischemic heart.")

Insufficiency, Mitral (Chronic or Acute)

Synonyms and Related Terms: Acquired mitral insufficiency; mitral incompetence; mitral regurgitation; congenital mitral insufficiency; floppy valve syndrome; mitral annular calcification; mitral valve prolapse; mitral regurgitation; myxomatous mitral valve disease; rheumatic mitral valve disease.

Possible Associated Conditions: Autoimmune connective tissue disorders; bicuspid aortic valve;* cardiomyopathy* (dilated, hypertrophic, or restrictive); infective endocarditis;* Marfan's syndrome;* metabolic/storage diseases, such as mucopolysaccharidoses;* ischemic heart disease;* rheumatic heart disease.*

Organs and Tissues	Procedures	Possible or Expected Findings
External examination	Prepare chest roentgenogram.	Cardiomegaly; calcification in and around mitral valve.
Blood	If infective endocarditis is suspected, submit sample for microbiologic study (p. 102).	Septicemia.
Heart and great vessels	For general dissection techniques in valvular and congenital heart disease, see p. 33.	See above under "Possible Associated Conditions."
	If infective endocarditis is suspected, follow procedures described on p. 103.	Infective endocarditis.*
	Record weight and measurements of heart. For dissection, tests for valvular insufficiency, and measurement of valve size, see p. 29.	Cardiomegaly; acute myocardial infarction, with or without rupture of papillary muscles; fibrosis of papillary muscles; myxomatous (floppy) mitral valve; rheumatic valvulitis; rupture of tendinous cords; other coexistent valve disease.
Other organs		See above under "Possible Associated Conditions."

Insufficiency, Pituitary

Synonym: Hypopituitarism.

Possible Associated Conditions: Diabetes mellitus;* pregnancy;* and other conditions listed below under "Brain, spinal cord, and pituitary gland."

Organs and Tissues	Procedures	Possible or Expected Findings
External examination	Record weight and length of body and distribution and intensity of hair growth.	Dwarfism in childhood cases.
	Prepare roentgenogram of skull.	Evidence of skull fractures or tumor.
Blood	Freeze sample for possible biochemical study.	
Extrapituitary endocrine organs	Dissect and record weights of all endocrine organs. Submit samples for histologic study.	Polyglandular atrophy.
Other organs	Procedures depend on expected findings or grossly identified abnormalities as listed in right-hand column.	Fatty changes of liver *(1)*. Manifestations of diabetes mellitus.* Systemic amyloidosis* or genetic hemochromatosis* with secondary infiltration of pituitary gland region.
Urine	Freeze sample for possible biochemical study.	
Brain, spinal cord, and pituitary gland	For removal and specimen preparation, see pp. 65, 67, and 71, respectively. For cerebral arteriography, see p. 80. Record weight of pituitary gland.	Developmental anomalies (pituitary aplasia or basal encephalocele). Postpartum necrosis of pituitary gland (Sheehan's syndrome*); lymphocytic hypophysitis; granulomatous inflammation (in sarcoidosis*); chromophobe pituitary adenoma; craniopharyngioma in childhood; other benign or malignant pituitary tumors; extrasellar cysts; effects of trauma or irradiation.
Base of skull	Expose venous sinuses (p. 71). Strip dura for inspection of bone.	Skull fractures; cavernous sinus thrombosis; primary or metastatic tumors.
Skeletal system		Bone fractures *(2)*.
Vitreous	Refrigerate sample for possible glucose and electrolyte determination (p. 85).	

References

1. Takano S, Kanzaki S, Sato M, Kubo T, Seino Y. Effect of growth hormone on fatty liver in panhypopituitarism. Arch Dis Childhood 1997;76:537–538.
2. Rosen T, Wilhelmsen L, Landin-Wilhelmsen K, Lappas G, Bengtsson BA. Increased fracture frequency in adult patients with hypopituitarism and GH deficiency. Eur J Endocrinol 1997;137:240–245.

Insufficiency, Pulmonary

Synonyms: Pulmonary incompetence; pulmonary regurgitation.

NOTE: Infective endocarditis due to *Strept. bovis*, especially when it involves the pulmonary valve, is often associated with an underlying adenocarcinoma of the colon.

Possible Associated Conditions: Carcinoid heart disease; congestive heart failure;* infective endocarditis;* pulmonary hypertension;* tetralogy of Fallot* with absent pulmonary valve (*not* the same as pulmonary atresia).

Insufficiency, Tricuspid (Chronic or Acute)

Synonyms: Tricuspid incompetence; tricuspid regurgitation.

Possible Associated Conditions: Cardiomyopathy* (dilated or restrictive); chronic congestive heart failure (any cause); chronic pulmonary hypertension (any cause)*. See also below under "Possible or Expected Findings."

Organs and Tissues	*Procedures*	*Possible or Expected Findings*
External examination		Cyanosis; edema.
Heart	If infective endocarditis is suspected, follow procedures described on p. 103. For dissection and histologic sampling, see pp. 23 and 30.	Infective endocarditis.* Carcinoid heart disease; Epstein's anomaly; rheumatic valve disease.
Lungs	Perfuse both lungs with formalin (p. 47). Request Verhoeff–van Gieson stain (p. 173).	Hypertensive pulmonary vascular changes (see "Hypertension, pulmonary").
Other organs		See "Failure, congestive heart."*

Interruption of Aortic Arch (See "Coarctation, aortic.")

Intolerance, Fructose

Synonyms: Hereditary fructose intolerance; hereditary fructosemia, deficiency of fructose-1-phosphate aldolase.

Organs and Tissues	*Procedures*	*Possible or Expected Findings*
External examination	Record body weight and length.	Signs of extreme weight loss; evidence of coagulopathy.
Eyes	Submit sample of vitreous for sodium, potassium, chloride, urea nitrogen, and glucose determination (p. 85).	Evidence of dehydration.* There is no reliable test for hypoglycemia.*
Blood	Submit plasma/serum for chemical study (see right-hand column).	Increased fructose and bilirubin concentrations.
Abdomen	Record volume of fluid.	Ascites.
Urine	Submit sample for chemical study.	Aminoaciduria;* fructosuria; proteinuria; urobilinuria.
Liver	Record weight. Snap-freeze tissue for histochemical or biochemical study. Submit samples for light microscopic and electron microscopic study (p. 132).	Hepatomegaly; steatosis; cholestasis; necrosis; fibrosis; cirrhosis; negative aldolase activity; "fructose holes" by electron microscopy *(1)*.
Spleen		Splenomegaly.
Other organs	Submit samples for histologic and histochemical study.	Evidence of coagulopathy.
Brain and spinal cord	For removal and specimen preparation, see pp. 65 and 67, respectively.	Cerebral edema.
Bone	Submit samples of epiphysis, if available, for histologic study (p. 95).	Rickets.

Reference

1. Phillips MJ, Poucell S, Patterson J, Valencia P. The Liver: An Atlas and Text of Ultrastructural Pathology, Raven Press, New York, 1987.

Intubation (See "Injury, intubation.")

Iodine (See "Poisoning, iodine.")

Ischemia, Cerebral (See "Attack, transient cerebral ischemic" and "Infarction, cerebral.")

Ischemic, Heart (See "Disease, ischemic heart.")

Isomorism (See "Syndrome, polysplenia and asplenia.")

K

Kala-Azar

Synonyms and Related Terms: *Leishmania donovani* infection; Dumdum fever; visceral leishmaniasis; infantile kala-azar.

NOTE: (1) Collect all tissues that appear to be infected. (2) Usually, cultures are not required, but direct examination for parasites is indicated. (3) Request Giemsa or Wright's stain (p. 172). (4) Usually, no special precautions are indicated. (5) Serologic studies are available from the Centers for Disease Control and Prevention, Atlanta, GA (p. 135). (6) This is not a reportable disease in the United States.

Organs and Tissues	*Procedures*	*Possible or Expected Findings*
External examination and skin	Photograph skin lesions; prepare histologic sections of normal and abnormal skin; request Giemsa or Wright's stain (p. 172).	Emaciation; jaundice or skin pigmentation from melanin accumulation; subcutaneous edema; petechiae; macular or nodular dermal leishmaniasis. Manifestations of vitamin C deficiency.*
Blood	Submit sample for bacterial culture (p. 102).	Superimposed bacteremia.
Oral cavity and other mucosal surfaces		Petechial hemorrhages and ulcers; noma.
Abdominal and pleural cavities	Record volume of effusions; centrifuge and prepare smears of sediment; request Giemsa or Wright's stain (p. 172).	Leishmanial infection or bacterial infection; pleural adhesions; intraperitoneal hemorrhages.
Heart	For histologic sampling, see p. 30; request Giemsa or Wright's stain (p. 172).	Infiltrates of lymphocytes and plasma cells with some eosinophils and mononuclear cells filled with *Leishmania* amastigotes.
Lungs	Submit a section for bacterial culture. Prepare smears; request Giemsa and Gram stains (p. 172).	Bacterial or leishmanial pneumonia, or both.
Liver	Record size and weight; photograph; submit samples for histologic study.	Hepatomegaly; diffuse leishmanial hepatitis, with or without cholestasis.
Spleen	Record size and weight; photograph; prepare smears of cut section; submit samples for histologic study.	Splenomegaly, often extreme, with possible hemorrhage from diagnostic puncture; infarctions; leishmanial splenitis.
Lymph nodes	Submit samples for histologic study.	Lymphadenopathy; see also above under "Heart."
Other organs	Procedures depend on expected findings or grossly identified abnormalities as listed in right-hand column.	See above under "Heart." Manifestations of anemia, agranulocytosis, or thrombocytopenia.
Bone marrow	For preparation of sections and smears, see p. 96.	Osteomyelitis with amastigotes present.
Brain and skeletal muscles		Not involved.

Ketoacidosis (See "Disorder, electrolyte(s)" and p. 115.)

Knife Wounds (See "Injury, stabbing.")

Kwashiorkor (See "Malnutrition...")

From: *Handbook of Autopsy Practice,* 3rd Ed. Edited by: J. Ludwig © Humana Press Inc., Totowa, NJ

L

Laryngitis

Synonyms and Related Terms: Acute infectious airway obstruction; croup; obstructive laryngitis with epiglottitis of infants.

NOTE: (1) Collect all tissues that appear to be infected. (2) Request aerobic bacterial and viral cultures. (3) Request Gram stain (p. 172). (4) Usually, no special precautions are indicated. (5) Serologic studies may be helpful in determining the etiologic agent. (6) This may be a reportable disease, depending on the etiologic agent.

Organs and Tissues	*Procedures*	*Possible or Expected Findings*
Blood and lungs	Submit for bacterial and viral cultures (p. 102). If diphtheria is suspected, see also under that heading.	*Hemophilus influenzae* (cannot always be isolated from larynx). Measles virus, myxovirus, parainfluenza virus, and other respiratory viruses that may affect infants and children.
Larynx and pharynx	Should be removed as soon as possible (before embalming), either from cervical midline incision or from chest (neck of cadaver must be well-extended). Photograph obstruction before larynx is opened, and inside of larynx and epiglottis after larynx is is opened in posterior midline.	Airway obstruction.*
	Make Gram-stained touch preparations (p. 172).	*Hemophilus influenzae* (small, pleomorphic, Gram-negative bacilli) in smear.
	Make histologic sections of larynx and epiglottis.	Other pathogenic and nonpathogenic microorganisms may be present. Acute laryngitis, often with ulcerations.

Lead (See "Poisoning, lead.")

Leishmaniasis (See "Kala-azar.")

Leprosy

Synonyms: Hansen's disease; lepromatous leprosy; *Mycobacterium leprae* infection; tuberculoid leprosy.

NOTE: (1) Collect all tissues that appear to be infected and submit for direct examination. (2) Cultivation of leprosy bacilli is not yet available for routine use. (3) Request Gram, Ziehl-Neelsen, Kinyoun, or fluorochrome stains (p. 172). (4) Usually, no special precautions are indicated. (5) Serologic studies are now available in some laboratories *(1)*. PCR assays are also available *(2)*. (6) This is a **reportable** disease.

Possible Associated Conditions: Amyloidosis;* tuberculosis.*

Organs and Tissues	*Procedures*	*Possible or Expected Findings*
External examination and skin	Photograph lesions, and record extent of skin involvement.	Hyperpigmented macules; annular plaques; nodules; erythematous lesions. In lepromatous leprosy, leonine face with enlarged earlobes and loss of eyebrows. Other mutilations and plantar ulcerations.

From: *Handbook of Autopsy Practice,* 3rd Ed. Edited by: J. Ludwig © Humana Press Inc., Totowa, NJ

Organs and Tissues	*Procedures*	*Possible or Expected Findings*
External examination and skin *(continued)*	Prepare sections of skin. For special stains, see above under "Note." Make touch preparations of skin specimens.	Skin and dermal nerves may be involved histologically.
Other organs	Submit samples of liver, spleen, kidneys, and bone marrow for histologic study.	Visceral involvement usually mild; amyloidosis;* tuberculosis;* erythema nodosum leprosum.
Lymph nodes	Submit samples for histologic study, particularly from drainage area of skin lesions.	Lepromatous lymphadenitis.
Peripheral nerves	For sampling and specimen preparation, see p. 79. Include ulnar, radial, median, and popliteal nerves.	Dermal nerves may be involved (see "External examination and skin"). Nerves may be thickened and fibrotic and may show obliteration of normal architecture. Nerve abscesses.
Eyes and extraglobal orbital tissues	For removal and specimen preparation, see pp. 85 and 73, respectively. Include ciliary nerves.	Iritis and keratitis; granulomas of anterior segment (in lepromatous leprosy) *(3)*; extraglobal granulomas, particularly in ciliary nerves (in tuberculoid leprosy).
Nasal cavity	For exposure, see p. 71. Submit tissue for histologic study.	Blockage of nasal cavity by lepromatous rhinitis.

References

1. Parkash O, Chaturvedi V, Girdhar BK, Sengupta U. A study on performance of two serological assays for diagnosis of leprosy. Leprosy Rev 1995;66:26–30.
2. Wichitwechkarn J, Karnjan S, Shuntawuttisettee S, Sornprasit C. Detection of *Mycobacterium leprae* infection by PCR. J Clin Micro 1995;33:45–49.
3. Job CK, Ebenezer GJ, Thompson K, Daniel E. Pathology of eye in leprosy. Ind J Leprosy 1998;70:79–91.

Leptospirosis

Synonyms: Canicola fever; Weil's disease; Fort Bragg Fever.

NOTE:

(1) Collect all tissues that appear to be infected. (2) Special culture media are required to cultivate the organisms. We recommend consultation with the microbiology laboratory before the postmortem examination is begun. (3) Direct dark-field examination by an experienced technologist is recommended for demonstrating the *Leptospira* organisms. Silver impregnation techniques are also useful. (4) Special **precautions** may be indicated, as this is a communicable disease (p. 146). (5) Serologic studies can be obtained from the state health department laboratories (p. 135). (5) This is not a reportable disease.

Organs and Tissues	*Procedures*	*Possible or Expected Findings*
External examination		Jaundice; skin hemorrhages.
Blood, urine, and cerebrospinal fluid	Submit samples for bacteriologic and serologic study (p. 102).	Pleocytosis of CSF early in the course.
Heart	Submit samples for histologic study (p. 30).	Myocarditis;* endocarditis;* hemorrhages.
Lungs	Submit samples for histologic study.	Hemorrhages; pneumonia.
Liver and spleen	Record sizes and weights; submit samples for histologic study.	Cholestatic hepatitis; hemorrhages; hepatomegaly and splenomegaly.
Stomach		Mucosal hemorrhages.
Kidneys	Submit samples for histologic and electron microscopic study (p. 132).	Hemorrhages; tubular degeneration and necrosis; hyaline and bile casts; interstitial nephritis; fusion of foot processes by electron microscopy.
Skeletal muscles	For sampling and specimen preparation, see p. 80.	Hemorrhages; necrosis.
Brain	For removal and specimen preparation, see p. 65.	Aseptic meningitis;* subarachnoid hemorrhages.*
Eyes	For removal and specimen preparation, see p. 85.	Optic neuritis; iridocyclitis; conjunctivitis; uveitis.

Leukemia, All Types or Type Unspecified

Synonyms and Related Terms: Acute or chronic lymphocytic leukemia, acute or chronic myelogenous leukemia, and hairy cell leukemia. Multiple subtypes have been identified; they are characterized by cell surface markers, chromosomal abnormalities, staining reactions, and morphologic features.

NOTE: At the time of autopsy, most leukemias have been properly classified and often treated. In these cases, the goal of the autopsy is to document the extent of the disease and the presence of complications. If the leukemia had not been classified or if the features might have changed from the time of the last work-up (e.g., in suspected cases of superimposed diffuse large cell lymphoma [Richter's syndrome]), material should be snap-frozen and studied in more detail. If the patient was treated by bone marrow transplantation,* see also under that heading.

The address of the appropriate registry is Hematologic and Lymphatic Pathology, Armed Forces Institute of Pathology (p. 148).

Possible Associated Conditions: Agnogenic myeloid metaplasia with myelofibrosis; Bloom's syndrome;* cutaneous mastocytosis; Down's syndrome;* immunodeficiency syndromes* (Bruton's disease; Louis-Bar syndrome; Wiskott-Aldrich syndrome); infantile genetic agranulocytosis; Klinefelter's syndrome;* lymphoma;* multiple myeloma;* polycythemia;* and many others.

Organs and Tissues	*Procedures*	*Possible or Expected Findings*
External examination, oral cavity, and skin	Record extent and character of skin lesions; photograph lesions and prepare histologic sections. Record appearance of oral cavity and eyes (see also below under "Eyes" and "Lacrimal glands; parotid and other salivary glands").	Nonspecific skin reactions; petechial and other types of hemorrhages; leukemic infiltrates; perianal ulcerations and abscesses; exophthalmos and salivary gland enlargement (Mikulicz's syndrome); gingival hemorrhages; mucosal ulcerations of mouth and nose; alopecia.
Blood and fascia lata	If chromosome study is intended, see p. 109.	Trisomy 21; Philadelphia chromosome; Christchurch chromosome; 47,XXY and less common variants of Klinefelter's syndrome.
	Submit sample of blood for bacterial, fungal, and viral studies (p. 102).	Septicemia. Blood most commonly positive for *Escherichia coli*, *Pseudomonas aeruginosa*, *Klebsiella pneumoniae*, *Staphylococcus aureus*, *Candida* spp., and *Aspergillus*.
Thymus	Record weight. See also below under "Lymph nodes."	Leukemic infiltrates.
Lungs	Submit one lobe for bacterial, fungal, and viral studies (p.103). Make touch preparation from cut sections and request Gram stain and Grocott's methenamine silver stain for demonstration of fungi and *Pneumocystis carinii* (p. 172). Perfuse one lung with formalin (p. 47).	Bacterial and fungal pneumonia; viral pneumonitis; hemorrhages and leukemic infiltrates. *Pneumocystis carinii* pneumonitis.
Gastrointestinal tract	Estimate volume of blood in lumen. If there are mucosal lesions, submit samples for histologic study.	Gastrointestinal hemorrhages; mucosal hemorrhagic necroses; leukemic infiltrates.
Liver and spleen	Record weight and size. Request Gomori's iron stain (p. 172).	Hepatosplenomegaly. Enlarged liver may be free of leukemic infiltrates.
Kidneys	Fix specimen in alcohol (p. 129) for preservation of urates.	Urate deposits.
Lymph nodes	Record average size. Fix specimens in B-5 fixative (p. 129). Make touch preparations. Request Giemsa or Wright stain (p. 172).	Leukemic lymphadenopathy; lymphadenitis.
Brain and spinal cord	For removal and specimen preparation, see pp. 65 and 67, respectively. Make touch preparations from meningeal lesions; request Gram and Grocott's methenamine silver stains for histologic sections (p. 172).	Meningeal leukemic infiltrates, particularly around brain stem; hydrocephalus; hemorrhages; meningitis* or meningoencephalitis.

Organs and Tissues	*Procedures*	*Possible or Expected Findings*
Middle and inner ears	For removal and specimen preparation, see p. 72.	Otitis media;* hemorrhages; leukemic infiltrates, particularly along eighth cranial nerve.
Eyes	For removal and specimen preparation, see p. 85. Include extrabulbar orbital tissue (p. 73).	Hemorrhages in conjunctiva and retina; leukemic infiltrate in uvea.
Lacrimal glands; parotid and other salivary glands	Remove for histologic study (p. 87). Parotid gland can be biopsied from scalp incision (p. 65). Submascillary gland can be removed with floor of mouth (p. 4).	Leukemic infiltrates (Mikulicz's syndrome).
Bone marrow	For preparation of sections and smears (imprints), see p. 96.	Leukemic infiltrates. Nonneoplastic proliferation of hematopoietic cells after bone marrow transplantation.
Joints	Remove synovial fluid for identification of crystals in secondary gout (p. 96). For removal, prosthetic repair, and specimen preparation of joints, see p. 96. If gout is suspected, fix tissue specimen in alcohol.	Leukemic infiltrates; gout.*
Other organs and tissues	Use Helly's (p. 131) or Bouin's (p. 129) fixative; request Wright stain (p. 173). For color preservation of chloroma, see p. 134.	Leukemic infiltrates, thromboses, infections, and hemorrhages may occur in all organs or tissues.

Leukemia, Eosinophilic ("Leukemia, all types or type unspecified.")

Leukemia, Mast Cell (See "Leukemia, all types or type unspecified" and "Mastocytosis, systemic.")

Leukodystrophy, All Types or Type Unspecified

NOTE: This term describes a group of diseases characterized by widespread and often symmetric bilateral demyelination or failure of myelin formation, or both, in the central nervous system. These conditions are thought to be caused by inborn errors of metabolism and enzymatic defects, which have been identified in at least two instances—namely, metachromatic leukoencephalopathy* and globoid cell leukodystrophy.* See also under "Degeneration, spongy, of white matter" and "Leukodystrophy, sudanophilic."

Leukodystrophy, Globoid Cell

Synonyms: Galactocerebroside lipidosis; Krabbe's disease.

Organs and Tissues	*Procedures*	*Possible or Expected Findings*
Cerebrospinal fluid	Submit sample for determination of protein concentration (p. 104).	Increased protein concentration.
Brain, spinal cord, and peripheral nerves	For removal and specimen preparation, see pp. 65, 67, and 79, respectively. Place samples of cerebral tissue into liquid nitrogen and submit for biochemical and histochemical studies. Submit tissue for electron microscopy (p. 132). Request Luxol fast blue stain for myelin (p. 172).	Areas of myelin loss in the central nervous system. Globoid cells containing cerebrosides in areas of demyelination. Segmental demyelination of peripheral nerves.

Leukodystrophy, Sudanophilic

Synonym: Pelizaeus-Merzbacher disease.

Organs and Tissues	*Procedures*	*Possible or Expected Findings*
Brain and spinal cord	For removal and specimen preparation, see pp. 65 and 66, respectively. Request Luxol fast blue stain for myelin (p. 172). Prepare frozen sections for Sudan stain (p. 173).	Demyelination in centrum ovale, cerebellum, and part of brain stem. Diffuse gliosis and perivascular sudanophilic lipid in white matter.

Leukoencephalopathy, Metachromatic

Synonyms: Sulfatide lipidosis; sulfatidosis.

Organs and Tissues	*Procedures*	*Possible or Expected Findings*
Cerebrospinal fluid	Submit sample for determination of protein concentration (p. 104).	Increased protein concentration.
Urine	Collect and stain sediment with toluidine blue (p. 173).	Material in sediment stains red with toluidine blue.
Other organs	Stain sections of liver, gallbladder, spleen, kidneys, lymph nodes, adrenal glands, and ovaries for metachromasia.	Metachromatic material.
Brain and spinal cord	For removal and specimen preparation, see pp. 65 and 67, respectively. Request Luxol fast blue and cresyl echt violet stain (p. 172).	Excessive loss of myelin with large amounts of metachromatic material (see above under "Urine") in white matter and also in some neurons.
Peripheral nerves	For sampling and specimen preparation, see p. 79.	Demyelination with metachromatic material (see above under "Urine").

Leukoencephalopathy, Progressive Multifocal

Possible Associated Conditions: AIDS* and other immunosuppressed states; carcinoma; malignant myeloproliferative or lymphoproliferative disorder; sarcoidosis;* tuberculosis.*

Organs and Tissues	*Procedures*	*Possible or Expected Findings*
Brain and spinal cord	For removal and specimen preparation, see pp. 65 and 67, respectively. Submit portion of fresh brain for viral culture. Fix remainder of brain and spinal cord in formalin and submit samples for histologic study. *In situ* hybridization for JC virus is available on paraffin-embedded tissue.	Small patches of demyelination with tendency to form confluent areas in the cerebral white matter. White matter necrosis may be present. Eosinophilic intranuclear inclusions occur in affected oligodendroglia cells. Subsequently, large, bizarre astrocytes develop. No inflammatory (lymphocyte) cell reaction is present.

Lightning (See "Injury, lightning.")

Lipoproteinemia (See "Hyperlipoproteinemia.")

Lipoproteinosis, Pulmonary Alveolar

Synonym: Idiopathic alveolar lipoproteinosis.

NOTE: The condition has been described in allografts *(1)*; in such cases, see also under "Transplantation, lung."

Organs and Tissues	*Procedures*	*Possible or Expected Findings*
External examination	Prepare chest roentgenogram.	"Butterfly" shadow on chest roentgenogram.
Lungs	Submit one lobe for bacterial, fungal, and viral cultures (p. 103). Prepare smears for identification of *Pneumocystis carinii*.	Superinfection with fungi (nocardiosis;* cryptococcosis*), viruses (cytomegalovirus infection*), or *Pneumocystis carinii.**
	Record weight of lungs; photograph. For perfusion fixation, see p. 47. Place some fresh tissue into Zenker's or Helly's fixative (p. 131).	Increased lung weights.
	Request PAS, toluidine blue, Gram, and Grocott's methenamine silver stains and fresh frozen sections for Sudan stain (p. 172).	Alveolar contents PAS-positive, meta chromatic, and positive for lipids. Microorganisms may be present.
	Prepare samples for electron microscopic study (p. 132). Snap-freeze tissue for histochemical study.	Osmiophilic densities; myelin figures.

Reference

1. Yousem AS. Alveolar lipoproteinosis in lung allograft recipients. Hum Pathol 1997;28:1383–1386.

Listeriosis

Synonyms: *Listeria monocytogenes* infection; listerosis.

NOTE: (1) Collect all tissues that appear to be infected. (2) Request aerobic bacterial cultures. Alert the laboratory that *Listeria* is suspected. (3) Request Gram stain (p. 172). (4) Usually, no special precautions are indicated. (5) Usually, serologic studies are not helpful. (6) This is not a reportable disease.

Possible Associated Conditions: Cirrhosis* of the liver; malignant neoplasms and other debilitating diseases, including human immunodeficiency virus infection *(1)*; previous steroid therapy.

Organs and Tissues	*Procedures*	*Possible or Expected Findings*
Placenta	Record weight and size; photograph. Prepare histologic sections.	Intervillous abscesses containing gram-positive, non-acid-fast bacilli.
External examination and skin	Record extent of skin lesions; prepare histologic sections of skin.	
Heart	If infective endocarditis is suspected, follow procedures described on p. 103.	Infective endocarditis* and, rarely, pericarditis *(2)*.
Lungs and trachea	Culture consolidated areas. Then, perfuse both lungs.	Tracheobronchitis and bronchopneumonia.
Liver and spleen	Record weights and submit samples for histologic study.	Hepatosplenomegaly; necrosis; granulomas; abscesses *(3)*. Bacteria are predominantly intracellular.
Intestine	Submit sample of meconium for culture.	Enterocolitis. *Listeria monocytogenes* can be cultured from meconium.
Lymph nodes	Prepare samples for histologic study.	Generalized lymphadenitis.
Other organs and tissues, including pharynx	Procedures depend on expected findings or grossly identified abnormalities as listed in right-hand column.	Disseminated abscesses and/or granulomas, particularly after transplacental infection; purulent conjunctivitis; uveitis; arthritis; osteomyelitis; peritonitis; cholecystitis.
Brain and spinal cord	For removal and specimen preparation, see pp. 65 and 67, respectively.	Meningitis;* brain abscess *(4)*; meningo encephalitis. The organism may appear coccoid in CSF.
Middle ears	Remove for histologic study (p. 72).	Otitis media.*

References

1. Marron A, Roson B, Mascaro J, Carratala J. Listeria monocytogenes empyema in an HIV infected patient. Thorax 1997;52:745–746.
2. Manso C, Rivas I, Peraire J, Vidal F, Richart C. Fatal Listeria meningitis, endocarditis and pericarditis in a patient with haemochromatosis. Scand J Inf Dis 1997;29:308–309.
3. Marino P, Maggioni M, Preatoni A, Cantoni A, Invernizzi F. Liver abscesses due to Listeria monocytogenes. Liver 1996;16:67–69.
4. Turner D, Fried M, Hoffman M, Paleacu D, Reider I, Yust I. Brainstem abscess and meningitis due to Listeria monocytogenes in an adult with juvenile chronic arthritis. Neurology 1995;45:1020–1021.

LSD (d-Lysergic Acid Diethylamide) (See "Abuse, hallucinogen(s).")

Lung, Farmer's (See "Pneumoconiosis.")

Lung, Honeycomb (See "Pneumonia, interstitial.")

Lupus Erythematosus, Systemic

Related Terms: Immune complex disease; immune connective tissue disease.

NOTE: The guide, *Pathology of Systemic Lupus Erythematosus, 1995* can be ordered from the American Registry of Pathology Sales Office, AFIP, Room 1077, Washington, DC 20306-6000.

Possible Associated Conditions: Rheumatoid arthritis;* Sjögren's syndrome.*

Organs and Tissues	*Procedures*	*Possible or Expected Findings*
External examination and skin; oral cavity		Malar, discoid, maculopapular, and other rashes; oral ulcers; alopecia.
	Prepare histologic sections of grossly abnormal and of unaffected skin.	Hyperkeratotic dermatitis with liquefaction necrosis. Vasculitis and panniculitis.
	Prepare histologic sections of subcutaneous nodules. If joints appear swollen, withdraw synovial fluid for cell count, and culture (p. 96).	Erosions and ulcers (including leg ulcers); ischemic changes of fingers. Rheumatoid granulomas (elbows, hands).
	Prepare skeletal roentgenograms.	Arthritis (see below under "Joints"); osteoporosis* and osteonecrosis* in steroid-treated patients.
Serosal cavities	Record volume of pericardial, pleural, or peritoneal exudates or effusions, and submit samples for culture (p. 102). Submit samples of serosal surfaces for histologic study.	Pleuritis; pericarditis;* ascites.
Blood	Submit sample for microbiologic and serologic study (p. 102).	Septicemia; circulating anticoagulant.
Heart	If infective endocarditis is suspected, remove vegetations for microbiologic study (p. 103).	Infective endocarditis.*
	Photograph valvular lesions and submit samples for histologic study. Include chordae tendineae, papillary muscles, and endocardium (where it borders on valves).	Libman-Sacks endocarditis (lupus endocarditis), with small vegetations on all valves and adjacent structures; myocarditis;* pericarditis.*
	For coronary arteriography, see p. 118. Submit samples of all coronary arteries for histologic study.	Coronary occlusion; coronary arteritis. Myocardial infarction. Cor pulmonale in cases with pulmonary hypertension *(1)*.
Lymph nodes	Submit axillary, tracheobronchial, and inguinal lymph nodes for histologic study.	Lymphadenitis.
Lungs	Submit one fresh lobe for microbiologic study (p. 103). Snap-freeze sample for possible special studies. Perfuse one lung with formalin (p. 47).	Interstitial pneumonitis and fibrosis; bronchopneumonia. Adult respiratory distress syndrome and pulmonary hemorrhages. Arterial and arteriolar thrombi and plexiform lesions *(1)*.
Gastrointestinal tract and mesentery	For mesenteric arteriography, see p. 55. Submit samples of all segments of gastrointestinal tract for histologic study. Dissect mesenteric vessels and submit sample, together with mesenteric lymph nodes, for histologic study.	Hemorrhagic necroses; ulcers; gastro intestinal vasculitis; mesenteric vasculitis.
Spleen, liver, and pancreas	Record weights; submit samples for histologic study.	Splenitis; nonspecific hepatic changes; rarely arteritis, infarctions, or nodular regenerative hyperplasia *(2)*. Chronic pancreatitis *(3)*.
Kidneys	Follow procedures described under "Glomerulonephritis."	Lupus glomerulonephritis. Kidney failure* is a common cause of death.
Neck organs	Submit thyroid, parathyroid, and submandibular glands and cervical lymph nodes for histologic study.	Manifestations of Sjögren's syndrome.*
Brain, spinal cord, and peripheral nerves	For removal and specimen preparation, see pp. 65, 67, and 79, respectively.	Subarachnoid hemorrhage; aseptic meningitis; perivascular necroses *(4)*; transverse myelitis; optic neuritis. Peripheral neuropathy.
Eyes and lacrimal glands	For removal and specimen preparation, see pp. 85 and 87, respectively.	Conjunctivitis; episcleritis; Retinal and choroidal hemorrhages. Dacryoadenitis in Sjögren's syndrome.*

Organs and Tissues	Procedures	Possible or Expected Findings
Blood vessels	For removal of femoral vessels, see p. 34. Submit samples of small blood vessels of extremities for histologic study.	Peripheral arteritis; arterial occlusions; thrombophlebitis.
Skeletal muscles	For sampling and specimen preparation, see p. 80. Refer to neurologic findings for proper sampling sites.	Myositis and vascultis *(5)*.
Joints	Remove affected diarthrodial joints, together with synovia, periarticular tissues, and tendon sheaths. For removal, prosthetic repair, and specimen preparation, see p. 96.	Arthritis, in decreasing order of frequency, in knees, small joints of hands, wrists, shoulders, ankles, elbows, and hips.
Bones and bone marrow	For removal, prosthetic repair, and specimen preparation, see p. 95.	Osteoporosis* and osteonecrosis.* (Ischemic necroses in hip joints *(6)*, femoral condyles, and small bones of hands.) These are complications of steroid therapy.
	Sample bone marrow for histologic study (p. 96).	Storage and hemophagocytic histiocytes *(7)*.

References

1. Yokoi T, Tomita Y, Fukaya M, Ichihara S, Kakudo K, Takahashi Y. Pulmonary hypertension associated with systemic lupus erythematosus: predominantly thrombotic arteriopathy accompanied by plexiform lesions. Arch Pathol Lab Med 1998;122:467–470.
2. Matsumoto T, Yoshimine T, Shimouchi K, Shiotu H, Kuwabara N, Fukuda V, Hoshi T. The liver in systemic lupus erythematosus: pathologic analysis of 52 cases and review of Japanese autopsy registry data. Hum Pathol 1992;23:1151–1158.
3. Borum M, Steinberg W, Steer M, Freedman S, White P. Chronic pancreatitis: a complication of systemic lupus erythematosus. Gastroenterology 1993;104:613–615.
4. Shintaku M, Matsumoto R. Disseminated perivenous necrotizing encephalomyelitis in systemic lupus erythematosus: report of an autopsy case. Acta Neuropathol 1998;95:313–317.
5. Lim KL, Lowe J, Powell RJ. Skeletal muscle lymphocytic vasculitis in systemic lupus erythematosus: relation to disease activity. Lupus 1995;4:148–151.
6. Aranow C, Zelicof S, Leslie D, Solomon S, Barland P, Norman A, Klein R, et al. Clinically occult avascular necrosis of the hip in systemic lupus erythematosus. J Rheumatol 1997;24:2318–2322.
7. Morales-Polanco M, Jimenez-Balderas FJ, Yanez P. Storage histiocytes and hemophagocytosis: a common finding in the bone marrow of patients with active systemic lupus erythematosus. Arch Med Res 1996;27:57–62.

Lye (See "Poisoning, lye.")

Lymphatics (See "Disease, lymphatic vascular.")

Lymphogranuloma Venereum

Synonym: Lymphogranuloma venereum *Chlamydia* infection.

NOTE: (1) Collect all tissues that appear to be infected. (2) Culture of tissues can be performed but requires special laboratory tests. Request consultation with a microbiology laboratory before a specimen is submitted. (3) Usually, special stains are not helpful. (4) Usually, no special precautions are indicated. (5) Serologic tests are available from the state health department laboratories (p. 135). (6) This is a **reportable** disease.

Organs and Tissues	Procedures	Possible or Expected Findings
External examination and skin	Record skin changes and prepare sections of affected skin. Record presence of perianal fistulas (see also below under "Pelvic organs and lymph nodes").	Elephantiasis of penis, scrotum, or vulva (in chronic cases); skin rash *(1)* and conjunctivitis (in acute cases); genital ulcers.
Blood	Submit serum for complement-fixation test.	
Pelvic organs and lymph nodes	If there are perirectal or lymphocutaneous fistulas, injection of dyes or contrast media (p. 138) may help for dissection.	Suppurative or fibrosing inguinal, iliac, or pelvic lymphadenitis, with or without sinus tracts. Rectal strictures and fistulas in chronic cases *(2)*.
	Prepare histologic sections of affected lymph nodes.	
Other organs	Procedures depend on expected findings or grossly identified abnormalities as listed in right-hand column.	Systemic involvement in the acute stage with pericarditis,* and arthritis,* and meningitis.*

References

1. Rosen T, Brown TJ. Cutaneous manifestations of sexually transmitted diseases. Med Clin North Am 1998;82:1081–1104.
2. Papagrigoriadis S, Rennie JA. Lymphogranuloma venereum as a cause of rectal strictures. Postgrad Med J 1998;74:168–169.

Lymphoma

Synonyms and Related Terms: AIDS-related lymphoma; adult T-cell leukemia/lymphoma; angioimmunoblastic lymphadenopathy; B-cell lymphoma; Burkitt's lymphoma; cutaneous T-cell lymphoma (includes mycosis fungoides and Sézary syndrome); Hodgkin's disease; non-Hodgkin's lymphoma (low grade, intermediate grade, high grade, all with multiple subtypes too numerous to list, which vary in natural history); natural killer cell neoplasms; post-transplant lymphoproliferative disorders (PTLD); T-cell lymphoma.

NOTE: At the time of autopsy, most lymphomas have been properly classified and often treated. In these cases, the goal of the autopsy is to document the extent of the disease and the presence of complications. If the lymphoma had not been classified or if the features might have changed from the time of the last work-up, material should be snap-frozen and studied in more detail. If the patient was treated by bone marrow transplantation,* see also under that heading.

The address of the appropriate registry is Hematologic and Lymphatic Pathology, Armed Forces Institute of Pathology (p. 148).

For current terminologies of Hodgkin's disease and non-Hodgkin lymphomas as well as for staging criteria, appropriate hematologic textbooks should be consulted.

Possible Associated Conditions: Acquired immunodeficiency diseases (e.g., after organ transplantation; human immunodeficiency virus-1 infection); autoimmune disease (e.g., celiac sprue,* rheumatoid arthritis,* systemic lupus erythematosus,* or Sjögren's syndrome*); chemotherapy with or without radiation treatment; Epstein-Barr virus infection; human T-cell leukemia virus infection; inherited diseases with immunodeficiency (e.g., Klinefelter syndrome;* common variable immunodeficiency disease, Wiskott-Aldrich syndrome); radiation.

Organs and Tissues	*Procedures*	*Possible or Expected Findings*
External examination, skin, and oral cavity	Record distribution of hair; record facial features and character and extent of skin lesions and of pigmentations. Record appearance of oral and nasal mucosa. Prepare histologic sections of skin.	Alopecia; disfigurement of face in Burkitt's lymphoma. Exophthalmos and salivary gland enlargement (Mikulicz's syndrome). Lymphomatous infiltrates of skin with or without ulcerations; herpes zoster;* jaundice.
	Prepare skeletal and chest roentgenograms.	Lymphomatous bone changes—for instance, skull defects in Burkitt's lymphoma. Calcifying lymphomatous tumors. Pulmonary infiltrates.
Blood and fascia lata	Submit sample of blood for bacterial, fungal, and viral cultures (p. 102).	Septicemia. Blood most commonly positive for *Escherichia coli*, *Pseudomonas aeruginosa*, *Klebsiella pneumoniae*, *Staphyloccus aureus*, *Candida* spp., and *Aspergillus*.
	If chromosomal abnormalities are suspected, submit sample of blood or fascia lata for chromosome analysis (pp. 108 and 109).	Chromosomal abnormalities.
	Collect serum for study of antibodies and of immunoglobulins.	Antibodies against reovirus type 3 or Epstein-Barr virus in Burkitt's lymphoma. Dysgammaglobulinemia.
Thymus	Record weight and submit samples for histologic study. See also below under "Lymph nodes."	Lymphomatous infiltrates.
Lungs	Submit one lobe for bacterial, fungal, and viral cultures (p. 103). Prepare smears of cut surface and request Grocott's methenamine silver stain for demonstration of fungi and *Pneumocystis carinii* (p. 172).	Bacterial, fungal, and viral pneumonia. *Pneumocystis carinii* infection.*
	Perfuse one lung with formalin (p. 47).	Lymphomatous infiltrates.
Lymph nodes	Record average size. Fix specimens in B5 (p. 129) fixative or Zenker's or Helly's solution (p. 131). Make touch preparations and request Giemsa or Wright stain. Snap-freeze lymphomatous tissue if immunophenotype studies are intended or for identification of surface markers for B- and T-lymphocytes and other lymphoreticular cells.	Lymphoma. Lymph nodes often unaffected in Burkitt's lymphoma.
Liver and spleen	Record size and weight. Submit samples for histologic study.	Spleen often unaffected in Burkitt's lymphoma; hepatosplenomegaly in most lymphomas.

Organs and Tissues	*Procedures*	*Possible or Expected Findings*
Other organs	Submit samples of all grossly abnormal tissues for histologic study. If systemic infection is suspected, collect appropriate specimens for microbiologic study.	All organs and tissues can be involved by lymphoma and by complicating infections. Retroperitoneal lymphoma with renal and ovarian involvement is common in Burkitt's lymphoma. Complications of radiation or cytostatic therapy also may be present.
Cerebrospinal fluid	Refrigerate sample for possible microbiologic study (p. 104), depending on cerebral changes. Prepare smear of sediment.	Lymphoma cells.
Brain and spinal cord	For removal and specimen preparation, see pp. 65 and 67, respectively. Make touch preparations of meningeal lesions. Request Giemsa, Gram, and Grocott's methenamine silver stains (p. 172).	Meningeal lymphomatous infiltrates. Hydrocephalus.* Meningitis* or meningoencephalitis.
Eyes and lacrimal glands	For removal and specimen preparation, see pp. 85 and 87, respectively. Include lacrimal glands and orbital soft tissue.	Burkitt's lymphoma may involve orbitae. Lacrimal lymphoma is found in Mikulicz's syndrome.
Middle and inner ears	For removal and specimen preparation, see p. 72.	
Salivary glands (parotid, submandibular)	Submit samples for histologic study. Parotid gland can be biopsied from scalp incision (p. 65). Submascillary gland can be removed with floor of mouth (p. 4).	Lymphomatous infiltrates in Burkitt's lymphoma and in Mikulicz's syndrome.
Thyroid gland		Often involved in Burkitt's lymphoma.
Bones and bone marrow	For sampling and specimen preparation of bones, see p. 95. For preparation of sections and smears of bone marrow, see p. 96.	Lymphomatous infiltrates. Involvement of maxilla and mandible in Burkitt's lymphoma.

M

Macroglobulinemia, Waldenström's

Synonyms and Related Terms: Dysproteinemia; monoclonal gammopathy; paraproteinemia; plasma cell dyscrasia.*

Organs and Tissues	*Procedures*	*Possible or Expected Findings*
External examination and oral cavity	Record extent of skin and oral mucosal lesions. Prepare histologic sections of affected tissues.	Vascular purpura. Gangrene after cold exposure.
Blood	Submit samples for microbiologic study and for protein electrophoresis (p. 102).	Increased IgM concentration. No evidence of hypercalcemia.
Lymph nodes	Record appearance and average size of lymph nodes. Snap-freeze tissue for immunophenotype study. Make touch preparations and request Wright stain (p. 173). Tissue for paraffin sections should be fixed in B-5 fixative (p. 129).	Lymphadenopathy. Follicular hyperplasia with proliferation of lymphocytes and plasma cells that exhibit IgM immunofluorescence.
Liver and spleen	Record size and weight; sample for histologic study.	Hepatosplenomegaly. Proliferation of lymphocytes and plasma cells that exhibit IgM immunofluorescence.
Other organs and tissues	Record size and weight of all parenchymatous organs. For further procedures, see above under "Lymph nodes." Request PAS and amyloid stains (p. 172; see also under "Amyloidosis"). Submit samples of all grossly abnormal tissues for histologic study.	Infiltrates of lymphocytes and plasma cells. Evidence of recurrent infections is common. Clinically, plasma hyperviscosity is a common complication. If features of other plasma cell disorders (amyloidosis,* heavy chain disease,* multiple myeloma*) are found, see under those headings.
Brain, spinal cord, and peripheral nerves	For removal and specimen preparation, see pp. 65, 67, and 79, respectively.	Cerebral hemorrhages. Peripheral neuropathy.*
Eyes	For removal and specimen preparation, see p. 85.	Retinal hemorrhages and exudates. Cyst of pars plana.
Skeletal muscles	For sampling and specimen preparation, see p. 80.	Myopathy.*
Bone marrow	For preparation of sections and smears, see p. 96.	Proliferation of lymphocytes and plasma cells with clasmacytosis, eosinophilia, and mast cell proliferation. No osteolytic lesions as in multiple myeloma.*

Malakoplakia

NOTE: Malakoplakia is a chronic inflammatory lesion with foamy macrophages, intracellular bacteria, and laminated, calcium-containg inclusions (Michaelis-Gutmann bodies). The lesions are found most commonly in the urinary bladder and other parts of the urinary tract, but may also occur at many other sites, including skin *(1)* and upper respiratory tract *(2)*.

From: *Handbook of Autopsy Practice,* 3rd Ed. Edited by: J. Ludwig © Humana Press Inc., Totowa, NJ

Organs and Tissues	*Procedures*	*Possible or Expected Findings*
Urinary tract, colon, or other tissues	Photograph gross lesions; record size and location. Submit samples for histologic and electron microscopic study (p. 132). Request PAS and von Kossa stains (p. 173).	Grayish nodular lesions with or without ulceration. Microscopic Michaelis-Gutmann bodies. Adenocarcinoma of the colon may be associated with malakoplakia *(3)*.

References

1. Barnard M, Chalvardjian A. Cutaneous malakoplakia in a patient with acquired immunodeficiency syndrome (AIDS). Am J Dermatol 1998;20:185–188.
2. Salins PC, Trivedi P. Extensive malakoplakia of the nasopharynx: management of a rare disease. J Oral Maxillofac Surg 1998;56:483–487.
3. Bates AW, Dev S, Baithun SI. Malakoplakia and colorectal adenocarcinoma. Postgrad Med J 1997;73:171–173.

Malaria

Synonyms and Related Terms: *Plasmodium falciparum* infection; *Plasmodium malariae* infection; *Plasmodium ovale* infection; *Plasmodium vivax* infection; malignant pernicious malaria; blackwater fever.

NOTE: (1) Collect all tissues that appear to be infected. (2) Usually, cultures are not indicated. (3) Request Giemsa or Wright stain (p. 172). Tissue blocks should be rinsed of blood and be as thin as possible before fixation in refrigerated buffered and neutral 10% formalin solution (p. 130). This is to avoid precipitation of formalin pigment that may be confused with malaria pigment. The formalin solution should be used in a ratio of 100 parts formalin to one part tissue and should be agitated every few hours. If one is dealing with tissues that contain formalin pigment, this pigment may be removed with a bleaching solution (p. 174). (4) Usually, no special precautions are indicated. (5) Serologic studies may be helpful and are available from the Centers for Disease Control and Prevention, Atlanta, GA (p. 135). (6) This is a **reportable** disease.

Organs and Tissues	*Procedures*	*Possible or Expected Findings*
Blood	Prepare "thick" and "thin" films.	Parasites; malaria pigment in erythrocytes.
Spleen	Record size and weight. Photograph cut section. For preparation of samples for histologic study, see above under "Note."	Splenomegaly with brown to gray discoloration because of malaria pigment; diffuse cellular hyperplasia and congestion; black opaque globules in histiocytes and in erythrocytes; parasitized red cells in sinusoids.
Liver	Record size and weight. Photograph cut section. For preparation of samples for histologic study, see above under "Note."	Hepatomegaly with congestion and centrilobular necrosis; malaria pigment in histiocytes; parasitized red cells in sinusoids.
Kidneys	For preparation of samples for histologic study, see above under "Note."	Ischemic cortex; congested medullary vessels; hemoglobin casts.
Other organs	Histologic sampling will depend on gross findings and clinical diagnosis of associated conditions. If placenta is present, prepare sections and smears. See also above under "Note."	Manifestations of disseminated intravascular coagulation;* parasitized red cells in any organ. Placenta may appear black; parasitized maternal cells; fetal cells rarely infected.
Brain and spinal cord	For removal and specimen preparation, see pp. 65 and 67, respectively.	Edema; "ring" hemorrhages; focal necrosis (acute cerebral malaria). Parasitized red cells in small vessels; reactive gliosis and malarial granulomas ("Dürck's" glial nodules).
Bone marrow	For preparation of sections and smears, see p. 96.	Erythroid and myeloid hyperplasia; parasitized red cells.

Malformation(s), Aortic Arch System (See "Artery, patent ductal," "Coarctation, aortic," and "Hypoplasia, tubular, of aortic arch.")

Malformation, Arnold-Chiari

Synonyms: Arnold-Chiari malformation, type I, adult form; Arnold-Chiari malformation, type II, infantile form; Arnold-Chiari malformation, type III (see below under "Note").

NOTE: In type I, relative frequent craniocervical bony malformations (platybasia,* basilar impression,* suboccipital dysplasia, Klippel-Feil syndrome*). For type II cases, see below. In type III, occipitocervical bony defect with cerebellar herniation into the encephalocele.

Possible Associated Conditions: Syringomyelia* (in 50% of type I cases); myelomeningocele, hydrocephalus,* and often craniolacunia in type II cases.

Organs and Tissues	Procedures	Possible or Expected Findings
External examination	Prepare roentgenograms of skull and cervix.	For bony malformations, see above under "Note."
Brain and spinal cord; base of skull and cervical spine	For removal and specimen preparation of brain, see p. 65. For removal of spinal cord, use combined approach (p. 71). If possible, prepare photographs to show bony malformations.	Downward displacement of cerebellar tonsils and vermis through foramen magnum; elongation and caudal displacement of brain stem (medulla and 4th ventricle). Herniated cerebellar tissue shows neuronal loss and gliosis. Beak-like deformity of quadrigeminal plate; upwards direction of the upper 4 to 6 cervical spinal roots. Aqueduct abnormalities may be present. Hydrocephalus* may occur in all forms of the disease.

Malformation, Arteriovenous, Cerebral or Spinal (or Both)

Synonyms and Related Terms: Arteriovenous aneurysm; arteriovenous anomaly; Foix-Alajouanine syndrome; hemangioma of brain or spinal cord; vascular malformation of brain or spinal cord.

NOTE: A group of abnormal vessels is fed by one or more arteries without intermediate capillary channels and emptying directly into one or more large veins; this anomaly is associated with compressive atrophy of intervening and adjacent nervous tissue or with evidence of recent or old hemorrhage, or with both. In the Foix-Alajouanine syndrome, enlarged, tortuous subarachnoid veins cover the cord, especially posteriorly, and are associated with patchy necrosis of the spinal cord tissue and small blood vessels with thickened collagenous walls, not clearly distinguishable as arteries or veins.

Organs and Tissues	Procedures	Possible or Expected Findings
Brain and spinal cord	For cerebral arteriography, see p. 80. For removal and specimen preparation, see pp. 65 and 67, respectively.	For expected findings, see above under "Note."
Spine and spinal canal		Vertebral hemangioma. Calcification of spinal canal.

Malformation(s), Biliary System (See "Atresia, biliary," "Cyst(s), choledochal," "Disease, Caroli's," "Disease, fibropolycystic, of the liver and biliary tract," and "Fibrosis, congenital hepatic.")

Malformation(s), Congenital, Cardiac and Vascular

NOTE: See under specific name of malformation.

Malformation(s), Coronary Artery (See "Anomaly, coronary artery.")

Malformation(s), Coronary Sinus

NOTE: See also "Defect, atrial septal, coronary sinus type."

Possible Associated Conditions: *Unroofed* coronary sinus with atrial septal defect* at site normally occupied by coronary sinus and with left superior vena cava terminating in the left atrium. *Absent* coronary sinus associated with asplenia syndrome or right isomerism.

Malformation, Ebstein's

Synonym: Ebstein's anomaly of tricuspid valve.

NOTE: The basic anomaly is a downward placement of functional tricuspid annulus, with adherent septal and posterior leaflets, and with redundant deformed anterior leaflet. Sudden death may occur in this condition. It may become symptomatic at any age and is often associated with cardiomegaly due to marked right atrial and right ventricular dilatation.

Possible Associated Conditions: Congenitally corrected transposition of the great arteries; interatrial communication; pulmonary atresia;* tricuspid insufficiency;* Wolff-Parkinson-White ventricular preexcitation syndrome.*

Malformation(s), Pulmonary Artery

Related Terms: Absence of one pulmonary artery; aortic origin of one pulmonary artery; connection of pulmonary artery with left atrium; ductal origin of one or both pulmonary arteries; idiopathic dilatation of pulmonary trunk; discrete pulmonary artery stenosis; supravalvular pulmonary stenosis.*

Possible Associated Conditions: Post-rubella syndrome; pulmonary atresia with a ventricular septal defect;* tetralogy of Fallot;* supravalvular aortic stenosis;* Williams-Beuren syndrome.

Malformation(s), Thoracic Vein

Related Terms: Atresia of common pulmonary vein; azygos continuation of inferior vena cava; connection of a vena cava or hepatic vein with left atrium; continuity of inferior vena cava with left atrium; levoatriocardinal vein; partial anomalous pulmonary venous connection; persistent left superior vena cava; polysplenia syndrome;* pulmonary arteriovenous fistula; stenosis of common pulmonary vein (triatrial heart); scimitar syndrome; stenosis of individual pulmonary vein; total anomalous pulmonary venous connection.

NOTE: Type of venous malformation usually must be determined before separartion of thoracoabdominal viscera, particularly the course and connections of the inferior vena cava, hepatic veins, and azygos and hemiazygos veins. En masse removal of organs is recommended (p. 3). Venography may be helpful.

Possible Associated Conditions: With anomalies of the pulmonary veins: asplenia syndrome (right isomerism), anomalous connections to the systemic veins, common atrium; complete atrioventricular septal defect;* polysplenia syndrome;* Scimitar syndrome. With connection of the inferior vena cava with the vena azygos: anomalous pulmonary venous return and polysplenia syndrome* (left isomerism). With intrapulmonary arteriovenous fistula: Osler-Weber-Rendu disease* or previous Glenn cavopulmonary venous anastomosis (p. 41). With levoatriocardinal vein between left atrium or left pulmonary vein and left innominate vein; stenotic oval foramen, or mitral or aortic stenosis* or atresia* or both. With persistent left superior vena cava: isolated or with various malformations of the heart and great vessels.

Malnutrition

Synonyms and Related Terms: Hypoproteinemic malnutrition (kwashiorkor); marasmus; protein-energy malnutrition; starvation.*

Possible Associated Conditions: Anemia, iron deficiency, and vitamin deficiencies are common complications of malnutrition. Gastrointestinal, infectious, renal, and other diseases, including malignancies of all types, are found in many cases and represent the likely causes of the malnutrition.

Organs and Tissues	*Procedures*	*Possible or Expected Findings*
External examination and skin	Record body weight and length (for body mass index, see p. 567). Photograph and record extent of skin lesions; prepare histologic sections of skin.	Weight loss (may be compensated by edema and ascites). Generalized pitting edema; pigmented, pellagra-type skin lesions, particularly of extremities and face; brittle hair. Atrophy of epidermis with hyperkeratosis and parakeratosis.
Vitreous	Submit sample for sodium, potassium, chloride, and urea nitrogen determination (p. 85).	Dehydration* and other electrolyte disorders.*
Abdomen	Record volume and character of fluid.	Ascites.
Liver	Record weight; request frozen sections for Sudan stain (p. 173).	Fatty changes, predominantly periportal.
Intestinal tract	Prepare for study under dissecting microscope (p. 54). Submit samples for histologic study.	Mucosal atrophy.
Other organs	Procedures depend on expected findings or grossly identified abnormalities as listed in right-hand column and above under "Note."	Atrophy, particularly of pancreas and endocrine glands. For possible underlying conditions, see also above under "Note."

Marasmus (See "Malnutrition" and "Starvation.")

Marihuana (See "Abuse, marihuana.")

Mast Cells (See "Mastocytosis, systemic.")

Mastocytosis, Systemic

Synonyms and Related Terms: Disease, mast cell; mastocytic leukemia; urticaria pigmentosa of childhood.

Possible Associated Conditions: Myelodysplastic or myeloproliferative disorders.

Organs and Tissues	*Procedures*	*Possible or Expected Findings*
External examination and skin	Record extent and character of skin lesions; photograph skin lesions. Fix skin specimens in formalin or alcohol (p. 129) and request Giemsa or toluidine blue stains for mast cells (p. 172). Prepare skeletal roentgenograms.	Macules with telangiectasias, papules, and nodules. Cachexia. Accumulation of mast cells in dermis. Multiple lytic bone lesions or new bone formation.

Organs and Tissues	*Procedures*	*Possible or Expected Findings*
Abdominal cavity		Ascites.
Gastrointestinal tract	Submit samples from all segments for histologic study.	Peptic ulcer* with perforation; gastroenteritis. See also under "Syndrome, malabsorption."
Liver, spleen, and lymph nodes	Record sizes and weights of liver and spleen and average size of lymph nodes. Submit tissue samples for histologic study (see above under "External examination and skin").	Hepatosplenomegaly; hepatic fibrosis; lymphadenopathy; mast cell infiltrates. Manifestations of portal hypertension.*
Other organs	If infection is suspected, submit appropriate material for microbiologic study. For staining of histologic sections, see above under "External examination and skin."	Hemorrhages and infections may complicate mast cell disease. Mast cell infiltrates may be leukemic (see "Leukemia, all types or type unspecified").
Bone and bone marrow	For removal, prosthetic repair, and specimen preparation of bone, see p. 95. Consult roentgenograms. For preparation of sections and smears of bone marrow, see p. 96.	Mast cell infiltrates with osteolysis and new bone formation. Eosinophils, lymphocytes, plasma cells and fibroblasts may be prominent. Osteomalacia* in patients with malabsorption syndrome.*

Measles

Synonyms: Morbilli; rubeola (the term rubeola is also used by some for "rubella").

NOTE: Various types of debilitating conditions may be complicated by measles—for instance, leukemia,* other neoplastic diseases and tuberculosis.*

(1) Collect all tissues that appear to be infected. (2) Request viral and aerobic bacterial cultures. (3) Request Gram stain (p. 172). Electron microscopy may demonstrate the virus (p. 132). (4) Special **precautions** are indicated (p. 146). (5) Serologic studies may be helpful. (6) This is a **reportable** disease.

Possible Associated Diseases: Adenovirus, parainfluenza virus, and other viral infections *(1)*.

Organs and Tissues	*Procedures*	*Possible or Expected Findings*
External examination and skin	If skin or oral lesions can be identified, submit samples for histologic study.	Maculopapular rash, Koplik spots; congestion; edema; perivascular lymphocytic infiltrates; thrombosis; red cell extravasation; multinucleated giant cells.
Thymus	Record weight; submit sample for histologic study.	Hyperplasia (see below under "Intestinal tract").
Urine	Submit sample for virologic culture.	
Heart		Myocarditis* (very rare).
Lungs	Perfuse one lung with formalin (p. 47). Submit areas of consolidation for bacterial and viral cultures (p. 103). Obtain areas of infected tissue for electron microscopy and place in suitable fixative (p. 132).	Bacterial pneumonia *(1) (Pneumococcus, Streptococcus pyogenes, Staphylococcus aureus, Hemophilus influenzae);* giant cells lining alveoli. Interstitial pneumonia* or giant cell pneumonia *(2)* and inclusion bodies in children with leukemia.*
Intestinal tract	Prepare histologic sections of Peyer's patches and appendix.	Lymphoid hyperplasia with Warthin-Finkeldey giant cells.
Kidneys, ureters, urinary bladder	Submit samples for histologic study.	Mononuclear cells with cytoplasmic and inclusions; giant cells.
Neck organs	Remove together with palatine tonsils and pharyngeal lymphatic tissue (p. 4). Prepare sections of lymphatic tissue and and larynx.	See above under "Intestinal tract."
Other organs and tissues		Thrombocytopenic hemorrhages at various sites.
Brain and spinal cord	For removal and specimen preparation, see pp. 65 and 67, respectively.	Subacute sclerosing panencephalitis with inclusion bodies.

Organs and Tissues	Procedures	Possible or Expected Findings
Middle ears	For removal and specimen preparation, see p. 72.	Otitis media;* mastoiditis.
Eyes	For removal and specimen preparation, see p. 85.	Optic neuritis; viral retinitis *(3)*; keratoconjunctivitis.

References

1. Quiambao BP, Gatchalian SR, Halonen P, Lucero M, Sombrero L, Paladin FJ, et al. Coinfection is common in measles associated pneumonia. Ped Inf Dis J 1998;17:89–93.
2. Rahman SM, Eto H, Morshed AS, Itakura H. Giant cell pneumonia: light microscopy, immunohistochemical, and ultrastructural study of an autopsy case. Ultrastr Pathol 1996;20:585–591.
3. Park DW, Boldt HC, Massicotte SJ, Akang EE, Roos KL, Bodnar A, et al. Subacute sclerosing panencephalitis manifesting as viral retinitis: clinical and histopathologic findings. Am J Ophthalmol 1997;123: 533–542.

Measles, German (See "Rubella.")

Mediastinitis, Chronic

Synonyms and Related Terms: Fibrosing mediastinitis; granulomatous mediastinitis; idiopathic sclerosing mediastinitis.

Possible Associated Conditions: Histoplasmosis* and other chronic fungal infections; immune connective tissue diseases such as rheumatoid arthritis* *(1)*; malignancies *(1)*; sarcoidosis;* silicosis;* tuberculosis* *(1)*.

NOTE: In rare instances, fibrosing mediastinitis appears to be associated with other chronic fibrosing conditions such as retroperitoneal fibrosis,* Riedel's thyroiditis (Riedel's struma), or sclerosing cholangitis.*

Organs and Tissues	Procedures	Possible or Expected Findings
Chest cavity and mediastinum	Dissect superior vena cava system, aorta, and trachea, either *in situ* or after en bloc removal of mediastinal organs. Horizontal slices may be informative.	Superior vena cava obstruction.
	Prepare histologic sections from sclerosing process around great vessels, right atrium, trachea, and pericardium and from mediastinal lymph nodes. Submit tissue sample for fungal culture, and request Grocott's methenamine silver stain (p. 172).	See above under "Possible Associated Conditions."
Other organs and tissues		See above under "Possible Associated Conditions."

Reference

1. Mole TM, Glover J, Sheppard MN. Sclerosing mediastinitis: a report of 18 cases. Thorax 1995;50:280–283.

Megacolon, Congenital

Synonyms: Hirschsprung's disease; idiopathic megacolon; megacolon.

Possible Associated Conditions: Atrial septal defect;* Down's syndrome;* meconium ileus;* megalobladder; megaloureter; ventricular septal defect.*

Organs and Tissues	Procedures	Possible or Expected Findings
External examination	Record weight, length, and abdominal circumference of body.	Manifestations of malnutrition;* abdominal distention; growth retardation.
Intestinal tract	Photograph *in situ*. Remove colon with rectum and anus; photograph colon before and after opening.	Necrotizing enterocolitis* and perforation of the colon or appendix (in neonates and infants). Narrow segment in distal colon.
	Submit samples for histologic study from all portions of intestinal tract, particularly from several portions of narrowed segment. Cut sections on edge, and prepare frozen sections *(2)*. For paraffin sections, request van Gieson's stain (p. 172).	Aganglionosis of narrow distal segment; intestinal neuronal dysplasia *(1)*.

References

1. Puri P, Wester T. Intestinal neuronal dysplasia. Sem Ped Surg 1998;7:181–186.
2. Kobayashi H, O'Brian DS, Hirakawa H, Wang Y, Puri P. A rapid technique of acetylcholinesterase staining. Arch Pathol Lab Med 1994;118:1127–1129.

Melioidosis

Synonyms and Related Terms: Glanders; *Pseudomonas mallei* infection; *Pseudomonas pseudomallei* infection.

NOTE: (1) Collect all tissues that appear to be infected. (2) Request aerobic bacterial cultures. (3) Request Gram stain (p. 172). Polyclonal antibodies can be used for the diagnosis. Formalin-fixed, paraffin embedded autopsy tissues can be stained with a modified immunoperoxidase technique *(1)*. (4) Usually, no special precautions are indicated. (5) Serologic studies are available through state and local health departments (p. 135). (6) This is not a reportable disease.

Organs and Tissues	*Procedures*	*Possible or Expected Findings*
Blood	Submit sample for aerobic bacterial culture (p. 102).	Septicemia.
Lungs	Submit consolidated areas for microbiologic study (p. 103). Perfuse at least one lung with formalin (p. 47).	Pneumonia, sometimes with cavitation and calcification, resembling tuberculosis.
Other organs	Procedures depend on expected findings or grossly identified abnormalities as listed in right-hand column.	Abscesses may occur in skin, lymph nodes, liver, lungs, heart, spleen, kidneys, and bones.

Reference

1. Wong KT, Vadivelu J, Puthucheary SD, Tan KL. An immunohistochemical method for the diagnosis of melioidosis. Pathology 1996;28:188–191.

Meningitis

Related Terms: Meningoencephalitis; meningoencephalomyelitis.

NOTE: If the infectious agent is known, follow procedures described under the name of the corresponding infectious disease. Meningitis may complicate many noninfectious diseases, such as carcinoma, lymphoproliferative or myeloproliferative disorders, sarcoidosis,* and other conditions, particularly if they require treatment with immunosuppressive agents.

Organs and Tissues	*Procedures*	*Possible or Expected Findings*
External examination	Prepare chest roentgenogram.	Pulmonary infiltrates—for example, in fungal pneumonia or tuberculosis.*
Cerebrospinal fluid	Submit sample for microbiologic study, cell count, and chemical analysis (p. 104).	
Brain and spinal cord	Submit samples for viral, fungal, and bacterial cultures (p. 102). For removal and specimen preparation, see pp. 65 and 67, respectively. Record distribution of exudate; photograph, and make smears, touch preparations, and sections. Request Gram, acid fast (see "Tuberculosis"), and Grocott's methenamine silver stains (p. 172). Make India ink preparations.	Bacterial (including tuberculous), fungal, and viral meningitis. Aseptic nonsuppurative inflammatory conditions. Uncal and cerebellar herniation; subdural effusion.
Blood	Submit sample for microbiologic study (p. 102).	Septicemia.
Other organs	Search for possible sites of primary infection. Procedures depend on expected findings or grossly identified abnormalities as listed in right-hand column.	Infective endocarditis,* with or without congenital heart disease; pulmonary infection (origin of infection in tuberculous meningitis in infancy); pulmonary fungal infection, with or without bronchiectasis and cavitation; purulent arthritis. Manifestations of disseminated intravascular coagulation.* Adrenal hemorrhages.

Meningocele

Related Terms: Complete rachischisis; meningomyelocele; spina bifida aperta; spina bifida occulta.

Possible Associated Conditions: Arnold-Chiari malformation;* diastematomyelia; diplomyelia; hydrocephalus;* hydromyelia; syringomyelia;* tethered cord.

Organs and Tissues	*Procedures*	*Possible or Expected Findings*
External examination	Record location and extent of skin changes or skin defects on back. Prepare skeletal roentgenograms. If meningitis is suspected, submit sample of cerebrospinal fluid for culture (p. 104).	Atrophic skin over meningocele, lacking rete pegs and skin appendages; skin defect in complete rachischisis. Bony defects of spine.
Brain and spinal cord	For removal and specimen preparation, see pp. 66 and 70, respectively.	In meningocele and spina bifida occulta, arachnoid and dura herniate through the vertebral defect. Spinal cord and roots are generally not involved. Lumbosacral mass in meningomyelocele, with a highly vascular mass (area medullovasculosa) in spina bifida aperta. Neural defects in complete rachischisis.
Other organs		Pyelonephritis;* enlarged urinary bladder ("neurogenic bladder").

Meningococcemia (See "Disease, meningococcal.")

Meningoencephalitis (See "Encephalitis, all types or type unspecified" and "Meningitis.")

Mercury (See "Poisoning, mercury.")

Metaplasia, Agnogenic Myeloid, With Myelofibrosis

Synonym: Idiopathic myelofibrosis.

Organs and Tissues	*Procedures*	*Possible or Expected Findings*
External examination	Prepare skeletal roentgenograms.	Osteosclerosis of vertebrae, ribs, clavicles, pelvic bones, scapulae, skull, and metaphyseal ends of femur and humerus.
Bones and bone marrow	For removal, prosthetic repair, and specimen preparation of bone, see p. 95. For preparation of sections and smears of bone marrow, see p. 96. See above (under "External examination) for selection of bones.	Osteomyelofibrosis or osteoreticulosis; rarely, panhyperplasia of bone marrow; increase of megakaryocytes.
	Request Giemsa, Masson's trichrome, and reticulum stains for bone marrow sections (p. 172). See also under "Leukemia."	Changes associated with chronic granulocytic leukemia* or with polycythemia vera* may imitate idiopathic myelofibrosis.
Other organs	Record weights of liver and spleen.	Widespread extramedullary hematopoiesis *(1)* with splenomegaly.
	Other procedures depend on expected findings or grossly identified abnormalities as listed in right-hand column.	Infectious diseases, including tuberculosis;* gouty arthritis; ascites and other manifestations of portal hypertension;* or hepatic vein thrombosis (Budd-Chiari syndrome*). Cardiac tamponade *(1)*.

Reference

1. Imam TH, Doll DC. Acute cardiac tamponade associated with pericardial extramedullary hematopoiesis in agnogenic myeloid metaplasia. Acta Haematol 1997;98:42–43.

Methanol (Methyl Alcohol) (See "Poisoning, methanol (methyl alcohol).")

Microangiopathy, Thrombotic Thrombocytopenic (See "Purpura, thrombotic thrombocytopenic.")

Microlithiasis, Pulmonary Alveolar

Organs and Tissues	*Procedures*	*Possible or Expected Findings*
External examination	Prepare chest roentgenogram.	Miliary mottling in lower lung fields.
Heart	Procedures depend on expected findings or grossly identified abnormalities as listed in right-hand column.	Mitral stenosis* may be a cause of microlithiasis (mostly intra-alveolar ossification).* Cor pulmonale and heart failure *(1)* may complicate chronic microlithiasis.
Lungs	Record weights. Prepare photographs and roentgenograms of fresh and fixed lung specimens. Specimens may have to be sawed (p. 95). Perfuse one lung with formalin (p. 47). For preparation of paper-mounted sections, see p. 49.	Increased weights and hardness. Miliary mottling, mainly in lower lobes.
	Submit one lobe for microbiologic and chemical study. Decalcify tissue for histologic study (p. 97). For preparation of undecalcified sections, see p. 97.	Calcospherites containing calcium, phosphate, iron, and magnesium. Reactive pulmonary fibrosis.
	Request van Gieson's, Hale's colloidal iron, PAS, and Sudan stains (pp. 172 and 173).	Center of calcospherites strongly positive with PAS and colloidal iron stains. Sudanophilic and doubly refractile fatty material in calcospherites.

Reference

1. Mariotta S, Guidi L, Mattia P, Torrelli L, Pallone G, Pedicelli G, Bisetti A. Pulmonary microlithiasis. Report of two cases. Respiration 1997;64: 165–169.

Mongolism (See "Syndrome, Down's.")

Mononucleosis, Infectious

Related Terms: *Cytomegalovirus* infection; *Epstein-Barr virus* (EBV) infection.

NOTE: If the EBV infection occurred after organ transplantation *(1)*, see also under that heading.

(1) Collect all tissues that appear to be infected. (2) Viral isolation, especially with EBV, is not diagnostically useful, due to long incubation periods. (3) No special precautions are indicated. (4) Serologic studies are the method of choice and are available from local or state health department laboratories (p. 135). (6) This is not a reportable disease.

Organs and Tissues	*Procedures*	*Possible or Expected Findings*
External examination		Jaundice; petechial rash.
Blood	Submit samples for bacterial and viral cultures and for serologic study (p. 102).	Septicemia. High Epstein-Barr virus antibody and heterophil titers.
	Prepare Giemsa-stained smear.	Atypical lymphocytes.
Heart	Record weight and submit samples for histologic study (p. 30).	Myocarditis.*
Lungs	Submit consolidated areas for bacterial culture (p. 103).	Edema and bacterial pneumonia.
Gastrointestinal tract		Hemorrhage.*
Spleen	Record size and weight. Submit sample for histologic study and make touch preparations. Request Giemsa stain (p. 172).	Splenomegaly; hematomas and rupture. Extensive hyperplasia of red pulp. See below, under "Lymph Nodes."
Liver	Record size and weight. Submit sample for histologic study.	Massive EBV necrosis *(2)*; granulomatous hepatitis; cytomegalovirus inclusions within hepatocytes and endothelial cells.

Organs and Tissues	Procedures	Possible or Expected Findings
Lymph nodes	Submit samples for histologic study and make touch preparations. Request azure-eosin stain (p. 172).	Generalized lymphadenopathy; abundant immunoblasts resembling Reed-Sternberg cells.
Neck organs	Make touch preparations and request sections of lingual, palatine, and pharyngeal lymphoid tissue (p. 4). Request azure-eosin stain (p. 172).	Nasopharyngeal hemorrhage. Glottis edema. Lymphoid hyperplasia (see also above under "Spleen" and "Lymph nodes").
Other organs	Procedures depend on grossly identified abnormalities as listed in right-hand column.	Manifestations of bleeding due to thrombocytopenia; lymphoid infiltrates in any organ.
Brain, spinal cord, and spinal ganglia	For removal and specimen preparation, see pp. 65, 67, and 69, respectively.	Meningoencephalitis; lymphocytic or serous meningitis;* polyradiculitis (clinically, Guillain-Barré syndrome*).
Peripheral nerves	For sampling and specimen preparation, see p. 79.	Peripheral neuritis.
Bone marrow	For preparation of sections and smears, see p. 96.	Agranulocytosis.

References

1. Hubscher SG, Williams A, Davison SM, Young LS, Niedobitek G. Epstein-Barr virus in inflammatory diseases of the liver and liver allografts: an in situ hybridization study. Hepatology 1994;20:899–907.
2. Papatheodoridis GV, Delladetsima JK, Kavallierou L, Kapranos N, Tassopoulos NC. Fulminant hepatitis due to Epstein-Barr virus infection. J Hepatol 1995;23:348–350.

Morphine (See "Dependence, drug(s), all types or type unspecified.")

Mucopolysaccharidosis

Synonyms and Related Terms: Mucopolysaccharidosis I H (gargoylism, Hurler's disease or syndrome, α-L-iduronidase deficiency, MPS I H); mucopolysaccharidosis I S (Scheie's syndrome α-L-iduronidase deficiency, MPS I S, MP V); mucopolysaccharidosis II (Hunter's disease or syndrome, MPS II); mucopolysaccharidosis III (heparitinuria, MPS III, polydystrophic oligophrenia, Sanfilippo's syndrome); mucopolysaccharidosis IV (Morquio's syndrome, keratosulfaturia, MPS IV); mucopolysaccharidosis VI (Maroteaux-Lamy syndrome, MPS VI, polydystrophic dwarfism); mucopolysaccharidosis VII (β-glucuronidase deficiency, MPS VII).

NOTE: These diseases are characterized by a deficiency of a variety of hydrolases, resulting in accumulation of glycosaminoglycans (mucopolysaccharides) and glycolipids within lysosomes of fibroblasts, macrophages, white cells, and parenchymal cells of many organs *(1,2)*. Mucopolysaccharides are also excreted in the urine. The general approach is similar in all types. Formalin may dissolve all of the stored material and leave empty vacuoles in the involved cells. Therefore, frozen sections should be utilized or tissues should be fixed in absolute alcohol (p. 129). The accumulated material will show intense metachromasia if stained with toluidine blue. It will also stain with PAS, alcian blue, and colloidal iron. Oil red O will also stain the material from frozen sections (p. 172). For specimen preparation for electron microscopy, see p. 132.

Characteristic external features include dwarfism; thickened long bones; coarse facial features; coarse hair; macrocephaly; prognathism; hypertelorism; malformed teeth, and scaphocephalic skull with hyperostosis of sagittal suture; short neck; chest deformity; umbilical and inguinal hernias; lower thoracic and lumbar gibbus; genu valgum and coxa valga; pes planus and other joint deformities; wide hands (clawhands) and feet. Coarse thickened skin, covered with lanugo-like hair. Hyperlordosis; ovoid deformities of vertebrae; odontoid hypoplasia; large, shoe-shaped sella turcica; kyphosis; hypoplasia of femoral heads; osteoporosis.*

If patient underwent bone marrow transplantation *(3)*, see also under that heading.

Organs and Tissues	Procedures	Possible or Expected Findings
External examination and extent and skin	Record body weight and length and type of deformities. Photograph head and deformities. Prepare sections of skin. Prepare skeletal roentgenograms.	Characteristic external features and possible roentgenographic features are listed above under "Note."
Placenta	Submit sections for histologic study.	Storage of material in Hofbauer cells and stromal cells.
Fascia lata	Submit sample for fibroblast tissue culture for enzyme assay (p. 109).	Increased intracellular mucopolysaccharides. Cultures are well-suited for special studies.
Blood	Prepare smears (see below under "Bone marrow"). Submit sample for microbiologic study (p. 102).	

Organs and Tissues	Procedures	Possible or Expected Findings
Urine	Submit sample for biochemical study.	Increased mucopolysaccharides.
Heart	Record weight. Prepare coronary arteriogram (p. 118).	Diffuse coronary narrowing because of the presence of intimal gargoyle cells (smooth muscle cells), elastic fiber proliferation, and other deformities. (Heart disease is a frequent cause of death.)
	Test competence of valves (p. 29).	Nodular thickening of mitral *(4)*, aortic *(4)*, tricuspid, and pulmonary valves (in this order of involvement).
	Prepare histologic sections of all valves and chordae tendineae.	Gargoyle cells in valves and chordae tendineae.
	Record thickness of ventricles and extent of myocardial necroses or scarring.	Hypertrophy of the heart. Myocardial infarction.
	Photograph valves and myocardium.	Endocardial fibroelastosis.
	Submit samples of epicardium, myocardium, coronary arteries, and conduction system for histologic study (p. 26).	Mucopolysaccharide deposits in epicardium and endocardium.
Aorta, pulmonary arteries, other great vessels, and peripheral muscular arteries	Request Verhoeff–van Gieson stain (p. 173).	Extensive intimal deposits, as in coronary arteries.
Tracheobronchial tree and lungs	For pulmonary arteriography, see p. 50.	Pulmonary vascular changes (see above).
	Submit consolidated areas for microbiologic study (p. 103).	Purulent bronchitis and bronchopneumonia. (Respiratory infection is a frequent cause of death).
	Perfuse one lung with formalin (p. 47). Submit samples of tracheal and bronchial cartilage for histologic study.	Gargoyle cells in cartilage.
Spleen	Record weight. Submit specimen for tissue culture (p. 108). Submit sample for histologic study.	Splenomegaly; gargoyle cells.
Liver	Record weight and submit samples for histologic study.	Hepatomegaly;* enlarged vacuolated hepatocytes with mucopolysaccharides; fibrosis.
Kidneys	Record weight and submit samples for histologic study.	Vacuolated cells in Bowman's capsule.
Endocrine organs	Record weight of all endocrine organs and submit samples for histologic study.	Gargoyle cells.
Brain, spinal cord, and peripheral ganglia	For removal and specimen preparation, see pp. 65, 67, and 69, respectively. Mucopolysaccharides may stain well with PAS reagent.	Hydrocephalus; cerebral cortical atrophy; storage of mucopolysaccharides in ganglion cells.
Eyes	For removal and specimen preparation, see p. 85.	Corneal clouding and retinal degeneration associated with storage of mucopolysaccharides in nuclear layer of retina.
Middle and inner ears	For removal and specimen preparation, see p. 72. (Study particularly indicated if patient was deaf.)	Chronic infections.
Sinuses and nasal cavities	Expose from base of skull, and submit samples of mucosa for histologic study (p. 71).	Chronic upper respiratory infections.
Bone marrow	For preparation of sections and smears, see p. 96. Prepare air-dried smears (without formalin fixation) for demonstration of metachromatic granules.	Large cytoplasmic granules in neutrophils.
Bones and joints, periosteum, tendons, and fasciae	For removal, prosthetic repair, and specimen preparation, see p. 95.	Storage of mucopolysaccharides in osteocytes, chondrocytes, and fibroblasts of periosteum, tendons, fasciae, and other connective tissues; dysostosis multiplex.

Organs and Tissues	Procedures	Possible or Expected Findings
Other tissues	Histologic sampling cannot be excessive.	Storage of mucopolysaccharides may occur anywhere.

References

1. Wraith JE. The mucopolysaccharidoses: a clinical review and guide to management. Arch Dis Child 1995;72(3):263–267.
2. Di Natale P, Annella T, Daniele A, De Luca T, Morabito E, Pallini R, et al. Biochemical diagnosis of mucopolysaccharidoses: experience of 297 diagnoses in a 15-year period (1997-1991). J Inher Metabolic Dis 1993;16(2):473–483.
3. Gatzoulis MA, Vellodi A, Redington AN. Cardiac involvement in mucopolysaccharidosis: effects of allogeneic bone marrow transplantation. Arch Dis Childhood 1995;73:259–260.
4. Wippermann CF, Beck M, Schranz D, Huth R, Michel-Behnke I, Jungst BK. Mitral and aortic regurgitation in 84 patients with mucopolysaccharidosis. Eur J Pediatr 1995;154:98–101.

Mucormycosis

Synonym: Phycomycosis; zygomycosis.

NOTE: Diseases that may be complicated by mucormycosis include burns,* diabetes mellitus,* leukemia,* lymphoma,* and tuberculosis.*

(1) Collect all tissues that appear to be infected. (2) Request fungal culture. (3) Request Grocott's methenamine silver stain (p. 172). (4) No special precautions are indicated. (5) Serologic studies are not available. (6) This is not a reportable disease.

Organs and Tissues	Procedures	Possible or Expected Findings
External examination and skin	Photograph all lesions attributable to this infection.	Skin ulcerations.
Lungs	Submit consolidated areas for fungal and bacterial culture (p. 103); make touch preparation of fresh lung. Perfuse both lungs with formalin (p. 47).	Necrotizing bronchopneumonia.
Gastrointestinal tract		Mucosal ulcers.
Other organs	Culture all tissues with gross evidence of thrombosis or infarction. Other procedures depend on expected findings or grossly identified abnormalities as listed in right-hand column.	Disseminated fungal arteritis with secondary thromboses and infarctions in heart, kidneys, and many other organs.
Skull with brain	For removal of brain and exposure of orbitae and paranasal sinuses, see pp. 65, 73, and 71, respectively. Prepare sections of abnormal tissues.	Primary infection in sinuses or orbitae; orbital cellulitis; fungal arteritis with cerebral infection; thrombosis of cavernous sinus and internal carotid artery.

Mucoviscidosis (See "Fibrosis, cystic.")

Mumps

NOTE: (1) Collect all tissues that appear to be infected. (2) Request viral cultures. (3) Usually, special stains are not helpful. (4) Special **precautions** are indicated (p. 146). (5) Serologic studies are available from state health department laboratories (p. 135). (6) This is not a reportable disease.

Organs and Tissues	Procedures	Possible or Expected Findings
External examination and skin	Prepare sections of skin.	Thrombocytopenic purpura.
Breasts	Submit tissue sample for histologic study.	Mastitis.
Blood	Submit samples for biochemical (serum amylase) and serologic study.	Complement-fixing antibodies.
Urine	Submit sample for viral cultures (p. 102).	
Heart	Submit samples for histologic study (p. 30).	Myocarditis* may be cause of death. Pericarditis* and endocardial fibroelastosis.*
Liver and pancreas	Record weights and submit samples for histologic study.	Hepatitis* and pancreatitis.*
Spleen	Record weight and size.	Splenomegaly.

Organs and Tissues	*Procedures*	*Possible or Expected Findings*
Kidneys	Record weights and submit samples for histologic study.	Nephritis.*
Male sex organs	Record weights of testes and epididymides; prepare histologic sections of testes, epididymides, seminal vesicles, and prostate, especially in postpubertal males.	Orchitis; epididymitis; seminal vesiculitis; prostatitis.
Female sex organs	Submit samples of ovaries and Bartholin's glands for histologic study.	Ovaritis (oophoritis); bartholinitis.
Neck organs	Prepare histologic sections of pharynx, submaxillary and sublingual glands (p. 4), and thyroid.	Sialadenitis; thyroiditis.
Brain, spinal cord, and spinal roots	For removal and specimen preparation, see pp. 65 and 67, respectively. Prepare sections of cranial nerves and spinal nerve roots (p. 69).	Meningitis or postinfectious encephalitis;* perivenous demyelination and mononuclear inflammation; neuritis of cranial nerves II, III, VI, VII, and VIII. Polyneuritis; meningoradiculitis. Myelitis.
Eyes and lacrimal glands	For removal and specimen preparation, see pp. 85 and 87, respectively.	Conjunctivitis; keratitis; uveitis; retinitis; dacryoadenitis.
Middle and inner ears	For removal and specimen preparation, see p. 72.	Labyrinthitis.
Parotid glands	Remove tissue from scalp incision (p. 65) with biopsy needle.	Parotitis.
Joints	For removal, prosthetic repair, and specimen preparation, see p. 96.	Arthritis.*

Murder (See "Homicide.")

Mushroom (See "Poisoning, mushroom.")

Myasthenia Gravis

Synonyms and Related Term: Acquired autoimmune myasthenic (due to anti-acetylcholine receptor antibodies, anti-AchR); myasthenic syndromes, aquired (Eaton-Lambert syndrome) or congenital.

NOTE: The acquired myasthenic syndrome is associated in 40–50% of cases with bronchogenic carcinoma.

Organs and Tissues	*Procedures*	*Possible or Expected Findings*
Thymus	Record size and weight. Submit sample for histologic studies. If a thymoma is present, prepare sections of tumor and of uninvolved thymus.	In early onset myasthenia (55% of cases), thymus shows hyperplasia with lymphoid follicles with germinal centers. In late onset myasthenia, thymus is atrophic. 10% of cases are associated with thymoma.
Blood	Submit sample for serologic study.	Serum concentrations of Anti Ach R (anti-acetylcholine receptor) autoantibodies are high in myasthenia. 85% of patients with myasthenia and thymoma have high anti-striated muscle autoantibodies.
Other organs	Search for tumors of any site (primarily lung small cell carcinoma) in acquired myasthenia syndrome (Eaton-Lambert); search for manifestations of "autoimmune" systemic diseases.	Manifestations of diabetes mellitus,* hyperthyroidism,* and rheumatoid arthritis* or other immune connective tissue diseases in myasthenia gravis. Thyroid abnormalities other than hyperplasia in myasthenia gravis. Tumors of lungs (small cell carcinoma), breast, and other sites in myasthenia syndrome (Eaton-Lambert).
Skeletal muscles	For sampling and specimen preparation, see p. 80. Respiratory musculature should always be included. Submit tissue samples for electron microscopic study (p. 132).	Abnormalities of postsynaptic membrane in myasthenia gravis.

Reference

1. Engel AG. Myasthenic syndromes. In: Myology, 2nd ed., vol. 2. Engel AG, Franzini-Armstrong C, eds. MacGraw-Hill, New York, 1994, pp. 1798–1835.

Mycosis (See under specific disease designation, such as "Candidiasis.")

Mycosis Fungoides

Related Terms: Lymphoma;* Sézary syndrome.

NOTE: If mycosis fungoides was the cause of death, the patient probably was in the tumor stage of the disease with lymph node and general organ involvement. Follow procedures described under "Lymphoma." Viscera most commonly involved in late mycosis fungoides are, in order of frequency, lungs, spleen, liver, kidneys, thyroid gland, pancreas, bone marrow, and heart. Almost all organs and tissues of the body may be involved.

Myelinosis, Central Pontine

Organs and Tissues	*Procedures*	*Possible or Expected Findings*
External examination		Malnutrition* or severe burns* may be causes of central pontine myelinosis.
Cerebrospinal fluid	Submit sample for microbiologic study (p. 104).	Sample should be sterile.
Brain and spinal cord	For removal and specimen preparation, see pp. 65 and 67, respectively. Request Luxol fast blue/PAS and Bielschowsky stains (p. 172).	Demyelination involving paramedian portion of the base of the pons, from just below the midbrain through the upper two-thirds of the pons. Myelin is lost and some axons may be fragmented while neurons in the nuclei pontis are preserved (unlike in centrale pontine infarct). Histiocytes may abound.
Other organs	Procedures depend on expected findings or grossly identified abnormalities as listed in right-hand column.	Manifestations of alcoholism;* electrolyte disorders* (including too rapid correction of hyponatremia); severe infections; liver disease (especially after liver transplantation*); neoplastic conditions; renal diseases.

Myelofibrosis with Myeloid Metaplasia (See "Metaplasia, agnogenic myeloid, with myelofibrosis.")

Myeloma, Multiple

Synonyms: Myeloma; osteosclerotic myeloma *(1)* (POEMS syndrome); plasma cell myeloma.

Possible Associated Condition: Acute myeloblastic or monocytic leukemia;* amyloidosis;* chronic myelogenous leukemia *(2)*; hyperviscosity syndrome.

Organs and Tissues	*Procedures*	*Possible or Expected Findings*
External examination, skin, and tongue	Record extent of skin lesions and size of tongue (may be accessible only after removal of neck organs). Take sections of skin lesions and tongue. Request amyloid stains (see "Amyloidosis").	Vascular purpura. Skin tumors. Macroglossia secondary to amyloid deposition.
	Prepare skeletal roentgenograms.	Osteolytic skeletal tumors. Calvarium may be involved. Tumors are rarely osteoblastic (osteosclerotic *[1]*). Generally, no lymphadenopathy.
Vitreous	Submit sample for sodium, potassium, chloride, urea nitrogen, and calcium determination (p. 85).	Evidence of electrolyte and other disorders (see under "Blood").*
Blood	Submit samples for bacterial and fungal cultures (p. 102) for serum electrophoresis, and for determination of calcium (post-mortem values not reliable) uric acid concentrations (p. 113).	Septicemia. Anemia (may be megaloblastic*). Hyperglobulinemia with hypogammaglobulinemia Hypercalcemia; hyperuricemia. Hyperviscosity of serum.

Organs and Tissues	Procedures	Possible or Expected Findings
Urine	Submit sample for determination of Bence Jones protein.	Bence Jones protein. Light-chain proteinuria.
Heart	Record weight. Request amyloid stains (see "Amyloidosis").	Cardiac amyloidosis.
Lungs	Submit one lobe for bacterial and fungal cultures (p. 103).	Various types of pneumonia.
	Make touch preparations of cut surface and request Grocott's methenamine silver stain (p. 172). Perfuse one lung with formalin (p. 47).	*Pneumocystis carinii* pneumonia.
	Histologic sections may need decalcification (p. 97).	Metastatic calcification.
Spleen and gastrointestinal tract	Request amyloid stains (see "Amyloidosis").	Amyloidosis.* Metastatic calcification in stomach. Tumor infiltrates generally are inconspicuous.
Kidneys	Submit sample for histologic study. Fix at least one specimen in alcohol (p. 129). Decalcify (p. 97).	Pyelonephritis.* Metastatic calcification; calcium and urate casts.
	Request amyloid stains (see "Amyloidosis").	Amyloidosis.*
Other organs	Submit samples of liver, pancreas, adrenal glands, thyroid, lymph nodes, and all grossly involved tissues for histologic study.	Amyloidosis;* myeloma infiltrates; evidence of infection. Lymph nodes are rarely involved.
Brain, spinal cord, and peripheral nerves	For removal and specimen preparation, see pp. 65, 67, and 79, respectively.	Cord compression after vertebral collapse.
	Request amyloid stains of peripheral nerves (see "Amyloidosis").	Amyloidosis of peripheral nerves. Demyelinating polyneuropathy in osteo sclerotic myeloma *(1)*.
Bones and bone marrow	For removal, prosthetic repair, and specimen preparation of bone, see p. 95. For decalcification, see p. 97; for maceration of bone, see p. 97. Also consult roentgenograms.	Osteolytic tumors (Chapter 8, Fig. 8-2, p. 98).
	For preparation of sections and smears of bone marrow, see p. 96. Snap-freeze bone marrow if immuno-phenotype study of immunoglobulin-producing cells is intended.	Plasmacellular bone marrow.

References

1. Lacy MQ, Gertz MA, Hanson CA, Inwards DJ, Kyle RA. Multiple myeloma associated with diffuse osteosclerotic bone lesions: a clinical entity distinct from osteosclerotic myeloma (POEMS syndrome). Am J Hematol 1997;56:288–293.
2. Tanaka M, Kimura R, Matsutani A, Zaitsu K, Oka Y, Oizumi K. Coexistence of chronic myelogenous leukemia and multiple myeloma. Case report and review of the literature. Acta Haematol 1998;99:221–223.

Myelomeningocele (See "Meningocele.")

Myelopathy/Myelitis

Synonyms and Related Terms: Acute transverse myelitis; acute or subacute necrotizing myelopathy; angiodysgenetic necrotizing myelopathy; compression myelopathy; encephalomyelitis;* infectious myelitis; ischemic myelopathy; traumatic myelopathy; postvaccinal/postinfectious myelitis.

Possible Associated or Underlying Conditions: Angiodysgenetic (subacute) necrotizing myelopathy results from arteriovenous malformations* (Foix-Alajouanine syndrome); compression myelopathy may complicate degenerative vertebral disease, rheumatoid arthritis* or ankylosing spondylitis,* bony abnormalities at the foramen magnum (basilar impression,* platybasia*), or infections (spinal epidural, tuberculous osteomyelitis), or neoplastic processes involving the vertebrae and meninges; subacute necrotizing myelopathy may be a manifestation of multiple sclerosis* or it may be a paraneoplastic condition, primarily associated with small cell carcinoma; traumatic myelopathy occurs with or without penetrating injury. Myelitis due to intramedullary infections may include bacterial or mycobacterial abscess, fungal or parasitic infections and viral infections, in particular, cytomegalovirus infection,* Herpes zoster,* poliomyelitis,* and human immunodeficiency virus (HIV) infection (acquired immunodeficiency syndrome*).

Organs and Tissues	Procedures	Possible or Expected Findings
Cerebrospinal fluid	Submit sample for microbiologic study (p. 104).	Bacterial, fungal, or viral infection.
Chest and abdominal organs; blood; spine	If the myelitis is thought to be infectious, submit samples of blood and appropriate tissues for microbiologic study. Procedures depend on expected findings and grossly identified abnormalities as listed in right-hand column.	Tuberculous osteomyelitis.* Cervical spondylitis in acute transverse myelitis. Rarely, parasitic disease. Neoplasm. Manifestations of nutritional deficiencies or vascular disease.
Brain, spinal cord, spinal roots, and sensory ganglia	For removal and specimen preparation, see pp. 65, 67, and 69, respectively.	
	If there are abscesses or other acute infectious lesions, submit material for culture, prepare smears, and request Gram and Grocott's methenamine silver stains (p. 172). Request Luxol fast blue stain for myelin and Bielschowsky's stain for axons (p. 172).	Bacterial or fungal epidural or subdural empyema or granuloma.

Myocardiopathy (See "Cardiomyopathy,...")

Myocarditis

Synonyms and Related Terms: Bacterial myocarditis; drug-induced myocarditis; fungal myocarditis; giant cell myocarditis; human immunodeficiency virus myocarditis; infectious myocarditis; interstitial myocarditis; Lyme carditis; protozoal myocarditis; rheumatic myocarditis; viral myocarditis.

Possible Associated Conditions: Bacterial, fungal, protozoal (toxoplasmosis) or viral infections (particularly coxsackievirus B); human immunodeficiency virus infection; hypersensitivity states (e.g., acute rheumatic fever); idiosyncratic or toxic reaction to drugs; irradiation; Lyme disease.

Organs and Tissues	Procedures	Possible or Expected Findings
Blood	Submit sample for microbiologic (p. 102) and, if, indicated, toxicologic and biochemical study (p. 16).	Septicemia; viremia; toxemia.
Pericardial sac	Submit sample of pericardial exudate for microbiologic study (p. 102). Record volume of exudate; centrifuge; prepare smear of pellet. Request Gram and Grocott's methenamine silver stains (p. 172).	Pericarditis.*
Heart	Record heart weight.	
	Excise apical portion of myocardium and submit for microbiologic study (p. 102).	Infectious myocarditis (for possible infectious agents, see above under "Possible Associated Conditions).
	If infective endocarditis is suspected, follow procedures described on p. 103. For histologic sampling, see p. 30.	Infective endocarditis.*
Other organs, tissues, and body fluids	Depending on clinical findings, submit samples of cerebrospinal fluid (p. 104), serosal exudates or transudates, intestinal contents, pulmonary tissue, liver, spleen, kidneys, and cerebral tissue for bacterial, fungal, and viral cultures.	Bacterial, mycotic, protozoal, or viral diseases. Postinfectious states. Manifestations of drug toxicity or hypersensitivity; Pheochromocytoma. Burns.* Manifestations of congestive heart failure.*

Myonecrosis, Clostridial (See "Gangrene, gas.")

Myopathy

Synonyms and Related Terms: Congenital myopathy (central core disease, centronuclear myopathy, mitochondrial myopathy (see also "Epilepsy, myoclonus"); myotubular myopathy, nemaline or rod myopathy); familial myoglobinuria; familial periodic paralysis; myositis ossificans; myotonia congenita (Thomsen's disease).

NOTE: Muscular dystrophy and motor neuron disease are listed separately.

Organs and Tissues	Procedures	Possible or Expected Findings
External examination		Kyphoscoliosis, pigeon breast, and pes cavus in congenital myopathy.
	Prepare soft tissue roentgenograms.	Myositis ossificans.
Heart	Submit samples for light microscopic (p. 30) and electron microscopic (p. 132) study. For study of the conduction system, see p. 26.	Cardiomyopathy;* conduction system abnormalities.
Skeletal muscles	For sampling and specimen preparation, see p. 80. Refer also to clinical findings. Prepare specimens for electron microscopic study (p. 132).	Variable changes, depending on disease entities.
Brain, spinal cord, and spinal ganglia	For removal and specimen preparation, see pp. 65, 67, and 69, respectively.	Should be normal in primary myopathies (important for differentiation from Werdnig-Hoffmann and other primarily (central) neurological disorders).
Eyes and gonads	If diagnosis is uncertain, prepare sections of eyes (p. 85) and gonads.	No cataracts and no gonadal atrophy (important for differentiation from muscular dystrophy).

Myotonia Congenita (Thomsen's Disease) (See "Myopathy.")

Myxedema (See "Hypothyroidism.")

Myxoma, Heart (See "Tumor of the heart.")

N

Narcotic(s) (See "Dependence, drug(s), all types or type unspecified.")

Necrolysis, Toxic Epidermal

Synonyms: Lyell's disease; scalded skin syndrome.

NOTE: Toxic epidermal necrolysis usually represent an adverse reaction to drugs or, rarely, other chemicals. If it appears linked to hyperacute graft-versus-host disease after allogeneic bone marrow transplantation *(1)*, see also under that heading.

Organs and Tissues	*Procedures*	*Possible or Expected Findings*
External examination and skin	Record extent of skin lesions and prepare photographs; prepare sections of affected and unaffected skin. Request Gram stain of sections and smears (p. 172).	Extensive epidermal necrosis. Shedding of granular and horny layers of epidermis.
Blood; other organs and tissues	Submit samples of blood (p. 102) and grossly affected organs or tissues for microbiologic study. Other procedures depend on expected findings or grossly identified abnormalities as listed in right-hand column.	Septicemia; staphylococcal infection of nose, throat, ears, eyes, heart valves, urogenital tract, and other sites. Bronchial epithelial detachment and bacterial pneumonia *(2)*.

References

1. Takeda H, Mitsuhashi Y, Kondo S, Kato Y, Tajima K. Toxic epidermal necrolysis possibly linked to hyperacute graft-versus-host disease after allogeneic bone marrow transplantation. J Dermatol 1997; 24:635–641.
2. Lebargy F, Wokenstein P, Gisselbrecht M, Lange F, Fleury-Feith J, Delclaux C, et al. Pulmonary complications in toxic epidermal necrolysis: a prospective clinical study. Intensive Care Med 1997;23:1237–1244.

Necrosis, Aseptic, of Bone (See "Osteonecrosis.")

Necrosis, Bilateral Renal Cortical (See "Coagulation, disseminated intravascular.")

Necrosis, Renal Tubular

Synonyms and Related Terms: Acute kidney failure;* acute tubular necrosis; lower nephron nephrosis.

NOTE: The morphologic diagnosis of this condition may be difficult. The autopsy should be performed as soon as possible after death (see p. 5). Needle specimens of the kidneys obtained in the immediate postmortem period may yield acceptable material. If nephrotoxic drugs or chemicals are thought to be responsible for tubular necrosis, submit samples for toxicologic study (p. 16; see also under "Poisoning,..." and under name of suspected drug or poison). If tubular necrosis occurred after transfusion of incompatible blood, see under "Reaction to transfusion." Autopsy procedures depend on suspected underlying condition, such as trauma or infection.

Neoplasia, Multiple Endocrine

Synonyms and Related Terms: Multiple endocrine neoplasia (MEN), **type 1** (parathyroid hyperplasia or adenoma; pancreatic islet cell hyperplasia, adenoma, or carcinoma; pituitary hyperplasia or adenoma); or **type 2A** (medullary thyroid carcinoma, parathyroid hyperplasia or adenoma; and pheochromocytoma); or **type 2B** (medullary thyroid carcinoma, pheochromocytoma, mucosal and gastrointestinal neuromas, and marfanoid features).

NOTE: In MEN, type 1, foregut carcinoids and subcutaneous and visceral lipomas also may be found. In type 2A, cutaneous lichen amyloidosis may be observed. Mixed syndromes include (1) familial pheochromocytoma and islet cell tumor, (2) von Hippel-Lindau syndrome, pheochromocytoma and islet cell tumor, (3) neurofibromatosis* with features of MEN1 or 2, and myxomas, spotty skin pigmentation, and generalized endocrine overactivity (Carney complex).

In all instances, the autopsy should be done as soon as possible after death so that tissues for biochemical study can be frozen without delay.

From: *Handbook of Autopsy Practice,* 3rd Ed. Edited by: J. Ludwig © Humana Press Inc., Totowa, NJ

Organs and Tissues	*Procedures*	*Possible or Expected Findings*
External examination	Record height, weight, habitus, and abnormal external features.	Marfanoid habitus; cushingoid features, features of acromegaly.*
	Record appearance of skin and oral cavity.	Spotty skin pigmentation. Thickened lips; nodules in anterior third of tongue. Cleft palate.
	Prepare skeletal roentgenograms. Studies should include long bones of extremities, bones of hands, feet, skull with calvarium, base of skull, and jaws.	Osteoporosis with osteoclastic cysts. Acromegalic features.
Blood	Snap-freeze specimen for hormone assay. Submit sample for determination of calcium concentration.	Hypercalcemia.
	If chromosome studies are intended, see p. 102.	Normal karyotype.
Urine	Snap-freeze specimen for hormone assays.	
	If pheochromocytoma is suspected, request catecholamine determination.	Increased catecholamine concentrations associated with pheochromocytoma.
Mediastinum	If a tumor is present, photograph *in situ* and after removal. See also under "Neck organs."	Thymoma and other mediastinal tumors or cysts. Cardiac myxoma.
Neck organs	Dissect, photograph, and weigh thyroid and all parathyroid glands. Snap-freeze tumor tissue for histochemical and biochemical study. Prepare tumor tissue samples for electron microscopy (p. 132). Submit samples of normal and abnormal endocrine tissue and cervical lymph nodes for histologic study.	Nodular (toxic) goiter; lymphocytic thyroiditis; multifocal hyperplasia of C cells of thyroid gland. Medullary carcinoma of thyroid with amyloid stroma. Chief cell hyperplasia of parathyroids. Parathyroid adenomas.
	Also submit samples of cervical sympathetic chain and vagus nerves.	Ganglioneuromatosis.
Small and large bowel	If tumors are present, prepare tissue for biochemical, histochemical, electron microscopic, and routine light microscopic study. See also above under "Neck organs."	Carcinoid tumors in small bowel. Diffuse ganglioneuromatosis of small and large bowel. Megacolon. Diffuse diverticulosis.
Stomach and duodenum	See above under "Small and large bowel."	Carcinoid tumors. Ganglioneuromatosis. Diffuse gastric polyposis. Peptic ulcer of stomach or duodenum.*
Pancreas	Prepare 2-mm sagittal slices throughout entire pancreas. If tumor is present, follow procedures suggested above under "Neck organs." Submit samples of parapancreatic lymph nodes for histologic study.	Islet cell adenomas or carcinomas, usually of non-beta cell type.
Adrenal glands	Record weights and photograph. If tumors are present, follow procedures described under "Tumor, of the adrenal glands" and above under "Neck organs."	Nodular hyperplasia of adrenal medulla; pheochromocytoms, frequently bilateral; primary pigmented nodular adrenal disease.
Ovaries	Submit samples for histologic study. Record size and contents of cysts.	Ovarian cysts.
Testes	Record number and size of tumors. Submit samples for histologic study.	Large-cell calcifying Sertoli cell tumor.
Other organs and tissues	Procedures depend on expected findings or grossly identified abnormalities.	See under "Synonyms and Related Terms" and under "Note."
Brain, spinal cord, and pituitary gland	For removal and specimen preparation, see pp. 65, 67, and 71, respectively.	Pinealoma.
	If tumor tissue is present, follow procedures suggested above under "Neck organs."	Pituitary hyperplasia or adenoma, usually chromophobe type.
Bones	For removal, prosthetic repair, and specimen preparation, see p. 95.	Osteoclastic osteoporosis secondary to hyperparathyroidism.* Benign cysts.

Nephritis

NOTE: See under specific designation, such as "Glomerulonephritis" and "Pyelonephritis," or under name of suspected underlying condition, such as "Gout" or "Lupus erythematosus, systemic."

Nephroblastoma (See "Tumor of the kidney(s).")

Nephrolithiasis

Synonyms and Related Terms: Renal stones; urolithiasis.

Possible Associated Conditions: Carcinomatosis; Cushing's syndrome;* Cystinuria;* Fanconi syndrome;* hyperoxaluria;* hypervitaminosis D;* gout;* multiple myeloma;* osteoporosis;* polycystic renal disease;* primary hyperparathyroidism;* rheumatoid arthritis* *(1)*; sarcoidosis* *(2)*.

Organs and Tissues	*Procedures*	*Possible or Expected Findings*
Kidneys	Remove kidneys, ureters, and urinary bladder en bloc. Excise kidneys from convexity to expose (but not cut) renal pelves and ureters. Record size, number, and appearance of stones, and save for chemical analysis.	Pyelonephritis;* nephrocalcinosis; granulomas; tumor infiltrates; manifestations of the conditions listed below under "Other organs." Calcium, cystine, struvite, and uric acid stones may form staghorn calculi.
Ureters, urinary bladder, and urethra		Obstructive uropathy with foreign bodies, stones, strictures, valves, or other lesions.
Other organs	Record heart weight.	Manifestations of hypertension *(3)*.
	Dissect and record weights of all parathyroid glands. Other procedures depend on suspected underlying conditions, as listed above under "Possible Associated Conditions."	Parathyroid hyperplasia.

References

1. Ito S, Nozawa S, Ishikawa H, Tohyama C, Nakazono K, Murasawa A, et al. Renal stones in patients with rheumatoid arthritis. J Rheumatol 1997;24:2123–2128.
2. Rizzato G, Colombo P. Nephrolithiasis as a presenting feature of chronic sarcoidosis: a prospective study. Sarcoidosis Vasculitis Diff Lung Dis 1996;13:167–172.
3. Madore F, Stampfer MJ, Rimm EB, Curhan GC. Nephrolithiasis and risk of hypertension. Am J Hypertension 1998;11:46–53.

Nephropathy

NOTE: See under name of suspected underlying condition, such as "Diabetes mellitus," "Disorder, electrolyte(s)" (hypercalcemia, potassium depletion), "Gout," "Hypertension (arterial), all types or type unspecified," or "Poisoning,..." (heavy metal). If kidney failure was present, procedures under that heading should also be followed. Renal tissue may need decalcification (p. 97) or fixation in water-free solution.

Nephrosis, Lipoid (See "Glomerulonephritis.")

Neuroblastoma (See "Tumor of the peripheral nerves.")

Neurofibromatosis

Synonyms and Related Terms: Neurofibromatosis type 1 (peripheral neurofibromatosis; von Recklinghausen's disease; von Recklinghausen's neurofibromatosis); neurofibromatosis, type 2 (bilateral acoustic neurofibromatosis).

NOTE: The term "von Recklinghausen's disease" should not be used for neurofibromatosis type 2. Because of the different manifestations, autopsy procedures for neurofibromatosis type 1 and type 2 are presented here separately.

Neurofibromatosis, type 1 *(1)*

Organs and Tissues	*Procedures*	*Possible or Expected Findings*
External examination, skin, soft tissues, and skeletal system		Short stature; bone deformities (see below).
	Sample skin tumors, pigmented areas of skin, and soft tissue tumors for microscopic study. Prepare roentgenograms of skeletal abnormalities.	Café au lait spots; axillary and/or inguinal freckling; dermal neurofibromas; rhabdo myosarcoma. Kyphoskoliosis; macrocephaly with asymmetry of facial and skull bones; sphenoid wing dysplasia; thinning, bending and pseudarthrosis of long bones (tibia).
Arteries	Prepare longitudinal sections and request Verhoeff-van Gieson stains (p. 173).	Fibromuscular dysplasia or renal and cervical arteries.

Organs and Tissues	Procedures	Possible or Expected Findings
Gastrointestinal tract	Search for tumors.	Duodenal carcinoid.
Adrenal glands	Record weights. If a tumor is present, see also under "Tumor, of the adrenal gland(s)").	Pheochromocytoma (more common on the left).
Brain, spinal cord, and spinal roots; base of skull	For removal and specimen preparation, see pp. 65, 67, and 69, respectively. Dissect cranial nerves (p. 66).	Optic nerve gliomas; pilocytic astrocytomas; glioblastomas; nerve sheath tumors. Hydrocephalus* (due to aqueduct stenosis).
Eyes and orbitae	For removal and specimen preparation, see p. 85.	Pigmented hamartomas, elevated on the surface of the iris (Lisch nodules). Neurofibromatosis of ciliary nerves; optic nerve gliomas.
Peripheral nerves, trunks, and plexuses	For removal and specimen preparation, see p. 79.	Benign neurofibromas and malignant peripheral nerve sheath tumors, including MPNST with divergent differentiation (malignant triton tumor). Peripheral neuropathy.
Other organs and tissues; bones and		Neurofibromas rarely in other organs such as the liver.
bone marrow	For removal of bones and prosthetic repair, see p. 95. For bone marrow preparations, see p. 96. If leukemia is expected, see also under that heading.	For skeletal abnormalitis, see above under "External examination, skin, soft tissues, and skeletal system." Bone marrow and other tissues may show features of juvenile chronic myeloid leukemia.*

Neurofibromatosis, type 2 *(2)*

NOTE: In this condition, lesions in the brain and cranial nerves, spinal cord, and spinal roots may be schwannomas (including bilateral vestibular schwannomas); multiple meningiomas; gliomas (generally of spinal cord), mostly ependymomas (75%) and pilocytic astrocytomas; or schwannosis of spinal dorsal root entry zones. Intracortical meningioangiomatosis; glial hamartia (intracortical, basal ganglia, thalamus, cerebellum, and dorsal horns of spinal cord) and cerebral calcifications also may be found.

Organs and Tissues	Procedures	Possible or Expected Findings
External examination and skin	Sample skin tumors for histologic study.	Schwannomas of skin.
Brain with cranial nerves, spinal cord, and spinal roots	For removal and specimen preparation, see pp. 65, 67, and 69, respectively.	A multitude of tumors or tumor-like lesions may be found, as listed above under "Note."
Eyes	For removal and specimen preparation, see p. 85.	Posterior lens opacities; retinal hamartomas.
Peripheral nerves	For removal and specimen preparation, see p. 79.	Peripheral neuropathy with focal schwannomatous changes or onion-bulb-like Schwann cell or perineural cell proliferation.

References

1. Von Deimling A, Krone W. Neurofibromatosis type 1. In: Pathology and Genetics of Tumours of the Nervous System. Kleihues P, Cavenee WK, eds. IARC, Lyon, 1997, pp. 172–174.
2. Louis DN, Wiestler OD. Neurofibromatosis type 2. In: Pathology and Genetics of Tumours of the Nervous System. Kleihues P, Cavenee WK, eds. IARC, Lyon, 1997, pp. 175–178.

Neuropathy

Synonyms and Related Terms: Multiple neuropathy; peripheral neuropathy; polyneuropathy; polyradiculoneuropathy; retrobulbar neuropathy (nutritional amblyopia).

Organs and Tissues	Procedures	Possible or Expected Findings
Spinal cord, dorsal root ganglia, and peripheral nerves	For removal and specimen preparation, see pp. 67, 69, and 79, respectively.	Fiber loss; segmental demyelination or wallerian degeneration, or both.

Organs and Tissues	Procedures	Possible or Expected Findings
Spinal cord, dorsal root ganglia, and peripheral nerves *(continued)*	Sural nerve is commonly used for peripheral nerve study. Stains for paraffin sections may include trichrome, LFB/PAS, methyl violet, and Congo red (p. 172). Stain semithin sections with toluidin blue.	Distribution of lesions depends on type of neuropathy. Vasculitis; amyloid deposition or other manifestations of the underlying condition may be present.
Other organs	Procedures depend on expected findings or grossly identified abnormalities as listed in right-hand column.	Manifestations of underlying conditions, such as alcoholism,* reliac sprue;* diabetes mellitus,* hormonal disorder, immune connective tissue disease, malignant tumor, malnutrition, pellagra,* peripheral vascular disease, megaloblastic anemia,* poisoning (with heavy metals, organo-phosphates, or drugs), post-gastrectomy syndrome, or uremia.

Neurosyphilis, Adult (See "Syphilis, acquired.")

Neurosyphilis, Congenital

NOTE: See also "Syphilis, congenital."

Organs and Tissues	Procedures	Possible or Expected Findings
External examination	Record presence or absence of abnormal external features, as listed in right-hand column. Prepare photographs.	Hydrocephalus;* dental deformities (Hutchinson's teeth); saddle nose; frontal bossing of skull; saber shins; nasal septal perforation; rhagades; ulnar deviation of fingers.
Cerebrospinal fluid	Submit samples for biochemical, cytologic, and microbiologic study (p. 104).	See below under "Brain and spinal cord."
Blood	Submit sample for serologic study.	
Brain and spinal cord	For removal and specimen preparation, see pp. 65 and 67, respectively. For histologic sections, request Warthin-Starry stain for spirochetes (p. 173).	Chronic syphilitic meningitis, encephalitis, and myelitis.
Eyes	For removal and specimen preparations, see p. 85.	Interstitial keratitis; chorioretinitis.

Nitrogen Oxide (See "Poisoning, gas.")

Nocardiosis

Synonym: *Nocardia* spp. infection.

NOTE: (1) Collect all tissues that appear to be infected. (2) Request culture for nocardiosis. (3) Request Gram and Ziehl-Neelsen stains (p. 172). (4) Usually, no special precautions are indicated. (5) Generally, serologic studies are not avail-able. (6) This is not a reportable disease.

Possible Associated Conditions: Acquired immunodeficiency syndrome (AIDS);* alveolar lipoproteinosis of lungs;* anthra-cosilicosis; asthma;* chronic obstructive pulmonary disease; leukemia,* post-transplantation, and other immunosuppressed or dysproteinemic states; systemic lupus erythematosus.*

Organs and Tissues	Procedures	Possible or Expected Findings
External examination	Sample involved skin for culture and histologic study.	Cutaneous abscess *(1)*.
Pleural cavities, pericardium, and lungs	Record presence (and sites) of pleural, pericardial, and chest-wall fistulas. Prepare smears from exudate or from caseating material. Culture consolidated areas. If diagnosis has already been confirmed, perfuse lungs with formalin (p. 47).	Acute necrotizing nocardial pneumonia with abscesses or sinus formation into surrounding tissues; empyema.

Organs and Tissues	Procedures	Possible or Expected Findings
Pulmonary and mediastinal lymph nodes	Submit samples for culture and histologic study (p. 102).	Regional lymphadenitis.
Other organs	Submit samples from all organs and tissues with suspicious gross lesions for culture and histologic study (p. 102).	Poorly encapsulated abscesses of any organ; endocarditis *(2)*.

References

1. Merigou D, Beylot-Barry M, Ly S, Deutre MS, Texier-Maugein J, Billes P, Beylot C. Primary cutaneous *Nocardia asteroides* infection after heart transplantation. Dermatol 1998;196:246–247.
2. Dhawan VK, Gadgil VG, Paliwal YK, Chavroshiya PS, Trivedi RR. Native valve endocarditis due to *Nocardia*-like organisms. Clin Inf Dis 1998;27:902–904.

Nutrition, Parenteral

Related Term: Total parenteral nutrition.

NOTE: Air embolism* or blood loss may have occurred if line became detached from the catheter hub. Metabolic complications such as fluid overload or disturbances of acid-base and electrolyte balance often cannot be diagnosed reliably at autopsy.

The disease(s) that may have necessitated parenteral nutrition therapy are not considered here; they include the acquired immunodeficiency syndrome (AIDS);* cancer cachexia; inflammatory bowel disease; liver or kidney failure;* severe pancreatitis;* short bowel syndrome, and others.

Organs and Tissues	Procedures	Possible or Expected Findings
External examination	Inspect skin site where catheter enters tunnel to venous access (e.g., subclavian or jugular vein; femoral vein).	Infection at any site along the catheter. Displacement of intravenous catheter; fractures or tears in catheter.
	Inspect gastrostomy or jejunostomy sites, if present.	Enteral nutrition may have been combined with parenteral nutrition. Infection and displacement of tube may occur.
	Prepare chest roentgenogram.	Pneumothorax.*
Vitreous	For removal, see p. 85.	Electrolyte disorders.*
Blood	Submit sample for culture (p. 102).	Septicemia (*Staphylococcus* or *Candida*).
Internal examination of major veins	Follow catheter from access site to its open end, generally in the superior vena cava. If clots are found, particulalry at the catheter tip, submit material for culture and prepare sections and smears (order Gram stain, p. 172).	Infection at any site along the catheter. Displacement of catheter with perforation of wall of vein; hemothorax; pneumothorax.*
Urine		Hypercalciuria
Trachea and lungs	If an enteral feeding tube is in place, search for feeding fluid in tracheobronchial tree and lungs.	Aspiration* and aspiration bronchopneumonia.
Gallbladder	Record nature of contens.	Cholelithiasis*
Liver	Record weight. Submit samples for histologic study.	Chronic liver disease with cholestasis and cirrhosis, particularly in children *(1,2)*.
Gastrointestinal tract	If feeding tube is in place, determine location.	Nasogastric, nasoduodenal, nasojejunal, and other tubes (see also above under "External examination").
Skeletal system		Osteoporosis.

References

1. Fein B, Holt P. Hepatobiliary complications of total parenteral nutrition. J Clin Gastroenterol 1994;18:62–66.
2. Mullock FG, Ishak KG. Total parenteral nutrition: a histopathologic analysis of the liver changes in 20 children. Mod Pathol 1994;7:190–194.

O

Obesity

Related Term: Morbid obesity; primary obesity; secondary obesity.

Organs and Tissues	*Procedures*	*Possible or Expected Findings*
External examination and subcutaneous tissue	Record body weight and length (for body mass index, see p. 567), distribution of fat, and thickness of subcutaneous fat layers.	Decubital ulcers; intertriginous infections.
Breast		Breast cancer *(1)*.
Blood		Hyperlipoproteinemia.
Heart and arteries	Record weight of heart and thickness of ventricular walls.	Cardiac hypertrophy* caused by pulmonary or systemic hypertension.* Cor pulmonale in Pickwickian syndrome. Atherosclerosis.
Liver	Record weight. Submit samples for histologic study. Request trichrome stain (p. 172).	Hepatomegaly and fatty changes; steatohepatitis with or without cirrhosis *(2)*.
Stomach	Record features of surgical procedures.	Weight-reducing surgery (gastroplasty or gastric bypass).
Pancreas	Cut in thin, sagittal slices.	Insulinoma (rare).
Other organs	Procedures depend on expected findings or grossly identified abnormalities as listed in right-hand column.	Manifestations of Cushing's syndrome,* type II diabetes mellitus,* hypothyroidism,* hypothalamic disorders (Laurence-Moon-Biedl syndrome* or Prader-Willi syndrome) and systemic hypertension.* Nephrotic syndrome* is a rare complication of obesity.

References

1. Pujol P, Galtier-Dereure F, Bringer J. Obesity and breast cancer risk. Hum Reprod 1997;12:116–125.
2. Ludwig J, McGill DB, Lindor KD. Nonalcoholic steatohepatitis. J Gastroenterol Hepatol 1997;12:398–403.

Obstruction, Acute Airway

Synonyms and Related Terms: Aspiration; bolus death; "café coronary"; croup; restaurant death.

NOTE: If permission has been obtained, remove neck organs through straight incision from chest to chin to avoid dislodging a foreign body. If dissection has to be accomplished from chest, neck of unembalmed cadaver should remain well extended during procedure. Inspect larynx and trachea from above and below, respectively, before opening them carefully along the posterior midline.

Organs and Tissues	*Procedures*	*Possible or Expected Findings*
Oral cavity		Edentulous mouth; malfitting dentures; food or other foreign body in oral cavity.
Blood	Submit sample for alcohol and other toxicologic studies (p. 16). If infectious airway obstruction is suspected, submit sample for microbiologic study (p. 102).	Evidence of alcohol intoxication.*

From: *Handbook of Autopsy Practice,* 3rd Ed. Edited by: J. Ludwig © Humana Press Inc., Totowa, NJ

Organs and Tissues	Procedures	Possible or Expected Findings
Larynx and pharynx	For dissection procedures, see above under "Note." Photograph larynx with foreign body or tumor. If infectious obstructive laryngitis is expected, follow procedures described under "Laryngitis."	Foreign body (food bolus; denture); malignant tumor of pharynx or larynx. Obstructive laryngitis* with epiglottiditis in infants.
Lungs	Record weights.	Acute pulmonary edema.
Brain and spinal cord	For removal and specimen preparation, see pp. 65 and 67, respectively.	Chronic neurologic disorder.

Obstruction, Arteriomesenteric

Organs and Tissues	Procedures	Possible or Expected Findings
External examination		Lax abdominal musculature.
Intestinal tract and mesentery	For mesenteric arteriography, see p. 54. Photograph obstruction *in situ*.	Superior mesenteric artery or abnormal arterial branch crosses and obstructs third portion of duodenum; dilatation of duodenum proximal to obstruction.

Obstruction, Biliary (See "Atresia, biliary," "Cholelithiasis," and "Tumor of the bile ducts (extrahepatic or hilar or of papilla of Vater.")

Obstruction, Chronic Airway (See "Asthma," "Bronchitis, chronic," and "Emphysema.")

Obstruction, Hepatic Vein (See "Syndrome, Budd-Chiari.")

Obstruction, Inferior Vena Cava

Organs and Tissues	Procedures	Possible or Expected Findings
Chest organs and abdominal organs	Remove thoracoabdominal viscera en masse (Letulle technique, p. 3) and dissect inferior vena cava from posterior aspect. Phlebography from lower extremities requires much contrast medium and interferes with clean dissection.	Adhesions; aortic aneurysm;* congenital malformation; enlargement of pancreas; annular pancreas; cirrhosis* and other conditions that may cause hepatomegaly (see also under "Syndrome, hepatorenal"); IVC filter with entrapped thromboembolus; surgical ligation; thrombosis; tumor (especially renal cell or hepatocellular carcinoma).

Obstruction, Portal Vein (See "Hypertension, portal.")

Obstruction, Pulmonary Venous

Synonyms and Related Terms: Congenital stenosis or atresia of pulmonary veins; pulmonary veno-occlusive disease; pulmonary venous hypertension.

Organs and Tissues	Procedures	Possible or Expected Findings
External examination	Prepare chest roentgenogram.	Mediastinal fibrosis or tumor.
Chest cavity	Record appearance of mediastinum and hilum of lungs. Remove chest organs en bloc. If an infectious process is suspected, submit samples for microbiologic study.	Idiopathic mediastinal or pulmonary hilar fibrosis; mediastinal radiation fibrosis; sclerosing mediastinitis;* mediastinal neoplasm; granulomas (histoplasma, sarcoid).

Organs and Tissues	Procedures	Possible or Expected Findings
Lungs	For pulmonary venography, see p. 50. Perfuse lungs with formalin (p. 47). Submit samples of tissues from periphery of lungs and from perihilar areas. Record sites from where tissues were sampled. Request Verhoeff–van Gieson stain (p. 173).	Congenital stenosis or atresia of pulmonary veins. Pulmonary veno-occlusive disease with old thrombi. Pulmonary venous hypertensive changes, most prominent in lower lobes.
Heart	Procedures depend on expected findings or grossly identified abnormalities as listed in right-hand column.	Thrombus or myxoma of left atrium; mitral or aortic stenosis;* chronic heart failure.*

Obstruction, Superior Mesenteric Artery (or Vein)

Organs and Tissues	Procedures	Possible or Expected Findings
Superior mesenteric artery system	For mesenteric arteriography, see p. 55. For dissection, en masse removal is recommended (p. 3). Open aorta posteriorly and record appearance of celiac and mesenteric artery orifices.	Atherosclerosis; emboli.
Superior mesenteric vein system	Dissect portal, splenic, and superior mesenteric vein branches *in situ*.	Thrombosis; migratory thrombophlebitis.
Intestine	Locate and photograph abnormalities *in situ*.	Infarction; strangulation; volvulus; intussesception.
Other organs	Procedures depend on expected findings or grossly identified abnormalities as listed in right-hand column.	Thromboembolic disease; atherosclerosis or vasculitis complicated by arterial occlusion; peritonitis;* tumor; previous operations or cirrhosis* complicated by venous thromboses.

Occlusion (See "Obstruction,...")

Ochronosis (See "Alkaptonuria.")

Onchocerciasis

Synonyms and Related Terms: Disseminated microfilariasis; *Onchocerca volvulus* infection; river blindness.

NOTE: (1) Collect cerebrospinal fluid, blood, urine, and all tissues that appear to be infected. (2) Request parasitologic examination. (3) Request Giemsa and PAS stains (p. 172). (4) No special precautions are indicated. (5) No serologic studies are available. (6) This is not a reportable disease.

Organs and Tissues	Procedures	Possible or Expected Findings
External examination, skin, subcutaneous tissue, and lymph nodes	Submit samples for histologic study.	Granulomatous inflammation with fibrosis; cutaneous lymphedema with leathery, depigmented, thickened skin; pendulous sacs of inguinal or femoral lymph nodes.
Cerebrospinal fluid	Submit sample for parasitologic study (p. 104). See also above under "Note."	Microfilariae may be present.
Abdomen	If ascitic fluid is present, record volume and submit sample for parasitologic study.	Microfilariae may be present.
Blood and urine	Prepare smears. Centrifuge urine prior to smear preparation.	Microfilariae may be present.
Other organs	Procedures depend on expected findings or grossly identified abnormalities as listed in right-hand column. Submit samples for histologic study.	Microfilariae or, in rare instances, adult *Onchocerca volvulus* may be found in internal organs, such as lungs, liver, spleen, pancreas, and kidneys.

Organs and Tissues	*Procedures*	*Possible or Expected Findings*
Eyes	For removal and specimen preparation, see p. 85.	Microfilariae, in anterior chamber and cornea of eyes as seen with a slit lamp; punctate keratitis; uveitis.

Opiate(s) (See "Dependence, drug(s), all types or type unspecified.")

Organophosphate(s) (See "Poisoning, organophosphate(s).")

Origin of Both Great Arteries from Right Ventricle (See "Ventricle, double outlet right.")

Ornithosis

Synonyms and Related Terms: *Chlamydia* infection; psittacosis; parrot fever.

NOTE: (1) Collect all tissues that appear to be infected. (2) Request cultures for ornithosis. Consult with microbiology laboratory before obtaining postmortem specimens. (3) Stains are not helpful in demonstrating the organism. (4) Special **precautions** are indicated (p. 146). (5) Serologic studies are available from the state health department laboratories (p. 135). (6) This is a **reportable** disease.

Organs and Tissues	*Procedures*	*Possible or Expected Findings*
External examination and skin	Photograph lesion.	Pale macular rash (Horder's spots); jaundice.
Chest	Record volume of effusions; submit samples for microbiologic and cytologic study.	Pleural effusions.*
Blood	Submit sample for serologic study.	
Heart	Submit samples for histologic study (p. 30).	Pericarditis* and myocarditis.*
Lungs	Perfuse one lung with formalin (p. 47). Submit multiple samples for histologic study.	Lymphocytic pneumonitis, which may be focally hemorrhagic and necrotizing; inclusion bodies.
Liver and spleen	Record weights and sample for histologic study.	Inclusion bodies in Kupffer cells; hepatosplenomegaly.
Other organs	Extensive histologic sampling is indicated.	Inclusion bodies may occur in kidneys, adrenal glands, brain and meninges, and other organs.

Osteitis Deformans (See "Disease, Paget's, of bone.")

Osteoarthritis

Related Term: Degenerative joint disease.

Possible Associated Conditions: Acromegaly;* acute and chronic trauma; alkaptonuria;* congenital or developmental bone diseases (e.g., congenital hip dislocation); diabetes mellitus;* Gaucher's disease;* hemochromatosis;* hyperparathyroidism;* hypothyroidism;* obesity;* Wilson's disease.*

Organs and Tissues	*Procedures*	*Possible or Expected Findings*
External examination		Heberden's nodes at interphalangeal joints of fingers.
	Prepare skeletal roentgenograms.	Degenerative changes, primarily of spine, hip joints, and knee joints.
Joints	For removal, prosthetic repair, and specimen preparation, see p. 96. Submit samples of osteocartilaginous and synovial tissues for histologic study; sagittal or frontal saw section through spine provides for best routine evaluation.	Histologic and macroscopic degeneration of cartilage; exposure of subchrondral bone; formation of marginal osteophytes; bone cysts; synovial fibrosis; hypertrophic synovitis.
	If artificial joints (e.g., hip or knee) had been implanted, record state of implant site.	Lose joint prostheses.

Osteoarthropathy, Hypertrophic

Synonyms: Hypertrophic pulmonary osteoarthropathy; pachydermoperiostosis (idiopathic hypertrophic osteoarthropathy *[1]*).

NOTE: In all instances, an underlying disease must be identified; they include cardiac disease (cyanotic congenital heart disease with right-to-left shunt; infective endocarditis*); gastroesophageal reflux *(3)*; neoplasms of lungs, esophagus, intestine, and liver; chronic liver disease; inflammatory bowel disease;* pulmonary disease (e.g., abscess;* bronchiectasis;* cystic fibrosis;* empyema;* emphysema;* lipoid pneumonia* *(4)*; *Pneumocystis* pneumonia; sarcoidosis;* tuberculosis*); hyperthyroidism.*

Organs and Tissues	*Procedures*	*Possible or Expected Findings*
External examination		Clubbing of fingers or toes (see below under "Elastic arteries"); swelling of extremities.
	Prepare roentgenograms of extremities.	Periosteal new bone formation in distal shafts of bones of forearms and legs. All bones of extremities may be involved (see Chapter 8, Fig. 8-3, p. 99).
Bones	For removal, prosthetic repair, and specimen preparation, see p. 95.	See above under "External examination."
Elastic arteries	Record presence of aneurysms (thoracic aorta, subclavian) or arteriovenous fistula of brachial vessels.	Unilateral clubbing.
	If abdominal aortic aneurysm had been surgically repaired, search for evidence of graft infection *(2)*.	Clubbing of toes but not of fingers.
Other organs	Procedures depend on expected findings or grossly identified abnormalities as listed above under "Note."	See above under "Note."

References

1. Sinha GP, Curtis P, Haigh D, Lealman GT, Dodds W, Bennett CP. Pachydermoperiostitis in childhood. Br J Rheum 1997;36:1224–1247.
2. Stevens M, Helms C, El-Khoury G, Chow S. Unilateral hypertrophic osteoarthropathy associated with aortofemoral graft infection. Am J Roentgenol 1998;170:1584–1586.
3. Greenwald M, Couper R, Laxer R, Durie P, Silverman E. Gastroesophageal reflux and esophagitis-associated hypertrophic osteoarthropathy. J Pediatr Gastroenterol Nutr 1996;23:178–181.
4. Hugosson C, Bahabri S, Rifai A, al-Dalaan A. Hypertrophic osteoarthropathy caused by lipoid pneumonia. Pediatr Radiol 1995;25:482–483.

Osteochondrodysplasia (See "Achondroplasia" and Dyschondroplasia, Ollier's.")

Osteodystrophy, Renal (See "Failure, kidney.")

Osteogenesis Imperfecta

Synonyms and Related Terms: Lobstein's syndrome; Osteogenesis imperfecta congenita; OI type I, II, and III; osteogenesis imperfecta cystica; osteogenesis imperfecta tarda; osteopsathyrosis; van der Hoeve's syndrome; Vrolik's disease (infantile form of OI).

NOTE: Contact the Osteogenesis Imperfecta Foundation, 804 W. Diamond Avenue, Suite 210, Gaithersburg, MD 20878, phone: (301) 947-0083.

Organs and Tissues	*Procedures*	*Possible or Expected Findings*
External examination and skin	Record body weight and length, shape of skull, shape of extremities, and appearance of eyes and teeth.	Soft skull bones (caput membranaceum); short and deformed long bones; blue sclerae (Lobstein's syndrome); abnormal teeth.
	Prepare sections of skin for histologic study.	Thin skin.
	Prepare skeletal roentgenograms. Submit fascia lata for tissue culture (p. 109) to reference laboratory for classification of collagen metabolism defect.	Narrow bones with multiple fractures in various phases of healing; exuberant callus formation; compression of vertebrae with weight bearing.
Blood	Obtain serum to assay for alkaline phosphatase activity. Postmortem and determination of calcium concentration is unreliable.	Normal values rule out hypophosphatasia. Hypercalcemia *(1)*.

Organs and Tissues	Procedures	Possible or Expected Findings
Urine	Submit urine for determination of phospho-ethanolamine concentration.	
Gastrointestinal tract	Photograph abnormalities *in situ*.	Fecal impaction due to pelvic deformity in OI, type III *(2)*.
Bones	For removal, prosthetic repair, and specimen preparation, see p. 95. Samples for histologic study should include areas of endochondral and periosteal bone formation.	Normal epiphysis; deficient ossification of metaphysis, diaphysis and cortex; multiple fractures with fibrosis and callus formation.
Tendons and ligaments	Submit samples for histologic study.	Thin, translucent structures that may have ruptured.
Eyes	For removal and specimen preparation, see p. 85.	Thin sclerae *(3)*.
Parathyroid glands	Record weights and submit samples for histologic study.	Normal parathyroid glands.
Middle ears	For exposure of middle ears, see p. 72. This procedure is particularly indicated if patient had been deaf.	Otosclerosis (van der Hoeve's syndrome).

References

1. Williams CJ, Smith RA, Ball RJ, Wilkinson H. Hypercalcemia in osteogenesis imperfecta treated with pamidronate. Arch Dis Child 1997;76: 169–170.
2. Lee JH, Gamble JG, Moore RE, Rinsky LA. Gastrointestinal problems in patients who have type-III osteogenesis imperfecta. J Bone Joint Surg 1995;77:1352–1356.
3. Mietz H, Kasner L, Green WR. Histopathologic and electron-microscopic features of corneal and scleral collagen fibers in osteogenesis imperfecta type III. Graefes Arch Clin Exp Ophthalmol 1997;235: 405–410.

Osteomalacia

Related Terms: Osteoporosis;* renal osteodystrophy; rickets.

NOTE: Many possible causes of osteomalacia may not be apparent at autopsy, e.g., sodium fluoride or diphosphonate toxicity or use of anticonvulsant drugs.

Possible Associated Conditions: Neurofibromatosis;* hypophosphatasia (inborn error of metabolism) and hypophosphatemic states *(1)*; parenteral nutrition;* vitamin D deficiency.* (See also below under "Other organs and tissues.")

Organs and Tissues	Procedures	Possible or Expected Findings
External examination	Prepare skeletal roentgenograms.	Pseudofractures (Looser's zones), most common at axillary borders of scapulae, ischial and pubic rami, femoral necks, and ribs.
Bones	For removal, prosthetic repair, and specimen preparation, see p. 95. Consult roentgenograms. Request cyanuric chloride stain (p. 172).	Abundant osteoid. May be associated with fibro-osteoclastic osteoporosis (renal osteodystrophy).
Other organs and tissues	Procedures depend on expected findings or grossly identified abnormalities as listed in right-hand column.	Changes secondary to chronic kidney failure* with phosphate depletion,* generalized renal tubular disorders (Fanconi syndrome*), vitamin D deficiency,* and chronic gastrointestinal, pancreatic or hepatobiliary diseases. Benign or malignant giant cell and other mesenchymal tumors or carcinoma of the prostate may cause (oncogenous) osteomalacia.
Parathyroid glands	Record weights and submit samples for histologic study.	If chronic renal disease was present, secondary parathyroid hyperplasia can be expected.

Reference

1. Clarke BL, Wynne AG, Wilson DM, Fitzpatrick LA. Osteomalacia associated with adult Fanconi syndrome: clinical and diagnostic features. Clin Endocrinol 1995;43:479–490.

Osteomyelitis

Organs and Tissues	*Procedures*	*Possible or Expected Findings*
External examination		Swelling; fistulas.
	Prepare skeletal roentgenograms.	Bone defect(s) and focal osteosclerosis.
Bones	For submission of material for microbiologic study, see p. 102. Record presence of contiguous infections.	Bacterial or fungal infections, most common in metaphyseal region of bones; paravertebral or psoas abscess in osteomyelitis of spine.
	Submit samples for histologic study. Request Gram stain and Grocott's methenamine silver stain for fungi (p. 172).	Bacterial or fungal osteomyelitis, with or without cavitation and fistulas.
Other organs	Procedures depend on expected findings or grossly identified abnormalities as listed in right-hand column.	Trauma, surgery, insertion of prosthesis, generalized *(1)* or contiguous infection, inflammatory bowel disease *(2)*, diabetes mellitus,* and peripheral vascular diseases.

References

1. Copie-Bergmann C, Niedobitek G, Mangham DC, Selves J, Baloch K, Diss TC, et al. Epstein-Barr virus in B-cell lymphomas associated with chronic suppurative inflammation. J Pathol 1997;183:287–292.
2. Freeman HJ. Osteomyelitis and osteonecrosis in inflammatory bowel disease. Can J Gastroenterol 1997;11:601–606.

Osteonecrosis

Synonyms and Related Terms: Aseptic necrosis of bone; avascular necrosis of bone; idiopathic osteonecrosis; Perthes' disease; postfracture osteonecrosis; renal transplant associated osteonecrosis.

NOTE: Possible underlying conditions include chronic alcoholism,* decompression sickness,* diseases that have been treated with high doses of corticosteroids *(1)*, Gaucher's disease,* human immunodeficiency virus infection* *(2)*, tuberculosis* *(1)*, sickle cell disease,* systemic lupus erythematosus,* tuberculosis* *(2)*, and other conditions.

Organs and Tissues	*Procedures*	*Possible or Expected Findings*
Blood	Submit sample for biochemical study.	Hyperlipidemia; hyperuricemia.
Bones and joints	For removal, prosthetic repair, and specimen preparation, see p. 95. If osteonecrosis is suspected because one of the possible underlying conditions (see above) is present, prepare saw sections through femoral heads, medial femoral condyles, and heads of humeri.	Fracture or traumatic dislocation of hip, causing avascular necrosis of bone.
Other organs	Procedures depend on suspected underlying conditions, as listed above under "Note."	See above under "Note."

References

1. Freeman HJ. Osteomyelitis and osteonecrosis in inflammatory bowel disease. Can J Gastroenterol 1997;11:601–606.
2. Rademaker J, Dobro JS, Solomon G. Osteonecrosis and human immunodeficiency virus infection. J Rheumatol 1997;24:601–604.

Osteopetrosis

Synonyms and Related Terms: Albers-Schönberg disease; autosomal-dominant osteopetrosis; carbonic anhydrase-II deficiency; malignant infantile osteopetrosis *(1)*; marble bone disease.

NOTE: Manifestations of renal tubular acidosis may have been a clinical complication.

Possible Associated Conditions: Bone marrow transplantation* (for infantile osteopetrosis). Anemia, recurrent infections, bleeding, and bruises may have resulted from myelophthisis associated with osteopetrosis. Upper airway obstruction in malignant infantile osteopetrosis may have necessitated tracheostomy *(1)*.

Organs and Tissues	*Procedures*	*Possible or Expected Findings*
External examination	Record weight and height.	Growth failure in infants; hypoplastic dentition.

Organs and Tissues	Procedures	Possible or Expected Findings
External examination *(continued)*	Prepare skeletal roentgenograms.	Increased density of all bones; bone deformities; narrowing of marrow spaces; malformation of the mastoid and paranasal sinuses; osteomyelitis* of jaws with facial fistulas. Exophthalmos.
Liver and spleen	Record weights and sizes; submit samples for histologic study.	Hepatosplenomegaly; extramedullary hematopoiesis.
Kidneys	Record weights and sizes; submit samples for histologic study.	Renal tubular acidosis in carbonic anhydrase II deficiency *(2)*.
Parathyroid glands	Record weights and submit samples for histologic study.	Normal parathyroid glands.
Brain	For removal and specimen preparation, see p. 65.	Hydrocephalus;* cerebral calcification. See also under "Skeletal system and skull."
Eyes	Remove for study in patients with visual disturbances (p. 85).	Retinal degeneration.
Skeletal system with skull	For removal, prosthetic repair, and specimen preparation of bones, see p. 95. Expose base of skull (p. 71) and record size of nerve foramina (optic, acoustic, and other cranial nerves). If there is evidence of infection, expose nasal cavities and prepare histologic sections. Histologic samples should include bone and bone marrow.	Spondylolysis in children *(3)*. Rhinogenic osteomyelitis; atrophy of cranial nerves after compression at foramina. (This may have caused optic atrophy or deafness, or both. See also above under "External examination.") Otitis media* *(1)*; osteomalacia* or rickets may complicate osteopetrosis. Myelophthisis secondary to osteopetrosis.

References

1. Stocks RM, Wang WC, Thompson JW, Stocks MC 2nd, Horwitz EM. Malignant infantile osteopetrosis: otolaryngological complications and management. Arch Otolaryngol Head Neck Surg 1998;124:689–694.
2. Nagai R, Kooh SW, Balfe JW, Fenton T, Halperin ML. Renal tubular acidosis and osteopetrosis with carbonic anhydrase II deficiency: pathogenesis of impaired acidification. Pediatr Nephrol 1997;11:633–636.
3. Martin RP, Deane RH, Collett V. Spondylolysis in children who have osteopetrosis. J Bone Joint Surg 1997;79:1685–1689.

Osteoporosis

Synonym and Related Terms: Drug-induced osteoporosis; idiopathic osteoporosis; juvenile osteoporosis; osteopenia; type I or type II osteoporosis; postmenopausal osteoporosis.

NOTE:
In heritable osteoporotic disorders of connective tissue (osteogenesis imperfecta,* Marfan's syndrome,* and others) are presented separately. For "osteomalacia," see above. For "osteodystrophy," see under "Failure, kidney."

Possible Associated Conditions: Acromegaly;* chronic alcoholism;* chronic obstructive pulmonary disease; chronic kidney failure* *(1)*; Cushing's syndrome;* debilitating disease (various kinds, often with immobilization); diabetes mellitus* *(2)*; epilepsy;* hyperthyroidism *(2)*;* hypogonadism; malabsorption syndrome;* malnutrition;* primary biliary cirrhosis;* rheumatoid arthritis;* scurvy;* steroid therapy or anticonvulsant medication.

Organs and Tissues	Procedures	Possible or Expected Findings
External examination	Record body length and shape of spine. Prepare skeletal roentgenograms.	Kyphosis or kyphoscoliosis. Gross deformities of bones; alveolar bone loss; fractures of vertebrae, wrist, hip, humerus, or tibia. Calvarium uninvolved in most uncomplicated cases. Malnutrition* and senility.
Other organs	Procedures depend on expected underlying conditions, as listed in right-hand column and above under "Possible Associated Conditions."	In acute cases, metastatic calcifications with nephrocalcinosis. For other findings, see above under "Possible Associated Conditions."
Parathyroid glands	Record weights and submit samples for histologic study.	Normal parathyroid glands in uncomplicated cases. Hyperparathyroidism* *(1)* (without osteitis fibrosa) may be present, however.

Organs and Tissues	Procedures	Possible or Expected Findings
Bones	For removal, prosthetic repair, and specimen preparation, see p. 95. Record appearance of saw sections of vertebral column, calvarium, and femur. Submit samples for histologic study.	Features of osteitis fibrosa (osteoclastic osteoporosis; see "Hyperparathyroidism") or osteomalacia* exclude the diagnosis of uncomplicated osteoporosis. Osteoporosis, which may be localized, occurs in various neoplastic (e.g., mastocytosis) and inflammatory diseases.

References

1. Nishizawa Y, Morii H. Osteoporosis and atherosclerosis in chronic renal failure. Osteoporos Int 1997;7 Suppl 3:S188–S192.
2. Rosen CJ. Endocrine disorders and osteoporosis. Curr Opin Rheumatol 1997;9:355–361.

Otitis Media

Organs and Tissues	Procedures	Possible or Expected Findings
External examination	Examine external ear canal.	Draining, foul-smelling greasy material associated with acquired cholesteatoma.
Brain and base of skull with middle ears	For removal and specimen preparation, see pp. 65 and 72, respectively. For microbiologic examination, see p. 102.	Bacterial or viral infection, with or without mastoid osteitis. Neck abscess, sinus thrombosis *(1)* and brain abscess* and meningitis* may complicate otitis media.

Reference

1. Garcia RD, Baker AS, Cunningham MJ, Weber AL. Lateral sinus thrombosis associated with otitis media and mastoiditis in children. Pediatr Inf Dis J 1995;14:617–623.

Otosclerosis

NOTE: Otosclerosis may be a measles-virus-associated disease *(1)* and therefore, studies to rule out a past infection may be indicated.

Organs and Tissues	Procedures	Possible or Expected Findings
Middle and inner ears	For removal and specimen preparation, see p. 72. For current methods of temporal bone studies, see ref. *(2)*.	Spongy bone in the capsule of the labyrinth. Trabeculae of woven bone show pagetoid changes. If stapedectomy had been done, a prosthesis may be in place.

References

1. Niedermeyer HP, Arnold W. Otosclerosis: a measles virus associated inflammatory disease. Acta Oto-Laryngol 1995;115:300–303.
2. Cherukupally SR, Merchant SM, Rosowski JJ. Correlations between pathologic changes in the stapes and conductive hearing loss in otosclerosis. Ann Otyol Rhinol Laryngol 1998;107:319–326.

Oxaluria (see "Hyperoxaluria.")

P

Palsy, Progressive Bulbar (See "Disease, motor neuron.")

Palsy, Progressive Supranuclear
Synonyms: Steele-Richardson-Olszewski syndrome.

Organs and Tissues	*Procedures*	*Possible or Expected Findings*
Brain	For removal and specimen preparation, see p. 65. Histologic samples should include all sites listed in right-hand column. Request Bielschowsky stain for paraffin sections (p. 172) and histochemical stains with ubiquitin and tau proteins.	Brain is externally normal or mildly atrophic. Characteristic is midbrain atrophy with aqueduct dilatation and depigmentation of the substantia nigra. Neuronal loss with reactive gliosis, associated with neurofibrillary tangles (globose tangles). Primarily affected are globus pallidus, subthalamic nucleus, red nucleus, substantia nigra, tectum, periaqueductal gray matter, and dentate nucleus (grumose degeneration).

Palsy, Pseudobulbar (See "Disease, motor neuron.")

Pancreatitis
Related Terms: Acute pancreatitis; alcoholic pancreatitis; chronic (or chronic fibrosing) pancreatitis; interstitial pancreatitis.
NOTE: Some causes of pancreatitis such as adverse drug reactions (e.g., due to azathioprine, furosemide, or estrogens) cannot be diagnosed at autopsy.
Possible Associated Conditions: Acute fatty liver of pregnancy; apolipoprotein CII deficiency; cystic fibrosis;* hyperparathyroidism;* kidney transplantation.* Status post endoscopic retrograde cholangiopancreatography.

Organs and Tissues	*Procedures*	*Possible or Expected Findings*
External examination and skin	Record appearance of subcutaneous fat tissue and prepare histologic sections.	Fat tissue necroses.
	Prepare skeletal roentgenograms.	Intraosseous calcification (femur and tibia).
Vitreous	Submit sample for determination of calcium, potassium, and sodium concentrations (p. 85).	Increased calcium concentration.
Abdominal cavity	If there are abscesses or other inflammatory changes, aspirate pus or exudate and submit sample for microbiologic study (p. 102).	Exudate or abscesses in lesser sac or other peritoneal pockets; ascites.
Chest cavity	Record volume of effusions. Submit sample for lipase and amylase determination.	Pleural effusions.*
Blood	Submit sample for microbiologic study (p. 102). Postmortem determination of calcium level is unreliable. Study of viral antibodies may be indicated.	Hypercalcemia or hypertriglyceridemia. Cultures or serologic studies may be positive for cytomegalovirus infection,* infectious mononucleosis,* mumps,* scarlet fever,* typhoid fever,* or viral hepatitis.

From: *Handbook of Autopsy Practice*, 3rd Ed. Edited by: J. Ludwig © Humana Press Inc., Totowa, NJ

Organs and Tissues	Procedures	Possible or Expected Findings
Heart and coronary arteries		Coronary thrombosis.
Lungs		Pulmomary embolism.*
Liver, gallbladder, extrahepatic bile ducts, and pancreas; splenic and portal veins	After removal of pancreas, open pancreatic ducts. Record type of entry of pancreatic ducts in relationship to common bile duct. Open common bile duct (including papilla of Vater) and splenic and portal veins *in situ*. For cholangiography and pancreatography, see pp. 56 and 57, respectively. Remove liver and gallbladder, and record contents of gallbladder. Sample pancreas, liver, and grossly identifiable abnormalities for histologic study.	Pancreatic and peripancreatic fat tissue necroses; abscesses; hemorrhages; pseudocysts; calcification. Pancreatolithiasis. Carcinoma of pancreas *(1)*. Stenosis of intrapancreatic common bile duct in chronic pancreatitis. Obstruction of ampulla by ulcer in Crohn's disease* or duodenal diverticulum. Ascariasis. Choledocholithiasis. Splenic vein thrombosis; may also involve portal vein. Cholecystitis* and cholelithiasis.* Alcoholic liver disease.
Other organs and tissues	Procedures depend on expected findings or grossly identified abnormalities as listed in right-hand column. If polyarteritis nodosa is suspected, study arteries of lower extremities. For possible systemic infections, see above under "Blood."	Extrahepatic manifestations of chronic alcoholism,* chronic renal failure; hyperparathyroidism* *(2)*, multiple myeloma,* polyarteritis nodosa,* thrombotic thrombocytopenic purpura *(3)*; sarcoidosis,* surgical and other types of trauma, systemic lupus erythematosus,* and other conditions.
Peripheral veins	For venography, see p. 120. For removal of peripheral veins, see p. 34.	Venous thromboses and thrombophlebitis.
Bones and bone marrow	For removal, prosthetic repair, and specimen preparation of bones, see p. 95. For preparation of sections and smears of bone marrow, see p. 96.	Necroses. Multilacunar osteolysis.
Eyes	For removal and specimen preparation, see p. 85.	Retinopathy (rare) *(4)*.

References

1. Andren-Sandberg A, Dervenis C, Lowenfels B. Etiologic links between chronic pancreatitis and pancreatic cancer. Scand J Gastroenterol 1997; 32:97–103.
2. Inabnet WB, Baldwin D, Daniel RO, Staren ED. Hyperparathyroidism and pancreatitis during pregnancy. Surgery 1996;119:710–713.
3. Silva VA. Thrombotic thrombocytopenic purpura/hemolytic uremic syndrome secondary to pancreatitis. Am J Hematol 1995;50:53–56.
4. Soledad Donoso Flores M, Narvaez Rodriguez I, Lopez Bernal I, del Mar Alcalde Rubio M, Galvan Ledesma A, et al. Retinopathy as a systemic complication of acute pancreatitis. Am J Gastroenterol 1995; 90:321–324.

Pancytopenia

Related Terms: Agranulocytosis;* aplastic anemia; Fanconi's anemia.*

NOTE: Some causes of pancytopenia such as adverse drug reactions (e.g., due to antimetabolites, sulfa drugs, or gold compounds) cannot be diagnosed at autopsy.

Possible Associated Conditions: Acquired immunodeficiency syndrome;* diffuse eosinophilic fasciitis; paroxysmal nocturnal hemoglobinuria;* pregnancy;* radiation injury;* systemic lupus erythematosus;* systemic viral infections and viral hepatitis; transfusion-related graft-versus-host disease.*

Organs and Tissues	Procedures	Possible or Expected Findings
External examination	Record skin abnormalities and prepare photographs.	Jaundice; ulcers of skin. Thrombocytopenic hemorrhages.
Other organs and blood	If toxicity of drugs or chemicals is suspected, submit appropriate tissue samples for toxicologic study. If viral infection is suspected as a cause, submit material for serologic or other diagnostic studies.	Manifestations of leukopenia or thrombocytopenia (infections, including septicemia; hemorrhages; various types of pneumonia*). Systemic viral infection; viral hepatitis.* Radiation injury.*

Organs and Tissues	Procedures	Possible or Expected Findings
Neck organs with oropharynx, tongue, tonsils, and soft palate	Request Gram and Grocott's methenamine silver stains for bacteria and fungi, respectively (p. 172); photograph lesions.	Ulcers in mouth and pharynx.
Lymph nodes and spleen	Record weight of spleen.	Reactive lymphadenitis and splenitis.
Rectum and vagina	See above under "Neck organs").	Rectal and vaginal ulcers.
Bone marrow	For specimen preparation, see p. 96.	Bone marrow may be hypocellular, normal, or hypercellular. Hematologic malignancies (myelodysplastic syndromes) or metastases may be present. Agnogenic myeloid metaplasia,* osteopetrosis,* or storage diseases are rare findings.

Panencephalitis, Subacute Sclerosing
(See "Encephalitis, all types or type unspecified.")

Panhypopituitarism (See "Insufficiency, pituitary.")

Panniculitis

Synonyms and Related Terms: Calcifying panniculitis; histiocytic cytophagic panniculitis; mesenteric panniculitis (mesenteric lipodystrophy); "sclerema neonatorum."

NOTE: The term Weber-Christian disease described systemic panniculitis with fever, bleeding, pulmonary and pancreatic lesions, and other abnormalities also involving lungs and pancreas, among others. However, this condition is not a specific entity and thus, the name has become obsolete. The term histiocytic cytophagic panniculitis is more descriptive and preferred.

Leukemia* and subcutaneous T-cell lymphoma* may closely simulate panniculitis.

Possible Associated Conditions: Alpha$_1$-antitrypsin deficiency;* dermatomyositis;* rheumatoid arthritis;* scleroderma and morphea; Sjögren's syndrome;* systemic lupus erythematosus.*

Organs and Tissues	Procedures	Possible or Expected Findings
External examination, skin, subcutaneous tissue, and breasts	Record extent and character of skin lesions. Record size, location, and gross appearance of subcutaneous nodules. Submit tissue samples for histologic study of grossly unaffected skin, skin lesions, and subcutaneous nodules. Request Verhoeff–van Gieson, Gram, and Grocott's methenamine silver stains (p. 172).	Dimpling of skin; necroses; fistulas. Panniculitis with subcutaneous nodules in trunk, breasts, and thighs. Calcification may occur in breast tissue but also at other sites (e.g., in kidney failure*). Pancreatic enzyme-induced fat necroses associated with severe pancreatitis. Widespread hardening of fat tissue with rupture of fat cells and crystal formation in "sclerema neonatorum." Focal traumatic panniculitis also may occur in newborns.
	Request S-100 protein stain. Ascertain that cell infiltrates are not leukemic or lymphomatous *(1)*.	S-100 stain negative in panniculitis but positive in Rosai-Dorfman disease (sinus histiocytosis with massive lymphadenopathy).
Chest	Submit tissue samples for histologic study of pretracheal and pericardial fat tissue.	Mediastinal panniculitis.
Heart	Record weight. For histologic sampling, see p. 30.	Pericarditis;* interstitial myocarditis.*
Lungs	Submit one lobe for microbiologic study (p. 103). Perfuse one lung with formalin (p. 47). Prepare frozen sections and request Sudan stain (p. 173).	Pneumonia;* pleuritis. Fat embolism.*
Liver and spleen	Record weights and submit samples for histologic study. Request PAS/diastase stain of liver (p. 173).	Features of alpha$_1$-antitrypsin deficiency* *(2)*. Fatty changes of liver; splenitis.
Mesentery and intestine	For mesenteric arteriography, see p. 55. For *in situ* fixation of small bowel, see p. 54. Submit tissue samples for histologic study of mucosal lesions and grossly uninvolved portions of intestine.	Intestinal mucosal erosions and ulcers, with or without perforation. Massive gastrointestinal hemorrhage in histiocytic cytophagic panniculitis. Blind intestinal loop *(3)*.

Organs and Tissues	Procedures	Possible or Expected Findings
Mesentery and intestine *(continued)*	Prepare thin slices of mesentery. Record size of nodules and appearance of vessels. Submit tissue samples for histologic study of nodules and vessels.	Mesenteric panniculitis.
Retroperitoneum with pancreas	Submit tissue samples for histologic study.	Retroperitoneal panniculitis. Necrotizing pancreatitis.*
Kidneys and adrenal glands	Dissect renal and adrenal vessels *in situ.* Record weights, prepare photographs, and sample for histologic study.	Vasculitis with thrombi; adrenocortical infarctions.
Other organs and tissues	Submit tissue samples for histologic study of large and small peripheral vessels. Request Verhoeff–van Gieson stain (p. 173). Samples should include all organs and tissues with gross lesions and also lymph nodes and bone marrow.	Vasculitis with thrombi and infarctions. Relapsing polychondritis *(4).* See also above under "Possible Associated Conditions."

References

1. Kumar S, Krenacs L, Medeiros J, Elenitoba-Johnson KS, Greiner TC, Sorbara L, et al. Subcutaneous panniculitic T-cell lymphoma is a tumor of cytotoxic T lymphocytes. Hum Pathol 1998;29:397–403.
2. O'Riordan K, Blei A, Rao MS, Abecassis M. Alpha 1-antitrypsin deficiency-associated panniculitis: resolution with intravenous alpha 1-antitrypsin administration and liver transplantation. Transplant 1997;63: 480–482.
3. Caux F, Halimi C, Kevorkian JP, Pinquier L, Dubertret L, Segrestaa JM. Blind loop syndrome: an unusual cause of panniculitis. J Am Acad Dermatol 1997;37:824–827.
4. Disdier P, Andrac L, Swiader L, Veit V, Fuzibet JG, Weiller-Merli C, et al. Cutaneous panniculitis and relapsing polychondritis: two cases. Dermatology 1996;193:266–268.

Paracoccidioidomycosis

Synonyms: *Paracoccidioides brasiliensis* infection; South American blastomycosis.

NOTE: (1) Collect all tissues that appear to be infected. (2) Request fungal cultures. (3) Request Grocott's methenamine silver stain for fungi (p. 172). A simple KOH mount of exudate or pus will demonstrate the organism in a majority of cases. (4) No special precautions are indicated. (5) Serologic studies are available from the Centers for Disease Control and Prevention, Atlanta, GA (p. 135). (6) This is not a reportable disease.

Organs and Tissues	Procedures	Possible or Expected Findings
External examination with mouth and nose; lymph nodes	Record and photograph skin lesions. Submit sample of exudate for fungal culture, and prepare smears.	
	Record appearance of mouth, nose and conjunctivas; record site of primary lesion. Excise regional lymph nodes and submit for histologic study.	Mucosal ulcerations (mulberry-like) of mouth and nose; cutaneous verrucous or ulcerated lesions; regional lymph-adenopathy. See below under "Other organs..."
Lungs	Submit samples of consolidated lung tissue for culture (p. 103).	Consolidation; cavitation; fibrosis; bullae.
Gastrointestinal tract	Submit samples of all segments for histologic study; include sample of anorectal mucosa.	Stomach and intestines are common sites of primary infection. Suppurative, ulcerative, and granulomatous lesions may occur.
Other organs and tissues; nasal cavities	For exposure of nasal cavities, see p. 71.	Nasal cavities may be the site of the primary infection; hematogenous dissemination to any organ, including the central nervous system.

Paralysis Agitans (See "Disease, Parkinson's.")

Paralysis, Familial Periodic

Synonyms and Related Terms: Hyperkalemic (hypokalemic, normokalemic) periodic paralysis; myotonia, paramyotonia congenita.

Organs and Tissues	*Procedures*	*Possible or Expected Findings*
Skeletal muscles	For sampling and specimen preparation, see p. 80. Prepare samples for electron microscopy (p. 132).	Vacuolar myopathy.

Paralysis, Landry's Ascending (See "Syndrome, Guillain-Barré.")

Paralysis, Spinal (See name of suspected underlying condition, such as "Poliomyelitis" and "Sclerosis, multiple.")

Paresis, General (See "Syphilis, acquired.")

Parkinsonism, All Types or Type Unspecified (See "Disease, Parkinson's.")

Parotitis, Epidemic (See "Mumps.")

Patent ductus arteriosus (See "Artery, patent ductal.")

Pellagra

Related Terms: Niacin deficiency; tryptophan deficiency.

Possible Associated Conditions: Chronic alcoholism;* chronic peritoneal dialysis;* hemodialysis; other vitamin deficiencies; refeeding after starvation.*

Organs and Tissues	*Procedures*	*Possible or Expected Findings*
External examination, skin, oral cavity, and tongue	Record extent of skin and mucosal lesions, photograph, and prepare histologic sections of skin and tongue.	Dermatitis with dark pigmentation; cheilosis (angular stomatitis); stomatitis; glossitis; necrotizing ulcerative gingivitis with Vincent's organsims.
Esophagus	Photograph and sample for histologic study.	Esophagitis *(1)*.
Liver	Record weight and submit samples for histologic study.	Alcoholic cirrhosis.*
Gastrointestinal tract	Submit samples of all segments (with and without ulcers) for histologic study.	Proctocolitis with or without ulcers and perianal excoriations *(2)*.
Urethra and vagina	Submit samples for histologic study.	Urethritis and vaginitis.
Brain and spinal cord	For removal and specimen preparation, see pp. 65 and 67, respectively. Request Luxol fast blue stain for myelin (p. 172).	Degeneration of large pyramidal cells (Betz's cells) of motor cortex. Demyelination in posterior and lateral columns of spinal cord.

References

1. Segal I, Hale M, Demetriou A, Mohamed AE. Pathological effects of pellagra on the esophagus. Nutr Canc 1990;14: 233–238.
2. Segal I, Ou Tim L, Demetriou A, Paterson A, Hale M, Lerios M. Rectal manifestations of pellagra. Int J Colorect Dis 1986;1:238–243.

Pemphigus

Synonyms: Paraneoplastic pemphigus; pemphigus erythematosus; pemphigus foliaceus; pemphigus neonatorum; pemphigus vegetans; pemphigus vulgaris.

Possible Associated Conditions: Leukemia,* lymphoma,* and other neoplastic disorders associated with paraneoplastic pemphigus *(1)*.

Organs and Tissues	*Procedures*	*Possible or Expected Findings*
External examination, skin, and mouth	Record extent of skin lesions; photograph; submit multiple samples for histologic study, preferably of areas that are free of secondary infection.	Bullous and other lesions of scalp, eyelids, nose, axillae, umbilicus, inframammary areas, back, hands, groins, genitalia, anus, knees, and feet. Similar lesions may occur in the mouth. Acantholysis is suprabasal or near granular layer.
	Prepare sections for immunofluorescent staining.	IgG deposits on the surfaces of keratinocytes.

Organs and Tissues	*Procedures*	*Possible or Expected Findings*
Blood	Submit sample for culture (p. 102).	Septicemia.
Heart	For histologic sampling, see p. 30.	Focal myocarditis.
Lungs	Submit one lobe for microbiologic study (p. 103).	Bronchopneumonia; thromboemboli after steroid therapy.
Esophagus	Sample for histologic study.	May be involved in pemphigus vulgaris *(2)*.
Kidneys and urinary bladder		Urinary tract infection.
Adrenal glands	Record weights; record appearance of cortex.	Cortical lipid depletion.
Neck organs	Sample for histologic study.	Pemphigus lesions of mucosa of pharynx and larynx.
Bones	For removal, prosthetic repair, and specimen preparation, see p. 95.	Osteoporosis* after steroid therapy.
Brain, spinal cord, and spinal ganglia	For removal and specimen preparation, see pp. 65, 67, and 69, respectively.	Degenerative changes in brain, spinal cord, and spinal ganglia.
Eyes	For removal and specimen preparation, see p. 85.	Pemphigus lesions of conjunctivas. Invasion of conjunctivas by connective tissue; possible conjunctival shrinkage.

References

1. Anhalt GJ. Paraneoplastic pemphigus. Adv Dermatol 1997;12:77–96.
2. Amichai B, Grunwald MH, Gasper N, Finkelstein E, Halevy S. A case of pemphigus vulgaris with esophageal involvement. J Dermatol 1996;23: 214–215.

Periarteritis Nodosa (See "Polyarteritis nodosa.")

Pericarditis

Organs and Tissues	*Procedures*	*Possible or Expected Findings*
External examination	Prepare chest roentgenogram.	Pericardial calcification; effusion.
Pleural cavities	If there are pleural exudates, follow procedures described below.	Pleuritis.
Pericardial sac	Aspirate exudate and submit for microbiologic study (p. 102). Record volume of pericardial fluid. Centrifuge fluid and prepare smear or section of pellet. Request Gram, Grocott's methenamine silver, and auramine-rhodamine stains (p. 172).	Infective pericarditis (pyogenic, tuberculous, or other bacterial infection; fungal or viral infection). (Gram-negative bacilli, *Staphylococcus aureus*, *Streptococcus*, and *Pneumococcus*.)
	If there is extensive calcification, see under "Syndrome, Budd-Chiari."	Constrictive pericarditis (idiopathic; irradiation; tuberculous; postoperative).
Blood	Submit sample for microbiologic study (p. 102).	Septicemia.
Heart	Histologic samples should include epicardium, pericardium, and myocardium.	Old or recent heart surgery; myocardial infarction.
	For coronary arteriography, see p. 118.	Coronary atherosclerosis with stenosis.
Other organs	Procedures depend on expected findings or grossly identified abnormalities as listed in right-hand column.	Neoplasm; trauma; manifestations of kidney failure* with uremia or of rheumatic fever;* sternal osteomyelitis (postoperative wound infection); rheumatoid arthritis* *(1)*; lupus erythematosus,* and other autoimmune diseases.

Reference

1. McRorie ER, Wright RA, Errington ML, Lugmani RA. Rheumatoid constrictive pericarditis (clinical conference). Br J Rheumatol 1997;36:100–103.

Peritonitis, Benign Paroxysmal (See "Fever, familial Mediterranean.")

Peritonitis, Infectious

NOTE: (1) Collect all tissues that appear to be infected. (2) Request aerobic, anaerobic, acid-fast, and fungal cultures. (3) Request Gram, Grocott's methenamine silver, and Kinyoun's stains (p. 172). (4) No special precautions are indicated. (5) Serologic studies are not available. (6) This is not a reportable disease.

Organs and Tissues	*Procedures*	*Possible or Expected Findings*
External examination	Prepare chest and abdominal roentgenograms.	Extraintestinal gas after perforation of hollow viscus; foreign body.
Vitreous	Request determination of sodium, chloride, and urea nitrogen concentrations (p. 85).	Manifestations of severe dehydration.*
Abdominal cavity	Aspirate fluid and submit for culture, particularly if cloudy.	Acute bacterial peritonitis (rarely, other infective agents); bile or chemical peritonitis.
	If cause of acute peritonitis is unknown, inspect *in situ* all intraperitoneal, pelvic, and extraperitoneal organs. If abscess is present, record location, size, and volume. Submit portion for culture.	Possible causes include appendicitis, colitis, diverticulitis, enteritis, infarction, peptic ulcer, trauma, tumor, surgical complication and pelvic disease (for instance, after attempted abortion).
	Absence of causative lesions must be documented.	Primary peritonitis, most commonly in female children.
	If exudate is milky, lymphangiography may be indicated (p. 34).	Chylous ascites.
Blood	Submit sample for aerobic, anaerobic, and fungal cultures (p. 102).	Septicemia.

Pertussis

Synonyms: *Bordatella pertussis* infection; whooping cough.

NOTE: (1) Collect all tissues that appear to be infected. (2) Request culture for *Bordatella*, as well as aerobic and anaerobic cultures. Special medium is required (see below) (3) Request Gram stain (p. 172). (4) No special precautions are indicated. (5) Serologic studies are not available in most institutions. (6) This is a **reportable** disease.

Organs and Tissues	*Procedures*	*Possible or Expected Findings*
External examination	Record body weight and length. If diagnosis had not been confirmed, prepare nasopharyngeal swabs, and culture immediately on Bordet-Gengou medium.	Manifestations of malnutrition;* petechiae, especially on face; scleral hemorrhages.
	Prepare chest roentgenogram.	Pneumothorax.*
Cerebrospinal fluid	Culture on Bordet-Gengou medium (p. 104).	Infectious meningitis.*
Blood	Submit sample for culture (p. 102) and above under "Note".	Septicemia.
Lungs	Submit one lobe for culture (see p. 103 and above under "Note"). Prepare Gram-stained smears from fresh cut section; perfuse one lung with formalin (p. 47).	Localized or interstitial pulmonary emphysema; atelectasis.
	Prepare histologic sections of bronchi, bronchioli, and pulmonary parenchyma.	Bronchitis; bronchiolitis; bronchopneumonia.
Neck organs and trachea	Prepare histologic sections of pharynx, larynx, and trachea.	Aspiration of vomitus; pharyngitis; laryngitis;* tracheitis.
Brain	For removal and specimen preparation, see p. 65.	Serous meningitis;* anoxic encephalopathy; epidural hematoma; petechial hemorrhages.
Middle ears	For removal and specimen preparation, see p. 72.	Bacterial otitis media.*

Pesticide (See "Poisoning, organophosphate(s).")

Phenylketonuria

NOTE: See also under "Aminoaciduria."

Organs and Tissues	*Procedures*	*Possible or Expected Findings*
Blood	If diagnosis had not been confirmed, submit plasma from a heparinized blood sample for ion-exchange test.	Hyperphenylalaninemia.
Urine	See above under "Blood."	Phenylketonuria. Urine may have a "mousy" odor.
Brain and spinal cord	For removal and specimen preparation, see pp. 65 and 67, respectively. Record brain weight. Request Luxol fast blue stain for myelin. Fresh material should be used for Sudan stain for fat (p. 173).	Microcephaly; delayed neuronal and myelin maturation; demyelinization with sudanophilic gitter cells; normal grey matter.

Pheochromocytoma (See "Tumor of the adrenal gland(s).")

Phlebitis

Related Terms: Migratory phlebitis; phlebothrombosis; phlegmasia alba dolens; phlegmasia cerulea dolens; thrombophlebitis migrans,* Trousseau's syndrome; venous thrombosis.*

NOTE: A clear distinction between phlebothrombosis and thrombophlebitis generally cannot be made.

Organs and Tissues	*Procedures*	*Possible or Expected Findings*
External examination	Describe discoloration of extremities, swelling or palpable venous lesions. Compare leg circumferences (measure above and below knees).	Stasis dermatitis of legs; varicous veins; gangrene of toes.
Lungs		Pulmonary embolism.*
Other organs	If systemic emboli and infarctions are present, record whether oval foramen was patent and whether there were other lesions with possible right-to-left shunt.	Paradoxic embolism. Carcinoma of pancreas, lung, stomach, colon, kidney, or other organs. Arteritis. Nonbacterial thrombotic endocarditis.*
Veins and arteries	For postmortem phlebography and ateriography, see p. 120. For removal of femoral vessels, see p. 34. If gangrene is present, demonstrate absence of concomitant arterial occlusion.	Thromboses are likely to be found (in decreasing order of frequency) in small saphenous veins, deep veins of calves, iliofemoral veins, great saphenous veins, superficial veins and varices of legs, and veins of arms. Other sites are rarely involved.

Phlegmasia Alba (or Cerulea) Dolens (See "Phlebitis.")

Phosgene ($COCl_2$) (See "Poisoning, gas.")

Phosphate Ester (Insecticide) (See "Poisoning, organophosphate(s).")

Phosphorus (See "Disorder, electrolyte(s)" or "Poisoning, phosphorus.")

Phycomycosis (See "Mucormycosis.")

Plague

Synonym: *Yersinia (Pasteurella) pestis* infection; Black Death; bubonic plague.

NOTE: (1) Collect all tissues that appear to be infected. (2) Request aerobic bacterial cultures. (3) Request Gram stain (p. 122). (4) Special **precautions** are indicated, as this is a highly communicable disease (p. 146). (5) Serologic studies are available from the Centers for Disease Control and Prevention, Atlanta, GA (p. 135). (6) This is a **reportable** disease.

Organs and Tissues	*Procedures*	*Possible or Expected Findings*
External examination and skin	Photograph and record extent of hemorrhages. Prepare histologic sections of skin.	Petechial and other types of hemorrhages in skin and subcutaneous tissues.
Blood	Submit sample for microbiologic (see p. 102) and above under "Note") and serologic study. Prepare smear and stain with Wright-Giemsa (p. 173).	Septicemia; bipolar staining rods.

Organs and Tissues	Procedures	Possible or Expected Findings
Lymph nodes	Collect inguinal, popliteal, axillary, and supraclavicular lymph nodes for aerobic culture. Photograph enlarged lymph nodes, and prepare smears of fresh cut surfaces.	Hemorrhagic necrosis; variable suppuration.
Lungs	Submit consolidated areas for microbiologic study (see p. 103 and above under "Note"). Perfuse both lungs with formalin (p. 47). Submit samples of pulmonary tissue and bronchial lymph nodes for histologic study.	Severe hemorrhagic edema; pneumonia with lobular to lobar features.
Other organs	Submit samples of grossly abnormal organs, exudates, or drainage fluids for culture and Gram stain.	Large areas of necrosis teeming with organisms and minimal to suppurative inflammation.

Plasmacytoma (See "Myeloma, multiple.")

Platybasia

NOTE: Possible causes or associated conditions include Arnold-Chiari malformation;* basilar impression* or invagination; fusion of atlas to the foramen magnum; Klippel-Feil syndrome;* malpositioning of odontoid process; osteitis deformans (Paget's disease of bone*); osteogenesis imperfecta;* osteomalacia;* rickets; syringobulbia, syringomyelia.*

Organs and Tissues	Procedures	Possible or Expected Findings
Skull and spine	Prepare roentgenograms of skull and cervical spine.	Flattening of the base of the skull (angle formed by the plane of the clivus and the plane of the anterior fossa exceeds 135°).

Pleuritis (See "Effusion(s) and exudate(s), pleural.")

Pleurodynia, epidemic

Synonyms: Bornholm disease; devil's grip; epidemic myalgia; epidemic myositis.

Organs and Tissues	Procedures	Possible or Expected Findings
Blood	Submit samples for viral culture (p. 102).	Coxsackie B virus infection.
Heart and pericardium	Sample for histologic study (p. 30) and for viral cultures (Coxsackievirus A and B; echoviruses). If pericardial fluid can be obtained, submit for viral culture also (p. 102). Cultures may be negative and search for viral RNA by *in situ* hybridization may be indicated.	Myocarditis* may be associated with Coxsackievirus B infection; may be rapidly fatal in infants.

Pneumatosis Cystoides Intestinalis

NOTE: Some potential causes such as steroid, chemo- or immunosuppressive therapy may not be apparent at autopsy.

Possible Associated Conditions: Acquired immunodeficiency syndrome* (AIDS) *(1)*; amyloidosis* *(2)*; primary combined immunodeficiency *(3)*; progressive systemic sclerosis;* organ or bone marrow *(4)* transplantation.*

Organs and Tissues	*Procedures*	*Possible or Expected Findings*
Abdomen	Expose serosal surfaces. Record location and size of cysts.	Gas cysts in stomach, small bowel, colon, mesentery, omentum, gastrohepatic ligament, gallbladder, retroperitoneal tissues, and renal capsule.
Chest organs	Dissect thoracic duct and its tributaries (see p. 34). Perfuse one or both lungs with formalin (p. 47).	Gas in thoracic duct. Emphysema* of lungs.
Gastrointestinal tract	Procedures depend on expected findings or grossly identified abnormalities as listed in right-hand column.	Necrotizing enterocolitis in premature infants. Pyloric stenosis, colitis *(5)*, redundant sigmoid colon, ischemic bowel disease. Mucosal pseudolipomatosis *(6)*.
	Submit samples of cystic lesions for histologic study.	Usually, cysts are subserosal in adults and located between muscularis mucosae and muscularis propria in infants and children. Mucosa may be inflamed.
Other organs	Submit samples of cystic lesions for histologic study.	Extraintestinal cysts, as listed above under "Abdomen." Cysts may also occur in vaginal mucosa.

References

1. Cunnion KM. Pneumatosis intestinalis in pediatric acquired immunodeficiency syndrome. Pediatr Inf Dis J 1998;17:355–356.
2. Pearson DC, Price LM, Urbanski S. Pneumatosis cystoides intestinalis: an unusual complication of systemic amyloidosis. J Clin Gastroenterol 1996;22:74–76.
3. Tang ML, Williams LW. Pneumatosis intestinalis in children with primary combined immunodeficiency. J Pediatr 1998;132:546–549.
4. Takanashi M, Hibi S, Todo S, Sawada T, Tsunamoto K, Imashaku S. Pneumatosis cystoides intestinalis with abdominal free air in a 2-year-old girl after allogeneic bone marrow transplantation. Pediatr Hematol Oncol 1998;15:81–84.
5. Pear BL. Pneumatosis intestinalis: a review. Radiol 1998;207:13–19.
6. Gagliardi G, Thompson IW, Hershman MJ, Forbes A, Hawley PR, Talbot IC. Pneumatosis coli: a proposed pathogenesis based on study of 25 cases and review of the literature. Intl J Colorect Dis 1996;11: 111–118.

Pneumoconiosis

Etiologic Types of Pneumoconiosis (With typical Examples): Collagenous inorganic dust pneumoconiosis, diffuse type: Aluminosis; asbestosis; chronic pulmonary berylliosis; talcosis; Collagenous inorganic dust pneumoconiosis, nodular type: Silicosis; Noncollagenous inorganic dust pneumoconiosis (includes mixed-dust fibrosis): Baritosis; China clay pneumoconiosis; chromite pneumoconiosis; coal worker's pneumoconiosis; fuller's earth pneumoconiosis; hematite or magnetite miner's lung; siderosis or welder's lung; stannosis; Organic dust pneumoconiosis: Byssinosis.

NOTE: In addition to the aforementioned classic forms of pneumoconiosis, many other airborne substances have been implicated in recent years, for example, cerium, manmade vitreous fibers, polyvinyl chloride, silicon carbide, and titanium *(1)*.

Chemical analysis of large samples of digested tissue is best suited for quantitative studies, particularly of trace substances. If only small tissue samples are available and if individual particles are to be analyzed and correlated with histologic lesions, *in situ* microanalysis must be done. Methods used include brightfield and polarized light microscopy, transmission electron microscopy, scanning or transmission electron microscopy with energy dispersive X-ray analysis *(2)* (p. 133), ion beam instrumentation, and secondary ion mass spectrometry. The last three methods are time-consuming, require much skill and expensive equipment, and do not lend themselves well to quantitation. Ideally, bulk analysis and *in situ* microanalysis should be used in combination. See also p. 52.

Analyses can be conducted in specialized laboratories at the following centers (for charges and other information, consult the appropriate laboratories):

Georgia Institute
of Technology
225 North Ave. N.W.
Atlanta, GA 30332

Medical University
of South Carolina
80 Barre St.
Charleston, SC 29401

Mount Sinai Hospital
5th Ave. E. 100th
New York, NY 10029

University of Utah
1400 East 2nd South
Salt Lake City, UT 84112

National Institute for
Occupational Safety & Health
Robert A. Taft Laboratories
4676 Columbia Parkway
Cincinnati, OH 45226

National Institute for
Occupational Safety & Health
1095 Willowdale Road
Morgantown, WV 26505

University of Wisconsin
3203 N. Downer
Milwaukee, WI 53201

An appropriate National Registry, "Pulmonary and Mediastinal Pathology," is located in the Armed Forces Institute of Pathology, Washington, DC (see p. 148).

Organs and Tissues	Procedures	Possible or Expected Findings
External examination		Clubbing of fingers.
	Prepare chest roentgenogram.	Diffuse or nodular pulmonary infiltrates.
Blood	Submit sample for microbiologic study (p. 102).	
	Refrigerate sample for possible immunologic study.	Rheumatoid factor in Caplan's syndrome.* Positive in vitro lymphocyte transformation test in berylliosis *(3)*.
Lungs	Submit one lobe or samples of all lobes for bulk analysis and for in situ microanalysis (see above under "Note"). Microincineration may permit preliminary dust analysis. For demonstration of asbestos fibers, see p. 52 and ref. *(4)*.	Large amounts of dust (up to 20 g) in coal worker's pneumoconiosis and other noncollagenous inorganic dust pneumoconioses. Small amounts of dust in silicosis (5–6 g).
	Submit one lobe or segment for microbiologic study.	Tuberculosis* (including infection with atypical mycobacteria *[5]*).
	For pulmonary arteriography and bronchography, see p. 50.	
	Prepare roentgenograms of entire lungs and slices. Perfuse one lung (or both, if only routine studies are intended) with formalin (p. 47). Submit samples for histologic study of nodular dust lesions, diffuse fibrotic lesions, grossly uninvolved areas, bronchi, and bronchopulmonary lymph nodes.	Asbestosis may be associated with pleural mesothelioma (see "Tumor, of the pleural") and carcinoma of lung (see "Tumor, of the lung or bronchus"). In silicotic lungs, squamous cell or small cell carcinomas are rather common *(6)*.
	For preparation of paper-mounted sections, see p. 49.	Chronic bronchitis.* Coniosis of lymph nodes.
	Prepare samples for transmission and scanning electron microscopic study (see p. 132)	Particle identification.
Joints	For removal, prosthetic repair, and specimen preparation, see p. 96.	Arthritis in Caplan's syndrome.*

References

1. Gong H Jr. Uncommon causes of occupational interstitial lung diseases. Curr Opin Pulm Med 1996;2:405–411.
2. McDonald JW, Ghio AJ, Sheehan CE, Bernhardt PF, Roggli VL. Rare earth (cerium oxide) pneumoconiosis: analytical scanning electron microscopy and literature review. Mod Pathol 1995;8:859–865.
3. Williams WJ. Diagnostic criteria for chronic beryllium disease (CBD) based on the UK registry 1945–1991. Sarcoidosis 1993;10:41–43.
4. King JA, Wong SW. Autopsy evaluation of asbestos exposure: retrospective study of 135 cases with quantitation of ferruginous bodies in digested lung tissue. South Med J 1996;89:380–385.
5. De Coster C, Verstraeten JM, Dumortier P, De Vuyst P. Atypical mycobacteriosis as a complication of talc pneumoconiosis. Eur Respir J 1996;9:1757–1759.
6. Honma K, Chiyotani K, Kimura K. Silicosis, mixed dust pneumoconiosis, and lung cancer. Am J Ind Med 1997;32:595–599.

Pneumocystis Carinii (See "Infection, Pneumocystis carinii.")

Pneumomediastinum

NOTE: This condition is diagnosed by inspection, palpation, and roentgenography. Tension pneumomediastinum may compromise venous return to the heart and may compress major bronchi. The condition is rapidly fatal and occurs after alveolar rupture with dissection of air into the mediastinum in neonates with respiratory distress (see "Syndrome, respiratory distress, of infant") and in adult patients ventilated on volume respirators.

Organs and Tissues	Procedures	Possible or Expected Findings
External examination	Prepare chest roentgenogram.	Roentgenograms provide the best permanent record of a pneumomediastinum.
Chest cavity	Photograph mediastinum. Explore major veins and record compression in cases of tension pneumomediatinum.	Air bubbles in mediastinal soft tissues.

Organs and Tissues	*Procedures*	*Possible or Expected Findings*
Lungs and mediastinum	Perfuse one lung with formalin (p. 47). Other procedures depend on expected findings or grossly identified abnormalities as listed in right-hand column.	Intubation injury *(1)*; perforation or rupture of major bronchus, trachea, or esophagus. Alveolar rupture, e.g., in asthma* *(2)*, may not be discernible. Bronchiolitis obliterans *(3)*, interstitial pneumonia* *(4)* and other lung conditions also may lead to pneumomediastinum.
Abdomen and neck organs	Search for evidence of trauma of other lesions that may have allowed air to enter soft tissues.	Dissection of air from lesions in abdomen (e.g., retroperitoneal colonic perforation *[5]*) or in neck area.

References

1. Vezina D, Lessard MR, Bussieres J, Topping C, Trepanier CA. Complications associated with the use of the Esophageal-Tracheal Combitube. Can J Anaesth 1998;45:76–80.
2. Van der Klooster JM, Grootendorst AF, Ophof PJ, Brouwers JW. Pneumomediastinum: an unusual complication of asthma in a young man. Netherl J Med 1998;52:150–154.
3. Galanis E, Litzow MR, Tefferi A, Scott JP. Spontaneous pneumomediastinum in a patient with bronchiolitis obliterans after bone marrow transplantation. Bone Marrow Transpl 1997;20:695–696.
4. Nagai Y, Ishikawa O, Miyachi Y. Pneumomediastinum and subcutaneous emphysema associated with fatal interstitial pneumonia in dermatomyositis. J Dermatol 1997;24:484–484.
5. Alvares JF, Dhawan PS, Tibrewala S, Shankaran K, Kulkarni SG, Rananavare R, et al. Retroperitoneal perforation in ulcerative colitis with mediastinal and subcutaneous emphysema. J Clin Gastroenterol 1997;453–455.

Pneumonia, All Types or Type Unspecified

NOTE: If the type of underlying infection is known, follow procedures suggested under the name of the infectious disease. If the etiologic agent of the pneumonia is unknown, proceed as follows: (1) Collect all tissues that appear to be infected. (2) Request aerobic, anaerobic, acid-fast, fungal, and viral cultures. (3) Request Gram, Kinyoun's acid-fast, and Grocott's methenamine silver stains (p. 172). (4) Special **precautions may be required** (p. 146). (5) Serologic studies may be helpful once a specific etiologic agent is suspected. Thus, collect serum at the time of autopsy or procure serum that was collected prior to death. (6) This **may be a reportable** disease.

Organs and Tissues	*Procedures*	*Possible or Expected Findings*
External examination		Herpes labialis; pyoderma; jaundice.
	Prepare chest roentgenogram.	Pneumothorax* or pneumatocele (in staphylococcal pneumonia of infancy); pleural effusions;* pulmonary infiltrates; abscesses.
Abdomen	Photograph abnormalities *in situ.*	Gastric dilatation and ileus; rarely, peritonitis.*
Pleural cavities	Puncture; submit samples of fluid for culture (p. 102).	Fibrinous pleuritis; pleural effusions and exudates.*
Blood	Submit sample for culture (p. 102).	Septicemia.
Heart	If infective endocarditis is suspected, follow procedures described on p. 103.	Infective endocarditis;* pericarditis.*
Lungs	Record weights. Submit consolidated areas for culture (p. 103). Prepare touch preps of fresh cut sections. Perfuse lungs with formalin (p. 47). For special stains, see above under "Note."	Bacterial, fungal, viral, or protozoal pneumonia; abscesses (*Staphylococcus aureus*) or hemorrhages (influenza, infection with *Pseudomonas* spp., and others). See also under name of suspected underlying infectious disease or underlying noninfectious disorder, such as rheumatoid arthritis.* Perifocal pneumonia around tumors.
	For bronchography, see p. 50.	Bronchiectasis;* bronchial obstruction.

Organs and Tissues	Procedures	Possible or Expected Findings
Mediastinum and neck organs	Submit samples of larynx, trachea, and major bronchi for histologic study.	Laryngotracheitis and tracheobronchitis.
Arteries and veins	For removal of femoral veins and arteries, see p. 34.	Infective vasculitis and thrombosis.
Brain and spinal cord	For appropriate microbiologic study, see p. 102.	Meningitis.*
Joints	For removal, prosthetic repair, and specimen preparation, see p. 96.	Rarely, septic arthritis.

Pneumonia, Eosinophilic
(See "Syndrome, eosinophilic pulmonary.")

Pneumonia, Interstitial

Related Terms: Acute interstitial pneumonia (Hamman-Rich syndrome); desquamative interstitial pneumonia (DIP); idiopathic organizing pneumonia (or "bronchiolitis obliterans with patchy organizing pneumonia [BOOP]" or "cryptogenic organizing pneumonitis"); idiopathic pulmonary fibrosis; lymphoid interstitial pneumonitis (LIP); nonspecific interstitial pneumonia (NSIP) (or "cellular interstitial pneumonia" [CIP]); usual interstitial pneumonia (UIP); fibrosing alveolitis; pulmonary alveolitis; and many others.

NOTE: The conditions listed under "Related Terms" are histologic variants of idiopathic interstitial pneumonia. UIP is synonymous with idiopathic pulmonary fibrosis (IPF) *(1)*. Diffuse alveolar damage is the histologic finding in patients with the adult respiratory distress syndrome* (ARDS) causing interstitial and intra-alveolar fibrosis. This is an acute condition, referred to as acute interstitial pneumonia when it occurs as an idiopathic form of rapidly progressive interstitial pneumonia.

Possible Associated Conditions: Acquired immunodeficiency syndrome* (AIDS) in patients with with LIP or nonspecific interstitial pneumonia *(2,3)*; trauma and shock in ARDS. Secondary pulmonary fibrosis from inhalants (extrinsic allergic alveolitis or pneumonia; pneumoconiosis*), in drug-induced pneumonia, hypersensitivity pneumonitis (microgranulomatous hypersensitivity reaction of lung), rheumatoid arthritis,* Sjögren's syndrome,* and other collagen-vascular diseases; primary biliary cirrhosis in patients with nonspecific interstitial pneumonia *(2)*.

Organs and Tissues	Procedures	Possible or Expected Findings
External examination	Prepare chest roentgenogram.	Clubbing of fingers. Distribution of densities may be important for determining the specific type of the condition. Pleural effusions.
Blood	Submit sample for bacterial, fungal, and viral cultures (p. 102) and protein electrophoresis. Snap-freeze sample for possible serologic studies.	Underlying or superimposed infections. Dysproteinemia in LIP *(2)*.
Lungs with hilar lymph nodes	Record weights and photograph both lungs. Submit one lobe for viral, bacterial, and fungal cultures (p. 102). Make touch preparations from cut surfaces. Leave one lung intact and perfuse with formalin (p. 47). For barium sulfate impregnation, see p. 47. Request Gram and Grocott's methenamine silver for microorganisms, and Verhoeff–van Gieson or other special stains to identify collagen and smooth muscle fibers (p. 172).	Interstitial pulmonary fibrosis, often with interstitial inflammatory infiltrates, alveolar edema, Masson bodies, and bronchiolitis obliterans. Minute noncaseating granulomas in extrinsic allergic alveolitis *(4)* and large granulomas in sarcoidosis.* Diffuse aggregates of lightly pigmented macrophages in DIP. Hyaline membranes in diffuse alveolar damage. LIP may be difficult to separate from lymphoma, with or without evidence of Epstein-Barr virus DNA *(2)*.
	Prepare samples of fresh lung for electron microscopy (see p. 132).	Tubuloreticular structures and electron-dense deposits in systemic lupus erythematosus;* identification of viruses, *Pneumocystis,* or particles in pneumoconiosis *(5)*.
	Prepare sections of hilar lymph nodes.	Granulomas in sarcoidosis.*
Other organs		Manifestations of conditions listed above under Possible Associated Conditions."

References

1. Katzenstein A-L, Myers J. Idiopathic pulmonary fibrosis: clinical relevance of pathologic classification. Am J Respir Crit Care Med 1998; 157:1301–1315.
2. Fishback N, Koss M. Update on lymphoid interstitial pneumonitis. Curr Opin Pulm Med 1996;2:429–433.
3. Schneider RF. Lymphocytic interstitial pneumonitis and nonspecific interstitial pneumonitis. Clin Chest Med 1996;17:763–766.
4. Coleman A, Colby TV: Histologic diagnosis of extrinsic allergic alveolitis. Am J Surg Pathol 1988;12:514–518.
5. Panchal A, Koss MN. Role of electron microscopy in interstitial lung disease. Curr Opin Pulm Med 1997;3:341–347.

Pneumonia, Lipoid

Related Terms: Exogenous lipoid pneumonia; inhalation lipoid pneumonia; lipid pneumonia; mineral oil pneumonia.

Organs and Tissues	*Procedures*	*Possible or Expected Findings*
Lungs	Submit one lobe for microbiologic study (p. 102). For bronchography, see p. 50. Dissect bronchial tree to demonstrate absence of bronchial obstruction. For formalin perfusion of lung, see p. 47. Request Verhoeff–van Gieson, Gram, and Kinyoun's stains (p. 172).	Saprophytic growth of acid-fast mycobacteria or, rarely, fungi *(1)*. Lipoid or liquid paraffin granulomas; foreign-body granulomas; endarteritis obliterans; pulmonary fibrosis. In rare instances, evidence of hemoptysis *(2)*.
Other organs	Procedures depend on expected findings or grossly identified abnormalities as listed in right-hand column.	Achalasia of esophagus* and other chronic esophageal or laryngopharyngeal diseases, including carcinoma. Hypertrophic pyloric stenosis. Parkinson's disease* or other chronic cerebrovascular and neurologic diseases.
Bones and joints		Rheumatoid arthritis.* Hypertrophic osteoarthropathy* may be a rare complication *(3)*.

References

1. Jouannic I, Desrues B, Lena H, Quinquenel ML, Donnio PY, Delaval P. Exogenous lipoid pneumonia complicated by Mycobacterium fortuitum and Aspergillus fumigatus infection. Eur Respir J 1996;9:172–174.
2. Haro M, Murcia I, Nunez A, Julia E, Valer J. Massive haemoptysis complicating exogenous lipid pneumonia. Eur Respir J 1998;11:507–508.
3. Hugosson C, Bahabri S, Rifai A, al-Dalaan A. Hypertrophic osteoarthropathy caused by lipoid pneumonia. Pediatr Radiol 1995;25:482–483.

Pneumothorax

Postmortem chest roentgenograms provide the only reliable and permanent record of a pneumothorax and its main complication, mediastinal shift due to a tension pneumothorax (Fig. II-4). If roentgenograms cannot be prepared, a reasonably reliable diagnosis still can be made if the prosector inserts a needle through the lateral chest wall. The needle should be connected to a water-filled flask. If a pneumothorax is present, gas bubbles appear in the flask as shown in Fig. II-5. One can also expose the intact parietal pleura and observe if the lung tissue is separated from the parietal pleura by gas. Incising the thorax at the base of a water-filled skin pocket is the least reliable method.

Infants can be totally submerged under water before the chest cavity is incised. However, care must be taken not to make an accidental incision into the underlying lung tissue.

Poisoning, All Types or Type Unspecified

NOTE: If a specific substance is suspected—for instance, arsenic or ethylene glycol—follow procedures described under the appropriate entry. Similar entries can be found for poisons whose general character or source is known—for instance, gas or mushroom poisoning. For some substances, the appropriate entry can be found under "Abuse,...," "Death,...," or "Dependence,..." In all instances, routine sampling of toxicologic material should be done as described in pp. 14–17. If no specific substances can be incriminated, the toxicologist must be provided with all available clinical information, as shown in Chapter 2.

In most cases of fatal poisoning, the coroner or medical examiner must be notified.

Poisoning, Alkaloid

NOTE: See under specific name of alkaloid—for instance, "Dependence, cocaine," "Poisoning, atropine," "Poisoning, digitalis," or "Poisoning, strychnine." Only a fraction of this large group of plant poisons has been listed. Whether the specific name of the alkaloid is known or unknown, complete toxicologic sampling (p. 16) is recommended.

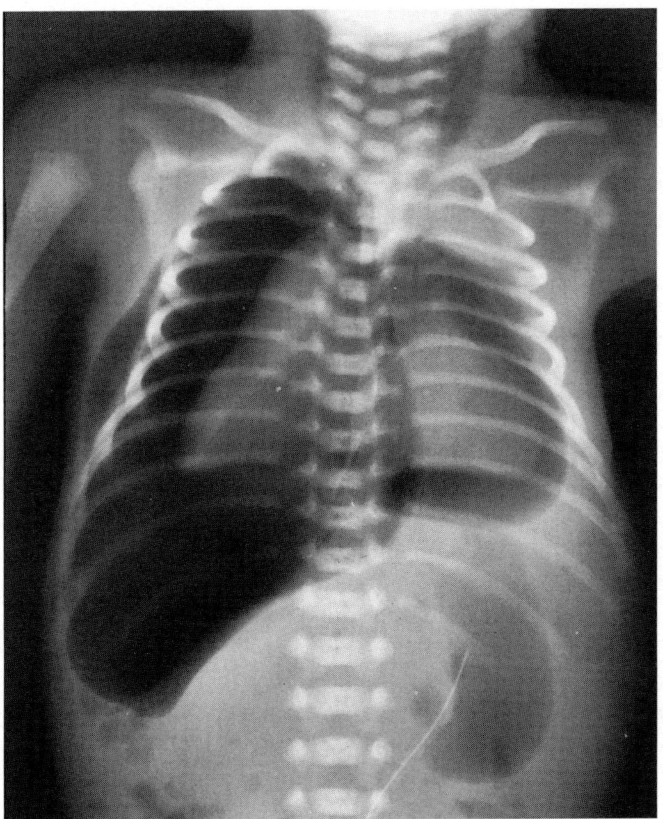

Fig. II-4. Tension pneumothorax. This premature newborn (26 wk gestation) had been intubated but died suddenly because of a pneumothorax on the left and a tension pneumothorax on the right. Pneumomediastinum was also present. These complications had not been recognized prior to death.

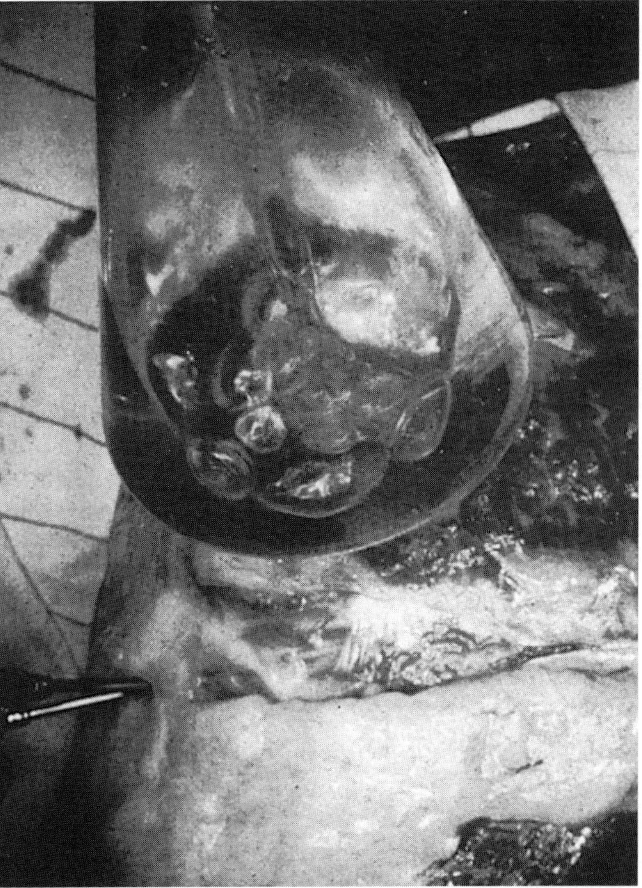

Fig. II-5. Tension pneumothorax. Skin has been dissected off right side of chest, and needle is inserted into chest wall. Rubber hose connects needle with glass tube. Note gas bubbles emerging from tip of glass tube at bottom of water-filled flask.

Poisoning, Ammonia

NOTE: The appropriate autopsy procedures are described under "Bronchitis, acute chemical" and under "Poisoning, gas." Blood ammonia concentrations are markedly increased. Formalin perfusion of lungs is not recommended; it may cause artifactual ballooning and internal ruptures of organ.

Poisoning, Antifreeze (See "Poisoning, ethylene glycol.")

Poisoning, Antimony

NOTE: Toxicologic material should be submitted for analysis, as suggested under "Poisoning, arsenic." Iatrogenic antimony toxicity may occur after treatment with antimony compounds for conditions such as filariasis, fungal infections, and schistosomiasis.*

Organs and Tissues	*Procedures*	*Possible or Expected Findings*
External examination and eyes	Record skin changes and eye abnormalities.	If exposure was from dust in smelting work, dermatitis and conjunctivitis may be present.
Pharynx and gastrointestinal tract	For toxicologic sampling of contents, see p. 16. Submit tissue samples for histologic study.	Severe gastroenteritis in acute poisoning. If victim drank antimony trichloride, ulcerative pharyngitis and gastritis may be present.
Heart, liver, and kidneys	Request frozen sections for Sudan stain (p. 173).	Fatty changes of myocardium and hepatic and renal parenchyma.

Poisoning, Arsenic

NOTE: Toxicologic material will be contaminated by bringing it in contact with fluids. Keratinized tissues take up arsenic from solutions. Put plastic bags over hands of victim.

If exhumed bodies are investigated for arsenic poisoning, include material from surrounding soil and coffin along with tissues submitted for chemical analysis.

Interpretation of toxicologic findings: After fatal poisoning, arsenic concentrations in the liver tend to exceed 0.5–1.0 mg/100 g wet tissue. In acute poisoning, arsenic concentrations in hair may reach 3 μg/g *(1)* and in nails 8 μg/g. Intervals between ingestion of a fatal dose of arsenic and death are given in Fig. 2-1, p. 15.

Organs and Tissues	*Procedures*	*Possible or Expected Findings*
External examination and skin	Pull (do not cut) 10 g of hair from scalp and tie in locks with cotton. The ends with the hair roots should be identified. Collect some whole fingernails and toenails. Collect skin for toxicologic study (p. 17). Record findings as listed in right-hand column; prepare photographs.	In chronic poisoning—manifestations of malnutrition,* alopecia, hyperpigmentation, eczematoid skin changes, hyperkeratosis of plantar and palmar surfaces, and white streaks (Mee's lines) on fingernails.
Blood	Submit sample for toxicologic study (p. 16). Prepare smear.	Basophilic stippling; immature cells.
Heart	For histologic sampling, see p. 30. Prepare frozen section of myocardium and request Sudan stain for fat.	Subendocardial ventricular hemorrhages; fatty changes and round cell infiltrates of myocardium; myocardial infarction.
Arteries	Request Verhoeff–van Gieson stain (p. 173) of samples from skin, heart, stomach, intestine, mesentery, liver, pancreas, spleen, and kidney.	Intimal thickening in chronic poisoning of infants.
Stomach	Submit all contents for toxicologic analysis (p. 16). Inspect wall with magnifying glass for identification of crystals.	Acute gastritis (in acute poisoning) with arsenous sulfide crystals in mucus coating wall of stomach.
Intestinal tract	Submit contents (feces) for toxicologic study (p. 16).	Congestion and inflammation of mucous membranes.
Liver	Record weight. Submit (together with bile) for toxicologic study (p. 16). Submit samples for histolgic study.	Cirrhosis. Fatty changes.
Kidneys	Submit samples for histologic study.	Fatty changes. Tubulo-interstitial nephritis *(2)*.
Urine	Submit sample for toxicologic and chemical study (p. 16).	Test for coproporphyrin positive.
Pharynx and larynx		Inflamed mucous membranes.
Other organs and tissues	For general toxicologic sampling, see p. 16.	
Bone	Submit sample for toxicologic study.	
Bone marrow	For preparation of sections and smears, see p. 96.	Toxic changes.

References

1. Pazirandeh A, Brati AH, Marageh MG. Determination of arsenic in hair using neutron activation. Appl Radiat Isot 1998;49:753–759.
2. Prasad GV, Rossi NF. Arsenic intoxication associated with tubulointerstitial nephritis. Am J Kidney Dis 1995;26:373–376.

Poisoning, Atropine

Synonyms and Related Terms: Belladonna; hyoscine (scopolamine); hyoscyamine; hyoscyamus; stramonium.

Organs and Tissues	*Procedures*	*Possible or Expected Findings*
External examination		Body dry and warm after death.
Eyes	Record diameter of pupils.	Mydriasis.
Blood and liver	Submit samples for toxicologic study (p. 16).	
Heart		Iatrogenic atrioventricular block *(1)*.
Gastrointestinal tract	Collect all contents (p. 16), particularly in accidental poisoning in children.	Fruits of *Atropa belladonna* or seeds of *Datura stramonium* may be found.
Other organs		No characteristic findings.

Reference

1. Brunner-La Rocca HP, Kiowski W, Bracht C, Weilenmann D, Follath F. Atrioventricular block after administration of atropine in patients following cardiac transplantation. Transplant 1997;63:1838–1839.

Poisoning, Barbiturate(s)

NOTE: This type of poisoning has become uncommon. Barbiturates may cause sudden death. In all instances, concomitant alcohol intoxication* must be ruled out. Standard toxicologic sampling is sufficient (p. 16).

Organs and Tissues	*Procedures*	*Possible or Expected Findings*
Blood	Submit samples of blood from portal vein and peripheral veins or heart for toxicologic study.	Evidence of alcohol intoxication.* Poisoning by other addictive drugs.
Bile	Refrigerate for possible toxicologic study.	
Urine	Record total volume and pH value. Request tests for protein, glucose, and ketones; request drug screen.	
Esophagus and stomach	Submit all contents and record their character. Analyze for barbiturates and alcohol.	Gritty residues of unabsorbed tablets, powder, or capsules. Mucosal corrosion, ulceration, and discoloration from capsules may occur.
Liver and brain	Submit samples for toxicologic study.	Concentration of barbiturate in parenchyma important for interpretation.

Poisoning, Bismuth

NOTE: Accidental poisoning is common (industrial exposure or drugs with soluble bismuth compounds). Search also for other heavy metals. Acute kidney failure* may be the cause of death. For toxicologic sampling, see p. 16.

Organs and Tissues	*Procedures*	*Possible or Expected Findings*
External examination and oral cavity	Record abnormalities as listed in right-hand column.	Stomatitis with bluish black discoloration of gums; loose teeth; sticky white membranous patches in mouth and throat. Jaundice.
Blood	Submit sample for toxicologic study.	
Urine	Submit sample for toxicologic study. Use one sample for preparation of sediment.	Protein casts and tubular epithelial cells in sediment.
Gastrointestinal tract	Submit contents for toxicologic study. Record appearance of mucosa. Submit samples for histologic study.	Gray or black mucosal membranes; swelling of mucosa; intestinal ulcers that may be perforated. Hemosiderosis.
Liver	Submit samples for toxicologic and histologic study. Request Gomori's iron stain (p. 172).	Fatty changes; hemosiderosis.
Spleen	Submit samples for toxicologic and histologic study.	Hemosiderosis.
Kidneys	Submit samples for toxicologic and histologic study.	Fatty changes; renal tubular degeneration with amorphic basophilic deposits in epithelium of convoluted tubules. Hemosiderosis.
Neck organs		See above under "External examination."
Peripheral nerves	For removal and specimen preparation, see p. 79.	Peripheral neuritis.

Poisoning, Bromide

Synonyms: Bromine poisoning; bromism.

NOTE: The lethal dose is about 0.2 g in children and 1 g in adults (ingested). After fatal methyl bromide poisoning, headspace gas chromatography revealed a subclavian blood concentration of 3.0 microgram/mL whereas inorganic bromide concentrations were 530 micrograms/mL in the blood *(1)*. Tissue concentrations were lower than those in the blood. For toxicologic sampling, see p. 16.

Organs and Tissues	*Procedures*	*Possible or Expected Findings*
External examination, skin, and eyes	Prepare photographs and histologic sections of skin lesions.	Chemical burns on face and conjunctivitis indicate direct exposure; skin pustules over body and nodose bromoderma of the legs indicate bromism.
Blood	Submit sample for toxicologic study.	Blood is best suited for bromide determination.
Urine	Submit sample for toxicologic study.	
Gastrointestinal tract	Submit gastric contents for toxicologic examination. Record appearance of gastrointestinal mucosa.	After ingestion of bromide, necrosis with brown discoloration of mucosa of upper gastrointestinal tract may be present.
Trachea, bronchi, and lungs	If possible, remove lungs together with neck organs; open major airways posteriorly.	After inhalation of bromide, swelling and inflammation of mucous membranes in upper and lower respiratory tracts may be present. There may be pulmonary edema. Pneumonia occurs in bromism.
Other organs	Toxicologic samples should include liver and kidneys.	

Reference

1. Michalodimitrakis MN, Tsatsakis AM, Christakis-Hampsas MG, Trikilis N, Christodoulou P. Death following intentional methyl bromide poisoning: toxicological data and literature review. Vet Hum Toxicol 1997;39:30–34.

Poisoning, Cadmium

Organs to be analyzed for Cd should have no contact with water or be contaminated with blood; they should be sealed in polyethylene bags. Cd leaks into fixation fluid. Postmortem blood concentrations are very high and no indicator of the antemortem values *(1)*. For toxicologic sampling, see p. 16.

Organs and Tissues	*Procedures*	*Possible or Expected Findings*
External examination and oral cavity		Yellow gingival line in chronic poisoning.
Blood	Submit sample for toxicologic study.	
Urine	Submit sample for determination of cadmium concentration.	Elevated urinary cadmium concentrations *(2)*.
Lungs	Submit sample for toxicologic study. and one lobe for microbiologic study (p. 103). Perfuse one lung with formalin (p. 47).	Pulmonary edema, alveolar wall damage, and interstitial pneumonia after acute inhalation. Severe pulmonary fibrosis may develop in chronic cases.
Gastrointestinal tract	For *in situ* fixation, see p. 54.	Gastroenteritis after nonlethal food poisoning.
Kidneys	Collect renal tissue for light microscopic and electron microscopic study (p. 132).	Degeneration of proximal tubules and proteinuria in acute poisoning; interstitial nephritis in chronic poisoning. Nephrolithiasis *(3)*.
Other organs	Sample for toxicologic study. Submit samples for histologic study also.	Degenerative changes of liver and myocardium.

References

1. Koizumi N, Hatayama F, Sumino K. Problems in the analysis of cadmium in autopsied tissues. Environm Res 1994;64:192–198.
2. Ando Y, Shibata E, Tsuchiyama F, Sakai S. Elevated urinary cadmium concentrations in a patient with acute cadmium pneumonitis. Scand J Work Environ Health 1996;22:150–153.
3. Savolainen H. Cadmium-associated renal disease. Ren Fail 1995;17:483–487.

Poisoning, Carbon Monoxide

NOTE: If the victim had been in a fire, see also under "Burns." Carbon monoxide poisoning may rarely be responsible for automobile accidents. Relatively low carboxyhemoglobin concentrations may contribute to death if there is concomitant poisoning—for instance, with alcohol or drugs, particularly sedatives. Anemia, atherosclerotic heart disease, and chronic pulmonary disease also increase sensitivity to carbon monoxide.

If blood had been withdrawn at time of hospital admission—for instance, for crossmatching—submit this for carboxyhemoglobin determination. If no blood can be obtained, see under "Heart, kidneys, and other organs." For quick-orienting qualitative tests, for quantitative methods of carbon monoxide determination, and for interpretation of toxicologic findings, see below. Request also determination of hemoglobin concentrations and of blood alcohol. Request drug screen. For shipping of blood and tissues for carbon monoxide determination, see p. 135. It should be noted that losses of up to 60% of the original saturation occurred when blood was kept in uncapped contained at room temperature for 2 ½ wk or at 4°C for 3 wk.

Organs and Tissues	*Procedures*	*Possible or Expected Findings*
External examination	Record color of fingernails, particularly in heavily pigmented persons in whom lividity is difficult to discern.	Pink skin and fingernails; bullous edema of skin; decubital ulcers.
Blood	Record appearance of blood and submit sample of postmortem blood for toxicologic study (p. 16). See also above under "Note."	Blood tends to be cherry red. For interpretation of toxicologic findings, see below.
Heart, kidneys, and other organs	If no blood can be obtained, prepare water extract of spleen, kidneys, or other organs. Request determination of carbon monoxide content and of carbon monoxide-binding capacity of this mixture. Submit tissue samples for histologic study.	Necrosis of papillary muscles in the heart or myocardial infarction may occur. Renal tubular degeneration may also be found. Acute kidney failure* has been observed after rhabdomyolysis complicated by compartment syndrome *(2)*.
Brain	For removal and specimen preparation, see p. 65.	Hemorrhagic necrosis of basal ganglia (lenticular nucleus in globus pallidus); diffuse petechial hemorrhages in white matter; cerebral edema. Acute hydrocephalus in infants *(3)*.

Methods of Carbon Monoxide Determination

Many methods of carbon monoxide determination have been described. Currently, carboxyhemoglobin is detected in most medical examiner toxicology laboratories by visible spectrophotometry or gas chromatography. In hospitals, carboxyhemoglobin is frequently detected and reported in the course of routine arterial blood gas analysis.

Pink discoloration of skin and organs usually indicates the presence of more than 30% carboxyhemoglobin (but rule out cyanide poisoning* and exposure to cold*).

In a healthy, middle-aged person, a carboxyhemoglobin concentration greater than 50–60% is usually fatal. If the victim was anemic or suffered from chronic lung disease, particularly emphysema* or atherosclerotic heart disease, the concentration may be lower. In association with alcohol, sedatives, and other drugs, carboxyhemoglobin levels may also be much lower and yet fatal.

A heavy cigarette smoker may have a carboxyhemoglobin concentration of 8–10%, and higher levels may occur in police officers and other persons exposed to automobile exhaust in dense traffic.

If the victim survived the carbon monoxide poisoning for several hours, postmortem blood samples usually will fail to show the presence of carboxyhemoglobin. In these instances, blood taken at the time of admission to the hospital may still be available and of particular value. If the victim had spent 1 h in fresh air before death, 40–50% of the carbon monoxide will have been removed, and 8–10% will have been removed during each subsequent hour. Even though clearance may be complete, death may still occur—primarily from brain damage and infectious complications in prolonged coma.

Physiologic Effects of Carbon Monoxide Poisoning[†]

% of carboxy-hemoglobin	*Clinical Signs/Symptoms*
10	No appreciable effect except shortness of breath on vigorous muscular exertion
20	In most cases, no appreciable effect except dyspnea, even on moderate exertion; slight headache in some cases
30	Decided headache; irritability; easy fatigability; disturbance of judgment
40–50	Headache; confusion; fainting and collapse on exertion
60–70	Unconsciousness, respiratory failure, and death if exposure is prolonged
80	Rapidly fatal
>80	Immediately fatal

[†]Modified from Henderson Y, Haggard HW. Noxious Gases. The Chemical Catalog Co., New York, 1927.

References

1. Ocak A, Valentour JC, Blanke RV. The effects of storage conditions on the stability of carbon monoxide in postmortem blood. J Anal Toxicol 1985;9:202–206.
2. Abdul-Ghaffar NU, Farghaly MM, Swamy AS. Acute renal failure, compartment syndrome, and systemic capillary leak syndrome complicating carbon monoxide poisoning. J Toxicol 1996;34:713–719.
3. So GM, Kosofsky BE, Southern JF. Acute hydrocephalus following carbon monoxide poisoning. Pediatr Neurol 1997;17:270–273.

Poisoning, Carbon Tetrachloride

Synonym: Tetrachloromethane poisoning.

NOTE: Toxicologic sampling of body fluids and organs should be done routinely in all cases (p. 16). In many instances, however, death occurs 1 wk to 10 d after exposure, and by this time no carbon tetrachloride is demonstrable. Death may be sudden or delayed by only a few hours, particularly after inhalation of carbon tetrachloride (see also Fig. 2-1, p. 15). Sudden death probably is caused by cardiac dysrrhythmia.

Alcohol concentrations should be determined in all cases or, if death was delayed, evidence of drinking at the time of exposure should be sought. Alcohol considerably increases the hazards of carbon tetrachloride.

Organs and Tissues	*Procedures*	*Possible or Expected Findings*
External examination		Jaundice; pedal edema.
Heart	Submit samples for histologic study, and request frozen sections for Sudan stain (p. 173).	Fatty changes of myocardium.
Liver	Record weight and photograph; submit samples for histologic study. Request frozen sections for Sudan stain.	Centrilobular or diffuse hepatic necrosis and fatty changes. Cirrhosis* after chronic exposure.
Kidneys	Photograph and submit samples for histologic study. Request frozen sections for Sudan stain.	Acute tubular necrosis (lower nephron nephrosis); fatty degeneration.
Adrenal glands	Sample for histologic study.	Necrosis in zona fasciculata and reticularis.
Brain	For removal and specimen preparation, see p. 65.	Perivenous necroses in cerebral white matter; cerebellar degeneration (Purkinje cells). Pontine necrosis.
Eyes	For removal and specimen preparation, see p. 85.	Optic neuritis in chronic cases.
Peripheral nerves	For sampling and specimen preparation, see p. 79.	Peripheral neuritis in chronic cases.

Poisoning, Chlorine or Hydrochloric Acid

Related Terms: Cl_2 poisoning; HCl poisoning.

NOTE: See also under "Bronchitis, acute chemical" and under "Poisoning, gas." Hydrochloric acid is sold by plumbing supply houses and pool supply companies as muriatic acid. It is a liquid. Chlorine is a water-soluble gas. As supplied for pool sanitation, liquid chlorine is usually acidic. For convenience, chlorine and hydrochloric acid are discussed here together.

Organs and Tissues	*Procedures*	*Possible or Expected Findings*
External examination and eyes	Prepare photographs of face.	Conjunctivitis and cyanosis in chlorine gas poisoning; burns of lips from hydrochloric acid.

Organs and Tissues	Procedures	Possible or Expected Findings
Lungs	Submit one lung for toxicologic study (p. 16; see also under "Poisoning, gas"). Record lung weights. Formalin perfusion of lungs is not recommended; it may cause artifactual ballooning and internal ruptures of organ.	Severe pulmonary edema, broncho pneumonia, and swelling of mucous membranes in chlorine poisoning. Arterial thrombosis may occur. Pulmonary fibrosis may develop after prolonged survival.
Larynx and trachea	Leave esophagus and stomach attached to neck organs. Open larynx anteriorly and check whether a perforation has occurred.	Swelling and ulceration of mucous membranes in chlorine poisoning; acute laryngotracheitis. Tracheoesophageal perforation.
Esophagus and stomach	See also above under "Larynx and trachea." Photograph opened esophagus and stomach.	Corrosion of mucosa with thickening, hemorrhage, and blackish discoloration after ingestion of hydrochloric acid.
	Sample for histologic study, particularly if there is doubt whether a perforation was antemortem or postmortem.	Antemortem and postmortem perforation may occur.
Kidneys		Glomerular capillary thromboses.
Brain	For removal and specimen preparation, see p. 65.	Hemorrhages in white matter *(1)*.

Reference

1. Adelson L, Kaufman J. Fatal chlorine poisoning: report of two cases with clinicopathologic correlation. Am J Clin Pathol 1971;56:430–442.

Poisoning, Cyanide

Synonym: Hydrocyanic acid (hydrogen cyanide) poisoning.

NOTE: Hydrocyanic acid (hydrogen cyanide, HCN) is a water-soluble gas. Its salts, sodium cyanide and potassium cyanide are sold as "eggs" to the jewelry industry. Hydrocyanic acid is formed when cyanide salts are dissolved in acidic solutions. Containers from which the poison might have been ingested or inhaled should also be submitted for toxicologic examination. For cyanide screening tests in the autopsy room and for interpretation of findings, see below. Caution: Stomach may still contain cyanide gas, formed by acidic reaction of cyanide salt. It may be best to open the stomach under a hood *(1)*. The odor is quite characteristic for cyanide poisoning but most persons are unable to smell this odor. It is helpful to know in advance if any person in an office or laboratory can smell cyanide. Forensic pathologists who can smell the compound state that it has its own specific odor, which differs from the often quoted smell of bitter almonds (see Chapter 2). Autopsies also can be done in a negatively pressured isolation room *(1)*. For toxicologic sampling, see p. 16.

Organs and Tissues	Procedures	Possible or Expected Findings
External examination and oral cavity	Record color of skin and possible corrosion marks, as listed in right-hand column.	For odor, see above under "Note." Bright red skin color is not always present. Corrosion around mouth and in oral cavity may be found after ingestion of potassium or sodium cyanide.
Blood	Submit sample for toxicologic study. For autopsy screening tests, see below.	Blood is fluid and sometimes bright red.
Stomach	See above under "Note." Submit contents for toxicologic study. Sample for histologic study.	If potassium or sodium cyanide was ingested, brown-red mucosal corrosion may be present in stomach or in upper digestive tract.
Pharynx and esophagus	See above under "Stomach."	
Lungs	Record lung weights and submit one lung for toxicologic study. Submit samples from other lung for histologic study.	Pulmonary edema.
Liver	Submit portion for toxicologic study.	
Brain	For removal and specimen preparation, see p. 65. Submit portion for toxicologic study.	For odor, see above under "Note." If death was not instantaneous, there may be hyaline thrombi in small blood vessels, minute hemorrhages, and necroses of lenticular nuclei.

Cyanide Screening Tests in the Autopsy Room

This test can be used for blood and gastric contents *(2)*. Dip squares of filter paper in a small amount of saturated picric acid. Let these squares dry until barely moist. Place a drop of the material to be tested—e.g., blood or gastric contents—on a piece of paper. Let material dry for a moment, and then place one drop of 10% sodium carbonate in the center of the material to be tested. If cyanide is present, a reddish purple color will chromatograph out from the material. The higher the concentration of cyanide the more blue the color will be. It is possible to recognize whole blood because the blood turns a rather dark brown and the reddish to purple color is clearly visible. High concentrations of sulfide interfere by giving a false-positive test.

Another screening test is done as follows *(3)*. Dip filter paper into normal blood. Then treat the paper with potassium chlorate, whereupon brown methemoglobin forms. Place this preparation into the fluid suspected of containing cyanide (e.g., blood, gastric contents, pulmonary edema fluid). If bright red cyanmethemoglobin forms, the reaction is positive.

Interpretation of Findings

If the concentration of cyanide in the stomach is high and the concentration in the lungs is low, cyanide was ingested. Alternatively, if the pulmonary cyanide concentration is high and the concentrtaion in the gastric contents is low, hydrogen cyanide most likely was inhaled. Occasionally, minimal cyanide levels will be present in decomposed bodies.

References

1. Nolte KB, Dasgupta A. Prevention of occupational cyanide exposure in autopsy prosectors. J Forens Sci 1996;41:146–147.
2. Camps FE. Gradwohl's Legal Medicine, 2nd ed. Williams & Wilkins Company, Baltimore, 1968, pp. 615–617.
3. Glaister J, Rentoul E. Medical Jurisprudence and Toxicology, 12th ed. E & S Livingstone, Edinburgh, 1966, p. 686.

Poisoning, Digitalis

Related Term: Digoxin toxicity.

NOTE: Certain drugs seem to interfere with correct digitalis determination.

Organs and Tissues	*Procedures*	*Possible or Expected Findings*
Blood	Submit sample of peripheral blood for digoxin radioimmunoassay (p. 16).	Digoxin values in digitalis toxicity are greater than 2 ng/mL *(1)*.
Heart	Freeze fresh myocardium for digitalis extraction.	Increased digitalis concentrations *(2)*.
Vitreous	Submit sample for digoxin radioimmunoassay (p. 16).	Digoxin concentration may be higher or lower than concentration in serum, depending on how long before death drug was taken *(1)*.

References

1. DiMaio VJM, Garriot JC, Putnam R. Digoxin concentrations in postmortem specimens after overdose and therapeutic use. J Forensic Sci 1975;20:340–347.
2. Jellifee RW, Stephenson RG. A fluorimetric determination of myocardial digoxin at autopsy, with identification of digitalis leaf, digitoxin and gitonin. Am J Clin Pathol 1969;51:347–357.

Poisoning, Drug(s) (See "Dependence, drug(s), all types or type unspecified" or under "Poisoning,..." followed by specific name of drug.)

Poisoning, Ethanol (Ethyl Alcohol) (See "Alcoholism and alcohol intoxication," "Cardiomyopathy, alcoholic," "Disease, alcoholic liver," "Syndrome, fetal alcoholic," and Syndrome, Wernicke-Korsakoff.")

Poisoning, Ethylene Glycol

Related Term: Antifreeze poisoning.

NOTE: Pulmonary and cerebral manifestations are the main findings in acute poisoning, and renal tubular necrosis is the primary finding in chronic poisoning. For general toxicologic sampling, see p. 16. Calcium oxalate crystals can be demonstrated in routine histologic sections but also in scanning electron micrographs of thick deparaffinized sections.

Organs and Tissues	*Procedures*	*Possible or Expected Findings*
Eyes	For removal and specimen preparation, see p. 85.	Papilledema; optic nerve atrophy.
Blood	In acute cases, submit sample for ethylene glycol determination (p. 16); in chronic cases, request determination of calcium concentrations.	Ethylene glycol in serum *(1)*.
Urine	Prepare sediment.	Protein casts; calcium oxalate crystals *(2)*. Crystals are light yellow and birefringent, arranged as sheaves, rhomboids, or prisms.

Organs and Tissues	Procedures	Possible or Expected Findings
Heart	Sample for histologic study.	Myocardial degeneration; petechial hemorrhages.
Blood vessels	Submit samples of small vessels from multiple sites for histologic study. Request Verhoeff–van Gieson stain (p. 173).	Oxalate crystals in media of small arteries, with associated ischemic lesions.
Lungs	Perfuse one lung with formalin (p. 47).	Congestion; petechial hemorrhages; bronchopneumonia; edema.
Gastrointestinal tract	Submit contents for toxicologic study (p. 16).	Petechial mucosal hemorrhages.
Liver	Record weight; submit samples for histologic study.	Hydropic hepatocellular degeneration; fatty changes and focal necroses.
Kidneys	See above under "Note."	Acute renal tubular necrosis;* intratubular crystals.
Brain	For removal and specimen preparation, see p. 65.	Petechial hemorrhages.

References

1. Eder AF, McGrath CM, Dowdy YG, Tomaszewski JE, Rosenberg FM, Wilson RB, et al. Ethylene glycol poisoning: toxicokinetic and analytical factors affecting laboratory diagnosis. Clin Chem 1998; 44:168–177.
2. Davis DP, Bramwell KJ, Hamilton RS, Williams SR. Ethylene glycol poisoning: case report of a record-high level and a review. J Emerg Med 1997;15:653–667.

Poisoning, Food

Related Terms: Bacillary dysentery* (*Shigella* food poisoning); botulism;* *Clostridium perfringens* food poisoning; favism; mushroom poisoning;* *Salmonella* food poisoning; staphylococcal food poisoning.

NOTE: If cause of food poisoning is unknown, submit suspected food for aerobic and anaerobic cultures, Gram stain of smears, and routine toxicologic study. This should include tests for heavy metals (antimony, cadmium, and lead) that may have leaked from old cooking utensils. Test for the presence of staphylococcal enterotoxin are done only in specialized laboratories. If botulism is suspected, follow procedures described under that heading. Mushroom poisoning also is listed as a separate entity. If *Salmonella* food poisoning is suspected, see under "Fever, typhoid." See also under "Enteritis" or "Enterocolitis" or under another specific heading such as "Dysentery, bacillary." Obtain sufficient material for microbiologic and histologic study to identify organisms such as *Chlamydia, Clostridium (type F strains), Salmonella, Shigella, verotoxic E. coli, Yersinia,* and others.

Organs and Tissues	Procedures	Possible or Expected Findings
External examination		Debilitated states; patients in extremes of life.
Gastrointestinal tract	Submit contents for aerobic and anaerobic cultures (p. 16 and above under "Note"); prepare smears of contents for Gram stain (p. 172). Submit samples for histologic study.	Enteritis or enterocolitis.

Poisoning, Gas

NOTE: Anesthesia-associated death,* carbon monoxide poisoning,* and sniffing and spray death* are presented under the appropriate headings. Procedures discussed here deal with other volatile substances, including chemical irritants such as ammonia (NH_3), chlorine or hydrochloric acid poisoning (see also under that heading); methylene chloride, phosgene ($COCl_2$), or sulfurous acid (H_2SO_3), sulfur dioxide (SO_2).

Gases from body cavities, heart chambers, or blood vessels can be removed as described under "Embolism, air." Gases can also be trapped with a rubber dam after cutting organs under water. Samples from various organs should be shipped in hermetically sealed nonplastic containers or in analyzing solutions.

Organs and Tissues	Procedures	Possible or Expected Findings
External examination, and oral cavity	Record extent of chemical burns.	Chemical burns in and around mouth or eyes of conjunctivas.
Blood	Submit sample for gas analysis (p. 16). In many instances, inhaled gases can be demonstrated chromatographically in gas from head space above sealed blood specimen.	
Larynx and trachea		Chemical burns.

Organs and Tissues	*Procedures*	*Possible or Expected Findings*
Lungs	If gas was inhaled and is to be analyzed, submit intact lungs with bronchi ligated in airtight, nonplastic container to laboratory that can conduct gas analysis. If survival was short, formalin perfusion of lungs is not recommended; it may cause artifactual ballooning and internal ruptures of organ. Submit samples of tissue for routine histologic study.	Chemical pneumonia; pulmonary edema. After longer survival, obliterating fibrous bronchiolitis, chronic bronchitis, and saccular bronchiectasis* may occur.
Other organs	See above under "Note."	

Poisoning, Glycol (See "Poisoning, ethylene glycol.")

Poisoning, Halogen (See "Fluorosis," "Poisoning, bromide," "Poisoning, chlorine or hydrochloric acid," "Poisoning, gas," and "Poisoning, iodine.")

Poisoning, Heavy Metal (See "Poisoning, antimony," "Poisoning, arsenic," "Poisoning, cadmium," "Poisoning, lead," Poisoning, mercury," "Poisoning, thallium.")

Poisoning, Insecticide (See "Poisoning, organophosphate(s)*)

Poisoning, Iodine

Related Terms: Lugol's solution; tincture of iodine. For toxicologic sampling, see p. 16.

Organs and Tissues	*Procedures*	*Possible or Expected Findings*
External examination and eyes	Record color of skin and extent of corrosive lesions.	Perioral corrosive lesions; yellow discoloration of skin; conjunctivitis after exposure to vapors.
Urine, blood, and parenchymal organs	Submit samples for toxicologic study.	
Lungs and upper respiratory tract	Submit samples for histologic study.	Acute inflammation of respiratory tract after inhalation of vapors.
Stomach	Submit contents for toxicologic study; photograph mucosa; prepare histologic sections.	Corrosive gastritis; if starch was used as antidote, gastric lining will be bluish. Histologically, well-preserved mucosa is present because of in vivo fixation.
Intestinal tract	See above under "Stomach."	Mucosa may show same changes as stomach.
Kidneys		Swelling of tubular epithelium.

Poisoning, Isopropyl Alcohol

Synonyms: Propanol; rubbing alcohol.

Organs and Tissues	*Procedures*	*Possible or Expected Findings*
All organs	See under "Alcoholism and alcohol intoxication."	Nonspecific autopsy findings: visceral congestion; pulmonary and cerebral edema.

Poisoning, Lead

NOTE: Lead-free syringes and lead-free polyethylene containers should be used. Blood lead concentrations can now be determined by inductively coupled plasma mass spectrometry *(1)*. For screening methods, see ref. *(2)*.

This is a **reportable** disease **in some states**.

Organs and Tissues	*Procedures*	*Possible or Expected Findings*
External examination, oral cavity, and hair		Bluish lead line at gingival margin in victims with poor oral hygiene.

Organs and Tissues	Procedures	Possible or Expected Findings
External examination, oral cavity, and hair *(continued)*	Prepare roentgenograms of long bones.	Densities at the ends of the shafts of long bones.
	For diagnosis of chronic plumbism, analysis of scalp hair may be useful (p. 17). Analysis is done by neutron activation (see also under "Poisoning, arsenic").	Lead content of hair may be used to estimate time and duration of exposure. Evidence of old shotgun injury may explain chronic lead poisoning *(3)*.
Blood	Remove samples with lead-free syringe (see above under "Note") or 20-mL Vacutainer tubes (Becton, Dickinson and Company). Do not add anti-coagulant or preservative.	Normal concentration in children is less than 0.04 mg/100 g; values for "safe" industrial exposure in adults vary from 0.01–0.07 mg/100 g.
Urine	For collection procedures, see above under "Blood" and under "Note." Request also determination of coproporphyrin concentrations.	Values for "safe" industrial exposure in adults vary from 0.01–0.15 mg/L. Aminoaciduria and glycosuria after lead poisoning in children *(4)*.
Liver	Submit sample for histologic study; submit remaining tissue for toxicologic analysis.	Intranuclear inclusion bodies in acute poisoning.
Small and large bowel	Submit with contents for toxicologic study, particularly in acute poisoning (p. 16).	
Kidneys	Submit sample from each kidney for histologic study; submit remaining tissue of both kidneys separately for toxicologic study.	Chronic nephritis; tubular degeneration with intranuclear inclusion bodies.
Bone	Submit at least 10 g of fresh bone for toxicologic study.	
Brain	For removal and specimen preparation, see p. 65.	Perivascular hemorrhages; cell necrosis; edema. Possibly increased risk of gliomas in chronic poisoning *(5)*.

References

1. Bergdahl IA, Schutz A, Gerhardsson L, Jensen A, Skerfving S. Lead concentrations in human plasma, urine and whole blood. Scand J Work Environ Health 1997;23:359–363.
2. Daher RT. Trace metals (lead and cadmium screening). Anal Chem 1995;67:405R–410R.
3. Wu PB, Kingery WS, Date ES. An EMG case report of lead neuropathy 19 years after a gunshot injury. Muscle Nerve 1995;18:326–329.
4. Loghman-Adham M. Aminoaciduria and glycosuria following severe childhood lead poisoning. Pediatr Nephrol 1998;12:218–221.
5. Anttila A, Heikkila P, Nykyri E, Kauppinen T, Pukkula E, Hernberg S, et al. Risk of nervous system cancer among workers exposed to lead. J Occup Environ Med 1996;38:131–136.

Poisoning, LSD (d-Lysergic Acid Diethylamide) (See "Abuse, hallucinogen(s).")

Poisoning, Lye

Related Terms: Ammonium hydroxide poisoning; calcium oxide or quicklime poisoning; poisoning by alkaline corrosives; potassium hydroxide poisoning; sodium hydroxide poisoning.

Organs and Tissues	Procedures	Possible or Expected Findings
External examination and oral cavity	Record extent of oral, perioral, and other facial corrosive injuries. Photograph lesions. Prepare histologic sections of tissue from inside of lips or mouth.	Lye burns on face and chest in acute cases; scars and manifestations of malnutrition* in chronic cases.
Blood	Submit sample for toxicologic study (p. 16).	
Neck organs, esophagus, trachea, and lungs	After removal of heart, remove neck organs with hypopharynx, esophagus, larynx, and trachea. Leave stomach attached to esophagus. Open pharynx and esophagus along posterior midline. In acute cases, formalin perfusion of lungs is not recommended; it may cause artifactual ballooning and internal ruptures of organ.	Swelling, edema, and necrosis of mucous membranes in acute poisoning. Fibrosis and strictures in chronic cases. Bronchitis* and bronchopneumonia.

Organs and Tissues	Procedures	Possible or Expected Findings
Stomach	Remove gastric contents carefully from *in situ* incision. Caution—tissues are very friable. Leave stomach attached to esophagus (see above under "Neck organs,...").	See below under "Intestinal tract."
Intestinal tract	Describe color of duodenal mucosa and odor of mucosa and contents.	Mucosal corrosion, with or without perforation.

Poisoning, Mercury

Related Term: Methylmercury poisoning (Minamata disease).

NOTE: For general toxicologic sampling, see p. 16. If kidney failure was present, see also under that heading. Analysis can be done by atomic absorption spectrophotometry *(1)*.

Organs and Tissues	Procedures	Possible or Expected Findings
External examination, skin, and oral cavity	Record extent of skin changes and prepare histologic sections.	Exfoliative dermatitis.
	Record appearance of oral cavity.	Blue line at gingival margin; hypertrophy of gum; acute and chronic gingivitis; exfoliation and loss of teeth *(2)*.
Blood	Submit sample for toxicologic study.	
Heart	Submit tissue for toxicologic study. Prepare histologic sections of myocardium (p. 30).	Degeneration of myocardium.
Lungs	Submit samples for toxicologic and histologic study.	Increased concentrations of mercury *(1)*.
Esophagus	Submit sample for histologic study.	Induration of mucosa.
Liver and spleen	Submit samples for toxicologic and histologic study.	Congestion.
Stomach and colon	Submit samples for histologic study. Submit sample of colon for toxicologic study.	Erosive gastritis and colitis.
Kidneys	Submit samples for toxicologic and histologic study.	Increased concentrations of mercury *(1)*. Degeneration of proximal tubules; calcifications. Chronic kidney failure* may be the cause of death.
Neck organs	Submit specimen from pharynx for histologic study.	Induration of mucosa.
Brain and spinal cord	For removal and specimen preparation, see pp. 65 and 67, respectively. Submit sample of brain for toxicologic study.	Increased concentrations of mercury *(1)*. Cortical hemorrhages.

References

1. Opitz H, Schweinsberg F, Grossmann T, Wendt-Gallitelli MF, Meyerman R. Demonstration of mercury in the human brain and other organs 17 years after metallic mercury exposure. Clin Neuropathol 1996;15:139–144.
2. Martin MD, Williams BJ, Charleston JD, Oda D. Spontaneous exfoliation of teeth following severe elemental mercury poisoning: case report and histological investigation for mechanism. Oral Surg Oral Med Oral Pathol 1997;84:495–501.

Poisoning, Metal (See "Poisoning, antimony," "Poisoning, arsenic," "Poisoning, cadmium," "Poisoning, lead," "Poisoning, mercury," and "Poisoning, thallium.")

Poisoning, Methanol (Methyl Alcohol)

Synonym: Wood alcohol.

NOTE: Autopsy findings are not diagnostic. Pulmonary and cerebral edema and edema of other viscera may be present. See also under "Alcoholism and alcohol intoxication."

Poisoning, Methylene Chloride (See "Poisoning, gas.")

Poisoning, Mushroom

NOTE: Fatalities usually are caused by members of the genus *Amanita*. The results of the autopsy may be less diagnostic than examination of the leftovers of the incriminated meal. If patient underwent liver *(1)* or kidney *(2)* transplantation, see also under these headings.

Organs and Tissues	*Procedures*	*Possible or Expected Findings*
Gastrointestinal tract	Submit gastric and intestinal contents for toxicologic study (p. 16).	Usually, study of gastrointestinal contents gives no meaningful results because of the long interval between consumption of the poisoned meal and death.
Liver	Record size and weight. Submit samples for histologic and toxicologic study.	Massive or submassive hepatic necrosis, involving primarily zones 2 and 3 *(3)*.
Kidneys	Sample tissue for toxicologic study, light microscopy, and electron microscopy (see p. 132).	Acute interstitial nephritis in *Cortinarius speciocissimus* poisoning. Acute tubular necrosis in *Amanita phalloides* poisoning *(3)* and in *Cortinarius speciocissimus* poisoning.
Other organs	For general toxicologic sampling, see p. 16. Histologic sections should include brain.	Hemorrhagic diathesis and cerebral edema in *Amanita phalloides* poisoning *(3)*.

References

1. Meunier B, Messner M, Bardaxoglou E, Spiliopoulos G, Terblanche J, Launois B. Liver transplantation for severe Lepiota helveola poisoning. Liver 1994;14:158–160.
2. Holmdahl J, Blohme I. Renal transplantation after Cortinarius speciocissimus poisoning. Nephrol Dialysis Transplant 1995;10:1920–1922.
3. Fineschi V, Di Paolo M, Centini F. Histological criteria for diagnosis of amanita phalloides poisoning. J Forens Sci 1996;41:429–432.

Poisoning, Organophosphate(s)

Synonyms and Related Terms: Compounds include diazinon, dichlorvos, malathion, and parathion. For updates, consult poison hotlines.

NOTE: Organophosphate insecticides may produce rapid and severe toxic affects leading to coma and pulmonary edema and respiratory insufficiency. Interpretation of toxicologic findings, see below. For toxicologic sampling, see p. 16.

Organs and Tissues	*Procedures*	*Possible or Expected Findings*
Blood and urine	Submit samples for toxicologic study and assay for cholinesterase activities.	Cholinesterase activity will be low.
Lungs	Record weights of lungs and contents of airways.	Pulmonary edema if poison was inhaled. Airways may contain aspirated material.
Gastrointestinal tract	Submit contents for toxicologic study.	
Liver and kidneys	Submit samples for toxicologic study.	
Skeletal muscles	Submit unfixed material for histochemical demonstration of reduced cholinesterase activity at motor end-plates.	Cholinesterase activity can be determined reliably even after decomposition and embalming.
Brain and spinal cord	For removal and specimen preparation, see pp. 65 and 67, respectively.	Clinically, Guillain-Barré syndrome has been observed after poisoning with organophosphate.

Interpretation of Toxicologic Findings (1)

In acute poisoning, the cholinesterase levels may be 25% of the normal values (see below). The cholinesterase levels in the blood are not affected by the duration of the postmortem interval; measurement may be attempted even on decomposed or exhumed bodies.

Normal Cholinesterase Levels in Red Blood Cells (RBC) and in Whole Blood, Measured in Micromoles of Acetylcholine Hydrolyzed

Substrate	*Males*	*Females*	*Children*
RBC	0.74–2.38	0.90–2.33	0.72–2.25
Whole blood	0.78–3.88	1.33–3.32	1.52–2.88

Reference

1. Fatteh A. Organophosphates (parathion). In: Handbook of Forensic Pathology. J.B. Lippincott Company, Philadelphia, 1973, pp. 310–312.

Poisoning, Pesticide(s) (See "Poisoning, organophosphate(s).")

Poisoning, Phosphorus

NOTE: Fatal dose is about 2–3 g. Phosphorus is used in some rat poisons. Phosphorus can be detected in exhumed bodies.

Organs and Tissues	*Procedures*	*Possible or Expected Findings*
External examination, skin, and hair	Submit skin and hair for toxicologic study (p. 16).	Jaundice (indicates subacute poisoning with severe hepatic changes).
Gastrointestinal tract	Tie stomach and various portions of intestinal tract and submit unopened for toxicologic study. If poisoning with yellow phosphorus is suspected, these viscera must be opened under nitrogen, just before analysis. Collect feces.	Gastric contents smell of garlic *(1)*.
Liver	Record weight. Photograph. Submit portion for toxicologic study. Request Sudan stain of frozen sections (p. 173).	Severe fatty changes; periportal necroses.
Other organs	For general toxicologic sampling, see p. 16. Samples should include kidneys and pancreas. Submit samples for histologic study, and request Sudan-stained frozen sections (p. 173).	Fatty changes in myocardium, skeletal muscles, and other organs.

Reference

1. Simon FA, Pickering LK. Acute yellow phosphorus poisoning: "smoking stool syndrome." JAMA 1976;235:1343–1344.

Poisoning, Strychnine

Organs and Tissues	*Procedures*	*Possible or Expected Findings*
External examination	Record extent and severity of rigor mortis and postmortem interval at time of recording.	Rigor mortis after fatal strychnine poisoning may occur very soon after death and may be very severe (opisthotonos); it may persist until decomposition sets in.
Organs and body fluids		Congestion of viscera; no characteristic morphologic autopsy findings. Acute pancreatitis has been observed *(1)*.
	For toxicologic sampling (gastric contents, urine, blood, brain, and other organs), see p. 16.	High strychnine concentrations (also demonstrable in exhumed bodies *[2]*).

References

1. Hernandez AF, Pomares J, Schiaffino S, Pla A, Villanueva E. Acute chemical pancreatitis associated with nonfatal strychnine poisoning. J Toxicol 1998;36:67–71.
2. Benomran FA, Henry JD. Homicide by strychnine poisoning. Med Sci Law 1996;36:271–273.

Poisoning, Thallium

NOTE: For toxicologic sampling, see below and p. 16.

Organs and Tissues	*Procedures*	*Possible or Expected Findings*
External examination and oral cavity	Record character and extent of skin and nail changes; record distribution of hair. Submit samples of skin for histologic study.	Dermatitis and trophic changes of fingernails; diffuse alopecia *(1)*. Stomatitis in acute poisoning.
	Examine hair under polarized light.	Dystrophic anagen hair with dark bands *(1)*.
Gastrointestinal tract	Submit samples of contents for toxicologic study (p. 16). Prepare histologic sections of all segments.	Gastroenteritis in acute poisoning.
Liver	Record weight. Submit samples for toxicologic and histologic study.	Centrilobular hepatic necrosis; fatty changes.

Organs and Tissues	Procedures	Possible or Expected Findings
Kidneys	Submit samples for toxicologic and histologic study.	Fatty changes.
Brain and spinal cord; optic nerves	For removal and specimen preparation, see pp. 65, 67, and 88, respectively. Submit brain for toxicologic study. Submit sections of brain and optic nerves for histologic study.	Retrobulbar neuritis.
Skeletal muscles	Submit specimens for toxicologic study (take from lower extremity).	
Bones and bone marrow	For removal, prosthetic repair, and specimen preparation of bones, see p. 95. For preparation of sections and smears of bone marrow, see p. 96. Submit samples for toxicologic study.	Osteomalacia;* osteomyelofibrosis.

Reference

1. Tromme I, van Neste D, Dobbelaere F, Bouffioux B, Courin C, Dugernier T, et al. Skin signs in the diagnosis of thallium poisoning. Br J Dermatol 1998;138:321–325.

Poliomyelitis

Synonym: Acute anterior poliomyelitis.

NOTE: The disease has been nearly eliminated in the USA but not in many other countries.

(1) Collect all tissues that appear to be infected. (2) Request viral cultures. (3) Usually, special stains are not helpful. (4) Special **precautions** are indicated (p. 146). (5) Serologic studies may be helpful and are available from the Centers for Disease Control and Prevention, Atlanta, GA (p. 135). (6) This is a **reportable** disease.

Organs and Tissues	Procedures	Possible or Expected Findings
External examination	If chronic paralysis had been present, record circumference of extremities on right and left sides.	Neurogenic atrophy of skeletal muscles in areas of paralysis.
Cerebrospinal fluid	In acute cases, submit for viral culture (p. 104) and cytologic study.	
Vitreous	If water or electrolyte disturbances are expected, submit for chemical study (p. 85).	Electrolyte disorder.*
Heart	Record weight; submit samples for histologic study (p. 30).	Hypertensive heart disease; myocarditis.*
Lungs	Submit one large sample for viral and bacterial cultures (p. 103). Perfuse one lung with formalin (p. 47).	Aspiration or bronchopneumonia (or both); edema; atelectasis; embolism;* alveolar wall necrosis (acute or organizing diffuse alveolar damage) after oxygen toxicity.
Esophagus		Acute ulcers.
Gastrointestinal tract	If there is blood in the lumen, record measured or estimated total volume.	Acute gastric dilatation; acute gastroduodenal ulcers; gastrointestinal erosions and hemorrhages. Dilatation of colon; perforation of cecum.
Kidneys and urinary bladder	Open renal pelves and ureters *in situ*; prepare photographs.	Urolithiasis and nephrolithiasis,* pyonephrosis and pyelonephritis.*
Veins	For removal of femoral veins, see p. 34.	Phlebothrombosis of legs, most commonly on left side.
Brain and spinal cord	For removal and specimen preparation, see pp. 65 and 67, respectively. In acute cases, submit portions of brain and spinal cord for viral culture.	Necrosis of anterior horn cells of spinal cord, with neuronophagia and perivascular inflammatory reaction. Old lesions show neuronal loss and gliosis. Medulla ("bulbar polio") and other areas of brain stem, cerebellum, and cerebrum, particularly the motor cortex, may be affected in various degrees.

Organs and Tissues	Procedures	Possible or Expected Findings
Bones and joints	For removal, prosthetic repair, and specimen preparation, see p. 95.	Arthritis* in acute cases; disuse osteoporosis* in chronic cases.
Skeletal muscles	For histologic sampling, see p. 80.	Neurogenic atrophy of affected muscles.
Eyes	For removal and specimen preparation, see p. 85.	Hypertensive retinopathy.

Polyarteritis Nodosa

Synonyms and Related Terms: Infantile polyarteritis nodosa; Kawasaki disease; mucocutaneous lymph node syndrome;* panarteritis nodosa; periarteritis nodosa. For other synonyms and related terms, see also under "Arteritis, all types or type unspecified."

Possible Associated Conditions: Acquired immunodeficiency syndrome* *(1)*; familial Mediterranean fever* *(2)*; polymyalgia rheumatica *(3)*; systemic lupus erythematosus* *(4)*; viral hepatitis B *(5)* or C *(6)*.* See also under "Arteritis, all types or type unspecified."

Organs and Tissues	Procedures	Possible or Expected Findings
External examination and skin	Record extent and character of skin lesions; submit samples of skin for histologic study.	Subcutaneous nodules (rare), sometimes with ulceration *(7)*.
Heart	For coronary arteriography, see p. 118. Record heart weight.	Coronary arteritis, with or without aneurysms and infarctions, primarily in childhood. Myocardial hypertrophy secondary to hypertension.*
Lungs	Perfuse with formalin (p. 47) and submit samples for histologic study.	Minimal or no involvement by polyarteritis nodosa; considerable involvement in other types of necrotizing vasculitis (see "Arteritis, all types or type unspecified").
Kidneys	Submit samples for light microscopic, electron microscopic (p. 132), and fluorescent microscopic study.	Polyarteritis nodosa; glomerulitis; deposition of γ-globulin, fibrinogen, and albumin.
Other organs	Submit samples of liver, gallbladder, spleen, pancreas, esophagus, gastrointestinal tract (all segments, including appendix), mesentery; adrenals; urinary bladder, epididymis, and endocrine glands, particularly testes. Submit samples of all other tissues with infarctions and related gross lesions. Request Verhoeff–van Gieson stain (p. 173). For special techniques, see above under "Kidneys."	Polyarteritis, with or without formation of aneurysms and infarctions, may occur in all organs. The liver may show bile duct injury and rarely, nodular regenerative hyperplasia *(8)*.
Aorta and other arteries	Submit samples for histologic study.	More frequently involved in giant cell elastic arteritis.*
Skeletal muscles	For removal and specimen preparation, see p. 80.	Polyarteritis of small muscular arteries, including vasa nervorum.
Joints	For removal, prosthetic repair, and specimen preparation, see p. 96. Submit samples of synovium for histologic study.	Arthritis* may rarely be present with swollen joints.
Brain and spinal cord	For removal and specimen preparation, see pp. 65 and 67, respectively. For cerebral arteriography, see p. 80.	Infarctions;* subarachnoid hemorrhage; arteritis of cerebral arteries.
Eyes	For removal and specimen preparation, see p. 85.	Papillitis; retinal hemorrhages; hypertensive retinopathy.

References

1. Libman BS, Quismorio FP Jr, Stimmler MM. Polyarteritis nodosa-like vasculitis in human immunodeficiency virus infection. J Rheumatol 1995;22:351–355.
2. Kocak H, Cakar N, Hekimoglu B, Atakan C, Akkok N, Unal S. The coexistence of familial Mediterranian fever and polyarteritis nodosa: report of a case. Pediatr Nephrol 1996;10:631–633.
3. Uematsu-Yanagita M, Cho M, Hakamata Y, Tanaka M, Ishii K, Kume N, et al. Microscopic polyarteritis during polymyalgia rheumatica remission. Am J Kidney Dis 1996;28:289–291.
4. Vivancos J, Soler-Carrillo J, Ara-del Rey J, Font J. Development of polyarteritis nodosa in the course of inactive systemic lupus erythematosus. Lupus 1995; 4:494–495.

5. Guillevin L, Lhote F, Cohen P, Sauvaget F, Jarrousse B, Lortholary O, et al. Polyarteritis nodosa related to hepatitis B virus. A prospective study with long-term observation of 41 patients. Medicine 1995; 74:238–253.
6. Pateron D, Fain O, Sehonnou J, Trinchet JC, Beaugrand M. Severe necrotizing vasculitis in a patient with hepatitis C virus infection treated by interferon. Clin Exp Rheumatol 1996;14:79–81.
7. Daoud MS, Hutton KP, Gibson LE. Cutaneous periarteritis nodosa: a clinicopathological study of 79 cases. Br J Dermatol 1997;136:706–713.
8. Goritsas CP, Repanti M, Papadaki E, Lazarou N, Andonopoulos AP. Intrahepatic bile duct injury and nodular regenerative hyperplasia of the liver in a patient with polyarteritis nodosa. J Hepatol 1997;26:727–730.

Polychondritis, Relapsing

Possible Associated Conditions: Dermatomyositis; myelodysplastic syndrome *(1)*; rheumatoid arthritis;* Sjögren's syndrome* *(2)*.

Organs and Tissues	*Procedures*	*Possible or Expected Findings*
External examination and skin	Photograph and record appearance of head, chest, hands, and feet.	Chondritis involving nose (saddle nose) and ears (floppy ears); flail chest. Arthritic changes at any site.
	Submit sections of skin lesions for histologic study.	Erythemata nodosum; erythema multiforme; panniculitis *(3)*; vasculitis; venous thromboses.
	Prepare skeletal roentgenograms.	See below under "Bones and joints."
Blood	Submit sample for antibody study.	Antibodies to type II collagen.
Heart	Record weight; test competence of valves (p. 29), and submit samples for histologic sudy (p. 30).	Pericarditis.* Myocarditis.* Dilatation of aortic ring and destruction of cusps with aortic regurgitation.* Other valves may be affected *(4)* (mitral regurgitation)
	For dissection of the conduction system, see p. 26.	Conduction system abnormalities *(4)* with atrioventricular block.
Aorta	If an aortic aneurysm appears to be present, follow procedures described under that heading.	Aneurysm* of proximal thoracic or abdominal aorta.
Lungs, trachea, and neck organs	Larynx and trachea are best removed together with other neck organs, mediastinum, and lungs. Open airways in posterior midline, photograph areas of collapse or obstruction, and record mechanical state (pliability) of cartilage. Submit samples of all segments for histologic study.	Degeneration and inflammation of larynx and tracheobronchial tree with tracheal stenosis or collapse, which may be the cause of sudden death and suffocation. Aspiration broncho pneumonia.
Kidneys	Follow procedures described under "glomerulonephritis."	Segmental necrotizing glomerulonephritis* with crescent formation.
Lymph nodes	Submit samples for histologic study.	Castleman-like lymphadenopathy *(5)*.
Other organs		Vasculitis of small vessels; manifestations of Sjögren's syndrome.*
Eyes	For removal and specimen preparation, see p. 85.	Conjunctivitis; episcleritis; iritis; keratitis; cataracts; optic neuritis; retinal vasculitis.
Base of skull with middle and inner ear	For removal of middle and inner ear, see p. 72.	Swelling and occlusion of Eustachian tube; otitis media.* Cochleo-vestibular system may be affected by polychondritic changes.
Bones and joints	For removal, prosthetic repair, and specimen preparation, see p. 95. For maceration techniques, see p. 97.	Eburnation of bones; periostitis; osteoarthritis;* degeneration of cartilage of costochondral junctions and peripheral joints, with joint deformities.
	Prepare sections of bone marrow (see p. 96).	Mylelodysplastic changes *(1)*.

References

1. Diebold L, Rauh G, Jager K, Lohrs U. Bone marrow pathology in relapsing polychonditis: high frequency of myelodysplastic syndrome. Br J Haematol 1995;89:820–830.
2. Harada M, Yoshida H, Mimura Y, Ohishi M, Miyazima I, Ichikawa F, et al. Relapsing polychondritis associated with subclinical Sjögren's syndrome and phlegmon of the neck. Intern Med 1995;34:768–771.
3. Disdier P, Andrac L, Swiader L, Veit V, Fuzibet JG, Weiller-Merli C, et al. Cutaneous panniculitis and relapsing polychonditis: two cases. Dermatology 1996:193:266–268.

4. Del Rosso A, Petix NR, Pratesi M, Bini A. Cardiovascular involvement in relapsing polychondritis. Semin Arthr Rheum 1997;26:840–844.

5. Manganelli P, Quaini F, Olivetti G, Savini M, Pileri S. Relapsing polychondritis with Castleman-like lymphadenopathy: a case report. Clin Rheumat 1997:16:480–484.

Polycythemia

Synonyms and Related Terms: Polycythemia vera; primary polycythemia; secondary polycythemia.

NOTE: If patient had recent radionuclide (^{32}P) treatment, special precautions are indicated (p. 125). Consult with radiation safety officer or other responsible person.

Possible Associated Conditions: For tumors producing erythropoietic substances and secondary polycythemia, see below under "Possible or Expected Findings." Certain drugs (androgens) or adrenal cortical hypersecretion also may cause polycythemia.

Organs and Tissues	*Procedures*	*Possible or Expected Findings*
Chest and abdomen	If large vessel thrombosis is suspected, remove chest and abdominal organs en masse (p. 3) and open posterior aspect of inferior vena cava and aorta.	Thrombosis of inferior vena cava or hepatic veins (or both); aortic thrombosis or thrombosis at other sites.
Heart	For coronary arteriography, see p. 118. Other procedures depend on expected findings or grossly identified abnormalities as listed in right-hand column.	Coronary thrombosis; myocardial infarction. Chronic cardiac disease and right-to-left shunt may cause secondary polycythemia.
Lungs	Dissect one lung fresh and perfuse one lung with formalin (p. 47).	Emboli;* chronic pulmonary disease with alveolar hypoventilation may cause secondary polycythemia.
Intestinal tract	Record volume of blood in lumen. Submit samples of all segments for histologic study.	Ulcer of the duodenum.* Gastrointestinal hemorrhage.* Venous infarction.
Esophagus and stomach	For demonstration of varices, see p. 53.	Esophageal varices;* gastric varices.
Liver; portal, mesenteric, and splenic veins	Dissect veins *in situ*.	Portal vein thrombosis (see also "Hypertension, portal").
	Record appearance of hepatic veins. Record weight of liver and submit samples for histologic study.	Budd-Chiari syndrome* (hepatic venous outflow obstruction); myeloid metaplasia or leukemic infiltrates (in primary polycythemia). Hepatocellular carcinoma may be a cause of secondary polycythemia.
Spleen	Record weight and submit samples for histologic study.	Congestive splenomegaly. Myeloid metaplasia or leukemic infiltrates (in primary polycythemia).
Lymph nodes	Record average size and submit samples for histologic study.	Infiltrative lymphadenopathy (see above under "Spleen").
Peripheral arteries and veins	For phlebography and removal of femoral vessels, see p. 34.	Venous thrombosis;* thrombophlebitis. Leriche's syndrome.* Thromboses may occur in any vessel.
Kidneys	Procedures depend on expected findings or grossly identified abnormalities as listed in right-hand column.	Chronic renal disease (hydronephrosis, parenchymal disease, nephrotic syndrome), kidney transplantation;* renal cell carcinoma and Wilms tumor *(1)* may be causes of secondary polycythemia.
Brain and spinal cord	For cerebral arteriography, see p. 80. For removal and specimen preparation, see pp. 65 and 67, respectively.	Thrombotic or embolic vascular occlusions. Cerebral infarction.* Rarely, cerebellar hemangioblastoma may be a cause of secondary polycythemia.
Bone marrow	For preparation of sections and smears, see p. 96.	Hyperplasia. Leukemic infiltrates in some patients with primary polycythemia. Rarely, multiple myeloma* may be a cause of secondary polycythemia. Myeloid fibrosis, myeloid metaplasia, and acute myeloid leukemia* are complications of polycythemia vera.

Organs and Tissues	Procedures	Possible or Expected Findings
Other organs	Sample tumor tissue for histologic and electron microscopic study. (Snap-freeze material for determination of erythropoietic material).	Tumors of the prostate,* rectum, ovary,* uterus (leiomyoma) or breast,* as well as pheochromocytoma or malignant melanoma, rarely may be causes secondary polycythemia.

Reference

1. Lal A, Rice A, al Mahr M, Kern IB, Marshall GM. Wilms tumor associated with polycythemia: case report and review of the literature. J Pediatr Hematol/Oncol 1997;19:263–265.

Polymyalgia Rheumatica

Possible Associated Condition: Giant cell arteritis* *(1)*.

Organs and Tissues	Procedures	Possible or Expected Findings
Blood	Submit sample for determination of rheumatoid factor, antinuclear factor, serum complement concentrations, immunoglobulins, and other serum proteins.	Immunologic tests are important for distinguishing polymyalgia rheumatica from systemic lupus erythematosus,* rheumatoid arthritis,* multiple myeloma,* and other diseases.
Other organs	Follow procedures described under "Arteritis, giant cell."	Giant cell arteritis* and polymyalgia rheumatica are commonly associated *(1)*. Other associations such as scleritis *(2)* or ankylosing spondylitis* *(3)* need further confirmation.
Skeletal muscles	For removal and specimen preparation, see p. 80.	No diagnostic changes.
Joints	For removal, prosthetic repair, and specimen preparation, see p. 96.	Focal synovitis, mostly in neck, shoulder, and hip area.

References

1. Hunder GG. Giant cell arteritis and polymyalgia rheumatica. Med Clin North Am 1997;81:195–219.
2. Simmons IG, Kritzinger EE, Murray PI. Posterior scleritis and polymyalgia rheumatica. Eye 1997;11:727–728.
3. Elkayam O, Paran D, Yaron M, Caspi D. Polymyalgia rheumatica in patients with ankylosing spondylitis: a report of 5 cases. Clin Exp Rheumatol 1997;15:411–414.

Polymyositis (See "Dermatomyositis.")

Polyneuritis (See "Syndrome, Guillain-Barré.")

Polyneuropathy (See "Beriberi.")

Polyposis, Familial, and Related Syndromes

Related Terms: Cowden's disease (multiple hamartoma syndrome); familial colonic polyposis; juvenile polyposis; Gardner's syndrome; non-polyposis syndrome (hereditary nonpolyposis colorectal cancer syndrome); Peutz-Jegher's syndrome; Turcot's syndrome.

NOTE: The conditions listed under "Related Terms" are hereditable (autosomal-dominant) polyp syndromes. The Cronkhite-Canada syndrome lacks a hereditary transmission.

Organs and Tissues	Procedures	Possible or Expected Findings
External examination and oral cavity	Record and photograph skin lesions, cutaneous tumors, and hair and nail abnormalities. Sampling for histologic study depends on expected findings or grossly identified abnormalities as listed in right-hand column. (See also below under "Soft tissues.")	Cachexia, edema, alopecia, hyperpigmentations and vitiligo, and onychodystrophy in Cronkhite-Canada syndrome; mucocutaneous pigmentations (buccal, perioral, priorbital, distal extremities) in Peutz-Jeghers syndrome;* papules in face and oral mucosa in Cowden's disease; tumors of skin and subcutis (see below under "Soft tissues...") in Gardner's syndrome.
	Prepare skeletal roentgenograms.	Osteomas or exostoses (mandible, calvara) in Gardner's syndrome.

Organs and Tissues	*Procedures*	*Possible or Expected Findings*
Soft tissues (skin, subcutis, mesentery, retroperitoneum)	Record size and distribution of tumors; submit samples for histologic study.	Epidermoid cysts, lipomas, desmoid tumors *(1)*, mesenteric fibromatosis, wound fibromatosis, other fibromas or leiomyomas, and fibrosarcomas in Gardner's syndrome.
Stomach	Prepare photographs of mucosa. Submit samples for histologic study.	Hamartomatous cystic-glandular polyps in Cronkhite-Canada syndrome and in Peutz-Jeghers syndrome.
Small bowel	For perfusion and specimen preparation, see p. 54. Photograph lesions. Submit samples for histologic study.	Hamartomatous cystic-glandular polyps in Cronkhite-Canada syndrome, in Peutz-Jeghers syndrome, and in juvenile polyposis. Adenomatous polyps in Gardner's syndrome.
Colon	Prepare photographs. Submit samples of several polyps for histologic study. Include regional lymph nodes for identification of metastases.	Adenomatous polyps in familial colonic polyposis, Gardner's syndrome, non-polyposis syndrome, and Turcot's syndrome. Colorectal carcinomas in familial polyposis, in Gardner's syndrome and in rare cases of juvenile polyposis *(2)*. Hamartomatous cystic-glandular polyps in Cronkhite-Canada syndrome, in Peutz-Jeghers syndrome, and in juvenile polyposis.
Liver and bile ducts	Open common bile duct *in situ*, prepare photographs and sample for histologic study.	Ampullary carcinoma *(3)* or adenoma of bile duct *(4)* in Gardners syndrome.
Other organs	Procedures depend on expected findings or grossly identified abnormalities as listed in right-hand column.	Tumors of the breast, pancreas, ovary, and endometrium in Peutz-Jeghers syndrome; breast and thyroid tumors in Cowden's disease; endometrial adenocarcinoma in nonpolyposis syndrome. Adrenocortical adenomas or carcinomas or bilateral nodular hyperplasia also may occur, rarely with hypercortisolism.
Brain	For removal and specimen preparation, see p. 65.	Brain tumor* (e.g., glioblastoma multiforme) in Turcot syndrome.
Eyes	For removal and specimen preparation, see p. 85.	Orbital osteoma in Gardner's syndrome *(5)*.

References

1. Clark SK, Philips RK. Desmoid in familial adenomatous polyposis. Br J Surg 1996;83:1494–1504.
2. Coburn MC, Pricolo VE, DeLuca FG, Bland KI. Malignant potential in intestinal juvenile polyposis syndromes. Ann Surg Oncol 1995;2: 386–391.
3. Tomia H, Fukunari H, Shibata M, Yoshinaga K, Iwama T, Mishima Y. Ampullary carcinoma in familial adenomatous polyposis. Surg Today 1996;26:522–526.
4. Futami H, Furuta T, Hanai H, Nakamura S, Baba S, Kaneko E. Adenoma of the common bile duct in Gardner's syndrome may cause relapsing acute pancreatitis. J Gastroenterol 1997;32:558–561.
5. McNab AA. Orbital osteoma in Gardner's syndrome. Austr NZ J Ophthalmol 1998;26:169–170.

Polyradiculoneuropathy (See "Encephalitis, all types or type unspecified," "Myelopathy/Myelitis," and "Syndrome, Guillain-Barré.")

Polyserositis, Familial Paroxysmal (See "Fever, familial Mediterranian.")

Porphyria, all Types or Type Unspecified (See "Porphyia,..." as listed in following entries, and "Protoporphria,...").

NOTE: A rare form of hepatic porphyria, delta-aminolevulinate dehydratase deficient porphyria, and the erythropoietic porphyria, X-linked sideroblastic anemia, have not been tabulated here.

Porphyria, Acute Intermittent

Related Terms: Hepatic porphyria; hydroxymethyl bilane synthase (HMB) deficiency; porphobilinogen deaminase deficiency *(1)*.

NOTE: Multiple drugs such as barbiturates or sulfonamides may precipitate attacks of the disease, which generally is not a fatal condition. Infections or surgery also may precipitate attacks.

Organs and Tissues	Procedures	Possible or Expected Findings
External examination	Record body weight and length. Record extent of pigmentation.	Pigmentation; emaciation.
Urine	Submit samples for determination of δ-aminolevulinic acid (ALA) and porphobilinogen (PBG).	Increased concentrations of ALA and PBG.
Heart and blood vessels	If hypertension is suspected, see under that heading.	Hypertensive cardiovascular disease.
Liver	Submit samples for histologic, electron microscopic (p. 132), toxicologic (p. 16), and porphyrin fluorescence study.	Porphyrin fluorescence usually not demonstrable. Hepatocellular carcinoma may be present.
Brain, spinal cord, and peripheral nerves	For removal and specimen preparation, see pp. 65, 67, and 79, respectively.	Peripheral motor neuropathy. Hypothalamic involvement may be a cause of hyponatremia.
Vitreous	If dehydration is suspected, submit sample for sodium, chloride, and urea nitrogen determination (p. 85).	Manifestations of dehydration.*

Reference

1. Grandchamp B. Acute intermittent porphyria. Semin Liv Dis 1998;18:17–24.

Porphyria, Congenital Erythropoietic

Synonyms: Günther's disease; uroporphyrinogen III (URO) cosynthase deficiency.

NOTE: If bone marrow transplantation *(1)* was done, see also under that heading. Cord blood stem cell transplantation also has been done for this condition *(2)*.

Organs and Tissues	Procedures	Possible or Expected Findings
External examination and skin	Record extent and character of changes of hair, skin, and teeth. Prepare histologic sections of skin.	Hypertrichosis; erythrodontia; scarring and mutilation of hands and face.
Blood and bone marrow	For preparation of sections and smears, see p. 96. Submit fresh samples for porphyrin studies.	Hemolytic anemia. Erythrocytes contain large amounts of uroporphyrin I; normoblasts and reticulocytes exhibit intense red fluorescence.
Urine	Submit sample for porphyrin study as listed in right-hand column.	Uroporphyrin I and coproporphyrin I in high concentrations.
Spleen	Record size and weight. Photograph spleen (with scale).	Splenomegaly (may have been treated by splenectomy).
Kidneys	Sample for histologic study; request Gomori's stain for iron (p. 172).	Glomerulosclerosis and iron deposits *(3)*.

References

1. Thomas C, Ged C, Nordmann Y, de Verneuil H, Pellier I, Fischer A, Blanche S. Correction of congenital erythropoietic porphyria by bone marrow transplantation. J Pediatr 1996;129:453–456.
2. Zix-Kieffer I, Langer B, Eyer D, Acar G, Racadot E, Schlaeder G, et al. Successful cord blood stem cell transplantation for congenital erythropoietic porphyria (Gunther's disease). Bone Marrow Transpl 1996;18:217–220.
3. Lange B, Hofweber K, Waldherr R, Scharer K. Congenital erythropoietic porphyria associated with nephrotic syndrome. Acta Pediatr 1995;84: 1325–1328.

Porphyria Cutanea Tarda

Synonyms and Related Terms: Hepatic porphyria; uroporphyrinogen decarboxylase deficiency.

Possible Associated Conditions: Adverse drug reaction; chronic alcoholism;* chronic hepatitis C *(1)*; human immunodeficiency virus infection (AIDS)* *(1)*.

Organs and Tissues	Procedures	Possible or Expected Findings
External examination and skin	Record extent and character of skin and hair changes. Prepare histologic sections of skin.	Vesicles and bullae in face and other sun-exposed areas. Thickening and scarring of skin, with or without calcifications; hyperpigmentation. Hypertrichosis.
Urine	Submit sample for porphyrin study as listed in right-hand column.	Increased concentrations of uroporphyrin and hepatocarboxylic porphyrin.
Liver	Submit fresh hepatic tissue for demonstration of porphyrin fluorescence in Wood's light. Record weight of liver and submit samples for histologic study. Request Gomori's iron stain (p. 172). Prepare sample for electron microscopy (p. 132). Needle-shaped inclusions are best seen by light microscopy in unstained paraffin sections or after staining with the ferric ferricyanide reduction test (p. 172).	Ultraviolet light reveals red hepatic porphyrin fluorescence. Fatty changes, fibrosis, cirrhosis,* and hepatocellular carcinoma. Hemosiderosis is commonly found. Chronic hepatitis C may be a cause of porphyria cutanea tarda *(2)*. Needle shaped cytoplasmic inclusions (visible by light, fluorescence-, and electron microscopy).

References

1. O'Connor WJ, Badley AD, Dicken CH, Murphy GM. Porphyria cutanea tarda and human immunodeficiency virus: two cases associated with hepatitis C. Mayo Clin Proc 1998;73:895–897.
2. Lacour JP, Bodokh I, Castanet J, Bekri S, Ortonne JP. Porphyria cutanea tarda and antibodies to hepatitis C virus. Br J Dermatol 1993; 128:121–123.

Porphyria, Variegate

Synonyms and Related Terms: Hepatic porphyria; protoporphyrinogen oxidase deficiency *(1)*.

NOTE: The manifestations of the disease closely resemble those in porphyria cutanea tarda and hereditary coproporphyria. Measurements of porphyrins and porphyrin precursors are the only clearly distinguishing features. For autopsy procedures, see under "Porphyria cutanea tarda."

Reference

1. Kirsch RE, Meissner PN, Hift RJ. Variegate porphyria. Semin Liv Dis 1998;18:33–41.

Potassium (See "Disorder, electrolyte(s) and p. 14.)

Preexcitation, Ventricular

Related Term: Aberrant atrioventricular conduction; Wolff-Parkinson-White syndrome.

Possible Associated Conditions: Ebstein's malformation of tricuspid valve.

Pregnancy

NOTE: For general autopsy procedures, see p. 60. In some instances, procedures described under "Death, abortion-associated," "Embolism, amniotic fluid," or "Toxemia of pregnancy" may be indicated.

Progeria

Synonym: Werner syndrome.

Organs and Tissues	Procedures	Possible or Expected Findings
External examination and skin	Record body weight and length; prepare histologic sections of skin. Prepare skeletal roentgenograms.	Growth retardation; short stature; alopecia; cutaneous atrophy; loss of subcutaneous fat. Premature fusion of epiphyses; large calvarium.
Cardiovascular system		Myocardial infarction; coronary and peripheral atherosclerosis.
Other organs	Record weights of endocrine organs and submit samples for histologic study. Other procedures depend on expected findings or grossly identified abnormalities as listed in right-hand column.	Manifestations of congestive heart failure;* normal endocrine system; osteoarthritis;* rare neoplasms, such as meningioma, soft tissue tumors, osteosarcoma, and myeloid tumors *(1)*.
Brain	For cerebral arteriography, see p. 80. For removal and specimen preparation, see p. 65.	Cerebral atherosclerosis and hemorrhage.

Reference

1. Goto M, Miller RW, Ishikawa Y, Sugano H. Excess of rare cancers in Werner syndrome (adult progeria). Cancer Epid Biomarkers Prev 1996;5: 239–246.

Propanol (See "Poisoning, isopropyl alcohol.")

Proteinosis, Pulmonary alveolar (See "Lipoproteinosis, pulmonary alveolar.")

Protoporphyria, Erythropoietic

Synonym: Ferrochelatase deficiency *(1)*.

Organs and Tissues	*Procedures*	*Possible or Expected Findings*
External examination and skin	Record character and extent of skin lesions and prepare histologic sections of skin. Request PAS stain, with diastase digestion (p. 173).	Chronic eczematous skin lesions or superficial scarring; nail changes. Perivascular PAS-positive hyaline *(2)*.
Blood	Submit sample for protoporphyrin study *(2)*.	High concentration of protoporphyrin IX in erythrocytes and plasma.
Feces and urine	Submit samples for protoporphyrin study.	High concentration of protoporphyrin IX in feces; normal concentration in urine.
Liver	Record weight. Submit samples for routine histologic study. Submit fresh material for biochemical study, and material for ultraviolet microscopy and transmission electron microscopy (p. 132).	Intrahepatic cholestasis. Cirrhosis* and liver failure* is a rare complication *(3)*. Brown protoporphyrin deposits with red to yellow birefringence with a maltese cross configuration in hepatocytes, Kupffer cells, and bile canaliculi.
Gallbladder and bile	Submit stones for protoporphyrin analysis.	Cholelithiasis.* Increased protoporphyrin in bile.

References

1. Cox TM. Erythropoietic protoporphyria. J Inherit Metab Dis 1997;20:258–269.
2. Schleiffenbaum BE, Minder EI, Mohr P, Decurtins M, Schaffner A. Cytofluorometry as a diagnosis of protoporphyria. Gastroenterology 1992; 102:1044–1048.
3. Sarkany RPE, Alexander GJMA, Cox TM. Recessive inheritance of erythropoietic protoporphyria with liver failure. Lancet 1994;343:1394–1396.

Pseudogout

Synonym: Calcium pyrophosphate dihydrate (CPPD) deposition disease.

Organs and Tissues	*Procedures*	*Possible or Expected Findings*
External examination	Prepare skeletal roentgenograms.	Punctate calcium deposits in knee joints and, less commonly, in joints of hips, ankles, shoulders, or wrists or in symphysis ossium pubis and intervertebral disks.
Joints	Puncture grossly affected joints and submit sample of synovial fluid for crystal analysis under compensated polarized light *(2)*. See also p. 96. For removal of joints, prosthetic repair, and specimen preparation, see p. 96. Consult roentgenograms (see above).	Arthritis* with synovitis. Crystals of calcium pyrophosphate dihydrate in periarticular tissue *(1)* and synovial fluid. Cartilage contains calcium salts of pyrophosphate, hydroxyapatite, and orthophosphate.
Other organs	Procedures depend on expected underlying disease, as listed in right-hand column.	Alkaptonuria;* gout;* hemochromatosis;* hyperparathyroidism.*

References

1. Luisiri P, Blair J, Ellman MH. Calcium pyrophosphate dihydrate deposition disease presenting as tumoral calcinosis (periarticular pseudogout). J Rheumatol 1996;23:1647–1650.
2. Joseph J, McGrath H. Gout or 'pseudogout': how to differentiate crystal-induced arthropathies. Geriatr 1995;50:33–39.

Pseudohyperparathyroidism

Synonyms: Ectopic hyperparathyroidism; hyperparathyroidism in malignancy.

NOTE: This condition is caused by pulmonary, renal, and other malignant tumors that secrete parathyroid hormone or a parathyroid hormone-like substance. If hormone assay is intended, snap-freeze tumor tissue. Other autopsy procedures are the same as in hyperparathyroidism. Parathyroid glands should be normal.

Pseudohypoparathyroidism

Related Term: Pseudopseudohypoparathyroidism.

Organs and Tissues	*Procedures*	*Possible or Expected Findings*
External examination and oral cavity	Record abnormalities of stature and appearance of teeth. Prepare roentgenograms of hands, feet, and skull.	Short stature, round face, brachydactyly with shortening of carpal and metatarsal bones and bowing of long bones, and heterotopic calcification (Albright's hereditary osteo dystrophy). Coxa vara or coxa valga. Exostoses and thickening of calvaria may be found.
	Inspect mouth.	Dental aplasia and enamel defects.
Vitreous and urine	Submit samples for calcium and phosphate determination (pp. 16 and 85).	Decreased calcium and increased phosphate concentrations.
Neck organs	Dissect and record weights of parathyroid glands; submit samples for histologic study.	Parathyroid glands are normal or hyperplastic.
Other organs	Soft tissue roentgenograms may reveal calcium deposits. Sample for histologic study and request van Kossa stain (p. 173).	Metastatic calcification or ossification in subcutaneous tissue, lungs, kidneys, basal ganglia of brain, and other organs.
Bones	For removal, prosthetic repair, and specimen preparation, see p. 95.	See above under "External examination and oral cavity."
Eyes	For removal and specimen preparation, see p. 85.	Cataracts.

Pseudomyxoma Peritonei

Related Terms: Disseminated peritoneal adenomucinosis *(1)*; peritoneal mucinous carcinomatosis *(1)*.

Organs and Tissues	*Procedures*	*Possible or Expected Findings*
Abdomen	Record volume of intraperitoneal fluid; prepare smears; submit samples of peritoneum for histologic study.	Colloid carcinoma of stomach or colon. Well-differentated adenocarcinoma of ovary or, rarely, of appendix; ruptured appendiceal mucinous adenoma is the most common cause of peritoneal adenomucinosis.

Reference

1. Ronnet BM, Shmookler BM, Sugarbaker PH, Kurman RJ. Pseudomyxoma peritonei: new concepts in diagnosis, origin, nomenclature, and relationship to mucinous borderline (low malignant potential) tumors of the ovary. Anat Pathol 1997;2:197–226.

Pseudotumor Cerebri

Synonym: Benign intracranial hypertension; meningeal hydrops.

NOTE: This condition, which generally affects young, obese females, is characterized by symptoms and signs of increased intracranial pressure without a demonstrable cause. Hence, intracranial mass lesions, infections, and related conditions should be excluded. Such conditions include adrenal insufficiency;* Guillain-Barré syndrome* (increased colloid-osmotic pressure); hyperadrenalism; hypervitaminosis A* (e.g., after treatment of acne); hypoparathyroidism;* hypothroidism;* infectious mononucleosis;* Lyme disease; pregnancy; Sydenham's chorea; thrombus of the lateral or superior sagittal sinus (otitic hydrocephalus); and Wiskott-Aldrich syndrome.

Organs and Tissues	*Procedures*	*Possible or Expected Findings*
External examination	Record body weight and external features.	Obesity* (pickwickian syndrome).
Lungs	Perfuse one lung with formalin (p. 47).	Emphysema.*
Genital organs	Procedures depend on expected findings or grossly identified abnormalities as listed in right-hand column.	Pregnancy* or postpartum changes.
Brain, spinal cord, base of skull	For removal and specimen preparation of brain and spinal cord, see pp. 65 and 67, respectively. For dissection of base of skull, see p. 71.	Mastoiditis; lateral sinus thrombosis; marantic sinus thrombosis; head trauma.
Peripheral nerves	For removal and specimen preparation, see p. 79.	Polyneuritis.

Pseudoxanthoma elasticum

Synonym: Grönblad-Strandberg syndrome.

NOTE: This disease has not been studied thoroughly. Each autopsy should be regarded as a research procedure.

Organs and Tissues	*Procedures*	*Possible or Expected Findings*
External examination and skin	Record extent and character of skin lesions, photograph, and prepare histologic sections. Request von Kossa's and Verhoeff–van Gieson stains (p. 173). For decalcification procedures, see p. 97.	Skin papules and plaques, particularly in neck, axillae, groins, and popliteal fossae. Telangiectases at edge of lesions. Hemorrhages (also in nose). Basophilic material and calcium deposits *(1)* in middle and lower dermis.
	Prepare soft tissue roentgenograms.	Calcifications in dermis; calcifications of blood vessels.
Abdomen		Diaphragmatic hernia.*
Heart	Record weight. Histologic samples should include pericardium, endocardium, and all valves. Photograph cardiac lesions. For special stains, see above under "External examination and skin."	Hypertensive cardiomegaly. Characteristic plaques in pericardium and endocardium, with or without mitral valve involvement. Coronary atherosclerosis may have been a cause of angina *(2)*. Coronary thrombosis and myocardial infarction may be present also.
Arteries	Submit samples of large and medium-sized arteries from various sites; request von Kossa's and Verhoeff–van Gieson stains (p. 173).	Accelerated atherosclerosis; calcification of peripheral vessels.
Gastrointestinal tract	Record estimated or measured amount of blood in lumen.	Gastrointestinal hemorrhage;* peptic ulcer;* ulcerative colitis.*
Kidneys	Dissect renal arteries. For renal arteriography, see p. 59.	Hemangiomas; abnormalities of renal arteries.
Urinary bladder and uterus		Hemorrhages.
Other organs	Submit samples of all accessible organs and tissues, with or without gross lesions. Submit material for electron microscopy (p. 132).	See above under "Note."
Brain	For removal and specimen preparation, see p. 65.	Subarachnoid and intracerebral hemorrhage; hypertensive cerebrovascular disease.
Eyes	For removal and specimen preparation, see p. 85.	Degeneration of Bruch's membrane with retinal hemorrhages; sclerosis of choroid vessels; angioid streaks; degenerative scleral changes, as in skin.
Joints	For removal, prosthetic repair, and specimen preparation, see p. 96.	Hemarthrosis.

References

1. Truter S, Rosenbaum-Fiedler J, Sapadin A, Lebwohl M. Calcification of elastic fibers in pseudoxanthoma elasticum. Mt Sinai J Med 1996;63:210–215.
2. Kevorkian JP, Masquet C, Kural-Menasche S, Le Dref O, Beaufils P. New report of severe coronary artery disease in an eighteen-year-old girl with pseudoxanthoma elasticum. Case report and review of the literature. Angiology 1997;48:735–741.

Psittacosis (See "Ornithosis.")

Psoriasis

Possible Associated Conditions: Acquired immunodeficiency syndrome* *(1)*; malabsorption syndrome.*

NOTE: The manifestations of psoriasis may be considerably aggravated if the patients have been infected with the human immunodeficiency virus.

Organs and Tissues	*Procedures*	*Possible or Expected Findings*
External examination	Record extent and character of skin lesions. Prepare histologic sections of skin.	Characteristic skin and nail changes.
	Prepare roentgenograms of joints.	Arthritis.*

Organs and Tissues	*Procedures*	*Possible or Expected Findings*
Heart	Procedures depend on expected findings or grossly identified abnormalities as listed in right-hand column.	Aortitis involving ascending aorta and aortic valve with regurgitation; mitral valve and adjacent myocardium and conduction system also may be involved.
Small bowel	For *in situ* fixation, see p. 54.	Sprue-like changes with loss of villi.
Liver	Record weight. Submit samples for histologic study.	Fibrosis or cirrhosis and other abnormalities, particularly in patients who had been taking methotrexate.
Bones and joints	For removal, prosthetic repair, and specimen preparation, see p. 95.	Psoriatic arthritis and spondylitis.

Reference

1. Weitzul S, Duvic M. HIV-related psoriasis and Reiter's syndrome. Semin Cut Med Surg 1997;16:213–218.

Purpura, Anaphylactoid (See "Purpura, Schönlein-Henoch.")

Purpura Fulminans

NOTE: This nonthrombocytopenic purpura occurs mainly in children, following an infectious disease, e.g., a staphylococcal infection. Skin hemorrhages, intravascular thromboses, and gangrene are major manifestations. For additional autopsy procedures, see under the name of the underlying infection.

Purpura, Schönlein-Henoch

Synonyms and Related Terms: Allergic purpura; anaphylactoid purpura; hypersensitivity vasculitis.

Organs and Tissues	*Procedures*	*Possible or Expected Findings*
External examination and skin	Record extent and character of skin lesions, and photograph lesions.	Macular, petechial, or vesicular purpura. Ulcers of skin and dermal nodules. Angioneurotic edema* of lips and neck.
	Prepare histologic sections of involved skin. Request Gomori's iron stain (p. 172).	Angiitis (necrotizing vasculitis) involving capillaries, venules, and arterioles of dermis.
Gastrointestinal tract	Record estimated or measured volume of blood in lumen. Submit samples of all segments for histologic study.	Gastrointestinal hemorrhage.* Intussusception. Angiitis, as in skin.
Kidneys	Follow procedures described under "Glomerulonephritis."	Swollen cortex with subcapsular petechial hemorrhages. Acute focal glomerulonephritis with IgG, IgA, complement, and fibrinogen in mesangium. Angiitis, as in skin.
Neck organs	Open trachea and larynx in posterior midline.	Angioneurotic edema.*
Other organs		Findings may be similar to those described under "Polyarteritis nodosa" and "Failure, kidney."
Joints	For removal, prosthetic repair, and specimen preparation, see p. 96. Submit samples of synovium for histologic study.	Swelling of joints. Synovial angiitis (histologic manifestations as in skin).

Purpura, Thrombotic Thrombocytopenic

Synonyms and Related Term: Hemolytic uremic syndrome;* thrombotic microangiopathy.

Possible Associated Conditions: Acquired immunodeficiency syndrome* *(1)*; angiotropic large cell lymphoma *(2)*; glomerulonephritis;* polyarteritis nodosa;* rheumatoid arthritis;* Sjögren's syndrome;* systemic lupus erythematosus;* systemic sclerosis.*

Organs and Tissues	*Procedures*	*Possible or Expected Findings*
External examination and skin	Prepare histologic sections of skin with purpura; for special stains, see below.	Purpura; jaundice.

Organs and Tissues	Procedures	Possible or Expected Findings
Blood	Submit sample for microbiologic and serologic study (p. 102).	
Other organs and tissues	Record extent of hemorrhages; submit samples from all viscera and tissues listed in right-hand column. Request phosphotungstic acid hematoxylin, PAS, and Verhoeff–van Gieson stain (p. 173). Snap-freeze tissue samples for immunofluorescent study. For preparation for electron microscopy, see p. 132.	Fibrin and platelet thrombi, with or without microaneurysms and purpura in kidneys, adrenal glands, pancreas, heart, and brain; lesions may also be present in liver; spleen *(3)*, lymph nodes, muscle, bone marrow, and synovium. Fibrin thrombi can be demonstrated with labeled antihuman fibrin antibodies. Lesions in precapillary arterioles.

References

1. de Man AM, Smulders YM, Roozendaal KJ, Frissen PH. HIV-related thrombotic thrombocytopenic purpura: report of 2 cases and a review of the literature. Netherl J Med 1997;51:103–109.
2. Sill H, Hofler G, Kaufmann P, Horina J, Spuller E, Kleinert R, Beham-Schmid C. Angiotropic large cell lymphoma presenting as thrombotic microangiopathy (thrombotic thrombocytopenic purpura). Cancer 1995;75:1167–1170.
3. Saracco SM, Farhi DC. Splenic pathology in thrombotic thrombocytopenic purpura. Am J Surg Pathol 1990;14:223–229.

Pyelonephritis

Synonyms and Related Terms: Acute ascending pyelonephritis; calculous pyelonephritis; chronic interstitial nephritis; chronic pyelonephritis; emphysematous pyelonephritis; obstructive uropathy.

NOTE: If chronic renal insufficiency was diagnosed, see under "Failure, kidney."

Possible Associated Conditions: Diabetes mellitus* *(1)*. See also below under "Possible or Expected Findings."

Organs and Tissues	Procedures	Possible or Expected Findings
Abdominal cavity	Identify and record site of obstruction before removal of retroperitoneal and pelvic organs. For renal angiography and urography, see p. 59.	Aberrant vessels; adhesions (postradiation lesions). Perirenal abscess in acute pyelonephritis. Retroperitoneal fibrosis.* Tumor.
Urine	Submit sample for microbiologic study (p. 102). Prepare smear of sediment.	Evidence of inflammation.
Urogenital system	Remove kidneys, ureters, and pelvic organs in one block. Record weight of both kidneys. If microbiologic study is intended, submit one-half of a kidney (p. 102).	Fistulas between kidney and other sites may be observed *(2,3)*.
	Record size of right and left renal pelves. Record character of contents. Cut kidneys in half and record number and size of abscesses and scars. Record appearance of papillae.	Hydronephrosis;* pyonephrosis; nephrolithiasis.* Necrotizing papillitis.
	Record width of ureters. Record size, contents, and degree of trabeculation of urinary bladder; record size and appearance of prostate.	Hydroureter; pyoureter. Urolithiasis; tumor of urinary bladder* or of adjacent organs; benign prostatic hyperplasia.
	If urethral valves are suspected to be present, see p. 60.	Urethral valves. A dilated bladder in a woman without obvious obstruction may indicate presence of descensus of uterus (which is difficult to demonstrate at autopsy).
Other organs	Procedures depend on suspected underlying conditions.	Amyloidosis* *(4)*. Manifestations of diabetes mellitus* or sickle cell disease.*
Neck organs	Dissect parathyroid glands, record weights, and submit samples for histologic study.	Hyperplasia or adenoma(s) of parathyroid glands.
Brain and spinal cord	For removal and specimen preparation, see pp. 65 and 67, respectively.	Abnormal findings may explain obstructive uropathy ("neurogenic bladder").
Bones	For sampling and specimen preparation, see p. 95.	Osteoclastic osteoporosis in primary or secondary hyperparathyroidism.*

References

1. Pontin AR, Barnes RD, Joffe J, Kahn D. Emphysematous pyelonephritis in diabetic patients. Br J Urol 1995;75:71–74.
2. O'Brien JD, Ettinger NA. Nephrobronchial fistula and lung abscess resulting from nephrolithiasis and pyelonephritis. Chest 1995;108:1166–1168.
3. Nayir A, Kadioglu A, Sirin A, Emre S, Oney V. A case of an enterorenal fistula and pyelonephritis with air in renal pelvis. Pediatr Radiol 1995;25: 229–230.
4. Mazuecos A, Araque A, Sanchez R, Martinez MA, Guesmes A, Rivero M, et al. Systemic amyloidosis secondary to pyonephrosis. Resolution after nephrectomy. Nephrol Dial Transplant 1996;11:875–878.

Pyothorax (See "Empyema, pleural.")

Q,R

Q Fever (See "Fever, Q")

Rabies

NOTE: (1) In most instances, an autopsy limited to the brain is sufficient to confirm the diagnosis. (2) Rabies virus is especially infectious and thus, universal **precautions** should be strictly followed (p. 146). Avoid the use of scalpels whenever possible. The generation of aerosols should be assiduously avoided. (3) Consult the state health department prior to commencing the autopsy. (4) Request viral cultures. (5) Request immunofluorescent stain for rabies. (6) Serologic studies are available from the state health department laboratories. (7) This is a **reportable** disease.

Organs and Tissues	*Procedures*	*Possible or Expected Findings*
External examination	Photograph possible sites of animal bite.	
Chest and abdomen	See above under "Note." If a complete autopsy is done, sample heart, lungs, kidneys, pancreas, submaxillary salivary glands, and adrenal glands; freeze or refrigerate sampled tissues and submit for viral study (see below under "Brain and spinal cord").	Myocarditis with necrosis of muscle fibers and infiltrates of lymphocytes and histiocytes.
Blood	Obtain serum for serologic studies.	
Brain and spinal cord	For removal and specimen preparation, see pp. 65 and 67, respectively. Freeze or refrigerate cerebral tissue immediately after removal and submit frozen to special laboratory for fluorescent antibody staining. Take these sections from hippocampus or brain stem. Place the refrigerated tissues in 50% neutral glycerol saline solution for preservation. Fix remaining brain and spinal cord tissue in 15% formalin and submit for histologic study. As an alternative to freezing of tissue, immunoperoxidase methods for detection of rabies viral antigens can now be applied to formalin-fixed tissue *(1)*. Viral particles can be revealed by ultrastructural examination.	Rabies encephalitis. Generally, no external abnormalities. Perivascular cuffing and microglial hyperplasia as well as neuronophagia, predominantly in gray matters (pons and medulla). Negri bodies in neurons are pathognomonic; they are found primarily in hippocampal pyramidal neurons and cerebellar Purkinje cells. Absence of Negri bodies does not exclude diagnosis of rabies encephalitis. Inflammatory reaction may be completely lacking. In paralytic rabies, changes are most evident in spinal cord, with anterior horn neuronal degeneration.
Lacrimal glands	For technique of removal, see p. 87. Submit refrigerated sample for virologic study and fluorescent antibody testing.	
Ganglia	Submit samples of cranial, spinal, and sympathetic ganglia for histologic study.	Neural degeneration with neuronophagia and lymphocytic infiltrates.

Reference

1. Mrack RE, Young L. Rabies encephalitis in humans: pathology, pathogenesis, and pathophysiology. J Neuropathol Exp Neurol 1994;53:1–10.

From: *Handbook of Autopsy Practice*, 3rd Ed. Edited by: J. Ludwig © Humana Press Inc., Totowa, NJ

Rachischisis (See "Meningocele.")

Radiation (See "Injury, radiation.")

Rape

Related Term: Sexual assault.

NOTE: In almost all instances, the procedures described under "Assault" and under "Homicide" must also be followed. See also refs. *(1)* and *(2)*. For the evaluation of bite marks, photographs with and without scales and black and white film should be used. The help of a forensic dentist may be required for proper evaluation. For possible sperm or other stains, wet mount smears are made by smearing a specimen swab onto a slide and then adding a drop of sterile saline and covering with a coverslip, or one can drop saline first and then mix with a specimen swab. One can also swirl a specimen swab in a test tube with 1–2 mL of sterile saline, aspirate some of the specimen-enriched fluid, and place on the slide. The remainder can be used for other tests.

Organs and Tissues	*Procedures*	*Possible or Expected Findings*
External examination	Comb pubic hair over a towel and then pull sample; also, pull samples of hair from head (p. 17). Collect fingernail clippings and place in containers marked "right" and "left."	Blood, hair, and other material on the victim's body may be the assailant's and thus may become important legal evidence.
	Collect blood, hair, fibers, and residues of urine or saliva and/or semen that may have stained the victim's clothing or that may be found on the skin of the victim. For study of stains and scrapings, see below.	Saline swab may reveal saliva, particularly on breasts (areola, nipples). Photographs of the decedent's teets, with and without scales, may be useful if the victim may have bitten the assailant.
	Introduce sterile dry cotton swab into the posterior vault of the vagina or—preferably—into the cervical canal. Prepare smear on glass slide and send to crime laboratory for identification of sperm (see also above under "Note").	
	Keep a second swab dry for acid phosphatase determination and other tests (fluorescence *in situ* hybridization, DNA fingerprinting, Southern blot analysis, and polymerase chain reaction).	Material may be positive for acid phosphatase or p30 glycoprotein. Nonsperm male cells may be present, identified by Y-chromosome specific DNA probes.
	Repeat above tests with two other sets of swabs for study of lower rectum and anus (smears should be as thin as possible) and of oral cavity.	Spermatozoa and acid phosphatase-positive material may be found in rectum and oral cavity.
	A Woods lamp can be used to illuminate semen stains on the body or clothing.	Due to the flavin residues, seminal fluid appears green-yellow.
	Photograph face and oral cavity, if indicated. If a photocolposcope is available, vaginal vault and cervix can be photographed *in situ.*	Lips and buccal surfaces of cheeks may show evidence of trauma. Bite marks may be present (see above under "Note") and may help to identify the assailant.
Blood	Submit sample in EDTA tube for determination of blood groups. Retain specimens through end of office retention period. Further testing, e.g., for HIV or syphilis, may be requested during this period.	The victim's blood groups are important for comparison with specimens from the alleged assailant. Evidence of acquired immunodeficiency syndrome,* syphilis,* or intoxication at time of rape may have legal implications.
Other organs and tissues	Submit samples for toxicologic study (p. 16).	
Genital organs	Photograph internal genitalia, anus, and vulva. Additional spermatic fluid may be retrieved from cervical canal during cervical dissection. Application of toluidine blue may enhance lacerations *(3)* (apply only after specimens for laboratory study have been obtained).	There may be perineal, perianal or vaginal lacerations, evidence of trauma to the cervix, or foreign bodies.
	Record appearance of all segments of genital tract. Prepare histologic sections of lacerations and wounds and of endometrium. If there is enough spermatic fluid, submit sample for microbiologic study.	Uterine contents and endometrium may reveal pregnancy.*

How Does One Examine Stains or Other Residues of Suspected Spermatic Fluid?

Using a sterile cotton swab moistened with sterile saline, lift suspected dried spermatic fluid from hair or skin of external genitalia, perineum, buttocks, or other sites. Stains on clothing will be extracted by forensic laboratory personnel. Let specimens air dry in absence of sunlight and then place in paper bags or envelopes and seal. Smears are made for the demonstration of spermatozoa, cytologic changes, bacteria, and other possible findings. Other samples are used for the determination of acid phosphatase, as described below.

How Is Acid Phosphatase Determined in Scrapings and Stains and What Does a Positive Test Mean?

Place frozen swab (see above) in 3 mL of isotonic saline and elute for one-half hour. Use 0.5 mL of this extract for acid phosphatase assay by the method of Shinowara, Jones, and Reinhart. For this, Harleco Dry-Pack Reagent is recommended. The presence of acid phosphatase indicates the presence of spermatic fluid. Determination of the acid phosphatase activity provides a guideline for a rough estimation of the time interval between intercourse and removal for freezing or testing of the specimen (see below).

How Can One Estimate the Time Interval Between Intercourse and Removal for Freezing or Testing of the Specimen?

Usually, the survival time of morphologically recognizable spermatozoa in the vagina is less than 24 h, but on occasion this may be much longer. Thus, within the first 24 h after coitus, 64% of cervical smears have been found to be positive for spermatozoa. At day 10, spermatozoa have been found in 13% of the smears. Obviously, if the assailant had had a vasectomy, spermatozoa will not be found at any time.

Spermatozoa have been found in the vagina of some women several days or weeks after death. Dried stains (see above) may give positive results after longer intervals. Acid phosphatase activities greater than 5 Bodansky units (for method, see above) indicate that probably less than 12 h have elapsed since the time of intercourse *(1)*. In another study, vaginal swab specimens showed acid phosphatase activities of more than 2,000 King-Armstrong units/dL during the first 12 h after intercourse. Vaginal acid phosphatase activities returned to normal (<201 King-Armstrong units/dL) within approx 48 h. Regardless of the methods used, only very rough estimates can be made.

References

1. Spitz WU, Platt MS. Medicolegal Investigation of Death. Charles C. Thomas Publisher, Springfield, IL, 1993, pp. 716–722.
2. Collins KA. The laboratory's role in detecting sexual assault. Lab Med 1998;29:361–365.
3. Bays J, Lewman LV. Toluidine blue in the detection at autopsy of perineal and anal lacerations in victimes of sexual abuse. Arch Pathol Lab Med 1992;116:620–621.

Acknowledgement

Julia Martin, M.D., Associate Medical Examiner, Hillsborough County Medical Examiner Department, has provided valuable advice on the procedures described in rape cases.

Reaction, Microgranulomatous Hypersensitivity, of Lungs (See "Pneumoconiosis" and "Pneumonia, interstitial.")

Reaction to Transfusion

NOTE: The autopsy should be done as soon as possible after death. Every attempt should be made to secure donor blood for typing and culture at 30°C and 37°C (see below).

Organs and Tissues	*Procedures*	*Possible or Expected Findings*
External examination	Record color of skin. If air embolism is suspected, follow procedures described under that heading.	Jaundice. Air embolism.*
Blood	Submit samples for microbiologic (p. 102) and serologic study and for typing.	Gram-negative rods or other endotoxin-producing bacteria may have been perfused accidentally. More reliable is culture from residual donor blood (see above) at 30°C and 37°C. Some contaminants do not grow at the higher temperature.
Lungs	Record weights; submit samples for histologic study.	Shock lungs (see under "Syndrome, adult respiratory distress").
Kidneys	Photograph, record weights, and submit samples for histologic study.	Fibrin thrombi and platelet thrombi in small vessels; hemoglobinuric nephrosis.
Other organs	Procedures depend on expected findings or grossly identified abnormalities as listed in right-hand column.	Fibrin thrombi and platelet thrombi in small vessels (see under "Coagulation, disseminated intravascular").
Urine	Prepare sediment.	Hematuria.
Neck organs and trachea	Open larynx and trachea along posterior midline.	Angioneurotic edema; aspiration of vomitus.

Regurgitation, Aortic (See "Insufficiency, aortic [chronic or acute].")

Regurgitation, Mitral (See "Insufficiency, mitral [chronic or acute].")

Regurgitation, Pulmonary (See "Insufficiency, pulmonary valvular.")

Regurgitation, Tricuspid (See "Insufficiency, tricuspid [chronic or acute].")

Reticulosis, Midline Malignant (See "Granuloma, midline.")

Rhabdomyoma, Cardiac (See "Tumor of the heart.")

Rickets (See "Deficiency, vitamin D" and "Syndrome, Fanconi.")

Ring, Lower Esophageal

Synonym: Schatzki's ring.

Organs and Tissues	*Procedures*	*Possible or Expected Findings*
External examination	Prepare chest roentgenogram or follow other procedures for diagnosis of pneumothorax (p. 430).	Pneumothorax.*
Esophagus	For postmortem demonstration of lower esophageal ring, see p. 53.	Bolus in esophagus; reflux esophagitis.

Rubella

Synonyms and Related Terms: Congenital rubella syndrome;* German measles; three-day measles.

NOTE: Congenital rubella syndrome is presented under "Syndrome, congenital rubella."

(1) The virus may be isolated from blood, urine, feces, tears, and CSF. (2) Collect any tissues that appear to be infected. (3) Usually, special stains are not helpful. (4) Serologic studies are available from local and state health department laboratories (p. 135). (5) This is a **reportable** disease.

Organs and Tissues	*Procedures*	*Possible or Expected Findings*
External examination, skin, and eyes	Prepare histologic sections of skin lesions.	Dermatitis and exanthema; subconjunctival hemorrhages; lymphadenopathy.
Blood	Obtain serum for serologic study.	
Cerebrospinal fluid	Submit sample for cell count and determination of protein concentrations (p. 104).	Increased cell count and elevated protein concentrations in presence of encephalitis.*
Gastrointestinal tract; kidneys		Hemorrhages.
Lymph nodes	Submit postauricular, suboccipital, and posterior cervical lymph nodes for histologic study.	Lymphadenitis.
Brain	For removal and specimen preparation, see p. 65. Submit sample for microbiologic study (see above under "Note" and p. 102).	Acute rubella encephalitis with nonspecific perivascular infiltrates, cerebral edema, and neuronal degeneration. Rarely, severe hemorrhages.
Joints	For removal, prosthetic repair, and specimen preparation, see p. 96.	Arthritis (polyarthritis and tenosynovitis) of fingers, wrists, and knees.

Rubeola (See "Measles.")

S

St. Louis Encephalitis (See "Encephalitis, all types or type unspecified.")

Sarcoidosis

NOTE: The typical noncaseating granuloma of sarcoidosis is not pathognomonic. Fungal or mycobacterial infections, brucellosis,* hypersensitivity pneumonitis, pneumoconiosis* (in rare instances, sarcoid granulomas may contain calcium oxalate crystals), and Wegener's granulomatosis* must be ruled out. Metastatic calcifications may occur *(1)*.

Organs and Tissues	*Procedures*	*Possible or Expected Findings*
External examination and skin	Prepare histologic sections of skin lesions.	Erythema nodosum; lupus pernio; maculopapular eruptions; scars and keloids.
	Prepare chest and skeletal roentgenograms.	Pulmonary and hilar infiltrates; cystic bone changes in phalanges of hands and feet.
Blood	Submit sample for determination of globulin concentrations.	Hyperglobulinemia; hypercalcemia.
Heart	Record weight. If there was a history of heart block, prepare histologic sections of conduction system (p. 26).	Cor pulmonale; myocardial sarcoidosis, particularly of left ventricular wall (cardiomyopathy*). The conduction system may be involved also *(1)*.
Lungs	Submit one lobe for microbiologic study (p. 103). Perfuse one lung with formalin (p. 47). If superinfection is expected, order Grocott's methenamine silver, acid fast, and Gram stain (p. 172).	Noncaseating, noninfectious granulomas. Pulmonary fibrosis with honeycombing; aspergillomas or other mycetomas may be found. Pleural sarcoidosis. See also above under "Note."
Lymph nodes	Record size of hilar (mediastinal), abdominal, and peripheral lymph nodes (cervical, axillary, inguinal). Submit samples for histologic study.	Granulomatous lymphadenitis with epithelioid cells and giant cells (with or without asteroid and conchoid or Schaumann bodies).
Liver	Record weight; submit samples for histologic study.	Granulomatous hepatitis. Granulomatous cholangitis (chronic cholestasis of sarcoidosis) resembling primary biliary cirrhosis.
Spleen	Record weight; submit samples for histologic study. If there is splenomegaly or other evidence of portal hypertension,* follow procedures described under that heading.	Granulomatous splenitis. For histologic features, see under "Lymph nodes."
Kidneys	If there is evidence of kidney failure,* see under that heading.	Nephrolithiasis;* nephrocalcinosis.
Other tissues	Procedures depend on expected findings or grossly identified abnormalities as listed in right-hand column. If metastatic calcifications are found *(1)*, order von Kossa stain (p. 173).	Manifestations of portal hypertension* or of kidney failure.* Granulomas and associated lesions may occur in many organs and tissues, such as nasal mucosa, tonsils, larynx with epiglottis, stomach, or rectum.

From: *Handbook of Autopsy Practice,* 3rd Ed. Edited by: J. Ludwig © Humana Press Inc., Totowa, NJ

Organs and Tissues	Procedures	Possible or Expected Findings
Brain and spinal cord	For removal and specimen preparation, see pp. 65 and 67, respectively.	Chronic meningitis; space-occupying lesions (submeningeal nodular granulomas).
Pituitary gland	If there is evidence of diabetes insipidus* or pituitary insufficiency,* see under those headings.	Granulomatosis.
Eyes, lacrimal glands, and other orbital tissues	For removal and specimen preparation, see pp. 85 and 87.	Iridocyclitis; chorioretinitis; papilledema; posterior uveitis; keratoconjunctivitis sicca; conjunctival follicles; cataracts. Involvement of lacrimal glands and other orbital tissues *(2)*.
Parotid gland	If there is evidence of parotid involvement, other salivary glands should also be studied. Parotid gland can be biopsied from scalp incision (p. 65). Submascillary gland can be removed with floor of mouth (p. 4).	Sarcoidosis of parotid gland is common.
Skeletal muscles and peripheral nerves	For sampling and specimen preparation, see pp. 80 and 79, respectively.	Sarcoid neuropathy and sarcoid myopathy.
Bones and joints	For removal, prosthetic repair, and specimen preparation, see p. 95.	Cystic changes, primarily of small bones of hands and feet. Sarcoidosis of joints *(3)*.

References

1. Nelson JE, Kirschner PA, Teirstein AS. Sarcoidosis presenting as heart disease. Sarcoidosis Vasculitis Diffuse Lung Dis 1996;13:178–182.
2. Smith JA, Foster CS. Sarcoidosis and its ocular manifestations. Int Ophthalmol Clin 1996;36:109–125.
3. Pettersson T. Rheumatic features of sarcoidosis. Curr Opin Rheumatol 1998;10:73–78.

Schistosomiasis

Synonyms and Related Terms: Bilharziasis; *Schistosoma haematobium* infection; *Schistosoma japonicum* infection; *Schistosoma mansoni* infection.

NOTE: Unless specifically stated, the changes listed below refer to chronic schistosomiasis mansoni and japonica.

(1) Collect all tissues that appear to be infected. (2) Request direct examination for *Schistosoma*. The following procedures have been described and recommended *(1)*. For demonstration of *Schistosoma* eggs, compress 4-mm tissue fragments—for instance, mucosa of the urinary bladder—between glass slides. If this gives negative results, digest a 5-g portion of tissue in potassium hydroxide.

For the recovery of adult worms of *Schistosoma mansoni* and *Schistosoma haematobium*, remove the viscera en bloc (p. 3) and rinse with water. Separate the intestines from the mesentery. Subsequently, perfuse the portal vein system, the liver, and one lung with saline *(2)*. Then pass the perfusion fluid through a monofilament nylon cloth with an aperture size of 180 µm. Submerge the cloth in water and examine with a dissecting microscope. Fix worms in formalin solution. Examine the intestinal mucosa directly.

From the urinary bladder, ureters, and surrounding connective tissue, worms can be recovered as follows. Inject water into the tissue until the tissue increases 2 or 3 times in thickness. Then compress the tissue gently with a glass plate. Cut slices 0.1–0.2 cm in thickness. Compress these slices between the glass plate and the stage of a dissecting microscope and examine for the presence of adult worms. Many worms also will be present in the fluid expressed from the tissue as it is cut. For the counting of eggs in tissues, urine, and feces, see ref. *(1)*. Immunodiagnostic methods (ELISA and immunoblot) also have been developed *(3)*. (3) Request Giemsa stain (p. 172). (4) Usually, no special precautions are indicated. (5) Serologic studies are available from the Centers for Disease Control and Prevention, Atlanta, GA (p. 135). (6) This is not a reportable disease.

Organs and Tissues	Procedures	Possible or Expected Findings
External examination and skin	Record extent and photograph skin lesions and prepare histologic sections.	Jaundice; edema and pyogenic infection of penis, scrotum, and perineum in *Schistosoma haematobium*. Clubbing of fingers and toes.
Blood	Collect serum for serologic studies.	
Heart	Record heart weight and thickness of ventricles.	Cor pulmonale.
Lungs	See above under "Note." For pulmonary arteriography, see p. 50. Perfuse one lung with formalin (p. 47). Request Verhoeff–van Gieson stain (p. 173).	Embolized eggs with obstructive arteriolitis, angiomatoid lesions, granulomas, and arteriovenous fistulas. Arteriosclerosis; hyaline emboli in small pulmonary arteries.
Peritoneal cavity	Submit samples with lesions for histologic study.	Subserosal granulomatous nodules; peritoneal and retroperitoneal fibrosis;* ascites.

Organs and Tissues	Procedures	Possible or Expected Findings
Intestinal tract and mesentery	See above under "Note." Submit samples of all segments for histologic study.	Submucosal granulomas and submucosal fibrosis; mucosal ulcers; esophageal varices; inflammatory polyps.
Portal and splenic veins	See above under "Note." Dissect *in situ* or after en bloc removal of abdominal organs (p. 3). If there is evidence of portal hypertension,* follow procedures described under that heading.	Thrombosis or cavernous transformation of portal vein system.
Liver	See above under "Note." For portal venography, see p. 56. Record weight, photograph, and submit samples for histologic study.	Hepatic fibrosis *(4)*. Hepatic thrombophlebitis.
Spleen	Record weight.	Congestive splenomegaly.
Kidneys, ureters, and pelvic organs	See above under "Note." Remove kidneys together with ureters and pelvic organs.	Hydronephrosis,* pyonephrosis, pyelonephritis,* granulomatous reaction to eggs and urinary bladder papillomas in *Schistosoma haematobium* infection.
	For *in situ* fixation of urinary bladder, see p. 59.	Ureteritis with strictures and scars; ureterolithiasis and urolithiasis; chronic constricting bilharzial cystitis and tumor of bladder in *Schistosoma haematobium* infection. The uterus and Fallopian tubes also may be involved *(5)*.
	For dissection of penis and urethra, see p. 60. Submit samples of prostate and seminal vesicles for histologic study.	Hyperplastic and fibrotic seminal vesiculitis and prostatitis; fibrotic granulomatous and suppurative infection of urethra and penis in *Schistosoma haematobium* infection.
	Submit samples of spermatic cord, epididymis, and testicles for histologic study.	Granulomatous infection by *Schistosoma haematobium.*
Other organs	Submit sections from all sites with grossly identifiable lesions.	*Schistosoma mansoni* infection may occur in every organ. Most frequent ectopic sites are spinal cord, brain, and genital tract.

References

1. Kamel IA, Cheever AW, Elwi AM, Mosimann JE, Danner R: *Schistosoma mansoni* and *S. haematobium* infections in Egypt. I. Evaluation of techniques for recovery of worms and eggs at necropsy. Am J Trop Med Hyg 1977;26:696–701.
2. Cheever AW. A quantitative post-mortem study of schistosomiasis mansoni in man. Am J Trop Med Hyg 1968;17:38–64.
3. Tsang VC, Wilkins PP. Immunodiagnosis of schistosomiasis. Screen with FAST-ELISA and confirm with immunoblot. Clin Lab Med 1991; 11(4):1029–1039.
4. Andrade ZA, Peixoto E, Guerret S, Grimaud JA. Hepatic connective tissue changes in hepatosplenic schistosomiasis. Hum Pathol 1992; 23(5):566–573.
5. Helling-Giese G, Kjetland EF, Gundersen SG, Poggensee G, Richter J, Krantz I, et al. Schistosomiasis in women: manifestations in the upper reproductive tract. Acta Trop 1996;62(4):225–238.

Scleroderma (See "Sclerosis, systemic.")

Sclerosis, Amyotrophic Lateral (See "Disease, motor neuron.")

Sclerosis, Diffuse (See "Sclerosis, Schilder's cerebral.")

Sclerosis, Multiple

Synonyms and Related Terms: Acute and subacute variants: Acute multiple sclerosis (Marburg type), acute necrotizing myelopathy; concentric sclerosis (Baló type); concentric lacunar leukoencephalopathy; encephalitis periaxialis diffusa (Schilder's type; see also next entry, "Sclerosis, Schilder's cerebral"*); neuromyelitis optica (Dèvic type).

Chronic Variants: Classic or Charcot type multiple sclerosis (relapsing and remitting, secondary progressive, arrested, benign, monosymptomatic and asymptomatic, primary progressive).

Possible Associated Conditions: Hypertrophic polyradiculoneuropathy.

Organs and Tissues	Procedures	Possible or Expected Findings
Brain and spinal cord	For removal and specimen preparation, see pp. 65 and 67, respectively. Record thickness of optic nerves. Request Luxol fast blue stain for myelin and Bielschowski's stain for axons (p. 172).	Changes most commonly in cerebral white matter (periventricular), spinal cord white matter, and optic nerves. Appearance of plaques varies, depending on whether they are active, chronic active, or inactive.

Organs and Tissues	Procedures	Possible or Expected Findings
Brain and spinal cord *(continued)*		Myelin loss, accompanied by a variable histiocytic infiltrate and gliosis, are characteristic findings. Perivascular lymphocytic cuffs are present.
Other organs and tissues	Procedures depend on expected findings or grossly identified abnormalities as listed in right-hand column.	Aspiration bronchopneumonia; disuse atrophy of skeletal muscles.

Sclerosis, Schilder's Cerebral

Synonyms: Encephalitis periaxialis diffusa; multiple sclerosis, Schilder's type.

NOTE: The pathologic changes in adrenoleukodystrophy may resemble those in Schilder's disease (see also under "Leukodystrophy,...").

Organs and Tissues	Procedures	Possible or Expected Findings
Brain and spinal cord	For removal and specimen preparation, see pp. 65 and 67, respectively. See also above under "Note."	Diffuse or large patches of demyelination in the cerebral white matter (>2 × 3 cm), with sudanophilic myelin breakdown products in macrophages.
	Submit wet tissue for determination of phospholipids and cholesterol esters.	Depletion of phospholipids and increase of cholesterol esters (nonspecific manifestations of myelin sheath breakdown).

Sclerosis, Systemic

Synonyms and Related Terms: Progressive systemic sclerosis; scleroderma.

Possible Associated Conditions: Sjögren's syndrome.*

Organs and Tissues	Procedures	Possible or Expected Findings
External examination	Record character and extent of skin lesions, photograph, and submit samples for histologic study, together with subcutaneous tissue.	Dermal sclerosis, primarily of face and fingers. Cutaneous calcium deposits with ulcerations. Ischemic ulcers of fingers.
	Prepare roentgenograms of jaws.	Thickening of periodontal membrane with replacement of the lamina dura.
Breast	If breast implants are present, record type and state whether they are intact.	Ruptured implants have been considered (probably erroneously) a possible cause of systemic sclerosis *(1)*.
Diaphragm		Diaphragmatic hernia.*
Blood	Freeze serum for possible serologic study.	
Heart	Measure volume of pericardial fluid. Record heart weight and measure thickness of ventricles.	Fibrinous pericarditis or hydropericardium. Cor pulmonale.
	For histologic study of the conduction system, see p. 26.	Interstitial fibrosis, which may involve the conduction system.
Lungs with hilar lymph nodes	Perfuse one lung with formalin (p. 47). Submit samples of lungs and hilar lymph nodes for histologic study.	Diffuse alveolar damage *(2)*. Interstitial pulmonary fibrosis with honey-combing. Vasculitis or intimal thickening of small pulmonary arteries and arterioles with pulmonary hypertension* (see "Heart"). Aspiration bronchopneumonia. Bronchioloalveolar carcinoma complicating advanced fibrosis.
Aorta and other elastic arteries		Rarely involved by vasculitis.
Esophagus	Leave esophagus attached to portion of stomach. Submit samples at various levels for histologic study.	Muscular fibrosis. Vasculitis. Dilatation and ulcers of lower esophagus; ulcers are secondary to systemic sclerosis or reflux.

Organs and Tissues	Procedures	Possible or Expected Findings
Gastrointesinal tract	For *in situ* fixation, see p. 54. Other procedures depend on expected findings or grossly identified abnormalities as listed in right-hand column.	Gastrointestinal fibrosis, most commonly of duodenum, jejunum, and colon; colonic muscular atrophy with large-mouth diverticula. Rarely, pneumatosis* of small intestine.
Kidneys	Follow procedures described under "Glomerulonephritis."	Intimal hyperplasia of interlobular arteries. Fibrinoid changes of afferent arterioles and glomeruli. Arteriolonecrosis. Cortical infarctions or ischemic scars. Hypertensive kidney failure* is a common cause of death.
Other organs	Procedures depend on expected findings or grossly identified abnormalities as listed in right-hand column.	Vasculitis in many organs and tissue—for instance, in pancreas, spleen, and central nervous system. Fibrosis of thyroid gland with hypothyroidism.*
Brain and spinal cord	For removal and specimen preparation, see pp. 65 and 67, respectively.	Generally not affected. Rare cases of cerebrovascular calcification have been reported *(3)*.
Skeletal muscles	For sampling and specimen preparation, see p. 80.	Polymyositis (overlap syndrome). Muscular fibrosis. Neurogenic changes also may occur *(4)*.
Bones and joints	For removal, prosthetic repair, and specimen preparation, see p. 95.	Osteoporosis.* Symmetric polyarthritis* with low-grade synovitis.

References

1. Anderson DR, Schwartz J, Cottrill CM, McClain AS, Ross JS, Magidson JG, et al. Silicone ganuloma in acral skin in a patient with silicone-gel implants and systemic sclerosis. Int J Dermatol 1996;35: 36–38.
2. Muir TE, Tazelaar HD, Colby TV, Myers JL. Organizing diffuse alveolar damage associated with progressive systemic sclerosis. Mayo Clin Proc 1997;72:639–642.
3. Heron E, Fornes P, Rance A, Emmerich J, Bayle O, Fiessinger JN. Brain involvement in scleroderma: two autopsy cases. Stroke 1998; 29:719–721.
4. Calore EE, Cavaliere MJ, Perez MN, Takayasu V, Wakamatsu A, Kiss MH. Skeletal muscle pathology in systemic sclerosis. J Rheumatol 1995;22:2246–2249.

Sclerosis, Tuberous

Synonyms and Related Terms: Bourneville's disease; Bourneville-Pringle disease; neurocutaneous syndrome; phacomatosis.

NOTE: There are probably more abnormalities than the ones listed below and some may have not yet been described *(1)*.

Organs and Tissues	Procedures	Possible or Expected Findings
External examination and skin	Prepare photographs of face and pigment abnormalities at other sites. If accessible, prepare sections of skin tumors.	Angiofibromas with characteristic facial distribution (so-called facial adenoma sebaceum). Peri- and subungual "fibromas." Rough yellow skin in lumbosacral region (shagreen patch). Hypopigmented spots (white spots; hypomelanotic macules) over trunk and limbs.
	Prepare skeletal roentgenograms.	See below under "Bones."
Heart	Prepare photographs and sample tumors for electron microscopic study (p. 132). See also under "Tumor, of the heart."	Rhabdomyomas, often multiple.
Lungs	Unless a large sample or samples need to be submitted for microbiologic study, perfuse both lungs with formalin.	Lymphangioleiomyomatosis characterized by multiple small cysts and honeycombing with proliferation of connective tissue and smooth muscle.
Liver	Record weight; perfuse with formalin (p. 56); photograph cut sections and sample possible abnormalities for histologic study.	Focal fatty change. Angioleiomyomas.

Organs and Tissues	*Procedures*	*Possible or Expected Findings*
Intestine	Fix intestinal wall samples on cork board and submit polyps for histologic study.	Microhamartomatous rectal polyps.
Kidneys	Record weights. Photograph outer surface and cut sections; submit tumor nodules for histologic study.	Angiomyolipomas; embryonal renal blastomas; microscopic cysts; cystic glomeruli; abnormal tubules.
Uterus	Sample for histologic study.	Abnormal proliferation of smooth muscle.
Neck organs	Open larynx in posterior midline.	Fibrous polyps of larynx.
Other organs and tissues	Procedures depend on expected findings or grossly identified abnormalities as listed in right-hand column.	Record size and character of all tumorous or other abnormal lesions. Angioleiomyomas in pancreas and adrenal glands.
Brain and spinal cord	For removal and specimen preparation, see pp. 65 and 67, respectively.	Cortical tuber; subependymal nodules; white matter hamartomas; subependymal giant cell astrocytoma.
Eyes	For removal and specimen preparation, see p. 85.	Retinal hamartoma; retinal giant cell astrocytoma; hypopigmented iris spot.
Bones	For removal, prosthetic repair, and specimen preparation, see p. 95.	Rarefaction of phalanges; periosteal thickening of metacarpals and metatarsals; focal sclerosis of calvaria; melorheostosis-type changes.

Reference

1. Wiestler OD, Lopex PS, Crino PB. Tuberous sclerosis complex and subependymal giant cell astrocytoma. In: Pathology and Genetics of the Nervous System. Kleihues P, Cavence WK, eds. IARC, Lyon, 1997, pp. 182–184.

Scopolamine (See "Poisoning, alkaloid.")

Scuba (See "Accident, diving [skin or scuba].")

Scurvy (See "Deficiency, vitamin C.")

Shigellosis (See "Dysentery, bacillary.")

Shingles (See "Infection, Herpes zoster.")

Shock

Related Terms: Anaphylactic shock; bacteremic shock; cardiogenic shock; electric shock; hypovolemic shock; septic shock; and many others.

NOTE: See also under name of suspected underlying condition, such as "Burns," "Death, anaphylactic," "Injury, electrical," and "Stroke, heat."

Organs and Tissues	*Procedures*	*Possible or Expected Findings*
Blood	Submit sample for bacterial culture (p. 102).	Bacteremia or septicemia may be either the cause or the effect of shock.
Heart	Dissection procedures depend on type of heart disease. Sample myocardium for histologic study (p. 30).	Heart disease causing cardiogenic shock. Other types of shock may cause subendocardial and subepicardial interstitial hemorrhages, minute necroses, and patchy contraction band changes.
Lungs	Record weights. Perfuse one lung with formalin (p. 47). Submit one lobe for bacteriologic study (p. 103).	Shock lungs (wet lungs). See also under "Syndrome, respiratory distress, of adult." Pulmonary embolism* may be the cause of shock.
Gastrointestinal tract	Record intestinal abnormalities and estimated amount of intraluminal blood.	Mucosal hemorrhages and necroses; erosions and ulcers.
Liver	Record weight and sample for histologic study.	Centrilobular (zone 3) necroses, with or without fatty changes.
Kidneys	Record weights. Submit samples of cortex and papillae for histologic study.	Acute tubular necrosis.
Adrenal glands	Record weights; record appearance of cortex.	Cortical lipid depletion and atrophy.
Brain	For removal and specimen preparation, see p. 65.	Hypoxic encephalopathy with neuronal damage.

Sickness, Decompression

Synonym: Caisson disease.

NOTE: See also "Accident, diving (skin or scuba)" and references below *(1–4)*.

Organs and Tissues	*Procedures*	*Possible or Expected Findings*
External examination	Prepare roentgenograms of chest, elbows, hips, and knees.	Subcutaneous and mediastinal emphysema; pneumothorax.* Osteonecrosis (aseptic necrosis of bone).
Chest and lungs	For tests for pneumothorax, see p. 430. Record lung weights. Prepare fresh-frozen sections of lung tissue and request Sudan stain (p. 173).	Pleural effusions; Tardieu's spots; pulmonary edema. Pulmonary fat embolism.
Liver and other organs	Procedures depend on expected findings or grossly identified abnormalities as listed in right-hand column.	Fatty changes of liver. Ischemic infarctions in many organs.
Brain	For removal and specimen preparation, see p. 65.	Air embolism;* cerebral edema.

References

1. Gallagher TJ. Scuba diving accidents: decompression sickness, air embolism. J Florida Med Assoc 1997;84:446–451.
2. Blanksby BA, Wearne FK, Elliott BC, Blitvich JD. Aetiology and occurrence of diving injuries. A review of diving safety. Sports Med 1997;23:228–246.
3. Arness MK. Scuba decompression illness and diving fatalities in an overseas military community. Aviation Space Environm Med 1997; 68:325–333.
4. Hardy KR. Diving related emergencies. Emerg Med Clin North Am 1997;15:223–240.

Sickness, Serum

Related Term: Immune complex disease.

NOTE: This is a nonfatal, self-limited disease, characterized by swelling of the face, rash, lymphadenopathy, and arthritis, mainly of large joints.* Globulin antibodies may be demonstrable. There may be proteinuria. Fatalities are caused by acute anaphylactic reactions, which may occur in the course of serum therapy. See under "Death, anaphylactic."

Sickness, Sleeping (See "Trypanosomiasis, African.")

Silicosis (See "Pneumoconiosis.")

Snakebite

Organs and Tissues	*Procedures*	*Possible or Expected Findings*
External examination and skin (wound)	Photograph and submit material from wound for histologic and possible toxicologic study. Use Gram stains if superinfection (e.g., with clostridia) appears to be present (p. 172).	Necrosis, edema, and hemorrhage around bite wound; bleeding from body orifices. Mild jaundice. Superinfection of wounds with or without gangrene.
Kidneys	Record weights, photograph, and sample for histologic study.	Renal cortical and tubular necrosis. Myoglobin or hemoglobin in tubules.
Other organs	Procedures depend on expected findings or grossly identified abnormalities as listed in right-hand column.	Features of disseminated intravascular coagulation.* Hemorrhages.

Sodium (See "Disorder, electrolyte(s)" and p. 114.)

Spherocytosis (See "Anemia, hemolytic.")

Sphingolipidosis (See "Gangliosidosis.")

Spina Bifida (See "Meningocele.")

Splenomegaly, Chronic Congestive (See "Hypertension, portal.")

Spondylitis, Ankylosing

Synonyms and Related Terms: Bechterew's disease; Marie-Strümpell spondylitis; rheumatoid spondylitis; spondylarthropathy *(1)*.

Possible Associated Conditions: Amyloidosis;* isolated heart block.

Organs and Tissues	*Procedures*	*Possible or Expected Findings*
External examination, skin, and subcutaneous tissue	Prepare skeletal roentgenograms.	Deformities of rheumatoid arthritis.* Kyphosis. See below under "Bones and joints."
Blood	There are no diagnostic laboratory tests but it still is advisable to save a blood sample.	The HLA-B27 gene is present in most cases. Rheumatoid factor and antinuclear antibodies are absent.
Heart and aorta	Record heart weight. Test competence of valves (p. 29). Open heart in line of blood flow. Photograph and measure valvular lesions. Prepare sections of valves, myocardium, conduction system (if there was a history of heart block), and ascending aorta.	Thickening of supravalvular aortic wall. Thickening of aortic cusps. Subaortic bump. Thickening of anterior mitral leaflet. Aortic and mitral insufficiency,* with signs of regurgitation. Aortitis.
Lungs	Perfuse one lung with formalin (p. 47). Submit abnormal lobe for microbiologic study (p. 103).	Interstitial fibrosis and cysts in upper lobes. Pleuritis, pleural effusions,* fibrobullous lesions, and cavitating lesions with fungal (Aspergillus) or bacterial infections.
Intestine	For *in situ* fixation, see p. 54. Other procedures depend on expected findings or grossly identified abnormalities as listed in right-hand column.	Chronic ulcerative colitis. Crohn's disease.* Microscopic inflammatory lesions may be the only manifestations *(2)*.
Kidneys and prostate	Sample for histologic study and request amyloid stains or renal parenchyma.	Amyloid nephropathy. Prostatitis.
Bones and joints	Prepare roentgenograms of spine, sacroiliac joints, symphysis ossium pubis, and manubriosternal, sternoclavicular, and humeroscapular joints. For removal of bones and joints, prosthetic repair, and specimen preparation, see p. 95. If spine cannot be removed in its entirety, it can be split in midline and one half can be removed, with costovertebral and costotransversal joints. Hip joints should be exposed. Maceration (p. 97) yields excellent specimens.	Fusion of sacroiliac and intervertebral joints and disks ("bamboo spine"). These changes often are associated with severe spinal osteoporosis.* The involvement of the sacroiliac joint is pathognomonic *(3)*. Cervical spinal fracture may be a cause of quadriplegia.
	Histologic sections should include synovia and periarticular tissue.	Secondary and peripheral osteoarthritis* may be present.
Bone marrow	For preparation of sections and smears, see p. 96.	Leukemia* developed in some patients who had had radiation treatment (1950 or earlier).
Eyes	For removal and specimen preparation, see p. 85.	Acute anterior uveitis.

References

1. Schumacher HR, Bardin T. The spondyloarthropathies: classification and diagnosis. Do we need new terminologies? Bailliers Clin Rheumatol 1998;12:551–565.
2. Porzio V, Biasi G, Corrado A, De Santi M, Vindigni C, Viti S, et al. Intestinal histological and ultrastructural inflammatory changes in spondyloarthropathy and rheumatoid arthritis. Scand J Rheumatol 1997;26:92–98.
3. Braun J, Sieper J. The sacroiliac joint in the spondyloarthropathies. Curr Opin Rheumatol 1996;8:275–287.

Sporotrichosis

Synonym: *Sporothrix (Sporotrichum) schenckii* infection.

NOTE: (1) Collect all tissues that appear to be infected. (2) Request fungal culture. (3) Request Grocott's methenamine silver stain (p. 172). (4) No special precautions are indicated. (5) Serologic studies are available on a research basis from the Centers for Disease Control and Prevention, Atlanta, GA (p. 135). (6) This is not a reportable disease.

Possible Associated Conditions: Sarcoidosis;* tuberculosis.*

Organs and Tissues	Procedures	Possible or Expected Findings
External examination and skin	Prepare sections of cutaneous and subcutaneous lesions. Prepare skeletal roentgenograms.	Acute or chronic skin infection, with or without granulomas and suppuration. Osteomyelitis* (metacarpals, phalanges, and tibiae) and arthritis.*
Lymph nodes	Dissect lymph nodes that drain cutaneous and subcutaneous infections. Submit samples for microbiologic (p. 102) and histologic study. See also above under "Note."	Lymphadenitis.
Chest cavity	Record volume of pleural effusions.	Pleural effusions* may be associated with pulmonary sporotrichosis.
Lungs	Submit consolidated areas for culture (see p. 103 and above under "Note"). Perfuse both lungs with formalin (p. 47).	Few sporadic cases with cavities and fungus ball. Pulmonary fibrosis.
Other organs	See above under "Note." Other procedures depend on expected findings or grossly identified abnormalities as listed in right-hand column.	Gastrointestinal tract, central nervous system, eyes, and skeletal system—among others—may be involved by hematogenous dissemination.

Sprue, Celiac

Synonyms and Related Terms: Adult celiac disease; collagenous sprue; gluten-sensitive enteropathy; idiopathic steatorrhea; nontropical sprue; protein-losing enteropathy; sprue syndrome.

Possible Associated Conditions: Chronic ulcerative colitis;* dermatitis herpetiformis; diabetes mellitus;* IgA deficiency; insufficiency, adrenal;* lipodystrophy *(1)*; lymphoma* *(2)*; primary biliary cirrhosis;* primary sclerosing cholangitis* (See also below under "Possible or Expected Findings.")

Organs and Tissues	Procedures	Possible or Expected Findings
External examination and skin	Submit samples of grossly normal and of abnormal skin for histologic study.	Baldness; perianal and perioral erosions; cutaneous vasculitis; dermatitis herpetiformis; eczema; psoriasis;* other skin diseases. Facial, upper extremity and truncal lipidystrophy *(1)*.
	Prepare skeletal roentgenograms.	Osteomalacia with compression fractures; kyphoskoliosis.
Heart		Ischemic heart disease.*
Lungs	Perfuse one lung with formalin (p. 47). Request Gomori's iron stain (p. 172).	Idiopathic pulmonary hemosiderosis; interstitial pneumonia.*
Esophagus and stomach	See "Tumor, of the esophageal" and "Tumor, of the stomach."	Carcinoma may be found in both organs.
Intestinal tract	For *in situ* fixation and preparation for study under the dissecting microscope, see p. 54. Record sites in small intestine from where histologic material was sampled (in centimeters from duodenojejunal junction or from ileocecal valve).	Volvulus; mucosal diaphragms; villous atrophy. Sprue-like changes in patients with carcinoma or lymphoma, with or without intestinal ulceration and perforation.
	Submit samples of colonic mucosa for histologic study. Request PAS and azure-eosin stains (p. 172).	Ulcerative colitis. Lymphocytic or microscopic colitis.
Other organs	Procedures depend on expected findings or grossly identified abnormalities as listed in right-hand column.	Manifestations of malabsorption syndrome* with osteomalacia.*

References

1. O'Mahony D, O'Mahony S, Whelton MJ, McKiernan J. Partial lipodystrophy in coeliac disease. Gut 1990;31:717–718.
2. Mathus-Vliegen EM. Coeliac disease and lymphoma: current status. Netherlands J Med 1996;49:212–220.

Sprue, Tropical

NOTE: This term is not well-defined and has been applied to a variety of diseases.

Organs and Tissues	*Procedures*	*Possible or Expected Findings*
Intestinal tract	For *in situ* fixation of small bowel and for preparation for study under dissecting microscope, see p. 54. Submit samples for histologic study.	Partial mucosal atrophy of whole length of the small bowel. Many geographic variations; probably infectious etiology in many instances.
Stomach		Atrophic gastritis.
Bone marrow	For preparation of sections and smears, see p. 96.	Macrocytic megaloblastic anemia.*

Stabbing (See "Injury, stabbing.")

Stannosis (See "Pneumoconiosis.")

Starvation

NOTE: In developed countries, psychiatric conditions such as anorexia nervosa* or organic diseases such as malignancies are the most common causes of starvation. See also under "Malnutrition."

Organs and Tissues	*Procedures*	*Possible or Expected Findings*
External examination and skin	Record body weight and length and location of edema. Prepare sections of skin lesions.	Hunger edema; skin changes secondary to vitamin deficiencies.
Blood	Submit sample for biochemical studies.	Hypoproteinemia.
Liver and spleen	Record weights.	Atrophy; hemosiderosis of spleen.
Other organs and tissues	Record weight of all organs (for expected weights, see Appendix, p. 571). Submit samples of all major organs, including endocrine glands, lymphatic and fat tissue, bone, and bone marrow for histologic study.	Degree of atrophy varies from organ to organ; atrophy of fat tissue, lymphoid tissue, and gonads usually is most pronounced. Severe infections, such as tuberculosis,* may be present without having been apparent clinically.

Steatohepatitis, Nonalcoholic (NASH)

NOTE: The morphologic findings in the liver are indistinguishable from those in alcoholic liver disease* *(1)*. Follow autopsy procedures described under "Disease, alcoholic liver." If the patient had received a liver transplant, procedures described under "Transplantation, liver" should be followed also.

Possible Associated Conditions: Celiac sprue (rare); diabetes mellitus* (type 2); hyperlipidemia; malnutrition* from bulemia (rare); morbid obesity with liver failure particularly after episodes of rapid weight loss (e.g., after recent gastroplasty); lipodystrophy; mild obesity;* short bowel syndrome (rare); total parenteral nutrition.*

Organs and Tissues	*Procedures*	*Possible or Expected Findings*
External examination and skin	Record body weight and length.	Obesity,* which may be mild or severe.
Liver	Record weight and sample for histologic study.	Chronic steatohepatitis with or without cirrhosis. Submassive hepatic necrosis.
Other organs	Procedures depend on expected findings or grossly identified abnormalities as listed in right-hand column.	Manifestations of portal hypertension.* See also above under "Possible Associated Conditions."
Brain and spinal cord	For removal and specimen preparation, see pp. 65 and 67, respectively.	Wernicke's encephalopathy *(2)*.

References

1. Ludwig J, McGill DB, Lindor KD. Review: nonalcoholic steatohepatitis. J Gastroenterol Hepatol 1997;12:398–403.
2. Yamamoto T. Alcoholic and non-alcoholic Wernicke's encephalopathy. Be alert to the preventable and treatable disease. Intern Med 1996;35:754–755.

Steatorrhea, Idiopathic (See "Sprue, celiac.")

Stenosis, Acquired Valvular Aortic

Related Terms: Acquired calcification of congenitally bicuspid aortic valve; degenerative (or senile) calcific aortic stenosis; rheumatic aortic stenosis.

NOTE: See also "Stenosis, congenital valvular aortic."

Organs and Tissues	*Procedures*	*Possible or Expected Findings*
Heart	Follow procedures described under "Stenosis, congenital valvular aortic."	Bicuspid aortic valve;* calcific nodular aortic stenosis. Chronic rheumatic mitral and tricuspid valvulitis.

Stenosis, Acquired Valvular Pulmonary

NOTE: For general dissection techniques, see p. 33. Record weight of heart, thickness of ventricles, and valve circumferences.

Possible Associated Conditions: Carcinoid heart disease (both the pulmonary valve and the tricuspid valve may be involved).

Stenosis, Congenital Supravalvular Aortic

Synonyms: Supravalvular aortic stenosis, diffuse type; supravalvular aortic stenosis, discrete; Williams-Beuren syndrome.

NOTE: Sudden death may occur, as may acute aortic dissection. For acquired forms, see "Arteritis, Takayasu's."

Possible Associated Conditions: Adhesions of aortic valve cusps; obstruction of coronary ostia and brachiocephalic branches of the aortic arch; supravalvular pulmonary stenosis; Williams-Beuren syndrome.

Organs and Tissues	*Procedures*	*Possible or Expected Findings*
External examination	Prepare photograph of face.	Unusual elfin-like facial features.
Blood	Submit sample of serum for microbiologic study (p. 102). Postmortem calcium values are unreliable.	Hypercalcemia; septicemia.
Heart	If infective aortitis is suspected, expose stenosed area through sterilized aortic wall (similar to procedure suggested for valvular aortic endocarditis, p. 103). Culture vegetations, prepare smears and sections, and request Gram stain (p. 172).	Infective aortitis.
	Remove heart together with aortic arch and adjacent great neck vessels. Measure diameters of stenosed and nonstenosed portions of aorta (calipers work best); record extent and nature of stenosis. For coronary arteriography, see p. 118. Prepare histologic sections of multiple segments of coronary arteries. Request Verhoeff–van Gieson stain (p. 173).	Diffuse or discrete type of aortic stenosis. Increased heart weight. Substantial thickening and stenosis of involved arteries. Microscopic arterial dysplasia with merged intima and media, and with haphazard interlacing of elastic layers.
Other organs		Manifestations of congestive heart failure.*

Stenosis, Congenital Supravalvular Pulmonary

Synonyms: Williams-Beuren syndrome.

NOTE: Follow procedures described under "Stenosis, congenital valvular pulmonary." For acquired forms, see "Arteritis, Takayasu's."

Possible Associated Conditions: Supravalvular aortic stenosis.*

Stenosis, Congenital Valvular Aortic

Synonyms: Acommissural (dome-shaped) aortic valve; unicommissural aortic valve; unicuspid aortic valve (either acommissural or unicommissural).

NOTE: Congenital aortic stenosis may cause sudden death in infancy and childhood. Most valves are unicommissural, hypoplastic, and dysplastic (thickened and malformed). Occasionally, bicuspid aortic valves are stenotic at birth.

Possible Associated Conditions: Coarctation of aorta;* endocardial fibroelastosis* of left ventricle; hypoplasia of left ventricle;* interrupted aortic arch;* tubular hypoplasia of aortic arch.*

Organs and Tissues	*Procedures*	*Possible or Expected Findings*
Heart	If infective endocarditis is suspected, follow procedures described on p. 103.	Infective endocarditis.*
	Remove heart with ascending aorta; record weight of heart and open in ventricular cross-sections (p. 22). Test competence of valves (p. 29). Leave aortic valve intact. Record size of valve orifice and thickness of heart chambers.	Hypertrophy of left and right ventricles; dilatation of left atrium.
	Histologic samples should include endocardium and area(s) of fusion of aortic cusp(s). Request Verhoeff–van Gieson stain (p. 173).	Endocardial fibroelastosis* of left ventricle. Infarction of mitral papillary muscles. Subendocardial fibrosis, biventricular.
Lungs	Perfuse one lung with formalin (p. 47). Request Verhoeff–van Gieson stain (p. 173).	Chronic pulmonary venous changes.

Stenosis, Congenital Valvular Pulmonary

Related Terms: Isolated (pure, simple, or dome-shaped) pulmonary stenosis.

NOTE: The pulmonary valve is usually acommissural in isolated congenital pulmonary stenosis. With other coexistant congenital heart disease (such as tetralogy), the pulmonary valve is usually bicuspid and hypoplastic, but may be unicommissural or dysplastic and tricuspid.

Organs and Tissues	*Procedures*	*Possible or Expected Findings*
Heart and great vessels; peripheral pulmonary arteries	If infective endocarditis is suspected, follow procedures described on p. 103.	Infective endocarditis* of pulmonary valve and tricuspid valve; infective endarteritis at bifurcation of pulmonary trunk.
	For general dissection techniques, see p. 33. Record weight of heart, thickness of ventricles, and annular circumferences.	Thickened and incompetent tricuspid valve; right ventricular hypertrophy; poststenotic dilatation of pulmonary trunk; peripheral pulmonary artery stenosis.
Brain	For removal and specimen preparation, see p. 65.	Cerebral abscess* (would indicate presence of right-to-left shunt).

Stenosis, Mitral

Synonyms and Related Terms: Acquired mitral stenosis; congenital mitral stenosis; rheumatic mitral stenosis.

Possible Associated Conditions: Acquired mitral stenosis generally is the result of rheumatic carditis (often decades earlier). Congenital mitral stenosis may be associated with bicuspid aortic valve;* coarctation of the aorta;* parachute mitral valve; Shone's syndrome; subaortic stenosis;* supravalvular stenosing ring of the left atrium; and ventricular septal defect.*

Organs and Tissues	*Procedures*	*Possible or Expected Findings*
External examination	Record color of skin.	Cyanosis.
	Prepare chest roentgenogram.	Cardiomegaly; calcification in and around mitral valve.
Blood	If infective endocarditis* is suspected, submit sample for microbiologic study (p. 102).	Septicemia.
Heart and great vessels	For general dissection techniques in congenital mitral stenosis, see p. 33.	See above under "Possible Associated Conditions."
	If infective endocarditis is suspected, see p. 103.	Infective endocarditis.*

Organs and Tissues	Procedures	Possible or Expected Findings
Heart and great vessels *(continued)*	Record weight and measurements of heart; record size of left atrium; record appearance and size of mitral orifice. For tests for stenosis and measurement of valve size, see p. 29.	Cardiomegaly; dilatation of left atrium; thrombi in atrial appendages. Rheumatic valvulitis.
Lungs	Perfuse lungs with formalin (p. 47); prepare sections of bronchi, pulmonary arteries, and pulmonary veins. Request Verhoeff–van Gieson stain (p. 173).	Pulmonary congestion, emboli, and infarctions; bronchopneumonia; manifestations of pulmonary venous hypertension.* Elevated left bronchus.
Other organs	Procedures depend on expected findings or grossly identified abnormalities as listed in right-hand column.	Manifestations of congestive heart failure;* systemic emboli; cholelithiasis* and chronic cholecystitis.*

Stenosis, Renal Artery

Organs and Tissues	Procedures	Possible or Expected Findings
Retroperitoneal organs	For renal arteriography, see p. 59. Open aorta lengthwise *in situ*; record width of renal artery orifices.	Dissection, embolus, or thrombus of renal artery. Fibromuscular renal artery dysplasia. Atherosclerotic plaques.
	Probe renal arteries, record width of lumen, and open lengthwise.	Some lesions may have been induced by previous percutaneous transluminal angioplasty.
	Photograph; submit samples for histologic study; request Verhoeff–van Gieson stain (p. 173).	Fibromuscular dysplasia with renal artery stenosis must beshown in longitudinal histologic sections ofthe artery.
Kidneys	Prepare histologic sections of both kidneys (it is important to identify the side, right or left, from which the sample was taken.	Ischemic damage with scarring in affected kidney. Hypertensive vascular changes in unprotected kidney. Abnormalities of juxtaglomerular apparatus.
Other organs		Manifestations of hypertension.*

Stenosis, Subvalvular Aortic

Synonyms and Related Terms: Discrete congenital subvalvular aortic stenosis; idiopathic hypertrophic subaortic stenosis (see "Cardiomyopathy, hypertrophic"); subaortic stenosis; subaortic stenosis of membranous type; subaortic stenosis of muscular type; tunnel subaortic stenosis.

Possible Associated Conditions: Accessory tissue (windsock deformity) of the mitral valve; age-related angled (sigmoid) ventricular septum; complete atrioventricular septal defect;* congenital rhabdomyoma; infundibular stenosis of right ventricle; mitral insufficiency;* supravalvular stenosis of left atrium, parachute mitral valve, and coarctation of aorta;* ventricular septal defect* (malalignment type); Shone's syndrome.

Organs and Tissues	Procedures	Possible or Expected Findings
Heart	For general dissection techniques, see p. 22. Before opening outflow tract, measure diameter of stenosis. Dissect by short axis (p. 22) or long-axis method (see p. 23). Compare septal thickness with thickness of lateral ventricular wall. Histologic samples should include ventricular septum. For fixation for electron microscopy, see p. 132.	Membranous or muscular subaortic (subvalvular) stenosis. Increased heart weight. Ventricular septum may be thicker than lateral wall of left ventricle (normal ratio <1.3).

Stenosis, Subvalvular Pulmonary

Synonyms: Right ventricular infundibular stenosis; stenosis of ostium infundibuli; double-chambered right ventricle; dynamic right ventricular outflow tract obstruction.

NOTE: Infective endocarditis* may occur on the wall of the right infundibular chamber above the localized area of infundibular stenosis. If this is suspected, follow procedures described on p. 103.

Stenosis, Subvalvular Pulmonary *(continued)*

Possible Associated Conditions: Congenital valvular pulmonary stenosis;* double outlet right ventricle;* tetralogy of Fallot;* ventricular septal defect.*

Stenosis, Tricuspid

NOTE: For general dissection techniques, see p. 22. Possible causes of tricuspid stenosis include carcinoid heart disease, chronic rheumatic valvulitis, and congenital anomaly.

Stillbirth

As stated in Chapter 1, it is preferable to have autopsies of fetuses, including stillbirth, performed by pathologists experienced in perinatal pathology. If such personnel are not immediately available, the attending pathologist may nevertheless collect important information. If attempts to induce abortion appear to have caused the death of the mother, see "Death, abortion-associated."

The placenta should be immediately procured from the delivery room should it not arrive in the laboratory with the fetus. This will avoid the possibility of the placenta being discarded by the delivery room staff. No fetal autopsy is complete without a careful examination of the placenta (for technical details, see Part I, Chapter 5, p. 60).

Fascia lata or other aseptically obtained tissue should be collected for tissue culture for karyotype analysis (p. 109). A portion of placenta and liver should be snap-frozen for possible molecular analysis.

The initial stage of the autopsy should include photography and radiography, taking anterior-posterior and lateral views. The photographs will record the degree of maceration, which can be roughly correlated with the duration of fetal demise before delivery (ref. *[1]*, pp. 270–273). External measurements should include body weight, circumference of head, chest and abdomen, crown-rump length, crown-heel length, and foot length. These measurements are compared with Tables of standards for normal fetuses (see Part III of this book and perinatal pathology texts quoted in Chapter 1). Assessment of growth retardation may be based on these data. A careful external examination should search for abnormalities such as jaundice, bulging fontanel, cranial bone softening, hyper- or hypotelorism, choanal atresia, external ear anomalies, cleft lip, cleft palate, macroglossia, micrognathia, colobomata, cystic hygroma, shortened neck, contractures, omphalocele, gastroschisis, abnormal external genitalia, anal atresia, absent vagina, sacral pits, open neural tube defects, hemihypertrophy, syndactyly, clinodactyly, simian creases, or incomplete descent of testes.

The organ bloc may be removed in the manner similar to the adult, using the technique of Letulle (see p. 3). If the thyroid gland is noted to be in its usual location and if it appears normal, then the tongue may be left in the body. In macerated fetuses, it is suggested that the organ bloc be fixed overnight in formalin solution prior to dissection. To aid adequate fixation, the following simple steps may be done: 1) wash the organ bloc thoroughly prior to fixation; 2) place multiple transverse cuts through the liver; 3) dissect the posterior leaves of the diaphragm away from the adrenal glands and kidneys; 4) bivalve the adrenal glands and kidneys in the coronal plane; 5) instill formalin in the lumen of the intestine, using a syringe; and 6) gently instill formalin into both ventricles of the heart, being careful to avoid the ventricular septum.

The procedure for dissection of the organs is similar to that of the adult except: 1) The venous and arterial connections of the heart, including the patency of the ductus arteriosus must be determined before the heart is removed; 2) The esophageal hiatus should be examined *in situ*. The esophagus must be opened posteriorly prior to its complete removal so that esophageal atresia or tracheo-esophageal fistula may be recognized and photographed prior to further dissection; 3) The location of the appendix and of the testes should be recorded. Until the intestine has been examined for stenosis or atresia, the mesentery should be left attached.

The degree of autolysis as seen with histologic examination can be used to estimate the duration of time between fetal death and delivery *(2)*. Trichrome stain is useful for better visualizing histologic features in severely autolyzed tissue.

To remove the brain, Benecke's technique of one of its modifications may be used (p. 66).

Stillbirth vs Livebirth. A decision has to be made whether the infant was born alive or was stillborn. The hydrostatic lung test, described in the previous edition, appears unreliable. The presence of gas in the lungs does not rule out stillbirth. After death, air can be introduced into the lungs, or putrefaction gases might be present. However, air artificially introduced after death will not distend the alveoli and can be squeezed out, whereas this does not seem to be the case after active ventilation. The distribution of fat in the fetal zone of the adrenal cortex may indicate whether intrauterine death was acute, more prolonged, or chronic *(3)*. This is particularly helpful if the stillborn baby is macerated. If the mother died also, see under "Death, abortion-associated."

References

1. Valdéz-Dapena MA, Huff, DS. Perinatal Autopsy Manual. Armed Forces Institute of Pathology, Washington, DC, 1983.
2. Genest DR, Williams MA, Greene MF. Estimating the time of death in stillborn fetuses: I. Histologic examination of fetal organs: an autopsy study of 150 stillborns. Obstet Gynecol 1992;80:575–584.
3. Becker MJ, Becker AE. Fat distribution in the adrenal cortex as an indication of the mode of intrauterine death. Hum Pathol 1976;7:495–504.

Stimulant(s) (See "Dependence, drug(s), all types or type undetermined.")

Sting, Insect (See "Death, anaphylactic.")

Strangulation

NOTE: In many instances, procedures described under "Homicide" must also be followed. If a rope or some other material had been used (see also under "Hanging"), leave ligature in place until autopsy can be done. See also under "Hypoxia." Toxicologic sampling, particularly for alcohol, should be done in all instances (p. 16).

Organs and Tissues	Procedures	Possible or Expected Findings
External examination and skin	If identity of victim is unknown, follow procedures described on p. 11.	
	If a ligature and knot are present, record and photograph their position. Do not disturb knot but cut ligature at some distance and bind ends together.	Strangulation ligatures tend to run horizontally.
	Photograph skin and neck and prepare histologic sections of strap muscles and fascia for demonstration of vital reaction. Collect fingernail scrapings.	Abrasions; fingernail marks; laceration. Defense marks.
Neck organs	Photograph sequentially during layer-wise dissection (see p. 14). Handle neck organs carefully.	
	Prepare roentgenogram of hyoid bone and submit tissues with evidence of trauma for histologic study.	Contusions in soft tissues. Fracture of hyoid bone; laryngeal injury.

Stroke, Cerebrovascular (See "Infarction, cerebral.")

Stroke, Heat (See "Heatstroke.")

Strychnine (See "Poisoning, strychnine.")

Sulfur (Dioxide or Sulfurous Acid) (See "Bronchitis, acute chemical" and "Poisoning, gas.")

Surgery (See following entries and under "Transplantation,..." See also under "Postoperative Autopsies," p. 4.)

Surgery, Aortocoronary Bypass

Organs and Tissues	Procedures	Possible or Expected Findings
Heart and ascending aorta	Record *in situ* appearance of heart and ascending aorta. Remove heart with ascending aorta and graft(s) attached.	Cardiomegaly. Injury to ascending aorta.
	Record weight of heart.	
	Prepare angiograms—first of saphenous vein or internal mammary artery graft(s) and and then of coronary arteries (p. 118).	Focal or diffuse graft obstruction. Aneurysm(s) of venous graft(s). Twisting or kinking of graft(s).
	Record patency of distal and proximal anastomoses of graft(s). Remove venous graft(s) for histologic study, including the distal anastomoses.	
	Prepare cross-sections of coronary arteries and graft(s). Request Verhoeff-van Gieson stain (p. 173). Decalcification (p. 97) of coronary arteries and of graft(s) may be required. Prepare 1-cm-thick transverse (coronal) slices of myocardium (p. 22).	Obstructive coronary atherosclerosis. Thrombosis, intimal proliferation, calcification, and atherosclerosis of venous graft(s). Scars, recent myocardial infarctions, myocardial aneurysm, mural thromboses.

Surgery, Cardiac Valvular Replacement

Organs and Tissues	Procedures	Possible or Expected Findings
External examination	Prepare chest roentgenogram.	Abnormal position of prosthesis or catheter. For identification of valve, see p. 33.
Blood	Submit sample for microbiologic study (p. 102).	Septicemia.

Organs and Tissues	Procedures	Possible or Expected Findings
Heart	If infective endocarditis is suspected, follow procedures described on p. 103.	Prosthetic infective endocarditis.* *Staphylococcus aureus* and Gram-negative bacilli are the most common microorganisms in early-onset endocarditis, and viridans streptococci and Gram-negative bacilli are the most com mon in late-onset cases. Poppet variance or dislodgement; paravalvular leak; thrombosed valve; calcification of bioprosthetic valve.
	Record weight of heart.	Cardiac hypertrophy.* Mural thrombi.
	For coronary arteriography, see p. 118.	Myocardial infarction.
	Open heart in cross sections (see p. 22). Leave valve prosthesis in place. For identification of valve type, see p. 33. Test function and record appearance of valves that had not been replaced.	Mechanical valve damage. Dislodged valve. Rheumatic and other diseases of valves that had not been replaced.
Lungs	Perfuse lungs with formalin (p. 47). Request Verhoeff-van Gieson stain (p. 173).	Emboli; diffuse alveolar damage. Chronic pulmonary venous hypertensive changes. Pneumonia.
Other organs	Procedures depend on expected findings or grossly identified abnormalities as listed in right-hand column.	Systemic emboli. Escaped poppet, usually at bifurcation of aorta. Hemorrhages secondary to coagulopathy or excessive anticoagulation.

Surgery, Heart Transplantation (See "Transplantation, heart.")

Surgery, Kidney Transplantation (See "Transplantation, kidney.")

Surgery, Liver Transplantation (See "Transplantation, liver.")

Surgery, Lung Transplantation (See "Transplantation, lung.")

Syndrome (See also under "Disease, . . ." and "Sickness,...")

Syndrome, Acquired Immunodeficiency (AIDS)

Synonyms: Human immunodeficiency virus (HIV) infection; HIV infection.

NOTE: For a general review of findings, see ref. *(1)*. Collect all tissues that appear to be infected. Tissue yields better culture results than body fluids. (2) Universal **precautions** should be strictly followed (p. 146).[a] The generation of aerosols should be minimized. To sterilize tissue surfaces in preparation for culture, swab the surface with povidone iodine. Avoid searing the tissue surface since this will produce an aerosol. Keep no more than one scalpel in the dissecting area at any one time. Have an assistant available with clean, gloved hands to receive specimens in containers, so as to minimize the degree of contamination on the outside of the containers. For cleaning procedures and related information, see Chapter 16. (3) HIV-1 in tissue may be demonstrated using polymerase chain reaction (PCR), immunohistochemistry, *in situ* hybridization, or immunofluorescence. (4) For immunocytochemical and molecular studies, fix tissue in ethanol (p. 129) or Carnoy's solution (p. 130). The virus can be identified using PCR in most tissues, whether fresh, frozen, or fixed in ethanol. (5) Serologic tests as well as direct fluorescent antibody tests are available for many of the expected infections. (6) This is not a reportable disease.

In Adults:

Organs and Tissues	Procedures	Possible or Expected Findings
External examination and skin	Record body weight and evidence of lipodystrophy following AIDS medications.	Cachexia. Severe loss of subcutaneous fat in face and extremities, associated with large fat deposits on upper back and upper abdomen ("protease paunch").
	Record and photograph any skin lesions. Examine oral cavity.	Cutaneous Kaposi's sarcoma *(1)*.
Blood and vitreous	If the diagnosis is in doubt, samples can be submitted for enzyme immunoassay.	Test may be positive for many weeks after death *(2)*.
Cardiovascular system	Procedures depend on expected findings or grossly identified abnormalities as listed in right-hand column.	Increased lipochrome deposition; toxoplasmosis of myocardium; *Cytomegalovirus* and atypical mycobacterial infections *(2)*.

Organs and Tissues	Procedures	Possible or Expected Findings
Respiratory tract	Culture any consolidated areas. If none can be identified, take a random section for viral culture.	Many routine and opportunistic infections; diffuse alveolar damage; diffuse interstitial fibrosis; malignant lymphoma;* foreign body granulomas (in parenteral drug users).
Gastrointestinal tract	Open and examine as soon as removed to minimize autolysis. Promptly fix any lesion. Submit sections for electron microscopy.	Villous atrophy and crypt hyperplasia of small bowel; cryptosporidiosis; microsporidiosis; *Mycobacterium avium-intracellulare* and other opportunistic infections; lymphoma.*
Liver	Record weight; sample for microbiologic and histologic study. If indicated, request acid fast stains, Grocott's methenamine silver stain, immunostains for hepatitis antigen, and Gomori's iron stain (p. 172).	Hepatitis *(3)* due to hepatitis A,B,C,delta, *Mycobacterium avium-intracellulare, Cytomegalovirus, Cryptococcus;* Kaposi's sarcoma; lymphoma; erythrophagocytosis; increased hemosiderin.
Pancreas	Sample for histologic study.	*Cytomegalovirus* pancreatitis.
Adrenal glands	Record weights. Sample for histologic study.	Medullary necrosis with *Cytomegalovirus*; lipid depletion.
Lymph nodes and bone marrow	Sample enlarged lymph nodes for histologic study. For preparation of sections and smears of bone marrow, see pp. 96 and 97, respectively.	Lymphadenopathy; follicular hyperplasia; absent germinal centers; sinus histiocytosis; hemophagocytosis. Bone marrow with plasmacytosis; variable cellularity; lymphoma;* lymphoproliferative disorder.
Spleen	Record weight and sample for histologic study.	Opportunistic infections; lymphoma;* depletion of white pulp with fibrosis; increased plasma cells; hemophagocytosis; increased hemosiderin in macrophages.
Brain	For removal and specimen preparation, see p. 65. The saw should be used within a plastic bag (p. 67) or it should be fitted with a vacuum to collect aerosolized bone particles. Other procedures, including requests for special stains, depend on expected findings or grossly identified abnormalities as listed in right-hand column.	Viral (HIV) encephalitis *(4)*; progressive herpes simplex, or varicella/zoster infection), multifocal leukoencephalopathy;* CMV, bacterial (*Mycobacterium avium intracellulare* infection; Whipple's disease; Nocardia), and fungal (*Aspergillus fumigatus; Candida albicans*; Coccidioidomycosis; Cryptococcosis; mucormycosis; histoplasmosis). Syphilis and infection with *Toxoplasma gondii* also may be found. Lymphoma;* Kaposi's sarcoma; vacuolar myelopathy; lymphocytic meningitis; cerebral hemorrhage or infarction.
Spinal cord	For removal, see p. 67. The saw should be fitted with a vacuum or used under a plastic cover sheet to collect aerosolized bone particles.	Demyelination of posterior columns and pyramidal tracts (vacuolar myelopathy) *(5)*; lymphoma; opportunistic infections.

[a]Vitreous tested up to 34 h postmortem and blood tested up to 58 d postmortem were consistently positive for HIV. No false-negatives *(6)*.

References

1. Fisher BK, Warner LC. Cutaneous manifestations of the acquired immunodeficiency syndrome. Intl J Dermatol 1987;26(10):615–630.
2. Lewis W. AIDS: cardiac findings from 115 autopsies. Prog Cardiovasc Dis 1989;32(3):207–215.
3. Schaffner F. The liver in HIV infection. Prog Liver Dis 1990;9:505–522.
4. Kanzer MD. Neuropathology of AIDS. Crit Rev Neurobiol 1990:5(4):313–362.
5. Hénin D, Smith TW, De Girolami U, Sughayer M, Hauw J-J. Neuropathology of the spinal cord in the acquired immunodeficiency syndrome. Hum Pathol 1992;23:1106–1114.
6. Klatt EC, Shibata D, Strigle SM. Postmortem enzyme immunoassay for human immunodeficiency virus. Arch Pathol Lab Med 1989;113:485–487.

In Children ***(1,2)*****:**

Organs and Tissues	*Procedures*	*Possible or Expected Findings*
External examination and skin	Obtain body weight and external measurements. Photograph all abnormalities. Perform whole body radiographs.	Developmental delay; cachexia.
Oral cavity	Obtain exudate of ulcers for smears and culture. Scrape ulcers for Tzanck prep and viral culture.	Candidal, cytomegalovirus and herpetic ulcers; EBV-induced oral hairy leukoplakia; oral warts due to papillomavirus; bacteria-induced necrotizing ulcerative gingivitis.
Salivary glands	Submit portion of parotid gland for histologic study. For sampling, see p. 382.	Lymphocytic infiltration; infectious sialoadenitis.
Thymus	Weigh and submit for histologic study.	Precocious involution *(3)*; dysinvolution (decrease or absence of Hassall's corpuscles); thymitis with giant cells.
Cardiovascular system	Procedures depend on expected findings or grossly identified abnormalities as listed in right-hand column.	Dilated cardiomyopathy;* myocarditis;* pericardial effusion; myocardial interstitial fibrosis; opportunistic infections; fibrocalcific vasculopathy; aneurysms.
	Prepare sections for electron microscopy (p.132).	Myelin-like figures within myocytes.
Respiratory tract	Culture any consolidated areas for viruses, fungi, and bacteria. Submit sections for histologic study. Photograph any lesion suspicious for neoplasm.	Bacterial, fungal, viral, and mycobacterial pneumonias; diffuse alveolar damage; lymphoid hyperplasia; malignant lymphoma;* lymphoproliferative disorder; Kaposi's sarcoma.
Gastrointestinal tract	Open and examine intestines as soon as they are removed, so as to limit autolysis. Promptly photograph and immerse lesions in fixative. Sample lesions for histologic study.	Infections due to parasites, viruses, fungi, bacteria, and mycobacteria; ulcers; necrotizing inflammation; lymphoproliferative disorder; lymphoma (including MALT [mucosea associated lymphoid tissue] lymphoma); Kaposi's sarcoma; calcific arteriopathy.
Liver	Photograph any grossly evident lesions. Submit lesions and grossly normal liver for histologic study.	Chronic hepatitis;* opportunistic infections; cholestasis; steatosis; Kupffer cell hyperplasia; lymphoproliferative disorder; Kaposi's sarcoma.
Pancreas	Submit for histologic study.	Drug-related acute pancreatitis; chronic pancreatitis; opportunistic infections.
Lymph nodes, bone marrow	For preparation of sections and smears, see p. 96.	Persistent generalized lymphadenopathy (hyperplasia, involution, or lymphoid depletion); lymphoproliferative disorder; Kaposi's sarcoma; opportunistic infections; hypercellular bone marrow with increased megakaryocytes, plasmacytosis, hematophagocytosis; increased iron stores; lymphoma;* leukemia.*
Spleen	Record weight and sample for histologic study.	Concentric vascular sclerosis; depletion of red/white pulp.
Urinary system	Submit kidney for histologic study. Follow procedures described under "Glomerulonephritis." Submit sections for electron microscopy (p. 132).	Focal segmental glomerulosclerosis; tubulo-Interstitial nephritis; mesangial hypercellularity; cytomegalovirus, candidal infection.
Brain and spinal cord	For removal and specimen preparation, see p. 66 and 70, respectively. For prevention of aerosolization of bone particles, see p. 479 under "Brain" and "Spinal Cord."	Micrencephaly *(4)*; enlarged ventricles; delayed myelination; interstitial mineralization of putamen, globus pallidus, frontal lobe white matter; mononuclear glial and microglial nodules with giant cells; leptomeningitis; lymphoma;* opportunistic infections. Spinal cord with pallor of corticospinal tracts; vacuolar myelopathy.

Organs and Tissues	Procedures	Possible or Expected Findings
Placenta	Record weight and photograph all gross lesions.	Retroplacental hematoma; infarcts; acute chorioamnionitis; funisitis; abnormal villous maturation; villitis due to *Cytomegalovirus, Toxoplasma.*

References

1. Systemic Pathology of HIV Infection and AIDS in Children. Moran C, Mullick FG, eds. Armed Forces Institute of Pathology. American Registry of Pathology, Washington, DC, 1997. (To order copies, call: 202-782-2100 or write to American Registry of Pathology Sales Office, AFIP, Room 1077, Washington, DC 20306-6000.)
2. Joshi W. Pathology of acquired immunodeficiency syndrome (AIDS) in children. Keio J Med 1996;45:306–312.
3. Grody WW, Fligiel S, Naeim F. Thymus involution in the acquired immunodeficiency syndrome. Am J Clin Pathol 1985;84:85–95.
4. Kozlowski PB, Brudkowska J, Kraszpulski M, Sersen EA, Wrzolek MA, Anzil AP, et al. Micrencephaly in children congenitally infected with human immunodeficiency virus—a gross-anatomical morphometric study. Acta Neuropathol 1997;93:136–145.

Syndrome, Adams-Stokes (See "Arrhythmia, cardiac.")

Syndrome, Adult Respiratory Distress [ARDS]

Related Term: Diffuse alveolar damage; shock lung.

NOTE: For related changes in infancy, see "Syndrome, respiratory distress, of infant."

Possible Associated Conditions: Amniotic fluid embolism;* aspiration (e.g., in near-drowning accidents*); burns;* inhalation of toxic gases; major trauma (with or without fat embolism*); malignancies; pancreatitis;* radiation injury;* severe infections, and many other potentially fatal conditions may cause ARDS, particularly if they are associated with shock.*

Organs and Tissues	Procedures	Possible or Expected Findings
External examination	Prepare chest roentgenogram.	Pneumothorax* (including tension pneumothorax); pneumomediatinum.
Blood	Submit sample for microbiologic study (p. 102), particularly if septicemia is suspected.	Septicemia.
	Toxicologic studies (drug screen) are indicated in some instances (p. 16).	Illicit drug use; paraquat or salicylate poisoning.
Heart	If the patient had cardiopulmonary surgery, see also under name of underlying condition.	Surgical procedures that required cardiopulmonary bypass may cause ARDS.
Trachea and lungs	Determine position of endotracheal tube.	Endotracheal tube may become dislodged.
	Record lung weights. Submit samples for microbiologic study (p. 103), particularly if septicemia is suspected. Perfuse one lung with formalin (p. 47). For the demonstration of edema, some samples should be fixed in Bouin's solution (p. 129).	Diffuse alveolar damage, with or without evidence of underlying condition such as trauma, fat embolism,* viral infection, damage from toxic inhalants (e.g., smoke, oxygen or nitrogen oxides), or aspiration (gastric acid or swimming pool water in near-drowning accidents).
Other organs	Procedures depend on expected associated conditions.	Manifestations of conditions listed above under "Possible Associated Conditions"

Syndrome, Afferent Loop

Possible Associated Conditions: Malabsorption syndrome* in patients with stasis and bacterial overgrowth in afferent loop.

Organs and Tissues	Procedures	Possible or Expected Findings
Stomach, duodenum, and jejunum	Dissect stomach and intestines *in situ.*	Previous Billroth II operation. Distension, lengthening, and kinking of afferent duodenal loop.

Syndrome, Albright's (See "Dysplasia, fibrous, of bone.")

Syndrome, Alport

Synonyms and Related Terms: Classic (X-linked) Alport syndrome; hereditary congenital hemorrhagic nephritis; hereditary nephritis with nerve deafness; nonclassic (autosomal) Alport syndrome without deafness or eye changes.

Organs and Tissues	Procedures	Possible or Expected Findings
All organs	Follow procedures described under "Glomerulonephritis" and "Failure, kidney."	Chronic glomerulonephritis* with foam cells.
Eyes	For removal and specimen preparation, see p. 85.	Conical deformation of the anterior surface of the lens (lenticonus) in classic Alport syndrome.

Syndrome, Aortic Arch (See "Arteritis, Takayasu's.")

Syndrome, Asplenia (See "Syndrome, polysplenia and asplenia.")

Syndrome, Ataxia-Telangiectasia

Synonym: Louis-Bar syndrome.

NOTE: See also under "Syndrome, immunodeficiency." Chronic pulmonary disease and malignancy (see below) are the most common causes of death.

Possible Associated Conditions: Malignant lymphomas* and, rarely, carcinomas.

Organs and Tissues	Procedures	Possible or Expected Findings
External examination and skin; oral cavity	Record body weight and height. Prepare photographs and histologic sections of skin lesions.	Growth retardation. Telangiectases of conjunctivas, face, ears, neck, and antecubital and popliteal fossae. Telangiectases of palate. Café au lait spots.
Thymus	Record weight and submit samples for histologic study.	Atrophy of thymus (embryonic appearance of thymus).
Blood	Submit sample for immunoglobulin determination.	IgA deficiency.
Lungs	Perfuse one lung with formalin (p. 47). Submit one lobe for microbiologic study (p. 103). Submit samples of all lobes for histologic study.	Bronchopulmonary infection, often with bronchiectasis. Characteristic cells in ataxia-telangiectasia (generalized nucleomegaly).
Small bowel	Record size of Peyer's plaques and prepare histologic sections.	Atrophy of Peyer's plaques.
Liver and kidneys	Record weights and sample for histologic study.	Characteristic cells in ataxia-telangiectasia (generalized nucleomegaly).
Lymph nodes	Submit samples for histologic study.	Atrophy.
Ovaries	Record presence or absence.	May be absent (agenesis).
Neck organs	Submit samples of tonsils and lymph nodes for histologic study. Record sizes.	Atrophy of tonsils and cervical lymph nodes.
Brain and spinal cord	For removal and specimen preparation, see pp. 66 and 70, respectively.	Atrophy of cerebellar cortex with loss of Purkinje and granular cells; irregular dendritic expansions and eosinophilic cytoplasmic inclusions in some of the remaining Purkinje cells. Degeneration of posterior columns (fasciculus gracilis more than fasciculus cuneatus) of spinal cord.
Peripheral nerves	For removal and specimen preparation, see p. 79.	Abnormal and large cells with bizarre nuclei.

Syndrome, Banti's (See "Hypertension, portal.")

Syndrome, Barrett's (See "Esophagus, Barrett's.")

Syndrome, Bartter's (See "Aldosteronism.")

Syndrome, Bassen-Kornzweig (See "Abetalipoproteinemia.")

Syndrome, Beckwith-Wiedemann

NOTE: This cellular overgrowth syndrome may be sporadic or autosomal dominant. In some patients, a duplication of chromosome 11p15.5 is present.

Organs and Tissues	Procedures	Possible or Expected Findings
External examination and skin	Record body weight, as well as head, abdomen, and chest circumference, crown-heel length, crown-rump length. Record and photograph all anomalies.	Hemihypertrophy; macroglossia; infraorbital hypoplasia; grooved ear lobules; capillary nevus flammeus; large fontanels; prominent occiput; malocclusion of teeth; cliteromegaly; hypospadias.
Abdominal organs	Carefully examine organs and photograph anomalies. Submit tissue for histologic study. Submit fascia (p. 109), tissue, such as liver or lung, or blood (p. 108) for karotype analysis.	Portal-biliary dysgenesis; hepatoblastoma; islet cell hyperplasia; cytomegaly of adrenal cortical cells; dysplastic renal medulla; Wilms tumor. Large ovaries, uterus, kidneys, and bladder; bicornuate uterus.
Brain	For removal and specimen preparation, see p. 66.	Brain stem gliomas.
Placenta and umbilical cord	Record weight. Submit sections away from periphery for histologic study.	Large placenta; edematous umbilical cord.

Syndrome, Behçet's

Organs and Tissues	Procedures	Possible or Expected Findings
External examination and skin	Record extent and character of skin and mucosal lesions. Prepare photographs; prepare sections of skin.	Ulcers *(1)* of oral mucosa; ulcers of perianal region and genitalia; erythema nodosum-like skin lesions; skin ulcers; subungual infarctions.
	Prepare roentgenograms of joints.	Monarthritis or polyarthritis (without deformations).
Central and peripheral and veins	For removal of femoral vessels, see p. 34.	Aortitis and other forms of arteritis;* arterial thromboses and peripheral arterial aneurysms; thrombophlebitis or thrombosis,* primarily of thigh and calf veins.
Lungs		Pulmonary embolism.*
Esophagus	Remove together with stomach.	Ulcers.
Colon, rectum, and pelvic organs	Open rectum in posterior midline.	Colitis; rectovaginal fistula.
Pancreas	Sample for histologic study.	Pancreatitis.*
Neck organs	Prepare sections of cricoarytenoid joint (p. 96), particularly if peripheral joints cannot be studied.	Ulcer of pharynx; scarring and stenosis of hypopharynx. Laryngeal arthritis.
Brain	For removal and specimen preparation, see p. 65.	Encephalitis;* pseudotumor cerebri.*
Base of skull	Expose venous sinuses (p. 71).	Thrombophlebitis of dural venous sinuses.
Eyes	For removal and specimen preparation, see p. 85.	Corneal ulceration; uveitis with hypopyon; iridocyclitis; thrombosis of central retinal vein. Eye changes may have caused blindness.
Peripheral nerves	For sampling and specimen preparation, see p. 79.	Peripheral neuropathy.
Skeletal muscles	For sampling and specimen preparation, see p. 80.	Vasculitis; inflammatory lesions; fibrosis.
Joints	For removal and specimen preparation, see p. 96. For proper sampling, consult roentgenograms and clinical records.	Monarthritis—for instance, of a sacroiliac joint—or polyarthritis.

Reference

1. Criteria for diagnosis of Behçet's Disease. International Study Group for Behçet's Disease. Lancet 1990;335:1078–1080.

Syndrome, Bloom's

Possible Associated Condition: Acute leukemia* and other malignancies.

Organs and Tissues	*Procedures*	*Possible or Expected Findings*
External examination, oral cavity, and skin	Record facial features and status of teeth; appearance of hands; body weight and length. Record and photograph skin abnormalities and prepare sections.	Small, narrow face with prominent nose and ears; telangiectases on face, hands, forearms. Defective dentition; polysyndactyly of hands. Stunted growth or dwarfism;* ichthyosis, café au lait spots.
Blood or fascia lata	Submit blood for immunoglobuliln study. For sampling for chromosome analysis, see pp. 108 and 109, respectively. Snap-freeze tissue for identification of BLM gene *(1)*.	Reduced immunoglobulin concentrations in blood. Chromatid breaks and gaps.
Other organs and tissues	Procedures depend on expected findings or grossly identified abnormalities as listed in right-hand column.	Multiple malignancies.

Reference

1. Straughen JE, Johnson J, McLaren D, Proytcheva M, Ellis N, German J, Groden J. A rapid method for detecting the predominant Ashkenazi Jewish mutation in the Bloom's syndrome gene. Hum Mutation 1998;11:175–178.

Syndrome, Bonnevie-Ullrich (See "Syndrome, Turner's.")

Syndrome, Budd-Chiari

Synonyms and Related Terms: Acute veno-occlusive disease of the liver; hepatic vein thrombosis; hepatic venous outflow obstruction.

Possible Associated Conditions: Antithrombin III deficiency; oral contraceptive use; paroxysmal nocturnal hemoglobinuria;* polycythemia rubra vera;* pregnancy;* protein C deficiency.

Organs and Tissues	*Procedures*	*Possible or Expected Findings*
External examination		Dilatation of abdominal veins. Edema of extremities.
Chest organs	In most cases, it seems best to remove chest organs together with abdominal organs (see below under "Portal and inferior vena cava system; heart").	Constrictive pericarditis or right atrial myxoma may be causes of hepatic venous outflow obstruction.
Abdominal and chest cavities	Measure volume of effusions and submit for culture (p. 102).	Ascites.
	For lymphangiography and dissection of the thoracic duct, see p. 34.	Dilatation of retroperitoneal, hepatic capsular, and anterior mediastinal lymphatics and of the thoracic duct.
	For hepatic phlebography, see p. 59 (under "Venography").	Dilatation (in suprahepatic obstruction) or intrahepatic obstruction of hepatic veins.
Portal and inferior vena cava system; heart	After removal of intestines, dissect mesenteric, splenic, and portal veins *in situ*. Remove chest and abdominal organs en masse (p. 3). Open inferior vena cava and its branches along posterior midline from iliac veins to right atrium.	Thromboses. Tumor of right atrium. Compression of intrathoracic inferior vena cava by constrictive (calcific) pericarditis.
Hepatic veins	Identify right, middle, and left hepatic veins. Record type and location of obstruction.	Thrombosis, tumor, or webs on or near hepatic ostia. Webs usually obstruct left and middle hepatic veins and the inferior vena cava just cephalad to the patent right hepatic vein.
	Record appearance of venous ostia of caudate lobe.	Veins of caudate lobe are not involved by disease process.

Organs and Tissues	Procedures	Possible or Expected Findings
Liver	Record weight and size. Photograph venous ostia and cut section of liver. Submit samples for histologic study. Request Verhoeff–van Gieson and Gomori's iron stains (p. 172). If condition was treated by liver transplantation,* search for thromboses in allograft.	Hepatic and portal vein thromboses. Congestive fibrosis with uninvolved or hypertrophic caudate lobe. Hemosiderosis. Tumor(s) of the liver;* amebic abscesses, and other lesions may have caused hepatic venous outflow obstruction.
Spleen	Record weight and size.	Congestive splenomegaly. Hemosiderosis.
Esophagus and stomach	Remove together. For demonstration of esophageal varices, see p. 53.	Esophageal varices.*
Bone marrow	For preparation of sections and smears, see p. 96.	Hyperplasia. See also under "Polycythemia."
Extremities	For phlebography and for removal of femoral and popliteal vessels, see pp. 120 and 34, respectively.	Phlebothrombosis or arterial thromboses. Thrombophlebitis migrans. Buerger's disease.*

Syndrome, Caplan's

Synonyms and Related Terms: Complicated pneumoconiosis;* conglomerate silicosis; progressive massive fibrosis of coal workers.

Organs and Tissues	Procedures	Possible or Expected Findings
External examination	Prepare roentgenograms of the chest and peripheral joints.	Pulmonary nodules, often perihilar. Joint changes of rheumatoid arthritis.*
Lungs	Submit one lobe for microbiologic study (p. 103). Perfuse one lung with formalin (p. 47). Photograph slices. Request Verhoeff–van Gieson stain (p. 173).	Rheumatoid-type pulmonary nodules (0.5–2.0 cm) often with necrotic center. Multiple small silicotic nodules.
Joints	For removal, prosthetic repair, and specimen preparation, see p. 96.	Rheumatoid arthritis.*
Other organs		Systemic manifestations of rheumatoid arthritis.*

Syndrome, Carcinoid

Synonyms and Related Terms: Argentaffinoma syndrome; carcinoid tumor; Cassidy-Scholte syndrome; malignant carcinoid syndrome.

NOTE: Autopsy should be performed as soon as possible, and tumor material should be removed first. Argentaffin cell reaction disappears within 3–6 h after death. If patient had undergone liver transplantation, see also under that heading.

Possible Associated Conditions: Cushing's syndrome;* multiple endocrine neoplasia.*

Organs and Tissues	Procedures	Possible or Expected Findings
External examination	Record extend of skin changes and prepare histologic sections of skin.	Hyperpigmentation and keratosis of skin (pellagra dermatosis).
Heart and inferior vena cava system	Remove chest and abdominal organs en masse (p. 3).	
	Open inferior vena cava posteriorly and expose hepatic vein orifices, right atrium of the heart, and tricuspid valve. Photograph intimal lesions and submit samples for histologic study. Request Verhoeff–van Gieson stain (p. 173). Test competence of tricuspid and pulmonary valves (p. 29). Open heart in direction of blood flow (p. 21).	Intimal fibrosis may involve hepatic veins, upper inferior vena cava, right atrium, coronary sinus, superior vena cava, tricuspid valve, right ventricle, pulmonary valve, and, rarely, the left heart chambers. Appreciable involvement of the left heart chambers indicates active pulmonary tumor or right-to-left shunt. Tricuspid stenosis* and insufficiency,* pulmonary stenosis,* and mild mitral and aortic fibrosis may occur.

Organs and Tissues	Procedures	Possible or Expected Findings
Lungs	If primary tumor is suspected in lungs, dissect and snap-freeze fresh tumor tissue for chemical analysis. For staining, see below under "Gastrointestinal tract."	Small cell (oat cell) carcinoma. Bronchial carcinoid.
	Perfuse tumor-free lung with formalin (p. 47). Request Verhoeff–van Gieson stain (p. 173).	Intimal fibrosis and fibroelastosis of small pulmonary arteries.
Peritoneum	Submit samples for histologic study.	Fibrosis (rare).
Urine	Submit sample for chemical analysis.	Increased concentration of 5-hydroxy indoleacetic acid (5-HIAA). Results are not always reliable.
Gastrointestinal tract		Endocrine-active carcinoid tumor may occur in all segments except in rectum. Most frequent in ileum; occurs also in Meckel's diverticulum.
	Freeze fresh tumor for chemical analysis. For formalin-fixed tissue, request Bodian stain for argyrophil cell reaction and Fontana-Masson stain for argentaffin cell reaction (p. 172). Prepare tumor samples for electron microscopy (p. 132).	High concentratios of 5-hydroxyindoles. Argyrophil cell reaction may persist for 24 h after death; argentaffin cell reaction disappears within 3–6 h. Autofluorescence in ultraviolet light.
		Peptic ulcer of stomach.* If malabsorption syndrome* was present, see under that heading.
Liver	Record weight. Photograph cut section and submit samples for histologic study.	Massive metastatic involvement in most instances.
Bile ducts and gallbladder	Dissect extrahepatic bile ducts *in situ*.	May contain active tumor tissue.
Pancreas	If tumor is present, submit samples as described above under "Gastrointestinal tract."	Carcinoid tumor. Islet cell tumor.
Lymph nodes	Submit samples for histologic and chemical study.	Massive para-aortic metastases may produce carcinoid syndrome in absence of hepatic metastases.
Ovaries	If ovaries appear abnormal, record sizes and weights and sample for histologic study.	Primary carcinoid tumors may occur in teratomas. Ovaries also may be site of metastases.
Testes		Rarely, primary carcinoid tumors may occur in teratomas.
Bones and joints	For removal, prosthetic repair, and specimen preparation, see pp. 65 and 67, respectively.	Osteogenic metastases (rare). Rheumatoid arthritis.*

Syndrome, Chédiak-Higashi

Synonyms and Related Terms: Chédiak-Higashi anomaly; Béguez-César disease; hereditary neutrophil granule dysfunction syndrome.

Possible Associated Condition: Lymphoma.*

Organs and Tissues	Procedures	Possible or Expected Findings
External examination and skin	Record extent of hypopigmented areas and of hemorrhagic and infected skin. Photograph and take sections of abnormal and of pigmented skin. Request Fontana-Masson silver stain (p. 172).	Decreased pigmentation of skin and hair (albinism). Pyoderma gangrenosum. Staphylococcal skin infection. Skin hemorrhages. Enlarged melanin granules in melanocytes of pigmented areas.
Blood	Submit sample for microbiologic study (p. 102) and for study of immunoglobulins. Prepare smears. If fresh specimens are available, submit sample for electron microscopic study (p. 132).	Bacteremia; septicemia. Hypogammaglobulinemia. Large azurophilic peroxidase-positive granules (giant lysosomes) in neutrophils. Granules in lymphocytes are peroxidase-negative and periodic acid–Schiff-positive.

Organs and Tissues	*Procedures*	*Possible or Expected Findings*
Lungs	Submit one lobe for bacterial culture (p. 103).	Bacterial pneumonia.
Liver and spleen	Record sizes and weights. Submit samples for histologic study.	Hepatosplenomegaly. Lymphohistiocytic infiltrates.
Lymph nodes	Request Wright stain for touch preparations. Use Zenker's or Helly's fixative for paraffin sections.	Lymphohistiocytic infiltrates.
Kidneys	Snap-freeze tissue for histochemical study.	Glycolipid inclusions in tubular epithelial cells.
Other organs	Procedures depend on expected findings or grossly identified abnormalities as listed in right-hand column.	Infections, particularly of upper respiratory tract, and hemorrhages caused bythrombo-cytopenia and coagulation factor deficiencies.
Bone marrow	For preparation of sections and smears, see p. 96. Snap-freeze material for histochemical study. Prepare sample for electron microscopy.	Large azurophilic granules in promyelocytes. Granules positive for acid phosphatase and myeloperoxidase. Lymphocytic infiltrates in accelerated phase of disease. Megaloblastic changes.
Brain and spinal cord	For removal and specimen preparation, see pp. 66 and 70, respectively. Snap-freeze material for histochemical study. Prepare sample for electron microscopy.	Lymphohistiocytic infiltrates. Glycolipid inclusions in neurons and histiocytes. Giant lysosomes.
Peripheral nerves	For sampling and specimen preparation, see p. 79. Prepare sample for electron microscopic study.	Lymphohistiocytic infiltrates. Degeneration of nerve tissue. Giant lysosomes.
Eyes	For removal and specimen preparation, see p. 85.	Decreased pigmentation (oculocutaneous albinism) of uvea and particularly of retina.

Syndrome, Churg-Strauss (See "Granulomatosis, allergic, and angiitis (Churg-Strauss syndrome).")

Syndrome, Congenital Rubella

Synonym and Related Term: Congenital rubella; rubella.*

NOTE: See also "Rubella." (1) Collect all tissues that appear to be infected. (2) Request viral cultures. (3) Usually, special stains are not helpful. (4) No special precautions are indicated. (5) Serologic studies are available from local or state health department laboratories (p. 135). (6) This is a **reportable** disease.

Organs and Tissues	*Procedures*	*Possible or Expected Findings*
External examination and umbilical cord; oral cavity	Record body weight and length. Record and photograph abnormalities as listed in right-hand column.	Intrauterine growth retardation; failure to thrive; purpura; jaundice; hypoplastic mandible; microcephaly; enamel hypoplasia; caries; delayed eruption of deciduous teeth; skin dimples; abnormal dermatoglyphics; skin pigmentation.
	Record appearance of external genitalia.	Hypospadias; cryptorchidism.
Cardiovascular system	Procedures depend on expected findings or grossly identified abnormalities as listed in right-hand column.	Congenital heart disease; myocarditis;* pulmonary artery branch stenosis; systemic arterial hypoplasia and stenosis due to intimal proliferation.
Lungs	Perfuse one lobe with formalin (p. 47).	Interstitial pneumonia.*
Liver	Record weight. Submit samples for histologic study. For cholangiography, see p. 56.	Giant cell hepatitis; cholestasis; fibrosis; cirrhosis;* necrosis; extramedullary hematopoiesis; bile duct proliferation mimicking biliary atresia.
Spleen	Record weight and sample for histologic study.	Splenomegaly with extramedullary hematopoiesis.
Blood	Submit sample for determination of IgM and IgG antibodies.	

Organs and Tissues	Procedures	Possible or Expected Findings
Lymph nodes	Submit samples for histologic study.	Lymphadenopathy with enlarged germinal centers or lymphoid depletion.
Kidneys	Submit samples for histologic study.	Extramedullary hematopoiesis; glomerulonephritis.
Pancreas	Submit samples for histologic study.	Lymphocytic infiltration of islets.
Brain and spinal cord	For removal and specimen preparation, see pp. 66 and 70, respectively.	Microcephaly; meningoencephalitis;* ischemic necrosis; later in life, progressive panencephalitis; perivascular mononuclear infiltrates; glial nodules in white matter.
Ears	For removal and specimen preparation, see p. 72.	Otitis media;* inflammation and scarring of cochlea.
Eyes	For removal and specimen preparation, see p. 85.	Microphthalmia; iridocyclitis; cataracts; chorioretinitis.
Skeletal muscles	For specimen preparation, see p. 80.	Myositis.
Bones	For removal and specimen preparation, see p. 95.	Metaphyseal osteoporosis;* retardation of ossification.
Placenta	Record weight and sample for histologic study.	Villus vessel necrosis; villus edema; necrosis of syncytiotrophoblast with fibrin accretion; plasma cell deciduitis. With infection late in gestation, villus sclerosis and small placenta.

Syndrome, Conn's (See "Aldosteronism.")

Syndrome, Cronkhite-Canada (See "Polyposis, familial, and related syndromes.")

Syndrome, Cushing's

Related Terms: Cushing's disease (associated with ACTH-producing pituitary tumor); hypercorticism.

NOTE: Glucocorticoid therapy is the most common cause of Cushing's syndrome and thus, the autopsy also may show the features of the condition that had been treated—for example, an allograft with signs of rejection.

Organs and Tissues	Procedures	Possible or Expected Findings
External examination and skin	Record body weight and length, abdominal circumference, skeletal muscle development, and hair distribution. Prepare sections of skin and smears of infectious skin lesions. Request Gram and Grocott's methenamine silver stains (p. 172).	"Moon face"; obesity of trunk; edema and striae of abdomen, hips, and shoulders. Muscle wasting. Virilism in women (acne and hirsutism) and children. Ecchymoses. Skin infections.
	Prepare skeletal roentgenograms.	Osteoporosis.*
Blood	Submit sample for biochemical study.	Increased concentrations of cortisol or adrenocorticotropic hormone (ACTH)-like substances. (This is not reliable because of diurnal variability.)
Heart	Record weight.	Hypertrophy secondary to hypertension.*
Lungs	Snap-freeze tumor tissue for determination of ACTH-like substances.	Bronchogenic carcinoma (oat cell type) or malignant bronchial carcinoid, producing ACTH-like substances.
Pancreas	See above under "Lungs."	Malignant islet cell tumor, producing ACTH-like substances.
Adrenal glands	Record weight, size, and thickness of cortex of both adrenal glands. Snap-freeze tumor tissue for biochemical study. See also under "Tumor, of the adrenal glands." Submit samples of both glands for histologic study.	Adrenal nodular hyperplasia; adrenal cortical adenoma or carcinoma. Pheochromocytoma, producing ACTH-like substances. Adrenocortical hypertrophy secondary to ACTH stimulation. Atrophy of adrenal cortex after steroid therapy or secondary to effects of adrenocortical tumor.

Organs and Tissues	Procedures	Possible or Expected Findings
Kidneys		Nephrolithiasis.*
Ovaries	Record sizes and weights. If tumor is present, snap-freeze sample for determination of ACTH-like substances. Submit samples for histologic study.	Ovarian tumor, producing ACTH-like substances.
Thyroid gland	See above under "Ovaries."	Carcinoma of thyroid gland, producing ACTH-like substances.
Other organs	See above under "Lungs," "Pancreas," "Ovaries," and "Thyroid gland."	ACTH-like substances may be produced by tumors at various sites.
Pituitary gland	For removal and specimen preparation, see p. 71. Submit samples for histologic study. Snap-freeze tumor tissue for biochemical study. See also under "Tumor, of the pituitary gland."	A normal pituitary gland is compatible with increased secretion of ACTH and with Cushing's disease. Pituitary micro- or macroadenoma (Cushing's disease), basophilic or chromophobic type. Crooke's hyaline degeneration in adenohypophysis indicates that excessive amounts of glucocorticoids had been present.
Bones	For removal and specimen preparation, see p. 95.	Osteoporosis.*
Skeletal muscles	For sampling and specimen preparation, see p. 80.	Steroid myopathy and atrophy.
Vitreous	Submit sample for glucose, sodium, and chloride determination (p. 114).	Hyperglycemia or electrolyte abnormalities may be present.

Syndrome, DiGeorge's

Synonyms and Related Terms: Harrington syndrome; 3rd and 4th pharyngeal pouch syndrome; thymic agenesis.

NOTE: See also "Syndrome, primary immunodeficiency."

Organs and Tissues	Procedures	Possible or Expected Findings
External examination	Record body weight and length. Record and photograph abnormalities as listed in right-hand column.	Growth retardation. Hypertelorism; anti-mongoloid slant of eyes; short philtrum; small and low set ears; notched pinnae; micrognathia. Eczema *(1)*.
Heart	See under specific lesion as listed in right-hand column.	Conotruncal and aortic arch anomalies.
Lungs	If any consolidated areas are identified, submit for culture (p. 103).	Pneumonia; pulmonary abscess.
Other organs and tissues	Record and photograph abnormalities and submit possible infectious lesions for culture (p. 102).	Infections at various sites.
Neck organs	Carefully search for thymus, parathyroid glands, and isthmus of thyroid.	Absence of thymus and parathyroid glands (3rd and 4th pharyngeal pouch derivatives) *(2)*. Absence of thyroid gland (rare) or of isthmus of thyroid.

References

1. Archer E, Chuang TY, Hong R. Severe eczema in a patient with DiGeorge's syndrome. Cutis 1990;45:455–459.
2. Robinson HB Jr. DiGeorge's syndrome or the III - IV pharyngeal pouch syndrome: pathology and a theory of pathogenesis. Perspect Pediatr Pathol 1975;3:773–206.

Syndrome, Down's

Synonyms and Related Terms: Mongolism; trisomy 21; trisomy G syndrome.

Possible Associated Conditions: Acute lymphocytic, myelocytic or megakaryocytic leukemia;* atresia of esophagus;* atresia or stenosis of duodenum;* congenital heart disease (especially ventricular septal defects and atrioventricular canal defects*).

Organs and Tissues	*Procedures*	*Possible or Expected Findings*
External examination and oral cavity	Record and photograph abnormalities as listed in right-hand column.	Epicanthal folds; cleft lip/palate; high arched palate; furrowed tongue; rhagades. Depressed nasal bridge; dysplastic ears; small, broad or flat nose; slanted palpebral fissures; flat occiput; brachycephaly; palmar "simian crease"; short fifth middle finger; short limbs; abnormal dermatoglyphics;
	Prepare radiographs of pelvis.	Horizontal acetabular roof.
Blood; fascia lata	Submit samples for chromosome study (p. 108).	Complete trisomy 21 or trisomy 12q due to a translocation.
Heart	Procedures depend on grossly identified abnormalities as listed in right-hand column.	Ventricular septal defect;* complete atrioventricular septal defect* *(1)*.
Gastrointestinal tract	Open stomach and duodenum *in situ*; if indicated, probe anus.	Duodenal stenosis and atresia; imperforate anus.
Brain and spinal cord	For removal and specimen preparation, see p. 66 and 70, respectively.	Microcephaly; poorly developed secondary gyri; open operculum; hypoplastic superior temporal gyrus *(2)*; short corpus callosum; hypoplastic brain stem, medulla and cerebellum; polymicrogyria; neurofibrillary tangles; meningomyelocoele.
Bone marrow	For preparation of sections and smears, see p. 96.	Acute lymphocytic leukemia; acute myelocytic leukemia; acute megakaryocytic leukemia.

References

1. Spicer RL. Cardiovascular disease in Down syndrome. Pediatr Clin North Am 1984;31(6):1331–1344.
2. Jay V. Brain and eye pathology in an infant with Down syndrome and tuberous sclerosis. Pediatr Neurol 1996;15:57–59.

Syndrome, Dystonia

Synonyms or Related Terms: Dopa-responsive dystonia (Segawa's syndrome); inherited or sporadic primary (or idiopathic) dystonia; primary torsion dystonia (dystonia musculorum deformans); secondary (or symptomatic) dystonia.

NOTE: Primary dystonia includes primary torsion dystonia (autosomal-dominant), an X-linked form, and Dopa responsive dystonia. The condition may be focal, multifocal, segmental, generalized, or appear as hemidystonia.

Organs and Tissues	*Procedures*	*Possible or Expected Findings*
Brain, spinal cord, and spinal ganglia	For removal and specimen preparation, see pp. 65, 67, and 69, respectively. Autopsy in cases of primary torsion dystonia should be considered a research procedure; extensive collection of tissue is indicated, including frozen samples.	No diagnostic pathologic changes in primary torsion dystonia. In hemidystonia, changes in the basal ganglia may be found, such as infarcts, tumors, or effects of trauma or toxic damage. These last findings may have medicolegal implications.

Syndrome, Eaton-Lambert (See "Myasthenia gravis.")

Syndrome, Ehlers-Danlos

NOTE: Nine subtypes have been distinguished, based primarily on the extent of the disease. However much overlap exists.

Organs and Tissues	*Procedures*	*Possible or Expected Findings*
External examination, skin, and oral cavity	Record body weight, length, stature; record and photograph all abnormal features, as listed in right-hand column.	Widely spaced eyes; epicanthal folds; broad nasal bridge; lop ears. Flatfeet or clubfeet; genu recurvatum; arachnodactyly; pigeon breast; kyphoscoliosis. Umbilical and inguinal hernias. Subcutaneous emphysema (see below under "Chest cavity"). Poorly formed teeth. High arched palate.

Organs and Tissues	Procedures	Possible or Expected Findings
External examination, skin, and oral cavity *(continued)*	Prepare sections of skin and request Verhoeff–van Gieson stain (p. 173). Submit samples of skin for electron microscopic study (p. 132).	Hyperelasticity of skin, bruises or scars, hemorrhages, and hyperpigmentation. Lipomatous pseudotumors that may be calcified or ossified. Normal or abnormal amounts and fragmentation of elastic tissue. Abnormalities of collagen.
	Prepare skeletal roentgenograms.	Dislocation of hip, shoulder, patella, radius, or clavicle. Loose-end clavicles; spondylolisthesis; osteolytic changes in distal phalanges. Degenerative arthritis.
Chest cavity	Record appearance of pleural surfaces *in situ*.	Rupture of lung with mediastinal and subcutaneous emphysema (see above).
Heart and great vessels	Procedures depend on grossly identified abnormalities as listed in right-hand column.	Congenital malformations of the heart. Mitral valve prolapse; aneurysm of aortic sinus.* Aortic insufficiency.* Dissecting hematoma of aorta.* Spontaneous rupture of arteries.
Lungs	Perfuse on lung with formalin (p. 47).	Various congenital anomalies.
Other organs and tissues	Procedures depend on expected findings or grossly identified abnormalities as listed in right-hand column.	Congenital anomalies of gastrointestinal and genitourinary tracts.
	Record size and location of hematomas. Prepare tissue samples with small vessels for electron microscopic study (p. 132).	Bleeding from various organ sites.
Joints	For removal, prosthetic repair, and specimen preparation, see p. 96.	Arthritis;* hemarthrosis. Effusions. Hyperextensibility of joints.

Syndrome, Ellis-Van Creveld

Synonyms and Related Terms: Chondrodysplasia;* chondroectodermal dysplasia; short-rib polydactyly chondrodysplasia.

NOTE: This syndrome belongs to a large family (with more than 30 subtypes) of chondrodysplasias. The suggested autopsy procedures are essentially the same in all chondrodysplasias.See also under "Chondrodysplasia."

Organs and Tissues	Procedures	Possible or Expected Findings
External examination	Record and photograph abnormal features as listed in right-hand column.	Short-limb dwarfism* with narrowing of the rib cage; polydactyly; dysplasia of fingernails; thin and sparse hair; premature eruption of teeth; defective dentition; eye abnormalities; upper lip bound down by multiple frenula.
	Record appearance of external genitalia.	Cryptorchidism; epispadias; hypospadias.
	Prepare skeletal roentgenograms.	Chondrodysplasia with acromelic micromelia (shortening of the distal segment of the limb); fusion of capitate and hamate bones of wrist; defects of lateral aspect of proximal tibia.
Heart		Congenital heart disease (atrial septal defect*).
Bones	For removal, prosthetic repair, and specimen preparation, see p. 95.	See lesions listed above under "External examination."

Syndrome, Empty Sella

Synonyms and Related Terms: Primary empty sella syndrome; secondary empty sella syndrome (e.g., after surgical removal or spontaneous infarction of pituitary adenoma).

Organs and Tissues	Procedures	Possible or Expected Findings
External examination	Record body weight and length.	Empty sella syndrome relatively common in obese females.
	Prepare roentgenogram of skull.	Enlargement of pituitary fossa visible on lateral roentgenograms of the skull.
Base of skull and pituitary gland	For exposure and specimen preparation, see p. 71. Photograph sella.	Flattening and postero-inferior displacement of the gland. Necrosis of pituitary gland (Sheehan's syndrome*) or of pituitary adenoma.
Other organs		Manifestations of pituitary insufficiency* (mostly in association with secondary empty sella syndrome).

Syndrome, Eosinophilic (Unspecified) (See "Cardiomyopathy, restrictive [eosinophilic type]," "Gastroenteritis, eosinophilic," and "Syndrome, eosinophilic pulmonary.")

Syndrome, Eosinophilic Pulmonary

Synonyms and Related Terms: Acute eosinophilic pneumonia with respiratory failure *(1)*; allergic bronchopulmonary aspergillosis; Carrington's chronic eosinophilic pneumonia; Churg-Strauss syndrome; eosinophilic pneumonia; hypereosinophilic syndrome; idiopathic acute eosinophilic pneumonia; Löffler's syndrome; pulmonary infiltration with eosinophilia (PIE syndrome); tropical pulmonary eosinophilia.

Organs and Tissues	Procedures	Possible or Expected Findings
External examination	Prepare chest roentgenogram.	Pulmonary infiltrates.
Lungs	Submit one lobe for culture (p. 103). Freeze portion of same lung for special studies. Prepare smears. Perfuse one lung with formalin (p. 47). Request Giemsa or azure-eosin stain for demonstration of eosinophilic leukocytes (p. 172).	Ascariasis and hookworm (pulmonary larval migration) infestation *(2)*; other parasitic diseases or fungal infections. Bronchiolitis obliterans; eosinophilic microabscesses *(3)*.
Other organs	Procedures depend on expected findings or grossly identified abnormalities as listed in right-hand column.	Systemic manifestations of eosinophilia; parasitic or other infectious or allergic disease.

References

1. Tazelaar H, Linz LJ, Colby TV, Myers JL, Limper AH. Acute eosinophilic pneumonia: Histopathologic features in nine cases. Am Rev Resp Crit Care Med 1997;155:296–302.
2. Sarinas PS, Chitkara RK. Ascariasis and hookworm. Semin Resp Inf 1997;12:130–137.
3. Jederlinic PJ, Sicilian L, Gaensler EA. Chronic eosinophilic pneumonia. A report of 19 cases and a review of the literature. Medicine 1988;67: 154–162.

Syndrome, Extrapyramidal (See "Chorea, acute," "Chorea, hereditary," and "Disease, Parkinson's.")

Syndrome, Fanconi

Related Terms: Aminoaciduria;* cystinosis;* familial hypophosphatemic vitamin D-resistant rickets; galactosemia;* proximal tubular transport defect; tyrosinemia.* Excludes Fanconi's anemia (sometimes also called Fanconi's syndrome) due to a defect in DNA repair.

Organs and Tissues	Procedures	Possible or Expected Findings
External examination	Record body weight and external measurements; record and photograph abnormalities as listed in right-hand column.	Red/blond hair, fair skin (diminished pigmentation); dehydration;* stigmata of hypothyroidism;* delay of sexual maturation.
	Prepare skeletal roentgenograms. Radiographs of long bones.	Rickets; osteomalacia.*
Fascia lata	Submit for tissue culture for possible enzyme analysis (p. 109).	

Organs and Tissues	Procedures	Possible or Expected Findings
Blood	Obtain sample for possible assay of heavy metals. Obtain sample for protein electrophoresis and parathyroid hormone assay.	Lead,* mercury,* cadmium,* uranium poisoning; myeloma;* parathyroid hyperplasia (primary or secondary).
Kidney	Photograph lesions. Submit for histologic study.	Cysts; nephrocalcinosis; pyelonephritis;* nephrolithiasis.*
Urine	Obtain sample for biochemical analysis.	Glucosuria; phosphaturia; aminoaciduria.

Syndrome, Felty's

Related Terms: Pseudo-Felty syndrome *(1)*; rheumatoid arthritis.*

Organs and Tissues	Procedures	Possible or Expected Findings
External examination, skin, and oral cavity	Record body weight and length.	Cachexia.
	Record extent and character of skin infections and ulcers, appearance of eyes and oral cavity, and character of pigmentation. Sample skin lesions for histologic study.	Infections involving skin, oral cavity, and eyes (corneas). Chronic leg ulcers. Brown pigmentation over exposed areas of extremities.
Subcutaneous tissues and lymph nodes	Submit samples of axillary, cervical, and other enlarged lymph nodes and all subcutaneous nodules for histologic study.	Lymphadenopathy. Rheumatoid nodules.
Blood	Submit sample for serologic study.	Positive rheumatoid factor.
Lungs	Submit one lobe for bacterial and fungal cultures (p. 103). Perfuse one lung with formalin (p. 47).	Various types of pneumonia. Bronchiectasis.*
Liver	Record weight and sample for histologic study.	Nodular regenerative hyperplasia *(2)*; sinusoidal lymphocytosis *(3)*.
Spleen	Record size and weight. If splenectomy had been done, record presence or absence of accessory spleens.	Splenomegaly *(4)*. After splenectomy, presence of accessory spleen may account for treatment failure.
Other organs		Manifestations of portal hypertension.*
Mediastinal and retroperitoneal lymph nodes	Submit samples for histologic study.	Lymphadenopathy of mediastinal and para-aortic lymph nodes.
Bone marrow, bones, and joints	For preparation of bone marrow sections and smears, see p. 96.	Anemia;* neutropenia; thrombocytopenia.
	For removal, prosthetic repair, and specimen preparation of bones and joints, see p. 95.	Rheumatoid arthritis.*

References

1. Rosenstein ED, Kramer N. Felty's and pseudo-Felty's syndrome. Semin Arthritis Rheum 1991;21:129–142.
2. Perez-Ruiz F, Orte Martinez FJ, Zea Mendoza AC, Ruiz del Arbol L, Moreno Caparros A. Nodular regenerative hyperplasia of the liver in rheumatic diseases: report of seven cases and review of the literature. Semin Arthritis Rheum 1991;21:47–54.
3. Cohen ML, Manier JW, Bredfeldt JE. Sinusoidal lymphocytosis of the liver in Felty's syndrome with a review of the liver involvement in Felty's syndrome. J Clin Gastroenterol 1989;11:92–94.
4. Fishman D, Isenberg DA. Splenic involvement in rheumatic diseases. Semin Arthritis Rheum 1997;27:141–155.

Syndrome, Fetal Alcoholic

Organs and Tissues	Procedures	Possible or Expected Findings
External examination and oral cavity	Record body weight and length, and head circumference. Record and photograph all abnormalities as listed in right-hand column.	Growth retardation; microcephaly; depressed nasal bridge; thin upper lip; smooth philtrum; epicanthal folds; small palpebral fissures; strabismus; midfacial hypoplasia; cleft palate; pectus excavatum; small nails; abnormal palmar creases; hirsutism; contractures; spina bifida; pigmented nevi.

Organs and Tissues	*Procedures*	*Possible or Expected Findings*
Diaphragm	Record location, character, and size of defects.	Anomalies of diaphragm.
Liver	Record weight and sample for histologic study.	Steatosis; fibrosis.
Heart		Ventricular and atrial septal defects.*
Brain	For removal, see p. 66.	Hydrocephalus; micrencephaly; small frontal lobes; irregular convolutions or microgyria; small third ventricle; arhinencephaly; abnormal lamination of cortical cells; malorientaton of neurons; cerebellar heterotopias *(1)*.
Eyes	For removal and specimen preparation, see p. 85.	Hypoplasia of optic nerve head; increased tortuosity of retinal vessels;.

Reference

1. Johnson VP, Swayze VW II, Sato Y, Andreasen NC. Fetal alcohol syndrome: craniofacial and central nervous system manifestations. Am J Med Genet 1996;61(4):329–339.

Syndrome, Fibrosing

Synonyms and Related Terms: Dupuytren's contracture; mediastinal fibrosis; multifocal fibrosclerosis; periureteral fibrosis; Peyronie's disease; pseudotumor of the orbit; retroperitoneal fibrosis,* Riedel's thyroiditis; sclerosing cholangitis;* sclerosing mediastinitis.*

NOTE: In rare instances, the conditions listed under "Synonyms and Related Terms" appear to occur together or overlap. Autopsy procedures in the most important conditions are listed under the specific title (see names with *). In all cases, other possible sites of fibrosis should be carefully studied.

Organs and Tissues	*Procedures*	*Possible or Expected Findings*
Mediastinum	If there is evidence of fibrosis, submit tissues for culture of *Histoplasma capsulatum*. Prepare horizontal sections through fixed tissues.	Superior vena cava obstruction. Sclerosing mediastinitis.* Histoplasmosis.*
Biliary system		Sclerosing cholangitis.*
Retroperitoneum		Retroperitoneal fibrosis.* Periureteral fibrosis.
Other organs and tissues	Procedures depend on expected findings or grossly identified abnormalities as listed in right-hand column. Use cultures and special stains to rule out underlying infection or tumor.	Dupuytren's contracture; pseudotumor of the orbit; Riedel's thyroiditis; Peyronie's disease; and possibly other fibrosing conditions.

Syndrome, Foix-Alajouanine (See "Malformation, arteriovenous, cerebral or spinal [or both].")

Syndrome, Gardner's (See "Polyposis, familial, and related syndromes.")

Syndrome, Gasser's (See "Syndrome, hemolytic uremic.")

Syndrome, Goodpasture's

Related Term: Goodpasture's disease.

NOTE: For a pertinent review, see ref. *(1)*.

Organs and Tissues	*Procedures*	*Possible or Expected Findings*
Lungs	Record weights. Photograph surface of lungs. Submit one lobe for general bacterial and viral cultures (p. 103).	Influenza virus infection.

Organs and Tissues	Procedures	Possible or Expected Findings
Lungs *(continued)*	Photograph cut surface of fresh lung. Snap-freeze tissue block for immunofluorescent study. Perfuse one lung with formalin (p. 47). Request Gomori's iron and Verhoeff–van Gieson stains (p. 172). Prepare samples for electron microscopic study (p. 132).	Pulmonary hemorrhages. Interstitial pulmonary fibrosis.
Kidneys	Follow procedures described under "Glomerulonephritis."	Anti-basement membrane antibody mediated nephritis (Goodpasture's disease). Glomeruli may appear normal or show focal proliferative or necrotizing changes. Linear immunofluorescence of glomerular basement membrane, indicating presence of IgG (or rarely IgA).
Urine	Submit sample for protein determination and study of sediment.	Proteinuria; hematuria; casts.
Other organs	Histologic samples should include heart, liver, spleen, lymph nodes, intestine, testes, and tissue from nasopharynx.	Histologic study of multiple organs may be needed to rule out other systemic diseases such as Wegener's granulomatosis.*

Reference

1. Bolton WK. Goodpasture's syndrome. Kidney Intl 1996;50:1753–1766.

Syndrome, Grönblad-Strandberg (See "Pseudoxanthoma elasticum.")

Syndrome, Guillain-Barré

Synonyms: Acute inflammatory polyradiculoneuropathy; Guillain-Barré-Strohl syndrome; idiopathic polyneuritis; Landry's ascending paralysis.

Organs and Tissues	Procedures	Possible or Expected Findings
Cerebrospinal fluid	For removal, see p. 104.	Increased proteins; normocellular.
Brain, spinal cord, dorsal and ventral roots of spinal cord, and spinal ganglia	For removal and specimen preparation, see pp. 65, 67, and 69, respectively. Request Luxol fast blue stain for demonstration of myelin and Bielschowky's stain for axons (p. 172). Embed samples in plastic for thick, toluidin-stained sections and for electron microscopic study (p. 132).	Segmental demyelination and mononuclear infiltrates in cranial and spinal nerve roots. If axons are involved, there is chromatolysis of lower motor neurons (spinal cord and brain stem).
Peripheral nerves	For sampling and specimen preparation, see p. 79 and above under "Brain, spinal cord,..."	Segmental demyelination and mononuclear infiltrates.
Eyes	For removal and specimen preparation, see p. 85.	Papilledema.
Urinary bladder and kidneys	Procedures depend on grossly identified abnormalities as listed in right-hand column.	Urinary retention with urocystitis and pyelonephritis.*

Syndrome, Hamman-Rich (See "Pneumonia, interstitial.")

Syndrome, Hand-Schüller-Christian (See "Histiocytosis, Langerhans cell.")

Syndrome, Hemolytic Uremic

Related Term: Thrombotic thrombocytopenic purpura *(1)*.

NOTE: If the patient underwent organ transplantation, see under "Transplantation,..."; use of cyclosporine may be a cause of hemolytic uremic syndrome *(2)*. Antineoplastics may have a similar effect.

Organs and Tissues	Procedures	Possible or Expected Findings
Kidney	Record weights, photograph, and sample for histologic study.	Renal cortical necrosis;* thromboses of glomerular arterioles and capillaries.
Gastrointestinal tract	If indicated, submit intestinal contents for microbiologic study.	Enterohemorrhagic *E. coli* 0157:H7 infection *(3)*.
Pancreas	Submit for histologic study.	Pancreatitis may be a complication or, rarely, a cause of the disease.
Other organs and tissues	Procedures depend on expected findings or grossly identified abnormalities as listed in right-hand column.	Childhood infection. Disseminated intravascular coagulation.* Toxemia of pregnancy.* Premature separation of placenta. Manifesfestations of HIV infection *(4)*. Malignancies such as carcinoma of prostate *(5)*.

References

1. Neild GH. Hemolytic uremic syndrome/thrombotic thrombocytopenic purpura: pathophysiology and treatment. Kidney Intl 1998;64:S45–S49.
2. Katznelson S, Wilkinson A, Rosenthal TR, Cohen A, Nast C, Danovitch GM. Cyclosporin-induced hemolytic uremic syndrome: factors that obscure its diagnosis. Transpl Proc 1994;26:2608–2609.
3. Koutkia P, Mylonakis E, Flanigan T. Enterohemorrhagic Escherichia coli 0157:H7: an emerging pathogen. Am Family Physician 1997;56: 853–856.
4. Badesha PS, Saklayen MG. Hemolytic uremic syndrome as a presenting form of HIV infection. Nephron 1996;72:472–475.
5. Muller NJ, Pestalozzi BC. Hemolytic uremic syndrome in prostatic carcinoma. Oncol 1998;55:174–176.

Syndrome, Hepatorenal

NOTE: Decompensated cirrhosis* of the liver with ascites is almost always present. Most possible causes of hepatorenal failure, such as intrarenal shunting or reduced plasma volume, have no anatomic substrate. A possible and demonstrable mechanical cause is enlargement of the caudate lobe, which may compress the hepatic fossa of the inferior vena cava. For roentgenologic demonstration of this system, see p. 59 (renal venography). See also under "Obstruction, inferior vena cava." The kidneys are often autolytic—particularly if jaundice is severe—but usually fail to show other morphologic abnormalities.

Syndrome, Heterotaxy (See "Syndrome, polysplenia and asplenia.")

Syndrome, Hunter-Hurler (See "Mucopolysaccharidosis.")

Syndrome, Hypereosinophilic (See "Cardiomyopathy, restrictive [with eosinophilia]," "Gastroenteritis, eosinophilic," and "Syndrome, eosinophilic pulmonary.")

Syndrome, Hypoplastic Left Heart (See "Atresia, aortic valvular.")

Syndrome, Immunodeficiency (See "Syndrome, acquired immunodeficiency (AIDS)" and "Syndrome, primary immunodeficiency.")

Syndrome, Intravascular Coagulation and Fibrinolysis (See "Coagulation, disseminated intravascular.")

Syndrome, Kimmelstiel-Wilson (See "Diabetes mellitus.")

Syndrome, Klinefelter's

Synonym: Seminiferous tubule dysgenesis.

Possible Associated Conditions: Carcinoma; chronic pulmonary disease; congenital malformations; diabetes mellitus* *(1)*; Down's syndrome;* leukemia;* malignant lymphoma;* Osler's disease;* progressive systemic sclerosis;* Sjögren's syndrome;* systemic lupus erythematosus.*

Organs and Tissues	Procedures	Possible or Expected Findings
External examination and breast tissue	Record body weight and length and length of lower extremities.	Tall person with long lower extremities; eunuchoidism; varicose veins.
	Record appearance of external genitalia.	Hypoplastic external genitalia; cryptorchidism; hypospadias.
	Prepare histologic sections of breast tissue.	Gynecomastia.
	Prepare skeletal roentgenograms.	Deformities—for instance, radioulnar synostosis.
Blood or fascia lata	Submit tissue or blood for chromosome analysis (p. 108). Refrigerate blood sample for possible hormone assay.	47, XXY and less common variants, including sex chromosome mosaicism.
Urine	Refrigerate specimen for possible hormone assay.	
Endocrine organs	Record weights and dimensions of both testes.	Germ cell deficiency or hyalinization of seminiferous tubules. Usually, longitudinal axis of testes is smaller than 2 cm.
	Record weights of all endocrine glands. Prepare histologic sections of adrenal glands and of pituitary gland (p. 71).	

Organs and Tissues	Procedures	Possible or Expected Findings
Other organs and tissues	Procedures depend on expected findings or grossly identified abnormalities as listed in right-hand column.	Suprasellar tumors of maldevelopmental origin *(2)*. Tumors at other sites such as prostate *(3)*.

References

1. Robinson S, Kessling A. Diabetes secondary to genetic disorders. Baillieres Clin Endocrin Metabol 1992;6:867–898.
2. Hamed LM, Maria BL, Quisling R, Fanous MM, Mickle P. Suprasellar tumors of maldevelopmental origin in Klinefelter's syndrome. A report of two cases. J Clin Neuro-Ophthalmol 1992;12:192–197.
3. Tay HP, Bidair M, Shabaik A, Gilbaugh JH 3rd, Schmidt JD. Primary yolk sac tumor of the prostate in a patient with Klinefelter's syndrome. J Urol 1995;153:1066–1069.

Syndrome, Klippel-Feil

Synonym: Congenital fusion of cervical vertebrae.

Organs and Tissues	Procedures	Possible or Expected Findings
External examination		Short neck. Disorders with dysraphia (see below).
	Prepare roentgenograms of chest, neck, and head.	Fusion of cervical vertebrae. Congenital elevation of the scapula (Sprengel's deformity).
Skull, spine, brain, and spinal cord	For removal and specimen preparation of brain and spinal cord, see pp. 65 and 67, respectively.	Arnold-Chiari malformation;* basilar impression;* meningomyelocele; platybasia;* spinal cord compression; syringomyelia.*

Syndrome, Korsakoff (See "Syndrome, Wernicke-Korsakoff.")

Syndrome, Lambert-Eaton (See "Myasthenia gravis.")

Syndrome, Laurence-Moon-Biedl

Related Term: Bardet-Biedl syndrome *(1)*.

Organs and Tissues	Procedures	Possible or Expected Findings
External examination	Record body weight and length; record and photograph abnormalities as listed in right-hand column.	Obesity;* polydactyly; developmental delay in infants. Dysmorphic extremities. Hypogonadism in males *(1)*.
Liver	Record weight and sample for histologic study.	Congenital hepatic fibrosis* *(2)*.
Kidneys	If renal transplantation *(3)* had been carried out, see also under that heading. Follow procedures described under "glomerulonephritis."	Multiple abnormalities, including renal, cysts, tubulointerstitial nephritis and focal sclerosing glomerulonephritis.
Gonads	Submit samples for histologic study.	Hypogonadism.
Eyes	For removal and specimen preparation, see p. 85.	Retinal dystrophy *(1)* and other retinal changes.

References

1. Green JS, Parfrey PS, Harnett JD, Farid NR, Cramer BC, Johnson G, et al. The cardinal manifestations of Bardet-Biedl syndrome, a form of Laurence-Moon-Biedl syndrome. N Engl J Med 1989;321:1002–1009.
2. Nakamura F, Sasaki H, Kajihara H, Yamanoue M. Laurence-Moon-Biedl syndrome accompanied by congenital hepatic fibrosis. J Gastroenterol Hepatol 1990;5:206–210.
3. Collins CM, Mendoza SA, Griswold WR, Tanney D, Liebermann E, Reznik VM. Pediatric renal transplantation in Laurence-Moon-Biedl syndrome. Pediatr Nephrol 1994;8:221–222.

Syndrome, Leriche's

NOTE: The morphologic substrate is isolated aortoiliac atherosclerosis. Remove aorta together with common and external iliac arteries. For arteriography of lower extremities, see p. 120.

Syndrome, Letterer-Siwe (See "Histiocytosis, Langerhans cell.")

Syndrome, Löffler's (See "Cardiomyopathy, restrictive [eosinophilic type] and "Syndrome, eosinophilic pulmonary.")

Syndrome, Louis-Bar (See "Syndrome, primary immunodeficiency.")

Syndrome, Malabsorption

NOTE: If malabsorption is suspected to have been caused by a systemic disease, see also under that entry. Such systemic diseases include abetalipoproteinemia,* amyloidosis,* Degos' disease, diabetes mellitus,* hyperthyroidism,* hypoparathyroidism,* hypothyroidism,* mastocytosis,* polyarteritis nodosa,* and systemic lupus erythematosus.*

Organs and Tissues	*Procedures*	*Possible or Expected Findings*
External examination and oral cavity	Record character and extent of skin and oral changes. Prepare histologic sections of affected skin. Prepare skeletal roentgenograms.	Brownish discoloration of skin; dermatitis; cheilosis; glossitis. Clubbing of fingers and toes. Osteomalacia;* rickets.
Intestinal tract	If an infectious or parasitic intestinal disorder is suspected, submit portions for microbiologic study (p. 102).	Bacterial, fungal, viral, or parasitic infection.
	For mesenteric angiography, see p. 55.	Mesenteric atherosclerosis,* vasculitis, thromboembolism, or other occlusive changes.
	For *in situ* formalin perfusion of small intestine, see p. 54. If there were surgical resections, anastomoses, or blind loops, record length of remaining intestine, size and location of anastomoses, and length of blind loops. Submit samples of all segment for dissecting microscopic (p. 54) and histologic study. Identify exact location of samples in relation to ligament of Treitz or other anatomic landmarks.	Previous intestinal resection ("short bowel syndrome"), anastomoses, and blind loops. Diverticula;* strictures; fistulas; carcinoid tumors. Granulomatous or nongranulamatous enteritis; eosinophilic enteritis; radiation enteritis; sprue;* Whipple's disease.* Intestinal lymphangiectasia. Lymphoma,* carcinoma, and many other diseases and conditions (see also above under "Note").
Mesentery	See also above under "Intestinal tract."	
	Prepare histologic sections of arteries, veins, and lymph nodes.	Lymphoma.* Granulomatous lymphadenitis. Vascular disease or other condition, as listed above under "Intestinal tract" and under "Note."
Liver and extrahepatic bile ducts	For postmortem cholangiography, see p. 56. Dissect extrahepatic bile ducts *in situ*.	Biliary obstruction. Pancreatitis.* Non-beta islet cell tumor.
Pancreas	For roentgenologic study of duct system, see p. 57. Prepare thin slices in order to detect minute lesions. If appropriate, see also under "Tumor, of the pancreas."	
Other organs and tissues	Procedures depend on expected findings or grossly identified abnormalities as listed above under "Note."	Manifestations of systemic diseases that may have caused malabsorption. See above under "Note."
Bones, bone marrow, and joints	For removal, prosthetic repair, and specimen preparation of bones and joints, see p. 95. For preparation of sections and smears of bone marrow, see p. 96.	Bone changes related to vitamin D deficiency.* Megaloblastic bone marrow.
Vitreous	Submit sample (p. 85) for sodium, calcium, chloride, magnesium phosphate, and urea nitrogen determination.	Manifestations of dehydration.* Electrolyte changes associated with vitamin D deficiency.*

Syndrome, Marfan's

Synonyms and Related Terms: Arachnodactyly; dolichostenomelia.

Organs and Tissues	Procedures	Possible or Expected Findings
External examination	Record body weight and length, arm span, pubis-to-sole distance, and pubis-to-vertex distance.	Typical skeletal proportions. Arachnodactyly; pectus excavatum; pigeon breast; dolichocephaly; kyphoscoliosis; genu recurvatum; dislocation of joints; striae of skin.
Diaphragm		Diaphragmatic hernia.*
Heart and aorta	If infective endocarditis is suspected, follow procedures described on p. 103. Leave aorta attached to heart. Test competence of mitral and aortic valves (p. 29). Record circumference of aorta and pulmonary artery just above valves and further distally.	Infective endocarditis.* Atrial septal defect.* Myxomatous transformation of mitral ring. Mitral valve prolapse. Aortic and pulmonary dilatation and valvular insufficiency.* Aortic dissection* with dissection of adjacent vessels. Ascending aortic aneurysm (rarely with aortopulmonary fistula *[1]*). Myocardial infarction *(2)*.
	Request PAS, toluidine blue, and Verhoeff–van Gieson stains of sections of vascular walls (p. 173).	Cystic change of media.
Lungs	Perfuse one or both lungs with formalin (p. 47).	Multiple cysts (see "Cyst(s), pulmonary").
Colon	Record extent of diverticulosis.	Diverticulosis.
Neck organs	Inspect carotid arteries.	Aneurysms *(3)*.
Eyes	For removal and specimen preparation, see p. 85.	Subluxation of lens.

References

1. Massetti M, Babatasi G, Rossi A, Kapadia N, Neri E, Bhoyroo S, et al. Aortopulmonary fistula: an uncommon complication in dystrophic aortic aneurysm. Ann Thor Surg 1995;59:1563–1564.
2. Santucci JJ, Katz S, Pogo GJ, Boxer R. Peripartum acute myocardial infarction in Marfan's syndrome. Am Heart J 1994;127:1404–1407.
3. Ohyama T, Ohara S, Momma F. Aneurysm of the cervical internal carotid artery associated with Marfan's syndrome—case report. Neurologia Medico-Chirrugica 1992;32:965–968.

Syndrome, Mucocutaneous Lymph Node

Synonyms and Related Terms: Infantile polyartritis nodosa;* Kawasaki disease.

NOTE: This syndrome is rarely fatal. The morphologic changes found at autopsy are identical to those seen in infantile polyarteritis nodosa.* The disease might be caused by an infectious agent *(1)*. The disease is reportable in some states.

Organs and Tissues	Procedures	Possible or Expected Findings
External examination and skin	Record and photograph abnormalities listed in right-hand column.	Congestion of conjunctivas. Fissuring of lips; protuberance of lingual papillae; edema of hands and feet; desquamation at junction of nails and skin of the fingers and toes; furrowing of the nails. Mild jaundice may be present.
Heart	For coronary arteriography, see p. 118. Submit samples of all coronary arteries for histologic study, and request Verhoeff–van Gieson' stain (p. 173).	Coronary thromboarteritis with coronary occlusion, indistinguishable from infantile polyarteritis nodosa.* Coronary artery aneurysms. Myocarditis and valvulitis in early phases of the disease *(1)*.
Other organs	Follow procedures described under "Polyarteritis nodosa."	Early in the disease, lymphocytic or mixed interstitial infiltrates in hilar area of liver, spleen, pancreas, and kidneys.
Neck organs	Remove together with tongue. Submit samples of tongue and of cervical lymph nodes for histologic study.	Protuberance of lingual papillae. Cervical lymphadenopathy.

Organs and Tissues	Procedures	Possible or Expected Findings
Urine	Submit sample for study of sediment.	Proteinuria; increased number of leukocytes.
Joints	For removal, prosthetic repair, and specimen preparation, see p. 96.	Arthritis.*
Brain	For removal and specimen preparation, see p. 66.	Aseptic meningitis.*

Reference

1. Landing BH, Larson EJ. Pathological features of Kawasaki disease (mucocutaneous lymph node syndrome). Am J Cardiovasc Pathol 1987;1: 218–229.

Syndrome, Myasthenia (See "Myasthenia gravis.")

Syndrome, Myelodysplastic

Synonyms and Related Terms: Chronic myelomonocytic leukemia;* refractory anemia; refractory anemia with excess of blasts; refractory anemia with excess of blasts in transformation; refractory anemia with ringed sideroblasts; refractory dysmyelopoietic anemias.

NOTE: The myelodysplastic syndromes are represented by a heterogeneous group of normocytic anemias, often with neutropenia, thrombocytopenia, and monocytosis. For expected bone marrow changes, see above under "Synonyms and Related Terms." Autopsy procedures are similar to those recommended for most cases of leukemia, with particular attention paid to intercurrent infections and thrombocytopenic hemorrhages. In all instances, material should be collected using aseptic technique for tissue culture for chromosome analysis (see Chapter 10). Common findings in these conditions are deletion of the long arm of chromosome 5, deletion of chromosome 5 or 7, or trisomy 8.

Syndrome, Nephrotic

NOTE: See under name of suspected underlying condition, such as amyloidosis,* anaphylactoid purpura,* diabetes mellitus,* glomerulonephritis,* Goodpasture's syndrome,* heavy metal poisoning, hemolytic uremic syndrome,* infective endocarditis,* polyarteritis nodosa,* syphilis,* or systemic lupus erythematosus.* If accelerated hypertension or constrictive pericarditis is the suspected underlying condition, see under "Hypertension (arterial), all types or type unspecified" or "Pericarditis," respectively.

In all instances, the renal veins and the inferior vena cava should be opened *in situ*. "En masse" removal of organs (p. 3) is recommended for this purpose. If thrombosis is found, record exact location and size of clot and submit sample of clot with wall of veins for histologic study. See also under "Thrombosis, venous." Coronary atherosclerosis and its complications seem to be increased in patients with the nephrotic syndrome.

Syndrome, Neurocutaneous (See "Disease, Sturge-Weber-Dimitri," "Disease, von Hippel-Lindau," "Neurofibromatosis," and "Sclerosis, tuberous.")

Syndrome, Neutrophil Dysfunction (See "Disease, chronic granulomatous," and "Syndrome, Chédiak-Higashi.")

Syndrome, Noonan's

Possible Associated Conditions: Acute leukemia *(1)*.

Organs and Tissues	Procedures	Possible or Expected Findings
External examination	Record body weight and length. Record and prepare photographs of all abnormalities listed in right-hand column.	Small stature; neck webbing; antimongoloid slant of palpebral fissures; micrognathia; hypertelorism; cubitus valgus; short curved fifth finger; broad, short fingernails; undescended testes. Hydrops fetalis* due to lymphatic dysplasia *(2)*.
	Prepare skeletal roentgenograms.	Pectus excavatum and other skeletal malformations;
Blood or fascia lata	These specimens should be collected using aseptic technique for tissue culture for chromosome analysis (see Chapter 10).	Normal karyotype in most instances.
Heart	Dissection techniques depend on expected abnormalities as shown in right-hand column.	Congenital valvular pulmonary stenosis.* Congestive obstructive or nonobstructive hypertrophic cardiomyopathy.* Left ventricular hypoplasia;* aneurysms of the sinuses of valsalva *(3)*.
	For coronary arteriography, see p. 118.	Congenital coronary anomalies.
Lungs	Perfuse lungs with formalin (p. 47).	Pulmonary lymphangiectasis.

Organs and Tissues	Procedures	Possible or Expected Findings
Kidneys	See "Cyst(s), renal."	Cystic renal disease.
Brain	For removal and specimen preparation, see p. 66. For cerebral angiography, see p. 80.	Cerebral arteriovenous malformation *(4)*.

References

1. Johannes JM, Garcia CR, De Vaan GA, Weening RS. Noonan's syndrome in association with acute leukemia. Pediatr Hematol Oncol 1995;12:571–575.
2. Bloomfield FH, Hadden W, Gunn TR. Lymphatic dysplasia in a neonate with Noonan's syndrome. Pediatr Radiol 1997;27:321–323.
3. Noonan J, O'Connor W. Noonan syndrome: a clinical description emphasizing the cardiac findings. Acta Pediatr Japn 1996;38:76–83.
4. Schon F, Bowler J, Baraitser M. Cerebral arteriovenous malformation in Noonan's syndrome. Postgrad Med J 1992;68:37–40.

Syndrome, Obesity-Hypoventilation (See "Obesity.")

Syndrome, Parkinson's (See "Disease, Parkinson's.")

Syndrome, Peutz-Jeghers

NOTE: For the gene location, see ref. *(1)*.

Organs and Tissues	Procedures	Possible or Expected Findings
External examination, skin, and oral cavity	Record extent of pigmentations; photograph and prepare histologic sections of skin.	Mucocutaneous pigmentations around lips and of buccal mucosa, forearms, hands, feet, and umbilical area.
Gastrointestinal tract and regional lymph nodes		Intussusception and hemorrhage.
	Record location and size of polypoid lesions. Leave polyps attached to wall of intestine until after fixation is completed. Histologic section should include polyps and wall of intestine. Request van Gieson's and mucicarmine stains (p. 173).	Hamartomatous polyps in jejunum and ileum and less commonly in stomach, duodenum, appendix, and colon. Adenocarcinomas may arise from the polyps.
	Submit samples of regional lymph nodes for histologic study.	Metastases in rare cases in which carcinoma had developed.
Other organs	Procedures depend on expected findings or grossly identified abnormalities as listed in right-hand column.	Rarely, hamartomatous polyps in pharynx, urinary bladder, and other sites. Gonadal tumors have been observed *(2,3)*.

References

1. Tomlinson IP, Houlston RS. Peutz-Jeghers syndrome. J Med Genet 1997;34:1007–1011.
2. Dreyer L, Jacyk WK, du Plessis DJ. Bilateral large-cell calcifying Sertoli cell tumor of the testes in Peutz-Jeghers syndrome: a case report. Pediatr Dermatol 1994;11:335–337.
3. Dozois RR, Kempers RD, Dahlin DC, Batholomew LG. Ovarian tumors associated with the Peutz-Jeghers syndrome. Ann Surg 1970;172:233–238.

Syndrome, Pickwickian (Obesity-Hypoventilation syndrome) (See "Obesity.")

Syndrome, Pierre Robin

Related Terms: Catel-Manzke syndrome (Pierre Robin complex with accessory metacarpal of index finger); Pierre-Robin sequence; Trisomy 18.

NOTE: The Pierre-Robin phenotype (i.e., micrognathia with resulting retroglossia and cleft palate) may be present in numerous other malformation complexes. Other abnormalities comprising these malformation complexes are listed below.

Organs and Tissues	Procedures	Possible or Expected Findings
External examination; oral and nasal cavities; soft tissues	Record and prepare photographs of all abnormalities as listed in right-hand column.	Micrognathia; cleft palate; bulging of upper rib cage; bivid uvula; choanal atresia; hypertelorism; hypertrophy of soft tissues of the neck.
	Prepare skeletal roentgenograms, including hands.	Rib defects; syndactyly; hypoplastic digits; extra metacarpal of index finger; hypoplastic femora.

Organs and Tissues	Procedures	Possible or Expected Findings
Chest		Pneumothorax.*
Blood or fascia lata	These specimens should be collected using aseptic technique for tissue culture for chromosome analysis (see Chapter 10). This is particularly important if condition must be distinguished from trisomy 18 or cri-du-chat syndrome.	Usually normal karyotype but chromosomal deletions may occur *(1)*.
Heart	For dissection techniques, see p. 33.	Congenital heart disease *(2)*. Cor pulmonale.
Liver	Record weight and sample for histologic study.	Congenital hepatic fibrosis.
Neck organs and tongue	Record size of tongue; record presence or absence of signs of asphyxiation from malformed organs and tissues.	Tongue size normal or decreased. Rarely, aglossia. Glossoptosis may lead to acute airways obstruction *(3)*.
Brain	For removal and specimen preparation, see p. 66.	Hypoxic encephalopathy.
Eyes	For removal and specimen preparation, see p. 85.	Glaucomatous cupping of optic disk; myopic disk changes; cataract; retinal detachment; microphthalmia.

References

1. Menk FH, Madan K, Baart JA, Beukenhorst HL. Robin sequence and a deficiency of the left forearm in a girl with a deletion of chromosome 4g33-gter. Am J Med Genet 1992;44:696–694.
2. Pearl W. Congenital heart disease in the Pierre Robin syndrome. Pediatr Cardiol 1982;2:307–309.
3. Cozzi F, Pierro A. Glossoptosis-apnea syndrome. Pediatr 1985;75:836–843.

Syndrome, Plummer-Vinson

Synonym: Sideropenic dysphagia.

Organs and Tissues	Procedures	Possible or Expected Findings
External examination		Koilonychia.
Esophagus and stomach	Request PAS-alcian blue stain of histologic samples (p. 173).	Squamous cell carcinoma of esophagus *(1)*. Chronic gastritis.
Neck organs	Remove together with base of tongue and oropharynx. Open esophagus in posterior midline, photograph, and take sections of grossly identifiable lesions and random sections at various levels.	Web formation; postcricoid carcinoma.
Other organs	For preparation of sections and smears of bone marrow, see p. 96.	Manifestations of hypochromic anemia.* Blood smears reveal microsytosis.

Reference

1. Ribeiro U Jr, Posner MC, Safatle-Ribeiro AV, Reynolds JC. Risk factors for squamous cell carcinoma of the esophagus. Br J Surg 1996;83:1174–1185.

Syndrome, Polysplenia and Asplenia

Synonyms: Heterotaxy syndrome; Ivemark's syndrome; visceral isomerism.

Possible Associated Conditions: With *asplenia*: Right isomerism (bilateral mirror-image right-sided symmetry) of heart, lungs, and abdominal viscera; common atrium; total anomalous pulmonary venous connection; absent coronary sinus; complete atrioventricular septal defect;* subpulmonary stenosis;* pulmonary valve atresia;* midline symmetric liver; malrotation of bowel; absent spleen.

With *polysplenia*: Left isomerism (bilateral mirror-image left-sided symmetry) of heart and lungs, with variable sidedness of abdominal viscera; anomalous pulmonary venous connection; ventricular inversion; subpulmonary stenosis;* transposition of the great arteries;* bilateral superior caval veins; azygos continuation of inferior vena cava; multiple spleens of variable size, all on same side as stomach and pancreas.

Organs and Tissues	Procedures	Possible or Expected Findings
Blood	Prepare smears.	Howell-Jolly bodies occur in asplenia syndrome and, rarely, in polysplenia.
Chest and abdominal cavity, cardiovascular system, and lungs	Procedures depend on expected findings or grossly identified abnormalities as listed in right-hand column and under "Possible Associated Conditions."	Two pulmonary lobes occur bilaterally in polysplenia, and three lobes in asplenia syndrome. If inferior vena cava is interrupted, hepatic veins unite to form a vessel or vessels that empty into either atrium. See also under "Possible Associated Conditions."
Spleen	Dissect splenic artery and vein *in situ*. For celiac arteriography, see p. 55.	In polysplenia, there are two or more splenic masses but no normal-sized spleen.
Liver, gallbladder, bile ducts	For postmortem cholangiography, see p. 56.	Rarely, absence of gallbladder; biliary atresia* in polysplenia. Large midline liver in asplenia.

Syndrome, Primary Immunodeficiency

Synonyms and Related Terms *(1)*: *T-cell defects*—Alymphocytosis (a severe combined immunodeficiency); ataxia telangiectasia; Bloom's syndrome;* deficit of T and NK cells (a severe combined immunodeficiency); DiGeorge's syndrome;* HLA-class I or II deficiency; hyper-IgM syndrome; Wiskott-Aldrich syndrome; xeroderma pigmentosum; reticular dysgenesis (a severe combined immunodeficiency); and several others. *B-cell defects*—Bruton's agammaglobulinemia; common variable immunodeficiency; hyper IgE syndrome; IgA deficiency or IgG subclass deficiency, lymphoproliferative syndrome (X-linked or autoimmunity); and several others. *Phagocytic defects*—Chédiak-Higashi syndrome;* chronic granulomatous disease;* leukocyte adhesion deficiency; and several others. *Complement deficiencies* also belong here.

NOTE:

For the usual complications, such as skin diseases, hematologic diseases, and various types of infections, see above under "Synonyms and Related Terms" and below under "Possible or Expected Findings." For the *acquired* immunodeficiency syndrome, see under "Syndrome, acquired immunodeficiency."

Possible Associated Conditions (syndromes associated with immunodeficiency): Chromosome abnormalities (Bloom's syndrome,* Down's syndrome,* or Fanconi syndrome*); hereditary metabolic defects (acrodermatitis enteropathica [zinc deficiency], biotin dependent carboxylase deficiency, transcobalamin II deficiency, and type I orotic aciduria); hypercatabolism of Ig (familial hypercatabolism of Ig, intestinal lymphangiectasia, and myotonic dystrophy); multiple organ system abnormalities (agenesis of the corpus callosum, cartilage hair hypoplasia, partial albinism, or short-limbed dwarfism); and other deficiences (chronic mucocutaneous candidiasis, hyper IgE syndrome, immunodeficiency following hereditarily determined susceptibility to Epstein-Barr virus, and thymoma).

Conditions that are more common in immunodeficient patients: Infectious mononucleosis (with or without B cell lymphoma in X-linked lymphoproliferative syndrome); rheumatoid arthritis;* systemic lupus erythematosus.*

Organs and Tissues	Procedures	Possible or Expected Findings
External examination, skin, and oral cavity	Record body weight and length; record and photograph abnormalities as listed in right-hand column. Prepare histologic sections of skin and oral mucosa, particularly of infected or eczematous areas.	Malformed ears, micrognathia, hypertelorism and short philtrum in Di George's syndrome.* Dermatomyositis* in immunoglobulin deficiency. Immunodeficiency may be associated with short-limbed dwarfism with absence of scalp hair, eyelashes, and eyebrows, ichthyosiform skin lesions, and erythroderma. Eczema in Wiskott-Aldrich syndrome; oculocutaneous telangiectasia (Louis-Bar syndrome); mucocutaneous infections, such as candidiasis* (chronic mucocutaneous candidiasis).
Thymus	Record weight of intact organ. Record presence or absence of ectopic thymic tissue in neck organs. Submit samples for histologic study, and snap-freeze fresh material for immunofluorescent study.	Thymus may be normal, hypoplastic (e.g., in ataxia telangiectasia), aplastic (for instance, in DiGeorge's syndrome*) or ectopic (see "Neck organs"). Spindle cell thymoma in hypogammaglobulinemia patients.

Organs and Tissues	*Procedures*	*Possible or Expected Findings*
Blood	Submit samples for microbiologic study (p. 102). Submit samples for determination of immunoglobulins in serum and for B and T lymphocyte counts.	Bacterial or fungal septicemia; viremia. Hypogammaglobulinemia; dysgammaglobulinemia; hyperimmunoglobulinemia.
	Blood or fascia lata should be collected using aseptic technique for tissue culture for chromosome analysis (see Chapter 10).	See above under "Possible Associated Conditions..."
Heart and great vessels		Malformations of aortic arch and/or conotruncus in DiGeorge's syndrome.
Lungs	Submit one lobe for microbiologic study (p. 103). Stain touch preparations for *Pneumocystis carinii*.* Perfuse one lung with formalin (p. 47). Request Gram and Grocott's methenamine silver stain (p. 172).	Bacterial, fungal, or viral pneumonia. *Pneumocystis carinii* infection.* Herpesvirus infection. Bronchiectasis,* e.g., in transient hypogammaglobulinemia of infancy or common variable immunodeficiency.
Gastrointestinal tract	For *in situ* fixation and preparation for study under the dissecting microscope, see p. 54. Submit contents for microbiologic study (p. 102). Submit samples of ileum, jejunum, appendix, and colon for histologic study.	Atrophy of intestinal villi and peripheral lymphoid tissue, most pronounced in Peyer's patches and appendix. Atrophic gastritis with megaloblastic anemia* or gastrointestinal infection, including giardiasis, may be present, e.g., in common variable immundeficiency.
Lymph nodes and spleen	Place specimens in omnifix fixative (p. 129). If lymphoma is suspected, follow procedures described under that heading.	T cells, primarily in paracortical zone of lymph nodes and in periarteriolar sheaths of the spleen. There may be generalized lymphadenopathy with or without lymphoma.*
Neck organs	Remove together with base of tongue, tonsils, soft palate, and pharyngeal wall (p. 4). Prepare histologic sections of lingual tonsils, palatine tonsils, and pharyngeal lymphatic tissue (see also above under "Thymus" and "Lymph nodes and spleen").	Upper respiratory infections. Ectopic thymus may occur near the base of the tongue, or in or around thyroid and parathyroid glands.
	Dissect and record weights of thyroid gland and parathyroid glands. Submit samples for histologic study.	Agenesis of parathyroid glands and—rarely—of thyroid gland in DiGeorge's syndrome.
Other organs	Procedures depend on expected findings or grossly identified abnormalities as listed in right-hand column.	Manifestations of malabsorption syndrome.* Infections. Ovarian agenesis in ataxia telangiectasia.
Middle ears and sinuses	For exposure and specimen preparation, see pp. 72 and 71, respectively.	Otitis media* and sinusitis.
Eyes	For removal and specimen preparation, see p. 85.	Oculocutaneous telangiectasias in ataxia telangiectasia.
Bone marrow	For preparation of sections and smears, see p. 95. If bone marrow had been transplanted (e.g., in severe combined immunodeficiency), see also under "Transplantation, bone marrow."	Hypoplasia (may be associated with agranulocytosis*). Leukemia* or related neoplastic disease. Megaloblastic anemia* in idiopathic late-onset immunoglobulin deficiency.
Joints	If infectious arthritis is suspected, submit exudate for microbiologic study (p. 102).	*Mycoplasma* infection in agammaglobulinemia.

Reference

1. Ten RM. Primary immunodeficiencies. Mayo Clin Proc 1998;73:865–872.

Syndrome, Reifenstein's

Related Term: Hereditary familial hypogonadism; male pseudohermaphroditism.

Organs and Tissues	*Procedures*	*Possible or Expected Findings*
External examination	Record and prepare photographs of all abnormalities as listed in right-hand column.	Microphallus; hypospadias; absent vas deferens; incomplete fusion of labioscrotal folds; gynecomastia.
Blood and fascia lata	These specimens should be collected using aseptic technique for tissue culture for chromosome analysis (see Chapter 10).	Normal karyotype.
Gonads	Record weights and prepare histologic sections.	Testicular atrophy; crytorchidism; germ cell neoplasia.

Syndrome, Reiter's

Synonym: Urethritis-arthritis-conjunctivitis syndrome.

NOTE: AIDS-related psoriasiform dermatitis may show clinical features of Reiter's syndrome *(1)*.

Possible Associated Condition: Ankylosing spondylitis.*

Organs and Tissues	*Procedures*	*Possible or Expected Findings*
External examination, skin, and oral cavity	Record character and extent of lesions of skin, external genitalia, and oral mucosa. Prepare photographs of lesions. Prepare histologic sections of skin and mucosal lesions.	Keratoderma (keratosis blennorrhagica) with vasculitis *(2)* of sole of feet, of palms, and of circumcised glans penis.
	Prepare roentgenograms of joints.	Arthritis* of knees, ankles, and metatarsal and midtarsal joints, with or without ankylosis. Osteoporosis.*
Blood	Submit sample for bacteriologic, viral, and serologic study (p. 102).	Usually, sterile culture.
Heart	Record weight and submit samples for histologic study (p. 30). If heart block was present, submit samples of conduction system for histologic study (p. 26).	Pericarditis;* myocarditis.* Aortic valve lesions.
Lungs	Submit consolidated areas for microbiologic study (p. 103). Perfuse one lung with formalin (p. 47).	Pleuritis and pneumonia.* Pulmonary fibrosis involving upper lobes.
Urinary bladder and urethra	For removal of urethra, see p. 60.	Erosions, papules, and plaques in urethral or bladder mucosa.
Other organs	Procedures depend on expected findings or grossly identified abnormalities as listed in right-hand column.	Enteritis. Thrombophlebitis.
Eyes	For removal and specimen preparation, see p. 85.	Conjunctivitis; multifocal choroiditis; acute anterior uveitis; iritis; keratitis.
Joints	For removal, prosthetic repair, and specimen preparation, see p. 96. Consult roentgenograms (see above under "External examination, skin, and oral cavity").	Arthritis* (see above under "External examination, skin, and oral cavity") resembling rheumatoid arthritis.* Nonspecific synovitis.

References

1. Romani J, Puig L, Baselga E, De Moragas JM. Reiter's syndrome-like pattern in AIDS-associated psoriasiform dermatitis. Intl J Dermatol 1996; 35:484–488.
2. Magro CM, Crowson AN, Peeling R. Vasculitis as the basis of cutaneous lesions in Reiter's disease. Hum Pathol 1995;26:633–638.

Syndrome, Respiratory Distress, of Adult (ARDS) (See "Syndrome, adult respiratory distress (ARDS).")

Syndrome, Respiratory Distress, of Infant

Related Terms: Hyaline membrane disease; bronchopulmonary dysplasia.

Organs and Tissues	*Procedures*	*Possible or Expected Findings*
External examination	Prepare chest and abdominal roentgenograms.	Pneumothorax;* pneumomediastinum;* pneumoperitoneum.
Blood	Submit sample for microbiologic study (p. 102) if sepsis is suspected.	Septicemia.
Heart	Record weight of heart and thickness of ventricles.	Right ventricular hypertrophy and/or dilatation.
Trachea, major bronchi, and lungs	Perfuse lungs with formalin at a pressure of 20 cm of water (p. 47). Submit multiple sections for histologic study. Submit a section for culture (p. 103).	Intubation trauma and mural edema and hemorrhage in trachea; hyaline membrane disease; pulmonary interstitial emphysema; bronchopulmonary dysplasia.
Neck organs	Prepare cross-sections that include larynx, thyroid, esophagus, and adjacent structures.	Intubation trauma.
Brain	For removal and specimen preparation, see p. 66.	Hemorrhages or other evidence of birth trauma; germinal matrix hemorrhages in premature infants; infarctions of subcortical white matter in term infants.
Eyes	For removal and specimen preparation, see p. 85.	Retinopathy of prematurity (a vasoproliferative disorder).

Reference

1. Stocker JT. Pathology of hyaline membrane disease and acute, reparative, and long-standing "healed" bronchopulmonary dysplasia. In: Pediatric Pulmonary Disease. Stocker JT, ed. Hemisphere, Washington, DC, 1989, p. 101.

Syndrome, Reye's

NOTE: Hypoglycemia* may have been present, but that condition is difficult or impossible to confirm after death. An immediate autopsy is indicated (see below under "Liver" and "Pancreas").

Organs and Tissues	*Procedures*	*Possible or Expected Findings*
Vitreous	Submit sample for sodium, chloride, and urea nitrogen determination (p. 85).	Manifestations of dehydration.*
Blood	Submit sample for microbiologic (viral) and serologic study (p. 102), for ammonia and bilirubin determination, and for determination of salicylate levels if there is a history of treatment with this drug.	Influenza;* varicella.* Manifestations of liver failure. Evidence of salicylate administration.
Urine	Obtain sample for biochemical and toxicologic analysis.	Assay for organic acids should rule out acyl-coenzyme A dehydrogenase deficiency, and toxicity, e.g., of acetaminophen and valproic acid *(1)*.
Heart	Record weight. Request frozen sections for Sudan stain (p. 173).	Cardiomegaly; fatty changes of myocardium and patchy myocytolysis.
Lungs	Submit fresh tissue for bacterial and viral culture (p. 103).	Viral pneumonia rarely present.
	Request paraffin sections and frozen sections for fat stain (see above under "Heart").	Acute interstitial pneumonia;* bronchitis;* hemorrhages. Lipid-laden histiocytes in alveoli.
Liver	Record weight and photograph; submit sample for microbiologic (viral) study (p. 102). Request frozen sections for fat stain (see above under "Heart").	Hepatomegaly; microvesicular fatty changes (they are not specific); zonal degeneration and necrosis *(2,3)*.

Organs and Tissues	Procedures	Possible or Expected Findings
Liver (continued)	If tissue can be obtained immediately after death, (p. 5), prepare sample for electron microscopic study (p. 132).	Increase of peroxisomes; proliferation of smooth endoplasmic reticulum; swelling of mitochondria.
Pancreas	If tissue can be obtained immediately after death, (p. 5), prepare sample electron microscopic study (p. 132).	Intranuclear inclusions *(4)*.
Kidneys	See above under "Liver."	Tubular fatty changes.
Brain and spinal cord	For removal and specimen preparation, see pp. 66 and 70, respectively. See also under "Encephalopathy, hepatic."	Hepatic encephalopathy.* Cerebral edema *(5)*.

References

1. Greene CL, Blitzer MG, Shapira E. Inborn errors of metabolism and Reye's syndrome: differential diagnosis. J Pediatr 11988;113:156–159.
2. Fraser JL, Antonioli DA, Chopra S, Wang HH. Prevalence and nonspecificity of microvesicular fatty changes. Mod Pathol 1995;8:65–70.
3. Kimura S, Kobayashi T, Tanaka Y, Sasaki Y. Liver histopathology in clinical Reye syndrome. Brain Dev 1991;13:95–100.
4. Collins DN. Ultrastructural study of intranuclear inclusions in the exocrine pancreas in Reye's syndrome. Lab Invest 1974;30:333–340.
5. Blisard KS, Davis LE. Neuropathologic findings in Reye syndrome. J Child Neurol 1991;6:41–44.

Syndrome, Sanfilippo's (See "Mucopolysaccharidosis.")

Syndrome, Scheie's (See "Mucopolysaccharidosis.")

Syndrome, Segawa's (See "Syndrome, dystonia.")

Syndrome, Sézary's (See "Lymphoma.")

Syndrome, Sheehan's

Synonyms: Postpartum pituitary necrosis; Sheehan's disease.

NOTE: Follow procedures described under "Insufficiency, pituitary." In early stages, the pituitary gland shows subtotal or total infarction; in late stages, fibrosis with residual small nests of normal chromophils is present. For *in situ* cerebral arteriography, see p. 81.

Syndrome, Shy-Drager (See "Atrophy, multiple system.")

Syndrome, Sick Sinus

Organs and Tissues	Procedures	Possible or Expected Findings
Heart	For histologic study of conduction system, see p. 26.	Excessive fibrosis of sinus node or adjacent myocardium.

Syndrome, Sipple's (See "Neoplasia, multiple endocrine.")

Syndrome, Sjögren's

Related Terms: Mikulicz's disease; sicca complex.

Possible Associated Conditions: Chronic hepatitis;* discoid lupus erythematosus; generalized or pulmonary amyloidosis* *(1)*; Hashimoto's thyroiditis; polyarteritis nodosa (necrotizing arteritis);* polymyositis; primary biliary cirrhosis; rheumatoid arthritis;* systemic lupus erythematosus* *(4)*; systemic sclerosis.*

Organs and Tissues	Procedures	Possible or Expected Findings
External examination and skin	Prepare histologic sections of skin.	Sweat gland atrophy.
Blood	Submit sample for determination of IgA, IgM, and IgG concentrations and of rheumatoid factor.	
Heart	Record volume and appearance of pericardial fluid.	Fibrinous or serofibrinous pericarditis.*
Trachea, bronchi, and lungs	Submit consolidated areas for microbiologic study (p. 103). Perfuse one lung with formalin (p. 47). If much inspissated mucus appears to be present, perfuse also through pulmonary artery. Submit samples for histologic study. Request Verhoeff–van Gieson and amyloid stains (p. 172).	Mucosal glandular atrophy. Inspissated mucous secretions. Pulmonary arterial hypertension;* lymphoma* or pseudolymphoma *(1)*; Bronchopneumonia. Bronchiolitis obliterans organizing pneumonia *(2)*; interstitial pulmonary fibrosis;* amyloidosis.*

Organs and Tissues	Procedures	Possible or Expected Findings
Esophagus	Submit samples for histologic study (pin on cork board, fix in formalin, and cut on edge).	Submucosal glandular atrophy. Atrophy of mucosa with infiltrates of lymphocytes and plasma cells.
Stomach and duodenum	Submit samples for histologic study (pin on cork board, fix in formalin, and cut on edge).	Chronic atrophic gastritis *(3)*; lymphocytosis of pyloric and Brunner's glands.
Liver and spleen	Record weights and sample for histologic study.	Hepatosplenomegaly. Primary biliary cirrhosis *(3)*.
Kidneys	Follow procedures described under "Glomerulonephritis."	Focal or membranous glomerulonephritis;* interstitial nephritis;* nephrocalcinosis; tubular atrophy.
Neck organs and tongue; salivary glands	Thyroid, submaxillary salivary gland, base of tongue, pharynx, and soft palate should be sampled for histologic study (p. 4).	Atrophic sialadenitis (see below under "Eyes and lacrimal glands"); loss of taste buds of tongue; thyroiditis.*
Eyes and lacrimal glands	For removal and specimen preparation of eyes, see p. 85. Submit samples of lacrimal glands (p. 87) for histologic study.	Keratoconjunctivitis. Lymphocytic, hyalinizing, atrophic dacryoadenitis with benign lymphoepithelial lesions (Mikulicz's disease).
Skeletal muscles	For sampling and specimen preparation, see p. 80.	Myopathy. Polymyositis *(2)*.
Other organs and tissues	Procedures depend on expected findings or grossly identified abnormalities as listed in right-hand column.	Lymphomas *(4)* and pseudolymphomas. See also under "Possible Associated Conditions."
Brain and spinal cord	For removal and specimen preparation, see pp. 65 and 67.	Transverse myelopathy *(5)*.

References

1. Quismorio FP Jr. Pulmonary involvement in primary Sjögren's syndrome. Curr Opin Pulm Med 1996;2:424–428.
2. Imasaki T, Yoshii A, Tanaka S, Ogura T, Ishikawa A, Takahashi T. Polymyositis and Sjögren's syndrome associated with bronchiolitis obliterans organizing pneumonia. Intern Med 1996;35:231–235.
3. Sheikh SH, Shaw-Stiffel TA. The gastrointestinal manifestations of Sjögren's syndrome. Am J Gastroenterol 1995;90:9–14.
4. Anaya JM, McGuff HS, Banks PM, Talal N. Clinicopathological factors relating malignant lymphoma with Sjögren's syndrome. Semin Arthritis Rheumat 1996;25:337–346.
5. Lyu RK, Chen ST, Tank LM, Chen TC. Acute transverse myelopathy and cutaneous vasculopathy in primary Sjögren's syndrome. Euro Neurol 1995;35:359–362.

Syndrome, Steele-Richardson (See "Disease, Parkinson's.")

Syndrome, Stevens-Johnson (See "Erythema multiforme.")

Syndrome, Stiff-Man

Related Terms: Armadillo disease; continuous muscle fiber activity; neuromyotonia; paraneoplastic opsoclonus *(1)*; quantal squander.

Organs and Tissues	Procedures	Possible or Expected Findings
Brain, spinal cord, and peripheral nerves	For removal and specimen preparation, see pp. 65, 67, and 79, respectively.	No diagnostic findings.
Skeletal muscles	For sampling and specimen preparation, see p. 80.	Variable but not diagnostic findings.

Reference

1. Dropcho EJ. Autoimmune central nervous system paraneoplastic disorders: mechanisms, diagnosis, and therapeutic options. Ann Neurol 1995; 37:S102–S113.

Syndrome, Sudden Infant Death (SIDS) (See "Death, Sudden unexpected, of Infant.")

Syndrome, Superior Vena Cava

Related Term: Superior vena cava obstruction.

Organs and Tissues	*Procedures*	*Possible or Expected Findings*
Chest cavity	Dissect superior vena cava and its tributaries *in situ*, with head and neck of deceased well-extended (place wooden block or some other support under scapulas). Continue dissection of veins into neck and axillas. Record and photograph site of thrombosis or of compression by surrounding pathologic conditions. Submit samples for histologic study.	Benign or malignant tumors; fibrosing mediastinitis;* postradiation fibrosis; infectious disease (tuberculosis,* histoplasmosis*); thoracic aortic aneurysm;* chronic constrictive pericarditis;* chest trauma; arteriovenous fistula between ascending aorta and superior vena cava; congenital anomaly of superior vena cava.

Syndrome, Toxic Shock

Synonyms and Related Terms: Staphylococcal scarlet fever.

NOTE: (1) Collect all tissues that appear to be infected. (2) Request aerobic and anaerobic cultures. (3) Request Gram stain (p. 172). (4) Usually, no special precautions are indicated. (5) Serologic studies are available from the Centers for Disease Control and Prevention, Atlanta, GA (p. 135). (6) This is a **reportable** disease.

Organs and Tissues	*Procedures*	*Possible or Expected Findings*
External examination, skin, oral cavity, and vagina	Record extent and character of skin and oral lesions; prepare photographs.	Erythematous, deep red "sun burn" rash; oral mucosal hyperemia; desquamation; conjunctival hyperemia.
	Culture vaginal discharge, if present. Culture cervix. Culture tampon, if present.	Infected tampon and vaginal discharge.
Other organs	Procedures depend on expected findings or grossly identified abnormalities as listed in right-hand column.	Periportal inflammation of liver; acute tubular necrosis of kidneys; hyaline membranes in lungs; evidence of coagulopathy.
Pelvic organs	Remove pelvic organs; open vagina and cervix with uterus in posterior midline; photograph and sample for histologic study.	Vaginal hyperemia; desquamation/ulceration of vaginal or cervical mucosa.

Syndrome, Turcot (See "Polyposis, familial, and related syndromes.")

Syndrome, Turner

Synonyms and Related Terms: Gonadal dysgenesis; primary ovarian failure.

Organs and Tissues	*Procedures*	*Possible or Expected Findings*
External examination	Record body weight and length, stature, and distribution of head, axillary, and pubic hair. Record and prepare photographs of features of face and neck. Prepare skeletal roentgenograms.	Premature aging; increased number of pigmented nevi; infantile sex organs; webbed neck; broad chest with wide spacing of nipples. Short fourth metacarpal; abnormal epiphyseal fusions; osteochondrosis-like changes of spine. Osteoporosis.
Breasts	Submit samples of breast tissues for histologic study.	Infantile breast tissue.*
Blood and fascia lata	These specimens should be collected using aseptic technique for tissue culture for chromosome analysis (see Chapter 10).	45, X(XO).
Heart and aorta	Procedures depend on expected findings or grossly identified abnormalities as listed in right-hand column.	Bicuspid aortic valve;* coarctation of aorta.* Rarely other anomalies *(1)*.

Organs and Tissues	*Procedures*	*Possible or Expected Findings*
Ovaries	Submit for histologic study.	Decreased/absent follicles.
Intestinal tract	Submit samples of all portions for histologic study.	Intestinal telangiectases.
Liver and extrahepatic bile ducts	If biliary atresia is suspected, follow procedures described under that heading.	Biliary atresia.*
Kidneys and ureters	Dissect kidneys and ureters *in situ* and record findings.	Horseshoe kidney; double ureters.
Pelvic organs	Submit samples of gonads or—if gonads cannot be identified—equivalent ridges on mesosalpinx for histologic study. Also submit samples of endometrium, cervix, and vagina.	Streak gonads without germ cells or follicles.
Thyroid gland	Record weight and submit sample for histologic study.	Hashimoto's thyroiditis.*
Other organs	Procedures depend on expected findings or grossly identified abnormalities as listed in right-hand column.	Manifestations of diabetes mellitus,* hypertension,* or thyrotoxicosis. Neuroblastoma and related tumors *(2)*.
Eyes	For removal and specimen preparation, see p. 85.	Keratoconus; retinal detachments *(3)*.

References

1. Oohara K, Yamazaki T, Sakaguchi K, Nakayama M, Kobayashi A. Acute aortic dissection, aortic insufficiency, and a single coronary artery in a patient with Turner's syndrome. J Cardiovasc Surg 1995;36:273–275.
2. Blatt J, Olshan AF, Lee PA, Ross JL. Neuroblastoma and related tumors in Turner's syndrome. J Pediatr 1997;131:666–670.
3. Mason JO III, Tasman W. Turner's syndrome associated with bilateral retinal detachments. Am J Ophthalmol 1996;122:742–743.

Syndrome, Waterhouse-Friderichsen (See "Disease, meningococcal.")

Syndrome, Weil's (See "Leptospirosis.")

Syndrome, Wernicke-Korsakoff

Related Terms: Alcoholic Wernicke's encephalopathy; Korsakoff's psychosis; nonalcoholic Wernicke's encephalopathy *(1,2)*; Wernicke's disease.

Organs and Tissues	*Procedures*	*Possible or Expected Findings*
Brain and spinal cord	For removal and specimen preparation, see pp. 65 and 67, respectively. For selection of histologic samples, see right-hand column. Request LFB stain to highlight areas of acute necrosis (p. 172).	Most characteristic lesions affect mammillary bodies, periventricular regions of 3rd (anterior fornices) and 4th ventricles (dorsal vagal nucleus) and aequeduct. Hemorrhage and necrosis are typical of acute stage; shrinkage and brown discoloration of mammillary bodies suggest chronic disease.
Other organs	Procedures depend on expected findings or grossly identified abnormalities as listed in right-hand column.	Other manifestations of chronic alcoholism (see under "Alcoholism and alcohol intoxication") or of nonalcoholic steatohepatitis *(1,2)*.
Peripheral nerves	For sampling and specimen preparation, see p. 79.	Peripheral neuropathy. See also under "Beriberi."

References

1. Christodoulakis M, Maris T, Plaitakis A, Melissas J. Wernicke's encephalopathy after vertical banded gastroplasty for morbid obesity. Eur J Surg 1997;163:473–474.
2. Yamamoto T. Alcoholic and non-alcoholic Wernicke's encephalopathy. Be alert to the preventable and treatable disease. Internal Med 1996;35: 754–755.

Syndrome, Wilson-Mikity (See "Syndrome, respiratory distress, of infant.")

Syndrome, Wiskott-Aldrich (See "Syndrome, primary immunodeficiency.")

Syndrome, Wolff-Parkinson-White (See "Malformation, Ebstein's" and "Preexcitation, ventricular.")

Syndrome, Zellweger

Synonyms and Related Terms: Adrenoleucodystrophy; cerebro-hepato-renal syndrome; infantile Refsum's disease.*

NOTE: This congenital familial cholestatic syndrome results from impaired assembly of peroxisomes and has its main manifestations in the brain, liver, and kidneys *(1)*. Craniofacial dysmorphia and hepatomegaly with siderosis are typical findings.

Reference

1. Lindhard A, Graem N, Skovby F, Jeppesen D. Postmortem findings and prenatal diagnosis of Zellweger syndrome. Case report. APMIS 1993;101:226–228.

Syndrome, Zieve (See "Alcoholism and alcohol intoxication" and "Disease, alcoholic liver.")

Syndrome, Zollinger-Ellison

Related Term: Endocrine hyperfunction and ulcer disease.

Possible Associated Condition: Multiple endocrine neoplasia.*

Organs and Tissues	*Procedures*	*Possible or Expected Findings*
Vitreous	Submit sample for sodium, chloride, urea nitrogen, and potassium determination (p. 85).	Manifestations of dehydration* and hypokalemia. Postmortem values of potassium are not reliable (p. 114).
Esophagus and gastrointestinal tract	Record character and location of ulcers. Histologic sections should include ulcers and all portions of stomach. Before samples are sectioned, pin stomach and other involved hollow viscera on corkboard for fixation.	Peptic ulcers in esophagus, stomach, duodenum, jejunum, and ileum. Usually, ulcers are at or near duodenal bulb. Parietal cells in corpus and fundus of stomach may be increased.
	Request PAS-alcian blue stain for sections of gastric mucosa (p. 173). If there is a tumor in the gastric or duodenal wall, follow procedures described below under "Pancreas."	Gastrinoma in cardia/fundus of stomach *(1)* or wall of duodenum *(2)*. Fundic argyrophil carcinoid tumors (in patients with type 1 multiple endocrine neoplasia) *(3)*.
Pancreas	If tumor is not immediately identifiable, prepare 2-mm sagittal slices of whole organ. Examine slices under dissecting microscope.	Gastrinoma or increased number of islets of Langerhans with high proportion of non-beta cells.
	Request aldehyde-thionin stain (p. 172), which stains islet B cells and frequently insulinoma cells. Request Grimelius silver stain (p. 172). Silver techniques for islet D or A (A_1 or A_2) cells are also indicated.	Insulinomas may give positive aldehyde-thionin stain. Gastrinomas give positive Grimelius silver stain.
	Snap-freeze fresh tumor tissue for immuno-histologic study. Submit tissue samples for electron microscopy (p. 132).	Peroxidase-labeled gastrin antibodies seem to react with cells in all gastrinomas.
Other organs	Submit extrapancreatic primary or metastatic tumor tissue for biochemical and other studies, as described above. Other procedures depend on expected findings or grossly identified abnormalities as listed in right-hand column.	Aberrant gastrinoma may occur at hilus of spleen. Metastases are found in regional lymph nodes and liver. There may be manifestations of multiple endocrine neoplasia.*

References

1. Gibril F, Curtis LT, Termanini B, Fritsch MK, Lubensky IA, Doppman JL, et al. Primary cardiac gastrinoma causing Zollinger-Ellison syndrome. Gastroenterology 1997;112:567–574.
2. Kisker O, Bastian D, Bartsch D, Nies C, Rothmund M. Localization, malignant potential, and surgical management of gastrinoma. World J Surg 1998;22:651–657.
3. Cadiot G, Vissuzaine C, Potet F, Mignon M. Fundic argyrophil carcinoid tumor in a patient with sporadic-type Zollinger-Ellison syndrome. Dig Dis Sci 1995;40:1275–1278.

Syphilis, Acquired

Synonym: *Treponema pallidum* infection.

NOTE: Congenital syphilis is presented below under a separate heading.

(1) Collect all tissues that appear to be infected. (2) Culture methods are not available, but animal inoculation can be performed. Consultation with a microbiology laboratory is recommended. (3) Special stains for *Treponema pallidum* rarely are positive except with material from fresh lesions of primary or secondary syphilis. Levaditi's stain or Warthin-Starry stain is recommended for paraffin sections (p. 172), and labeled fluorescent antibody techniques are recommended for frozen sections. India ink preparations or the Fontana-Masson silver stain has been used for the study of fresh lesions, and electron microscopy has also been employed. (4) In adult autopsies, no special precautions are indicated (see below under "Liver"). (5) Serologic studies are available from local and state health department laboratories (p. 135). (6) This is a **reportable** disease.

Organs and Tissues	*Procedures*	*Possible or Expected Findings*
External examination	Record and prepare photographs of all abnormalities listed in right-hand column.	Hunterian chancre in primary syphilis; condylomata lata. Noduloulcerative gummas and scarring in later stages.
	Prepare smears and sections of acute lesions; prepare sections of older skin lesions or anogenital mucosal lesions.	
	Prepare skeletal roentgenograms.	Syphilitic periostitis; gummas; arthritis (Charcot joints of knees, hips, ankles, and lumbar and thoracic spine).
Cerebrospinal fluid	Obtain sample for laboratiory study (see p. 104).	Lymphocytosis and increased protein concentrations.
Lymph nodes		Syphilitic lymphadenitis.
Heart and aorta	For coronary arteriography (p. 118), inject contrast medium into the clamped, ascending aorta to show takeoff of coronary arteries.	Intimal proliferation with narrowing of coronary orifices; myocarditis.
	Record competence of aortic valve (p. 29). Leave aorta attached to heart. Request Verhoeff–van Gieson stain for histologic sections of aorta (p. 173).	Syphilitic aortic valvulitis and aortic insufficiency.* Syphilitic aortitis with arteritis of vasa vasorum. Saccular thoracic aortic aneurysm.*
Other organs and tissues	Procedures depend on expected findings or grossly identified abnormalities. Submit samples for histologic study of small arteries.	
Brain and spinal cord	For removal and specimen preparation, see pp. 65 and 67, respectively.	Meningitis with mononuclear cells mainly in adventitial/perivascular distribution. Infarcts; focal cortical atrophy; gliosis of floor of 4th ventricle. Tabes dorsalis.*
Bones and joints	For removal, prosthetic repair, and specimen preparation, see p. 95.	See above under "External examination and skin."

Syphilis, Congenital

Related Term: Congenital neurosyphilis.*

NOTE: Prior to 20 wk gestation, the destructive effects of syphilis may not be seen. Gummata are rare in neonates. Tabes dorsalis is also uncommon. Serologic diagnosis is difficult in the neonate because of transplacental transfer of maternal IgG antibodies. Acquired syphilis (syphilis in adulthood) is presented above under a separate heading.

(1) Collect all tissues that appear to be infected. (2) Culture methods are not available, but animal inoculation can be performed. Consultation with a microbiology laboratory is recommended. (3) Special stains for *Treponema pallidum* rarely are positive except with material from fresh lesions of primary or secondary syphilis and of syphilitic hepatitis of the newborn. Levaditi's stain or Warthin-Starry stain is recommended for paraffin sections (p. 172), and labeled fluorescent antibody techniques are recommended for frozen sections. India ink preparations or the Fontana-Masson silver stain has been used for the study of fresh lesions, and electron microscopy has also been employed. (4) In neonates, special **precautions** are indicated (see below under "Liver") (5) Serologic studies are available from local and state health department laboratories (p. 135). (6) This is a **reportable** disease.

Organs and Tissues	*Procedures*	*Possible or Expected Findings*
Placenta	Record weight and submit samples for histologic study.	Villous edema; plasma cell villitis and chorioamnionitis.
External examination, skin, oral and nasal cavity	Record and prepare photographs of all abnormalities listed in right-hand column.	Growth retardation; jaundice; maculopapular rash; bullae; condylomata lata;

Organs and Tissues	Procedures	Possible or Expected Findings
External examination, skin, oral and nasal cavity *(continued)*	Prepare histologic sections of skin lesions.	hydrocephalus;* dental deformities (Hutchinson's teeth); saddle nose; frontal bossing of skull; saber shins; snuffles; nasal septal perforation; rhagades; ulnar deviation of fingers; hydrops fetalis *(1)*.
	Prepare skeletal roentgenograms.	Irregular radiolucencies in the metaphyses and diaphyses *(2)*.
Cerebrospinal fluid	Submit samples for serologic biochemical, cytologic, and microbiologic study (p. 104).	A detectable fluorescent antitreponemal antibody (absorbed) titer.[a]
Blood	Submit sample for serologic study.	A detectable fluorescent antitreponemal antibody (absorbed) titer.[a]
Liver	Record weight and sample for histologic study. For special stains and infectious precautions, see above under "Note."	Syphilitic hepatitis. Histologic sections show abundance of *Treponema* organisms.
Other organs	Procedures depend on expected findings or grossly identified abnormalities as listed in right-hand column. Submit samples for histologic study.	Fibrosing pneumonia; thymic abscesses; splenomegaly; thickening of bowel wall by inflammation and fibrosis *(2)*; splenomegaly; interstitial fibrosis and inflammation of pancreas *(2)*.
Brain and spinal cord	For removal and specimen preparation, see pp. 66 and 70, respectively. For histologic sections, request Warthin-Starry stain for spirochetes (p. 173).	Chronic meningitis, encephalitis, and myelitis. For details, see under "Neurosyphilis, congenital."
Eyes	For removal and specimen preparations, see p. 85.	Interstitial keratitis; choroiditis; uveitis; optic atrophy.
Bones and joints	For removal, prosthetic repair and specimen preparation, see p. 95.	Mononuclear periostitis; osteochondritis; "Clutton's joints" (fused joints).

[a]Immunofluorescent antigen testing is more sensitive than silver staining for the detection of Treponema pallidum *(3)*.

References

1. Levine Z, Sherer DM, Jacobs A, Rotenberg O. Nonimmune hydrops fetalis due to congenital syphilis associated with negative intrapartum maternal serology screening. Am J Perinatol 1998;15:233–236.
2. Oppenheimer EH, Dahms BB. Congenital syphilis in the fetus and neonate. Perspectives Pediatr Pathol 1981;6:115–138.
3. Rawstron SA, Vetrano J, Tannis G, Bromberg K. Congenital syphilis: detection of Treponema pallidum in stillborns. Clin Infect Dis 1997;24:24–27.

Syringomyelia

Synonyms and Related Term: Hydromyelia; idiopathic syringomyelia; secondary syringomyelia; syringobulbia.

Possible Associated Conditions: With idiopathic syringomyelia—Arnold Chiari malformation, type I;* basilar impression;* Klippel-Feil syndrome;* spina bifida. With secondary syringomyelia—Intramedullary gliomas (ependymoma, pilocytic astrocytoma) and vascular tumors; spinal arachnoiditis and pachymeningitis; traumatic myelopathy.

Organs and Tissues	Procedures	Possible or Expected Findings
External examination	Record and prepare photographs of all abnormalities as listed in right-hand column.	Hypertrophy of body parts. Muscle atrophy of upper extremities and hands. Cyanosis, hyperkeratosis, and other trophic changes of hands.
	Prepare roentgenograms of spine and joints.	Kyphoscoliosis. Clubfoot deformities. Cervical rib. Traumatic osteoarthropathy (Charcot joints).
Brain and spinal cord	For removal and specimen preparation, see pp. 66 and 70, respectively. For histologic sampling, see right-hand column.	Hydrocephalus.* Cervical spinal cord is swollen and tense, with cavitation (syrinx) containing clear fluid. Wall of cavity consists of degenerated glial and neural elements, with marked gliosis. Spinal cord parenchyma is markedly compressed. See also above under "Possible Associated Conditions."

T

Tabes Dorsalis

Related Terms: General paralysis; locomotor ataxia; parenchymatous neurosyphilis; taboparesis.

Possible Associated Conditions: Acquired immunodeficiency syndrome.*

Organs and Tissues	*Procedures*	*Possible or Expected Findings*
External examination		Ulcers of feet.
	Prepare roentgenograms of major joints.	Degenerative arthritis (Charcot joints).
Cerebrospinal fluid	Submit sample for serologic study, cell count, and determination of protein concentrations (p. 104).	Late in the disease, serologic tests for syphilis* may be negative. Pleocytosis and increased protein concentrations may indicate presence of meningitis.*
Brain, spinal cord, spinal ganglia, and nerves of lumbar plexus	For removal and specimen preparation of brain, spinal cord, and spinal ganglia, see pp. 65, 67, and 69, respectively. Request Luxol fast blue stain for myelin and Bielschowsky's stain for axons (p. 172).	Syphilitic meningoencephalitis (general paresis) may also be present. Degeneration of dorsal root ganglia and posterior nerve roots (mainly lumbosacral) with Wallerian degeneration of posterior columns. Posterior roots are grey and shrunken and the spinal cord is atrophic with excavated posterior surface.
Eyes and optic nerves	For removal and specimen preparation, see p. 85.	Optic nerve atrophy.

Talcosis (See "Pneumoconiosis.")

Telangiectasia, Hereditary Hemorrhagic (See "Disease, Osler-Rendu-Weber.")

Tetanus

Synonym: *Clostridium tetani* infection; lockjaw.

NOTE: (1) Collect all tissues that appear infected. (2) Request aerobic and anaerobic cultures. However, the presence of tetanus bacilli established in culture is not diagnostic, since spores of *C. tetani* frequently contaminate wounds. (3) Request Gram stain (p. 172). (4) Usually, no special precautions are indicated. (5) Serologic studies are available from the Centers of Disease Control and Prevention, Atlanta, GA (p. 135). (6) This is a **reportable** disease.

Organs and Tissues	*Procedures*	*Possible or Expected Findings*
External examination	Record body weight and length and appearance of wound(s); photograph and excise wound(s) for histologic study.	Evidence of weight loss; subcutaneous abscesses.
	Record evidence of parenteral drug abuse, especially subcutaneous injection (i.e., "skin popping").	Tetanus may occur in drug addicts.
	Prepare chest roentgenogram.	Tension pneumothorax* after mechanical ventilation.
Cerebrospinal fluid	Submit sample for microbiologic study (p. 104).	Bacterial meningitis must be ruled out.

Organs and Tissues	Procedures	Possible or Expected Findings
Lungs	Submit one lobe for microbiologic study (p. 103).	Aspiration and bronchopneumonia; embolism;* atelectasis.

Tetany

NOTE: See under name of suspected underlying conditions, such as hyperparathyroidism,* malabsorption syndrome,* or vitamin D deficiency.* For interpretation of calcium concentrations in blood and vitreous, see p. 347. Respiratory or metabolic alkalosis* cannot be confirmed after death; determination of blood pH is not helpful because acidity increases rapidly after death. The concentration of serum phosphates also increases after death.

Tetralogy of Fallot

Synonym: Large ventricular septal defect with pulmonary stenosis* or atresia.*

NOTE: The basic anomaly consists of subpulmonary stenosis, ventricular septal defect, overriding aorta, and secondary right ventricular hypertrophy. For general dissection techniques, see p. 33. Surgical interventions include modified Blalock-Taussig subclavian-to-pulmonary arterial shunt; complete repair with patch closure of ventricular septal defect, and reconstruction of right ventricular outflow tract (with a patch or with an extracardial conduit).

Possible Associated Conditions: Origin of left pulmonary artery from aorta; minor abnormalities of the tricuspid valve; absent ductal artery (25%); atrial septal defect* (in 20%; pentalogy of Fallot); bicuspid pulmonary valve;* dextroposition of aorta; double aortic arch; hypoplastic pulmonary arteries; patent ductal artery;* patent oval foramen; complete atrioventricular septal defect* (usually with Down's syndrome*); persis-tent left superior vena cava; pulmonary valve atresia (see "Atresia, pulmonary valve, with ventricular septal defect"); right aortic arch (25%); second ventricular septal defect; origin of left anterior descending (LAD) or right coronary artery (RCA) from contralateral aortic sinus or coronary artery (5%); syndrome with absent pulmonary valve and massively dilated pulmonary arteries (rare).

Organs and Tissues	Procedures	Possible or Expected Findings
Chest cavity	Record course of superior vena cava and of its tributaries.	Persistent left superior vena cava.
	Record course of thoracic aorta and of its main branches.	Right aortic arch with or without right-sided ductal artery; double aortic arch; absent ductal artery.
	Record origin of pulmonary arteries.	Origin of the left pulmonary artery from ascending aorta. For possible additional findings, see above under "Note" and under "Possible Associated Conditions."
Heart	If infective endocarditis is suspected, follow procedures described under that heading (p.103). For coronary arteriography, see p. 118.	Infective endocarditis* (usually of pulmonary or aortic valve). See also above under "Possible Associated Conditions." Marked right ventricular hypertrophy. Right ventricular dilatation and fibrosis with late postoperative right-sided heart failure or sudden death due to arrhythmia.
Lungs	Perfuse one lung with formalin (p. 47). Request Verhoeff–van Gieson stain (p. 173).	Old *in situ* thrombosis of small pulmonary artery branches.
Other organs	Procedures depend on expected findings or grossly identified abnormalities as listed in right-hand column.	Paradoxic embolism; cerebral abscess.*

Thalassemia

Synonyms and Related Terms: Congenital hemolytic anemia; alpha-thalassemia; beta-thalassemia major (Cooley's anemia); beta thalassemia minor (beta-thalassemia trait).

NOTE: The changes described below are observed primarily in beta-thalassemia major.

Organs and Tissues	Procedures	Possible or Expected Findings
External examination	Record body weight and length; record and prepare photographs of other abnormalities as listed in right-hand column.	Evidence of wasting with peculiar brownish skin pigmentation. Hydrops fetalis *(1)* and limb deformities *(2)* in rare forms of alpha-thalassemia.

Organs and Tissues	Procedures	Possible or Expected Findings
External examination (continued)	Prepare roentgenogram of skull and, if indicated, of deformed extremities.	Malocclusion of jaws due to enlargement of malar bones; bone deformities of calvaria. Deformed extremities.
All organs	Procedures depend on expected findings or grossly identified abnormalities as listed in right-hand column. See also under "Anemia, hemolytic."	Cardiomegaly and myocardial hemosiderosis with manifestations of congestive heart failure.* Pancreatic hemosiderosis (with or without diabetes mellitus); hepatosplenomegaly.

References

1. Chui DH, Waye JS. Hydrops fetalis caused by alpha-thalassemia: an emerging health care problem. Blood 1998;91:2213–2222.
2. Chitayat D, Silver MM, O'Brien K, Wyatt P, Waye JS, Chiu DH, et al. Limb defects in homozygous alpha-thalassemia: report of three cases. Am J Med Genet 1997;68:162–167.

Thallium (See "Poisoning, thallium.")

Thirst (See "Dehydration.")

Thromboangiitis Obliterans (See "Disease, Buerger's.")

Thrombocytopenia (See "Purpura, thrombotic thrombocytopenic" and "Syndrome, hemolytic uremic.")

Thrombophlebitis, Ileofemoral (See "Thrombosis, venous.")

Thrombophlebitis Migrans (See "Phlebitis.")

Thrombosis, Cavernous Sinus (See "Thrombosis, cerebral venous sinus.")

Thrombosis, Cerebral Venous Sinus

Related Term: Cavernous sinus thrombosis.

NOTE: Idiopathic recurrent venous thrombosis also may affect the cerebral venous sinuses.

Organs and Tissues	Procedures	Possible or Expected Findings
External examination	Record body weight and length and skin turgor. Prepare photograph of face.	In infants, manifestations of marasmus and dehydration.* Head injury;* infection of skin in upper half of face. Presence of edema of forehead and eyelids, proptosis, and chemosis indicate cavernous sinus thrombosis.
Vitreous and eyes	If dehydration is suspected, submit samples of vitreous for electrolyte studies (p. 85). For removal and specimen preparation of eyes, see p. 85.	In infants, manifestations of dehydration.* Thrombosis of angular and superior ophthalmic veins may be associated with cavernous sinus thrombosis.
Cerebrospinal fluid	Submit sample for microbiologic study (p. 104).	See below under "Brain and meninges."
Brain and meninges	For removal and specimen preparation, see p. 65.	Cerebral abscess* or tumor; meningitis.* Venous infarction of brain may be caused by superior sagittal sinus thrombosis. Epidural and subdural empyema* may be present.
Calvaria and base of skull with venous sinuses	For exposure of venous sinuses, see p. 71. Submit contents of affected sinuses for microbiologic study. Prepare smears of contents and submit samples of sinus walls for histologic study.	Superior sagittal sinus thrombosis may be associated with terminal diseases with marasmus, with osteomyelitis,* or a tumor of the skull. (See also below under "Systemic veins.") Thrombosis and thrombophlebitis may occur in all venous sinuses.

Organs and Tissues	Procedures	Possible or Expected Findings
Pituitary gland	For dissection and specimen preparation, see p. 71.	Infarction or abscess of pituitary gland may be caused by cavernous sinus thrombosis.
Paranasal sinuses, middle ears, and mastoid cells	For exposure of middle ears and paranasal sinuses, see pp. 72 and 71, respectively. If there is evidence of infection, prepare smears of contents and submit for microbiologic study.	Acute and chronic otitis media* and interna; mastoiditis; paranasal sinusitis.
Systemic veins	Procedures depend on expected findings or grossly identified abnormalities as listed in right-hand column.	Thrombosis—for instance, of pelvic veins in presence of pelvic infection. Pelvic infections and pregnancy may be associated with superior sagittal sinus thrombosis.

Thrombosis, Lateral Sinus

NOTE: Possible causes include cholesteatoma, infections in the neck or pharynx, mastoiditis, and otitis media.* For general autopsy procedures, see "Thrombosis, cerebral venous sinus."

Thrombosis, Portal Vein (See "Hypertension, portal.")

Thrombosis, Renal Vein

NOTE: In infants, inquire about birth injury, maternal diabetes mellitus,* toxemia,* or anoxia.

Organs and Tissues	Procedures	Possible or Expected Findings
Vitreous	Submit samples of vitreous of infants for determination of sodium, chloride, and urea nitrogen concentrations.	In infants, manifestations of dehydration.*
Lungs		Pulmonary embolism.*
Retroperitoneal space and femoral veins	Procedures depend on expected findings or grossly identified abnormalities as listed in right-hand column. For renal venography, see p. 59. Open veins *in situ*. Dissect testicular or ovarian veins—particularly on left—and adrenal veins. For removal of femoral vessels, see p. 34.	Tumor of the kidney* (renal cell carcinoma); aortic aneurysm; lymphadenopathy; other mass lesions. Inferior vena cava thrombosis involving orifice or whole length of renal veins. Tumor thrombus (e.g., from renal cell carcinoma). Femoral vein thrombosis. Rare venous malformations also may cause renal vein thrombosis *(1)*.
Kidneys	Unless the cause of the renal vein thrombosis and the nature of the complicating or underlying renal disease are known, follow procedures described under "Glomerulonephritis."	Hemorrhagic infartion. Parenchymal renal disease with nephrotic syndrome,* including amyloidosis* and vasculitis* (these last conditions may be associated with renal vein thrombosis).
Other organs	Procedures depend on expected findings or grossly identified abnormalities as listed in right-hand column.	Acute gastroenteritis in infancy. Hyperparathyroidism,* pregnancy,* trauma, and other conditions.

Reference

1. Lash C, Radhakrishnan J, McFadden JC. Renal vein thrombosis secondary to absent inferior vena cava. Urol 1998;51:829–830.

Thrombosis, Venous

NOTE: For peripheral venous thrombosis, the autopsy procedures are essentially similar to those described under "Phlebitis." See also under "Hypertension, portal," "Syndrome, Budd-Chiari," "Thrombosis, cerebral venous sinus," "Thrombosis, lateral sinus," and "Thrombosis, renal vein."

Thymoma (See "Tumor of the thymus.")

Thyroiditis

Synonyms and Related Terms: Chronic fibrosing thyroiditis (Riedel's struma); chronic thyroiditis with transient thyrotoxicosis; Hashimoto's thyroiditis; pyogenic thyroiditis; subacute (granulomatous, giant cell, de Quervain's) thyroiditis.

Possible Associated Conditions: With Hashimoto's thyroiditis—autoimmune (chronic) hepatitis,* megaloblastic anemia,* rheumatoid arthritis,* Sjögren's syndrome,* and systemic lupus erythematosus.* With Riedel's struma—retroperitoneal fibrosis,* sclerosing cholangitis,* sclerosing mediastinitis,* and other conditions with idiopathic fibrosis. With subacute thyroiditis—viral infection.

Organs and Tissues	*Procedures*	*Possible or Expected Findings*
Blood	Submit sample for serologic study (p.102).	Viral antibodies in subacute (de Quervain) thyroiditis; tissue antibodies in Hashimoto's thyroiditis.
Thymus	Record weight and submit sample for histologic study.	Enlarged thymus with multiple germinal centers with Hashimoto's thyroiditis.
Neck organs	Remove together with tongue (p. 4). If there is evidence of pyogenic infection, submit material for culture. Record weight of thyroid and of parathyroid glands and submit samples for histologic study, together with cervical lymph nodes. Record presence or absence of compression of trachea by struma.	Acute suppurative thyroiditis. Acute nonsuppurative thyroiditis after irradiation. Struma and lymphadenopathy in Hashimoto's thyroiditis. Fibrosis with tracheal compression associated with Riedel's struma.
Other organs	Submit samples of all endocrine glands for histologic study.	If hypothyroidism* is suspected, see also under that entry.

Thyrotoxicosis (See "Hyperthyroidism.")

Torticollis, Spasmodic

Related Terms: Dystonia musculorum deformans; torsion dystonia.

Organs and Tissues	*Procedures*	*Possible or Expected Findings*
Brain	For removal and specimen preparation, see p. 65.	No diagnostic pathologic lesions.

Torulosis (See "Cryptococcosis.")

Toxemia of Pregnancy

Related Terms: Eclampsia or preeclampsia; postpartum hemolytic uremic syndrome; postpartum renal failure.

NOTE: See also "Failure, kidney."

Organs and Tissues	*Procedures*	*Possible or Expected Findings*
External examination	Record body weight, extent and location of edema, and level of fundus of uterus.	Edema involving periorbital region, hands, and ankles; hemorrhagic foci in conjunctivas and fingernails.
	Prepare chest roentgenogram.	Infiltrates.
Blood	Submit sample for microbiologic study (p. 102). Refrigerate sample for possible serologic, toxicologic, or biochemical study.	Evidence of infection, poisoning, electrolyte abnormalities, and other conditions.
Heart	Record weight; submit samples for histologic study.	Cardiac hypertrophy; hemorrhagic necroses caused by small-vessel thromboses.
Lungs	Submit one lobe for microbiologic study (p. 103); perfuse one lung with formalin (p. 47).	Hemorrhagic necroses.

Organs and Tissues	Procedures	Possible or Expected Findings
Liver	Record weight; submit samples for histologic study. For the demonstration of fibrin depositis, request phosphotungstic acid hematoxylin (PTAH) stain (p. 173).	Periportal fibrin deposition with hemorrhages; centrilobular and midzonal necroses or cell dropout. Infarction *(1)* and one-time or recurrent hemorrhages *(2)*.
Adrenal glands	Submit samples for histologic study (see also "Liver").	Hemorrhagic necroses.
Kidneys	Follow procedures described under "Glomerulonephritis."	Thromboses of small vessels. Glomerulonephritis.* Hemorrhagic necroses.
Urine	Submit sample for determination of protein concentration; record appearance of sediment.	Proteinuria; abnormal sediment.
Pelvic organs	For dissection, fixation, and removal for preservation of the pregnant uterus, see p. 60.	Abruptio placentae may be present; also thrombotic vascular occlusions.
Brain and spinal cord; pituitary gland	For removal and specimen preparation, see pp. 65, 67, and 71, respectively.	Thrombotic occlusion of small vessels with hemorrhagic necroses; anterior lobe of pituitary gland may contain necroses (see also "Syndrome, Sheehan's").

References

1. Krueger KJ, Hoffman BJ, Lee WM. Hepatic infarction associated with ecclampsia. Am J Gastroenterol 1990;85:588–592.
2. Greenstein D, Henerson JM, Boyer TD. Liver hemorrhage: recurrent episodes during pregnancy complicated by eclampsia. Gastroenterol 1994; 106:1668–1671.

Toxoplasmosis

Synonyms: Adult toxoplasmosis; congenital toxoplasmosis; disseminated toxoplasmosis; latent toxoplasmosis; *Toxoplasma gondii* infection.

NOTE: (1) Collect all tissues that appear to be infected. (2) Culturing requires animal inoculation in specialized laboratories. Consult microbiology laboratory before performing autopsy. (3) Request Giemsa stain (p. 172) and *Toxoplasma* immunoperoxidase or immunofluorescent stain. (4) No special precautions are indicated. (5) Serologic studies are available from local and state health department laboratories (p. 135). (6) This is not a reportable disease.

Possible Associated Conditions: Acquired immunodeficiency syndrome (AIDS)* *(1,2)*.

Organs and Tissues	Procedures	Possible or Expected Findings
External examination	Record head circumference of infant. Prepare radiograph of cranium of infants.	Jaundice and hydrocephalus* in congenital toxoplasmosis.
Blood	Submit sample for serologic study.	See above under "Note."
Heart	Record weight; submit samples for histologic study (p. 30) and request PAS stain (p. 173). Snap-freeze myocardium for immuno-fluorescent study.	Myocarditis* in adult form of toxoplasmosis. Trophozoites of *Toxoplasma* stain well with PAS.
Lungs	Prepare smears and request Giemsa (p. 172) and immunofluorescent stains. Perfuse one lung with formalin (p. 47).	Interstitial pneumonitis* in adult toxoplasmosis *(1)*.
Liver	Record weight. Submit sample for histologic study.	*Toxoplasma* hepatitis, with hepatocellular giant cell transformation in congenital toxoplasmosis.
	In diagnostically difficult cases, submit material for electron microscopic study (p. 132).	Electron micrographs allow distinction between *Toxoplasma* and *Sarcocystis,* oval yeasts, and other organisms.
Spleen	Record weight.	Splenomegaly in congenital toxoplasmosis.
Lymph nodes	Submit samples for histologic study.	Marked follicular hyperplasia with histiocytes inside and around follicles *(3)*.
Skeletal muscles	For sampling and specimen preparation, see p. 80.	Myositis occurs in adult toxoplasmosis.

Organs and Tissues	Procedures	Possible or Expected Findings
Placenta	Record weight and sample for histologic study.	Diffuse lymphoplasmacytic villitis with sclerosis of villi. Cysts may be found.
Other organs and tissues	Procedures depend on expected findings or grossly identified abnormalities as mentioned in right-hand column.	Infections may occur in many organs and tissues.
Brain and spinal cord	For removal and specimen preparation, see pp. 65 and 67, respectively.	Cerebral calcifications; periventricular necrosis. Hydrocephalus* in congenital toxoplasmosis; meningoencephalitis in adult form.
Eyes	For removal and specimen preparation, see p. 85.	Chorioretinitis; uveitis.

References

1. Nash G, Kerschmann RL, Herndier B, Dubey JP. The pathological manifestations of pulmonary toxoplasmosis in the acquired immunodeficiency syndrome. Hum Pathol 1994;25:652–658.
2. Bertoli F, Espino M, Arosemena JR 5th, Fishback JL, Frenkel JK. A spectrum in the pathology of toxoplasmosis in patients with acquired immunodeficiency syndrome. Arch Pathol Lab Med 1995;119:214–224.
3. Rose I. Morphology and diagnostics of human toxoplasmosis. General Diagn Pathol 1997;142:257–270.

Transfusion (See "Reaction to transfusion.")

Transplantation, Bone Marrow

NOTE: If the patient had symptoms of acute or chronic graft-versus-host disease (GVHD), see "Disease, graft-versus-host." If the patient developed recurrent leukemia, see under "Leukemia,..." Cytogenetic and other techniques can be used in such cases to determine whether the leukemic cells are of donor or host origin. If the patient developed post-transplant lymphoproliferative disease (PTLD), see under "Lymphoma."

Organs and Tissues	Procedures	Possible or Expected Findings
External examination and skin	Record skin abnormalities and sample for histologic study.	Manifestations of graft-versus-host disease (e.g., scleroderma-like changes).*
Blood	Submit sample for microbiologic study (p. 102).	Septicemia.
Lungs	Submit samples for microbiologic (bacterial, fungal, and viral) and histologic studies (p. 103). Request Grocott's methenamine silver stain (p. 172) to detect *Pneumocystis carinii* organisms. If complicating toxoplasmosis is suspected, see under that heading.	Interstitial pneumonia* and cytomegalovirus infection* or human herpesvirus 6 infection *(1)*. Bacterial, fungal, or protozoal infections. Pulmonary veno-occlusive disease (see "Hypertension, pulmonary") *(2)*.
Liver	Record weight; sample for histologic study.	Hepatic veno-occlusive disease. Viral hepatitis (hepatitis C; herpesvirus hepatitis). Cholangitis or ductopenia and other manifestations of GVHD.
Kidneys	If indicated, see also "Failure, kidney."	Kidney failure* associated with tumor lysis syndrome, hepatorenal syndrome,* cyclosporine nephrotoxicity, or bone marrow-transplant associated nephropathy *(3)*.
Other organs and tissues	If there is evidence of infection, submit material for microbiologic studies. If there is evidence of recurrent leukemia or lymphoma, sample as described under those headings.	Bacterial or fungal infections in GVHD.* Other manifestations of GVHD.* Recurrent leukemia,* lymphoma* (including post-transplant, Epstein-Barr virus associated lymphoproliferative disorder). Recurrent solid tumor, e.g., carcinoma of breast, lung (small cell carcinoma), ovary, or testis.
	If the patient had symptoms of thrombotic thrombocytopenic purpura (TTP) or hemolytic uremic syndrome (HUS), see these headings.	Manifestations of TTP, HUS *(4)*, or thrombotic microangiopathy *(5)*.

Organs and Tissues	Procedures	Possible or Expected Findings
Lymph nodes	Record average size. Fix specimens in B-5 fixative (p. 129). Make touch preparations. Request Giemsa or Wright stain (p. 172).	Lymphomatous or leukemic infiltrates.
Bone marrow	For preparation of sections and smears (imprints), see p. 96.	Myeloid cells may be absent in marrow graft rejection or nonimmunologic marrow graft failure.
Brain and spinal cord; peripheral nerves	For removal and specimen preparation, see pp. 65, 67, and 79, respectively.	Hematomas; hemorrhagic necroses; infarcts; bacterial or fungal infections; leukoencephalopathy; vascular siderocalcinosis; neuroaxonal spheroids *(6)*. Peripheral neuropathy.

References

1. Kadakia MP. Human herpesvirus 6 infection and associated pathogenesis following bone marrow transplantation. Leukemia Lymphoma 1998;31:251–266.
2. Williams LM, Fussell S, Veith RW, Nelson S, Mason CM. Pulmonary veno-occlusive disease in an adult following bone marrow transplantation. Case report and review of the literature. Chest 1996;109:1388–1391.
3. Pulla B, Barri YM, Anaissie E. Acute renal failure following bone marrow transplantation. Renal Failure 1998;20:421–435.
4. Schriber JR, Herzig GP. Transplantation-associated thrombotic thrombocytopenic purpura and hemolytic uremic syndrome. Semin Hematol 1997;34:126–133.
5. Moake JL, Byrness JJ. Thrombotic microangiopathies associated with drugs and bone marrow transplantation. Hematol Oncol Clin North Am 1996:485–497.
6. Mohrmann RL, Mah V, Vinters HV. Neuropathologic findings after bone marrow transplantation: an autopsy study. Hum Pathol 1990;21:630–639.

Transplantation, Heart

Organs and Tissues	Procedures	Possible or Expected Findings
External examination	Record abnormalities, e.g., after high-dose steroid therapy.	Cushingoid features (see "Syndrome, Cushing's") after steroid therapy.
Chest cavity	Record status of all vascular anstomoses. If there are hemorrhages, record volume and site.	Suture dehiscence. Hemothorax or hemomediastinum in recent cases.
Heart	Record weight, ventricular thickness, and valve circumferences. For sampling of myocardium, see p. 30. Cut coronary arteries in cross sections; request Verhoeff–van Gieson stain (p. 173).	Left ventricular hypertrophy, from cyclosporine-related hypertension. Acute transplant rejection (for grading, see ref. *1*). Chronic transplant vasculopathy with coronary artery stenosis *(2)*. Old or recent myocardial infarction. Recurrence of native cardiac disease (e.g., amyloidosis* or giant cell myocarditis). Infection.
Other organs	Procedures depend on expected findings or grossly identified abnormalities as listed in right-hand column.	Post-transplant lymphoproliferative disorder *(1)*. Opportunistic infection *(1)*. Pneumonia; septicemia.

References

1. Billingham ME, Cary NRB, Hammond ME, Kemnitz J, Marboe C, McCallister HA, et al. A working formulation for the standardization of nomenclature in the diagnosis of heart and lung rejection: Heart and Lung Rejection Study Group. J Heart Transplant 1990;9:587–593.
2. Graham A. Autopsy findings in cardiac transplant patients: a 10-year experience. Am J Clin Pathol 1992;97:369–375.

Transplantation, Kidney

Organs and Tissues	Procedures	Possible or Expected Findings
External examination	Record abnormalities, e.g., after high-dose steroid therapy.	Cushingoid features (see "Syndrome, Cushing's") after steroid therapy.
Blood	Submit sample for bacterial, fungal, and viral cultures (p. 102). Submit samples for tests for hepatitis B and C antigens.	Septicemia (see below under "Other organs").

Organs and Tissues	Procedures	Possible or Expected Findings
Other organs	If systemic infection is suspected, sample material for microbiologic study. Other procedures depend on expected findings or grossly identified abnormalities as listed in right-hand column.	Bacterial, fungal, or viral infections may be observed. There may be evidence of post-transplant lymphoproliferative disorder.
Kidneys	Dissect renal allograft *in situ* and record whether vascular and ureteral anastomoses were competent. For renal arteriography, see p. 59. For the processing of samples from the allograft and the native kidneys (if they had been left *in situ*), follow procedures described under "Glomerulonephritis."	Leaking anastomoses; infection; acute or chronic graft rejection. Recurrent primary disease.
Lymph nodes and bone marrow	Fix samples in B-5 solution (p. 129). For preparation of sections and smears of bone marrow, see p. 96.	Post-transplant lymphoproliferative disorder.

Transplantation, Liver

Organs and Tissues	Procedures	Possible or Expected Findings
External examination	Record abnormalities, e.g., after high-dose steroid therapy.	Cushingoid features (see "Syndrome, Cushing's") after steroid therapy.
Chest organs	Open right atrium *in situ* and probe sub-diaphragmatic inferior vena cava anastomosis; leave thoracic inferior vena cava with sleeve of right atrium attached to liver.	Dehiscence or stricture of subdiaphragmatic vena cava anastomosis. Leave esophagus attached to stomach, particularly if varices might be present.
Liver, hepatic artery, portal vein, hepatic vein, and bile ducts	Dissect *in situ* hepatic artery anastomosis, portal vein anastomosis, and bile duct anastomosis. Remove abdominal organs en block (intestines can be removed earlier to debulk organ block) and partially open inferior vena cava to inspect anastomoses with the graft.	Dehiscence or stricture of anastomoses.
	If there is evidence of hepatic infection, sample material for microbiologic and histologic study. Perfuse entire liver with formalin (p. 56) or slice fresh organ horizontally with long-bladed knive. Obtain multiple samples for histologic study.	Ascending biliary infections; hematogenous infections; ischemic lesions, including infected infarcts; recurrent primary disease such as primary biliary cirrhosis, viral hepatitis, or tumors. Acute-cellular or chronic-ductopenic rejection (for grading of rejection, see ref. *1*).
Other organs and blood	If systemic infection is suspected, sample material for microbiologic study (p. 102). Other procedures depend on expected findings or grossly identified abnormalities as listed in right-hand column.	Bacterial, fungal, or viral infections may be observed. Septicemia. Post-transplant lymphoproliferative disorder.

Reference

1. Anonymous. Banff schema for grading liver allograft rejection: an international consensus document. Hepatology 1997;25:658–663.

Transplantation, Lung

Organs and Tissues	Procedures	Possible or Expected Findings
External examination	Record abnormalities, e.g., after high-dose steroid therapy.	Cushingoid features (see "Syndrome, Cushing's") after steroid therapy.

Organs and Tissues	Procedures	Possible or Expected Findings
Chest cavity	Record status of all vascular anstomoses. If there are hemorrhages, record volume and site.	Suture dehiscence. Hemothorax or hemomediastinum in recent cases.
Lungs	Record lung weights separately. If lung infection is suspected, submit material for microbiologic study (p. 103). For perfusion of lungs with formalin, see p. 47. Cut lungs in frontal sections. Submit sections of proximal airways and of distal parenchyma for histologic study. Request Verhoeff–van Gieson and Gomori's methenamine silver stains (p. 173).	Opportunistic infection (in patients with a single lung transplant, infections may involve the nontransplant lung, as well). Chronic bronchitis* and bronchiectasis.* Acute rejection (rare); chronic airway rejection (obliterative bronchiolitis); chronic vascular rejection. (For grading of rejection, see ref. *1*.) Post-transplant lymphoproliferative disorder. Recurrence of primary disease (e.g., sarcoidosis,* lymphangioleiomyomatosis).
Kidneys	Submit samples for histologic study.	Manifestations of cyclosporine toxicity.
Other organs	If infection is expected, submit material for microbiologic study. Other procedures depend on expected findings or grossly identified abnormalities as listed in right-hand column.	Infection *(1)* or septicemia. Post-transplant lymphoproliferative disorder.

References

1. Billingham ME, Cary NRB, Hammond ME, Kemnitz J, Marboe C, McCallister HA, et al. A working formulation for the standardization of nomenclature in the diagnosis of heart and lung rejection: Heart and Lung Rejection Study Group. J Heart Transplant 1990;9:587–593.
2. Tazelaar HD, Yousem SA. The pathology of combined heart-lung transplantation: an autopsy study. Hum Pathol 1988;19:1403–1416.

Transposition, Complete, of the Great Arteries

NOTE: The basic anomaly is the origin of the aorta from the right ventricle, and of the pulmonary artery from the left ventricle, with a shunt, and usually with a right anterior aorta. There are four major types: (1) with an intact ventricular septum (65%), (2) with a ventricular septal defect* (20%), (3) with a ventricular septal defect and subvalvular pulmonary stenosis* (10%), and (4) with an intact ventricular septum and subvalvular pulmonary stenosis* (5%). For general dissection techniques, see p. 33. Interventions include atrial septostomy or septectomy; Mustard or Senning atrial switch procedure; Rastelli-type repair with a valved extracardiac conduit; and Jatene arterial switch procedure with LeCompte maneuver.

Possible Associated Conditions: Abnormal origin of coronary arteries (10%); atrial septal defect* (5%); coarctation of the aorta;* interrution of the aortic arch;* juxtaposition of atrial appendages (4%); overriding aorta (5%); overriding pulmonary artery (10%); patent ductal artery;* patent oval foramen; subvalvular pulmonary stenosis* (15%); tubular hypoplasia of the aortic arch;* ventricular septal defect* (30%), often malalignment type (50%).

Transposition, Congenitally Corrected, of the Great Arteries

Synonyms: Atrioventricular and ventriculoarterial discordance; L-transposition.

NOTE: The basic anomaly is a mirror-image ventricular inversion, with a left anterior aorta, and with blood flow from right atrium to left ventricle to pulmonary artery, and from left atrium to right ventricle to aorta. For general dissection techniques, see p. 33. Interventions include patch closure of the ventricular septal defect; relief of pulmonary stenosis; relief of tricuspid insufficiency; and insertion of pacemakers.

Possible Associated Conditions: Anterior and posterior AV nodes (100%), prone to develop complete heart block; dysplasia or Epstein's malformation* of left-sided tricuspid valve (40%); mirror-image epicardial coronary artery distribution (100%); right-sided mitral valve anomalies; subvalvular pulmonary stenosis* (40%); ventricular septal defect* (65%).

Trichinosis

Synonyms: *Trichinella spiralis* infection; trichinelliasis; trichiniasis.

NOTE: (1) Collect all tissues that appear infected. (2) Request direct examination for *Trichinella.* (3) Request Giemsa stain (p. 172). (4) No special precautions are indicated. (5) Serologic studies are available from local and state health department laboratories (p. 135). (6) This is a **reportable** disease.

Organs and Tissues	Procedures	Possible or Expected Findings
External examination and skin	Record abnormalities and photopgraph edema and hemorrhages.	Palpebral and facial edema; splinter hemorrhages under the nails.
Blood	Obtain sample for quantification of IgE and eosinophils.	Increased IgE concentration and eosinophilia.
Heart	Record weight and submit samples of myocardium for histologic study (p. 30).	Interstitial myocarditis early in the disease; focal necroses; no cysts can be seen.

Organs and Tissues	Procedures	Possible or Expected Findings
Duodenum, jejunum, and ileum	For *in situ* fixation and preparation for study under the dissecting microscope, see p. 54. Submit samples for histologic study.	Mild partial villous atrophy; acute and chronic infiltrate with eosinophils in mucosa and submucosa; mucosal edema; punctate hemorrhages; prominent Peyer's plaques.
Lungs, kidney, liver, pancreas, and soft tissues	Submit samples for histologic study. In older infections, decalcification of cysts and larvae may be required.	Resorption granulomas around migrating larvae.
	Prepare roentgenograms of organs and soft tissues.	Calcified cysts.
Kidneys	Follow procedures described under "Glomerulonephritis."	Immune-mediated glomerulonephritis.*
Lymph nodes	Submit samples for histologic study.	Resorption granulomas around migrating larvae.
Brain and spinal cord	For removal and specimen preparation, see pp. 65 and 67, respectively. For decalcification, see p. 97.	Mononuclear meningitis; tiny foci of gliosis around capillaries; encephalitis.
Skeletal muscles	Submit samples for histologic study, especially from diaphragm, gastrocnemius, intercostal, deltoid, gluteus, and pectoral muscles. For decalcification, see p. 97.	Encysted larvae; cysts in varying stages of lymphocytic and eosinophilic inflammation and degeneration.
	Prepare roentgenograms.	Calcified cysts.
Bone marrow	For preparation of sections and smears, see p. 96.	Hyperplasia and eosinophilia.

Trisomy 21 (See "Syndrome, Down's.")

Truncus Arteriosus (See "Artery, persistent truncal.")

Trypanosomiasis, African

Synonyms: African sleeping sickness; *Trypanosoma brucei gambiense* infection (West African trypanosomiasis); *Trypanosoma brucei rhodesiense* infection (East African trypanosomiasis).

NOTE: (1) Collect all tissues that appear infected. (2) Request direct examination for trypanosomes. (3) Request Giemsa stain (p. 172). (4) No special precautions are indicated. (5) Serologic studies are available from the Centers for Disease Control and Prevention, Atlanta, GA (p. 135). (6) This is not a reportable disease.

Organs and Tissues	Procedures	Possible or Expected Findings
External examination	Record abnormalities and photograph skin changes.	Cachexia. Facial edema; rash, especially on rump.
Cerebrospinal fluid	Submit sample for biochemical analysis and prepare sediment (p. 104).	Increased IgM protein concentrations; trypanosomes may be present, especially in late Gambian disease; plasma cells with Russell bodies (Mott cells).
Chest and abdomen	Record volume of effusions and prepare smears of sediment.	Ascites; pleural* and pericardial effusions with trypanosomes.
Blood	Prepare thick, unfixed film and request Giemsa stain (p. 102).	Trypanosomes may be present, particularly in Rhodesian disease.
Heart	Record weight and submit samples for histologic study (p. 30).	Acute and chronic pancarditis, or both, with cardiac hypertrophy* and dilatation.
Lymph nodes	Submit touch preparations and material in B-5 fixative (p. 129) for histologic study.	Reactive hyperplasia in early stages; perivascular mononuclear infiltration; fibrosis in later stages.
Brain and spinal cord	For removal and specimen preparation, see pp. 65 and 67, respectively. Histologic sections should include cortex, basal ganglia, cerebellum, brain stem, and spinal cord.	Cerebral edema; diffuse perivascular lymphoplasmacytic meningoencephalitis in cortex; characteristic are Mott cells (see above) in brain and spinal cord; inflamed choroid plexus; hydrocephalus.*

Trypanosomiasis, American (See "Disease, Chagas.")

Tuberculosis

Synonyms and Related Terms: *Mycobacterium tuberculosis, M. bovis, M. africanum* infection; scrofula; lupus vulgaris.

NOTE: (1) Collect all tissues that appear infected. (2) Request mycobacterial cultures. (3) Request Ziehl-Neelsen, Kinyoun's, or other acid-fast stains (p. 172). Polymerase chain reaction for mycobacterial DNA may be helpful in the differential diagnosis of granulomas *(1)*. (4) Universal **precautions** should be strictly followed and aerolization should be avoided (p. 146). (5) Reliable serologic studies are not available. A definite diagnosis requires isolation of the organism. (6) This is a **reportable** disease.

Organs and Tissues	*Procedures*	*Possible or Expected Findings*
External examination and skin	Record abnormalities and prepare photographs. Submit sections of skin lesions for histologic study; if there are fistulas, obtain curettings for smears for acid fast stains (see "Note" above) and for culture. Fill fistulas with contrast medium and prepare roentgenograms.	Tuberculosis of skin (lupus vulgaris).
	Prepare chest and skeletal roentgenograms.	Pulmonary infiltrates and cavities; effusions; manifestations of tuberculous osteomyelitis and arthritis.
Chest and abdomen	Record volume of effusions or exudates; submit sections of serosal surfaces for histologic study.	Tuberculous pleuritis, pericarditis,* and peritonitis.
Lungs with hilar lymph nodes	If diagnosis was confirmed clinically, perfuse both lungs with formalin (p. 47); if not, submit consolidated or cavitated areas for culture (p. 103) and histologic study with acid-fast stains. For decalcification procedures, see p. 97.	Cavitary, fibrocalcific, miliary, bronchial, and other types of pulmonary tuberculosis; granulomas in hilar lymph nodes.
Other organs	Procedures depend on expected findings or grossly identified abnormalities as listed in right-hand column. See also above under "Lungs with hilar lymph nodes."	Most organs and tissues may be involved, including liver, pancreas, spleen, kidneys, adrenal glands and other endocrine glands, gonads, and lymph nodes.
Brain and spinal cord	For removal and specimen preparation, see pp. 65 and 67, respectively. If material is to be submitted for culture, follow procedures described on p. 389 (meningitis).	Tuberculous meningitis; tuberculoma.
Eyes	For removal and specimen preparation, see p. 85.	Iridocyclitis or panophthalmitis.
Bones and joints	Submit sample of synovial fluid for culture (p. 102). For removal, prosthetic repair, and specimen preparation, see p. 96.	Tuberculous arthritis and synovitis (hips, spine, knee); tuberculous osteomyelitis (anterior aspect of vertebrae; metaphysis of long bones).

Reference

1. Trauner M, Grasmug E, Stauber RE, Hammer HF, Hoefler G, Reisinger EC. Recurrent Salmonella enteritidis and hepatic tuberculosis. Gut 1995; 37:136–139.

Tularemia

Synonyms and Related Terms: *Francisella tularensis* infection; *Pasteurella tularensis* infection; typhoidal tularemia; ulceroglandular tularemia; rabbit fever.

NOTE: (1) Collect all tissues that appear infected. (2) Request aerobic bacterial cultures. (3) Request Gram stain (p. 172). (4) Special **precautions** are indicated (p. 146). (5) Serologic studies are available from local and state health department laboratories (p. 135). (6) This is not a reportable disease.

Organs and Tissues	*Procedures*	*Possible or Expected Findings*
External examination, skin, and eyes	Record abnormalities and photograph skin changes; submit for histologic study.	Skin ulcers of hands, feet or perineal area; necrotizing lesions of eye and purulent conjunctivitis.

Organs and Tissues	Procedures	Possible or Expected Findings
Chest and abdomen	Submit samples of serosal surfaces for histologic study.	Peritonitis;* perisplenitis; pleural effusions.*
Heart	If infective endocarditis is suspected, follow procedures described on p. 103.	Infective endocarditis;* pericarditis.*
Lungs	Record lung weights. Submit consolidated areas for bacterial culture (p. 103).	Necrotizing bronchopneumonia.
Liver and spleen	Record weights. Submit samples for histologic study.	Hepatosplenomegaly; characteristic granulomas.
Lymph nodes	Submit enlarged lymph nodes (particularly those with draining skin lesions) for histologic and microbiologic study (p. 102). Prepare smears for Gram stain (p. 172).	Lymphadenopathy; granulomatous lymphadenitis.
Brain and spinal cord	For removal and specimen preparation, see pp. 65 and 67, respectively.	Meningitis.*
Nasopharynx	Remove neck organs together with portions of pharynx. Nasal cavities will be accessible after removal of brain (p. 71).	Necrotizing nasopharyngeal lesions.
Bones		Osteomyelitis.*

Tumor, Carcinoid (See "Syndrome, carcinoid.")

Tumor, Endocrine (See "Neoplasia, multiple endocrine," "Syndrome, carcinoid," and "Tumor, of the [name of affected gland].")

Tumor, Malignant, Any Type

NOTE: If the tumor had been treated by surgery, irradiation, chemotherapy, or other means (the most common situation at autopsy), record possible adverse treatment effects and presence or absence of recurrent or metastatic malignancy. If patient had participated in a treatment trial, contact investigator or consult study protocol to provide optimal autopsy documentation.

For classification and terminology of tumors and their histologic features, the tumor fascicles of the Armed Forces Institute of Pathology are recommended references. Of course, many other excellent textbooks of tumor pathology are available.

For some tumors, possible associated or underlying conditions are listed. However, many additional associations do or might exist and therefore, careful documentation of all autopsy findings is recommended, even if abnormalities do not appear clearly tumor-related.

Tumor of the Adrenal Gland(s)

NOTE: See also "Tumor, malignant, any type."

Possible Associated Conditions: With adrenocortical adenoma—Conn's syndrome (primary hyperaldosteronism); Cushing's syndrome* with virilization. With adrenocortical carcinoma—Cushing's syndrome;* hypoglycemia;* virilization. With pheochromocytoma—cerebellar hemangioblastoma; erythrocytosis; hypercalcemia; hypertension,* multiple endocrine neoplasia* (with medullary carcinoma of the thyroid in types 2a and 2b and with hyperparathyroidism in type 2a); neurofibromatosis* (von Recklinghausen's disease); von Hippel-Lindau disease.*

Organs and Tissues	Procedures	Possible or Expected Findings
External examination	Record body weight and abnormal features. Photograph skin changes.	Cachexia. Virilization or cushingoid features (see above under "Possible Associated Conditions.")
Heart and arteries	Record heart weight and thickness of ventricles. For histologic sampling of myocardium, see p. 30.	Focal myocarditis.* Hypertensive cardiovascular disease (See "Hypertension [arterial], all types or type unspecified"). Myocardial infarction without severe coronary artery disease (with pheochromocytoma).
Gallbladder	Record contents of gallbladder.	Cholelithiasis* with pheochromocytoma.
Urine	Refrigerate sample for biochemical study—for instance, of catecholamines in cases with pheochromocytoma, or 17-ketosteroids and 17-hydroxy-corticosteroids with adrenocortical carcinoma.	Abnormal metabolites.

Organs and Tissues	Procedures	Possible or Expected Findings
Retroperitoneal space	Photograph and record size of tumor(s). Snap-freeze portion of fresh tumor tissue for biochemical study. Submit samples of both tumor and adjacent tissues for histologic study. For fixation in Orth's solution and gross staining procedures for pheochromocytoma, see pp. 131 and 134, respectively.	Pheochromocytoma may be bilateral and multiple. The tumor may also occur in other sites of the retroperitoneal space (organ of Zuckerkandl) and pelvis.
Other organs and tissues	Chemodectomas and carotid body tumors rarely may produce large amounts of catecholamines. Tumors of this type must be searched for if adrenal glands appear normal.	Pheochromocytoma may occur in paravertebral areas of thorax and neck and, rarely, in the urinary bladder. Widespread metastases may occur with pheochromocytoma and with adrenocortical carcinoma.
Bone marrow	For preparation of sections and smears, see p. 96.	Hyperplasia in association with pheochromocytoma. Extramedullary hematopoiesis may also be present. Hyperplasia would indicate the presence of an erythropoiesis-stimulating factor in tumor and plasma.

Tumor of the Bile Ducts (Extrahepatic or Hilar or of Papilla of Vater)

NOTE: The address of an appropriate Registry is Hepatic and Gastrointestinal Pathology, Armed Forces Institute of Pathology (p. 148). See also "Tumor, malignant, any type."

Possible Associated Conditions: Clonorchiasis;* fibropolycystic disease of the liver and biliary tract;* inflammatory bowel disease;* primary sclerosing cholangitis.*

Organs and Tissues	Procedures	Possible or Expected Findings
External examination	Record body weight.	Cachexia; jaundice.
Duodenum	Open *in situ* for inspection and cholangiography (p. 56).	Tumor of papilla of Vater.
Bile ducts	Expose extrahepatic bile ducts *in situ.* Record width of lumen at area of obstruction and proximal and distal to it. Record and collect contents of bile duct (sludge, concrements, parasites).	Usually, bile ducts proximal to the obstruction are dilated. Choledochal cyst* *(1).* Primary sclerosing cholangitis.* Infestation with *Clonorchis sinensis* or *Opisthorchis viverrini* (rarely observed in North America) *(2).*
Lymph nodes	Dissect all hepatoduodenal lymph nodes and submit samples for histologic study, even if no metastatic tumor is grossly evident.	Lymph nodes seldom compress bile ducts to such an extent that they cause bile duct obstruction.
Portal vein	Dissect vein *in situ.*	Thrombosis* (blood clot or tumor or both); pylephlebitis.
Gallbladder	Record volume and character of contents. Search for primary tumor (with or without cholelithiasis) or tumor infiltration of gallbladder.	Dilatation of gallbladder (Courvoisier's sign); cholecystitis;* cholelithiasis.* White bile.
Liver	Record weight. Submit samples for histologic and microbiologic study (p. 102).	Ascending cholangitis. Cholangitic and pylephlebitic abscesses; cholestasis. Primary sclerosing cholangitis* (PSC) with or without biliary cirrhosis. Secondary (obstructive) biliary cirrhosis without PSC. Intrahepatic metastases.
Colon	Procedures depend on expected findings or grossly identified abnormalities as listed in right-hand column.	Chronic ulcerative colitis may be associated with carcinoma of bile ducts, typically arising in PSC.*
Other organs	Procedures depend on expected findings or grossly identified abnormalities as listed in right-hand column.	Metastases common in regional lymph nodes and lungs.

References

1. Fieber SS, Nance FC. Choledochal cyst and neoplasm: a comprehensive review of 106 cases and presentation of two original cases. Am Surgeon 1997;63:982–987.
2. Elkins DB, Mairiang E, Sithithaworn P, Mairiang P, Chaiyakum J, Chamadol N, et al. Cross sectional patterns of hepatobiliary abnormalities and possible precursor conditions of cholangiocarcinoma associated with Opisthorchis viverrini infections in humans. Am J Trop Med Hyg 1996;55: 295–301.

Tumor of Bone or Cartilage

NOTE: The address of an appropriate registry is Orthopedic Pathology, Armed Forces Institute of Pathology (p. 148). See also "Tumor, malignant, any type."

Possible Associated Conditions: Bone infarction; chronic osteomyelitis;* fibrous dysplasia of bone; Paget's disease of bone.*

Organs and Tissues	*Procedures*	*Possible or Expected Findings*
External examination	Record body weight.	Cachexia.
Vitreous	Submit for determination of electrolyte concentrations. Postmortem calcium in blood is unreliable.	Evidence of hypercalcemia (particularly in presence of osteolytic metastases).
Bones and joints	Prepare roentgenograms or review clinical films. For removal, prosthetic repair, and specimen preparation, see p. 85. For decalcification procedures, see p. 97. If *osteoblastic* metastases appear to be present, search for primary tumor in prostate and breast, carcinoid tumors and Hodgkin's lymphoma.	Metastases to bone (e.g., from carcinoma of prostate, breast, bronchi, thyroid gland, kidney, or urinary bladder) usually involve red bone marrow. Therefore, distal extremities are rarely involved by metastatic tumors in adults.
Other organs	Procedures depend on expected findings or grossly identified abnormalities as listed in right-hand column.	Metastases, commonly in lungs.

Tumor of the Brain

NOTE: The address of an appropriate registry is Neuropathology, Armed Forces Institute of Pathology (p. 148). See also "Tumor, malignant, any type." For pituitary tumors or tumors of the spinal cord, see under these headings.

Possible Associated Conditions: Neurofibromatosis;* tuberous sclerosis;* von Hippel-Lindau Disease.*

Organs and Tissues	*Procedures*	*Possible or Expected Findings*
External examination	Record body weight.	Cachexia.
Brain and spinal cord	For removal and specimen preparation, see pp. 65 and 67, respectively. For cerebral arteriography, see p. 80.	
	If tumor showed endocrine activity, submit fresh sample (snap-freeze) for biochemical study.	Cerebellar hemangioblastoma with erythropoiesis-stimulating factor. Other endocrine-active tumors. See also "Tumor, of the pituitary gland."

Tumor of the Breast

NOTE: The address of an appropriate registry is Gynecologic/Breast Pathology, Armed Forces Institute of Pathology (p. 148). See also "Tumor, malignant, any type."

Possible Associated Conditions: Acanthosis nigricans; cerebellar cortical degeneration;* dermatomyositis;* subacute spinocerebellar degeneration.* See also below under "Possible or Expected Findings."

Organs and Tissues	*Procedures*	*Possible or Expected Findings*
External examination and skin	Record body weight. Record skin abnormalities, prepare photographs of these lesions, and sample for histologic study.	Cachexia. Acanthosis nigricans; herpes zoster infection;* dermatomyositis.* Carcinoma metastases to skin.
Breasts and axillary lymph nodes	Record size and location of tumor. Submit tumor tissue for histologic study. Grossly uninvolved breast tissue as well as sentinel and other axillary lymph nodes of both sides should be cut into thin slices to detect tumor.	Metastases or secondary primary tumor may occur in opposite breast.

Organs and Tissues	Procedures	Possible or Expected Findings
Breasts and axillary lymph nodes *(continued)*	If a mastectomy or other breast surgery had been done, explore site for local recurrence.	Local recurrence of breast tumor.
Other organs	Histologic samples should include right and left supraclavicular and retrosternal lymph nodes, lungs, liver, bone marrow, and endocrine (pituitary) glands.	Regional and systemic metastases frequent at sites listed in middle column. Eosinophilic infiltrates may be present in many tissues.
Brain and spinal cord	For removal and specimen preparation, see pp. 65 and 67, respectively.	Cerebellar cortical degeneration.* Subacute spinocerebellar degeneration.*
Skeletal muscles	For sampling and specimen preparation, see p. 80.	Myopathy;* dermatomyositis.*

Tumor of the Colon

NOTE: The address of an appropriate registry is Hepatic and Gastrointestinal Pathology, Armed Forces Institute of Pathology (p. 148). See also "Tumor, malignant, any type."

Possible Associated Conditions: With adenocarcinoma of the colon—Barrett's esophagus *(1)*; chronic ulcerative colitis; Crohn's disease;* familial colonic polyposis;* Gardner's syndrome; juvenile polyposis; non-polyposis syndrome; Peutz-Jeghers syndrome;* Turcot's syndrome.

Organs and Tissues	Procedures	Possible or Expected Findings
External examination	Record body weight.	Cachexia.
Blood and vitreous	Submit blood sample for microbiologic study (p. 102). Submit vitreous for determination of calcium and glucose concentration. Postmortem calcium values in blood are unreliable.	Increased incidence of colonic cancer in the presence of *S. bovis* bacteremia. Hypercalcemia. Hypoglycemia* may be present but usually cannot be diagnosed at autopsy.
	Circulating carcinoembryonic antigen can be determined in blood sample.	Carcinoembryonic antigen not specific for carcinoma of the colon.
Heart	If endocarditis is suspected, see under that heading.	Increased incidence of colonic cancer in the presence of *S.bovis* endocarditis.
Colon	Record exact location, size, and shape of tumor and width of lumen in area of tumor and proximal and distal to it.	See above under "Possible Associated Conditions." Muscular hypertrophy of colon proximal to tumor.
	Record presence of ureterosigmoidostomy (for congenital extrophy of bladder).	Increased incidence of colon cancer after ureterosigmoidostomy.
Other organs	Procedures depend on expected findings or grossly identified abnormalities as listed in right-hand column. For decalcification methods, see p. 97.	Metastatic calcification in patients with hypercalcemia. Eosinophilia. Myopathy.* Metastases in liver and regional lymph nodes. See also above under "Possible Associated Conditions." Malakoplakia (rare) *(2)*.

References

1. Howden CW, Hornung CA. A systematic review of the association between Barrett's esophagus and colon neoplasm. Am J Gastroenterol 1995;90: 1814–1819.
2. Bates AW, Dev S, Baithun SI. Malakoplakia and colorectal adenocarcinoma. Postgrad Med J 1997;73:171–173.

Tumor of the Esophagus

NOTE: The address of an appropriate registry is Hepatic and Gastrointestinal Pathology, Armed Forces Institute of Pathology (p. 148). See also "Tumor, malignant, any type."

Possible Associated Conditions: Barrett's esophagus;* Plummer-Vinson syndrome;* tylosis of palms and soles. See also below under "Possible or Expected Findings."

Organs and Tissues	Procedures	Possible or Expected Findings
External examination and skin	Record body weight.	Cachexia.
	Record skin changes, prepare photographs, and sample for histologic study.	Congenital hyperkeratosis and pitting of the palms and soles (tylosis of palms and soles).

Organs and Tissues	Procedures	Possible or Expected Findings
Chest	Record volume and character of fluid in pleural cavities.	Pleural empyema.*
	For demonstration of tracheoesophageal fistula, see p. 45 and Fig. 4-1, p. 46. See also below under "Esophagus with neck organs. Submit lymph nodes for histologic study.	Tracheoesophageal fistula. Mediastinitis, with or without mediastinal emphysema. Metastases.
Esophagus with neck organs and stomach	Remove neck organs with tongue together with esophagus (p. 4). Open pharynx and esophagus in posterior midline. If fistulas and abscesses are suspected, dissect esophagus but leave attached to mediastinum, stomach and diaphragm.	Esophageal web and glossitis in Plummer-Vinson syndrome.*
	Record width of lumen of esophagus at various levels. Photograph and record size and location of tumor; sample tumor and uninvolved esophagus for histologic study. Request PAS stain (p. 173) of uninvolved esophagus (sample from all levels).	Esophagus dilated proximal to obstruction, with or without retained food or medications. Stricture or total luminal occlusion by tumor. Reflux esophagitis (distal) and Barrett's esophagus* with low-grade and high-grade dysplasia (distal or at all levels).
Other organs	Procedures depend on expected findings or grossly identified abnormalities as listed in right-hand column.	Metastases in regional lymph nodes and lungs.

Tumor of the Gallbladder

NOTE: Follow procedures described under "Tumor, of the bile ducts (extrahepatic or hilar or of papilla of Vater").

Tumor of the Heart

NOTE: The address of an appropriate registry is Cardiovascular Pathology, Armed Forces Institute of Pathology (p. 148). See also "Tumor, malignant, any type."

Possible Associated Conditions: Carney's syndrome with cardiac myxomas; LAMB syndrome (lentigines, atrial myxoma, blue nevi); NAME syndrome (pigmented nevi, atrial myxoma, myxoid neurofibroma, and ephelids); also with myxoma of the heart: Adrenal cortical nodules with or without Cushing's syndrome;* pituitary adenomas; and testicular tumors. With cardiac rhabdomyoma(s): Adenoma sebaceum; benign kidney tumors;* tuberous sclerosis.*

Organs and Tissues	Procedures	Possible or Expected Findings
External examination	Record and prepare photographs of skin lesions.	Freckles (ephelides); pigmented spots (lentigines) or pigmented nevi; clubbing of fingers (with cardiac myxoma).
Heart	If rhabdomyoma(s) are suspected, submit tumor samples in absolute alcohol (p. 129) or other water-free fixative for demonstration of glycogen. Record size and location of tumor(s). If tumor is within a heart chamber (usually a myxoma), record extent of mobility and capability of tumor to obstruct a valvular orifice. Submit samples of tumor(s) for histologic study and, particularly if the tumor is of unknown type, for immunohistochemical study and electron microscopy (p. 132).	Glycogen in rhabdomyoma is extractable with dilute trichloracetic acid. Tumor types include fibroma, lipoma, myxoma; primary or metastatic sarcoma; lymphoma;* metastatic carcinoma or melanoma. Secondary cardiac effects by tumors include carcinoid heart disease, amyloid heart disease in multiple myeloma, and lymphocytic myocarditis in pheochromocytoma. Treatment effects such as adriamycin cardiotoxicity may be noted also.
Other organs and peripheral arteries	Procedures depend on expected findings or grossly identified abnormalities as listed in right-hand column.	Tumor (myxoma) emboli in pulmonary or peripheral vessels. Multiple aneurysms* of cerebral and other arteries may rarely be associated with atrial myxomas.

Tumor of the Hematopoietic or Lymphatic Tissue (See "Leukemia" or "Lymphoma.")

Tumor of the Intestines (See "Tumor, colon" and "Tumor, of the small intestine.")

Tumor of the Kidney(s)

NOTE: The address of an appropriate registry is Genitourinary Pathology, Armed Forces Institute of Pathology (p. 148). See also "Tumor, malignant, any type."

Possible Associated Conditions: With adult renal cell carcinoma—amyloidosis,* hepatomegaly (Stauffer's syndrome), von Hippel Lindau disease;* also leukemoid reaction and plasmacytosis; with either adult renal cell carcinoma or nephroblastoma—manifestations of hypertension* or polycythemia;* with Wilms tumor—polycythemia* *(1)*; with renal medullary carcinoma—sickle cell disease* *(2)*. See also below under "Possible or Expected Findings."

Organs and Tissues	*Procedures*	*Possible or Expected Findings*
External examination and skin	Record body weight. Record skin changes, prepare photographs, and sample for histologic study.	Cachexia. Excematoid dermatitis with adult renal cell carcinoma. Cushing's syndrome,* galactorrhea or feminization or masculinization in some cases of renal cell carcinoma.
Blood	Submit sample for biochemical study.	Evidence of hyperalcemia.
Lungs	Inspect lumen of pulmonary arteries prior to dissection (fresh emboli may fall out).	Pulmonary tumor embolism after invasion of renal vein and inferior vena cava.
Retroperitoneal space and kidneys	Renal veins and inferior vena cava should be opened *in situ* or after removal of organ block. For dissection technique, see p. 59 and Fig. 5-8, p. 60. Photograph tumor; record size of tumor and extent of tumor invasion.	Acquired renal cystic disease (mainly in dialysis patients) with renal cell carcinoma *(3)*. Tumor thrombus in renal vein and inferior vena cava.
	Snap-freeze portion of tumor tissue for possible biochemical study. For arteriography of kidneys, see p. 59.	Erythropoietin, gonadotropins, parathyroid hormone, prolactin, renin, and prostaglandins in some renal cell carcinomas.
Other organs	Procedures depend on expected findings or grossly identified abnormalities as listed above and in right-hand column.	See above under "Possible Associated Conditions." Metastases are common in lungs and regional lymph nodes.

References

1. Lal A, Rice A, al Mahr M, Kern IB, Marshall GM. Wilms tumor associated with polycythemia: case report and review of the literature. J Pediatr Hematol/Oncol 1997;19:263–265.
2. Wesche WA, Wilimas J, Khare V, Parham DM. Renal medullary carcinoma: a potential sickle cell nephropathy of children and adolescents. Pediatr Pathol Lab Med 1998;18:97–113.
3. Levine E. Acquired cystic kidney disease. Radiol Clin North Am 1996;34:947–964.

Tumor of the Liver

NOTE: The address of an appropriate registry is Hepatic and Gastrointestinal Pathology, Armed Forces Institute of Pathology (p. 148). See also "Tumor, malignant, any type."

Possible Associated Conditions: With hepatocellular carcinoma (HCC)—Alagille's syndrome (arteriohepatic dysplasia), alpha$_1$-antitrypsin deficiency,* alpha-fetoproteinemia, ataxia telangiectasia, Byler's disease, carcinoid syndrome,* cirrhosis* of any type (mostly nonbiliary), congenital hepatic fibrosis,* Cushing's syndrome,* erythrocytosis, genetic hemochromatosis,* glycogen storage disease (type I),* hepatitis B or C virus infection, hereditary tyrosinemia (type I),* hypercalcemia, hypercholesterolemia, hypoglycemia,* neurofibromatosis,* Osler-Rendu-Weber disease* (hereditary hemorrhagic telangiectasia), polycythemia,* porphyria (acute intermittent and porphyria cutanea tarda),* pseudohyperparathyroidism,* and thorium (thorotrast) deposition.

With bile duct carcinoma (cholangiocarcinoma)—*Clonorchis sinensis* or *Opisthorchis viverrini* infection, fibropolycystic liver and biliary tract disease,* hepatolithiasis, hypercalcemia, primary sclerosing cholangitis,* and thorium (thorotrast) deposition.

With hepatoblastoma—Alpha-fetoproteinemia, cardiac and renal malformations, cleft palate, diaphragmatic hernia,* Down's syndrome,* familial colonic polyposis,* hemihypertrophy, nephroblastoma.

With angiosarcoma—Thorium (thorotrast) deposition.

See also below under "Possible or Expected Findings."

Organs and Tissues	*Procedures*	*Possible or Expected Findings*
External examination and skin	Record body weight. Record abnormal features as listed in right-hand column; prepare photographs.	Cachexia. Precocious puberty. Feminization and gynecomastia in rare cases of HCC. Spider angiomas; clubbing of fingers.
Blood	Refrigerate sample for possible biochemical study.	See above under "Possible Associated Conditions."

Organs and Tissues	Procedures	Possible or Expected Findings
Abdominal cavity	Record volume and character of contents; determine hematocrit of hemorrhagic fluid.	Hemoperitoneum or ascites (which may be hemorrhagic).
Liver	For hepatic angiography, see p. 56. Record weight and size of liver and size and location of tumor(s). Describe and photograph cut surfaces.	Tumor thrombi or thromboses in hepatic and portal veins. Hemorrhages after rupture of tumor (HCC and angiosarcoma).
	Sample tumor and nonneoplastic liver for histologic study. If thorium deposition is suspected, prepare roentgenograms of liver slices and submit samples for energy-dispersive x-ray microanalysis of paraffin sections.	Evidence of chronic viral hepatitis B or C;* cirrhosis* of any type (mostly nonbiliary). Thorotrast storage may cause cirrhosis, HCC, bile duct carcinoma, or angiosarcoma.
Other organs	Procedures depend on expected findings or grossly identified abnormalities as listed above and in right-hand column.	See above under "Possible Associated Conditions." Metastases most common in lungs and regional lymph nodes.

Tumor of the Lung or Bronchus

NOTE: The address of an appropriate registry is Pulmonary and Mediastinal Pathology, Armed Forces Institute of Pathology (p. 148). See also "Tumor, malignant, any type."

Possible Associated Conditions: Abnormal concentrations of hormons or other metabolites in blood and tumor tissue (adrenocorticotropic, antidiuretic, growth hormone, parathyroid-like substances, or 5-hydroxyindolacetic acid); acanthosis nigricans; acromegaloid features; carcinoid syndrome;* Cushing's syndrome;* dermal hyperpigmentation; feminization; hyperglycemia; hypercalcemia; hypoglycemia;* hypokalemia; hyponatremia; precocious puberty. For syndromes affecting the brain, peripheral nerves or muscles, see below under "Possible or Expected Findings." (Most paracarcinomatous syndromes are associated with small cell or other types of bronchogenic carcinoma.)

Organs and Tissues	Procedures	Possible or Expected Findings
External examination and skin	Record body weight. Record abnormal features as listed in right-hand column; prepare photographs. Prepare histologic sections of normal and grossly abnormal skin. Prepare skeletal roentgenograms.	Cachexia. Skin metastases. Clubbing of fingers; spider angiomas. For other rare tumor-related changes, see above under "Possible Associated Conditions." Hypertrophic osteoarthropathy;* pachydermoperiostosis. Bone marrow metastases.
Blood and vitreous	Submit samples of vitreous for study of electrolyte and sugar concentrations. Submit sample of serum for possible hormon assay.	See above under "Possible Associated Conditions." Note that hypoglycemia* generally cannot be confirmed at autopsy.
Heart	Inspect valves and prepare photographs and sections of vegetations.	Nonbacterial thrombotic endocarditis.*
Lungs	For pulmonary arteriography and bronchography, see p. 50. Record size and location of tumor(s). If there was evidence of endocrine activity (see above), snap-freeze portion of fresh tumor for hormone assay. For demonstration of asbestos bodies, see p. 52. Perfuse lungs with formalin (p. 47). Sample neoplastic and non-neoplastic tissue for histologic study.	Carcinoma may be associated with asbestosis or other types of pneumoconiosis,* chronic bronchitis,* emphysema,* interstitial pneumonia,* and many other bronchopulmonary diseases.
Other organs and tissues	Procedures depend on expected findings or grossly identified abnormalities as listed above and in right-hand column.	See above under "Possible Associated Conditions." Metastases (regional lymph nodes, liver, bones, brain, and many other sites) and metastatic calcification.
Peripheral veins	For removal and specimen preparation, see p. 34.	Migratory thrombophlebitis.*
Brain and spinal cord	For removal and specimen preparation, see pp. 65 and 67, respectively.	Encephalomyelitis;* cerebellar corticoid degeneration;* subacute spinocerebellar degeneration.*

Organs and Tissues	Procedures	Possible or Expected Findings
Pituitary gland	For removal and specimen preparation, see p. 71.	Crooke cell hyperplasia.
Skeletal muscles and peripheral nerves	For removal and specimen preparation, see p. 80 and 79, respectively.	Myasthenic syndrome (Eaton-Lambert syndrome); myopathy;* dermatomyositis.* Peripheral neuropathy.
Bones	For removal and specimen preparation, see p. 95.	See above under "External examination and skin." Bones (with red marrow) are common sites of metastases.

Tumor of the Ovary (or Ovaries)

NOTE: The address of an appropriate registry is Gynecologic/Breast Pathology, Armed Forces Institute of Pathology (p. 148). See also "Tumor, malignant, any type."

Possible Associated Conditions: Cushing's syndrome,* dermal hyperpigmentation; dermatomyositis.* See also below under "Possible or Expected Findings."

Organs and Tissues	Procedures	Possible or Expected Findings
External examination and skin	Record body weight.	Cachexia.
	Record and prepare photographs of abnormal features as listed in right-hand column. Prepare histologic sections of normal and grossly abnormal skin.	Dermal hyperpigmentation; dermatomyositis.* Cushingoid features. Gangrene of fingers *(1)*.
Vitreous	Submit samples for electrolyte analysis. Postmortem calcium values in blood are unreliable.	Hypercalcemia.
Abdominal cavity and pelvic organs	Record appearance of peritoneum and volume and character of intraabdominal fluid.	Peritoneal carcinomatosis; ascites.
	If possible, remove pelvic organs with tumor(s) en block. Record size, weight, and appearance of ovarian tumor.	Tumors may be bilateral or may be so large (e.g., cystadenocarcinoma) that they are difficult to remove with pelvic organs.
Other organs and tissues, including skeletal muscles	For sampling and specimen preparation, see p. 80.	See above under "Possible Associated Conditions."
Peripheral veins	For phlebography and removal of femoral veins, see pp. 120 and 34, respectively.	Venous thromboses.*
Brain and spinal cord	For removal and specimen preparation, see pp. 65 and 67, respectively.	Cerebellar cortical degeneration.*

Reference

1. Chow SF, McKenna CH. Ovarian cancer and gangrene of the digits: case report and review of the literature. Mayo Clin Proc 1996;71:253–258.

Tumor of the Pancreas

NOTE: The address of an appropriate registry is Hepatic and Gastrointestinal Pathology, Armed Forces Institute of Pathology (p. 148). See also "Tumor, malignant, any type."

Possible Associated Conditions: With carcinoma of the exocrine pancreas—Cushing's syndrome;* diabetes mellitus* (rare); hypercalcemia; hyperglycemia; dermal hyperpigmentation; pemphigus* *(1)*; Peutz-Jeghers syndrome* *(2)*; venous thromboses or thrombophlebitis.

With islet cell tumor—Abnormal concentrations of hormons in blood and tumor tissue (see below under "pancreas"); carcinoid syndrome;* Cushing's syndrome;* diabetes mellitus;* hypoglycemia;* hypokalemia; Zollinger-Ellison syndrome.*

Organs and Tissues	Procedures	Possible or Expected Findings
External examination and skin	Record body weight.	Cachexia; jaundice.
	Record abnormal features as listed in right-hand column; prepare photographs. Prepare histologic sections of normal and grossly abnormal skin.	Cushingoid features. Dermal hyperpigmentation. For other rare tumor-related changes, see above under "Possible Associated Conditions."

Organs and Tissues	Procedures	Possible or Expected Findings
Blood and vitreous	Submit samples of vitreous for determination of electrolyte and glucose concentrations (p. 114) Blood values are often unreliable. Snap-freeze serum for possible hormone assay.	See above under "Possible Associated Conditions." Note that hypoglycemia generally cannot be confirmed at autopsy.
Heart	Inspect valves and prepare photographs and sections of vegetations.	Nonbacterial thrombotic endocarditis.*
Esophagus and gastrointestinal tract	Record or estimate volume of blood in lumen.	Esophageal varices.* Gastrointestinal hemorrhage.
Pancreas	For pancreatography, see p. 57. Dissect common bile duct *in situ*. Record size and location of tumor in relationship to head, body, and tail of pancreas.	Biliary obstruction caused by tumor in head of pancreas.
	Portions of primary or metastatic endocrine tumors should be snap-frozen for biochemical and histochemical study and for hormone assay. For preparation of tissue for electron microscopy, see p. 132.	Islet cell tumor with adrenocorticotropic hormone, gastrin, glucagon, insulin, or other peptide hormones.
Other organs	Procedures depend on expected findings or grossly identified abnormalities as listed above and in right-hand column.	See above under "Possible Associated Conditions." Regional lymph nodes and liver are common sites of metastases.
Veins	For phlebography and removal of femoral veins, see pp. 120 and 34, respectively.	Venous thrombosis or migratory thrombophlebitis associated with carcinoma of exocrine pancreas.

References

1. Matz H, Milner Y, Frusic-Zlotkin M, Brenner S. Paraneoplastic pemphigus associated with pancreatic carcinoma. Acta-Dermato-Venereol 1997;77:289–291.
2. Pauwels M, Delcenserie R, Yzet T, Duchmann JC, Capron JP. Pancreatic cystadenocarcinoma in Peutz-Jeghers syndrome. J Clin Gastroenterol 1997;25:485–486.

Tumor of the Peripheral Nerves

NOTE: The address of an appropriate registry is Neuropathology, Armed Forces Institute of Pathology (p. 148). See also "Tumor, malignant, all types."

Possible Associated Conditions: Abnormal concentrations of metabolites in urine and tumor tissue (with ganglioneuroma or neuroblastoma); neurofibromatosis;* pheochromocytoma.

Organs and Tissues	Procedures	Possible or Expected Findings
External examination and skin	Record abnormal pigmentations and presence of skin tumors.	Manifestations of neurofibromatosis.*
Urine	If ganglioneuroma or neuroblastoma is suspected, submit sample for determination of catecholamin concentration.	Abnormal concentrations of catecholamine in association with ganglioneuroma or neuroblastoma.
Peripheral nerves and tumor tissue	Record size and location. If biochemical study is intended, snap-freeze tumor tissue. For removal and specimen preparation of peripheral nerves, see p. 79.	Catecholamine may be found in ganglioneuroma or neuroblastoma.
Other organs and tissues	Procedures depend on expected findings or grossly identified abnormalities as listed above.	See above under "Possible Associated Conditions."

Tumor of the Pituitary Gland

NOTE: See also "Tumor, malignant, any type."

Possible Associated Conditions: Acromegaly;* Cushing's syndrome.* See also below under "Possible or Expected Findings."

Organs and Tissues	Procedures	Possible or Expected Findings
External examination	Record abnormal features as listed in right-hand column.	Features of acromegaly* or of Cushing's syndrome.*

Organs and Tissues	*Procedures*	*Possible or Expected Findings*
Pituitary gland	For removal and specimen preparation, see p. 71. Record size, weight, and boundaries of tumor; photograph tumor *in situ* and after removal. If hormone assay is intended, snap-freeze portion of tumor. Prolactin and growth hormone cells can be localized by the immunoperoxidase method. If an adenoma of unknown type is suspected, submit sample for electron microscopic study (p. 132).	Carcinoma metastases in the pituitary gland most commonly originate from breast carcinoma. Usually, metastases are found in the posterior lobe, whereas adenomas are anterior lobe tumors.
Other organs and tissues	Procedures depend on expected findings or grossly identified abnormalities as listed in right-hand column.	Manifestations of pituitary insufficiency* or of excessive hormone production (acromegaly,* Cushing's syndrome*).

Tumor of the Pleura

NOTE: The address of an appropriate registry is Pulmonary and Mediastinal Pathology, Armed Forces Institute of Pathology (p. 148). See also "Tumor, malignant, any type."

Organs and Tissues	*Procedures*	*Possible or Expected Findings*
External examination	Record abnormal features as listed in right-hand column. Prepare roentgenograms of chest and extremities.	Hypertrophic osteoarthropathy* (with pleural mesothelioma).
Chest cavity	Record character and volume of pleural effusions. Record size and location of tumor(s).	Pleural effusions.*
	Submit sample of tumor tissue and of non-neoplastic lung tissue for analysis of asbestos bodies (p. 52).	Asbestosis may be complicated by pleural mesothelioma.
Other organs and tissue	Document absence of tumor that might have metastasized to pleurae.	Pleural metastases from distant primary tumors may mimic mesothelioma.

Tumor of the Prostate

NOTE: The address of an appropriate registry is Genitourinary Pathology, Armed Forces Institute of Pathology (p. 148). See also "Tumor, malignant, any type."

Possible Associated Conditions: Cushing's syndrome;* disseminated intravascular coagulation;* hemolytic uremic syndrome* *(1)*; osteomalacia* *(2)*.

Organs and Tissues	*Procedures*	*Possible or Expected Findings*
External examination	Record body weight.	Cachexia.
	Record abnormal features as listed in right-hand column.	Dermal hyperpigmentation; Cushingoid features.
	Prepare roentgenograms of chest, thoracic and lumbar spine, and extremities.	Osteomalacia *(2)*. Osteoblastic bone metastases.
Pelvic organs with prostate; testes	For dissection of pelvic organs, see p. 59.	Infiltrating carcinoma of prostate may cause obstructive uropathy and other complications.
	Record presence or absence of testes.	Testes may have been surgically removed to achieve androgen deprivation.
Other organs	Procedures depend on expected findings or grossly identified abnormalities as listed in right-hand column.	Urinary obstruction and hydronephrosis.* Osteoblastic metastases, particularly in vertebral bodies. See also above under "Possible Associated Conditions."

References

1. Muller NJ, Pestalozzi BC. Hemolytic uremic syndrome in prostatic carcinoma. Oncol 1998;55:174–176.
2. Reese DM, Rosen PJ. Oncogenic osteomalacia associated with prostatic cancer. J Urol 1997;158:887.

Tumor of the Small Intestine

NOTE: The address of an appropriate registry is Hepatic and Gastrointestinal Pathology, Armed Forces Institute of Pathology (p. 148). See also "Tumor, malignant, any type."

Possible Associated Conditions: Acquired immunodeficiency syndrome* (AIDS) in patients with small bowel lymphoma;* Carcinoid syndrome;* familial polyposis and related syndromes* (Cronkhite-Canada syndrome; Gardner's syndrome); Peutz-Jeghers syndrome.*

Organs and Tissues	*Procedures*	*Possible or Expected Findings*
External examination	Record body weight. Record abnormal features as listed above.	Cachexia. Mucocutaneous pigmentations associated with Peutz-Jeghers syndrome.*
Small and large bowel	For mesenteric angiography, see p. 55. For *in situ* fixation of small intestine, see p. 54.	
	If there is a history of carcinoid syndrome,* see under that entry. A frozen section diagnosis of the tumor may help to determine how to process the tumor tissue and what stains to order. Submit sample of non-neoplastic small bowel for histologic study.	Carcinoid tumor. Lymphoma (see also above under "Possible Associated Conditions"). Familial polyposis or related syndrome.* Celiac sprue.* Crohn's disease.*
Other organs and tissues	Procedures depend on expected findings or grossly identified abnormalities as listed above.	See above under "Possible Associated Conditions." Regional lymph nodes and liver are common sites of metastases.

Tumor of the Soft Tissues

NOTE: The address of an appropriate registry is Soft Tissue Pathology, Armed Forces Institute of Pathology (p. 148). See also "Tumor, malignant, any type."

The possible sites and characteristics of soft tissue tumors vary so much that no universally applicable autopsy techniques can be presented. In all instances, the size, weight, and location of the tumor(s) must be recorded and tissue must be sampled for histologic study. If the tumor had not been classified prior to death, samples should be snap-frozen for immunohistochemical study. Other samples should be prepared for electron microscopic study (p. 132). Evidence of paraneoplastic syndromes (see below) may require additional procedures.

Possible Associated Conditions: Only a few paraneoplastic syndromes or systemic complications can be presented here. For the type of soft tissue tumor that was associated with each condition, see title of reference. Kasabach-Merritt syndrome *(1)* (thrombocytopenia, microangiopathic hemolytic anemia, and acute or chronic coagulopathy associated with a rapidly enlarging hemangioma); liver function abnormalities *(2)*; neurofibromatosis *(3)*; osteomalacia *(4)*.

References

1. Esterly NB. Kasabach Merritt syndrome in infants. J Am Acad Dermatol 1983;8:504–513.
2. Sharara AI, Panella TJ, Fitz JG. Paraneoplastic hepatopathy associated with soft tissue sarcoma. Gastroenterol 1992;103:330–332.
3. Hartley AL, Birch JM, Marsden HB, Harris M, Blair V. Neurofibromatosis in children with soft tissue sarcoma. Pediatr Hematol Oncol 1988;5:7–16.
4. Zura RD, Minasi JS, Kahler DM. Tumor-induced osteomalacia and symptomatic looser zones secondary to mesenchymal chondrosarcoma. J Surg Oncol 1999;71:58–62.

Tumor of the Spinal Cord

NOTE: The address of an appropriate registry is Neuropathology, Armed Forces Institute of Pathology (p. 148). See also "Tumor, malignant, any type."

Possible Associated Conditions: With angioma—cerebellar hemangioblastoma; segmental cutaneous vascular nevi; with hemangioblastoma—von Hippel-Lindau disease;* with arteriovenous malformation—vertebral hemangioma(s).

Organs and Tissues	*Procedures*	*Possible or Expected Findings*
External examination and skin	Record abnormal features; photograph and submit nevi for histologic study.	Segmental cutaneous vascular nevi (associated with spinal cord angiomas).
Brain and spinal cord	For removal and specimen preparation, see pp. 65 and 67, respectively. See also below under "Vertebral column." Describe gross appearance, location, and size of spinal cord tumor and status of adjacent spinal cord.	Subarachnoid hemorrhage.* Spinal cord compression; ischemic spinal cord changes. See also above under "Possible Associated Conditions."

Organs and Tissues	Procedures	Possible or Expected Findings
Vertebral column	Record and photograph changes listed in right-hand column.	Bone erosion and calcification of spinal canal. Vertebral hemangiomas may be associated with arteriovenous malformation of spinal cord.
Other organs and tissues	Procedures depend on expected findings or grossly identified abnormalities as listed in right-hand column.	Manifestations of von Hippel-Lindau disease.*

Tumor of the Stomach

NOTE: The address of an appropriate registry is "Hepatic and Gastrointestinal Pathology, Armed Forces Institute of Pathology (p. 148). See also "Tumor, malignant, any type."

Possible Associated Conditions: Hypoglycemia;* megaloblastic anemia;* skin changes (as listed under "Possible or Expected Findings); venous thromboses.

Organs and Tissues	Procedures	Possible or Expected Findings
External examination and skin	Record body weight.	Cachexia.
	Record abnormal features; photograph and submit samples of normal and abnormal skin for histologic study.	Acanthosis nigricans; hyperkeratosis palmaris and plantaris *(1)*. Pyoderma gangrenosum. Dermatomyositis;* herpes zoster.* Periumbilical metastases.
Blood and vitreous	In most instances, determination of vitreous sugar concentration and of blood group is not indicated.	Hypoglycemia may have been present but this condition generally cannot be confirmed at autopsy. Blood group A is more common in patients with carcinoma of stomach than in controls.
Heart	Inspect valves and prepare photographs and sections of vegetations.	Nonbacterial thrombotic endocarditis.*
Esophagus, stomach, and duodenum	Leave esophagus and part of duodenum attached to stomach.	Acanthosis of the esophagus *(1)*.
	For specimen preparation of stomach, see p. 53.	
	Submit samples of tumor and of grossly uninvolved stomach for histologic study. Request PAS stain and Warthin-Starry stain (p. 173) for identification of *H. pylori.*	Chronic gastritis with or without intestinal metaplasia. Infection with *H. pylori* (with carcinoma or lymphoma *[2]*).
	Portions of endocrine gastric tumor should be snap-frozen for immunohistochemical study and possible hormone assay.	Gastric carcinoid tumors; neuroendocrine carcinoma (rare).
Other organs and tissues		Eosinophilia. Manifestations of paraneoplastic syndromes as listed above under "Possible Associated Conditions."
	Record location of tumor metastases.	Metastases common in liver, retroperitoneal and supraclavicular lymph nodes (Virchow's node), ovaries (Krukenberg tumor), and peritoneal cul de sac (Blumer's shelf").

References

1. Murata I, Ogami Y, Nagai Y, Furuma K, Yoshikawa I, Otsuli M. Carcinoma of the stomach with hyperkeratosis palmaris and plantaris and acanthosis of the esophagus. Am J Gastroenterol 1998;93:449–451.
2. Wotherspoon AC. Gastric lymphoma of mucosa-associated lymphoid tissue and Helicobacter pylori. Ann Rev Med 1998;49:289–299.

Tumor of the Testis

NOTE: The address of an appropriate registry is Genitourinary Pathology, Armed Forces Institute of Pathology (p. 148). See also "Tumor, malignant, any type."

Possible Associated Conditions: Demyelinating neuropathy *(1)*; dermatomyositis* *(2)*; Down's syndrome;* eosinophilia; herpes zoster;* megaloblastic anemia.*

Organs and Tissues	Procedures	Possible or Expected Findings
External examination	Record body weight. Record genital abnormalities as listed in right-hand column. Submit breast tissue for histologic study.	Cachexia. Cryptorchism; hypospadia. Gynecomastia.
Blood and urine	Freeze samples for hormone assay.	Increased concentrations of alpha-fetoprotein and human chorionic gonadotropin.
Kidneys	If indicated, follow procedures described under "glomerulonephritis."	Glomerulonephritis;* developmental anomalies *(3)*.
Testes	Record location, size, and weight of both testes and of testicular tumor. Submit samples of tumor and of ininvolved testis and epididymis for histologic study. Snap-freeze tumor tissue for hormone assay.	Cryptorchid testis with tumor or contralateral to testicular tumor. Testicular microlithiasis. Secondary testicular tumors (metastases to the testes) are rare, except in association with leukemia* in children.
Other organs	Procedures depend on expected findings or grossly identified abnormalities as listed in right-hand column. For dissection of the thoracic duct (for search of tumor cell clusters), see p. 34.	Pulmonari embolism.* Paraneoplastic diseases as listed above under "Possible Associated Conditions." Metastases are found primarily in retroperitoneal lymph nodes, left supraclavicular lymph nodes, and lungs.

References

1. Greenspan BN, Felice KJ. Chronic inflammatory demyelinating polyneuropathy (CIDP) associated with seminoma. Eur Neurol 1998;39:57–58.
2. Hayami S, Kubota Y, Sasagawa I, Suzuki H, Nakada N, Motoyama T. Dermatomyositis associated with intratubular germ cell tumor and metastatic germ cell cancer. J Urol 1998;159:2096–2097.
3. Klein EA, Chen RN, Levin HS, Rackley RR, Williams BR. Testicular cancer in association with developmental renal anomalies and hypospadias. Urol 1996;47:82–87.

Tumor of the Thymus

NOTE: The address of an appropriate registry is Hematologic and Lymphatic Pathology, Armed Forces Institute of Pathology (p. 148). See also "Tumor, Malignant, any type."

Possible Associated Conditions: Anemia (autoimmune hemolytic or aplastic);* Cushing's syndrome;* dermal hyperpigmentation; hypogammaglobulinemia (and other immunoglobulin abnormalities); myasthenia gravis;* pancytopenia;* pemphigus foliaceus; polymyositis;* Sjögren's syndrome;* thrombotic thrombocytopenic purpura* *(1)*. See also below under "Other organs."

Organs and Tissues	Procedures	Possible or Expected Findings
External examination	Record body weight. Record and prepare photographs of skin abnormalities; sample for histologic study.	Cachexia. Dermal hyperpigmentation. Pemphigus foliaceus (rare).
Blood	Submit samples for protein analysis.	Hypogammaglobulinemia and other immunoglobulin abnormalities.
Chest	Photograph and dissect tumor *in situ*. Record size, weight, gross appearance, and relationship to thoracic veins, pericardium, lungs, and other tissues. Sample for histologic and electron microscopic study (p. 132).	Usually, thymoma presents as an infiltrating, anterior mediastinal mass that rarely metastasizes. Carcinoid tumor, malignant lymphoma* (Hodgkin's disease), and metastases from carcinoma of the breast* and other tumors also may occur in this location.
Heart	Record weight. Submit samples for histologic study (p. 30).	Idiopathic granulomatous myocarditis.*
Kidneys	Follow procedures described under "Glomerulonephritis."	Minimal-change or membranous nephropathy; extracapillary glomerulonephritis* *(2)*.
Other organs	Submit samples of lymph nodes, spleen, Peyer's plaques, and bone marrow (p. 96) for histologic study.	Viral (e.g., herpes simplex*) and fungal infections (e.g., candidiasis*) due to thymoma-related immunodeficiency *(3)*.

Organs and Tissues	*Procedures*	*Possible or Expected Findings*
Other organs *(continued)*	Other procedures depend on expected findings or grossly identified abnormalities as listed in right-hand column.	Manifestations of paraneoplastic diseases and conditions as listed above under "Possible Associated Conditions."

References

1. Hatama S, Kumagai H, Iwato K, Fujiwara M, Fujishima M. Thrombotic thrombocytopenic purpura accompanied by transient pure red cell aplasia and thymoma. Clin Nephrol 1998;49:193–197.
2. Valli G, Fogazzi GB, Cappelari A, Rivolta E. Glomerulonephritis associated with myasthenia gravis. Am J Kidney Dis 1998;31:350–355.
3. Sicherer SH, Cabana MD, Perlman EJ, Lederman HM, Matsakis RR, Winkelstein JA. Thymoma and cellular immune deficiency in an adolescent. Pediatr Allergy Immunol 1998;9:49–52.

Tumor of the Thyroid Gland

NOTE: See also "Tumor, malignant, any type."

Possible Associated Conditions: With papillary carcinoma—Familial adenomatous polyposis* *(1)*; with medullary thyroid carcinoma—Multiple endocrine neoplasia (MEN, type 2A or 2B).*

Organs and Tissues	*Procedures*	*Possible or Expected Findings*
External examination	Record abnormal features.	Acromegaly* *(2)*.
Neck organs with thyroid organs	Leave thyroid gland and tumor attached to trachea until degree of tracheal compression can be recorded. Identify exact location of cervical lymph nodes that are submitted for histologic study.	Upper airway obstruction *(3)*. Benign nodular goiter or adenoma(s); carcinoma or lymphoma. Hashimoto's thyroiditis with lymphoma.
	If medullary carcinoma is suspected, snap-freeze portion of fresh tumor for hormone assay.	Thyrocalcitonin in medullary carcinoma of thyroid.
Other organs	Samples of thymic tissue, lymph nodes, and endocrine glands should be submitted for histologic study. Other procedures depend on expected findings or grossly identified abnormalities as listed in right-hand column.	Manifestations of hyperthyroidism,* which may be associated with metastasizing follicular carcinoma. Manifestations of MEN (see above under "Possible Associated Conditions").

References

1. Cetta F, Toti P, Petracci M, Montalto G, Disanto A, Lore F, Fusco A. Thyroid carcinoma associated with familial adenomatous polyposis. Histopathology 1997;31:231–236.
2. Balkany C, Cushing GW. An association between acromegaly and thyroid carcinoma. Thyroid 1995;5:47–50.
3. Carter N, Milroy CM. Thyroid carcinoma causing fatal laryngeal obstruction. J Laryngol Otol 1996;110:1176–1178.

Tumor of the Urinary Bladder

NOTE: The address of an appropriate registry is Genitourinary Pathology, Armed Forces Instituite of Pathology (p. 148). See also "Tumor, malignant, any type."

Organs and Tissues	*Procedures*	*Possible or Expected Findings*
External examination	Record body weight.	Cachexia.
Kidneys and ureters	Leave these organs attached to urinary bladder, particularly if hydronephrosis and hydroureter are noted. En block removal of abdominal organs generally is the best approach (p. 3).	Hydronephrosis* (obstructive uropathy) and hydroureter, usually caused by distal ureteral obstruction. Recurrent nephrolithiasis* or pyelitis may have been present and is a risk factor for urinary bladder carcinoma.
Pelvic organs with urinary bladder	For *in situ* fixation and dissection of the urinary bladder, see p. 59.	
	Sample bladder tumor and uninvolved urinary bladder for histologic study.	Chronic urocystitis; infestation with *Schistosoma haematobium (1)* (uncommon in North America).
Other organs		Manifestations of uremia (see "Failure, kidney").

Reference

1. Bedwani R, Renganathan E, El Kwhsky F, Braga C, Abu Seif HH, Abul Azm T, et al. Schistosomiasis and the risk of bladder cancer in Alexandria, Egypt. Br J Canc 1998;77:1186–1189.

Tumor of the Uterus (with Cervix)

NOTE: The address of an appropriate registry is Gynecologic/Breast Pathology, Armed Forces Institute of Pathology (p. 148). See also "Tumor, malignant, any type."

Possible Associated Conditions: Acquired immunodeficiency syndrome* (AIDS) *(1)*. With carcinoma of the uterus—Cerebellar cortical degeneration;* with carcinoma of the cervix—Myopathy.*

Organs and Tissues	*Procedures*	*Possible or Expected Findings*
External examination	Record body weight.	Cachexia.
Vitreous	Submit samples for determination of calcium concentrations. Postmortem calcium values in blood are unreliable.	Evidence of hypercalcemia.
Kidneys and ureters	Leave these organs attached to urinary bladder, particularly if there is evidence of hydronephrosis and hydroureter. En block removal of abdominal organs generally is the best approach (p. 3).	Hydronephrosis* (obstructive uropathy) and hydroureter, usually caused by distal ureteral obstruction.
Pelvic organs	Record size and location of tumor; sample tumor and non-neoplastic uterus and cervix for histologic study. If indicated, submit samples for electron microscopic study.	Fistulas to urinary bladder or rectum or both. Human papilloma virus infection *(2)* or herpesvirus infection *(3)* with invasive cervical carcinoma.
	If hormone assay is intended, snap-freeze portion of tumor.	Erythropoietin may be found in some tumors.
Veins	For removal of femoral veins, see p. 34.	Thrombosis.*
Skeletal muscles	For sampling and specimen preparation, see p. 80.	Myopathy* may be associated with carcinoma of the cervix.
Brain and spinal cord	For removal and specimen preparation, see pp. 65 and 67, respectively.	Cerebellar cortical degeneration* may be associated with carcinoma of the uterus.
Other organs	Procedures depend on expected findings or grossly identified abnormalities as listed in right-hand column.	Manifestations of uremia (see "Failure, kidney"). Manifestations of acquired immunodeficiency syndrome* (AIDS).

References

1. Chin KM, Sidhu JS, Janssen RS, Weber JT. Invasive cervical cancer in human immunodeficiency virus-infected and uninfected hospital patients. Obstetr Gynecol 1998;92:83–87.
2. Ursic-Vrscaj M, Kovacic J, Poljak M, Marin J. Association of risk factors for cervical cancer and human papilloma viruses in invasive cervical cancer. Eur J Gynaecol Oncol 1996;17:368–371.
3. Koffa M, Koumantakis E, Ergazaki M, Tsatsanis C, Spandidos DA. Association of herpesvirus infection with the development of genital cancer. Intl J Canc 1995;63:58–62.

Tumor, Wilms (See "Tumor of the kidney(s).")

Tyrosinemia

Synonyms and Related Terms: Fumarylacetoacetate hydrolase deficiency; aminoaciduria.*

Organs and Tissues	*Procedures*	*Possible or Expected Findings*
External examination and skin	Record body weight. Note odor.	Growth delay. The body may have a "fishy" odor.
	Sample skin for histologic study.	Hyperkeratosis of skin *(1)*.
	Prepare skeletal roentgenograms (especially of epiphyses).	Hypophosphatemic rickets.
Fascia lata	Specimens should be collected using aseptic technique for tissue culture for biochemical studies (see Chapter 10).	Enzyme deficiency (see above under "Synonyms and Related Terms").

Organs and Tissues	*Procedures*	*Possible or Expected Findings*
Blood	Submit samples for culture (p. 102) and biochemical analysis.	Sepsis. Increased concentrations of methionine, tyrosine, alpha-fetoprotein, and delta-aminolevulinic acid.
Urine	Submit sample for biochemical analysis.	Evidence of aminoaciduria (see above under "Blood"); tyrosine metabolites.
Liver	Record weight, photograph cut surfaces, and sample for histologic study (include nodules that might be neoplastic).	Enlarged liver with lobular disarray, fibrosis or cirrhosis;* steatosis; cholestasis; hepatocellular carcinoma *(2)*.
Kidneys	Weigh both kidneys and submit for histologic study.	Tubular ectasia; tubular calcification.
Other organs	Procedures depend on expected findings or grossly identified abnormalities as listed in right-hand column.	Evidence of bleeding. Islet cell hyperplasia and mineralization of pancreas; hepatic encephalopathy.*
Bones	Prepare sections of epiphyses for histologic study (p. 95).	See above under "External examination."

References

1. Benoldi D, Orsoni JB, Allegra F. Tyrosinemia type II: a challenge for ophthalmologists and dermatologists. Ped Dermatol 1997;14:110–112.
2. Dehner LP, Snover DC, Sharp HL, Ascher N, Nakhleh R, Day DL. Hereditary tyrosinemia type I (chronic form): Pathologic findings in the liver. Hum Pathol 1989;20:149–158.

U

Ulcer, Peptic, of Stomach or Duodenum

Possible Associated Conditions: Multiple endocrine neoplasia;* rheumatoid arthritis;* Zollinger-Ellison syndrome.*

Organs and Tissues	*Procedures*	*Possible or Expected Findings*
External examination	Prepare roentgenograms of chest and abdomen.	Free air in abdomen suggests perforation of ulcer.
Peritoneal cavity	If peritonitis is present, submit exudate for bacteriologic study (p. 102). Record volume of exudate and location of perforation.	Peritonitis.* Perforation of ulcer.
Heart	See "Disease, ischemic heart."	Coronary atherosclerosis and manifestations of coronary insufficiency are commonly associated with peptic ulcer disease.
	Other procedures depend on grossly identified abnormalities as listed in right-hand column.	In rare instances, pericardial fistula may be present from ulcer in hiatus hernia.
Lungs	Procedures depend on expected findings or grossly identified abnormalities as listed in right-hand column. Perfuse on lung with formalin (p. 47).	Peptic ulcers may be associated with emphysema,* tuberculosis,* and other chronic pulmonary diseases.
Stomach and duodenum	For celiac arteriography, see p. 55. Open stomach and duodenum *in situ* and record site of perforation or penetration. Record measured or estimated volume of blood in gastrointestinal tract. Rinse ulcer with saline to locate eroded vessel(s).	Perforating or penetrating peptic ulcer. Infiltrating and ulcerating carcinoma or lymphoma of stomach.* Gastrointestinal hemorrhage.*
	Pin stomach and duodenum on corckboard (serosa toward board) and fix specimen in formalin before sectioning. Prepare histologic sections of ulcer(s) and of remainder of stomach. Request Warthin-Starry stain (p. 173) for *H. pylori.*	Chronic gastritis (with *H. pylori* infection) and duodenitis.
Other organs	Procedures depend on expected findings or grossly identified abnormalities as listed in right-hand column.	Manifestations of multiple endocrine neoplasia;* Zollinger-Ellison syndrome,* and rheumatoid arthritis.*

Uncinariasis (See "Ancylostomiasis.")

Uremia (See "Failure, kidney.")

Uropathy, Obstructive (See "Hydronephrosis.")

Urticaria Pigmentosa of Childhood (See "Mastocytosis, systemic.")

From: *Handbook of Autopsy Practice,* 3rd Ed. Edited by: J. Ludwig © Humana Press Inc., Totowa, NJ

V–X

Valve, Congenitally Bicuspid Aortic

Possible Associated Conditions: Acute aortic dissection;* aneurysma(s) of cerebral arteries; aortic insufficiency;* calcific aortic stenosis,* coarctation of the aorta;* infective endocarditis;* Shone's syndrome; Turner's syndrome.*

Organs and Tissues	*Procedures*	*Possible or Expected Findings*
Heart	If infective endocarditis is suspected, see p. 103. Open heart in cross-sections (p. 22). Photograph aortic valve and test valvular competence (p. 29). Prepare histologic section of aortic valve, if infected; request Gram and Grocott's methenamine silver stains (p. 172).	Infective endocarditis* of bicuspid aortic valve. Aortic valvular insufficiency* may be present.

Valve, Congenitally Bicuspid Pulmonary

Possible Associated Conditions: Double outlet left ventricle; tetralogy of Fallot;* complete or congenitally corrected transposition of the great arteries;* tricuspid atresia;* congenitally bicuspid aortic valve.*

Valve, Congenitally Quadricuspid Aortic

NOTE: The condition may be complicated by infective endocarditis.* Follow procedures described under that heading.

Varicella

Synonyms and Related Terms: Chickenpox; congenital varicella syndrome; varicella gangrenosa; varicella-zoster virus infection.

NOTE:

Reye's syndrome* is a possible postviral complication of varicella that must be distinguished from varicella encephalitis. Varicella may also cause exacerbation of tuberculosis.*

(1) Collect all tissues that appear infected. (2) Request viral cultures. (3) Usually, special stains are not helpful. (4) Special **precautions** are indicated (p. 146). (5) Serologic studies are available from state health department laboratories (p. 135). (6) This is not a reportable disease.

Possible Associated Conditions: Human immunodeficiency virus (HIV) infection *(1)*; leukemia;* lymphoma;* other immunodeficient conditions. See also above under "Note."

Organs and Tissues	*Procedures*	*Possible or Expected Findings*
External examination, skin, and oral cavity	Record extent and character of skin and oral mucosal lesions; photograph lesions and submit samples for histologic study (preferably lesions without evidence of superinfection).	Vesicular crusting rash; vesicles with type A intranuclear inclusions in surrounding epithelial cells, endothelial cells and fibroblasts; evidence of disseminated intravascular coagulation;* purpura fulminans.* (See also below under "Eyes, orbitae, and surrounding skin.")
Cerebrospinal fluid	Submit sample for viral culture and for cell count (p. 104).	Evidence of meningitis.
Chest cavity	Record volume of fluid.	Pleural effusions.*
Blood	Submit sample for microbiologic study (p. 102).	Septicemia (e.g., group A beta-hemolytic streptococcus; *Staphylococcus aureus*).
Heart	Submit samples for histologic study (p. 30).	Pancarditis (usually mild).

From: *Handbook of Autopsy Practice,* 3rd Ed. Edited by: J. Ludwig © Humana Press Inc., Totowa, NJ

Organs and Tissues	Procedures	Possible or Expected Findings
Lungs	Record weights. Submit consolidated areas for bacterial and viral cultures (p. 103). Perfuse lungs with formalin (p. 47).	Varicella pneumonia, with or without bacterial superinfection; intranuclear inclusions in epithelial, mesothelial, and endothelial cells; pulmonary edema; hemorrhages and abscesses; fibrosis and calcification in late stages.
Liver	Record weight and submit samples for histologic study.	Varicella hepatitis.
Spleen	Inspect carefully *in situ* to detect evidence of rupture. Record weight and consistency; sample for histologic study.	Splenitis, with or without rupture of spleen.
Stomach	Examine as soon as possible to minimize autolysis. Submit sections for histologic study.	Ulcerative gastritis.
Kidneys	Follow procedures described under "Glomerulonephritis."	Glomerulonephritis.*
Testes	Record weights; submit samples for histologic study.	Orchitis.
Neck organs	Open in posterior midline. (See also under "Laryngitis.")	Bacterial epiglottitis *(2)*.
Brain and spinal cord	For removal and specimen preparation, see pp. 65 and 67, respectively.	Encephalitis with cerebral edema; petechial hemorrhages; perivenous demyelination; acute cerebellitis; aseptic meningitis;* transverse myelitis.*
Eyes, orbitae, and surrounding skin	For removal and specimen preparation, see p. 85.	Keratitis; vesicular conjunctivitis; optic neuritis *(3)*. Periorbital varicella gangrenosa *(4)*.
Peripheral nerves	For removal and specimen preparation, see p. 79.	Acute motor axonal neuropathy *(5)*.
Skeletal muscles and soft tissues	Procedures depend on expected findings or grossly identified abnormalities as listed in right-hand column. For specimen preparation of muscles, see p. 80.	Rhabdomyolysis; necrotizing fasciitis (varicella gangrenosa).
Joints	For removal, prosthetic repair, and specimen preparation, see p. 96.	Arthritis.*

References

1. Gershon AA, Mervish N, LaRussa P, Steinberg S, Lo SH, Hodes D, et al. Varicella-zoster virus infection in children with underlying immunodeficiency virus infection. J Infect Dis 1997;176:1496–1500.
2. Belfer RA. Group A beta-hemolytic streptococcal epiglottitis as a complication of varicella infection. Pediatr Emerg Care 1996;12:202–204.
3. Lee CC, Venketasubramanian N, Lam MS. Optic neuritis: a rare complication of primary varicella infection. Clin Infect Dis 1997;24:515–516.
4. Tornervy NR, Fomsgaard A, Nielsen NV. HSV-1-induced acute retinal necrosis syndrome presenting with severe inflammatory orbitopathy, proptosis, and optic nerve involvement. Opthal 2000;107:397–400.
5. Picard F, Gericke CA, Frey M, Collard M. Varicella with acute motor axonal neuropathy. Euro Neurol 1997;38:68–71.

Varices, Esophageal

NOTE: See also under "Hypertension, portal."

Organs and Tissues	Procedures	Possible or Expected Findings
Chest	Dissect major veins *in situ.*	Superior vena cava obstruction; other venous abnormalities such as unilateral pulmonary vein atresia.
Esophagus and stomach	Remove esophagus and stomach together as one specimen. Record volume and character of blood in stomach. For demonstration of esophageal varices, see p. 53.	Gastric varices; blood in stomach. Esophageal varices with or without evidence of rupture.

Organs and Tissues	*Procedures*	*Possible or Expected Findings*
Esophagus and stomach *(continued)*	Record effects of sclerotherapy or evidence of surgical esophageal transection.	Evidence of sclerotherapy or esophageal transection surgery may be found.
Intestinal tract	Record measured or estimated amount of blood in lumen.	Blood in intestinal tract.
Portal vein system	Dissect all accessible veins *in situ*. Submit samples of veins for histologic study. Request Verhoeff–van Gieson stain (p. 173). If surgical shunts had been created, record type, location, and patency of anastomoses.	Portal vein thrombosis; other conditions causing portal vein obstruction. Sclerosis associated with idiopathic portal hypertension. Shunt surgery (portacaval and proximal or distal splenorenal shunts.)
Liver	Record weight and submit samples for histologic study. If a transjugular intrahepatic portasystemic shunt had been placed, document location and patency. For portal venography, see p. 56.	Cirrhosis;* chronic alcoholic hepatitis; congenital hepatic fibrosis* and other fibropolycystic liver diseases;* nodular regenerative hyperplasia, veno-occlusive disease, and other liver diseases.
Spleen	Record weight.	Congestive splenomegaly.

Vasculitis (See "Aortitis," "Arteritis, ...," "Phlebitis," and "Purpura,...")

Ventricle, Double Inlet Left

Synonyms: Single functional ventricle; univentricular heart; univentricular atrioventricular connection; Holmes heart.

NOTE: The basic anomaly is the connection of both atrioventricular valves to the left ventricle, often with transposed great arteries and a restrictive ventricular septal defect. There are four major types, based on the ventriculoarterial connection: (1) with congenitally corrected transposition (60%); (2) with complete transposition (30%); (3) with normally related great arteries (Holmes heart; 5%); and (4) double outlet, persistent truncal artery, or pulmonary atresia (5%). For general dissection techniques, see p. 33.

Possible Associated Conditions: Bicuspid pulmonary valve; bilateral mirror-image mitral valves (without tricuspid morphology); subvalvular aortic stenosis,* often with hypoplasia, coarctation, or interruption of the aortic arch; subvalvular pulmonary stenosis;* dual AV nodes and progressive heart block in patients with congenitally corrected transposition.

Ventricle, Double Outlet Right

Synonym: Origin of both great arteries from right ventricle; Taussig-Bing anomaly.

NOTE: The basic anomaly is the origin of the aorta and pulmonary artery primarily from the right ventricle, usually with a ventricular septal defect, and often with subpulmonary stenosis. For general dissection techniques, see p. 33.

Possible Associated Conditions: Complete atrioventricular septal defect (often with asplenia syndrome); muscular discontinuity between aortic and mitral valves; right ventricular infundibular stenosis; ventricular septal defect* that may be subaortic, subpulmonary, doubly committed, or remote.

Virus, Respiratory Syncytial (See "Pneumonia, all types or type unspecified.")

Virus, Salivary Gland (See "Infection, cytomegalovirus.")

Vitamin A (See "Deficiency, vitamin A" and "Hypervitaminosis A.")

Vitamin B1 (Thiamine) (See "Syndrome, Wernicke-Korsakoff.")

Vitamin B6 (See "Beriberi.")

Vitamin B12 (See "Anemia, megaloblastic.")

Vitamin C (See "Deficiency, vitamin C.")

Vitamin D (See "Deficiency, vitamin D" and "Hypervitaminosis D.")

Whooping Cough (See "Pertussis.")

Xanthoma Tuberosum (See "Hyperlipoproteinemia.")

NORMAL WEIGHTS AND MEASUREMENTS

III

Weights and Measurements

HAGEN BLASZYK, JURGEN LUDWIG, AND WILLIAM D. EDWARDS

Conversion Factors

To convert from	*To*	*Multiply by*
Metric to English		
Centimeters (cm)	Inches (US) (in)	0.394
Centimeters (cm)	Feet (US) (ft)	0.033
Square meters (m^2)	Square feet (US) (ft)	10.753
Grams (g)	Ounces (avoirdupois) (oz)	0.035
Grams (g)	Pounds (avoirdupois) (lb)	0.002
Kilograms (kg)	Ounces (avoirdupois) (oz)	35.274
Kilograms (kg)	Pounds (avoirdupois) (lb)	2.205
Milliliters (mL)*	Ounces (US fluid) (fl oz)	0.034
Liters (L)	Quarts (US liquid) (qt)	1.057
Liters (L)	Gallons (US) (gal)	0.264
English to Metric		
Inches (US) (in)	Centimeters (cm)	2.54
Feet (US) (ft)	Centimeters (cm)	30.480
Square feet (US) (ft)	Square meters (m^2)	0.093
Ounces (avoirdupois) (oz)	Grams (g)	28.350
Pounds (avoirdupois) (lb)	Grams (g)	453.592
Ounces (avoirdupois) (oz)	Kilograms (kg)	0.454
Pounds (avoirdupois) (lb)	Kilograms (kg)	29.574
Ounces (US fluid) (fl oz)	Milliliters (mL)*	473.179
Quarts (US liquid) (qt)	Liters (L)	0.946
Gallons (US) (gal)	Liters (L)	3.785
Pressure Conversion		
cm H_2O	mm Hg	0.760
mm Hg	cm H_2O	1.316
	Temperature Conversion	
°C	°F	$°F = (1.8 \times °C) + 32$
°F	°C	$°C = \frac{(°F - 32)}{1.8}$

Concentration Conversion for Ethyl Alcohol:

1,000 ug/mL = 100 mg/dL = 21.74 mmol/Liter = 1.0 promille = 0.1%

*For most purposes, cubic centimeter (cc) is equal to milliliter (mL).

From: *Handbook of Autopsy Practice,* 3rd Ed. Edited by: J. Ludwig © Humana Press Inc., Totowa, NJ

WEIGHTS AND MEASUREMENTS IN FETUSES, INFANTS, CHILDREN, AND ADOLESCENTS

Body Weight, Body Length, and Head Circumference in Relation to Age: Boys, Birth to 28 Mo of Age*

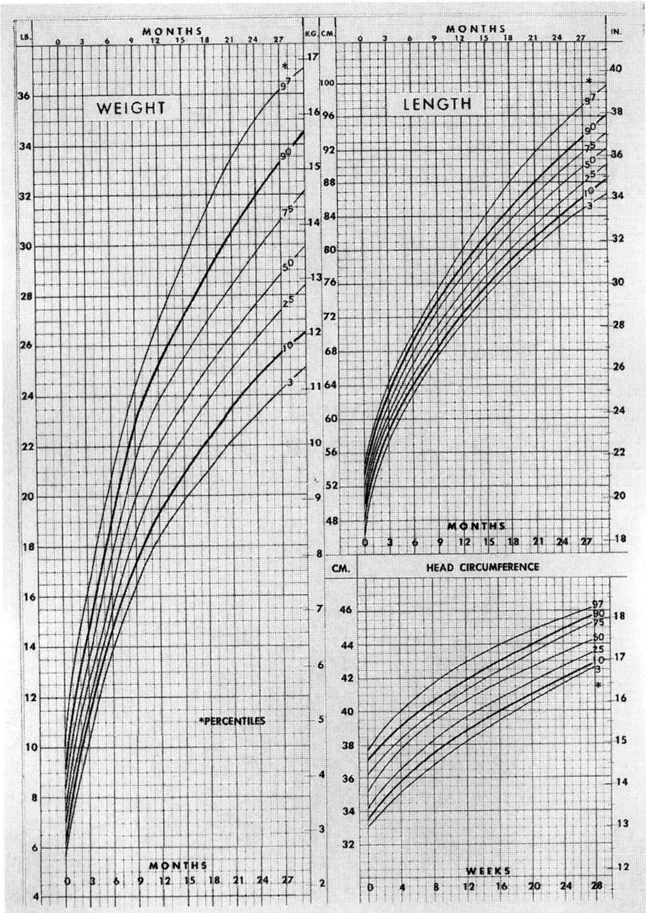

*Adapted with permission from: Stuart HC. Anthropometric charts of infant boys and girls from birth to 28 mo. Harvard School of Public Health, Department of Maternal and Child Health. Children's Medical Center, Boston.

Body Weight, Body Length, and Head Circumference in Relation to Age: Girls, Birth to 28 Mo of Age*

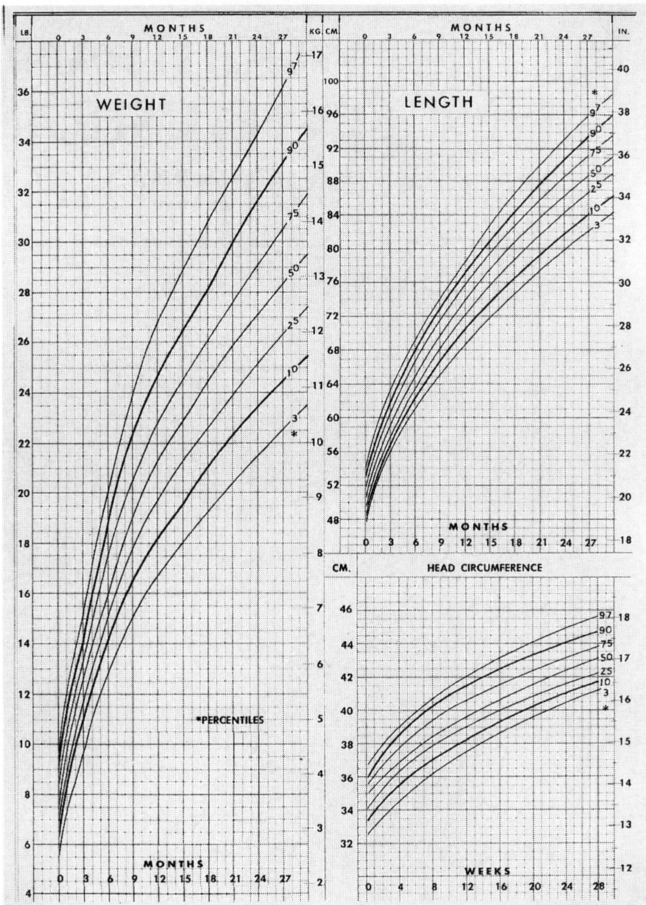

*Adapted with permission from: Stuart HC. Anthropometric charts of infant boys and girls from birth to 28 mo. Harvard School of Public Health, Department of Maternal and Child Health. Children's Medical Center, Boston.

Body Weight and Length in Relation to Age: Boys, 2–13 Yr of Age*

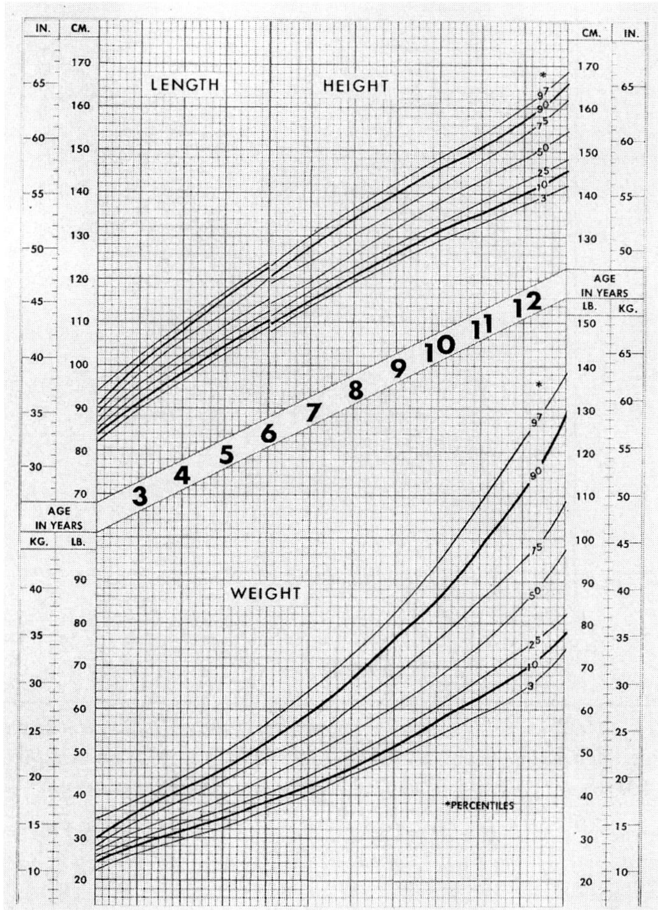

*Adapted with permission from: Stuart HC. Anthropometric charts for boys and girls from 2–13 yr. Harvard School of Public Health, Department of Maternal and Child Health. Children's Medical Center, Boston.

Body Weight and Length in Relation to Age: Girls, 2–13 Yr of Age*

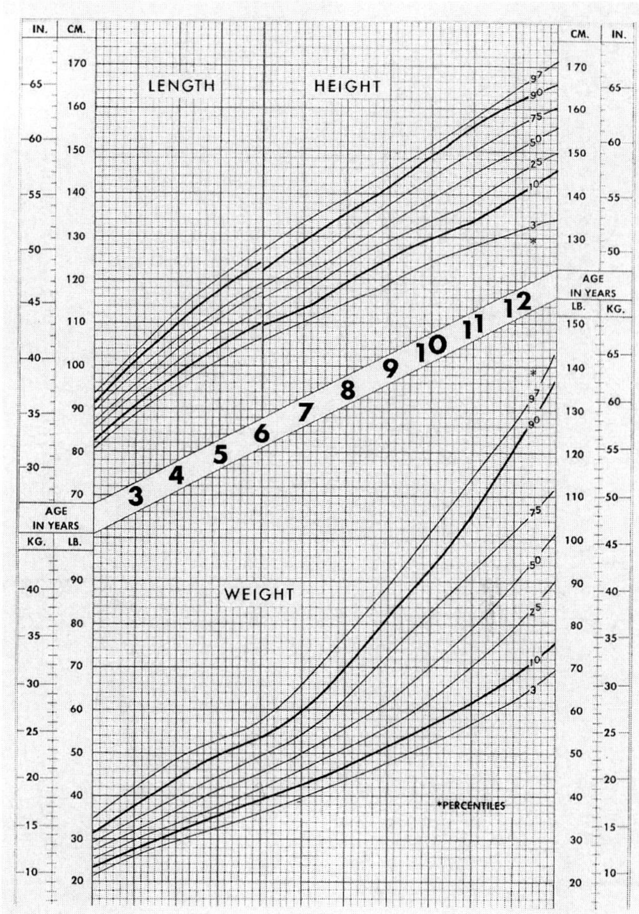

*Adapted with permission from: Stuart HC. Anthropometric charts for boys and girls from 2–13 yr. Harvard School of Public Health, Department of Maternal and Child Health. Children's Medical Center, Boston.

Body Surface Area from Height and Weight: Children*

Height | Body surface area | Weight

cm 120 – 47 in ... cm 25 – 10 in | 1.10 m^2 ... 0.074 m^2 | kg 40.0 – 90 lb ... kg 1.0 – 2.2 lb

*Adapted with permission from: Diem K. Documenta Geigy. Scientific Tables, 7th ed. Geigy Pharmaceuticals, New York, 1970, p. 538.

Body Surface Area from Age: Children*

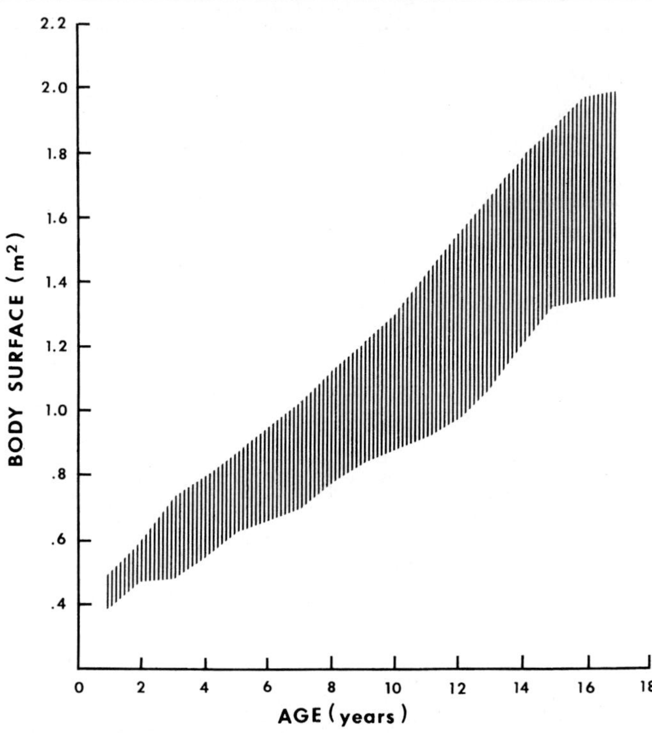

*Modified with permission from Dhom G, Piroth M. Das Wachstum der Nebennierenrinde im Kindesalter. Verh Dtsch Ges Pathol 1969; 53:418–422. Limits of hatched area indicate the 95th percentiles.

Growth Characteristics of Placenta and Fetus*

Gestation (wk)	*Placental weight (g)*	*Expected term weight (%)*	*Fetal weight (g)*	*Expected term weight (%)*
24	195	41	680	21
26	220	47	880	27
28	280	58	1,070	33
30	290	60	1,330	41
32	320	68	1,690	52
34	370	77	2,090	62
36	420	87	2,500	77
38	450	93	2,960	91
40	480	100	3,250	100
42	495	103	3,410	105

*Data adapted with permission from Wigglesworth JS, Singer DB. Textbook of Fetal and Perinatal Pathology. Blackwell Scientific Publications, Boston, 1991.

Weights and Measurements of Stillborn Infants*

Gest. age (wk)	*Body weight (g)*	*Crown rump (cm)*	*Crown heel (cm)*	*Toe heel (cm)*	*Brain (g)*	*Thymus (g)*	*Heart (g)*	*Lungs (g)*	*Spleen (g)*	*Liver (g)*	*Kidneys (g)*	*Adrenals (g)*	*Pancreas (g)*
20	313 (139)	18.0 (2.0)	24.9 (2.3)	3.3 (0.6)	41 (24)	0.4 (0.3)	2.4 (1.0)	7.1 (3.0)	0.3 (1.0)	17 (9)	2.7 (2.9)	1.3 (0.6)	0.5 (0.1)
21	353 (125)	18.9 (4.8)	26.2 (3.6)	3.5 (0.6)	48 (18)	0.5 (0.3)	2.6 (0.9)	7.9 (3.8)	0.4 (0.6)	18 (7)	3.1 (1.3)	1.4 (0.7)	0.5 (0.4)
22	398 (117)	19.8 (9.6)	27.4 (2.5)	3.8 (0.4)	55 (15)	0.6 (0.4)	2.8 (0.9)	8.7 (3.1)	0.5 (0.4)	19 (10)	3.5 (0.8)	1.4 (0.6)	0.6 (0.5)
23	450 (118)	20.6 (2.3)	28.7 (3.3)	4.0 (0.5)	64 (18)	0.8 (0.5)	3.0 (1.4)	9.5 (5.7)	0.7 (0.5)	21 (7)	4.1 (1.7)	1.5 (0.8)	0.7 (0.3)
24	510 (179)	21.5 (3.1)	29.9 (4.3)	4.2 (0.8)	74 (25)	0.9 (0.7)	3.3 (1.8)	10.5 (5.6)	0.9 (0.7)	22 (8)	4.6 (2.4)	1.5 (0.8)	0.7 (0.3)
25	581 (178)	22.3 (4.0)	31.1 (6.5)	4.4 (0.8)	85 (31)	1.1 (0.8)	3.7 (1.3)	11.6 (4.9)	1.2 (0.4)	24 (35)	5.3 (2.4)	1.6 (0.8)	0.8 (0.7)
26	663 (227)	23.2 (4.1)	32.4 (5.3)	4.7 (0.9)	98 (37)	1.4 (1.4)	4.2 (2.2)	12.9 (8.7)	1.5 (1.1)	26 (16)	6.1 (3.6)	1.7 (0.9)	0.8 (0.7)
27	758 (227)	24.1 (2.9)	33.6 (3.2)	4.9 (1.4)	112 (37)	1.7 (1.1)	4.8 (3.6)	14.4 (9.7)	1.9 (1.0)	29 (24)	7.0 (3.1)	1.9 (1.5)	0.9 (0.3)
28	864 (247)	24.9 (2.2)	34.9 (5.6)	5.1 (1.2)	127 (39)	2.0 (2.1)	5.4 (2.6)	16.1 (7.0)	2.3 (1.1)	32 (32)	7.9 (2.5)	2.1 (1.6)	1.0 (0.3)
29	984 (511)	25.8 (4.1)	36.1 (5.9)	5.3 (1.2)	143 (57)	2.4 (2.6)	6.2 (2.4)	18.0 (13.6)	2.7 (2.0)	36 (23)	9.0 (4.5)	2.4 (1.2)	1.1 (1.2)
30	1115 (329)	26.6 (2.4)	37.3 (3.6)	5.6 (0.7)	160 (72)	2.8 (4.2)	7.0 (2.8)	20.1 (8.6)	3.1 (1.5)	40 (22)	10.1 (6.0)	2.7 (1.3)	1.2 (0.2)
31	1259 (588)	27.5 (3.0)	38.6 (2.7)	5.8 (0.7)	178 (32)	3.2 (1.9)	8.0 (3.1)	22.5 (10.1)	3.6 (4.0)	46 (38)	11.3 (4.1)	3.0 (1.8)	1.4 (1.4)
32	1413 (623)	28.4 (2.8)	39.8 (5.4)	6.0 (0.6)	196 (92)	3.7 (2.2)	9.1 (4.1)	25.0 (10.7)	4.2 (2.4)	52 (32)	12.6 (8.0)	3.5 (1.8)	1.6 (0.6)
33	1578 (254)	29.2 (3.5)	41.1 (3.1)	6.2 (0.4)	216 (51)	4.3 (1.5)	10.2 (2.0)	27.8 (5.8)	4.7 (2.3)	58 (17)	13.9 (3.5)	3.9 (1.4)	1.8 (0.8)
34	1750 (494)	30.1 (3.5)	42.3 (4.3)	6.5 (0.8)	236 (42)	4.8 (5.6)	11.4 (3.2)	30.7 (15.2)	5.3 (2.5)	66 (22)	15.3 (5.1)	4.4 (1.3)	2.0 (0.5)
35	1930 (865)	30.9 (3.9)	43.5 (5.8)	6.7 (0.9)	256 (70)	5.4 (3.4)	12.6 (5.3)	33.7 (14.3)	5.9 (6.8)	74 (46)	16.7 (7.1)	4.9 (1.9)	2.3 (0.7)
36	2114 (616)	31.8 (4.0)	44.8 (7.2)	6.9 (0.8)	277 (94)	6.1 (4.1)	13.9 (5.8)	36.7 (16.8)	6.5 (2.9)	82 (36)	18.1 (6.3)	5.4 (2.4)	2.6 (2.6)
37	2300 (647)	32.7 (5.1)	46.0 (7.9)	7.2 (0.9)	297 (69)	6.7 (3.9)	15.1 (9.9)	39.8 (11.1)	7.2 (6.3)	91 (57)	19.4 (9.7)	5.8 (6.2)	2.9 (3.1)
38	2485 (579)	33.5 (2.6)	47.3 (3.9)	7.4 (0.8)	317 (83)	7.4 (6.1)	16.4 (4.4)	42.9 (15.7)	7.8 (5.9)	100 (44)	20.8 (6.0)	6.3 (2.1)	3.2 (1.6)
39	2667 (596)	34.4 (3.7)	48.5 (4.9)	7.6 (0.5)	337 (89)	8.1 (4.7)	17.5 (3.9)	45.8 (15.2)	8.5 (4.5)	109 (53)	22.0 (5.8)	6.7 (5.3)	3.5 (1.9)
40	2842 (482)	35.2 (6.4)	49.7 (3.2)	7.8 (0.7)	355 (57)	8.9 (4.3)	18.6 (9.9)	48.6 (19.4)	9.2 (4.1)	118 (49)	23.1 (8.6)	7.0 (2.9)	3.9 (1.7)
41	3006 (761)	36.1 (3.7)	51.0 (5.4)	8.1 (0.8)	373 (98)	9.6 (5.6)	19.5 (4.9)	51.1 (17.0)	9.9 (4.5)	126 (53)	24.1 (10.5)	7.1 (3.0)	4.2 (2.2)
42	3156 (678)	36.9 (2.0)	52.2 (3.0)	8.3 (0.5)	389 (36)	10.4 (5.0)	20.3 (4.5)	53.2 (10.1)	10.6 (3.7)	135 (54)	24.9 (8.1)	7.2 (2.9)	4.5 (2.3)

*Data given as mean (standard deviation). Adapted with permission from Wigglesworth JS, Singer DB. Textbook of Fetal and Perinatal Pathology. Blackwell Scientific Publications, Boston, 1991.

Weights and Measurements of Liveborn Infants*

Gest. age (wk)	*Body weight (g)*	*Crown rump (cm)*	*Crown heel (cm)*	*Toe heel (cm)*	*Brain (g)*	*Thymus (g)*	*Heart (g)*	*Lungs (g)*	*Spleen (g)*	*Liver (g)*	*Kidneys (g)*	*Adrenals (g)*	*Pancreas (g)*
20	381 (104)	18.3 (2.2)	25.6 (2.2)	3.6 (0.7)	49 (15)	0.8 (2.3)	2.8 (1.0)	11.5 (2.9)	0.7 (0.3)	22.4 (8.0)	3.7 (1.3)	1.8 (1.0)	0.5 (0.5)
21	426 (66)	19.1 (1.2)	26.7 (1.7)	3.8 (0.1)	57 (8)	1.0 (0.3)	3.2 (0.4)	12.9 (2.8)	0.7 (0.2)	24.1 (4.2)	4.2 (0.7)	2.0 (0.5)	0.5 (0.5)
22	473 (63)	20.0 (1.3)	27.8 (1.6)	4.0 (0.4)	65 (13)	1.2 (0.3)	3.5 (0.6)	14.4 (4.3)	0.8 (0.4)	25.4 (5.2)	4.7 (1.5)	2.0 (0.6)	0.6 (0.3)
23	524 (116)	20.8 (1.9)	28.9 (3.0)	4.2 (0.5)	74 (11)	1.4 (0.7)	3.9 (1.3)	15.9 (4.9)	0.8 (0.4)	26.6 (8.0)	5.3 (1.8)	2.1 (0.8)	0.7 (0.4)
24	584 (92)	21.6 (1.4)	30.0 (1.7)	4.4 (0.3)	83 (15)	1.5 (0.7)	4.2 (1.0)	17.4 (5.9)	0.9 (0.5)	28.0 (7.1)	6.0 (1.8)	2.2 (0.8)	0.8 (0.5)
25	655 (106)	22.5 (1.6)	31.1 (2.0)	4.6 (0.4)	94 (25)	1.8 (1.2)	4.7 (1.2)	19.0 (5.3)	1.1 (1.6)	29.7 (9.8)	6.8 (1.9)	2.2 (1.4)	0.9 (0.3)
26	739 (181)	23.3 (1.9)	32.2 (2.4)	4.8 (0.7)	105 (21)	2.0 (1.1)	5.2 (1.3)	20.6 (6.3)	1.3 (0.7)	32.1 (10.9)	7.6 (2.5)	2.4 (1.1)	1.0 (0.5)
27	836 (197)	24.2 (2.5)	33.4 (3.5)	5.0 (0.5)	118 (21)	2.3 (1.2)	5.8 (1.9)	22.1 (9.7)	1.7 (1.0)	35.1 (13.3)	8.6 (3.0)	2.5 (1.1)	1.2 (0.5)
28	949 (190)	25.0 (1.7)	34.5 (2.3)	5.2 (0.6)	132 (29)	2.6 (1.5)	6.5 (1.9)	23.7 (10.0)	2.1 (0.8)	38.9 (12.6)	9.7 (12.0)	2.7 (1.2)	1.4 (0.5)
29	1077 (449)	25.9 (2.8)	35.6 (4.4)	5.4 (0.8)	147 (49)	3.0 (1.9)	7.2 (2.7)	25.3 (12.6)	2.6 (0.9)	43.5 (15.8)	10.9 (4.4)	3.0 (1.2)	1.5 (1.0)
30	1219 (431)	26.7 (3.3)	36.7 (4.2)	5.7 (0.7)	163 (38)	3.5 (2.6)	8.1 (2.6)	26.9 (20.3)	3.3 (2.0)	49.1 (18.8)	12.3 (8.5)	3.3 (2.7)	1.7 (1.0)
31	1375 (281)	27.6 (3.8)	37.8 (3.1)	5.9 (0.7)	180 (34)	4.0 (3.4)	9.0 (2.8)	28.5 (13.2)	4.0 (1.2)	55.4 (17.3)	13.7 (5.2)	3.7 (1.3)	1.8 (0.6)
32	1543 (519)	28.4 (9.5)	38.9 (5.7)	6.1 (1.1)	198 (48)	4.7 (3.6)	10.1 (4.4)	30.2 (19.0)	4.7 (5.4)	62.5 (30.0)	15.2 (7.4)	4.1 (1.7)	2.0 (0.8)
33	1720 (580)	29.3 (3.3)	40.0 (3.5)	6.3 (0.7)	217 (49)	5.4 (3.2)	11.2 (4.0)	31.8 (13.5)	5.5 (3.5)	70.3 (25.4)	16.8 (7.7)	4.6 (1.5)	2.1 (0.8)
34	1905 (625)	30.1 (4.3)	41.1 (4.0)	6.5 (0.6)	237 (53)	6.1 (3.8)	12.4 (2.8)	33.5 (16.5)	6.4 (3.0)	78.7 (30.2)	18.5 (9.3)	5.1 (2.2)	2.3 (1.1)
35	2093 (309)	30.9 (2.0)	42.3 (2.9)	6.7 (0.4)	257 (45)	6.9 (4.5)	13.7 (3.6)	35.2 (20.5)	7.2 (5.2)	87.4 (30.6)	20.1 (10.9)	5.6 (2.8)	2.5 (0.6)
36	2280 (615)	31.8 (3.9)	43.4 (5.9)	6.9 (1.1)	278 (96)	7.7 (5.0)	15.0 (5.1)	36.9 (17.5)	8.1 (3.1)	96.3 (33.7)	21.7 (6.8)	6.1 (3.1)	2.6 (0.7)
37	2462 (821)	32.6 (5.0)	44.5 (7.0)	7.1 (1.2)	298 (70)	8.4 (5.6)	16.4 (5.7)	38.7 (22.9)	8.8 (6.4)	105.1 (33.7)	23.3 (9.9)	6.6 (3.3)	2.8 (0.9)
38	2634 (534)	33.5 (3.2)	45.6 (5.1)	7.3 (0.8)	318(106)	9.0 (2.8)	17.7 (5.4)	40.6 (17.1)	9.5 (3.5)	113.5 (34.7)	24.8 (7.2)	7.1 (2.9)	3.0 (1.1)
39	2789 (520)	34.3 (1.9)	46.7 (4.4)	7.5 (0.5)	337 (91)	9.4 (2.5)	19.1 (2.8)	42.6 (14.9)	10.1 (3.5)	121.3 (39.2)	26.1 (4.9)	7.4 (2.5)	3.3 (0.5)
40	2922 (450)	35.2 (2.8)	47.8 (4.2)	7.7 (0.8)	356 (79)	9.5 (5.0)	20.4 (5.6)	44.6 (22.7)	10.4 (3.3)	127.9 (35.8)	27.3 (11.5)	7.7 (3.0)	3.6 (1.3)
41	3025 (600)	36.0 (3.1)	48.9 (5.4)	7.9 (0.8)	372 (65)	9.1 (4.8)	21.7 (10.9)	46.8 (26.2)	10.5 (4.5)	133.1 (55.7)	28.1 (12.7)	7.8 (2.8)	3.9 (1.5)
42	3091 (617)	36.9 (2.4)	50.0 (3.8)	8.1 (1.1)	387 (61)	8.1 (3.8)	22.9 (6.2)	49.1 (14.6)	10.3 (3.6)	136.4 (38.9)	28.7 (9.7)	7.8 (3.2)	4.3 (1.9)

*Data given as mean (standard deviation). Adapted with permission from Wigglesworth JS, Singer DB. Textbook of Fetal and Perinatal Pathology. Blackwell Scientific Publications, Boston, 1991.

Fetal Organ Weights as a Function of Body Weight*

	Total Body Weight (g)								
	500–999	*1,000–1,499*	*1,500–1,999*	*2,000–2,499*	*2,500–2,999*	*3,000–3,499*	*3,500–3,999*	*4,000–4,499*	*>4,500*
Brain	109	180	256	308	359	403	421	424	406
Heart	5.8	9.4	12.7	15.5	19	21.2	23.4	28	36
Lungs, combined	18.2	27.1	37.9	43.6	48.9	54.9	58	65.8	74
Liver	38.8	59.8	76.3	98.1	127.4	155.1	178.1	215.2	275.6
Spleen	1.7	3.4	4.9	7	9.1	10.4	12	13.6	16.7
Pancreas	1	1.4	2	2.3	3	3.5	4	4.6	6.2
Kidneys, combined	7.1	12.2	16.2	19.9	23	25.3	28.5	31	33.2
Adrenals, combined	3.1	3.9	5	6.3	8.2	9.8	10.7	12.5	15.1
Thymus	2.1	4.3	6.6	8.2	9.3	11	12.6	14.3	17.3
Thyroid Gland	0.8	0.8	0.9	1.1	1.3	1.6	1.7	1.9	2.4

*Data adapted with permission from Potter EL. Pathology of the Fetus and Infant, 2nd ed. Year Book Medical Publishers, Chicago, 1961.

Organ Weights in Fetuses from 8–19 Wk of Development*

Gestational age (d)	*Body weight (g)*	*Crown-rump length (cm)*	*Crown-heel length (cm)*	*Foot length (cm)*	*Brain (g)*	*Heart (g)*	*Lungs (g)*	*Liver (g)*	*Adrenals (g)*	*Kidneys (g)*
56	10	–	2	–	–	–	–	–	–	–
63	11	3	3	–	1.2	0.1	0.1	0.2	0.1	0.1
67	13	4	–	–	1.5	0.2	0.3	0.7	0.1	0.1
71	15	6	4	–	2.6	0.2	0.4	0.8	0.1	0.1
73	20	7	–	–	4.3	0.3	0.4	1.1	0.1	0.2
76	25	7	6	0.9	4.8	0.4	0.7	1.1	0.2	0.2
79	30	8	–	–	5.4	0.4	1.0	1.3	0.2	0.2
84	35	9	7	1.1	6.2	0.5	1.4	2.0	0.2	0.3
89	45	9	–	–	7.4	0.5	1.9	2.5	0.4	0.4
90	50	10	–	–	8.5	0.5	1.9	3.0	0.5	0.5
91	60	10	9	1.4	10	0.5	2.5	3.4	0.6	0.6
92	70	11	–	–	11	0.6	3.0	3.6	0.6	0.8
96	80	11	10	1.7	12	0.7	3.0	4.3	0.6	0.8
100	90	12	–	–	14	0.9	3.0	4.7	0.7	0.9
105	100	12	13	2.1	17	1.1	3.9	5.6	0.7	1.4
109	125	13	–	–	23	1.3	4.1	7.4	0.7	1.4
115	150	14	14	2.2	23	1.4	5.3	9.2	0.8	1.4
117	175	14	–	–	23	1.4	5.6	11	0.8	1.8
118	200	15	17	2.4	33	1.7	7.2	12	1.1	2.2
124	250	16	19	2.6	39	2.2	9.1	15	1.2	2.7
130	285	17	–	–	46	2.4	10	17	1.5	3.1
133	350	18	20	2.9	54	2.9	11	21	2.0	3.8

*Data adapted with permission from Gilbert-Barness E. Potter's Pathology of the Fetus and Infant. Mosby (now Elsevier), New York, NY, 1997.

Organ Weights in Children*

Age	Body Length (cm)	Brain (g)	Heart (g)	Right lung (g)	Left lung (g)	Spleen (g)	Liver (g)	Right Kidney (g)	Left Kidney (g)	Combined Adrenals (g)	Thymus (g)	Pancreas (g)
Birth–3 d	49	335	17	21	18	8	78	13	14	–	–	–
3–7 d	49	358	18	24	22	9	96	14	14	–	–	–
1–3 wk	52	382	19	29	26	10	123	15	15	–	–	–
3–5 wk	52	413	20	31	27	12	127	16	16	4.9	5.5–8.5	5.7
5–7 wk	53	422	21	32	28	13	133	19	18	–	–	–
7–9 wk	55	489	23	32	29	13	136	19	18	4.9	5.0–10.0	7.2
2–3 mo	56	516	23	35	30	14	140	20	19	4.9	10.0	8.0
4 mo	59	540	27	37	33	16	160	22	21	4.8	9.5	10.0
5 mo	61	644	29	38	35	16	188	25	25	5.0	12.5	11.0
6 mo	62	660	31	42	39	17	200	26	25	4.9	10.0	11.0
7 mo	65	691	34	49	41	19	227	30	30	5.5	11.0	11.0
8 mo	65	714	37	52	45	20	254	31	30	5.4	9.0	12.0
9 mo	67	750	37	53	47	20	260	31	30	5.4	9.5	15.0
10 mo	69	809	39	54	51	22	274	32	31	5.7	20–38	13.5
11 mo	70	852	40	59	53	25	277	34	33	6.1	20–38	15.0
12 mo	73	925	44	64	57	26	288	36	35	6.2	20–38	14.5
14 mo	74	944	45	66	60	26	304	36	35	–	20–38	–
16 mo	77	1,010	48	72	64	28	331	39	39	–	20–38	–
18 mo	78	1,042	52	72	65	30	345	40	43	–	20–38	–
20 mo	79	1,050	56	83	74	30	370	43	44	–	20–38	–
22 mo	82	1,059	56	80	75	33	380	44	44	–	20–38	–
24 mo	84	1,064	56	88	76	33	394	47	46	–	20–38	–
3 yr	88	1,141	59	89	77	37	418	48	49	–	25	–
4 yr	99	1,191	73	90	85	39	516	58	56	–	25	–
5 yr	106	1,237	85	107	104	47	596	65	64	–	25	–
6 yr	109	1,243	94	121	122	58	642	68	67	–	25	–
7 yr	113	1,263	100	130	123	66	680	69	70	–	25	–
8 yr	119	1,273	110	150	140	69	736	74	75	–	25	–
9 yr	125	1,275	115	174	152	73	756	82	83	–	25	–
10 yr	130	1,290	116	177	166	85	852	92	95	–	25	–
11 yr	135	1,320	122	201	190	87	909	94	95	–	25	–
12 yr	139	1,351	124	–	–	93	936	95	96	–	25	–

*Data adapted with permission from Sunderman FW, Boerner F. Normal Values in Clinical Medicine. W.B. Saunders Company, Philadelphia, 1949, and from Schulz DM, Giordano DA, Schulz DH. Weights of organs of fetuses and infants. Arch Pathol 1969;74:244–250.

Heart Weight as a Function of Body Height: Infants and Adolescents*

Body Weight		*Heart Weight*			
		Females		*Males*	
		Mean	*Range*	*Mean*	*Range*
(Kg)	*(Lbs)*	*(g)*		*(g)*	
40	16	12	8–19	14	8–26
45	18	15	10–24	18	10–32
50	20	19	12–29	22	12–39
55	22	24	14–35	26	14–46
60	24	27	17–42	35	20–63
70	28	36	23–56	40	23–72
75	30	41	26–64	46	26–81
80	31	46	30–72	51	29–92
85	33	52	33–81	58	32–103
90	35	58	37–90	64	36–114
95	37	64	41–100	71	40–126
100	39	71	45–111	78	44–138
105	41	78	50–122	85	48–151
110	43	85	55–133	93	52–165
115	45	93	59–145	100	56–179
120	47	101	64–157	109	61–194
125	49	109	70–170	117	66–209
130	51	117	75–183	126	71–224
135	53	126	81–197	135	76–240
140	55	135	87–211	144	81–257
145	57	145	93–226	154	86–274
150	59	154	99–241	164	92–292
155	61	165	105–257	174	98–310
160	63	175	112–273	184	103–329
165	65	185	119–290	195	109–348
170	67	196	126–307	206	116–367
175	69	208	133–324	217	122–388
180	71	219	140–342	229	128–408
185	73	231	148–361	241	135–429
190	75	243	156–380	253	142–451
195	77	256	164–399	265	149–473
200	79	268	172–419	278	156–495

*Data adapted with permission from Scholz DG, Kitzman DW, Hagen PT, Ilstrup DM, Edwards WD. Age-related changes in normal human hearts during the first 10 decades of life. Part I (Growth): A quantitative anatomic study of 200 specimens from subjects from birth to 19 years old. Mayo Clin Proc 1988;63:126–136.

Heart Weight as a Function of Body Weight: Infants and Adolescents*

Body Height		*Heart Weight*			
		Females		*Males*	
		Mean	*Range*	*Mean*	*Range*
(cm)	*(in)*	*(g)*		*(g)*	
3	7	19	13–29	16	11–24
4	9	24	16–37	21	14–31
5	11	29	19–44	26	18–38
6	13	33	22–51	30	21–45
7	15	38	25–58	35	24–51
8	18	42	28–64	39	27–58
9	20	46	30–71	44	30–64
10	22	50	33–77	48	33–71
12	26	58	38–89	57	39–83
14	31	66	43–101	65	45–96
16	35	74	48–113	74	50–108
18	40	81	53–124	82	56–120
20	44	88	58–135	90	61–132
22	49	95	62–146	98	67–143
24	53	102	67–156	106	72–155
26	57	109	71–166	114	78–167
28	62	116	76–177	122	83–178
30	66	122	80–187	130	89–190
32	71	129	84–197	137	94–201
34	75	135	88–207	145	99–212
36	79	148	97–226	160	110–235
40	88	154	101–236	168	115–246
42	93	160	105–245	175	120–257
44	97	166	109–254	183	125–268
46	101	172	113–264	190	130–279
48	106	179	117–273	198	135–289
50	110	184	121–282	205	140–300
55	121	199	130–304	224	153–327
60	132	214	140–326	242	165–354
65	143	228	149–348	260	178–380
70	154	242	158–370	278	190–406
75	165	256	167–391	295	202–432
80	176	269	176–412	313	214–458
85	187	283	185–432	331	226–484
90	198	296	194–453	348	238–509
95	209	309	202–473	365	250–535
100	220	322	211–493	383	262–560

*Data adapted with permission from Scholz DG, Kitzman DW, Hagen PT, Ilstrup DM, Edwards WD. Age-related changes in normal human hearts during the first 10 decades of life. Part I (Growth): A quantitative anatomic study of 200 specimens from subjects from birth to 19 years old. Mayo Clin Proc 1988;63:126–136.

Heart Valve Circumferences (cm) as a Function of Age: Infants and Adolescents*

Age	Aortic valve				Mitral valve				Pulmonary valve				Tricuspid valve			
	Female		*Male*		*Female*		*Male*		*Female*		*Male*		*Female*		*Male*	
(yr)	*Mean*	*Range*	*Mean*	*Range*	*Mean*	*Range*	*Mean*	*Range*	*Mean*	*Range*	*Mean*	*Range*	*Mean*	*Range*	*Mean*	*Range*
0	2.2	1.33–3.00	2.2	1.35–3.02	2.8	1.31–4.31	2.6	0.83–4.44	2.2	1.13–3.23	2.1	0.83–3.32	3.0	1.11–4.88	2.5	0.66–4.38
1	3.0	2.11–3.79	3.0	2.20–3.87	4.1	2.57–5.57	4.1	2.24–5.86	3.0	1.97–4.07	3.0	1.78–4.27	4.7	2.80–6.56	4.5	2.67–6.39
2	3.4	2.53–4.21	3.5	2.65–4.32	4.7	3.25–6.24	4.8	3.00–6.62	3.5	2.42–4.52	3.5	2.29–4.78	5.6	3.70–7.46	5.6	3.75–7.47
3	3.7	2.82–4.50	3.8	2.96–4.63	5.2	3.71–6.70	5.3	3.52–7.13	3.8	2.72–4.82	3.9	2.64–5.13	6.2	4.31–8.08	6.3	4.48–8.20
4	3.9	3.04–4.72	4.0	3.20–4.87	5.6	4.06–7.06	5.7	3.91–7.53	4.0	2.96–5.06	4.2	2.91–5.40	6.7	4.78–8.55	6.9	5.04–8.77
5	4.1	3.22–4.89	4.2	3.39–5.06	5.8	4.34–7.34	6.0	4.23–7.85	4.2	3.14–5.24	4.4	3.12–5.61	7.1	5.17–8.93	7.4	5.50–9.22
6	4.2	3.37–5.04	4.4	3.55–5.22	6.1	4.58–7.58	6.3	4.50–8.12	4.4	3.30–5.40	4.6	3.30–5.79	7.4	5.48–9.25	7.7	5.88–9.60
7	4.3	3.49–5.17	4.5	3.69–5.36	6.3	4.79–7.78	6.5	4.73–8.35	4.5	3.49–5.54	4.7	3.46–5.95	7.6	5.76–9.53	8.1	6.21–9.93
8	4.5	3.61–5.28	4.7	3.81–5.48	6.5	4.97–7.96	6.7	4.93–8.55	4.6	3.56–5.66	4.8	3.59–6.08	7.8	6.00–9.77	8.4	6.50–10.2
9	4.6	3.71–5.38	4.8	3.92–5.59	6.6	5.13–8.13	6.9	5.12–8.73	4.7	3.67–5.77	5.0	3.71–6.21	8.1	6.22–9.98	8.6	6.75–10.5
10	4.6	3.88–5.47	4.9	4.02–5.69	6.8	5.27–8.27	7.1	5.28–8.89	4.8	3.76–5.86	5.1	3.82–6.32	8.3	6.41–10.2	8.9	6.99–10.7
11	4.7	3.92–5.56	4.9	4.11–5.78	6.9	5.40–8.40	7.2	5.43–9.04	4.9	3.85–5.95	5.2	3.92–6.42	8.5	6.59–10.3	9.1	7.20–10.9
12	4.8	3.96–5.63	5.0	4.19–5.86	7.0	5.53–8.52	7.4	5.56–9.18	5.0	3.93–6.03	5.3	4.02–6.51	8.6	6.75–10.5	9.3	7.39–11.1
13	4.9	4.03–5.70	5.1	4.27–5.93	7.1	5.64–8.64	7.5	5.69–9.31	5.1	4.01–6.11	5.4	4.10–6.59	8.8	6.90–10.7	9.4	7.57–11.3
14	4.9	4.09–5.77	5.2	4.34–6.00	7.2	5.74–8.74	7.6	5.81–9.42	5.1	4.07–6.17	5.4	4.18–6.67	8.9	7.04–10.8	9.6	7.74–11.5
15	5.0	4.15–5.83	5.2	4.40–6.07	7.3	5.84–8.84	7.7	5.92–9.53	5.2	4.14–6.24	5.5	4.25–6.74	9.1	7.17–10.9	9.8	7.89–11.6
16	5.1	4.21–5.89	5.3	4.46–6.13	7.4	5.93–8.93	7.8	6.02–9.64	5.3	4.20–6.30	5.6	4.32–6.81	9.2	7.29–11.1	9.9	8.04–11.8
17	5.1	4.26–5.94	5.4	4.52–6.19	7.5	6.02–9.02	7.9	6.12–9.73	5.3	4.26–6.36	5.6	4.39–6.88	9.3	7.41–11.2	10.0	8.18–11.9
18	5.2	4.32–5.99	5.4	4.58–6.25	7.6	6.10–9.10	8.0	6.21–9.83	5.4	4.31–6.41	5.7	4.45–6.94	9.4	7.52–11.3	10.2	8.31–12.0
19	5.2	4.36–6.04	5.5	4.63–6.30	7.7	6.18–9.17	8.1	6.30–9.91	5.4	4.36–6.46	5.8	4.51–7.00	9.5	7.62–11.4	10.3	8.43–12.1

*Data adapted with permission from Scholz DG, Kitzman DW, Hagen PT, Ilstrup DM, Edwards WD. Age-related changes in normal human hearts during the first 10 decades of life. Part I (Growth): A quantitative anatomic study of 200 specimens from subjects from birth to 19 years old. Mayo Clin Proc 1988;63:126–136.

Urogenital Organ Weights of Infants and Children*

Age (yr)	*Uterus (g)*	*Ovaries combined (g)*	*Testes combined (g)*	*Seminal vesicles combined (g)*	*Prostate (g)*
Birth	4.6	0.4	0.4	0.05	0.9
1	2.3	1.0	1.4	0.08	1.2
2	1.9	0.9	1.8	0.09	–
3	2.5	1.4	1.8	0.09	1.1
4	–	1.4	1.8	0.09	–
5	2.9	2.1	1.8	0.09	1.2
6	2.9	2.2	–	–	–
7	2.6	–	–	–	–
8	2.6	3.1	1.6	0.1	1.3
9	3.4	3.1	1.6	0.1	–
10	3.4	3.1	1.6	0.1	1.4
11	5.3	4.3	2.5	–	2.3
12	5.3	4.3	3.0	0.12	2.8
13	15.9	–	–	–	3.7
14	–	–	3.0	0.15	3.5
15	–	–	13.6	1.5	5.1
16	43.0	4.0	–	–	6.1
17	–	–	–	–	11.4

*Data adapted with permission from Sunderman FW, Boerner F. Normal Values in Clinical Medicine. W.B. Saunders Company, Philadelphia, 1949.

Brain Weight as a Function of Age in Children and Adolescents*

	Females		*Males*	
Age	*Body Height (cm)*	*Brain Weight (g)*	*Body Height (cm)*	*Brain Weight (g)*
0 mo	49	372	51	448
1 mo	54	516	54	523
2 mo	57	560	58	609
4 mo	60	645	62	718
7 mo	66	755	68	871
9 mo	71	935	72	999
13 mo	75	961	79	1,141
16 mo	78	1,117	83	1,176
19 mo	82	1,121	83	1,109
22 mo	87	1,063	83	1,088
2 yr	87	1,176	90	1,249
3 yr	98	1,213	99	1,317
4 yr	99	1,243	107	1,419
5 yr	109	1,284	114	1,480
6 yr	118	1,286	117	1,437
7 yr	123	1,328	128	1,424
8 yr	130	1,400	133	1,457
9 yr	132	1,360	138	1,489
10 yr	135	1,550	135	1,501
11 yr	145	1,380	148	1,397
12 yr	157	1,356	154	1,483
13 yr	163	1,453	159	1,564
14 yr	164	1,322	166	1,484
15 yr	166	1,378	168	1,483
16 yr	164	1,383	175	1,547
17 yr	166	1,380	174	1,528
18 yr	166	1,359	176	1,491

*Data adapted with permission from Voigt J, Pakkenberg H. Brain weight of Danish children. Acta Anat 1983;116:290–301.

WEIGHTS AND MEASUREMENTS IN ADULTS

BODY MASS INDEX (BMI)

Body size, shape, and composition influence susceptibility and resistance to disease. To understand how body composition relates specifically to morbidity and mortality, many measures of fat distribution pattern have been applied. Considerable variability in body composition is due to effects of age, sex, and ethnicity. The most accurate methods are expensive and are primarily useful in nutritional and metabolic studies. For routine use, the body mass index (BMI [kg/m^2]) can be applied as a measure of fatness, because it is easily determined and remembered; it predicts morbidity and mortality in many populations.

$$\text{BMI} = \frac{\text{Body Weight [kg]}}{(\text{Body Height})^2\ [\text{m}^2]}$$

A simplified scheme for the interpretation of BMI in adults is provided below:*

BMI (kg/m^2)	*Body Stature*	*Risk for Morbidity/Mortality*
<15	Anorectic	Moderate to high
15–20	Underweight/lean	Low
20–25	Normal	Low
25–30	Overweight	Low to moderate
>30	Morbidly obese	High

*Data modified with permission from Baumgartner RN, Heymsfield SB, Roche AF. Human body composition and the epidemiology of chronic disease. Obesity Res 1995;3:73–95.

In children, recommendations for weight control should be focused primarily on those with a BMI above the 95th percentile, and those with a BMI above the 85th percentile who show even minimal signs of physical impairment.

Body Surface Area from Height and Weight: Adults*

Height cm. in.
cm: 200 195 190 185 180 175 170 165 160 155 150 145 140 135 130 125 120 115 110 105 100
in.: 79 78 76 74 72 70 68 66 64 62 60 58 56 54 52 50 48 46 44 42 40 39

Body surface area sq.m.
2·80 2·70 2·60 2·50 2·40 2·30 2·20 2·10 2·00 1·95 1·90 1·85 1·80 1·75 1·70 1·65 1·60 1·55 1·50 1·45 1·40 1·35 1·30 1·25 1·20 1·15 1·10 1·05 1·00 0·95 0·90 0·86

Weight kg. lb.
kg: 150 145 140 135 130 125 120 115 110 105 100 95 90 85 80 75 70 65 60 55 50 45 40 35 30
lb.: 330 320 310 300 290 280 270 260 250 240 230 220 210 200 190 180 170 160 150 140 130 120 110 105 100 95 90 85 80 75 70 66

*Adapted with permission from Furbank RA. Conversion data, normal values, nomograms and other standards. In: Modern Trends in Forensic Medicine. Simpson K, ed. Appleton-Century-Crofts, New York, NY, 1967, pp. 344-364.

Heart Weight as a Function of Body Weight: Adults*

Body Weight		*Heart Weight*			
		Females		*Males*	
		Mean	*Range*	*Mean*	*Range*
(kg)	*(lbs)*	*(g)*		*(g)*	
30	66	196	133–287	213	162–282
32	71	201	137–295	220	167–291
34	75	206	141–302	227	172–300
36	79	211	144–310	234	177–309
38	84	216	148–317	240	182–317
40	88	221	151–324	247	187–325
42	93	226	154–331	253	191–334
44	97	230	157–337	259	196–341
46	101	234	160–344	265	200–349
48	106	239	163–350	270	205–357
50	110	243	166–356	276	209–364
52	115	247	169–362	281	213–371
54	119	251	171–368	287	217–379
56	123	255	174–374	292	221–386
58	128	259	177–379	297	225–392
60	132	262	179–385	302	229–399
62	137	266	182–390	307	233–406
64	141	270	184–395	312	237–412
66	146	273	187–401	317	240–419
68	150	277	189–406	322	244–425
70	154	280	191–411	327	248–431
72	159	284	194–416	331	251–437
74	163	287	196–420	336	255–444
76	168	290	198–425	341	258–450
78	172	293	200–430	345	261–455
80	176	297	202–435	349	265–461
82	181	300	205–439	354	268–467
84	185	303	207–444	358	271–473
86	190	306	209–448	362	275–478
88	194	309	211–453	367	278–484
90	198	312	213–457	371	281–489
92	203	315	215–461	375	284–495
94	207	318	217–465	379	287–500
96	212	320	219–470	383	290–506
98	216	323	221–474	387	293–511
100	220	326	222–478	391	296–516
102	225	329	224–482	395	299–521
104	229	331	226–486	399	302–526
106	234	334	228–490	403	305–531
108	238	337	230–494	406	308–536
110	243	339	232–497	410	311–541
112	247	342	233–501	414	314–546
114	251	345	235–505	418	316–551
116	256	347	237–509	421	319–556
118	260	350	239–513	425	322–561
120	265	352	240–516	429	325–566
125	275	359	244–525	437	331–577
130	287	364	249–534	446	338–589
135	297	370	252–542	455	345–600
140	309	376	257–551	463	351–611
145	320	382	260–560	472	357–622
150	331	387	264–567	479	363–633

*Data adapted with permission from Kitzman DW, Scholz DG, Hagen PT, Ilstrup DM, Edwards WD. Age-related changes in normal human hearts during the first 10 decades of life. Part II: (Maturity): A quantitative anatomic study of 765 specimens from subjects 20 to 99 years old. Mayo Clin Proc 1988;63:137–146.

Heart Measurements in Adults*

	Age 20–60 yr		*Age > 60 yr*	
	Men	*Women*	*Men*	*Women*
1. Valve Circumference (cm)	*mean (range)*	*mean (range)*	*mean (range)*	*mean (range)*
Aortic Valve	6.7 (6.0–7.4)	6.3 (5.7–6.9)	8.3 (8.1–8.5)	7.6 (7.3–7.9)
Pulmonary Valve	6.6 (6.1–7.1)	6.2 (5.7–6.7)	7.3 (7.2–7.5)	7.1 (6.8–7.4)
Mitral Valve	9.6 (9.4–9.9)	8.6 (8.2–9.1)	9.5 (9.2–9.8)	8.6 (8.2–9.0)
Tricuspid Valve	11.4 (11.2-11.7)	10.6 (10.2-10.9)	11.6 (11.4-11.8)	10.5 (10.0-11.1)
2. Wall Thickness (cm)	*mean*	*range*	*mean*	*range*
Left Ventricle	1.25	1.00–1.50	1.15	1.05–1.25
Right Ventricle	0.40	0.25–0.50	0.38	0.35–0.40
Ventricular Septum	1.35	1.20–1.60	1.35	1.20–1.60
Atrial Muscle	0.20	0.10–0.30	0.20	0.10–0.30

*Modified with permission from Sunderman FW, Boerner F. Normal Values in Clinical Medicine. W.B. Saunders Company, Philadelphia, 1949; and from Kitzman DW, Scholz DG, Hagen PT, Ilstrup DM, Edwards WD. Age-related changes in normal human hearts. Part II: (Maturity): A quantitative anatomic study of 765 specimens from subjects 20 to 99 years old. Mayo Clin Proc 1988;63:137–146.

Factors for Calculation of Cardiac Muscle Mass from Specific Gravity*

Spec Grav	*x*	*Spec Grav*	*x*	*Spec Grav*	*x*	*Spec Grav*	*x*	*Spec Grav*	*x*
1.055	1.000	1.032	0.798	1.009	0.569	0.986	0.395	0.963	0.193
1.054	0.991	1.031	0.789	1.008	0.588	0.985	0.386	0.962	0.184
1.053	0.982	1.030	0.781	1.007	0.579	0.984	0.377	0.961	0.175
1.052	0.974	1.029	0.772	1.006	0.570	0.983	0.368	0.960	0.167
1.051	0.965	1.028	0.763	1.005	0.561	0.982	0.360	0.959	0.158
1.050	0.956	1.027	0.754	1.004	0.553	0.981	0.351	0.958	0.149
1.049	0.947	1.026	0.746	1.003	0.544	0.980	0.342	0.957	0.140
1.048	0.939	1.025	0.737	1.002	0.535	0.979	0.333	0.956	0.132
1.047	0.930	1.024	0.728	1.001	0.526	0.978	0.325	0.955	0.123
1.046	0.921	1.023	0.719	1.000	0.518	0.977	0.316	0.954	0.114
1.045	0.912	1.022	0.711	0.999	0.509	0.976	0.307	0.953	0.105
1.044	0.904	1.021	0.702	0.998	0.500	0.975	0.298	0.952	0.096
1.043	0.895	1.020	0.693	0.997	0.491	0.974	0.289	0.951	0.088
1.042	0.886	1.019	0.684	0.996	0.482	0.973	0.281	0.950	0.079
1.041	0.877	1.018	0.675	0.995	0.474	0.972	0.272	0.949	0.070
1.040	0.868	1.017	0.667	0.994	0.465	0.971	0.263	0.948	0.061
1.039	0.860	1.016	0.658	0.993	0.456	0.970	0.254	0.947	0.053
1.038	0.851	1.015	0.649	0.992	0.447	0.969	0.246	0.946	0.044
1.037	0.842	1.014	0.640	0.991	0.439	0.968	0.237	0.945	0.035
1.036	0.833	1.013	0.632	0.990	0.430	0.967	0.228	0.944	0.026
1.035	0.825	1.012	0.623	0.989	0.421	0.966	0.219	0.943	0.018
1.034	0.816	1.011	0.614	0.988	0.412	0.965	0.211	0.942	0.009
1.033	0.807	1.010	0.605	0.987	0.404	0.964	0.202	0.941	0.000

*The Heart is weighed in isotonic saline for this determination. From the table above, one uses the specific gravity to find the factor that, when multiplied by heart weight, gives the cardiac muscle mass. *Example:* A heart weighing 700 g has a specific gravity of 1.032. The table shows a factor (X) of 0.798, or 79.8%. The muscle mass of this heart is 79.8% of 700 g, or 558.6 g.

Data adapted with permission from: Masshoff W, Scheidt D, Reimers HF. Quantitative Bestimmung des Fett- und Myokardgewebes im Leichenherzen. Virchows Arch [Pathol Anat] 1967;342:184–189.

Extent of Left Ventricular Hypertrophy and Dilatation in Adult Hearts*

Extent of left ventricular hypertrophy	*Percent increase in total heart weight*[a]
None	0–25
Mild	26–50
Moderate	51–100
Severe	>100

[a]Based on the expected normal mean value for the subject's gender and body size. For example, if the expected mean heart weight is 300 g, then hearts weighing 375–450 g have mild left ventricular hypertrophy (LVH), those weighing 451–600 g show moderate LVH, and hearts weighing >600 g have severe LVH. (Note: There may be some overlap between the upper range of normal heart weight and the lower range of mild hypertrophy.)

Extent of left ventricular dilatation	*Left ventricular short-axis diameter (cm)*[b]
None	0–2.5
Mild	2.6–4.0
Moderate	4.1–5.5
Severe	>5.5

[b]For an adult of average size, with rigor mortis. (Note: Once rigor mortis has abated, artifactual dilatation of all four cardiac chambers commonly occurs and may be substantial, such that this table no longer applies.)

*Data adapted with permission from Edwards WD. Applied anatomy of the heart. In: Mayo Clinic Practice of Cardiology, 3rd ed. Giuliani ER, et al., eds. Mosby, St. Louis, 1996, pp. 422-489.

Spleen Weight as a Function of Age in Adults*

Spleen weight (g) in men				*Spleen weight (g) in women*			
Age (yr)	*Race*	*Mean*	*Range*	*Age (yr)*	*Race*	*Mean*	*Range*
15–24	White	190	105–280	15–59	White	120	60–185
25–39	White	155	75–250	60+	White	110	55–195
40–54	White	145	75–230	All	White	115	55–190
55+	White	145	70–225				
15–39	White	170	85–275				
40+	White	145	70–225				
All	White	145	75–245				
15–24	Black	120	60–190	15–36	Black	100	35–190
25–39	Black	115	50–225	37+	Black	95	45–150
40–54	Black	110	50–210	All	Black	95	35–190
55+	Black	90	40–135				
15–39	Black	115	55–220				
40+	Black	105	45–190				
All	Black	105	40–200				

*Data adapted with permission from Myers J, Segal RJ. Weight of the spleen. Range of normal in a nonhospital population. Arch Pathol 1974;98:33–38.

Brain Weight as a Function of Age in Adults*

	Brain Weight (g)			
	Men		*Women*	
Age (yr)	*Mean*	*Range*	*Mean*	*Range*
17–19	1,340	1,170–1,527	1,242	1,120–1,420
20–29	1,396	1,158–1,620	1,234	1,057–1,565
30–39	1,365	1,075–1,685	1,233	1,038–1,440
40–49	1,366	1,069–1,605	1,240	995–1,543
50–59	1,375	1,113–1,665	1,200	820–1,447
60–69	1,323	1,018–1,610	1,178	920–1,372
70–85	1,279	1,039–1,485	1,121	832–1,370

*Data adapted with permission from Sunderman FW, Boerner F. Normal Values in Clinical Medicine. W.B. Saunders, Philadelphia, 1949.

Miscellaneous Weights and Measurements of Adults*

	Weight (g)		*Weight*	*Size or Length*
	mean	*range*	*(% of Body Weight)*	*(cm)*
Adrenal glands, combined	11.5	8.3–16.7	–	–
Bones	–	–	11.6	–
Brain	–	–	1.4	–
Carotid bodies, combined	0.02	0.004–0.034	–	–
Colon	–	–	–	150–170
Duodenum	–	–	–	30
Esophagus	–	–	–	25
Heart	–	–	0.40–0.45	–
Kidneys, combined	–	–	0.3	11.5 × 5.5 × 3.5
Male	313	230–440	–	–
Female	288	240–350	–	–
Liver				
Male	–	–	1.9–3.0	–
Female	–	–	2.2–2.9	–
Lung				
Combined	–	–	1	–
Right	450	360–570	–	–
Left	375	325–480	–	–
Ovary	7	–	–	3.4 × 1.5 × 0.8
Pancreas	110	60–135	0.1	23 × 4.5 × 3.8
Parathyroid glands, combined	0.15	0.12–0.18	–	–
Pineal gland	0.14	0.10–0.18	–	0.7 × 0.45 × 0.4
Pituitary gland	–	–	–	2.1 × 1.4 × 0.5
Ages 10–20 yr	0.56	–	–	–
Ages 20–70 yr	0.61	–	–	–
Pregnancy	0.95	–	–	–
Placenta	500	–	–	18 × 2.8
Prostate	–	–	–	3.6 × 2.8 × 1.9
Ages 21–25 yr	18	–	–	–
Ages 51–60 yr	20	–	–	–
Ages 71–80 yr	40	–	–	–
Seminal vesicle	–	–	–	4.3 × 1.7 × 0.9
Skeletal muscle	–	–	28.7	–
Small intestine	–	–	–	550–650
Spinal cord	27	–	–	45
Spleen	–	–	0.16	–
Testis	25	20–27	–	4.5 × 3.0 × 2.4
Thymus				
Ages <25 yr	25	–	–	–
Ages 26–35 yr	20	–	–	–
Ages >65 yr	6	–	–	–
Thyroid gland	40	30–70	–	6.5 × 3.5 × 2.0
Uterus				
Multiparus	110	102–117	–	9.0 × 5.7 × 3.4
Nulliparus	35	33–41	–	7.9 × 3.9 × 2.3

*Modified with permission from Furbank RA. Conversion data, normal values, normograms and other standards. In: Modern Trends in Forensic Medicine. Simpson K, ed. Appleton-Century-Crofts, New York, 1967, pp. 344–364; and Sunderman FW, Boerner F. Normal Values in Clinical Medicine. W.B. Saunders, Philadelphia, 1949.

Weight Changes of Organs after Formalin Fixation*

Organ	*Weight after fixation*	*% Weight change*	
		Mean	*Range*
Heart			
Adults	Decreased	4.0	0.4–9.0
Children	Decreased	5.8	0.9–19.2
Lung	Increased or decreased	6.6	0.4–17.1
Liver			
Adults	Decreased	4.0	0.5–7.6
Children	Decreased	4.0	0.7–6.6
Spleen			
Adults	Increased or decreased	2.1	0.1–6.2
Children	Decreased	3.1	0.2–6.6
Kidney			
Adults	Increased or decreased	1.9	0.1–6.4
Children	Decreased	3.3	0.2–6.0
Thyroid gland	Increased	14.8	6.2–34.0
Testis	Increased or decreased	3.2	0.0–8.8
Placenta	Increased	9.9	0.7–23.0
Skeletal muscle	Decreased	7.0	0.8–13.3
Adipose tissue	Increased	2.2	0.1–4.8
Brain			
Adults	Increased	8.8	3.3–19.2
Children	Increased	14.1	8.0–22.3
Dura mater cerebri	decreased	3.9	0.2–10.0

*Weight changes were determined after 10 d of fixation in 10% buffered formalin. Adapted with permission from Schremmer C-N. Gewichtsänderungen verschiedener Gewebe nach Formalinfixierung. Frankf Z Pathol 1967;77:299–304.

Index

A
Abdominal aorta
anterior view of, 60f
Abetalipoproteinemia, 175, 195, 245, 354, 482, 498
Abortion, 9, 14, 107–109, 159, 175, 239, 290–291, 300, 423, 476
Abortuses
chromosome studies and, 107–108
Abscess
cerebral, *See* Cerebral abscess
collection of, 103
epidural, 176, 296
lung, 171, 176, 458
Abuse
hallucinogen, 327
marihuana, 177, 185, 327, 386
Acanthocytosis, 175
Accident
aircraft, 177
diving, 178, 283, 468–469
vehicular, 178, 180
Accidental death
definition of, 7
Achalasia, esophageal, 182
Achondroplasia, 183, 228, 286, 411
Acidosis, 115, 183, 284, 413–414
postmortem chemical changes in, 115t
Acquired immunodeficiency syndrome (AIDS), 1, 6, 83, 99, 133, 146, 148–149, 177, 185, 191–192, 208, 215, 225, 234–235, 249, 257, 287, 321, 324, 325, 330, 336, 357, 362, 367–368, 377, 381, 384, 397, 405–406, 418, 425–426, 429, 446, 451, 455–456, 478–479, 481, 496, 503, 515, 520–521, 537, 541
Acquired syphilis, 512
Acquired valvular aortic stenosis, 262, 473
Acromegaly, 29, 183–184, 205, 251, 287, 321, 347, 402, 410, 414, 535–536, 540
Acromioclavicular joints, 96
Acrylic museum jars, 137
Actinomycosis, 184
Acute chorea, 492
Acute intermittent porphyria, 451
Addison's disease, 367
Adipocere, 11
Adolescents
weights and measurement of, 563t–565t
Adrenal insufficiency, 194, 254, 367–368, 454, 471
Adult autopsies
techniques of, 3–4
Adult respiratory distress syndrome (ARDS), 7, 239, 308, 368, 429, 481, 505
Afferent loop syndrome, 481
AFIP, 147
American Registry of Pathology, 148
African trypanosomiasis, 525
Agenesis, renal, 185
Agnogenic myeloid metaplasia, 390, 419
AIDS, *See* Acquired immunodeficiency syndrome
Aircraft accident, 177
Air embolism, 3, 10, 117, 179–182, 239–240, 249, 290–292, 292f, 294, 406, 461, 469
Air volumes
measurements of, 51–52
Alagille's syndrome, 210
Albers-Schonberg disease, 413
Alcohol, 129
Alcohol amblyopia, 191
Alcoholic cardiomyopathy, 186, 216, 224, 254, 306
Alcoholic cerebellar degeneration, 247
Alcoholic cirrhosis, 186
Alcoholic liver disease, 186, 189, 197, 230, 249, 254–255, 299–300, 418, 472
Alcoholic liver disease, 254, 331, 438, 472, 511
Alcohol intoxication, 17, 177, 180, 185–186, 249, 255, 285, 306, 364, 407, 433, 438, 442, 511
Alcoholism, 17, 147, 151, 177, 180, 185–186, 191, 197, 216, 220, 230, 241, 247, 255, 272, 285, 304, 306, 322, 396, 405, 413–414, 418, 421, 438, 440, 442, 451, 510–511
Aldosteronism, 189
Algor mortis, 10
Alkaloid poisoning, 345, 430, 468
Alkalosis, 115, 190, 516
postmortem chemical changes in, 115t
Alkaptonuria, 190, 409–410

f: figure
t: table

Alpha-lipoprotein deficiency, 278
Alport, 321–322, 481–482
Aluminum tube, 35f
Alzheimer's disease, 7, 74, 193, 200, 248, 255, 304
Amaurosis fugax, 191
Amblyopia, nutritional, 191, 197
Ambulance run sheet, 180
Amebiasis, 191–192, 247, 290, 297
American Registry of Pathology
  Armed Forces Institute of Pathology, 148
Aminoaciduria, 192, 231, 237, 271, 319, 343, 345, 370, 424, 441, 492–493, 541–542
Ammonia poisoning, 431
Amniotic fluid embolism, 232, 293–294, 481
Amphetamine dependence, 193, 248
Amyloidosis, 21, 193–194, 200, 205–206, 218, 225, 261, 268, 270, 282, 286, 310–311, 317, 321, 351, 353, 368–369, 373–374, 383, 396–397, 401, 425–426, 457–458, 470, 498, 500, 507, 518, 522, 532
Amyloid stains, 133
Anal atresia, 211–212, 476
Anaphylactic death, 241
Ancylostomiasis, 194, 268, 543
Andersen's disease, 265
Anemia
  Fanconi's, 194–195, 251, 418, 492
  hemolytic, *See* Hemolytic anemia
  iron deficiency, 196, 386
  megaloblastic, *See* Megaloblastic anemia
  refractory, 500
Anencephaly, 197
Anesthesia-associated death, *See* Death, anesthesia-associated
Aneurysm, 117
  aortic sinus, 198
  ascending aorta, 198
  atherosclerotic aortic, 198
  cerebral artery, 151, 198–199, 236, 330–331
  measurement of, 34
  mycotic aortic, 199
  syphilitic aortic, 199
  traumatic aortic, 200
Angina pectoris, 200
  coronary atherosclerosis microscopic features, 31t
Angioedema, 289
Angiography, 81f, 117, 118–121
  preparation for, 58f
Ankylosing spondylitis, 96, 205–206, 261–262, 268–269, 368, 397, 449, 470, 505
Anomaly, coronary artery, 200
Anorexia nervosa, 201, 472
Anthrax, 201
Antimony poisoning, 202, 431, 440, 442
Anus, imperforate, 202, 210
Aorta
  atherosclerosis of, 34
  evaluation of, 34
Aortic aneurysm, 199
Aortic arch syndrome, 204
Aortic coarctation, 212, 244
Aortic disease, 199, 283, 328, 510
Aortic dissection, 2, 21, 34, 204, 241, 270, 359, 368, 473, 510, 545
Aortic insufficiency, 204, 212, 270, 368, 461, 491, 510, 545
Aorticopulmonary septal defect, 243
Aortic sinus aneurysm, 198
Aortic stenosis
  and heart weight, 29
Aortitis, 199, 202–203, 232, 269, 283, 368, 456, 473, 483, 512, 547
Aortocoronary bypass surgery, 221, 477
Arachnodactyly, 498
Arachnoiditis, spinal, 202
Arch, aortic, interrupted, 203
ARDS, *See* Adult respiratory distress syndrome
Argentaffinoma syndrome, 485
Armed Forces Institute of Pathology (AFIP), 147
  American Registry of Pathology, 148
Arm lesions, 5–6
Arnold-Chiari, 3, 68, 71, 246, 343, 357, 384, 390, 425, 497
Arrhythmia, cardiac, 203, 217, 316, 481
Arsenic poisoning, 203, 431–432, 432, 440–441, 442
Arterial embalming, 14
Arteries
  patent ductal, 204, 286, 421
  persistent truncal, 204, 525
Arteries
  evaluation of, 34
Arteriosclerosis, 203, 210, 223, 252, 276, 464
Arteriosclerosis obliterans, 210
Arteriovenous malformations, 117, 385, 494, 501, 537–538
Arteritis, 34, 198, 200, 202–204, 206, 233, 241, 250, 269–271, 276, 278, 294, 312–313, 324, 326, 368, 379–380, 394, 424, 446, 449, 473, 482–483, 507, 512, 547
  giant cell, 203, 449
  Takayasu's, 203–204, 278, 473, 482
Arthritis, 45, 96, 184, 193–194, 202–203, 205–208, 218–220, 225, 229, 250, 260, 266, 268–269, 271, 273, 278, 280, 287, 310, 312–314, 321–323, 326, 334, 349, 353, 356, 357, 378–381, 388–390, 395, 397, 403, 414, 419, 422, 427–430, 446–447, 449, 453, 455–456, 462, 469–471, 483, 485–486, 491, 493, 500, 503–505, 507–508, 512, 515, 519, 526, 543, 546
Arthritis, rheumatoid, *See* Rheumatoid arthritis
Arthrogryposis multiplex congenita, 207–208
Asbestosis, 52, 208, 426–427, 533
  quantitative evaluation of, 52
Ascending aorta aneurysm, 198
Ascites, chylous, 208
Aspergillosis, 208, 218, 252, 324, 492
Asphyxia, 114, 181, 188, 209, 327, 356
Aspiration, 9, 16, 45, 85–86, 104, 124, 146, 180, 182, 186, 198, 209, 217–218, 240, 242, 249, 291, 306, 354, 356, 406, 407, 423, 445, 447, 461, 466, 481, 516
Asplenia, 212, 244, 370, 385–386, 482, 496, 502–503, 547
Assault, 8, 209, 337, 460–461
Asthma, 209–210, 241, 323–324, 405, 408, 428
Ataxia-telangiectasia, 107, 482

Atherosclerosis, 33, 61, 103, 115, 120, 202–204, 209–210, 213, 224, 232, 241, 251, 259, 269–270, 285, 295, 301, 307, 345, 348, 351, 355, 359, 407, 409, 415, 422, 452, 455, 477, 497–498, 500, 543
Atherosclerotic plaques
  correlated with coronary artery disease, 31t
Atlanto-occipital joints, 96
Atomic absorption spectroscopy, 115
Atresia
  biliary, 210, 385, 408
  duodenal, 211–212
  esophageal, 211
  mitral valvular, 211–212
  pulmonary valvular
    with ventricular septal defect, 211
  small intestinal, 211–212
  tricuspid valvular, 212
  urethral, 213
Atrial septal defect, 205, 210, 212–213, 213, 243–244, 244, 303, 385, 388, 491, 499, 516, 524
Atrioventricular conduction system
  dissection of, 26, 28f
Atrophy, multiple system, 213, 247, 507
Atropine, 213, 345, 430, 432–433
  poisoning, 213, 430, 432
Attack, transient cerebral ischemic, 213, 370
Attorneys, 7
Authorization, 159, 160–161
  restricted, 162
Authorization form, 161f
Autolysis, 11
Autopsies by permission, 160–162
Autopsy
  indications for, 160
Autopsy chemistry, 113–115
  definition of, 113
  indications for, 113
  limitations of, 113
  specimen collection for, 113–114
Autopsy diagnoses, 151
Autopsy facilities
  maintenance of, 143–145
Autopsy laboratory, 145f
Autopsy material
  shipping of, 134–135
Autopsy microbiology, 101–104
  processing equipment, 102f
  specimen collection, 102–104
  specimen submission and culture, 102
Autopsy photography, 140–141, 140f
Autopsy protocols, 153–154
Autopsy records
  institutional, 154–155
Autopsy roentgenology, 117–121
  applications of, 117
Autopsy room
  cleaning of, 143–144
  equipment in, 118
  safety features of, 144f
Autopsy techniques, 3–4
Autopsy toxicology, 14
Autoradiography, 133
Avitaminosis, 213

B

Bacillary dysentery, 205, 439
Bagassosis, 215
Band saws, 95
Barbiturate poisoning, 215, 353, 433
Barbiturates, 17, 304, 433, 450
Baritosis, 215, 426
Barium sulfate mixtures, 138
Barrett's esophagus, 183, 530
Bartonellosis, 215
Basedow's disease, 350
Base of heart method
  of cardiac dissection, 23–24, 25f
Basilar impression, 357, 384, 397, 425, 513
Bassen-Kornzweig syndrome, 175
Bechterew's disease, 470
Beckwith-Wiedemann, 482
Beguez-Cesar disease, 486
Belladonna, 432
Beneke's technique, 68f
Beriberi, 216, 245, 449, 510, 547
Bertrand-van Bogaert disease, 247
Berylliosis, 216, 322, 426–427
B-5 fixative, 129–130
Bile
  sampling of, 16
Bilharziasis, 216, 464
Biliary atresia, 56, 210–211, 235, 245–246, 357, 487, 510
Bilirubin
  postmortem changes in, 114t
Binswanger's disease, 299
Bismuth, 17, 51, 216, 364, 433
Blackwater fever, 384
Blalock-Hanlon shunt, 41
Blalock-Taussig shunt, 41
Blastomycosis
  North American, 216
  South American, 217
Blood
  for carbon monoxide determination
    shipping of, 135
  collection of
    for autopsy chemistry, 113
  sampling of, 16
Blood cultures
  collection of, 102–103
Blood typing, 11
Bloom's syndrome, 375, 484, 503
BMI, 567t
Bodies, foreign, 217, 338
Body
  donation of, 162–163
  identification of, 11–12
  transportation of, 164
Body fluids
  for microbiologic study
    shipping of, 135

Body mass index (BMI), 567t
Bolus, 217, 240–241, 407–408, 462
Bolus death, 407
Bone marrow
  chromosome studies, 109
  preparation of, 96–97
Bone marrow transplantation, 266–267, 267, 277, 375–376, 381, 392, 394, 401, 413, 426, 428, 451, 504, 521, 522
Bones
  of extremities
    sawing, 96
  maceration of, 97–98
Bone specimens
  dissection and removal of, 95
  preparation of, 95
Bornholm disease, 425
Borreliosis, 312
Botulism, 217, 439
Bouin's fixative, 129
Bourneville's disease, 467
Brain
  detachment of, 65–66
  dissection of, 74
    in infants and fetuses, 74
  fibers of
    staining of, 133
  perfusion of, 74
  removal of, 65
    in infants and fetuses, 66–67
  tissue blocks
    for histologic examination, 79
  ventriculography of, 81–82
  weight and measurement of, 565t, 570t
Brain abscess, 176
Brain stem
  dissection of, 77f
  sectioning of, 75f
Brain stem encephalitis, 297–298
Breast carcinoma, 99f
Brill-Zinsser disease, 315
Bromide, 109, 130, 218, 433–434, 440
Bronchi
  dissection of, 45
Bronchial arteriography, 50, 51f
Bronchial casts
  preparation of, 51
Bronchiectasis, 176, 193, 206, 208, 218–219, 225, 233–234, 258, 267, 316, 389, 411, 428, 440, 482, 493, 504, 524
Bronchitis
  acute chemical, 218, 289, 431, 436, 477
  chronic, *See* Chronic bronchitis
Bronchocentric granulomatosis, 208–209, 324
Bronchography, 50
Bronchopneumonia, 7, 13, 153, 182, 217, 219, 221, 223–224, 236, 260, 271, 273, 287, 305, 313–314, 378–379, 393–394, 406, 422–423, 439, 441, 445, 466, 475, 507, 516, 527
Brucellosis, 205, 219, 226, 463
Budd-Chiari, 279, 349, 390, 408, 422, 448, 484, 518
Buerger's disease, 203, 255, 276, 517
Bullet
  skull base, 118f
Bullet wounds
  appearance of, 365f
Burns, 9, 14, 220–221, 242, 247, 318, 327, 346, 363, 366, 394, 396, 398, 434–436, 439, 441, 468, 481
Bypass, aortocoronary, 221
Byssinosis, 221, 426

C

Cadmium, 51, 223, 434, 439–442, 493
Cadmium poisoning, 223, 434, 440, 442
Caisson disease, 469
Calcium pyrophosphate dihydrate deposition disease, 453
Calcium stains, 134
Calvarium
  macerated, 98f
  opening of
    in neonate and fetus, 68f
  sawing, 96
Canavan's disease, 247
Candidiasis, 223, 354, 396, 503, 539
Canicola fever, 374
Cannabis, 177
CAP, 155
Carbon monoxide
  detection of, 17
Carbon monoxide poisoning, 223, 435–436
Carbon monoxide rejuvenation, 132
Carcinoid syndrome, 485–486, 532–533, 537
Cardiac chamber
  sizes of, 29
Cardiac conduction system
  dissection of, 26–28
Cardiac dilatation, 29
Cardiac dissection
  methods of, 21–28
Cardiac hypertrophy, 29, 35, 251, 275, 407, 478, 519, 525
Cardiac valves
  circumference of, 29
  diameter of, 29
  size of, 29
Cardiac valvular vegetations, 103f
  collection of, 103–104
Cardiac wall
  thickness of, 29
Cardiomegaly, 33
Cardiomyopathy, 33
  alcoholic, 224, 306
  dilated, 224, 368, 370
  and heart weight, 29
  hypertrophic, 224, 475
  restrictive, *See* Restrictive cardiomyopathy
Cardiospasm, 182
Cardiovascular system, 21–35
  Latin terms for, 40
Care coronary, 407
Carnoy's fixative, 130
Caroli's disease, 117, 236, 256, 263, 316, 385
Carotid arteries, 83

Carrion's disease, 215
Cassidy-Scholte syndrome, 485
Cat scratch disease, 215, 257
Cause of death
  definition of, 7
  immediate, 152
Celiac arteriography
  partitioned abdominal viscera for, 55f
Central pontine myelinosis, 396
Cerebellar cortical degeneration, 186, 247, 529–530, 534, 541
Cerebellum
  dissection of, 77f
Cerebral abscess, 8, 192, 205, 218, 249, 365, 474, 516–517
Cerebral arteries
  arteriography of, 80–81
Cerebral hemispheres
  sectioning of, 76f
Cerebral infarction, 263, 448
Cerebral venous sinus thrombosis, 176, 269, 359, 517–518
Cerebrospinal fluid
  collection of, 104
  sampling of, 16
Cerebrovascular disease, 214
Cervical spinal cord
  removal of, 69
Cervical spine
  removal of, 71f
Cervical vertebrae
  congenital fusion of, 245, 497
Chagas disease, 182, 257–258, 526
Chain of custody, 13, 17
Chediak-Higashi syndrome, 503
Chickenpox, 545
Child abuse
  vitreous sampling, 85
Children
  chromosome study
    indications for, 107
  weights and measurement of, 554t–565t, 563t–565t
Chinese liver fluke infection, 231
Chlamydia, 410
Chloride
  postmortem changes in, 114t
Chlorine poisoning, 436, 440
Chloroma
  stains for, 134
Cholangiography, 56–57, 59f, 117
  preparation for, 58f
Cholangitis
  sclerosing, 225, 317, 494, 519
  suppurative, 226
Cholecystitis, 196, 220, 226–227, 235, 277, 296, 314, 317, 321, 378, 418, 475, 528
Choledocholithiasis, 196, 227, 256, 277, 418
Cholelithiasis, 196, 211, 226–227, 231, 252, 256, 262, 277, 314, 317, 332, 347, 406, 408, 418, 453, 475, 527–528
Cholera, 227
Cholesterol
  postmortem changes in, 114t
Cholesteryl ester storage disease, 258
Cholinesterase
  postmortem changes in, 114t
Chondrodysplasia, 228, 344, 490, 491
Chondrodystrophia fetalis, 183
Chorea
  acute, 229, 492
  hereditary, 229, 268, 492
Chromosome analysis
  methods of, 109
Chromosome study, 107–110
  costs of, 108
  indications for, 107–108
  specimen collection, transport and processing, 108–109
Chronic bronchitis, 188, 219, 244, 295, 362, 427, 440
Chronic heart failure
  coronary atherosclerosis microscopic features, 31t
Chronic hepatitis, 253, 308, 451–452, 480, 507, 519
Chronic mediastinitis, 317
Churg-Strauss syndrome, 323–324, 487, 492
Chylothorax, 208, 229–230, 344
Chylous ascites, 423
Cirrhosis, liver, 230, 234, 308, 329
Classic autopsy techniques, 3
Classification
  in death certificates, 152
Clearing techniques, 139
Clinical disease
  and postmortem culture results, 101
Clonorchiasis, 231, 308, 318, 528
Closed head injury
  in vehicular accidents, 181
Clostridial infection, 310
Clostridium botulinum, 217
Clostridium tetani, 515
Coagulation, disseminated intravascular, 231–232, 281–282, 353, 496
Coarctation, aortic, 232, 370, 384
Cocaine dependence, 233, 248, 430
Coding manuals, 155
Colitis, collagenous, 234
Collagen disease, 260, 305
College of American Pathologists (CAP), 155
Colorado tick fever, 309
Common atrium, 244, 386, 502
Complete atrioventricular septal defect, 23, 244, 475, 502
Complete transposition, 547
Computerized tomography, 121
Conception
  products of
    chromosome studies, 109
Confidentiality
  of records, 163–164
Congenital bicuspid aortic valve, 283, 368, 473
Congenital cardiac left-to-right shunts
  plexogenic pulmonary hypertension in
    modified Heath-Edwards classification of, 33t
Congenital coronary abnormalities, 117
Congenital erythropoietic porphyria, 451

Congenital heart disease, 33–34
  and heart weight, 29
  standardized form for, 42–43
  synonyms for diagnostic terms in, 39
Congenital hepatic fibrosis, 235–236, 263, 497, 502, 547
Congenitally bicuspid aortic valve, 545
Congenitally bicuspid pulmonary valve, 545
Congenitally corrected transposition, 547
Congenital malformations
  surgical procedures for
    eponyms for, 41
Congenital megacolon, 357
Congenital neurosyphilis, 512
Congenital rubella, 210–211, 462, 487
Congenital supravalvular aortic stenosis, 473
Congenital supravalvular pulmonary stenosis, 473
Congenital syphilis, 357, 512–513
Congenital urethral valves
  urogram of, 62f
Congenital valvular aortic stenosis, 473–474
Congenital valvular pulmonary stenosis, 500
Congestive heart failure, 121, 193, 196, 204, 233, 270, 275, 278, 290, 303, 307, 355, 370, 398, 473
Congophil cerebral angiopathy, 193
Conn's syndrome, 189, 488, 527
Consent form, 162
Contaminated equipment
  warning label for, 144f
Contrast media, 138
Cori's disease, 265
Cornea
  rcmoval of, 86
Coronary abnormalities
  congenital, 117
Coronary angiogram, 120f
Coronary arteries
  atherosclerosis of, 34
  contrast medium injection into, 120f
  dissection of, 21
  evaluation of, 21
Coronary artery bypass graft
  schematic diagram of, 32f
Coronary artery disease, 117
  correlated with atherosclerotic plaques, 31t
Coronary obstruction
  grading of, 21
Coroners, 7
Corpora cavernosa
  fixation of, 60
Corrosion casts
  preparation of, 57
Corrosion methods, 139
Cranial nerves, 66
Cranium
  Paget's disease, 98f
  sawing of, 65
Creatinine
  postmortem changes in, 114t
Cremation
  radioisotopes contaminating, 126
Cretinism, 355
Creutzfeldt-Jakob disease, 65, 83, 146, 149, 260–261, 276, 304
Crib death, 242
Cri du Chat syndrome, 107
Crohn's disease, 193, 196–197, 225, 230, 261–262, 265, 268–269, 301, 303, 418, 470, 530
Cronkhite-Canada, 449–450, 488, 537
Croup, 373, 407
Cryptococcosis, 216, 234, 252, 368, 377, 479, 519
Cryptosporidiosis, 234–235, 479
Cushing's, 252, 262, 287, 345, 403, 407, 414, 485, 488–489, 522–523, 527, 531–536, 539
Custody, 160
Cyanide
  detection of, 18
Cyanide poisoning, 235, 435, 437
Cystic fibrosis, 115, 211–212, 218, 317, 324, 357, 411, 417
Cystinosis, 236–237, 492
Cysts, renal, 279
Cytochemistry
  immediate autopsy for, 5
Cytomegalovirus infection, 237, 262, 359–360, 391, 397, 417, 547

D

Damus-Kaye-Stansel procedure, 41
Data processing
  planning of, 155
Data retrieval
  methods of, 154–155
Davies' endomyocardial fibrosis, 225
Death
  abortion-associated, 175, 239, 452, 476
  accidental
    definition of, 7
  anaphylactic, 194, 239, 241, 289, 468–469, 476
  anesthesia-associated, 198, 239–240, 240, 327, 439
  bolus, 407
  chemical evidence of, 11
  circumstances of, 8–10
  crib, 242
  definition of, 7–8
  entomologic evidence of, 11
  manner of
    definition of, 7
  natural, 8
  from natural causes, 8
  postoperative, 240, 244
  pronouncement of, 8
  restaurant, 407
  sniffing and spray, 240, 439
  spray, 209
  sudden, *See* Sudden death
    of adult, 241
    of infant, 240, 242, 508
  time of
    estimation of, 10–11

Death certificates, 8, 151–153
admissibility as evidence, 163–164
delayed, 152–153
problems with, 153
Death masks, 6
Death scene evaluation, 8–10
Decalcifying procedures, 97
Decedent
permission from, 160
Decompression sickness, 178, 180, 243, 256, 413, 469
Decontamination
of instruments, clothing, and waste products
in radioactive deceased person, 127
Degeneration
spongy
of white matter, 247, 263, 376
Dehiscence
in postoperative autopsies, 4
Dehydration, 9, 114–115, 131, 134, 223, 227–228, 234, 242, 247–248, 251, 261, 287, 302, 319, 328, 348, 358, 367, 370, 386, 423, 451, 492, 498, 506, 511, 517–518
postmortem chemical changes in, 115t
Dental roentgenograms, 117
Deoxyribonucleic acid
postmortem changes in, 114t
Dermatomyositis, 203, 206, 250, 260, 262, 321, 419, 428, 447, 449, 503, 529–530, 534, 538–539
De Toni-Debre-Fanconi syndrome, 236
Devil's grip, 425
Diabetes insipidus, 251, 464
Diabetes mellitus, 114–115, 184, 193, 210, 234, 242–243, 250–251, 253, 270, 307, 317, 321, 367, 369, 394–395, 403, 405, 407, 410, 413–414, 457, 471–472, 496, 498, 510, 517–518, 534
postmortem chemical changes in, 115t
Dialysis, 9, 17, 193, 216, 253, 256, 290, 307, 322, 333, 421, 443, 532
Diaphragmatic hernia, 196, 306, 334, 455, 466, 499, 532
Diatom
detection of, 286
Diffuse alveolar disease, 263
DiGeorge's syndrome, 489, 503–504
Digestions
at time of death, 10–11
Digitalis poisoning, 203, 254, 430, 438
Dilated cardiomyopathy, 24, 33, 224, 316, 324, 368, 370, 480
Diphtheria, 229, 254, 373
Disseminated intravascular coagulation, 195, 232, 272–273, 285, 300, 307, 315, 389, 536
Diverticula, 55, 196–197, 283, 336, 344, 467, 498
Diving accident, 178, 283, 468–469
Documents
flow of, 143
Donation, 162–163
Double inlet left ventricle, 547
Down syndrome, 107
Drowning, 34, 45, 178–179, 284–285
Drug dependence, 249, 321, 334, 353
Drug screening, 17
Dumdum fever, 371
Dupuytren's contracture, 494
Dura, 71
Dwarfism, 183, 228, 286, 369, 392, 484, 491, 503
Dysentery, bacillary, 287, 302, 468
Dyskinesia, 287
Dystrophy, muscular, 288

E

Ear, 72
Ebstein's malformation, 201, 385, 452, 511
Echinococcosis, 268, 289, 297
Edema, 7, 32, 46, 129, 176, 179–182, 189, 201, 216, 218, 221, 224, 228, 240–242, 249–250, 257, 261, 268, 270–271, 278, 280, 284–285, 289, 295, 299, 305–306, 307–308, 310, 320, 328, 334, 356, 359, 363, 366, 370, 371, 384, 386–387, 391–392, 408, 425, 429, 434–443, 445, 449, 456, 461–462, 464, 469, 472, 481, 484, 488, 499, 506–507, 512, 517, 519, 524–525, 546
Edwards syndrome, 107
Effusions, 2, 14, 201, 219–220, 224, 229–230, 254, 257, 259, 270–271, 284, 344, 355, 361, 371, 379, 410, 417, 428–429, 469–471, 484, 491, 525–527, 536, 545
Electrical injury, 220, 290, 363, 366, 468
Electric burns, 363
Electric shock, 363
Electrolyte, 97, 183, 189–190, 221, 223, 225, 242, 247, 261, 282, 290, 328, 345–346, 348, 351, 353–354, 367, 369, 371, 386, 396, 403, 406, 424, 445, 452, 469, 489, 498, 517, 519, 529, 533–535
Electron microscopy
fixation for, 132–133
immediate autopsy for, 5
sample collection for, 5
ELISA, 16, 17
Ellis-van Creveld syndrome, 228, 287, 491
Embalming, 14, 164
obtaining vessels after, 34
of radioactive deceased person, 124–125
Embolism
air, *See* Air embolism
amniotic fluid, *See* Amniotic fluid embolism
arterial, 293
fat, *See* Fat embolism
gas, 117
pulmonary, *See* Pulmonary embolism
EMIT, 16, 17
Emphysema, 9, 47, 52, 103, 179–180, 188, 209, 219, 240, 242, 244, 250, 260, 285, 295, 316, 324, 350, 362, 366, 408, 411, 423, 426, 428, 435, 454, 469, 490–491, 506, 531, 533, 543
Empty sella, 491–492
Empyema, epidural, 176–177, 296
Encephalitis
brain stem, 297
limbic, 297–298
Encephalomyelitis, 263, 297–298, 353, 360, 380, 397, 533
Encephalopathy
hepatic, 298, 507
hypertensive, 299
Encephalotrigeminal angiomatosis, 278

Enchondromatosis
multiple, 286
Endocardial cushion defect, 244
Endocarditis, infective, *See* Infective endocarditis
Endocrine disorders
postmortem chemical changes in, 115t
Endoscopic autopsies, 5
Energy-dispersive x-ray microanalysis, 133
Entamoeba histolytica, 191
Enteritis, necrotizing, 301
Enterocolitis
ischemic, 301–302
neutropenic, 301–302
pseudomembranous, 302, 321
staphylococcal, 301–302
Enteropathy, protein-losing, 302
Enzyme-linked immunosorbent assay (ELISA), 16, 17
Enzyme-multiplied immunotechnique (EMIT), 16, 17
Eosinophilic gastroenteritis, 321
Eosinophilic pneumonia, 324
Eosinophilic pulmonary syndrome, 303, 324, 429, 492, 496, 498
Eosin stains, 133
Epidural abscess, 176, 296
Epidural empyema, 176, 249
Epilepsy
idiopathic, 303–304
myoclonus, 303–304, 398
symptomatic, 303–304
Equipment
cleaning of, 143–144
contaminated
warning label for, 144f
Erythema multiforme, 261, 304–305, 447, 508
Erythroblastosis fetalis, 305
Erythropoietic porphyria
congenital, 451
Esophageal achalasia, 183
Esophageal atresia, 212
Esophageal varices, 53–54, 54f, 121, 151, 254, 264, 274, 316, 330, 349, 448, 465, 485, 535, 546
demonstration of, 53
Esophagus, 46f, 53–62
Esophagus, Barrett's, 306, 482
Ethanol intoxication, 186
Ethyl alcohol
gas chromatography of, 17
Ethylenediamine tetraaceticacid (EDTA) decalcification fluid, 97
Ethylene glycol poisoning, 202, 431, 438, 439–440, 440
European blastomycosis, 234
Exhumation, 14, 164–165
Exposure, cold, 233, 277, 306, 355
External examination, 13–14
Extrapyramidal, 492
Eye, 85–93
for corneal transplantation, 87f
on dental wax, 90f, 91f
enucleated, 89f
removal of, 73f, 85–86
Eyelids
held apart, 86f

F

Fabry's disease, 33, 263, 282, 321
Face
protective garments for, 145
Facial lesions, 5–6
Factor IX deficiency, 259
Familial Mediterranean fever, 311, 446, 450
Familial periodic paralysis, 398, 421
Familial polyposis, 450, 537
Fanconi's anemia, 194–195, 251, 418, 492
Fanconi syndrome
infantile, 234
Fat embolism, 34, 254, 294, 365, 367, 419, 469, 481
Fat stains, 133
Feminization, testicular, 308
Femoral arteries
obtaining after embalming, 34
Femoral-popliteal vessels, 35f
Femur
sawing, 96
Ferrochelatase deficiency, 453
Ferruginous bodies, 52
Fetal alcoholic syndrome, 186
Fetalis
erythroblastosis, 344
Fetus
brain
dissection of, 74
removal of, 66–67
calvarium
opening of, 68f
weights and measurement of, 554t, 556t, 559t–561t
Fibroblasts
chromosome studies, 109
Fibropolycystic disease
of the liver and biliary tract, 235, 263, 276
Fibropolycystic liver disease, 256
Fibrosing syndrome, 494
Fibrosis
congenital hepatic, 316, 385
cystic, 316, 394
retroperitoneal, 317
Fibrous dysplasia, 529
Fingerprinting, 11
Firearm injury, 217, 326, 336, 363, 365
FISH, 109, 110f
Fistulas
in postoperative autopsies, 4
Fixation mixtures, 129–132
color preserving, 131–132
Fixed brain
dissection of, 74–75
Fixed lungs, 46–47
slicing of, 47
Flavivirus infection, 315
Floppy valve syndrome, 368
Fluorescence in situ hybridization (FISH), 109, 110f

Fluorosis, 318, 440
Foix-Alajouanine syndrome, 385
Fontan procedure, 41
Food poisoning, 434, 439
Foramen ovale
  patency of, 29–30
Forbe's disease, 265
Foreign bodies, 117, 179, 217, 239, 281, 284, 320, 403, 460
Forensic autopsy protocol, 12–13
Forensic pathologists, 7
Formalin fixation
  of lungs, 46–47
  organ weight changes after, 372f
Formalin-fixed specimens
  rejuvenation of, 132
Formalin pigment
  removal from histological sections, 174
Formalin replacements, 130–131
Formalin solutions, 130
Formic acid decalcification fluid, 97
Fort Bragg fever, 374
Four-chamber method
  of cardiac dissection, 23, 24f
Fractures
  in vehicular accidents, 181
Francisella tularensis, 526
Franklin's disease, 267
Friedreich's ataxia, 224, 247, 251
Fructose intolerance, 370
Fructosemia
  hereditary, 370
Funeral director, 161–162

G
Galactosemia, 231, 319, 333, 492
Gallbladder, 57
  stains for, 134
Gallstones, 57
Ganglia, 71
Gangliosidosis, 279, 282, 303, 319–320, 469
Gangrene, gas, 320, 398
Gas chromatography, 17
Gas chromatography linked to mass spectrometry (GC/MS), 17–18
Gas embolism, 117
Gastric arteriography, 53
Gastroenteritis
  clostridial, 301
Gastrointestinal hemorrhage, 151, 230, 264, 270, 274, 315–316, 455–456, 535, 543
Gastrointestinal tract
  sampling of, 16
Gaucher's disease, 264–265, 282, 286, 410, 413
GC/MS, 17–18
Genetic hemochromatosis, 56
Genital system, 59–61
German measles, 462
Ghon technique, 3
Giant cell arteritis, 203–204, 449
Glanders, 389
Glass slides
  shipping of, 134
Glenn anastomosis, 41
Globe
  measurement of, 90f
  roentgenogram of, 91f
  sectioned, 92f
    instruments for, 93f
  sectioning of, 91f
Globoid cell leukodystrophy, 263, 270, 376
Glomerulonephritis, 225, 236, 245, 269, 307–308, 311, 313, 317, 321–322, 331, 348, 379, 403, 447, 456, 467, 480, 482, 488, 497, 500, 508, 518, 520, 523, 525, 539–540, 546
Gloves, 145–146
Glucose
  postmortem changes in, 114t
Glutaraldehyde, 130–131
Glycogen storage disease, 265, 279, 322, 532
Goodpasture's syndrome, 203, 263, 321, 331, 494–495, 500
Gout, 96, 99, 134, 205, 251, 265, 308, 322, 347, 376, 403, 453
  stains for, 134
Graft-*versus*-host disease, 266–267, 401, 418, 521
Gram stain, 101
Granuloma, midline, 323, 462
Granulomatosis
  allergic
    and angiitis, 323, 487
  bronchocentric, 324
  lymphomatoid, 324
Graves' disease, 350
Gronblad-Strandberg syndrome, 455
Gross tissues
  staining, 133–134
Group B arbovirus infection, 315
Gunther's disease, 451

H
Hair
  sampling of, 17
Hands
  lesions of, 5–6
  in peritoneal cavity
    dose to, 125t
Hand-Schuller-Christian disease, 335
Hanging, 327, 476
Hansen's disease, 373
Harrington syndrome, 489
Hashish, 177
HCOM, 224
Head injury, 176, 181, 251, 303–304, 330–331, 364–365, 517
Heart
  description of, 21
  dissection methods of, 21–28
  gross examination of, 30
  microscopic examination of, 30
  perfusion fixation of, 28
  quantitative measurements of, 28–30
  removal from chest, 21

tomographic dissection of
repairing mistakes in, 23
weight and measurement of, 562t–564t, 568t–570t
weight of, 28–29
Heart block, 26, 470, 505, 524, 547
Heart concussion
in vehicular accidents, 181
Heart transplantation, 406, 478, 522
Heatstroke, 327–328, 350, 477
Heavy chain disease, 282
Heavy metals
detection of, 17–18
in media, 138
Helly's fixative, 131
Hematoma
spinal epidural, 328
subdural, 328, 331
Hematoxylin stains, 133
Hemochromatosis, 33, 56, 133, 224, 230, 245, 251–252, 269, 328–329, 331, 351, 369, 410, 453, 532
Hemolytic anemia, 9, 175, 195–197, 215, 225, 277–278, 281, 305, 451, 516, 537
Hemolytic uremic syndrome, 456
Hemophilia, 231, 254, 259, 280–282, 330
Hemorrhage, gastrointestinal, 230, 330
Hemorrhagic fever
with renal syndrome, 310, 360
Hemorrhagic fever syndrome, 315
Hemorrhagic telangiectasia
hereditary, 274
Hemosiderin, 133
Hemosiderosis, idiopathic pulmonary, 331
Hemothorax
in vehicular accidents, 181
Hepatic arteriography, 56–57
Hepatic coma
postmortem chemical changes in, 115t
Hepatic encephalopathy, 231, 298, 507
Hepatitis
chronic, 330–331, 333–334, 367
neonatal, 225, 332
viral, 171, 234, 240, 308, 332–333
Hepatoduodenal ligament, 55–56
Hernia
diaphragmatic, *See* Diaphragmatic hernia
Herpes simplex infection, 298, 334, 360
Herpes zoster infection, 334, 360, 361, 397, 468
Hers' disease, 265
Heterotaxy syndrome, 502
High-performance liquid chromatography (HPLC), 17, 114
High-risk autopsies
policies for, 146
Hilus
dissection from, 45
Hirschsprung's disease, 388
Histiocytosis, Langerhans cell, 323, 335, 495, 498
Histochemistry
fixation for, 132–133
Histological sections
removal of formalin pigment from, 174
Histological stains, 172t–173t
Histoplasmosis, 336, 368, 388, 479, 494, 509
HIV, 478
Hoeve's syndrome, 412
Holmes heart, 547
Homicide, 7–9, 11, 152, 159, 164–165, 209, 336, 339, 358, 363, 366, 395, 444, 460, 476
definition of, 7
Homocystinuria, 192, 343
Hospital risk managers, 7
HPLC, 17, 114
Human immunodeficiency virus (HIV), 478
Humeroscapular joints, 96
Humerus
macerated, 98f
sawing, 96
Hunter disease, 282
Huntington's chorea, 229
Hurler's disease, 282, 392
Hydatid disease, 289
Hydrocephalus, 75, 183, 228, 234, 272, 300, 314, 343, 352, 375, 382, 384–385, 390, 393, 404–405, 414, 435–436, 454, 494, 513, 520–521, 525
Hydrochloric acid poisoning, 439–440
Hydromyelia, 513
Hydronephrosis, 213, 262, 317, 343, 448, 457, 465, 536, 540–541, 543
Hydrops fetalis, 320, 500, 513, 516–517
Hypereosinophilic syndrome, 225
Hyperglycemia
postmortem chemical changes in, 115t
Hyperlipoproteinemia, 251, 286, 345–346, 377, 407, 547
Hyperoxaluria, 346, 403, 415
Hyperparathyroidism, 118, 184, 277, 280, 322, 346–347, 349, 402–403, 410, 414–415, 417–418, 453, 457, 516, 518, 527
Hyperpituitary gigantism, 183
Hypertension, *See* specific disease
Hypertensive encephalopathy, 299
Hyperthermia, 327
Hyperthyroidism, 229, 267, 270, 287, 350, 395, 411, 414, 498, 519, 540
Hypertrophic cardiomyopathy, 24, 29, 33, 263, 500
Hypertrophic obstructive cardiomyopathy (HCOM), 224
Hypertrophy
cardiac, 224, 351
Hyperuricemia, 322
Hypervitaminosis A, 454, 547
Hypervitaminosis D, 403, 547
Hypofibrinogenemia, 232
Hypogammaglobulinemia, 353, 362, 503–504, 539
Hypoglycemia, 114–115, 252, 265, 304, 348, 353–355, 370, 506, 527, 530, 532–535, 538
postmortem chemical changes in, 115t
Hypoparathyroidism, 197, 354, 367, 454, 498
Hypoplasia, 355
Hypoplastic left heart syndrome, 210
Hypothyroidism, 194, 234, 270, 286, 322, 345, 355–356, 366–368, 399, 407, 410, 467, 492, 498, 519
Hypovitaminosis A, 245

Hypovitaminosis C, 245
Hypovitaminosis D, 245
Hypoxanthine
  postmortem changes in, 114t
Hypoxia, 178–179, 181, 188, 209, 217, 277, 284, 356, 476

I

ICD9CM, 155
Ileus, meconium, 357
Iliac crest
  sawing, 96
Immediate autopsies, 5
Immunochemistry, 114
Immunocompromised patients, 101
Immunohistochemistry, 114–115
  fixation for, 133
Imperforate anus, 211
Impression, basilar, 318, 357
Inborn errors of metabolism
  postmortem chemical changes in, 115t
Incisions
  in postoperative autopsies, 4
India ink, 138
Infanticide, 177, 240, 242, 336, 358
Infantile Fanconi syndrome, 236
Infantile obstructive cholangiopathy, 210
Infants
  brain
    dissection of, 74
    removal of, 66–67
  chromosome study
    indications for, 107
  spinal cord
    removal of, 70–71
  weights and measurement of, 557t–558t, 563t, 564t–565t
Infarction, cerebral, 213, 257, 294, 330–331, 359, 370, 477
Infectious arthritis, 96
Infectious mononucleosis, 454, 503
Infectious peritonitis, 423
Infective endocarditis, 103, 176–177, 198–199, 205, 213, 219, 226–227, 232, 249, 253, 272, 293, 300, 312, 321, 359, 368–370, 378–379, 389, 398, 411, 428, 474–475, 478, 499–500, 516, 527, 545
Inferior vena cava
  anterior view of, 60f
Infiltration, 139
Inflammatory bowel disease, 233, 235, 245, 250, 261, 268–269, 302, 411, 413, 528
Inflow-outflow method
  of cardiac dissection, 21–22, 22f
Influenza, 153, 362, 428, 494, 506
Injectable media, 138–139
Injection-corrosion method
  of cardiac dissection, 26
Injury
  at autopsy facility, 146
In situ hybridization
  fixation for, 133
Institutional tissue registry, 146
Instruments
  safety for, 146
Insurance
  unauthorized autopsies, 162
Internal carotid artery
  intracranial freeing of, 82f
International Classification of Diseases (ICD9CM), 155
Interrupted aortic arch, 205, 474
Interstitial pneumonia, 191, 250, 317, 359, 378, 387, 428–429, 434, 461, 471, 487, 495, 506, 521
Intestinal tract, 53–54
Intolerance, fructose, 318, 370
Intraocular prosthesis (IOL), 93
Intubation injury, 366, 370, 428
Iodine poisoning, 370, 440
IOL, 93
Iron
  stain for, 133
Irradiation
  protection from, 146
Ischemic enterocolitis, 301
Ischemic heart disease, 29–32, 180, 188, 200, 255, 269–270, 345, 359, 366, 368, 370, 471, 543
Isopropyl alcohol poisoning, 185, 440, 453
Ivemark's syndrome, 502

J

Jatene procedure, 41
JCAHO, 155
Joint Commission of Accreditation of Health Care Organizations (JCAHO), 155
Joints
  dissection and removal of, 96
Jores' solution, 132
Juvenile rheumatoid arthritis, 206

K

Kaiserling's solutions, 132
  modified after Lundquist, 132
Kala-Azar, 371, 373
Kawasaki disease, 446, 499
Keratomalacia, 245
Kernohan's extraction technique, 69–70
Kidneys, 59
  anterior view of, 60f
  vinyl plastic cast of, 139f
Klinefelter's syndrome, 107, 287, 375, 496–497
Klippel-Feil deformity, 246, 357, 384, 425, 497, 513
Konno procedure, 41
Krabbe's disease, 282

L

Lacrimal gland
  removal of, 87
Lactic acid
  postmortem changes in, 114t
Lafora's disease, 303
Langer-Giedion syndrome, 107
Langerhans cell histiocytosis, 96, 286
Laryngeal joints, 96
Laryngitis, 209, 234, 243, 275, 303, 305–306, 373, 408, 423, 546

Larynx, 46f
  dissection of, 45
Lassa fever, 310–311
Latex injection, 51
Latin terms
  for cardiovascular structures, 40
Laurence-Moon-Biedl, 407, 497
Law, 159–164
Lead poisoning, 196, 297, 299, 304, 322, 373, 440–441, 442
Left orbit view
  diagram of, 88f
Left ventricular hypoplasia, 500
Left ventricular region
  schematic diagram of, 31f
Legionnaires' disease, 270, 271
Leishmania donovani, 371
Leprosy, 193, 321, 323, 373–374
Leptospirosis, 297, 374, 510
Letulle technique, 3
Leukemia, 9, 86, 195, 208, 223, 225, 232, 234, 264, 266–267, 282, 286, 330, 344, 361–362, 366, 375–376, 381, 386–387, 390, 394, 396–397, 404–405, 419, 421, 448, 470, 480, 484, 489–490, 496, 500–501, 504, 521–522, 531, 539, 545
Leukodystrophy, 247, 275, 466
  globoid cell, 270, 376
  sudanophilic, 263, 376
Libman-Sacks verrucous nonbacterial endocarditis, 300
Life insurance companies, 7
Light microscopy
  fixation for, 129
Lightning injury, 366, 377
Lipidosis
  sulfatide, 377
Lipoid pneumonia, 263, 411, 430
Lipoid stains, 133
Lipoproteinosis, pulmonary alveolar, 263, 377, 453
Lipoproteins
  postmortem changes in, 114t
Lipshaw autopsy saw, 95
Liquid radioisotopes
  and autopsy, 125–126
  and embalming, 124–125
Listeriosis, 378
Liver, 55–56
  fixation of, 56
  gross staining for iron, 56
  posterior view of, 56f
  sampling of, 16–17
  slicing, 56, 57f
Liver cirrhosis, 121, 265
Liver disease
  postmortem chemical changes in, 115t
Liver mortis, 10
Liver transplantation, 230, 245, 396, 420, 443, 472, 478, 485, 523
Lobstein's syndrome, 412
Lockjaw, 515
Loffler's eosinophilic endomyocarditis, 225
Loffler's syndrome, 492
Long-axis method
  of cardiac dissection, 23, 25f
Louis-Bar syndrome, 482
Lower esophageal rings
  demonstration of, 53
Low-salt pattern
  postmortem chemical changes in, 115t
Lumbar roots
  freeing of, 70f
Lungs, 45–52
  abscess, 171, 176, 458
  arteriogram of, 50f
  cultures
    collection of, 103
  cut surface of, 46f–47f
  dissection of, 45–46
  formalin perfusion techniques, 47
  histologic sampling of, 45–46
  paper-mounted sections of, 49–50
  perfusion system for, 48f
  wet fixation of, 46–47
Lung slices, 49f
  barium sulfate impregnation of, 47–49
  perfusion fixed, 49f, 51f
  in plastic bags
    heat sealing for, 147f
  storage of, 49
Lung transplantation, 377, 478, 523
Lyell's disease, 401
Lye poisoning, 380, 441
Lyme disease, 271, 398, 454
Lymphangiography, 35, 50, 121f
Lymphatic channels, 35
Lymphatic vascular disease, 380
Lymphatic vessels
  evaluation of, 34–35
Lymphogranuloma venereum, 302, 380
Lymphoma, 86, 103, 182, 193, 195, 202, 208, 234, 250, 262, 264, 267–269, 275, 303, 305, 317, 323–325, 335, 343, 361–362, 366, 368, 375, 381–382, 394, 396, 419–421, 429, 456–457, 471–472, 479–480, 486, 496, 498, 503–504, 507–508, 521–522, 529, 531, 537–540, 543, 545
Lymphomatoid granulomatosis, 325
Lysosomal storage, 282, 320

M

Maggots, 11
Magnetic resonance imaging, 121
Malabsorption syndrome, 175, 196, 245, 246, 303, 316, 321, 387, 455, 471, 481, 486, 498, 504, 516
Malakoplakia, 344, 383–384, 530
Malaria, 249, 297, 384
Malnutrition, 9, 186, 191, 196–197, 216, 227, 247, 249, 272, 299, 316–317, 319, 357, 371, 386, 388, 396, 405, 414, 423, 432, 441, 472
Malta fever, 219
Manner of death
  definition of, 7
Maple syrup urine disease, 115, 271

Marble bone disease, 413
Marchiafava-Bignami disease, 186, 272
Marfan's syndrome, 283, 343, 368, 414, 498–499
Maroteaux-Lamy syndrome, 392
McArdle's disease, 265
Measles, 297, 373, 387–388, 415, 462
Measurements, *See* Weights and measurements
Measuring devices
  calibrated, 30f
Mechanism of death, 152
  definition of, 7
Meckel's diverticulum, 283
Meconium ileus, 316, 357, 388
Mediastinitis, chronic, 317, 388
Medical examiners, 7
Medical malpractice, 7
Medicolegal autopsies, 7
Medicolegal cases
  death certificates in, 152
Medicolegal investigation
  errors in, 7–8
    caused by, 8
Medicolegal material
  shipping and labeling for, 135
Mediterranean fever, 219
Megacolon
  congenital, 268, 357, 388
Megaloblastic anemia, 197, 304, 405, 472, 504, 519, 538
Melanoma
  stains for, 134
Melioidosis, 389
Meningeal hydrops, 454
Meningococcal disease, 241, 272, 390, 510
Mercury poisoning, 390, 440, 442
Mesenteric angiography, 55
Mesenteric arteries
  atherosclerosis of, 34
Mesenteric arteriography
  partitioned abdominal viscera for, 55f
Metal casts, 139
Metal cone, 30f
Metal probes, 30f
Metaplasia, agnogenic myeloid, 390, 396
Microfilariasis
  disseminated, 409
Microlithiasis, pulmonary alveolar, 391
Microradiography, 97
Microscopic slides
  abbreviations for labeling, 38
Microwave heating
  fixation by, 131
Middle ear
  removal of, 73f
Middle ear joints, 96
Midline granuloma, 323
Mitral insufficiency, 368, 461, 470, 475
Mitral regurgitation, 368
Mitral stenosis, 171, 232, 391, 474
Mitral valve, 104f
Mitral valve prolapse, 368
Mitral valvular atresia, 211
Mongolism, 489
Moniliasis, 223
Mononucleosis, infectious, 391
Morquio disease, 282, 392
Motor neuron disease, 194, 213, 273, 280, 398, 417, 465
Mucocutaneous lymph node syndrome, 446, 499, 500
Mucopolysaccharidosis, 392, 394, 496, 507
Mucormycosis, 253, 394, 424, 479
Mucoviscidosis, 316
Multiple endocrine neoplasia, 183–184, 185, 401, 485, 507, 511, 527, 540, 543
Multiple myeloma, 98, 193, 286, 307, 361, 375, 383, 397, 403, 418, 448–449, 531
  cancellous bone, 98f
Multiple sclerosis, 263, 397, 421, 465–466
Multiple system atrophy, 275
Mummification, 11, 139
Mummified tissues
  rehydration of, 137
Mumps, 394, 417, 421
Murexide test, 134
Muscles
  for sampling, 80t
Mushroom poisoning, 299, 395, 430, 439, 442
Mustard procedure, 41
Myasthenia gravis, 395, 490, 497, 500, 539–540
Mycobacterium leprae, 373
Mycobacterium tuberculosis, 526
Mycotic aortic aneurysm, 199
Myelinosis, central pontine, 396
Myeloma, multiple, 282, 396, 425
Myelopathy/myelitis, 298, 397, 450
Myocardial infarction
  age-related features of, 32t
  coronary atherosclerosis microscopic features, 31t
Myocarditis, 21, 34, 200, 203, 208, 219, 224–225, 241–242, 248, 254, 258, 271, 308, 312, 314–315, 333, 344, 360, 362, 374, 379, 387, 391, 394, 398, 410, 419, 422, 425, 445, 447, 459, 480, 487, 499, 505, 512, 520, 522, 524, 527, 531, 539
Myoclonus epilepsy, 303–304
Myopathy, 184, 186, 253, 255, 280, 298, 304, 308, 329, 354, 383, 398–399, 421, 464, 489, 508, 530, 534, 541

N

Narrative protocols, 153
Nasopharynx, 71–72
National registries, 147
Natural death, 8
  definition of, 7
Natural diseases
  possible violent antecedents of, 9t
Neck
  vertebral arteries in, 83f
Neck vessels
  removal of, 82
Necrotizing enteritis, 301
Needle autopsies, 5
Neisseria meningitidis, 272

Neonates
calvarium
opening of, 68f
chromosome study
indications for, 107
Nephrolithiasis, 178, 184, 190, 216, 223, 236, 269, 322, 346–347, 403, 434, 445, 457–458, 463, 489, 493, 540
Nephropathy, 190, 193, 252, 266, 282, 321–322, 346, 348, 403, 470, 521, 532, 539
Nervous system, 65–83
fixation of, 72–74
tissue blocks
for histologic examination, 79–80
selection of, 79f
venography of, 81
Neurocutaneous syndrome, 467
Neurofibromatosis, 277, 280, 401, 403–404, 412, 500, 527, 529, 532, 535, 537
Neuropathy, 186, 191, 193, 216, 253, 255, 267, 277, 298, 332, 344, 346, 379, 383, 404–405, 441, 451, 464, 483, 510, 522, 534, 538, 546
Neurosyphilis
congenital, 405, 512, 513
Neutropenic enterocolitis, 301–302
Next-of-kin, 7, 160
interview with, 147–149
Niemann Pick disease, 273, 282
Nocardiosis, 368, 377, 405
Nonalcoholic steatohepatitis, 407, 473, 510
Noonan's syndrome, 500–501
Norwood procedure, 41
Nutritional amblyopia, 253, 272, 404

O

Obesity, 11, 251, 322, 345, 348, 407, 410, 454, 472, 488, 497, 501, 510, 567
Obstruction
acute airway, 209, 217, 240–241, 407
arteriomesenteric, 408
inferior vena cava, 408, 496
pulmonary venous, 276, 408
superior mesenteric, 409
Obstructive cholangiopathy
infantile, 210
Ocular specimens
documentation of, 87–88
and electron microscopy, 93
fixation of, 87–88
orientation of, 87–88
processing of, 87–88
staining procedures for, 93
Ollier's syndrome, 274, 286, 299, 411
Onchocerciasis, 409
Orbital contents
removal of, 85–86
Organ models, 139–140
Organophosphate poisoning, 367, 410, 423–424, 440, 443–444
Organs
donation of, 162–163
retention for study, 162
Oriental liver fluke infection, 231
Oroya fever, 215
Orthochromatic leukodystrophy, 275
Orth's solution, 131
Oscillating saws, 95
Osler-Rendu-Weber disease, 274, 515, 532
Osteitis deformans, 275
Osteoarthritis, 275, 281, 329, 352, 410, 447, 452, 470
Osteoarthropathy, 99, 230, 269, 316–317, 411, 430, 513, 533, 536
Osteochondrodysplasia, 286
Osteogenesis imperfecta, 280, 357, 411–412, 425
Osteomalacia, 174, 230, 246, 303, 308, 318, 354, 357, 387, 412, 414–415, 425, 445, 471, 492, 498, 536–537
Osteomyelitis, 176, 185, 193–194, 217, 219–220, 257, 259–260, 272–273, 278, 296, 300, 314, 326, 362, 365, 371, 378, 397–398, 413–414, 422, 471, 517, 526–527, 529
Osteonecrosis, 180, 186, 195–196, 264, 272–273, 276–277, 379–380, 401, 413, 469
Osteopetrosis, 254, 272, 413–414, 419
Osteoporosis, 184, 195, 205, 207, 230, 246, 268–269, 308, 329, 332, 346, 350–352, 379–380, 392, 402–403, 406, 412, 414–415, 422, 446, 457, 467, 470, 488–489, 505, 509
Otitis media, 176, 228, 243, 272, 287, 313–315, 326, 361, 376, 378, 388, 414–415, 423, 447, 488, 504, 518
Otosclerosis, 412, 415
Oxalosis, 346

P

Paget's disease, 98, 275, 322, 357, 410, 425, 529
cranium, 98f
Pancreas, 57–59
arteriography, 57–59
posterior view of, 56f
Pancreatitis, 186, 225, 227, 231, 245, 252, 255, 262, 269, 290, 296, 306, 321, 330, 333, 345, 347, 350, 360, 379–380, 394, 406, 417–420, 444, 450, 479–481, 483, 496, 498
Pancytopenia, 185, 194–195, 323, 334, 366, 418, 539
Panniculitis, 244–245, 250, 280, 379, 419–420, 447
Paraffin blocks
shipping of, 134
Paranasal sinuses, 71–72
Parenchymatous cerebellar degeneration, 247
Parenteral nutrition, 406, 412, 472
Parkinson's disease, 275, 420–421, 430, 492, 501, 508
Parrot fever, 410
Parrot syndrome, 183
Partial atrioventricular septal defect, 244
Partial hydatidiform moles, 108
Particles
histologic analysis of, 52
identification of, 52
quantitative studies of, 52
Partition method
of cardiac dissection, 26
Pasteurella tularensis, 526
Patau syndrome, 107
Patent ductal artery, 26, 203, 210, 212, 243–244, 516, 524

Patent ductus arteriosus, 204
Pathological conditions
postmortem chemical changes in, 115t
Pathology museum, 137
specimens for, 137–138
Pedestrians
in vehicular accidents, 181
Pediatric autopsies
techniques of, 4
Pelizaeus-Merzbacher syndrome, 275, 376
Pellagra, 247, 405, 421, 485
Pelvic organs, 59–61
Pemphigus, 421–422, 534–535, 539
Penis, 60
Peptic ulcer, 209, 295, 387, 402, 455, 486, 543
Pericarditis, 191, 205–206, 208, 217, 259, 268, 272, 280, 303, 305, 308, 311–312, 331, 336, 351, 378–380, 394, 410, 419, 422, 428, 447, 466, 484, 500, 507, 509, 526–527
Peripheral lymphatics, 35
Peripheral nerves
tissue blocks
for histologic examination, 79–80
Peritonitis
infectious, 423
Persistent truncal artery, 200, 203, 547
Perthes' disease, 413
Pertussis, 229, 423, 547
Peutz-Jeghers syndrome, 449–450, 501, 530, 534–535, 537
Peyronie's disease, 494
Phacomatosis, 467
Phenylketonuria, 192, 424
Pheochromocytoma
stains for, 134
Phlebitis, 250, 294, 424, 517–518, 547
Phosphorus poisoning, 424, 444
Photographs
in external examination, 13
Phthisical eye, 87
Phycomycosis, 394
Physicians' Current Procedural Terminology, 155
Phytanoyl-coenzyme A hydroxylase deficiency, 277
Pick's lobar atrophy, 276
Pick's syndrome, 213, 276
Pictorial protocols, 153
Pierre-Robin syndrome, 501
Pigment cirrhosis, 330
Pituitary gland, 71
removal of, 72f
tumor of, 529
Pituitary insufficiency, 184, 194, 277, 286, 306, 355–356, 369, 419, 464, 492, 536
Placentas
in multiple pregnancies, 61
Plague, 424
Plasma cell dyscrasia, 383
Plastic casts
preparation for, 59
Plastination, 137–138
Platybasia, 246, 357, 384, 397, 425, 497
Pleurodynia
epidemic, 255, 425
Plexogenic pulmonary hypertension
in congenital cardiac left-to-right shunts
modified Heath-Edwards classification of, 33t
Plummer-Vinson syndrome, 196, 287, 502, 530
Pneumomediastinum, 117, 179, 250, 427–428, 431, 506
Pneumonia, 9, 33, 101, 103, 176, 185–186, 191, 201, 206, 216–219, 239, 249–250, 252, 267, 270, 272, 277, 290, 293, 296–297, 308, 311, 313, 316–317, 321, 335–336, 350, 359, 362, 371, 374–375, 378, 381, 387–389, 391, 397, 401, 405, 411, 418–419, 425, 428–429, 434, 437, 440, 447, 461, 471, 478, 487, 489, 492–493, 495, 504–508, 513, 521–522, 533, 546–547
eosinophilic, 324
interstitial, *See* Interstitial pneumonia
lipoid, 263, 411, 430
Pneumoperitoneum, 117
Pneumothorax, 2–3, 9, 14, 46, 117, 179, 182, 206, 209, 218, 295–296, 316, 325, 338, 406, 423, 428, 430–431, 462, 469, 481, 502, 506, 515
detection of
in postoperative autopsies, 4
Poisoning, 8, 14–17, 114, 132, 165, 177, 179–180, 185, 188, 193–196, 202–203, 213, 215–216, 218, 223, 229, 235, 241, 248–249, 251, 254, 275, 286, 289, 297, 299, 304, 306, 307, 322, 345–346, 348, 353, 356, 361, 367, 370, 373, 380, 390, 395, 401, 403, 405, 410, 423–424, 430–445, 453, 468, 477, 481, 500, 517, 519, *See also* names of specific agents
average time of death in, 15f
investigation of circumstances, 14–15, 15t
Poliomyelitis, 277, 397, 421, 445
Polyarteritis nodosa, 203, 226–227, 260–261, 270, 313, 324, 418, 422, 446–447, 456, 498–500, 507
Polychondritis, relapsing, 447
Polycythemia, 236, 270, 275, 282, 322, 350, 375, 390, 448–449, 484–485, 532
Polymerase chain reaction, 115
Polymyalgia rheumatica, 198, 203, 446, 449
Polyposis
familial, 449, 488, 494, 509
Polysplenia, 210–212, 244, 370, 385–386, 482, 496, 502–503
Polyvinyl chloride corrosion, 51
Pompe's disease, 265
Popliteal arteries
obtaining after embalming, 34
Porphyria
acute intermittent, 450, 532
congenital erythropoietic, 451
variegate, 452
Porphyria cutanea tarda, 451–452, 532
Portal hypertension, 193, 231, 235, 237, 256, 264, 316, 387, 390, 463, 465, 472, 493
Portal venography, 56–57
Posterior neck dissection
in vehicular accidents, 181
Postmortem chemical data
interpretation of, 114
Postmortem chemical values
changes of, 114t

Postmortem chemistry, *See* Autopsy chemistry
Postmortem cooling, 10
Postmortem coronary angiography, 118–121
Postmortem lividity, 10
Postmortem rigidity, 10
Postmortem roentgenograms
autopsy rack for, 119f
clinical conditions demonstrable by, 117–118
Postmortem samples
advanced analytical methods applied to, 114–115
Postoperative autopsies, 4–5
Postoperative death, 244
Potassium
postmortem changes in, 114t
Potts shunt, 41
Prague solution, 137
Preexcitation, ventricular, 452, 511
Pregnancy, 9, 190, 197, 229, 239, 283, 285, 289–290, 299, 322, 347–348, 369, 417–418, 452, 454, 460, 484, 496, 518–520, 571
Pregnant uterus, 60
Primary immunodeficiency, 185, 202, 288, 302, 357, 489, 496, 498, 503, 511
Problem-oriented protocols, 154
Progeria, 452
Progressive supranuclear palsy, 275, 417
Pronouncement of death, 8
Prostheses, 97
Prosthetic heart valves
types of, 33t
Protective devices, 67f
Protective garments, 145–146
Protein-losing enteropathy, 321, 471
Proteins
postmortem changes in, 114t
Protocols
admissibility as evidence, 163–164
Protoporphyria, erythropoietic, 453
Pseudogout, 96, 99, 134, 228, 322, 347, 453
stains for, 134
Pseudohyperparathyroidism, 453, 532
Pseudohypoparathyroidism, 454
Pseudomembranous enterocolitis, 302
Pseudomyxoma, 454
Pseudotumor cerebri, 454, 483
Pseudoxanthoma, 270, 455, 495
Psittacosis, 410
Psoriasis, 206, 322, 455–456, 471
Pulmonary alveolar microlithiasis, 263
Pulmonary angiography, 50
Pulmonary artery malformation, 385
Pulmonary blood
measurements of, 51–52
Pulmonary embolism, 7, 9, 152–153, 204, 220, 424, 468, 483, 518
Pulmonary hypertension, 23, 29, 33, 204, 244, 264, 270, 370, 379–380, 466
Pulmonary insufficiency, 370, 462, 485
Pulmonary vascular casts
preparation of, 51
Pulmonary venography, 50
Pulseless disease, 204
Pupil/optic disc (PO) section, 88
Purpura, thrombotic thrombocytopenic, 391, 456, 517
Putrefaction, 11, 98
Pyelonephritis, 9, 236, 252, 269, 317, 322, 347–348, 390, 397, 403, 445, 457–458, 465, 493, 495

Q

Q fever, 311–312, 459
Quality assurance, 155–156

R

Rabies, 86, 297, 459
Radiation enterocolitis, 366
Radiation injury, 194, 366, 418, 460, 481
Radiation nephritis, 366
Radiation pneumonitis, 366
Radioactive deceased person
embalming of, 124–125
instruments use for
decontamination of, 127
precautions for, 125–126
tag for, 124f
Radioactive implants
radiation exposure rates from, 126t
Radioactive materials, 123–127
hazard types, 123–124
unshielded dose rates for, 124t
Radioactive tissues
sectioning and storage of, 127–128
Rape, 221, 284–285, 337, 358, 460–461
Rastelli procedure, 41
Raynaud's syndrome, 276
Reaction to transfusion, 461, 521
Recombinant immunoblot assay (RIBA), 114
Records
confidentiality of, 163–164
Refsum's syndrome, 511
Regaud's fixative, 131
Regional enteritis, 261
Rejuvenation solution, 132
Relapsing fever, 312, 314
Relapsing polychondritis, 420, 447–448
Renal agenesis, 3, 212
Renal arteries
atherosclerosis of, 34
Renal arteriograms
in situ, 61f
Renal arteriography, 59
Renal artery stenosis, 475
Renal cysts, 235, 264, 316
Renal tubular necrosis, 9, 254, 401, 438–439
Renal vein thrombosis, 117, 193, 518
Renal vein thrombosis, 518
Renal venogram, 62f
Renal venography, 59
Respiratory distress syndrome, 308, 427, 506, 510
Restaurant death, 407
Restrictive cardiomyopathy, 24, 33, 225, 263, 300, 492, 498

Retrobulbar neuropathy, 191
Retroperitoneal fibrosis, 225, 388, 457, 464, 494, 519
Reusable items
 cleaning of, 145
Reye's syndrome, 298–299, 362, 506–507, 545
Rheumatic fever, 229, 312, 313, 398, 422
Rheumatoid arthritis, 96, 193–194, 202–203, 205–207, 218, 225, 250, 260, 271, 321–322, 357, 378, 381, 388, 395, 397, 403, 419, 422, 428–430, 447, 456, 470, 485, 493, 503, 505, 507, 519, 543
RIBA, 114
Ribonucleic acid
 postmortem changes in, 114t
Ribs
 sawing, 95
Rickets, 245
Rickettsia rickettsii, 313
Riedel's thyroiditis, 494
Right ventricular dysplasia, 225
Right ventricular region
 schematic diagram of, 31f
Rigor mortis, 10
Ring, lower esophageal, 462
River blindness, 409
Rocky Mountain spotted fever, 313–314
Roentgenographs
 in external examination, 13
 shielded autopsy room for, 119f
Rokitansky technique, 3
Rubella, 205, 210–211, 333, 387–388, 462, 487
 congenital, 210–211, 462, 487
Rubeola, 387

S

Safety, 145–146
Salivary gland virus disease, 359
Sandhoff's disease, 319
Sanfilippo disease, 282
San Joaquin fever, 233
Sarcoidosis, 34, 208, 216, 234, 251, 321–323, 326, 343, 356, 369, 377, 388–389, 403, 411, 418, 427, 429, 463–464, 470, 524
Scalded skin syndrome, 401
Scalp
 incision of, 66f
Scanning electron microscopy
 fixation for, 132
Scarlet fever, 314, 417, 509
 staphylococcal, 509
Schatzki rings
 demonstration of, 53
Scheie's syndrome, 392
Schilder's syndrome, 263, 277, 465–466
Schistosomiasis, 216, 297, 349, 431, 464–465, 541
Schuknecht temporal trephine, 95
Sclera
 removal of, 87
Scleral tissue
 for transplantation, 88f
Scleroderma, 466
Sclerosing cholangitis, 225–226, 230, 235, 262, 268, 388, 471, 494, 519, 528, 532
Scopolamine, 432
Scurvy, 245
Seeds
 radiation exposure rates from, 126t
Segawa's syndrome, 490
Seligmann's disease, 267
Senning procedure, 41
Serum sickness, 321, 469
Sex determination, 11
Sharps
 disposal of, 144–145
Shipping
 for carbon monoxide determination, 135
 containers for, 134–135
 of medicolegal materials, 135
 for microbiologic study, 135
Shock, 9, 27, 149, 181, 301–302, 310, 321, 363, 429, 461, 468, 481, 509
Short-axis method
 of cardiac dissection, 22, 23f
Shy-Drager syndrome, 213
Sickle cell, 115, 195–197, 234, 270, 277–278, 413, 457, 532
Sick sinus, 507
Silicosis, 388, 426–427, 469, 485
Sinuses
 draining
  collection of, 104
Sinus node
 dissection of, 26, 27f
Sjogren's syndrome, 225
Skeletal muscle, 80
Skeletal system, 95–99
Skin incisions
 restriction of, 5
 sampling of, 17
Skull
 base of, 71
Skullcap
 removal of, 67f
Small intestinal atresia, 212
Small intestinal mucosa
 preservation of, 54
Sniffing and spray death, 439
SNOMED International, 155
Sodium
 postmortem changes in, 114t
Sodium hydroxide, 98
Source material, 159160
South American blastomycosis, 420
Spalteholz
 clearing method after, 139
Specimens
 containers, 15–16
 flow of, 143
Sphingomyelinase deficiency, 273
Spinal arachnoiditis, 202, 513

Spinal cord
  anterior approach to, 68–70, 69f
  dissection of, 77–79, 78f
  posterior approach to, 67–68, 68f
  removal of, 67–69
    in infants, 70–71
  tissue blocks
    for histologic examination, 79
Spinal epidural infection, 362
Spinocerebellar degeneration, 210, 247, 529–530, 533
Spleen, 59
  posterior view of, 56f
  weight and measurement of, 570t
Spontaneous abortions
  chromosome studies and, 107–108
Sporotrichosis, 470–471
Spouse, 160
Spray death, 209
Sprue
  celiac, 257, 302, 471, 473
  tropical, 472
Stabbing injury, 336, 366, 371, 472
Starvation, 201, 243, 386, 421, 472
Statutes, 159–160
Statutory autopsies
  objections to, 159
Steatohepatitis, nonalcoholic, 472
Steele-Richardson-Olszewski syndrome, 417
Sternoclavicular joints, 96
Sternum
  sawing, 95–96
Stevens-Johnson syndrome, 304
Stiff-man syndrome, 508
Stillbirth, 3, 6, 60, 110, 121, 175, 239–240, 358, 476
  products of
    chromosome studies, 109
Still's disease, 205
Stomach, 53
  contents of
    at time of death, 10–11
  tumor of, 397
Storage requirements
  minimal, 143, 144t
Strachan's syndrome, 191
Stramonium, 432
Strangulation, 2, 13, 45, 221, 242, 285, 338, 356, 409, 476–477
Striatonigral degeneration, 213
Strychnine poisoning, 430, 444, 477
Stryker autopsy saw, 95
Sturge-Weber-Dimitri, 200, 278, 500
Subdural hematoma, 8
Subphrenic empyema, 227, 259, 290, 296
Subvalvular aortic stenosis, 475, 547
Subvalvular pulmonary stenosis, 475–476, 524
Sudanophilic leukodystrophy, 263, 275, 376
Sudden death, 33, 181, 201, 204, 206, 221, 240–242, 265, 433, 473–474, 516
  coronary atherosclerosis microscopic features, 31t
  unexplained, 34
Suicide, 180
Sulfatidosis, 377
Superior vena cava syndrome, 509
Suppurative cholangitis, 226–227, 231, 256
Sural nerve, 80
Syphilis
  acquired, 405, 421, 512
  congenital, 357, 405, 512–513
Syphilitic aortic aneurysm, 199
Syringomyelia, 246, 277, 384, 390, 425, 497, 513
Systemic hypertension
  and heart weight, 29
Systemic lupus erythematosus, 203, 206, 208, 225, 229, 260, 301, 321, 378, 380–381, 403, 405, 413, 418–419, 429, 446, 449, 456, 496, 498, 503, 507, 519
Systemic mastocytosis, 272, 376, 386, 543
Systemic sclerosis, 202–203, 225, 250, 260, 277, 303, 425, 456, 465–467, 496, 507

T

Tabes dorsalis, 512, 515
Takayasu's arteritis, 202–203, 269, 368
Tangier's syndrome, 245, 354
Tarui disease, 265
Taussig-Bing anomaly, 547
Temporal arteries
  obtaining after embalming, 34
Temporal bones
  removal of, 95
Tension pneumothorax, 431f
Terminology
  in death certificates, 152
Testicular feminization, 309
Tetanus, 249, 367, 515
Tetralogy of Fallot, 200, 212, 243–244, 370, 385, 516, 545
Thalassemia, 96, 195, 329, 516
Thallium poisoning, 18, 440, 442, 444, 445, 517
Thin-layer chromatography (TLC), 17
Thoracic duct
  removal of, 36f
Thrombocytopenic, 195–196, 225, 309, 321, 331, 387, 391, 394, 418, 456–457, 495–496, 500, 517, 521–522, 539–540
Thrombotic thrombocytopenic purpura, 196, 321, 418, 457, 495–496, 539–540
Thrush, 223
Thyroiditis, 197, 217, 317, 321, 328, 331–332, 351, 355, 367, 388, 395, 402, 494, 507–508, 510, 519, 540
Thyrotoxicosis, 350
Tibia
  macerated, 99f
Time of death
  estimation of, 10–11
Tissue culture
  immediate autopsy for, 5
Tissues
  for carbon monoxide determination
    shipping of, 135
  donation of, 162–163
  for microbiologic study
    shipping of, 135
  retention for study, 162

TLC, 17
Tobacco amblyopia, 191
Torticollis, 519
Torulosis, 234
Toxemia of pregnancy, 190, 289, 452, 496, 519
Toxic epidermal necrolysis, 304–305, 401
Toxic fumes
  monitoring for, 146
  protection from, 146
Toxicologic material
  routine sampling of, 16–17
Toxic shock, 509
Toxoplasmosis, 297, 332, 343, 398, 478, 520–521
Trachea
  with carina, 46f
  dissection of, 45
Tracheobronchial tree, 45–52
Transient cerebral ischemia, 213
Transient stroke, 213
Transmission electron microscopy
  fixation for, 132
Transmittal sheet, 17, 18t
Transplantation, 86–87
Transportation
  of body, 164
Traumatic aortic aneurysm, 200
Treponema pallidum, 512
Trichinosis, 297, 524
Tricuspid insufficiency, 212, 370, 385, 462, 524
Tricuspid stenosis, 212, 476, 485
Triglycerides
  postmortem changes in, 114t
Trisomy 21, 489
Trocar embalming, 14
Tropical sprue, 303
Trypanosoma brucei, 515
Trypanosoma cruzi, 257
Trypanosomiasis, African, 469, 525
Tuberculosis, 118, 145–146, 149, 186, 191, 193–194, 202, 205, 208, 218, 223, 229, 234, 296, 302–303, 323, 343, 361, 367, 373–374, 377, 387–390, 394, 411, 413, 427, 470, 472, 509, 526, 543, 545
Tuberous sclerosis, 255, 467, 468, 490, 500, 529, 531
Tubular hypoplasia of aortic arch, 474
Tularemia, 526
Tumors
  adrenal gland, 404, 424, 527
  bile ducts, 269, 408, 528, 531
  bone, 229, 275, 529
  brain, 191, 450, 529
  chromosome studies, 109
  esophagus, 303, 530
  heart, 399, 462, 467, 531
  kidney, 403, 518, 532, 541
  liver, 329, 532
  lung, 533
  ovarian, 489, 534
  pancreas, 498, 534
  peripheral nerves, 319, 535
  pituitary gland, 234, 489, 529, 535
  pleura, 536
  prostate, 497, 536
  small intestine, 531, 537
  soft tissue, 537
  spinal cord, 537
  staining, 133–134
  stomach, 303, 471, 538
  testis, 538
  thymus, 519, 539
  thyroid gland, 540
  urinary bladder, 540
  uterus, 541
Turner syndrome, 107
Typhoid fever, 301, 314, 417, 439
Typhus fever, 315
Tyrosinemia, 192, 492, 532, 541–542

U

Unauthorized autopsies, 162
Unrolling method
  of cardiac dissection, 26
Unverricht-Lundborg disease, 303
Urea nitrogen
  postmortem changes in, 114t
Uremia
  postmortem chemical changes in, 115t
Ureters, 59
Urethra
  with congenital valves, 63f
  male, 60
Urethral valves
  congenital
    urogram of, 62f
Urinary bladder, 59
Urinary system, 59–61
Urine
  radioactivity of, 125
  sampling of, 16
Urogenital organs
  weight and measurement of, 565t
Urography, 59
Uterus, 60

V

Valley fever, 233
Valvular aortic stenosis
  congenital, 473
Valvular heart disease, 32–33
Valvular pulmonary stenosis
  congenital, 500
Variegate porphyria, 452
Vasculature
  evaluation of, 34–35
Vehicular accident, 178, 180
Veno-occlusive disease, 276, 279, 350, 408–409, 484, 521–522, 547
Venous air embolism
  in vehicular accidents, 181
Venous sinuses, 71
Venous thrombosis, 35f

Ventricular preexcitation, 385
Ventricular septal defect, 198–199, 204, 211–212, 232, 234, 243–244, 244, 327, 368, 385, 388, 474–476, 490, 516, 524, 547
Vertebrae
  sawing, 96
Vertebral arteries, 83
  dissection of, 82–83
  intracranial freeing of, 82f
  in neck, 83f
Viral hepatitis, 171, 196, 230, 245, 249, 321, 417–418, 446, 521, 533
Virchow technique, 3, 74
Vital statistics registration system, 154f
Vitamin A deficiency, 175, 245, 356, 547
Vitamin C deficiency, 245, 468, 547
Vitamin D deficiency, 243, 246, 354, 356, 412, 462, 516, 547
Vitreous
  aspiration of, 86f
  collection of
    for autopsy chemistry, 113–114
  sampling of, 16, 85
Volume hypertrophy, 29
Von Gierke's disease, 265
Von Hippel-Lindau, 268, 279, 401, 500, 527, 529, 537–538
Von Recklinghausen's disease, 403
Vrolik's disease, 412

W

Waste disposal, 144–145
Waterhouse-Friderichsen syndrome, 272
Waterston shunt, 41
Wegener's granulomatosis, 321, 325, 326, 463, 495
Weights and measurements, 12, 551t–572t
  of body, 554t–555t, 557t–561t, 567t
  of body surface area, 556t, 567t
  of brain, 565t
  conversion factors for, 551t
  of hearts, 562t–564t, 568t–570t
  of spleen, 570t
  of urogenital organs, 565t
Weil's disease, 374
WELD-ON, 137
Wernicke-Korsakoff syndrome, 186
Wet fixation
  of lungs, 46–47
Wet material
  shipping containers for, 134–135
Whipple's disease, 193, 280–281, 303, 479, 498
Whooping cough, 423
Williams-Beuren syndrome, 473
Wilson's disease, 247, 281, 331–332, 410
Window method
  of cardiac dissection, 25, 26f
Wiskott-Aldrich syndrome, 503
Wolf-Hirschhorn syndrome, 107
Wooden spokes, 97
Wood's metal, 51
Wounds
  measurement of, 12
Wrongful autopsy
  prevention of, 163

X–Z

Xerophthalmia, 245
X-ray microanalysis, 133
Yellow fever, 315
Zamboni's solution, 131
Zenker's fixative, 131
Zollinger-Ellison, 511, 534, 543
Zygomycosis, 394